SELLERS' MIDWIFERY

Third edition

Editors:

Joan Dippenaar

Dicky da Serra

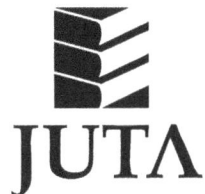

JUTA

Sellers' Midwifery

First published 1993
Second edition 2012
Third edition 2018

Juta and Company (Pty) Ltd
First floor, Sunclare building, 21 Dreyer street, Claremont 7708
PO Box 14373, Lansdowne 7779, Cape Town, South Africa

ISBN 978 1 48512 102 2

Project manager: Seshni Kazadi
Editor and Proofreader: Simone Chiara van der Merwe
Cover designer: Waterberry Designs
Typesetter: Lebone Publishing Services
Indexer: Lexinfo
Cover image: Pamela Soeharno
Illustrations: Anne Westoby, *Sellers' Midwifery Volumes 1 and 2*, Pamela Soeharno

Acknowledgements:
Sandton Radiology
Life Fourways Hospital
Oula family
Allan family

Typeset in Adobe Text Pro 9.5 on 12

Disclaimer
In the writing of this book, every effort has been made to present accurate and up-to-date information from the best and most reliable sources. However, the results of healthcare professionals depend on a variety of factors that are beyond the control of the authors and publishers. Therefore, neither the authors nor the publishers assume responsibility for, nor make any warranty with regards to, the outcomes achieved from the procedures described in this book.

The authors and publisher have exerted every effort to ensure that drug selections and dosages set forth in this text are in accord with current recommendations and practice at the time of publication. However, readers are urged to check the package insert for each drug for any change in indications of dosage and for added warning and precautions. The information in this book is provided in good faith and the authors and publisher cannot be held responsible for errors, individual responses to drugs and other consequences.

This book has been independently peer-reviewed by academics who are experts in this field.

Contents

About the editors

J M Dippenaar

RN (General, Midwifery and Psychiatry); B Soc Sc (Hon) (UFS), RM; Dip Nursing Education and Administration and (UJ) Community (UNISA); M Cur (RAU) Clinical Specialist (Advanced Midwifery and Neonatal Science); D Cur (Nursing Administration) (UJ)

Dr Dippenaar has 30 years of clinical experience in both the public and private healthcare sectors, which includes experience as a midwife and unit manager in labour wards and maternity sections, a case manager and a clinical auditor. She was a post-basic midwifery moderator for the South African Nursing Council (SANC) for 10 years as well as a midwifery moderator for nursing colleges and master's and doctoral students. Dr Dippenaar lectured theory and clinical midwifery (basic and post-basic) at the Ann Latsky Nursing College, the University of Pretoria and Medunsa, and was a senior lecturer at the University of Limpopo from 2004 to 2013. She was part of a team at the University of the Witwatersrand that trained post-graduate midwives in reproductive health for the CHENA ICASA Mozambique project 2012–2013. In 2013, she joined Health Systems Trust and entered the public health field as DCST facilitator in the RMCH programme for the re-engineering of the three streams of PHC. She then worked as a researcher and is currently a technical advisor for training and e-learning.

As a midwife in private practice, she has delivered more than 100 babies in natural birth units or in the home setting and provided both ante- and postnatal care. She was instrumental in establishing and managing the first natural birth unit in the private sector in Gauteng.

DGJ da Serra

RN (General and Psychiatry); RM; Dip Nursing Education; Dip Nursing Administration and Community Nursing; Clinical Specialist in Advanced Midwifery and Neonatal Nursing Science; B Soc. Sc (Hon) (UFS); M Cur Clinical Advanced Midwifery and Neonatal Nursing (RAU); D Cur Advanced Midwifery and Neonatal Nursing Science (RAU)

Dr Da Serra has more than 30 years of practical experience in both the public and private healthcare sectors, in both managerial and educational roles. This includes experience as a midwife and unit manager in labour wards and maternity sections, a clinical lecturer, a clinical auditor, a nursing manager and an educator. Dr Da Serra lectured theory and clinical midwifery as well as research and community health at the SG Lourens Nursing College from 1984 until 1996. She was head of department for Community Nursing Science as well as Research. She was a nursing manager at Mediclinic Gyneacological Hospital from 1996 until 2007. Dr Da Serra lectured theory and clinical midwifery (basic and post-basic) at the SG Lourens Nursing College (basic), the University of Pretoria and Medunsa. Dr Da Serra was formerly a senior lecturer at the University of Pretoria, where she lectured basic and master's students in midwifery and was the programme manager for the B Cur students. She currently moderates post-basic midwifery for Garankuwa Nursing College and works as an independent midwifery consultant.

About the contributors

MR Digamela (sections of chapters 2, 21, 22 and 32)
RN; RM; Dip Community Health Nursing Science; B Cur (I et A) (UP); Dip Nursing Education (UP); M Cur Clinical (Advanced Midwifery and Neonatal Nursing Science) (UP); PhD (UP). Manager of the skill centre at SMU.

DW du Plessis (chapters 3, 9, 39 and sections of the clinical procedures)
RN; RM; (General, Midwifery Psychiatry); Advanced Midwife; Dip Community Health Nursing Science (UFS); Dip Nursing Education (UFS); Dip Nursing Administration (UFS); Dip Operating Room (SANC); M Cur Clinical (Advanced Midwifery and Neonatal Nursing Science) (UJ) PhD Midwifery and Neonatology (UJ).

T Heyns (Chapter 35)
RN; RM; Dip Nursing Education (UP); B Soc Sc (Hon) (General, Midwifery & Psychiatry) Critical Care (UFS); M Cur Clinical Emergency Nursing (UP); PhD (Unisa). Senior lecturer, Critical Care, University of Pretoria.

Dr P Kocheleff (Chapter 49)
M. Dr, Physician (ULB/Belgium), Technical Adviser HST.

Prof P Kuswayo (Chapter 51)
B Sc (Dietetics); Postgraduate Diploma in Hospital Dietetics (UKZN); B Sc (Hon) Dietetics (Medunsa); MPH (University of North Carolina, Chapel Hill, USA). Former Head of Department, Human Nutrition and Dietetics, University of Limpopo, Medunsa campus.

Prof U MacIntyre (Chapter 51)
B Sc (Dietetics) (UKZN); Postgraduate Dip Hospital Dietetics (UP); B Sc (Hon) (Dietetics) (UP); M Sc (Dietetics) (Medunsa), Diploma in Datametrics (Unisa), PhD (Nutrition) (PUCHE). Formerly Director of the Institute for Human Nutrition at the University of Limpopo, Medunsa campus. Lecturing at University of Pretoria.

L Paramor (Chapter 52)
RN; RM; B. Cur Nursing (University of Stellenbosch); Dip Midwifery; Cert Reflexology (International Institute of Reflexology); Cert of Ayurvedic Medicine (Rajan Coopan, India). Sister Lilian Paramor owns a successful and well-known company in the private sector.

G Schellack (Chapter 53)
RN; B Cur (UP); Adv Univ Dip Nurs Sc (HSM) (Unisa); B Sc (Hon) (Pharmacology) (NWU). Training specialist in the pharmaceutical industry, with a special interest in clinical research and applied pharmacology.

N Schellack (Chapter 53)
B Cur (UP); B Pharm (Medunsa); PhD (Pharmacy) (Medunsa). Senior lecturer, Department of Pharmacy, University of Limpopo, Medunsa campus.

OB Tagutanazvo (sections of chapters 17, 18 and 19)
RN; RM; Dip Nursing Science; Dip Midwifery; Cert HIV/AIDS; BA Cur (Education and Administration) (Unisa); M Sc (Maternal and Child Health) (Zimbabwe); D Cur Maternal and Child Nursing: Advanced Midwifery and Neonatal Nursing Science (UJ). Senior lecturer, Department of Midwifery Science, University of Swaziland.

A Truter (Chapter 48)
RN; RM; B Nursing (General, Midwifery, Psychiatry and Community) (US); BA Cur (Nursing Education and Nursing Administration) (SA); M Cur (SA); D Litt et Phil (SA). Senior lecturer, Community Nursing Science, Western Cape College of Nursing in conjunction with Cape Peninsula University of Technology.

A van den Heever (chapters 10, 12 and 13)
RN; RM (General, Midwifery, Psychiatry and Community); Dip Nursing Education, RM; Dip Psychosocial Nursing (UK); M Cur Advanced psychiatric and mental health nurse (UJ). Lecturer, University of the Witwatersrand.

List of figures

List of tables

List of statutes

Basic Conditions of Employment Act 75 of 1997
The Batho Pele Principles
Births and Deaths Registration Act 51 of 1992
Births and Deaths Registration Amendment Act 18 of 2010
Children's Act 38 of 2005 (CA)
Choice on Termination of Pregnancy Act 92 of 1996
Domestic Violence Act 116 of 1998
Marriage Act 25 of 1961
Medicines and Related Substances Act 101 of 1965
Mental Health Care Act 17 of 2002
National Health Act 61 of 2003 (NHA)
National Health Amendment Act 12 of 2013
National Policy for Health Act 116 of 1990
Nursing Act 33 of 2005 (NA)
Traditional Health Practitioners Act 22 of 2007

List of abbreviations

3TC	lamivudine	CAM	complementary and alternative medicine
ABC	abacavir	CBF	cerebral blood flow
ADH	antidiuretic hormone	CEmONC	comprehensive emergency obstetric and neonatal care
ADHD	attention deficit hyperactivity disorder		
AFIS	amniotic fluid infection syndrome	CHC	community health clinics
AFP	alpha-fetoprotein	ChildPIP	Child Healthcare Problem Identification Programme
AGA	appropriate for gestational age		
AHPCSA	Allied Health Professions Council of South Africa	CHW	community health workers
		CIN	cervical intraepithelial neoplasia
AMTSL	active management of the third stage of labour	CMV	cytomegalovirus
AOP	apnoea of prematurity	CNS	central nervous system
AP	anteroposterior	CO	cardiac output
APH	antepartum haemorrhage	COC	continuum of care; combined oral contraceptive
ARDS	acute respiratory distress syndrome		
AROM	artificial rupture of membranes	CPAP	continuous positive airway pressure
ARV	antiretroviral	CPD	cephalopelvic disproportion; continuing professional development
ART	antiretroviral therapy		
ASD	atrial septal defect	CRL	crown–rump length
ATC	Anatomical Therapeutic Chemical	CRP	C-reactive protein
ATLS	Advanced Trauma Life Support	CRS	congenital rubella syndrome
AZT	zidovudine	CSF	cerebrospinal fluid
BANC	Basic Antenatal Care	CTG	cardiotocography
BBI	Better Birth Initiative	CTOP	choice of termination of pregnancy
BCE	before the Common Era	CuIUCD	copper-containing/-bearing intrauterine contraceptive device
BCG	Bacilli Calmetti-Guérin vaccine		
BFC	baby-friendly care	CVP	central venous pressure
BFHI	Baby-Friendly Hospital Initiative	CVS	chorionic villus sampling
BMI	basic metabolic index; body mass index	CYPR	couple year protection rate
BMR	basal metabolic rate	d4T	stavudine
BNBAS	Brazelton Neonatal Behaviour Assessment Scale	D&C	dilatation and curettage
		DCST	district clinical specialist team
BPD	biparietal diameter; bronchopulmonary dysplasia	ddI	didanosine
		DENOSA	Democratic Nursing Organisation of South Africa
BSA	body surface area		
BV	baseline variability; bacterial vaginosis	DHA	Department of Home Affairs; docosahexaenoic acid
CARMMA	Campaign on Accelerated Reduction of Maternal and Child Mortality in Africa		
		DHB	District Health Barometer

DHIS	District Health Information System	GI	gastrointestinal
DHMIS	District Health Management Information System	GIF	gastric intrinsic factor
		GnRH	gonadotrophin-releasing hormone
DHP	district health plan	GORD	gastro-esophageal reflux disease
DHS	district health system	GSV	gestational sac volume
DIC	disseminated intravascular coagulation	GTT	glucose tolerance test
DMB	donor milk banks	Hb	haemoglobin
DMPA	depot medroxyprogesterone acetate	HBB	Helping Babies Breathe
DNA	deoxyribonucleic acid	HBsAg	Hepatitis B surface antigen (test)
DoH	Department of Health	HBV	Hepatitis B virus
DOTS	direct observation treatment short-course	hCG	human chorionic gonadotrophin
DSC	developmental supportive care	HCS	human chorionic somatomammotropin
DVT	deep vein thrombosis	HCT	HIV counselling and testing
EBF	exclusive breastfeeding	HDN	haemolytic disease of the newborn
EBM	expressed breast milk	HELLP	haemolytic anaemia, elevated liver enzymes, low platelet count
EBP	evidence-based practice		
EC	emergency contraception	HGH	human growth hormone
ECG	electrocardiogram	HIE	hypoxic-ischaemic encephalopathy
ECP	emergency contraceptive pills	HITT	Health Information Task Team
ECV	external cephalic version	HPL	human placental lactogen
EDD	estimated date of delivery	HPV	human papillomavirus
EEG	electroencephalography	HMD	hyaline membrane disease
EFV	efiravenz	HST	Health Systems Trust
eGFR	estimated glomerular filtration rate	HSV	herpes simplex virus
ELBW	extremely low birth weight	ICDM	Integrated Chronic Disease Management
EOC	essential obstetric care	ICEA	International Childbirth Education Association
EOST	Emergency Obstetric Simulation Training		
EPDS	Edinburgh Postnatal Depression Scale	ICM	International Confederation of Midwives
EPI	expanded programme on immunisation	ICN	International Council of Nurses
ESMOE	Essential Steps in the Management of Obstetric Emergencies	IgA	immunoglobulin A
		IgD	immunoglobulin D
FAM	fertility awareness method	IgE	immunoglobulin E
FAS	fetal alcohol syndrome	IgG	immunoglobulin G
FASD	fetal alcohol spectrum disorder	IgM	immunoglobulin M
FBC	full blood count	IMCI	Integrated Management of Childhood Illnesses
FDA	Food and Drug Administration		
FDC	fixed-dose combination	iMMR	institutional maternal mortality ratio
FGM	female genital mutilation	INSTI	integrase strand transfer inhibitor
FHR	fetal heart rate	IOL	induction of labour
FI	fusion inhibitor	IPT	isoniazid preventive therapy
FIGO	International Federation of Gynaecology and Obstetrics	IRDS	infant respiratory distress syndrome
		IUCD	intrauterine contraceptive device
FISH	fluorescent *in situ* hybridisation test	IUD	intrauterine death
FSH	follicle-stimulating hormone	IUGR	intrauterine growth restriction
FTC	emtricitabine	IVCS	inferior vena cava syndrome
GA	gestational age	IVH	intraventricular hemorrhage
GAD	general anxiety disorder	IVP	internal podalic version
GBS	Group B Streptococcus	KMC	kangaroo-mother-care
GFR	glomerular filtration rate	LAM	lactational amenorrhea method

LBW	low birth weight		NTD	neural tube defect
LDH	lactate dehydrogenase		NVP	nevirapine
LGA	large for gestational age		OA	occipitoanterior
LH	luteinising hormone		OFC	occiput frontal circumference
LMP	last menstrual period		OP	occipitoposterior
LOA	left occipitoanterior		OT	occipitotransverse
LOP	left occipitoposterior		OTC	over-the-counter
LPV/r	lopinavir/ritonavir		$PaCO_2$	carbon dioxide tension
LSA	left sacroanterior		PaO_2	oxygen tension
LS	lecithin sphingomyelin		PAPP	pregnancy-associated plasma protein
MAS	meconium aspiration syndrome		PAHIV	perinatally acquired HIV
MCR	maternity case record		PCO_2	partial carbon dioxide
MC&S	microscopy, culture and sensitivity		PCP	*Pneumocystis carinii* pneumonia
MDGs	Millennium Development Goals		PCR	polymerase chain reaction
MDR-TB	multi-drug-resistant TB		PCV	packed cell volume
MLC	midwifery-led care		PDA	patent ductus arteriosus
MMR	maternal mortality rate; measles, mumps and rubella		PGL	persistent general lymphadenopathy
MNCWH	Maternal, Newborn, Child and Women's Health		PHC	primary healthcare
			PI	protease inhibitor
MODS	multi-organ dysfunction syndrome		PID	pelvic inflammatory disease
MOU	midwife obstetrics unit		PIH	pregnancy-induced hypertension
MRC	Medical Research Council		PJP	*Pneumocystis jiroveci* pneumonia
MSE	mental status examination		PKU	phenylketonuria
MTOP	medical termination of pregnancy		PMNCH	Partnership for Maternal, Newborn and Child Health
MUAC	mid-upper-arm circumference		PMTCT	prevention of mother-to-child transmission
MVA	manual vacuum aspiration		PND	postnatal depression
MVU	Montevideo units		PNMR	perinatal mortality rate
NaPEMMCo	National Perinatal Morbidity and Mortality Committee		POC	progesterone-only oral contraceptive
			POP	progesterone-only pill
NCCEMD	National Committee on Confidential Enquiries into Maternal Deaths		POPSAMSS	psychiatric history, obstetric history, partner relations, support network, attitude, mental status, self-concept, suicide risk
nCPAP	nasal continuous positive airway pressure			
NE	neonatal encephalopathy		PPCM	peripartum cardiomyopathy
NEC	necrotising enterocolitis		PPH	postpartum haemorrhage
NHA	National Health Act 61 of 2003		PPIP	Perinatal Problem Identification Programme
NHC	National Health Council		pPROM	pre-premature rupture of membranes
NIDS	National Indicator Data Set		PROM	premature rupture of membranes
NIMART	nurse-initiated management of antiretroviral therapy		PTSD	post-traumatic stress disorder
			PTT	partial thromboplastin time
NMR	neonatal mortality rate		QIP	Quality Improvement Plan
NNRTI	non-nucleoside/-nucleotide reverse transcriptase inhibitor		RBC	red blood cell
			RDA	recommended dietary allowance
NPRI	non-pregnancy-related infections		RDS	respiratory distress syndrome
NRTI	nucleoside/nucleotide reverse transcriptase inhibitor		REM	rapid eye movement
			Rh	rhesus
NSAID	non-steroidal anti-inflammatory drug		ROM	rupture of membranes
NST	non-stress test		ROP	right occipitoposterior

RPR	rapid plasma reagin
RMCH	Reducing Maternal and Child Mortality through Strengthening Primary Health Care
RSA	right sacroanterior
SADHS	South African Demographic Health Survey
SAM	severe acute malnutrition
SANC	South African Nursing Council
SBAR	situation, background, assessment, recommendation
SCD	sickle cell disease
SDGs	Sustainable Development Goals
SFH	symphysis fundal height
SG	specific gravity
SGA	small for gestational age
SIDS	sudden infant death syndrome
SIRS	systemic inflammatory response syndrome
SMI	Safe Motherhood Initiative
SPLEN	skin, plantar creases, labia or male, ear, nipple
STI	sexually transmitted infections
TBA	traditional birth attendant
TBV	total blood volume
TCA	tricyclic antidepressant
TDF	tenofovir
TEF	trachea-oesophageal fistula
TENS	transcutaneous electrical nerve stimulation
TMP/SMX	trimethoprim/sulfamethoxazole
TOP	termination of pregnancy
TORCH	toxoplasmosis, other, rubella, cytomegalovirus, herpes simplex
TTN	transient tachypnoea of the newborn
TSB	total serum bilirubin
TSH	thyroid-stimulating hormone
TSI	thyroid-stimulating immunoglobulin
UTI	urinary tract infection
VAS	vitamin A supplementation
VBAC	vaginal birth after Caesarean section
Vd	volume of distribution
VDRL	venereal disease research laboratory (test)
VDS	vaginal discharge syndrome
VLBW	very low birth weight
VSD	ventricular septal defect
VVC	vulvo-vaginal candidiasis
VZV	*Varicella zoster* virus
WBC	white blood cells
WBOT	ward-based outreach team
WCC	white cell count
XDR-TB	extreme drug-resistant TB

Preface

The writing of *Sellers' Midwifery* third edition has been influenced by the integrated nursing education model that includes midwifery in the South African Qualifications Authority higher education and training band. The proposed changes to the nursing curricula (South African Nursing Council, Education and Training Quality Assurance body) have also been considered in this updated version.

The content has been further influenced by:
- the transformation of the South African healthcare system, with reference to the district health system
- maternal and perinatal mortality in South Africa and the recommendations of the *Saving Mothers* and *Saving Babies* reports (1998–2015)
- evidence-based care principles to improve clinical care (RMCH, LINC, ESMOE and other initiatives in SA)
- ongoing initiatives by the WHO, International Council of Midwives (ICM) and International Council of Nurses (ICN) to strengthen the practice of midwifery
- the Scope of Practice of Basic Midwifery (focusing on normal pregnancy and childbirth) with reference to common disorders, recognition of such and care of specific conditions and situations.

A post-basic diploma in midwifery is required to be registered as an additional qualification with SANC. In this book, basic midwifery is emphasised and reference is made to the advanced knowledge and functions in midwifery, roles, and task shifting. New pathways and specialisation options are being developed for South African needs in line with international standards.

This third edition of the popular and well-established *Sellers' Midwifery* has been updated by a variety of specialists in their fields, who have considered both the contextual realities as well as scientific principles within the framework of the latest scientific developments in the field.

We hope you enjoy the new format, which also includes 25 basic procedures with more illustrations. Each chapter considers the core objectives for learning, with tasks, activities and highlights that link the learner to local and international references and information. Attention is given to the psychosocial aspects important in obstetrics and, as usual, also to applied anatomy and the physiology of pregnancy, birth and the newborn.

An additional electronic material and workbook, based on the ICM's core competencies for midwives, is available free of charge from www.juta.co.za (click on the Student Support Material link). This allows lecturers to adapt activities in line with their own curricula.

We trust that lecturers and learners will find the references and support material useful.

Joan Dippenaar
Dicky da Serra
(Editors)

Acknowledgements

The valuable contribution of the following people to the first edition of *Sellers' Midwifery* is acknowledged: Prof B Chalmers, Dr J Parkes, L Scott, J Lund, Prof S Ross, B Haddad, K Dorkein, G Green, Dr P Moore, Dr L Middleton and S Adendorff.

Numerous people also assisted with reviews at various stages of the development of this book. Their contributions are appreciated and their time and valuable input acknowledged:

- The midwifery lecturers at the SG Lourens Nursing College, who reviewed the first edition and gave input on necessary updates: Mpho Satekge, Martha Ditshego and Wilhemina Qofela.
- Mrs Maureen de Kock from the Western Cape College of Nursing and Mrs Soobamah Naicker, Vice Principal, KwaZulu-Natal College of Nursing, who reviewed the draft manuscript.
- Professor Anna Nolte of the University of Johannesburg, who reviewed the final draft of this book.
- Contributors to the second edition are acknowledged for their contribution and input: Dr M Madumo, Dr ML Modiba, and S M Naude.
- Dr D du Plessis reviewed chapters 5, 6, 7, 8, 9, 27, 45, 46 and 47 of the third edition and is mainly responsible for the procedure development.
- Prof Christa van der Walt reviewed chapters 1 to 15 of the third edition (RN, RM, RNE, RNA, RCN. B Art et Science [Potc], M Soc Sc [UFS], B Ed [UFS], M Ed [UFS], D Cur [UJ] Midwifery and Neonatal Nursing Science [Standards for antenatal care].

The following consultants are acknowledged and thanked for their dedication, time and valuable contribution in reviewing all the relevant chapters as experts in the fields of obstetrics and advanced midwifery:

- Prof Eckhart J Buchmann: PhD, MSc (Med), MB BCh, FCOG (SA). Obstetrician, clinician and researcher at the Department of Obstetrics and Gynaecology, University of the Witwatersrand. Chairperson of Priorities in Perinatal Care Association of South Africa 2004–2017.
- Dr Elizabeth Kay-Petersen: RPN, Diploma in Advanced Midwifery and Neonatal Nursing Science; Diploma in Nursing Education, B. Cur (Nursing Admin and Community Health); M Cur in Midwifery; D Cur in Professional Nursing Science. Title of Thesis: 'A Continuing Professional Development System for Nurses and Midwives in South Africa'. Nursing and midwifery lecturer for 20 years, 10 of which were as HOD for midwifery theory and practice. Dr Kay-Petersen's last 10 working years were spent at the GDOH as Director of Public Health for five years; Maternal, Neonatal, Child, and Woman's Health and Nutrition for two years; and Acting Chief Nursing and Midwifery Officer for Public Service in Gauteng for three years. She is passionate about ethically based leadership and striving for excellence in service delivery.

Section One

Maternal and child healthcare

The history of midwifery

LEARNING OBJECTIVES

On completion of this chapter, you must be able to:
- explain the meaning of the word 'midwife'
- differentiate between 'traditional midwife' and 'professional midwife'
- explain the events that have influenced the development of midwifery, both globally and in South Africa
- identify and explain the global trends in midwifery.

KNOWLEDGE ASSUMED TO BE IN PLACE

Background knowledge of the history of South Africa

KEYWORDS

midwifery • obstetrics • Safe Motherhood Initiative (SMI) • Partnership for Maternal, Newborn and Child Health (PMNCH) • traditional midwife • technical/professional midwifery • obstetrics • United Nations Educational, Scientific and Cultural Organisation (UNESCO)

1.1   Introduction

This chapter focuses on the highlights of the development of midwifery, as recorded in history. The history of humankind contains within it the reproductive care of women in pregnancy and birth as an essential aspect for the survival of a community or nation. For much of history, women were assisted by other women, often referred to as 'traditional midwives', for reproductive care.

The original word for a woman was 'wifman' or 'wif'. In the old English language, 'mid' also meant middle, indicating that the midwife was an intermediary between the mother, baby and family. 'Midwife' literally means 'with woman' or 'together with' or 'standing by'. In the Hebrew Old Testament, the word 'yalad' appears 497 times, referring among other things to both the concept of 'born' (make to) or 'prevail, attend or assist' the birth (Biblesoft, 2006).

This short overview of midwifery acknowledges both the formal and informal forms of care that existed and still exist today for women in pregnancy and birth. It also seeks to explain the recorded historical events that led to the development of midwifery as a formal profession.

1.2   How is history remembered?

History is the narrative or stories of humankind as verbally transmitted or written down in various forms. Written history only extends for about 5 000 years (starting with the Sumerians in Mesopotamia, then Egypt, Greece and others). Some ancient writings are not understood, because the language cannot be deciphered and there is always the risk of misinterpretation. Verification of historical facts is usually done through scientific research and archaeological evidence and artefacts.

Historical occurrences, developments and events always need to be judged against the background of the time period and context in history. For example, in many regions and in many time periods, women did not have rights and were not allowed to study as doctors. Therefore, many historical events mentioned in documents refer to men only. Currently there is a move towards a new narrative, where people want their 'truths', not previously recorded or verified, to be known. Women today have more rights, status and independence in most societies.

It is against this historical background that midwifery as a profession developed. It is not known how many women died in childbirth over time, but the training and regulation of midwives were seen as an effort to improve care for women and newborn babies for better health outcomes. Although midwifery has become a regulated profession, many births worldwide are still supported by traditional midwives, as is the case in Africa. In Canada, midwifery has been regulated only since 1999, and in many parts of the country 'traditional midwives' assist at what is known as midwifery-led births (CAM ACSF, 2017).

1.3 Africa as the origin of humankind

The 'Taung child', discovered in 1924 in the North West in South Africa, is estimated to be 2,8 million years old (Maropeng, 2009). It has been speculated that this skull can explain the evolution of *homo sapiens* and that humankind originated from Africa. In 1947, 'Mrs Ples', a fossil 2,3 million years old (Maropeng, 2017), was discovered 50 km northwest of Johannesburg at the Cradle of Humankind, declared a World Heritage Site by UNESCO in 1999. In 2010, the third species of human relative, named *Homo naledi*, was discovered. These discoveries stimulate questions regarding the evolution of humankind and the practices around birth in prehistoric and ancient times.

Birth is considered the most vulnerable time for a human female. Throughout history women have been attended to and supported by other women, those trusted and appointed by communities, during birth. In African cultures, people view birth as spiritual and African women were always surrounded by trusted helpers.

1.4 Medicine and care in Africa

The continent of Africa has a rich history in terms of medicine and care.

Africa played an important role in the history of the world in terms of the development of medicine and midwifery. It is acknowledged that Western medicine originated in the ancient civilisations that developed through the 30 Egyptian dynasties (3100 BCE – 332 BCE). The advanced knowledge of the Egyptians in medicine, ointments, chemistry and surgery (around 1800 BCE) influenced the development of Western medicine. Hippocrates (460–370 BCE), considered to be the 'father of modern medicine', studied at the temple of Amenhotep in Egypt. The Kahun Gynaecological Papyrus, which dates back to 1800 BCE, is the oldest surviving medical text. It describes the diagnosis and treatment of women's complaints, including problems of conception.

Libraries and universities in Africa

The library in Alexandria in Egypt, which contained 700 000 scrolls, was the largest and most important library in the ancient world. It unfortunately burnt down in 48 BCE. Another important city in Africa was Timbuktu, situated on the edge of the Sahara desert near the Niger river (today the Republic of Mali). The city existed from the fifth century, but during the 11th century it developed into a well-known centre of scholarship, with universities and a library with manuscripts on art, medicine, philosophy and astronomy, mainly in Arabic. Some of these manuscripts have been preserved and still exist today.

Although the scientific basis for medical practice originated in Egypt, in the rest of Africa traditional healthcare services provided care according to the philosophy of *ubuntu* or *unhu*. Norms, taboos, tradition and culture are the cornerstones of African traditional medicine. Pregnancy and the birth process are included in these practices.

1.5 Traditional and professional midwifery

Women as caregivers

'Midwives' have cared for women during pregnancy and birth in most communities since ancient times. For example, in the Hebrew Old Testament, in Exodus 1:14, midwives were ordered to kill baby boys at birth in Egypt, and Genesis 38:28 describes the death of a woman during the birth of twin boys, assisted by a midwife (*yalad*). These recorded stories, as well as stories in the texts of other religions and civilisations, indicate that the concept 'midwife' is found since the beginning of the recorded history of humankind. This practice was transferred from woman to woman in ancient societies through tradition and experience.

Professional midwifery

Professional midwifery refers to the science of how to best take care of women in pregnancy and birth. The importance of technical development and improved care in midwifery is reflected in the technical and scientific training of women as carers. Unfortunately, globally it is felt that the caring side of midwifery has been affected by the technical approach, although this approach has brought many benefits for mothers and children.

The rest of this chapter gives a brief overview of how midwifery developed to become a registered profession. First, midwifery is discussed in a global context, after which the development of midwifery in South Africa is explained, in order to give you a better understanding of your chosen profession.

1.6 The global development of midwifery as a profession

The profession of midwifery preceded the medical and nursing professions by millennia. As discussed above, references to midwives exist in the writings of many ancient civilisations. Limited historical records exist of birth practices on the African continent, but rich childbirth practices and traditions existed within African societies and had been maintained for centuries.

Midwifery up to the 17th century

Up until the 17th century, community or traditional midwives were the main carers of women and newborns, with little or no male involvement. Midwifery care was informal and babies were born at home. The midwife who was called to support the woman in labour was usually an older woman from the community who was experienced and trusted. This midwife is still known as a 'traditional midwife' in many parts of Africa.

The development of midwifery as a profession was influenced by changes in social structure, industrialisation, urbanisation and modernisation, as well as increasing scientific and medical knowledge. At this time, women in most societies were not allowed to study medicine. There were cases of women who disguised themselves as men in order to practise professionally. Thus, up to a few centuries ago, nearly all developments in the medical field were spearheaded by men.

The written records that provide reliable accounts of past events are limited to certain countries or areas. In cases where written records do not exist, there is an oral history, for example of the contributions of informal community birth attendants, both in Africa and in the rest of the world. This oral history is often less clear or verifiable.

The following recorded historical events are some of the significant developments that shaped midwifery as a profession before the 17th century:

- **10th century:** The first medical school in the world was founded in Salerno, Italy.
- **12th century:** At the abovementioned medical school, a female doctor named Trotula de Ruggeiro wrote a number of books, now called *The Trotula*, which gave guidelines on women's medicine, including information on a retained placenta, puerperal care and the management of third-degree perineal tears (De Divitiis, Cappabianca & De Divitiis, 2004).
- **1500:** Jakob Nufer successfully operated on his wife to deliver their baby.
- **1530:** Eucharius Rösslin, a German physician, wrote a book about childbirth that became the standard medical text for the next 200 years.

- **1561:** Gabriele Fallopio, who studied medicine at the University of Ferrara, described the female reproductive organs and named the Fallopian tubes, vagina and placenta.
- **1501–1590:** Ambroise Paré (a French surgeon to kings such as Henry III) sutured the perineum.
- **1598:** Peter Chamberlain (a French man who fled to London in 1596 and became surgeon to Queen Anne) developed the obstetric forceps (currently there are 600 types).

Midwifery in the 17th and 18th century

Until the 19th century, childbirth in most parts of the world remained informal and pregnant women were supported exclusively by other women. Hospital births were uncommon. The care of women was one-on-one, with a traditional midwife as caregiver. Some of the highlights of this period include the following:

- **1616:** William Harvey (an English physician) described human blood circulation as well as the embryo and the fetus in all its stages.
- **1637–1709:** A French obstetrician by the name of Francois Mauriceau described the mechanism of labour. He also developed the birth chair.
- **1697–1763:** William Smellie, a Scottish obstetrician, developed techniques in midwifery such as a manoeuvre to facilitate the birth of a baby in the breech position, known as the Smellie–Veit breech delivery manoeuvre.
- **1718:** The first maternity hospital was opened in England.
- **1718–1783:** William Hunter, an anatomist, described the gravid uterus and the placenta.
- **1768:** A young French student performed a symphysiotomy.
- **1768:** Margaret Stephens, a midwife herself, became the first tutor in midwifery. She later wrote a thesis entitled *The domestic midwife*.

Midwifery during the 19th century

During the 19th century, women in Europe began giving birth in institutions, in 'lying-in' wards, rather than at home. This period was marked by problems associated with puerperal fever, later identified as sepsis, which was directly related to infections acquired in hospitals. Mortality rates increased dramatically. Even though puerperal sepsis had first been described in the 1600s, it reached epidemic proportions in Europe between 1770 and 1846 and remained a problem until the role of microorganisms was discovered by Semmelweis and Oliver Holmes. Charles White (1728–1813) provided guidelines on the prevention of sepsis, and the development of the magnifying glass by Anthony van Leeuwenhoek (1632–1723) continued to add to the understanding of pathological microorganisms.

During the 19th century, both medical practitioners and midwives developed and used models to demonstrate and teach midwifery. The most important advances in midwifery during this period were pioneered in the USA. Some of the highlights include the following:

▶ **1808:** Dr John Stearns (an American physician) introduced ergot alkaloid in clinical practice. Ergot is the resting phase of a fungus, *Claviceps purpurea*, found on plant leaves. (Ergot poisoning, called St Anthony's fire, was common in populations that consumed affected grain.) Ergot was used by midwives for many centuries and caused powerful contractions of the uterus, particularly useful in postpartum haemorrhage (PPH). The drug still exists today, as ergometrine in tablet and injectable form and as syntometrine, a combination of ergometrine and oxytocin, used mainly after birth or in gynaecology practice.

▶ **1812:** Madame Marie Anne Boivin (1773–1841) published the first edition of her *Memorial of Deliveries* (second edition 1817). She was later awarded the degree of Doctor of Medicine and she contributed greatly to the medical literature of her day.

▶ **1819:** The German obstetrician Professor Franz K Naegele devised Naegele's rule to determine the estimated date of delivery (EDD). He published his research for the use of midwives in 1830; this book is still relevant today.

▶ **1822:** Gregor Mendel, an Austrian scientist and monk, described the science of genetics.

▶ **1824:** James Blundell, an English obstetrician, completed the first successful blood transfusion.

▶ **1846:** William Morton, an American dentist, demonstrated the use of chloroform as an anaesthetic agent, which changed the face of surgery. Chloroform soon found application in childbirth.

▶ **1850:** James Young Simpson, Professor of Midwifery at the University of Edinburgh, promoted chloroform for use in labour. Queen Victoria agreed to use it during her labour, making it a popular practice for that time.

▶ **1853:** Florence Nightingale started the reformation of nursing in England to improve hospital conditions and training for nurses and midwives.

▶ **1860:** Louis Pasteur, a French chemist and microbiologist, showed that the microorganism *Streptococcus* was the cause of puerperal sepsis.

▶ **1861:** A training school for midwives was opened by Florence Nightingale in London called The King's College. It was the first nursing school continuously connected to a fully serving hospital and medical school, St Thomas' hospital.

▶ **1872:** John Braxton Hicks, an English obstetrician, described the uterine action during labour.

▶ **1879:** Albert Neisser, a German physician and bacteriologist, described the causative organism of gonorrhoea, the microorganism *Neisseria gonococcus*.

▶ **1881:** The Trained Midwives' Registration Society was founded in the UK, which raised standards in the profession. Midwifery started to develop into a formal, independent profession.

Midwifery in the 20th century

Midwifery in the 20th century was still unsophisticated, but the foundations for change were laid by the introduction of 'pro-maternity' care to make giving birth safer for mothers and newborns. Some important developments in midwifery during this period include the following:

▶ **1928:** Selmar Aschheim and Bernard Zondek (a German gynaecologist) developed the pregnancy test.

▶ **1939:** Alexander Weiner and Dr Karl Landsteiner discovered the Rh factor in blood group typing.

▶ **1940:** Alexander Fleming (a Scottish pharmacologist) developed penicillin after he accidently discovered it in fungi.

▶ **1955:** Vincent du Vigneaud, an American biochemist, received the Nobel Prize for the synthesis of polypeptide hormones, particularly oxytocin.

Medical developments stretched over the Western world and included rapid advances in healthcare through anaesthetics and analgesia, surgery, X-rays, early diagnosis of pregnancy, antibiotics, the development of antenatal care, advances in nutrition and the artificial feeding of babies, phototherapy, ultrasound, contraception, infertility care, genetics and preterm intensive care. At the same time, improvements in maternal care practice and services were recognised and investigated.

In 1979, during the International Year of the Child, the WHO and 33 member states recognised unresolved issues in maternal healthcare. A five-year study was conducted in Europe, called 'Having a baby in Europe'. The conclusions from this study showed that the fragmentation of care of women in childbirth and the high level of interventions in healthcare systems were having a negative impact on midwifery practice (WHO, 1985). It was recognised that midwives had become the sole providers of care only when a medical practitioner was not present, mainly to the poor.

As a way of recognising the important role of the midwife globally, the Safe Motherhood Initiative (SMI) was established in 1987. This initiative was supported by the International Council of Nurses (ICN), the International Confederation of Midwives (ICM), the United Nations Children's Fund (UNICEF) and the World Bank. The original aim was to strengthen midwifery practice in order to reduce maternal mortality by 50 per cent globally by the year 2000. A civil organisation, the White Ribbon Alliance for Safe Motherhood (an international voice for women), also joined the movement to make childbirth safer.

Acknowledging that 80 per cent of births globally were still conducted by midwives, the SMI recognised problems in terms of human resources and in healthcare systems that affected the delivery of maternal healthcare. The SMI published several documents that advocated for the value of midwives as key care providers and that made recommendations to strengthen the midwifery profession. Midwifery is now on the global agenda and several partnerships have been formed to strengthen midwifery and healthcare systems.

The following are the major activities undertaken by the SMI, some of which are still ongoing:

- **1987:** The SMI was launched in Nairobi. In the same year, the partogram was launched as a quality care tool in labour.
- **1989:** The first global study and fact book on maternal mortality was released (Zhar & Royston, 1991).
- **1991–1992:** The ICM conference decided on actions to strengthen the midwifery curriculum, with a move to more community-based learning and a better understanding of obstetric emergencies (Resolution WHA 42.27) (Broad, 1991).
- **1994:** Mother–baby packages were produced, with appropriately trained midwives as key healthcare providers.
- **1995:** Resolution WHA 45.5, by the 45th World Health Assembly, was published for implementation (De la Santé, 1995).
- **1996:** Education modules were produced for midwives.
- **1996:** The WHO led a working group to define 'normal birth'.
- **2005:** Safe motherhood came to be considered as a fundamental human rights issue and researchers concluded that interventions for maternal and newborn health at community and primary care level are the most beneficial and cost-effective way to reduce mortality. (For more about the SMI, see Islam, 2007, or go to http://www.who.int/bulletin/volumes/85/10/07-045963/en/.)

Midwifery in the 21st century

At the beginning of the 21st century, there was global reflection on the role and function of the midwife in healthcare. It was apparent from research that midwives were carrying the burden of care during childbirth and that, often, nurses and midwives were the main and only caregivers for the poor. The WHO expressed concern about the recruitment and retention of skilled and motivated nurse-midwives and midwives for the healthcare workforce. In May 2001, the 54th World Health Assembly adopted Resolution WHA 54.12, which aimed to strengthen nursing and midwifery.

Several strategies were adopted to improve maternal healthcare in various contexts. In the USA, the Pew Commission accepted the midwifery model of care as the official model for the 21st century. Similar initiatives in Europe referred to midwifery-led care (MLC) as a model to improve and strengthen standards of care in midwifery. The new models of care sought to improve the quality of care through improved continuity of the carer, thereby avoiding fragmentation of care.

Between 2000 and 2005, the SMI launched and promoted the Making Pregnancy Safer campaign. One of the objectives was the promotion of the skilled attendance approach to reduce maternal mortality. The SMI identified the indicators required for the reduction of maternal deaths. The ICM developed several documents to strengthen midwifery, including the definition of a midwife and an outline of core competencies, as determined by research that involved all members. In addition, the ICN published the standards of education for nurses and midwives. The research and developmental support of the SMI and ICM is ongoing.

An additional international collaboration was developed to support maternal, newborn and child health and healthcare professionals, namely the WHO's Partnership for Maternal, Newborn and Child Health (PMNCH), launched in 2005 (visit www.who.int/pmnch/ to read more about this partnership). Membership is available only for groups and institutions that support the cause.

1.7 The development of midwifery in South Africa

As previously mentioned, there are not many historical records of the practices related to birth in African societies prior to a certain point in time. For example, it is not clear how many women died in childbirth in African societies and how this was handled. It is known that women were mainly involved in the birthing process and older women and family members took care of birthing women. These assisting women were not initially called midwives, but were later referred to as traditional midwives. Some still exist in Africa, but not many remain in South Africa.

Beverly Chalmers (1990) explores African birth traditions, emphasising their sacredness and their natural approach, with an emphasis on deeply rooted cultural beliefs and the reverence for new life, spirituality and traditions that is the hallmark of African societies. The exposure of African cultures to European people and European medical doctors played a role in the transition of birth traditions in the African population in South Africa. Western medicine became accepted alongside traditional practices.

From the time of European settlement in South Africa, midwives were brought from Europe to Africa. Among the European settlers, private nursing and midwifery services were available. Mothers outside the European settlements either gave birth on their own or were assisted within the community by traditional midwives or helpers.

The early days

The recorded history of midwifery in South Africa starts with the establishment of a halfway post at the Cape by the Dutch East India Company (DEIC). The post was a stopping point for ships on the trade route between Europe and India and included medical care for those who became ill on the long journey at sea.

The DEIC endeavoured to provide sworn midwives in the Cape Colony, the first of which arrived from Europe and was appointed in 1703. These sworn midwives usually came from the Netherlands, but sometimes local women were sworn in as well, for example Marie Buisset (1676–1708). These sworn midwives enjoyed some status in the community of European settlers. They were employees of the DEIC and received a monthly salary. The midwives were 'skilled attendants' and one of their tasks was to name the father of the child, as many were the children of soldiers in service of the DEIC.

During the 17th and 18th centuries, medical practitioners in Europe were drawn from a variety of occupations, but unfortunately not all were well qualified. Towards the close of the 18th century, a university-educated medical professional, Dr JHFCL Wehr, settled in the Cape. Dr Wehr would play a significant role in the development of midwifery in South Africa.

In 1807, during the second British occupation of the Cape, further controls for midwives were instituted. Hospitals were established which compared favourably with European hospitals. Beds were only available for the use of midwives in emergencies. Maternal deaths were uncommon and puerperal sepsis was unheard of, because women did not give birth in institutions.

The 19th century

Dr Wehr started the first midwifery school in 1810. On 2 August 1813, the first seven European midwives who graduated took an oath, which had been developed from an ethical code of conduct. The first midwives from non-European ethnic groups in the area were also trained and registered later in this period. As mentioned, women from non-European population groups in South Africa at that time gave birth with the assistance of traditional helpers, mainly a trusted woman in the family or community.

Other highlights of this period include the following:
- **1809:** The first midwifery handbook was completed by Dr Kemp.
- **1816:** Dr James Barry performed the first Caesarean section in the Cape.
- **1858:** Beds were made available for midwifery cases in Albany Hospital, Grahamstown.
- **1876:** Sr Henrietta Stockdale (a pioneer from Britain) was trained by Dr Prince (a Canadian) as a midwife in Kimberley. She went on to establish southern Africa's first training school for nurses at the Carnarvon Hospital.
- **1887:** Mary Hirst Watkins, a nurse and midwife, became the founder of modern midwifery in South Africa. She founded district midwifery and became famous throughout South Africa and Britain.
- **1891:** South African midwives were the first in the world to obtain state registration. This took place through the Medical and Pharmacy Act 34 of 1891, which regulated their practice. (This registration is still applicable today for nurses and midwives through the Nursing Act 33 of 2005.) The Act was extended to non-European territories.
- **1892:** Regulations for the certification of midwives were gazetted on 31 May 1892. Section A made provision for recognising overseas qualifications. The first seven midwives to register, on 6 September 1892, held qualifications from Stockholm, the City of London, Dublin and Edinburgh.
- **End of the 19th century:** Midwifery education and registration were well established in South Africa. Midwives also worked in other regions of southern Africa.

The 20th century

The development of midwifery in South Africa continued in the 20th century, with ever-increasing formalisation for candidates from all population groups. For example, the late Albertina Sisulu studied to become a nurse and midwife in 1939. In 1954 she obtained her midwifery qualification and worked in the city of Johannesburg as a professional midwife

(Littlejohn, 2014). The following were other important events that took place in the 20th century:

▶ **1904:** The Orange Free State made provision for the registration of health professionals, including nurses and midwives.

▶ **1908:** Cecilia Makiwane was registered as the first black professional nurse in South Africa.

▶ **1910:** With the Union (merging) of the colonies, all laws were consolidated. This led to the establishment of the Medical, Dental and Pharmacy Council Act 13 of 1928.

▶ **1927:** Beatrice Msimeng was registered as the first black general nurse and midwife in South Africa.

▶ **1944:** The Nursing Act 45 of 1944 was approved, making nursing and midwifery in South Africa self-regulated. Two statutory bodies were created: the Nursing Council (to safeguard the public) and the South African Nursing Association (to look after the interests of the profession). The Nursing Act 69 of 1957 replaced Act 45 of 1944 in an attempt to address the diverse needs of the population, with the aim of increasing the number of nurses from ethnic population groups and replacing white nurses in hospitals that existed for different racial groups at the time.

▶ **1947:** Courses for midwifery educators and lecturers were established at the University of the Witwatersrand and the University of Pretoria, followed by courses at other universities.

▶ **1955:** Thirty scholarships were made available for nursing students to enrol in the first Faculty of Arts and the Faculty of Science at the University of Pretoria. Other universities followed suit.

▶ **1960:** Midwifery was offered as a one-year post-basic diploma following three years of basic general training. Direct entry to midwifery allowed students to do only midwifery over a two-year period.

▶ **1968:** The training of nurses and midwives became integrated in a four-and-a-half-year programme and, later, a four-year degree or diploma.

▶ **1971:** Nurses from all ethnic groups gained access to B Cur I et A education in nursing administration and education at the University of the North.

▶ **1972:** Direct entry to midwifery was ruled out by the South African Nursing Council (SANC) and only people with previous professional qualifications could be admitted to a one-year midwifery diploma.

▶ **1977:** By this time, 18 362 nurses from other ethnic population groups were registered with the SANC, with 60 nursing schools offering midwifery for nurses from ethnic population groups.

▶ **1977:** Male students were admitted to midwifery training. They were called accoucheurs.

▶ **1980:** The first nurses from population groups other than white nurses gained admission to study nursing at the University of the Witwatersrand.

▶ **1985:** The four-year basic nursing programme diploma or degree (R425) became comprehensive and students were registered for general, midwifery, psychiatry and community nursing. Professionals in this category are considered to be nurse-midwives today according to the ICN (see www.icn.ch) because they were trained in general nursing and midwifery care through an integrated training programme.

▶ **1993:** An additional advanced midwifery qualification became available as a post-basic diploma or degree.

The 21st century: The democratic Republic of South Africa

After the democratic elections of 1994, the political landscape of South Africa changed. All political, legal and management structures were transformed. The following are important developments that took place after the advent of democracy:

▶ **2005:** The Nursing Act 33 of 2005 (NA) was enacted. The transformation of the healthcare system and nursing was initiated, with the South African Nursing Association becoming the Democratic Nursing Organisation of South Africa (DENOSA). The transformation of all systems continues.

▶ **2009:** The Collaboration in Higher Education for Nursing and Midwifery in Africa (CHENMA): Through NEPAD funding, selected South African universities supported post-basic specialist education and training for nurses in Africa at master's degree level. These were the Muhimbili College of Health Sciences and the Kilimanjaro Christian Medical Centre at universities in Tanzania, and the Moi, East Africa (Baraton) and Nairobi universities in Kenya as well as ISCISA in Mozambique in 2010 (Bruce et al, 2017).

▶ **2011:** Recognising the growing challenges confronting nurses and midwives in South Africa, the Department of Health (DoH) convened a National Nursing Summit from 5 to 7 April 2011 in Johannesburg to 'reconstruct and revitalize the nursing profession' (DoH, 2013a).

▶ **2013:** The *National Strategic Plan for Nurse Education, Training and Practice 2012/13–2016/17* was launched in March 2013 to give direction to decisions for nursing and midwifery. The first Chief Nursing Officer (CNO) was appointed in December 2013 to provide leadership and stewardship.

Seven strategic priorities were established, namely (DoH, 2013a):

1. declaring nursing colleges as higher education institutions
2. developing a core curriculum for nursing
3. developing leadership and management structures
4. creating positive practice environments
5. improving ethos
6. setting national norms and standards
7. setting staffing norms.

▶ **2015:** New nursing curricula were instituted for 2018 and midwifery remained in the basic nursing programme. Midwives are registered on a separate roll at the SANC, indicating the professional status of midwives and nurse-midwives in South Africa. Specialist nurse programmes are approved by the Minister of Health and will be developed in line with local needs and international trends.

▶ **2016:** The NA makes provision for continuing professional development (CPD) for all categories of nurses and midwives. A CPD system was developed and piloted in 2016.

1.8   Conclusion

Midwifery practice, including technical, pharmaceutical and surgical practice, developed and changed over time to adapt to the contextual realities of countries around the world, including South Africa. Midwifery has stood the test of time and is still considered the best practice to care for women, newborns and children. It is supported and strengthened internationally through research and international guidelines (visit www.who.int/pmnch/ for more details).

Strategies to improve maternal and perinatal care and reduce mortality and morbidity

LEARNING OBJECTIVES

On completion of this chapter, you must be able to:

▶ describe the causes of maternal and perinatal deaths in South Africa
▶ know and apply the relevant recommendations of the tri-annual reports *Saving Mothers* and *Saving Babies*
▶ explain the strategies, programmes and interventions developed to improve maternal and neonatal health outcomes in South Africa.

KNOWLEDGE ASSUMED TO BE IN PLACE

Basic knowledge of the nursing process regarding maternal and child healthcare
The principles of observation, management, referral and record keeping

KEYWORDS

maternal morbidity and mortality • perinatal morbidity and mortality • *Saving Mothers* reports • *Saving Babies* reports • National Committee on Confidential Enquiries into Maternal Deaths (NCCEMD) • Perinatal Problem Identification Programme (PPIP)

2.1   Introduction

This chapter provides an overview of the status of maternal and newborn healthcare. The surveillance, analysis and interpretation of critical indicators show the effectiveness and performance of the healthcare system. The reports generated form the basis for the development of interventions and strategies aimed at improving maternal and perinatal healthcare outcomes in South Africa.

This chapter is an introduction to the indicators and data that are gathered in the South African healthcare system.

2.2   Birth statistics

Vital statistics are gathered by the government and a database is kept of data such as the births and deaths registered in the country (see www.statssa.gov.za). Birth statistics are important, as they facilitate the analysis of demographic trends for the

assessment and planning of reproductive health services, and for antenatal and neonatal healthcare services. The birth certificate is one way of gathering information.

The value of a birth certificate is unfortunately not widely understood, and a child without a birth certificate is vulnerable. In 2013 it was reported that, globally, the existence of one in three children (or 60 per cent) under five years is not legally acknowledged, because they do not have birth certificates (UNICEF, 2013a). This makes these children vulnerable, as without a birth certificate, it is not possible to obtain an identity document for a child, nor is it possible to access welfare grants or other social services. The failure to register a child's birth is therefore considered a violation of the child's human rights (OHCHR, 2014).

In South Africa, the Births and Deaths Registration Amendment Act 18 of 2010 regulates the registration of births and deaths in the country, to ensure the protection of the population's human rights. However, birth statistics in South Africa are incomplete and inconsistent because of missing or incomplete birth notification forms. The district health system and district management teams are responsible for recording and reporting the birth notifications of all births in the different districts. This includes home births or out-of-hospital births under their jurisdiction. Although the Department of Home Affairs (DHA) instituted a system to register births in facilities in the public health system, not all facilities have officials to assist mothers to register the baby. Midwives should therefore take responsibility to complete birth notifications for the births they attend.

Birth notification and registration: DHA-24

The birth notification is an official record completed by the professional attending the birth on behalf of the local authority, for the purpose of monitoring and planning for future services.

Birth registration as a statutory requirement

All live or stillborn children (viable after 28 weeks), born of permanent or non-permanent South African citizens, must be registered by parents, guardians or any legal person with the DHA within 30 days after birth (form B1-24, completed in black ink). An abridged birth certificate is issued free of charge. If a birth is not registered within the first 30 days of life, that birth is considered as a late registration. There are two categories of late registration, namely after 30 days but before one year, and after one year up to 15 years.

In South Africa, there has been a vast improvement in the registration of births. In 2015, 84.8 per cent of births were registered (Stats SA, 2016a).

2.3 Health statistics

Health statistics are a numeric expression of aspects of health in a population. Maternal and newborn outcomes are important indicators of how well a healthcare system is functioning. These statistics include an evaluation of mortality and morbidity data. Data such as birth rates and maternal, perinatal and neonatal morbidity and mortality are important indicators of maternal healthcare services. The accurate measurement of these remains a challenge.

Birth rate

The crude birth rate is the number of live births per 1 000 people in a population per year. The birth rate for South Africa in 2016 was 20.5 live births per 1 000 of the population (Index Mundi, 2017). In 2016, the average crude birth rate for the world was 19/1 000 of the population (World Bank, 2017). This is 15 000 births per hour. According to the CIA's World Factbook (2016), the country with the highest birth rate in 2016 was Niger, at 44.8/1 000 of the population, and the country with the lowest birth rate was Monaco, at 6.6/1 000. A birth rate ranging from 10 to 20/1 000 is considered low and a birth rate ranging from 40 to 50/1 000 is considered high (The World Factbook, 2016).

Birth weight

Birth weight is an important indicator of the health of mothers and babies. It can indicate long-term maternal malnutrition, ill health or strain, and sub-standard or poor antenatal care. Low birth weight (LBW) is a global concern and is associated with higher infant mortality. LBW is defined by the WHO as babies born alive below the birth weight of 2 500 g. Globally, 15–20 per cent of babies are born with LBW according to the estimated date of birth. The World Health Assembly (WHA) set a target to reduce LBW by 30 per cent by the year 2025 (WHO, 2014a). The prevalence varies between regions, with most cases occurring in low- and middle-income countries. The incidence of LBW is estimated at 13 per cent in sub-Saharan Africa (WHO 2014a). The *Saving Babies 2012–2013* report indicated that district hospitals deliver a live LBW baby every five days and that 12 per cent (one in eight) will be an early newborn death (Pattinson & Rhoda 2014). UNICEF has indicated that in 2008–2013, 46 per cent of babies were not weighed at birth in eastern and southern Africa (UNICEF, 2016a).

Maternal mortality

The maternal mortality rate is defined as the death of a woman while pregnant, during childbirth or within 42 days after termination of pregnancy, from any cause related to or provoked by pregnancy or its management, expressed per 100 000 live births during a particular time period. The causes of maternal deaths are categorised as follows:

▶ *Direct causes* of maternal mortality are factors associated with complications in pregnancy and birth, and management.
▶ *Indirect causes* are pre-existing conditions, such as cardiac conditions, which are aggravated by pregnancy and birth.

Coincidental deaths are unrelated to pregnancy – for example deaths from cancer or other conditions – and are therefore are not included in the statistics.

Perinatal mortality

The perinatal period is from 154 days of gestation (22 weeks) until seven days after birth. The perinatal mortality rate

(PNMR) is expressed as the number of deaths and stillbirths occurring from 22 weeks of gestation up to the first week of life per 1 000 live births.

Stillbirth

A stillbirth is the birth of a fetus that died *in utero* (macerated fetus) or had a heartbeat in labour but showed no signs of life after birth (fresh stillbirth). The statistics are expressed per 1 000 live births. Stillbirths are under-reported (WHO, 2017a). The stillbirth rate is included in the PNMR, but considered separately it was estimated at 32/1 000 live births in developing countries versus 5/1 000 live births in developed countries in 2009 (WHO, 2011a).

Abortion/miscarriage

An abortion refers to the termination of a pregnancy before the fetus is viable, whether spontaneous or induced. When the process occurs spontaneously, it is referred to as a miscarriage in common language. In South Africa, a fetus is considered viable after 28 weeks of gestation. Viability refers to the ability to exist physiologically separate from the mother and is based on the maturity of the lungs.

Neonatal mortality

The neonatal period is from birth until 28 days after birth. A neonate is therefore defined as a newborn under 28 days of life. The neonatal mortality rate (NMR) is defined as the total number of neonatal deaths expressed per 1 000 live births. It is divided into early neonatal death (within seven days after birth) and late neonatal death (8–28 days after birth).

Maternal, perinatal and neonatal morbidity

Morbidity refers to complications and long-term health problems that result from pregnancy and birth. For every maternal death, there are 30 women who will develop illnesses that result in long-term health problems. Neonatal morbidity has both short- and long-term effects on the infant's or baby's development, some of which may carry over into childhood and adulthood.

2.4 Maternal mortality in South Africa

Since 1990, South Africa has followed best practice guidelines as set out by the WHO and other countries (such as the UK) in gathering information to determine the rates and causes of maternal and perinatal deaths. These data are used to identify the causes of death and to develop strategies to prevent them.

Since 1 October 1997, in South Africa the death of a woman during pregnancy or in childbirth has been declared a notifiable condition in terms of the National Policy for Health Act 116 of 1990, when the Minister of Health appointed the National Committee on Confidential Enquiries into Maternal Deaths (NCCEMD). The first report, entitled *Maternal Deaths in South Africa 1998*, was published in 1998. Since then, South Africa has measured maternal deaths and has reported on these deaths every three years in a report referred to as *Saving Mothers*. (You can view the latest report, *Saving Mothers 2011–2013*, at https://www.health-e.org.za/wp-content/uploads/2016/05/Saving-Mothers-2011-2013-short-report.pdf. You can also follow new reports as they are published.)

Main causes of maternal deaths in South Africa

Most maternal deaths are preventable. According to *Saving Mothers 2011–2013*, five factors are the main causes of maternal deaths in South Africa (DoH, 2014):

▸ Two-thirds of all maternal deaths are due to three factors:
  • The most common cause of maternal death is non-pregnancy-related infections (NPRIs). Most women in this group die of HIV and TB infections. A decline in HIV-related deaths since the monitoring of maternal mortality in 1998 is most likely due to HIV screening and treatment programmes.
  • Ante- and postpartum haemorrhage during or after pregnancy is the second most common cause of maternal death in South Africa. *The Saving Mothers 2011–2013* report indicates that more than half of women who died from obstetric haemorrhage during this period had Caesarean sections (DoH, 2014: v).
  • The third most common cause of maternal death is complications due to hypertension in pregnancy.
▸ Medical and surgical conditions and pregnancy-related sepsis are also indicated as causes of maternal death.

Other risk factors to be considered include:
▸ a maternal age of under 20 years (which carries a risk for hypertensive conditions)
▸ an advanced maternal age of 35 years and older (which carries a risk for obstetric haemorrhage and other direct and indirect causes of maternal death)
▸ administrative problems such as transport problems and a lack of facilities and staff
▸ patient problems, such as non- or delayed health-seeking behaviour
▸ healthcare provider problems, such as poor assessment and the failure to recognise obstetric emergencies and to follow treatment protocols.

Recommendations

The ten recommendations contained in the first to fifth *Saving Mothers* reports are summarised in the latest, sixth report as the five Hs and five Cs (DoH, 2014).

The five Hs are focused on ease of implementation. These refer to:
1. HIV
2. haemorrhage
3. hypertension
4. health professional training
5. health system strengthening.

The five Cs are:
1. care and commitment to quality
2. coverage of programme delivery and emergency management systems (EMS), waiting areas and MomConnect (an electronic SMS programme for improved communication with pregnant women)
3. Ceasarean section safety – to ensure skills and facilities
4. contraception – to improve uptake of contraception
5. community involvement – to encourage involvement through health committees.

The *Saving Mothers 2011–2013* report, published in 2014, indicated the key areas for improvement in maternal health outcomes (see Table 2.1). The report addresses quality of care in the prevention of pregnancy (contraception), early antenatal care (before 20 weeks), quality service delivery (including appropriate facilities, skilled attendance, effective emergency transport and safe Caesarean section) and community involvement. Monitoring and evaluation are essential and audit cycles and maternal mortality reviews (including near-miss events) are needed at district and facility level.

Table 2.1

Summary of the strategy to reduce maternal deaths (adapted from DoH, 2014)

Essential aspects of the strategy (five Hs and five Cs)	
HIV	Care and commitment to quality of care
Hypertension	Coverage of care
Haemorrhage	Community participation
Human resources (healthcare provider [HCP]): Knowledge and skill development (Essential Steps in the Management of Obstetric Emergencies/Emergency Obstetric Simulation Training [ESMOE/EOST])	Contraception
Health systems: Appropriate resource facilities (maternity waiting rooms)	Caesarean section safety
Functional, reliable 24-hr emergency and transport system	
Monitoring and evaluation systems	
Audit cycles and review meetings	
↓	
REDUCTION IN MATERNAL MORTALITY	

2.5 Perinatal mortality in South Africa

The National Perinatal Morbidity and Mortality Committee (NaPeMMCo) reports triennially and provides recommendations on perinatal care (see Pattinson & Rhoda, 2014). The Medical Research Council's (MRC) Maternal and Infant Health Care Strategy Research Unit in Kalafong was initiated on 1 October 1999. The programme under the MRC is called the Perinatal Problem Identification Programme (PPIP) (see www.ppip.co.za). In 2014, the PPIP collected 75.6 per cent of birth data at district level through the District Health Information System (DHIS), thereby enhancing the quality of data collected in South Africa (Pattinson & Rhoda, 2014: 2).

Important indicators as reflected at district level are indicted in Table 2.2.

Table 2.2

Perinatal and neonatal indicators (HST, 2016: 83, 88, 108)

Indicator	Target	South African average 2015–16
Stillbirth ratio	Set by district	20.7 %
In-patient early neonatal death	Facility-based	10.1 per 1 000 live births
Infant's first PCR* DNA or RNA test 6 weeks uptake	To be determined at district level	100 %
Infant's first PCR test positive at 6 weeks	1.8 %	1.5 %

*Polymerase chain reaction

Causes of perinatal deaths

The main causes of perinatal deaths are hypoxia and immaturity. The transmission of HIV from mother to child and TB are also critical factors for poor maternal and neonatal outcomes in South Africa. It is clear from the nine PPIP reports that the health system and human resource issues are pivotal factors to improved health outcomes for babies in South Africa.

NaPEMMCo and the Child Health Cluster's strategies: HHAPI-Ness for improved health outcomes for newborns

The following are considered:

H = Health systems for mothers and babies must be appropriate and effective.

H = Healthcare providers must be skilled and there must be enough healthcare providers.

A = Asphyxia must be prevented and reduced.

P = Prematurity must be prevented and reduced.

I = Infections must be prevented and reduced.

Ness = Newborn Survival Strategy

The effective implementation of these strategies include the five Hs detailed in the *Saving Mothers 2011–2013* report, as mentioned on page 14.

Recommendations

In 2013, the Child Health Cluster of the South African national Department of Health (DoH) developed a plan of action for newborn care. This plan is called the *HHAPI-Ness Road Map for Healthy Babies in South Africa* (DoH, 2013b) and it summarises national key findings and recommendations for newborns (see www.childhealthpriorities.co.za for more information). The plan sets out clear steps, roles and responsibilities for all levels of healthcare.

2.6 Conclusion

It is important to consider maternal and perinatal mortality jointly, as the mother's health influences that of the fetus and the newborn.

The *Saving Mothers* and *Saving Babies* reports are ongoing documents and new and improved implementation strategies are introduced after each report. Midwives need to stay abreast of these changes.

Midwifery practice and care

3.1 Introduction

Chapter 1 gave a brief overview of the development of midwifery in South Africa. This chapter will look at the current and future roles and functions of midwives, benchmarked against international trends in midwifery.

3.2 Description: Midwives and midwifery as a profession

The most recent South African Nursing Act 33 of 2005 (NA) defines a midwife – in Chapter 2(30)(2) – as 'a person who is qualified and competent to independently practise midwifery in the manner and to the level prescribed and who is capable of assuming responsibility and accountability for such practice'. This is in line with the international definition of midwifery. In South Africa, midwifery is acknowledged as a separate discipline, as the NA refers to nursing as well as midwifery.

South Africa is a member of the International Confederation of Midwives (ICM), and practice in the country is aligned to the principles, definitions and practices for midwives as presented by that body. The ICM's definition of a midwife is the following (ICM, 2017):

A midwife is a person who has successfully completed a midwifery education programme that is recognised in the country where it is located and that is based on the ICM Essential Competencies for Basic Midwifery Practice and the framework of the ICM Global Standards for Midwifery Education; who has acquired the requisite qualifications to be registered and/or legally licensed to practice midwifery and use the title 'midwife'; and who demonstrates competency in the practice of midwifery.

The ICM's definition is expanded to recognise the following scope of practice (ICM, 2017):

The midwife is recognised as a responsible and accountable professional who works in partnership with women to give the necessary support, care and advice during pregnancy, labour and the postpartum period, to conduct births on the midwife's own responsibility and to provide care for the newborn and the infant. This care includes preventative measures, the promotion of normal birth, the detection of complications in mother and child, the accessing of medical care or other appropriate assistance and the carrying out of emergency measures. The midwife has an important task in health counselling and education, not only for the woman, but also within the family and the community. This work should involve antenatal education and preparation for parenthood and may extend to women's health, sexual or reproductive health and childcare. A midwife may practise in any setting including the home, community, hospitals, clinics or health units.

In 2008, at the Glasgow council meeting, 67 of the 200 members of the ICM voted in favour of making abortion care part of the practice of midwives (ICM, 2014c).

Categories of midwives

There are different categories of midwives in formal and informal healthcare settings, namely traditional midwives, lay midwives and professional midwives or nurse-midwives. The term 'nurse-midwife' refers to midwives trained in general nursing and in midwifery. Around the world, 60 per cent of nurses are also trained as midwives.

In the third version of the International Standard Classification of Occupations (ISCO-88[2]), as agreed upon by the International Labour Organisation (ILO) in 1987, nurses and midwives are classified as one category, namely code 223. Together with medical practitioners (ISCO code 222), they are classified as healthcare workers. Midwifery is not regarded as a separate discipline or healthcare professional in the ISCO-88.

South Africa has only two categories of midwives registered with the South African Nursing Council (SANC): professional midwives and enrolled midwives. In South Africa, approximately 50–60 per cent of midwives are nurse-midwives, trained in both general nursing and midwifery. There are separate rolls for the registration of nurses (general, community and psychiatry) and midwifery. There is no database of the number of midwives actively and directly involved in maternal child care. This makes it difficult to know the midwifery workforce needed for the future.

The SANC's rolls of 2015 reflected a total number of 102 085 registered midwives. These included:
- 8 306 accoucheurs
- 93 739 midwives (165 without general nursing)
- 46 enrolled midwives.

Strategies to strengthen the midwifery profession

The midwife is the primary and preferred provider for 80 per cent of care of mothers and babies in pregnancy and birth globally. Since 1987, the Safe Motherhood Initiative (SMI) has developed strategies to make pregnancy safer and to strengthen midwifery.

The ICM supports, represents and works towards strengthening professional associations of midwives. The ICM

is organised into four regions: Africa, the Americas, Asia Pacific and Europe. Currently, there are 131 midwives' associations, representing 113 countries across every continent. These organisations include the WHO, the Federation of Gynaecology and Obstetrics (FIGO), the International Paediatric Association (IPA), the International Council of Nurses (ICN) and bilateral civil societies. Although the transformation of nursing and midwifery is still in progress, South African midwives, through the Society of Midwives of South Africa (SOMSA), subscribe to the principles of the ICM.

The core functions of midwives

The midwife has the knowledge and skill to care for women and their newborns.

Styles or forms of midwifery practice vary greatly between healthcare systems due to contextual differences, and midwifery practice may be different in different settings.

On the other hand, there is consensus on the tasks of the midwife globally, but not on the optimal provision and form of midwifery care to the community. The midwife's practice ranges from being the only practitioner a woman will ever see (independently or as an employee in an institution), to being a referral practice or part of a multidisciplinary team within a tertiary healthcare setting.

Midwifery in the South African context

In South Africa, the transformation of the healthcare system and higher education has had an impact on the role and function of the midwife. The development of the district health system (DHS) placed the care of mothers and babies in the hands of midwives for the population that use the public healthcare system.

Midwifery is an integral part of the healthcare system in South Africa. This means that most women will receive care from a midwife during childbirth in some form or other.

Traditionally, midwives were seen as a separate profession in South Africa, with separate rolls. Today there are separate rolls for the registration of professional nurses (general, community and psychiatry) and midwives. In South Africa, midwives complete a prescribed SANC-approved programme with associated practical experience before they are registered on the SANC roll for midwives.

Data on the number of midwives vary, depending on the source of information. Approximately 50–60 per cent of midwives in South Africa are dually qualified as general nurses and midwives.

Midwives who are also qualified as general nurses may find themselves doing many other tasks assigned to them by the workplace. Most midwives in South Africa work within the national healthcare system at different levels of care. The *South African Demographic Health Survey* (SADHS) (DoH, 1998) indicated that in 1998 only three out of 10 women in the public sector saw a medical practitioner at least once in pregnancy and labour. In other words, 70 per cent of the care of mothers and babies in the public sector is in the hands of midwives. This makes maternal and newborn care in South Africa a nurse-based system.

The number of midwives working in private maternity hospitals is unknown but is always reported as insufficient. It is estimated that only 300 midwives are providing private ante- and postnatal care, of whom only 30 are doing home and hospital deliveries as private one-to-one caregivers.

3.3   The competencies of midwives

The definition of competency by Knol and Van Linge (2009: 361) indicates that competency can be explained as more than knowledge, skills, attitude and attributes; it also includes the level of confidence a person has in his or her ability to perform a job well in a given environment.

If the environment is well resourced and supportive, the practitioner's performance is enhanced. The competency required of midwives, as determined globally, therefore needs to be grounded in different contexts for healthcare professionals to perform effectively.

The following discussion on competency refers to both the science and art of midwifery, and ways in which these aspects are integrated.

Core competencies: The science of midwifery

The core competencies of midwives have been defined by the ICM in a document entitled *Essential Competencies for Basic Midwifery Practice* (ICM, 2013). The ICM promotes guidelines for evidence-based midwifery practice and has established clearly defined core competencies for midwives. These guidelines are used around the globe to guide the practice in different contexts.

The ICM's standards for midwifery

Read more about international standards of midwifery. The following documents are available from the ICM at www. internationalmidwives.org (accessed June 2017):
▶ *ICM Global Standards for Midwifery Education* (2010–2013)
▶ *ICM Global Standards for Midwifery Regulation* (2011)

continued

▶ *ICM Model Curriculum Outlines for Professional Midwifery*
▶ *ICM Midwifery Service Framework*
▶ *ICM Essential Competencies for Basic Midwifery Practice* (2010–2013)
▶ *ICM Standard Equipment List for Competency-Based Skills Training in Midwifery Schools* (2012)
▶ *ICM Competency Self-Assessment Tool* (2013).

The scope of midwifery practice and basic competencies

The SANC's regulation R2488, dated 26 October 1990, clearly indicates the scope of practice for midwives in South Africa as the 'normal pregnancy, postnatal and newborn care' (SANC, 1990). However, midwives need to be skilled and competent to identify and refer risks and manage complications and abnormalities in an emergency where necessary.

Life-saving skills and competency (skilled attendance)

The SMI and WHO made a call to save the lives of mothers during pregnancy and birth 22 years ago. The best way to save women's lives is through skilled birth attendance in an accredited heath facility. The SMI considers skilled attendance as one of the main ways to improve skills and competency to save lives for improved maternal healthcare outcomes. These competencies exceed the scope of 'normal' and require midwives to be competent in more advanced skills focused on pregnancy and birth. In South Africa, this necessitates training at post-basic or post-graduate diploma level.

A *skilled attendant* is defined as an accredited professional nurse, doctor or midwife with emergency and midwifery skills who attends a birth. This concept therefore refers to the skill of the clinician. *Skilled attendance*, on the other hand, is care given in a well-resourced environment, backed by political will. This concept refers to the environment for practice and indicates the need for a positive practice environment for quality care.

A positive practice environment is a setting that supports excellence and decent work; is fair and manageable; is effectively managed; has reasonable workloads; offers job security and a decent salary; has safe staff levels; offers support, supervision and mentoring; and is well-resourced for service (ICN et al, 2008).

The SMI's plan to improve maternal health outcomes requires 72 per cent skilled attendance as the critical aspect to reduce maternal mortality (PMNCH, 2011). In 2003, 91 per cent of births in South Africa were attended by skilled healthcare professionals (Stats SA, 2015). Clearly, skilled attendance alone cannot reduce maternal mortality.

Midwifery education for competency

The democratic transformation of the South African healthcare system and the transformation of higher education in South Africa influenced changes in nursing education.

The new nursing education will be offered from 2024 through a four-year bachelor's degree in the higher education band (Level 8) according to SANC Regulation 175, published on 1 January 2016. Accordingly, midwifery is integrated in the programme and candidates will exit as registered nurse-midwives. New regulations to be promulgated will allow for specialisation in midwifery.

In the South African context, all midwives working in the public sector are required to attend various up-skilling programmes (four to five days each) or in-service training in basic antenatal care (BANC), Essential Steps in the Management of Obstetric Emergencies (ESMOE), Integrated Management of Childhood Illnesses (IMCI), HIV counselling and testing (HCT), nurse-initiated management of antiretroviral therapy (NIMART) or PC101, prevention of mother-to-child transmission (PMTCT) of HIV, and the Integrated Chronic Disease Management (ICDM) programme.

Research competencies

There is insufficient research focused on midwifery practice in South Africa. Most research focuses on maternal healthcare and the healthcare system or clinical care. Research on factors that could influence policies around maternal healthcare planning in general and by midwives in particular is limited in South Africa. The role and function of the midwife are unique but still undervalued, a fact which is reflected by this lack of research.

The principal researchers in maternal healthcare come from related disciplines, such as sociology, anthropology, economics and medicine. There is thus a particular need for midwives to be involved in or spearhead relevant research that can affect policy decisions impacting on midwifery practice.

Global midwifery research

Since 1987, the SMI has undertaken global research with the objective of strengthening midwifery globally. This research has led to the development of global guidelines to support midwifery. The ICM's *Philosophy and Model of Midwifery Care* (CD2005_001) (ICM, 2014a) contains a statement of belief and model for midwifery care which guide midwifery practice globally. This model will be discussed in the next section.

The art of midwifery: The competency of caring

The USA's Pew Commission described the midwifery model of care that the USA sees as the model for the 21st century (Paine, Dower & O'Neill, 1999). This model supports the three Cs: choice, continuity of carer and control of pregnancy, birth and newborn-care events by the birthing woman. This model aims to restore woman-centred or humane care to the community, as well as a focus on normal pregnancy, birth and care for mother and the newborn. The model is explained in Table 3.1 on the next page.

The midwifery model of care

The midwifery model of care is in contrast to the medical model of care and has been widely researched and described.

It includes the mother in decision making and requires a continuous one-to-one caregiver in ideal circumstances with hands-on assistance, care and support during birth. This has also been referred to as midwifery-led care (MLC) or humane care. The midwifery model may look different in different settings, but it always subscribes to the same principles. The ICM's position statement, *Philosophy and Model of Midwifery Care* (ICM, 2014a), lists the principles and guidelines for midwifery practice.

Activity

Read the following article for details on the full development and value of the midwifery model: Hatem, M, Sandall, J, Devane, D, Soltani, H & Gates, S. 2008. 'Midwife-led versus other models of care for childbearing women'. Cochrane Database Syst Rev(4): CD004667. DOI: 10.1002/14651858.CD004667. pub2.

Table 3.1

The three Cs of the midwifery model of care (Rooks, 1999)

Choice	The essence of the midwifery model is the recognition of the following: • The (pregnant or labouring) woman can make decisions. This gives choice and control back to the woman. • The birthing process is a normal physiological process until proven otherwise. • The role of the midwife is to identify problems, give information, provide options and give support for the choices made, using scientific principles. • Midwives are partners that form an alliance with the woman, family and environment through trust, mutual control and shared decision making. • The dynamic relationship between the midwife and the woman focuses on the normal and supportive environment.
Continuity of carer	Continuity of carer suggests the following: • When midwives know the women for whom they provide care, interventions are minimised through the early detection of potential problems. • Continuous care by one caregiver throughout pregnancy, birth and the postnatal period, particularly when in labour, is ideal. • Care is a time-, education- and relationship-intensive practice. • Midwives use their own energy to encourage, support and comfort women in normal pregnancy, labour and during the postnatal period. • The continuous presence of a known carer using scientifically grounded clinical processes allows for early identification of potential complications and referral. • Continuity of carer is also practised in collaborative practice, where teams of midwives work together and are known to the women they take care of, with medical back-up.
Control (autonomy)	In terms of control by the birthing woman, the midwifery model is described as follows: • The model provides comprehensive emotional, social and cultural care. • It views birth as a meaningful experience that empowers the woman and strengthens bonds between father, mother, baby and siblings. • The model views birth as a critical developmental phase for the woman and portrays the transition to motherhood as a positive experience. • It supports women to make informed choices about the care they prefer and about the place of birth; the choice of provider; the choice of inductions, Caesarean section and other interventions such as pain relief; the presence of a significant person during labour; breastfeeding and other important aspects of care.

The philosophy of *humane care* and the midwifery model of care are evidence-based practices (EBPs) (Sandall et al, 2016) that have not been established in South Africa as an official policy. However, the midwifery model of care is practised by independent private midwives who conduct deliveries at home or in natural birthing centres in larger cities.

The role of midwives as part of a caring profession can be strengthened in the South African cross-cultural society. In the public health sector, the quality of care and the relationship between midwives and the public have been criticised (Honikman, Fawcus & Meintjes, 2015).

The unique role of the midwife in a therapeutic relationship offering support in childbirth receives attention in the following section, based on the scientific explanation of 'caring'.

The therapeutic relationship

The midwife, as the instrument of care (Kennedy, Rousseau & Low, 2003a) and through her presence and care, makes a difference in the experience of birth for the woman.

It is important to maintain a person-centred approach and to keep professional boundaries at all times when in a therapeutic relationship. The nurse–patient therapeutic relationship focuses on meeting the healthcare needs of the patient and can be plotted on a continuum of professional behaviour: from under-involvement (disinterested and neglectful), to the zone of helpfulness (the therapeutic relationship) and over-involvement (boundary violations) (Nursing Council of New Zealand, 2012).

Activity

Read the following article:
Hunter, B. 2010. 'Mapping the emotional terrain of midwifery: What can we see and what lies ahead?'. *Int J Work Organisation and Emotion* 3(3): 253–269.

The person-centred approach was first described by Carl Rogers (1902–1987) (BAPCA, 2015) in the 1950s and later by Hildegard Peplau, seen as the mother of psychiatric nursing, when she published her theory on the stages of the interpersonal relationship (Currentnursing.com, 2012). This was followed by the caring theory of Jean Watson (2008), who describes the 'caring moment' and the caritas processes. The caritas processes are guidelines that describe 10 factors for love- or heart-centred care and mindfulness.

Midwives need to develop the art of *therapeutic communication* and the science of creating a caring and mindful relationship. The core conditions of the approach (Rogers, 1967) are:

- empathy (to understand the patient's point of view)
- congruence (being a genuine person)
- unconditional positive regard (being non-judgemental).

These conditions do not exist in a vacuum. Verbal and non-verbal communication skills enable the midwife to facilitate a therapeutic relationship and may prevent misunderstanding and unhappiness with care. Table 3.2 lists the principles of verbal and non-verbal communication that should be observed during therapeutic communication.

Table 3.2

Communication (Ford, Byrt & Dooher, 2010)

Verbal communication	Non-verbal communication
The content and tone of speech should convey respect and concern.	Practise active, attentive listening to convey interest in the person and avoid interrupting him or her.
Set verbal limits to ensure safety, but do this in a respectful and polite manner.	Use silence. Develop the ability to assess whether the person needs space or periods of silence and enable this as necessary.
Adapt communication to the patient's needs, but without being patronising. Consider the patient's abilities, language and culture.	Control facial expressions to convey interest and concern – mirror the patient's emotions (apart from aggression).
Assess language needs and provide an interpreter as needed.	Use gestures such as nods of the head, which convey interest and understanding (not excessive), but avoid finger pointing.
Avoid medical jargon to ensure understanding.	Develop an open and relaxed posture, which demonstrates perceptiveness and availability for communication (sitting or standing).
Moderate the pitch of speech and speak clearly, but not too loudly or too softly. Adopt a pleasant and professional tone and pitch.	Maintain eye contact in a non-threatening way to convey interest and enhance communication.
Avoid talking about the patient rather than with the patient.	Use touch therapeutically only. Anything more than this may be seen as inappropriate, for example due to gender and culture norms.

The caring moment and mindfulness

A caring moment involves an action and choice by both the nurse and the woman. They both have the opportunity to decide how to be in the moment and in the relationship and what to do during the moment (Watson, 2008). Being in the caring moment is to be present, mindful and 'being at ease' in the moment (Nghiem, 2008).

Mindfulness is a state of active, open attention on the present. When a person is mindful, they observe their thoughts and feelings from a distance, without judging them as good or bad. Mindfulness means living in the moment and awakening to experience.

Theory of human caring
The core concepts of the theory of human caring and caritas processes in a transpersonal caring relationship in midwifery go beyond the ego and the self, because of the deeper connections to birth and new beginnings in life (Cara, 2003).

Competency in caring and empowerment

Personal empowerment

Midwives who develop competency in caring and learn to set aside their egos and own emotional needs, and who learn to be present and mindful, may also experience personal empowerment.

Personal empowerment is a process of change that has both internal and external aspects. Internally, it is reflected in an individual's sense or belief in his or her decision-making and problem-solving abilities. Externally, change finds expression in a person's ability to act and to implement the practical knowledge, information, skills, capabilities and other new resources acquired in the process (Sadan, 2004).

Woman-centred practice (the midwifery model of care) is the event and outcome of importance for the empowerment of midwifery. An empowerment scale was developed that included conditions of control, support, recognition and skills that are important in the facilitation of midwifery empowerment (Matthews, Scott & Gallagher, 2009). It asserts that midwives themselves need to be empowered if they are to empower women. In South Africa, the process of empowering midwives is still ongoing.

Structural organisational empowerment

Competency and work performance are not just technical knowledge and skills, but also express the influence a work environment has on work satisfaction and performance, referred to as empowerment.

Kanter's structural theory of organisational empowerment (1993) (see Table 3.3) is a useful framework to explain the relationship between the work environment/organisation and workforce behaviour, attitude and performance. There are several studies in nursing that investigate the work environment and employees in the organisation. The expanded model of Laschinger, Finegan and Shamian (2001) added the psychological empowerment dimensions described by Spreitzer (1996). Psychological dimensions reflect aspects of meaning, confidence, autonomy and the impact of the work environment on work behaviour as described by Knol and Van Linge (2009).

Table 3.3

Kanter's structural empowerment framework (1993)

Opportunity	Growth, mobility and the chance to increase knowledge and skills in the organisation (competence)
Structure of power	The ability to access resources, information and support from the organisation to get the job done: • *Information* is the data, technical knowledge and expertise required for the job. • *Resources* is the ability to get the materials, supplies, money and staff for the task. • *Support* is feedback and guidance from peers, subordinates and supervisors to enhance effectiveness.
Formal power	The level of flexibility, visibility and creativity allowed in the organisation, as well as the level at which participatory decision making is allowed
Informal power	Derived from networks and relationships with peers, subordinates and supervisors within and outside the organisation, including internal direction and motivation

Kanter's expanded framework assists in describing the organisational workplace and the attitudes, behaviours and performance of staff. Midwives can employ the framework to solve work-related issues to improve performance.

3.4 The regulatory framework for midwifery

Midwives, as independent practitioners, practice within the regulatory framework of the country in which they function. The aspects detailed in the following sections should be considered in professional practice.

The regulation of midwifery professional practice in South Africa

The registration of midwives takes place through the SANC after completion of a prescribed programme in midwifery. Licensing refers to the unique legal requirements that permit midwifery practice by a midwife, agent or institution, according to set standards. These license structures are the official structures in a healthcare system (WHO, 1985: 5) recognised by law and government. The SANC is the legal structure for licensing in South Africa.

Acts and regulations relevant to midwifery practice

- The South African Patient's Rights Charter
- The National Health Act 61 of 2003, as amended by the National Health Amendment Act 12 of 2013
- The Nursing Act 33 of 2005
- The Choice on Termination of Pregnancy Act 92 of 1996
- The Medicines and Related Substances Act 101 of 1965
- Section 47 of the Medicine and Related Substances Act, published in Regulation 24727 of 10 April 2003: 'Obtaining of pethidine or preparations or mixtures thereof by registered midwives' (Government Gazette 7636). (This was previously controlled by Regulation 777, dated 10 April 1981.)
- The Births and Deaths Registration Act 51 of 1992, as amended by the Births and Deaths Registration Amendment Act 18 of 2010
- Form DHA 1663: Notification of Maternal Death
- Death Certification/Stillbirth

continued

Professional regulations

- SANC Regulation 2418, dated 2 November 1984: Regulations regarding registered nurses keeping, supplying, administering or prescribing medicines
- SANC Regulation 2488, dated 26 October 1990: Conditions under which registered/enrolled midwives may carry on their profession
- SANC Regulation 2489, dated 26 October 1990: Regulations concerning the control of the practice of the enrolled midwife
- Regulation 786, dated 15 October 2013: Regulations regarding the scope of practice for nurses and midwives. (Nursing Act 33 of 2005, Government notice 36935, DoH).
- The Births and Deaths Registration Act 51 of 1992, as amended by the Births and Deaths Registration Amendment Act 18 of 2010)
- SANC Regulation 767, dated 1 October 2014: Regulations setting out the acts or omissions in respect of which the SANC may take disciplinary steps.

Ethical considerations/code of ethics

The ICM developed a code of ethics for midwives, which was revised in 2014. This code acknowledges women as people with human rights, seeks justice for all people and equity in access to healthcare, and is based on mutual relationships of respect, trust, and the dignity of all members of society.

The ICM's code of ethics

The ICM's code of ethics (ICM, 2014b) is available online. It is divided into the following chapters:
1. Midwifery relationships
2. Practice of midwifery
3. The professional responsibilities of midwives
4. Advancement of midwifery knowledge and practice

Standards of midwifery

The standards for midwifery practice are set and monitored by the SANC. Registration and licensing is granted and maintained by the SANC after a practitioner has completed a prescribed programme in midwifery. In addition, the Department of Health's (DoH) *Guidelines for Maternity Care in South Africa* (DoH, 2015a) is regularly updated and serves as a manual for clinics, community health clinics (CHCs) and districts as to the minimum technical, organisational and operational standards for the healthcare of mothers and babies.

Professional accountability and midwifery

There has been a steady increase in the number of malpractice claims brought against healthcare providers in South Africa, specifically in maternity care, and in the monetary damages awarded to plaintiffs. The delivery of babies is one of the most complicated areas of healthcare practice, because midwives and doctors share a monopoly over the right to attend to a woman in childbirth. Birth is unpredictable and even under controlled circumstances things can go wrong.

Accountability

As registered, competent practitioners, midwives must have the knowledge, skills, attitudes and values to deliver safe care. They are thus personally accountable for their acts and omissions, even when practising within a multidisciplinary team. Every healthcare professional has an ethical obligation to act in the interests of the mother and baby.

During pregnancy, labour and birth, the patient, family and community expect quality care by a competent midwife who possesses all the necessary abilities to perform care. In turn, the employer expects quality care in a cost-effective manner, in accordance with the service agreement between employer and employee.

The employer is responsible for providing a positive practice environment for quality healthcare services in order to facilitate safe maternity nursing care of high quality. The manager and healthcare practitioners share responsibility in respect of the outputs of the health service, namely quality care, staff management and cost-effectiveness. This means that the manager accepts vicarious liability for the events within healthcare services.

A lack of accountability, the failure to supervise maternity staff, the failure to adhere to standard protocols for maternity care, breaches in ethical practice (including physical and emotional abuse) and other risky practices by healthcare professionals during maternity care compromise the quality of care offered to women. They also contribute to violations of the right to life, health and the right to freedom from cruel, inhumane and degrading treatment.

Obstetric negligence

Obstetric negligence by a healthcare professional (obstetrician, general medical practitioner or midwife) is the failure to follow policies, clinical guidelines and safety or standard principles in practice. This may put a mother and baby at risk or cause harm, loss or death.

Malpractice

Malpractice is the failure to exercise an ordinary degree of professional judgement and skill.

Midwives have a duty to care for women during pregnancy, labour, birth and the early neonatal period. SANC Regulations 2488, 2598 and 767 determine midwives' legal obligation to take reasonable care and to avoid harm. In South Africa, registered nurses and midwives are recognised as practitioners in their own right.

While there is a shared responsibility for healthcare, there is also individual liability for the consequences thereof. There has been an increase in health litigation in South Africa, much of which is related to claims of misdiagnosis, practising outside the scope of practice, and refusal to treat patients. Malpractice claims have devastating outcomes for health professionals and can cripple the healthcare system financially.

Negligence

Negligence is an act with any element of carelessness or lack of regard, resulting in injury, harm or loss. It is any act or omission that falls short of the standard expected from 'the reasonable person'.

The concept 'negligence' is referred to in two ways, namely:
1. to describe a *particular type of fault* or wrongdoing (with characteristics that are defined by a number of legal decisions). Negligence in this respect can be either criminal (resulting in prosecution) or civil (leading to an action in the civil court for compensation)
2. to describe that which must *be proven* in order for a claimant to succeed in recovering money (damages) in respect of damage that was caused by the fault.

The vast majority of medico-legal cases concern the civil law of negligence. These are tried in court by a judge sitting alone. Only a small amount of cases will ever get to court, as most are settled or abandoned before trial. Of those that do get to trial, most are decided in the defendant's favour.

There are three civil wrongdoings that must be proven for a successful claim of negligence (Brennan et al, 1991):
1. A duty of care was owed (eg a duty to do something that should have been done, or a duty not to do something that had been done).
2. The duty of care was breached.
3. The breach was the direct cause of the person's damage in the form of injury or loss.

Litigation

Litigation is typically settled by agreement between the parties, but may also be heard and decided by a jury or judge in court. In such cases, professionals are equally vulnerable to being sued for malpractice or negligence. A complaint can be made to the professional bodies for midwives (eg the SANC), or the Health Professions Council of South Africa (HPCSA) for medical practitioners. Litigation through a civil suit is a possible occurrence when a woman approaches a court through an attorney to claim damages for harm or loss due to medical or midwifery actions or practice. Litigation and professional conduct investigations are very taxing and time-consuming, and may lead to the practitioner losing her or his registration to practice.

Indemnity

The indemnity insurance that is needed for protection against malpractice and negligence is the highest for obstetricians and medical practitioners, especially paediatricians. This insurance is usually obtained through the relevant professional body.

For the South African registered nurse and midwife, midwifery clinical practice carries the highest risk of litigation. It is rare for midwives to be sued individually, unless they are practising in their private capacity as independent practitioners. It is thus of utmost importance for a midwife who wishes to start a private or independent practice to be insured against potential lawsuits. Insurance is hard to come by and very few agencies are prepared to insure a midwife in private practice. Midwives are therefore affiliated through nursing associations or unions (eg the Democratic Nursing Organisation of South Africa [DENOSA] and the Health and Other Service Personnel Trade Union of South Africa [HOSPERSA]) to protect themselves against litigation.

If a midwife has been negligent, a claim may be brought against her, but generally her employer – the DoH, private hospital or clinic – will be sued. This is a consequence of the doctrine of vicarious liability (Brennan et al, 1991), which states that employers are liable for the wrongdoings of their employees. This does not absolve the employee from responsibility; the claimant can sue the employee instead of or as well as the employer.

Documentation and record keeping

One of the most important aspects in litigation is the keeping of accurate records. Clinical record keeping in nursing is a professional responsibility that is often neglected, resulting in litigation. However, it can also provide evidence to exonerate the practitioner of wrongdoing. The midwife must provide evidence of the care that has been provided. This evidence can only be found in the documentation.

Problems commonly encountered in record keeping include (Geyer, 2005):

▶ inadequate or incomplete documentation
▶ a lack of dates and times

▶ an absence of important documentation, especially blood results and CTG tracings
▶ missing records or missing parts of the clinical record
▶ altered records or evidence of falsification in the clinical record.

The partogram provides an overview of what transpired during birth and many cases can be settled or dropped because of the documented evidence on the partogram, even if the progress reports were not up to standard.

Health services and working conditions

The norms and standards for practice include a positive practice environment, with enough staff and equipment to perform tasks. Many claims arise when midwives supervising the birthing mother are under pressure because of insufficient resources, high staff turnover, a lack of morale, inadequate infrastructure or a lack of transfer support from the midwife obstetrics units (MOUs) to higher levels of care via emergency services.

On analysis of documents, it appears that acts of negligence or malpractice often occur after hours, at shift changes or in the early hours after midnight, when a call for an urgent Caesarean section necessitates support staff coming back to the hospital. Under these circumstances babies are often born with some form of neurological damage due to hypoxia.

The outcomes of litigation

In many cases, an agreement is reached between the plaintiff and the practitioner. Most medical negligence and malpractice claims result in a damages award. These are usually calculated to cover various losses, such as medical bills, hospital payments and lost wages. In cases involving serious injuries or losses, such as in the case of a child being physically disabled, the damages awards can be quite substantial.

Other legal consequences, such as a loss of operating license or civil fines, may occur in connection with obstetric negligence. In cases involving gross or severe negligence, criminal consequences may also result.

The purpose of malpractice litigation is not only to seek compensation in cases of malpractice or negligence; it is intended, in part, to make substandard care leading to injuries widely known, in the hope of improving the quality of the healthcare system and thereby reducing mother and child morbidity and mortality rates.

3.5   Conclusion

This chapter defined the midwife as an accountable professional who provides support and care during pregnancy, labour and postpartum. The different categories of midwives found globally and in South Africa were discussed.

It is important for a midwife to understand both the science and the art of midwifery. The midwife is called upon to be a skilled attendant and also needs to be competent in more advanced skills focused on pregnancy and birth.

The midwifery model of care and the philosophy of humane care are significant developments that the midwife needs to stay abreast of and apply in her practice. This chapter also discussed the maintenance of a therapeutic relationship for the best outcomes. In order to achieve this, the midwife needs communication skills and skills in mindfulness.

Lastly, the regulatory framework for midwives in South Africa was discussed. The midwifery clinical practice is especially vulnerable and at risk for litigation, and the cost of litigation is crippling to a country where essential and basic services are needed. The individual midwife cannot absolve herself from responsibility and should take the lead in practising according to the norms and standards for midwifery practice.

Maternal and newborn healthcare in South Africa

LEARNING OBJECTIVES

On completion of this chapter, you must be able to:

▶ demonstrate and understand the context of healthcare in South Africa
▶ explain international and national strategies to improve maternal, child and women's healthcare
▶ explain the South African healthcare system and the care provided for mothers, newborns, children and women
▶ explain the programmes aimed at improving healthcare for women and children in South Africa
▶ identify and explain the signal functions in obstetrics and neonatal care.

KNOWLEDGE ASSUMED TO BE IN PLACE

Knowledge of the South African healthcare system

KEYWORDS

healthcare system • reproductive healthcare • Essential Steps in the Management of Obstetric Emergencies (ESMOE) • Emergency Obstetric Simulation Training (EOST) • signal functions

4.1 Introduction

This chapter gives an overview of the South African healthcare system. Chapter 2 explained the terminology and guidelines used to collect statistics on maternal, perinatal and neonatal mortality in South Africa. Chapter 3 gave an overview of the global and South African legal frameworks for midwifery practice. This chapter will contextualise midwifery practice in the South African context of primary healthcare (PHC).

Midwives, as the key healthcare providers for maternal and child care, work within this context. It is therefore necessary to know and understand the healthcare context (WHO, 2012).

4.2 Structural factors: The South African healthcare context

In South Africa, an estimated 80 per cent of a population of 51.77 million (according to the 2011 census) depend on the public healthcare system for health services. About 16 per cent of people have private health insurance. Approximately 30 per cent of the population can access private healthcare by paying for it directly (CMS, 2015).

The South African healthcare system

South Africa has a two-tier healthcare system that delivers healthcare through both the private and the public health sector. In addition, there are various non-governmental organisations (NGOs) that deliver services.

The private health sector

As of 2016, South Africa had more than 83 registered medical schemes, with 7.8 million beneficiaries (CMS, 2016). There are 238 private hospitals in the country: 188 in urban areas and 50 in rural areas (SA Private Hospitals, 2017).

The public health sector

There are 376 public hospitals in South Africa (Jobson, 2015). The public health sector has been transformed since 1992. The health system has a three-layered structure, as established through the National Health Act 61 of 2003 (NHA), run by different administrations:

1. *The national Department of Health (DoH):* The DoH is responsible for the development and implementation of

national health policy in collaboration with the National Health Council (NHC).

2. *The nine provincial departments of health:* These are responsible for the implementation of healthcare in the provinces, as specified by Chapter 4 of the NHA. The provincial departments of health are responsible for the financial management of healthcare, for the planning and governance of public healthcare institutions and the certification and regulation of private institutions, according to the NHA (Chapter 6, Reg 45, 46 and 47) in compliance with the quality requirements of the Office of Standard Compliance.

3. *The district health system (DHS):* This system is governed by Chapter 5 of the NHA and is responsible for South Africa's 52 health districts, which are further divided in sub-districts. Comprehensive PHC and community hospital services are part and parcel of the DHS.

Local governments do not form part of the healthcare system. There are three types of municipalities: metropolitan, district and local municipalities. There are eight metropolitan municipalities, 44 district municipalities and 226 local municipalities. The 52 health districts are linked to metropolitan and district municipalities, and in many cases more than one local municipality is included in one health district.

Health districts are responsible for comprehensive PHC as delivered through service delivery platforms, as per Table 4.1.

Table 4.1

Service delivery platforms for the 52 health districts in South Africa as of 2014 (compiled by the author)

Type of facility	Number of facilities (2014)
PHC	3 310
Mobile clinics	1 068
Community health clinics (CHCs)	278
Special clinics	31
Health posts	30
District hospitals	257
Total	**4 974**

The role and functions of municipal health services, according to the NHA, are expressed in several regulations as published in the *Government Gazette* No 36849, dated 20 September 2013, vol 579. These include various regulations on food and environmental issues, such as:

▶ health surveillance of premises for identification of environmental health risks
▶ surveillance and prevention of communicable diseases, excluding vaccination
▶ environmental population control
▶ water quality
▶ noise management
▶ vector control
▶ community participation and involvement
▶ disposal of the dead
▶ chemical safety
▶ client information service centres.

NGOs

Multiple NGOs contribute to the health sector through focusing on specific illnesses such as HIV/AIDS and TB. As supportive partners, NGOs assist with developing skills and priority programmes, as well as other tasks as required.

4.3 Levels of healthcare in the public sector

The three levels of care in the public healthcare system deliver primary, secondary and tertiary care. Hospitals are categorised accordingly. Levels of care are published in the DoH's policy regulation R655 (2011a). The types of care offered at each level of the public healthcare system are stipulated in service packages. The efficient functioning of all levels of care requires effective management, finance, appropriate staff, resources and support services.

The national Department of Health

The 10 major teaching hospitals in South Africa are managed by the DoH. Of these, the Chris Hani Baragwanath Hospital in Johannesburg is the third-largest hospital in the world. These institutions are highly specialised.

Provincial health departments (levels 2 and 3)

Currently, there are 115 public hospitals in the country's provinces, including specialised regional hospitals on levels 2 and 3.

Regional hospitals are Level 2 facilities that provide care requiring the intervention of specialists and general practitioners. A hospital providing a single specialist service would be classified as a specialised Level 2 hospital. A general Level 2 hospital would need to provide and be staffed permanently in at least five of the following eight basic specialties: surgery, medicine, orthopaedics, paediatrics, obstetrics and gynaecology, psychiatry, diagnostic radiology and anaesthetics.

A Level 3 facility provides specialist and sub-specialist care, such as:

- Speciality 1: neonatal care and obstetrics and 24 others
- Speciality 2: paediatrics and 13 others
- Speciality 3: liver transplants.

Specialised hospitals are mainly for mental health and TB-related care.

The district healthcare system and primary healthcare, Level 1

South Africa is a signatory to the 2008 Ouagadougou Declaration on Primary Healthcare and Health Systems in Africa (30th anniversary of the Alma Ata Declaration). A commitment to PHC is expressed in the National Health Insurance White Paper (DoH, 2015b), including the re-engineering of PHC.

Primary healthcare services

PHC services are the first point of entry for healthcare. PHC is at the centre of the strategy to transform health services in South Africa, bringing the services closer to the receiver of the care, within the community. The PHC service package and the district hospital service package indicate the services that are offered at the district level for PHC. This essential package of PHC services is the foundation for a unified health system.

The essential elements of PHC that are relevant to the South African context are:

- education concerning prevailing health problems and methods to prevent and control them
- the promotion of food supply and proper nutrition
- an adequate supply of safe water and basic sanitation
- maternal and child healthcare, including family planning
- immunisation against major infectious diseases
- the prevention and control of locally endemic diseases
- the appropriate treatment of common diseases and injuries
- the provision of essential drugs and laboratory tests.

PHC involves both the physical facilities as well as the care provided by healthcare professionals, both of which are regulated. PHC programmes are designed for care within a context and can be delivered by what the WHO refers to as primary care teams. A primary care team is defined as 'a group of fellow professionals with complimentary contributions to give patient care' (WHO, 2004). A team can be made up of up to 30 professionals, including community nurses, midwives, dentists, physiotherapists, social workers, psychiatrists, speech therapists, pharmacists, administrative staff and managers.

District health systems and health facilities

Provinces and districts develop the number and type of facilities needed in each particular province. Districts receive finances through the provinces for service delivery. The health districts include all service delivery platforms, as indicated in Table 4.1.

Hospitals are classified, according to the levels of care in the NHA, as district, regional, tertiary, central and specialised hospitals.

The following sections detail the facilities that exist in districts.

Primary healthcare clinics

PHC clinics vary in size depending on the size of the population they serve. There should be one clinic for about 50 000–80 000 people. The norms and standards for clinics constituted in the *Ideal Clinic Manual* (DoH, 2016) gives the standards that clinics need to meet for quality of care.

The comprehensive PHC package for South Africa describes PHC norms and standards for each component to be rendered at a PHC clinic. The new comprehensive and integrated package of essential health services to be provided by PHC services (DoH, 2105c) is guided by the principle of dealing with the whole life cycle, from pre-birth to death. PHC services are provided across the continuum of care in three streams of care:

1. *Acute:* This stream includes the treatment of minor ailments, emergency treatment as well as the treatment of violence and injuries. It covers both children and adults.
2. *Chronic:* This stream includes all non-communicable diseases, such as diabetes, hypertension and asthma, and communicable diseases such as HIV (pre-antiretroviral treatment and antiretroviral treatment [ART]) and TB. Mental health is also included, as is the treatment of persistent physical impairments such as strokes and cerebral palsy.
3. *Maternal, women and child health:* This includes:
   - immunisation
   - antenatal care
   - postnatal care
   - school health/early childhood development (ECD).

Community health clinics

CHCs are facilities that render a broad range of PHC services 24 hours a day, 7 days a week. CHCs also offer accident and emergency and midwifery services, but not surgery under general anaesthesia. There is a medical doctor at the centre 24 hours a day.

When births are conducted, CHCs need to be staffed by midwives or advanced midwives and supportive categories of staff. In South Africa, births are planned to take place mainly at CHCs and district hospitals. Complicated cases and women with risk factors will deliver in regional facilities and in academic centres.

Midwife obstetrics units (MOUs) exist mainly in Gauteng and the Western Cape. These focus only on obstetric care.

District hospitals

District hospitals support PHC. Community members receive Level 1 care as in-patients or out-patients and can access the district hospital directly or may be referred from PHC clinics or CHCs. District hospitals render Level 1 care – that is, basic care – and surgery that is commonly required and should be readily available for all. These hospitals have 30–200 beds, 24-hour emergency services and an operating theatre.

The range of hospital services includes family medicine and PHC, obstetrics, psychiatry, eye care, rehabilitation, surgery, paediatrics and geriatrics.

District hospitals are able to perform basic surgery, including Caesarean sections, emergency and critical care and the management of complications and referrals. District hospitals and specialists are responsible for specialist care outreach to clinics. There is a written, agreed-upon referral system for obstetric complications between clinics and the district hospital, with a dedicated obstetric ambulance operating either from the district hospital or from the CHC.

Primary healthcare programmes

The type and content of care, as well as norms and standards of care, are stipulated in the comprehensive PHC package of SA (Bettercare, 2000). This covers women's health, Integrated Management of Childhood Illnesses (IMCI), immunisation, adolescent health, HIV/AIDS, sexually transmitted infections (STIs), cholera and diarrhoea, communicable conditions, hearing, oral health, mental health, geriatrics, non-communicable conditions and rehabilitation. The *District Hospital Service Package* (DoH, 2002) covers women's health, childhood illnesses, infants and children, trauma and emergency care, surgical services, oral health, adult medical care, mental health, rehabilitation and pharmaceutical services.

The key priority programmes that are guided by policy for maternal and infant care are briefly highlighted in Table 4.2. They will be further discussed and referenced in the rest of this book.

Table 4.2

Key priority PHC programmes for maternal and child care

Policy and programme	Prevention, treatment and healthcare guidelines or policy for maternal and infant care
Basic Antenatal Care (BANC Plus)	BANC Plus promotes early attendance before 20 weeks and eight antenatal visits at an antenatal clinic to ensure the provision of high-quality antenatal care and to integrate prevention of mother-to-child-transmission (PMTCT) of HIV and TB screening into routine antenatal provision.
Intrapartum standards of care	Intrapartum care is focused on low risk or normal birth and is available at some clinics, but only CHCs give 24-hour services. High-risk and complicated cases are referred to the district hospital. The use and audit of the partogram in labour is routine and is enforced.
Postnatal care	Postnatal care is included in community services where the ward-based outreach teams (WBOTs) render services to mothers and babies.
Reproductive services and contraception (see Chapter 48)	All PHC facilities should provide a full range of contraceptive services and promote the use of dual methods (contraceptive, sub-dermal implant and condom use). It is especially important to ensure that adolescents have access to reproductive health services, including family planning and pregnancy testing services.

continued

Reproductive services and contraception (continued)	Termination of pregnancy (TOP) is legal and should be readily available. TOP by a professional nurse trained in this service can only be done in the first trimester. Extending access to emergency contraception (EC) and promoting early confirmation of pregnancy (through improved knowledge of sexual and reproductive health, and by promoting pregnancy testing) are important measures for reducing second-trimester terminations and unintended pregnancies. However, it is also important to ensure that services are accessible in all districts for both first- and second-trimester terminations.
Cancer screening (see Chapter 48)	Screening is done for cervical and other cancers according to the *National Guidelines for Cervical Cancer Screening Programme* (DoH, nd [a]). Women and teenagers are educated on the correct way to examine their breasts. The Human Papilloma Virus Prevention Programme for Cervical Cancer was launched in 2015 for Grade 4 girls who are older than 9 years. It is also included in the cervical cancer screening policy.
Genetic services	The goal of genetic services is to prevent birth defects and improve the management of genetic disorders, birth defects and disabilities. Of the 52 districts, 32 have at least one nurse trained in genetics to implement the standardised birth defects collection tool.
Child and youth health	The provision of health services for the youth is guided by the *Draft Policy Guidelines for Adolescent and Youth Health* (DoH, 1999), which outlines five intervention strategies: promoting a safe and supportive environment, providing information, building skills, counselling and access to health services.
IMCI	IMCI starts at birth. All mothers or families with babies receive the Road to Health chart at birth to monitor the baby's care and well-being. IMCI has a strong preventative focus. The case management process for each child should include an assessment of the child's immunisation and nutritional status. Counselling on appropriate feeding during health and illness should be provided where necessary.
Expanded programme on immunisation (EPI)	South Africa has achieved high cover of routine immunisation, with the aim of achieving 100 % cover. Polio and TB immunisations are given before the baby leaves the healthcare system after birth. South Africa was declared free of the polio virus in 2006, and neonatal tetanus has also been eliminated. The number of measles cases has been dramatically reduced. The routine EPI schedule has been updated to include immunisation with tetanus toxoid at 6 and 12 years. This should mean, in the long term, that pregnant women do not require tetanus toxoid. Vaccines against pneumococcal and rotavirus infections are also being introduced as part of the routine immunisation programme. These vaccines are expected to have a positive impact on under-five mortality rates; their introduction needs to be as rapid as possible.
PMTCT of HIV	PMTCT of HIV is one of the key goals of the *National Strategic Plan on HIV, TB and STIs 2017–2022* (SANAC, 2017). The four pillars of the strategy are primary prevention of HIV infections, the prevention of unwanted pregnancies among HIV-infected women, the provision of ART to mothers and infants to prevent transmission and ensuring that eligible mothers receive ART.
Nurse-initiated management of antiretroviral therapy (NIMART)	The NIMART rollout guidelines are focused on improving access to treatment with antiretrovirals (ARVs). All women are tested at first contact and started on ART as per the guidelines. Women who have tested positive for HIV should be referred for medical care in pregnancy and are no longer supposed to get BANC. Early diagnosis and management of children with HIV/AIDS is key to improved outcomes (see Chapter 50).

continued

Growth monitoring and promotion	The early identification and appropriate classification of stunted growth, malnutrition and severe acute malnutrition (SAM) are pivotal to appropriate and timely intervention, especially in children below 5 years of age. Regular correct weighing as well as plotting and interpretation of the growth curve on the child's Road to Health chart form the core of the growth monitoring and promotion strategy.
	Growth monitoring also provides an opportunity for assessment of the child's development. Children with poor eyesight, hearing loss and other developmental and behavioural problems can be identified and referred for the appropriate remedial support.
	The eradication of poverty is the biggest challenge facing South Africa. Stunted growth in children under 5 years of age is an indicator of the level of equity in healthcare (WHO, 2015a). The Index for Equity in Health (WHO, 2015a) suggested a reduction of 20 % of cases of malnutrition, with South Africa only achieving 11.6 % for malnutrition and 8 % for SAM. Malnutrition is a severe problem in South Africa.
The Baby-Friendly Hospital Initiative (BFHI) and infant feeding	The *Infant and Young Child Feeding Policy* (DoH, 2013c) aims to harmonise infant and young child feeding messages and practices. Key components of the policy include the promotion of exclusive breastfeeding (EBF) (Tshwane Declaration of Support for Breastfeeding in South Africa, 2011), supporting appropriate and safe infant feeding choices for mothers who are HIV-infected and the promotion of appropriate complementary feeding. The BFHI (Henney, 2013) recognises the special role of maternity services in early support and protection of breastfeeding, while promoting safe infant feeding for breastfeeding and non-breastfeeding babies. It aims to ensure early initiation of breastfeeding, provide an enabling environment for safe infant feeding and ensure that all mothers receive continued support irrespective of their feeding choice. Hospitals that meet the BFHI criteria can apply to be accredited as being baby-friendly.
	The follow-up process once women leave maternity facilities is often not optimal and needs to be strengthened (the provision of early postnatal care provides an opportunity for this). In particular, improved support for breastfeeding at community and household levels is urgently needed. There is also a need to strengthen mechanisms for monitoring and scaling up the BFHI.
Vitamin A supplementation (VAS)	Vitamin A deficiency contributes to as many as one out of four childhood deaths (WHO, 2009a). Deficiency may result from inadequate dietary intake of vitamin A or from rapid utilisation of vitamin A during illness, pregnancy and lactation and during phases of rapid growth in young children. Children between 6 and 59 months experience more serious effects from vitamin A deficiency than other groups. Although the vast majority of children with vitamin A deficiency have no clinical signs, even moderate vitamin A deficiency significantly increases a child's risk of dying from an infectious disease. Routine VAS for children younger than five years was introduced in South Africa in 2003. Children between 12 and 59 months receive vitamin A every six months, as well as de-worming, catch-up vaccination and nutritional screening on contact. The recommended dosage is 100 000 IU at 6–11 months and 200 000 IU at 12–59 months every 4–6 months when the baby is making contact with healthcare (including HIV-related services) (WHO, 2009a). This is part of the package of services offered to households by the WBOTs. The national target for vitamin A administration is 55 %. The District Health Barometer (DHB) of 2015/16 (HST, 2016) indicated that coverage was 52.2 %. Vitamin A deficiency is common in children under five years. Those with measles, SAM and diarrhoea of more than 14 days are given high doses of vitamin A on medical prescription or as per clinical guideline.
	A combination of interventions is usually used to prevent and eliminate vitamin A deficiency. These include breastfeeding protection and promotion, food fortification, VAS and dietary diversification.
Maternal healthy lifestyle promotion	A healthy lifestyle among pregnant women can play an important role in improving the health of mothers and their newborn babies.

continued

Maternal healthy lifestyle promotion (continued)	Adequate nutrition (see Chapter 51) and moderate exercise are particularly important during pregnancy. The WHO (2009a) recommends a daily intake of fresh vegetables and fruit (including green leafy and other vegetables, legumes and fruit in adequate quantities) to reduce the risk of coronary heart disease, stroke and high blood pressure. Other important interventions include the promotion of safe sex and avoiding smoking and alcohol intake during pregnancy (see Chapter 51).
Micronutrient control	All pregnant women should receive supplementation with iron and folate during pregnancy, and one dose of vitamin A (200 000 IU) in the postpartum period. All pregnant women should be given calcium supplementation (at least 800–1 200 mg per day).
Kangaroo-mother-care (KMC)	KMC is currently being implemented in all provinces, although coverage data for facilities are not yet available. KMC has the potential to reduce mortality and morbidity in low birth-weight (LBW) infants and needs to be implemented in all facilities that provide newborn care. Incorporating KMC assessments into BFHI assessments would ensure that more facilities implement both strategies. Data from the Perinatal Problem Identification Programme (PPIP) have shown that hospitals that implemented KMC reduced their mortality rates among small babies (weighing 1–2 kg) by 30 % (Pattinson & Rhoda, 2014).
Post-rape services	South Africa's National Sexual Assault Policy (DoH, 2005) and the accompanying clinical management guidelines have been developed and implemented nationally. The guidelines emphasise both the medical and psychological management of rape survivors as well as the medico-legal responsibilities of health professionals. Continued efforts are needed to ensure that services meet the physical and mental health needs of adult and child victims. Standardising training using the recently developed national curriculum for training sexual assault care providers is important in improving service quality, and this needs to be extended to all post-rape service providers. Continued efforts are needed to strengthen service infrastructure, and to ensure 24-hour access to all post-rape services.

4.4 Quality improvement strategies for maternal and newborn care and health outcomes

The improvement of maternal, newborn and child healthcare and health outcomes has been a global priority since 1985. Several initiatives have led to the development of strategies to reduce maternal, newborn and child mortality and morbidity.

Initiating international strategies to improve maternal and newborn care

International strategies are presented in Table 4.3 on page 34. These include the Safe Motherhood Initiative (SMI) and the Millennium Development Goals (MDGs) 2000–2012. Both of these placed a global focus on mothers and babies, developed monitoring tools and reported on global progress. The MDGs, published in 2000, aimed at the improvement of health for all and included clear targets for the improvement of maternal and newborn health outcomes. Although there was an improvement in many areas, several developing countries (including South Africa) did not achieve the targets for 2015.

In 2012, the Sustainable Development Goals (SDGs) were announced by the United Nations General Assembly. The SDGs replaced the MDGs and set 169 targets aimed at reducing poverty and improving environmental sustainability by 2030. Poverty is still the main reason for poor health outcomes, with women and children being the most vulnerable. The MDGs and SDGs are strategies with targets focused on many indicators, such as poverty and equity, gender equality, hunger, HIV/AIDS and also maternal and child care.

In 2005, the WHO established the Partnership for Maternal, Newborn and Child Health (PMNCH). This global organisation focuses mainly on strengthening maternal, newborn and child healthcare globally. The Every Woman, Every Child movement 2010 (UN, nd) originated from the PMNCH.

Table 4.3

Global strategies for the improvement of quality care and health outcomes for mothers and children (UN, 2015)

International strategies	Purpose, targets and global progress made
SMI, WHO, 1987	The SMI is an international strategy that was launched in 1987 to advocate for safer care for mothers and babies. In 2004, this initiative broadened its mandate to focus on the most vulnerable groups of mothers and children, and particularly on maternal deaths in developing countries.
MDGs 2000–2012	MDG 1: *Reduce and eradicate extreme poverty and hunger.* This was reduced from 49 % to 14 % globally. MDG 3: *Promote gender equality and empower women.* Inequality still persists. MDG 4: *Reduce child deaths by two-thirds (60 %) between 1990 and 2015.* MDG 5: *Reduce maternal deaths by three-quarters (75 %) between 1990 and 2015 and provide universal access to reproductive health services.* MDG 6: *Combat diseases, especially HIV/AIDS and malaria.* Twelve million people in low- and middle-income countries received ARVs by 2013. (Seventy-five per cent of HIV-positive patients live in sub-Saharan Africa). On average, malaria still kills a child every minute (UNICEF, nd).
SDGs 2012–2030	The six elements of the SDGs include dignity, people, prosperity, our planet, justice and partnership. The targets set are: • ending poverty in all its forms, everywhere • ending hunger • achieving gender equality • ensuring healthy lives and promoting well-being for all people at all ages • ensuring access to affordable, reliable, sustainable and modern energy for all.
PMNCH (WHO, 2017b)	The PMNCH is an alliance of more than 700 organisations (in 77 countries) from the sexual, reproductive, maternal, newborn, child and adolescent healthcare communities. It was established to advocate for and agree on evidence-based interventions to improve maternal, newborn, child and adolescent health. Their mandate is to engage, align and hold accountable multi-stakeholder action to improve the health and well-being of women, newborns, children and adolescents. The movement gives support to partners to work together to achieve the Global Strategy for the Every Woman Every Child movement by 2030.
UNICEF: Education of girls and protection of children	UNICEF is committed to supporting the African Union (AU) on the education of girls and the protection of children within the framework of Africa's agenda.

The integration guidelines for improving maternal and child outcomes

To improve the quality of care, the WHO (2007d) presented the continuum of maternal and newborn care (Kerber et al, 2007). The continuum of care (COC) is a public health framework that advocates for the integration of service delivery for women and children throughout the reproductive life cycle. The aim is for the individual to receive a package of care that will allow the right person to provide the right care, at the right time and in the right place, throughout the patient's lifespan. The COC is a core principle in improving the quality of care provided to women, newborns and children in reproductive health. It calls for an integrated approach to deliver evidence-based care as a package.

The COC package offers 190 interventions that can be scaled up through combined clinical care, outpatient, community and household levels to improve health outcomes for mothers and children. Each healthcare context is encouraged to develop a package suited to its particular system. The package should include the 190 interventions throughout the life cycle in order to meet the needs of women and children and thereby reduce maternal and child mortality and morbidity.

These interventions include services at household level, in the community, at outreach level and in health facilities, as shown in Figure 4.1. Some of these services in the South African context are reflected in Table 4.2 on pages 30–33.

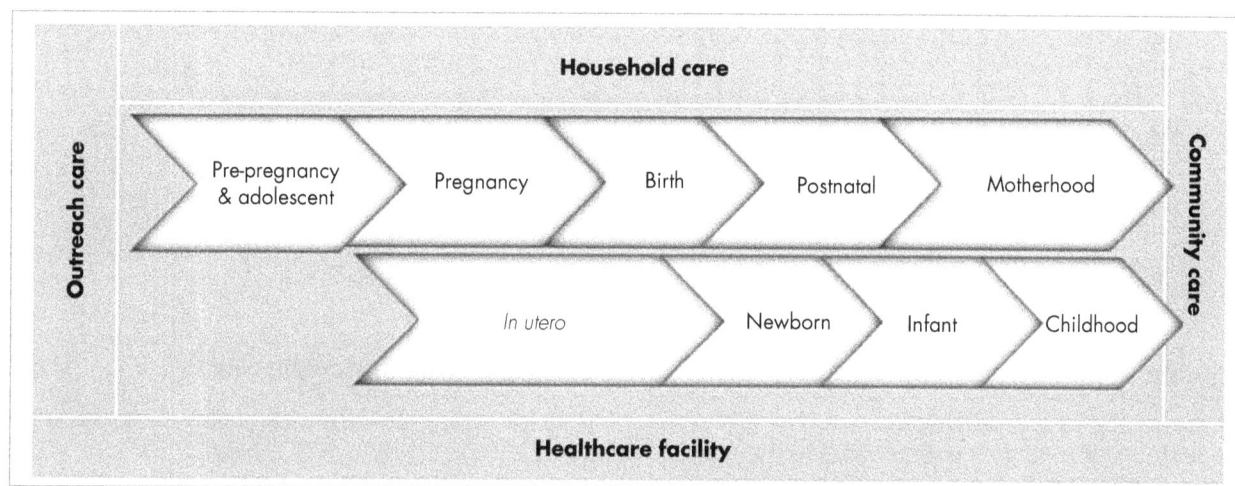

Figure 4.1 The COC and integrated service platforms (adapted from WHO, 2007d; WHO, 2011b)

Policy development: CARMMA

In response to international strategies, the AU launched the Campaign on Accelerated Reduction of Maternal, Newborn and Child Mortality in Africa (CARMMA) in Africa on 7 May 2009, during the fourth session of the conference of AU Ministers of Health (Banda, 2012). It was asserted that Africa accounts for 53 per cent of women who die annually due to pregnancy and birth. The CARMMA campaign called for increased action towards improving maternal and newborn health and survival in Africa in view of the MDGs.

The CARMMA website (see www.carmma.org) releases statistics for Africa, including the country scorecard on countries in Africa that have launched CARMMA. By 2010, 44 countries in Africa had launched CARMMA, three more were preparing to launch and five countries were outstanding. South Africa launched CARMMA in 2012.

Implementation of South African strategies to improve maternal and newborn care and outcomes

In addition to many policies already in place, since 2011 the South African government has made a concerted effort to improve healthcare for South Africans. The Maternal,

Newborn, Child and Women's Health and Nutrition (MNCWH and N) Directorate was instituted in 1995 to develop strategy, guide policies and programmes in the public sector and to continuously set priorities for maternal healthcare. The DoH develops policy and the MNCWH directorate implements these policies.

Besides MNCWH policy, the South African government has developed priority strategies and campaigns to reduce maternal, newborn and child mortality. These include the re-engineering of PHC, the launch of CARMMA, the National Strategic Plan for Maternity Care in South Africa and the strengthening of health systems, including monitoring of progress. These guidelines are briefly described in the sections that follow.

MNCWH and nutrition in South Africa: Strategic Plan 2012–2016

The main goal of the MNCWH and N Strategic Plan is to reduce maternal, newborn and under-five mortality against set targets and indicators. The development of action plans to implement the targeted initiatives takes place at all levels of district healthcare to meet the set targets. These strategies and targets are presented in Table 4.4 on page 36.

Table 4.4

Specific implemented targeted interventions for MNCWH and N 2012–2016 (Cadegan, 2012)

Maternal health interventions	Newborn health interventions
BANC: four visits for every pregnant woman, to be started before 20 weeks Initiation of HIV testing and ART in accordance with appropriate guidelines, to support the PMTCT of HIV Introduction of dedicated obstetric ambulances and the establishment of maternity waiting homes Improved intrapartum care, focusing on the correct use of the partogram and standard protocols for management of complications Postnatal care within six days of delivery	Promotion of early and exclusive breastfeeding to ensure the safety of newborns exposed to HIV Providing PMTCT services Resuscitation of newborns Caring for small or ill newborns according to standardised protocols Promoting KMC for stable and LBW infants Ensuring a postnatal visit within six days to offer newborn care and support for EBF
Community interventions	**Women's health interventions**
The provision of a package of community-based MNCWH care services by ward-based PHC outreach teams (community health workers [CHWs]) Multi-sectoral action to reduce poverty and inequity and to improve access to services such as water and sanitation Developing MNCWH communication with the community and women	Increased access to contraceptive services, including but not limited to pregnancy confirmation and EC Post-rape care for adults and children Youth-friendly counselling and reproductive health services at health facilities and through school health services Improving coverage of cervical screening and strengthening follow-up mechanisms

Child health

Promoting EBF and complementary feeding practices for infants and young children

Preventive services such as immunisation, growth monitoring and promotion, VAS and regular de-worming

Correct management of childhood illnesses using the IMCI case management process

Early identification and appropriate management of all HIV-infected children

Improved hospital care using standardised protocols for children with conditions such as pneumonia, diarrhoea and malnutrition

Expanding and increasing school health services

Initiating services for children with long-term health conditions

The re-engineering of primary healthcare

In 2011, the South African government launched a policy to re-engineer PHC in South Africa. As a result, the Negotiated Service Delivery Agreement Charter (NSDA) 2010–2014 (DoH, nd[c]) was negotiated between the MECs of the nine provinces and the president to deliver quality and accessible services to increase life expectancy, decrease maternal and child mortality, combat HIV/AIDS and the burden of disease for TB, and strengthen the healthcare system.

By 2012, this policy was ready for implementation (see Figure 4.1 on page 35). This integrated care system also incorporated and focused on maternal and child care at PHC level. The model has three streams that are additional programmes aimed at improving the quality of clinical care, access and service delivery. The three streams are as presented in the following sections. Figure 4.2 illustrates the PHC model.

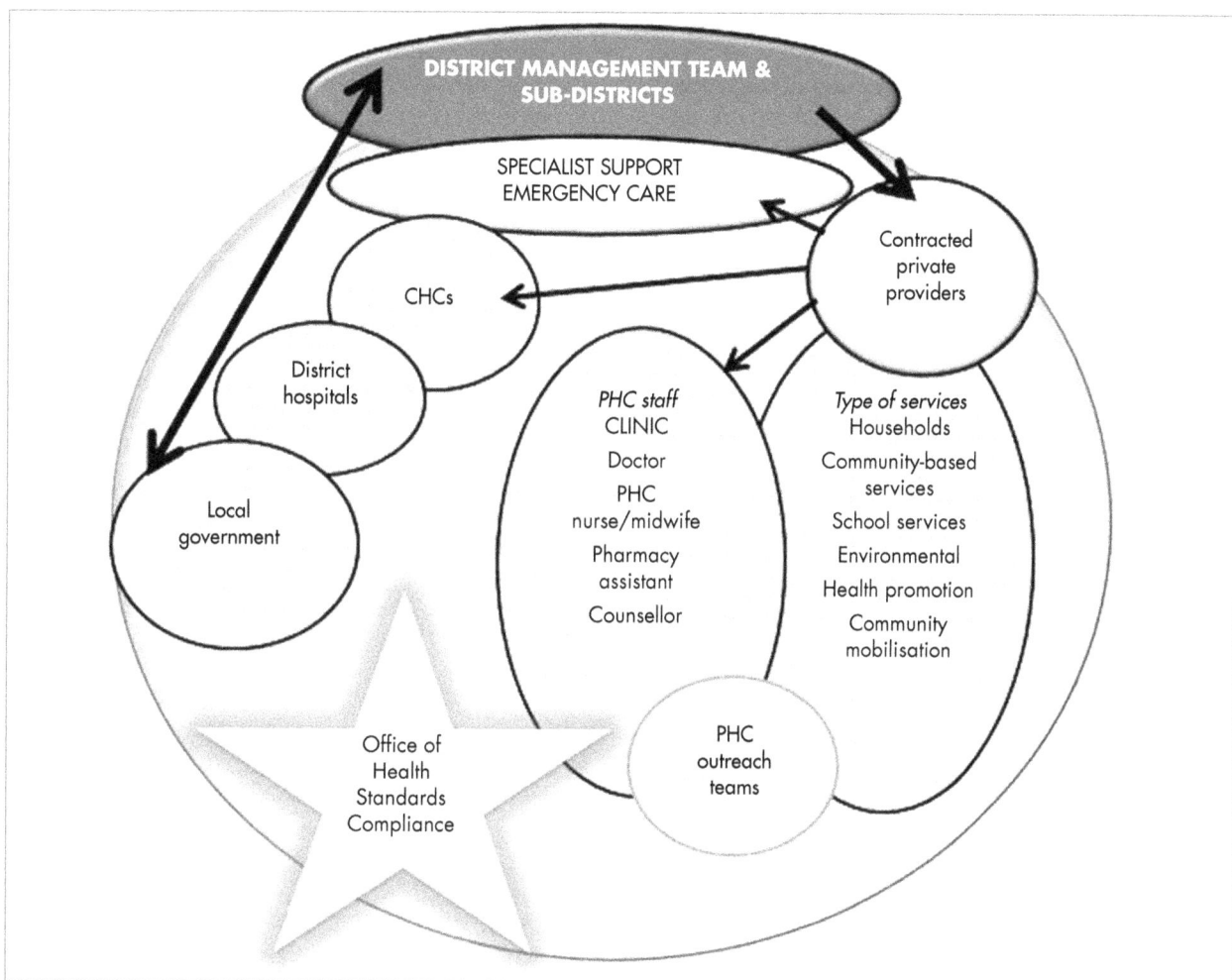

Figure 4.2 PHC model (adapted from Naledi, Barron & Schneider, 2011)

Stream 1: Ward-based primary healthcare outreach teams

Ward-based PHC outreach teams (also called WBOTs), led by a professional nurse, consist of six to eight trained CHWs. Each team takes care of 1 500 households in the community they serve. The aim is to reduce the pressure on clinics and improve care for individuals and communities. Home- and community-based health services are linked to a fixed clinic to make care more accessible, to identify problems and refer those needing care to the clinic.

The WBOTs are trained in:
▶ identifying and registering households
▶ conducting household assessments
▶ providing education on the promotion of good health and the prevention of illness (maternal and child health, HIV/AIDS, TB).

Identifying chronic diseases is an essential element of all home visits and other community-based activities of the CHW. Specific functions include:
▶ providing health-related information on immunisation, antenatal and postnatal care, HIV/AIDS, TB and chronic diseases
▶ conducting simple screenings for potential health problems
▶ providing adherence support and counselling
▶ referring patients to other health services and receiving referrals from other health services
▶ providing basic first aid and emergency interventions.

Stream 2: School health services

A policy for school health services was developed by the DoH. The Department of Basic Education (DBE) and the Department of Social Development (DSD) collaborated

37

on the development and implementation of the Integrated School Health Programme (ISHP) (DoH, 2012) and School Health Package. Although implementation and progress have been slow, it is desirable for each school to have a health nurse. The focus is on the improvement of the health of children, early detection of health problems, malnutrition and the sexual healthcare needs of teenagers for improved health outcomes among young people.

Stream 3: District clinical specialist teams

Each district clinical specialist team (DCST) consists of seven specialist clinicians who are appointed in each district to give clinical oversight, support and training, particularly in maternal, newborn and child care. The team is made up of three dyads (teams of two: a doctor and a nurse who are specialists in the same field) and an anaesthetist. The proposed composition of each team is as follows:

- PHC: a family physician and a PHC professional nurse
- Obstetrics: an obstetrician and an advanced midwife
- Child care: a paediatrician and a specialist paediatric professional nurse
- An anaesthetist.

Because of a shortage of categories of staff such as paediatricians, obstetricians and anaesthetists, not all vacancies have been filled. Where a medical doctor could not be appointed, an advanced nurse practitioner is responsible for this function in the districts.

The main tasks of the DCSTs are clinical governance, training, monitoring of quality of care and assisting districts to set standards, identify gaps in care and take corrective measures. The main function of the DCSTs is reduction of maternal and child mortality and morbidity.

The DCSTs have been instrumental in training doctors and midwives on the Essential Steps in the Management of Obstetric Emergencies (ESMOE) programme and Emergency Obstetric Simulation Training (EOST), as well as in the improvement of neonatal care. Further progress has been made in the development and maintenance of maternal and perinatal review committees, the improvement of data management and the reduction of maternal, neonatal and under-five mortality rates. Undertaking research and developing standards, policy and quality improvement plans in collaboration with the district clinical and management teams are essential activities for implementing best practices. The DCSTs continue to support the districts.

CARMMA South Africa

South Africa responded to the AU by launching CARMMA locally on 4 May 2012. In addition, a campaign entitled

Reducing Maternal and Child Mortality through Strengthening Primary Healthcare (RMCH) was developed to orientate the DCSTs in their new role and function and to assist areas that perform the worst in maternal and child care. Several interventions were included to improve maternal and infant care and outcomes in priority districts.

The RMCH was a collaborative intervention between the DoH, stakeholders and partners to implement PHC re-engineering and CARMMA, in order to transform the maternal and child health outcomes in 25 priority districts across nine provinces, as agreed by the NHC.

Activity

Read more about some of the policies and guidelines that were implemented through CARMMA and the RMCH between 2010 and 2014:

- Robertson-Sutton, A. 2011. Improving newborn care in South Africa: Lessons learned from the Limpopo Initiative for Newborn Care (LINC). UNICEF, DoH and Save the Children.
- DoH. 2013. *Essential newborn care quality improvement toolkit.* http://www.lincare.co.za/wp-content/uploads/2016/06/Essential-Newborn-Care-Quality-Improvement-Toolkit-2013-1.pdf (Accessed 2 October 2017).
- DoH. 2014. *Newborn care charts. Routine care at birth and management of the sick and small newborn in hospital.* http://www.kznhealth.gov.za/kinc/Newborn_care_charts_March_2014.pdf (Accessed 2 October 2017).
- DoH. 2015. *Guidelines for Maternity Care in South Africa. A manual for clinics, community health centres and district hospitals.* https://www.health-e.org.za/wp-content/uploads/2015/11/Maternal-Care-Guidelines-2015_FINAL-21.7.15.pdf (Accessed 2 October 2017).

The DoH, donors, partners, NGOs, stakeholders and districts all worked together to develop contextual and evidence-based solutions to improve maternal, newborn and child mortality in South Africa and its districts. The box above highlights only a few of the clinical and service guidelines that were published for implementation to guide practitioners and managers with regard to clinical standards and protocols.

All provinces and districts are required to implement the policies at all levels of healthcare.

The National Strategy for Maternity Care in South Africa

The National Strategy for Maternity Care in South Africa gives the important broader aspects to improve maternal and newborn care in South Africa, as reflected in the *Guidelines for Maternity Care in South Africa* (DoH, 2015a:15). Table 4.5 summarises the strategic aspects for intervention, mainly focused on community, government and management

factors, to strengthen the healthcare system. The national strategy recognises that improvement of quality in healthcare is multifactorial. Healthcare staff function within a system and are dependent on the system to provide quality care.

Table 4.5

Adapted summary of the National Strategy for Maternity Care (DoH, 2015a:15)

Strategy	Required actions
Community participation	Engage and empower the community for change. Develop and implement community outreach teams.
A supportive legal framework	Legislation and policies must be in place to support the national strategies.
Adaptation to local realities	Underlying causes, such as poverty and illiteracy, need attention.
Quality of care	A quality framework that considers all aspects to improve quality, including caring behaviour on the part of health workers, must be in place.
Improvement in the status of women	Improve the status of women through education and employment and preventing abuse.
Provision of skilled midwifery and obstetric services	There must be a fully functional healthcare system with enough skilled midwives and doctors to support women during their reproductive lives, which is referred to as *skilled attendance*. All hospitals must offer Caesarean sections and blood must be available at all times to save lives.
Clinical guidelines	Knowledge and practice of maternal and neonatal standards and guidelines for low- and high-risk pregnancies must be in place and must be of a high standard.
Regionalised care and referral systems	A fully functional referral system with safe transport is critical for optimal care.
Management capacity	Effective management of staff and resources is key to a functional system.
Continuing audit of services	Reviews and audits at all levels of healthcare are essential to identify gaps, risks and adverse events and to take remedial action.
Research	Research is important to find solutions that are specific for the context.

4.5 Quality, standards, targets and monitoring of data and outcomes

The setting of standards and targets is essential for quality improvement. Monitoring and measuring are important to view trends, needs, gaps and performance against standards and targets. What follows is a brief discussion on the standards to improve care and the current programmes to collect, analyse and measure outcomes in healthcare, with particular reference to maternal and child care.

Standards of health establishments

The Office for Health Standards Compliance (OHSC) established the National Core Standards 2011 (DoH, 2011b)

for all health establishments in South Africa, based on international standards (McKenzie et al, 2016). As per the NHA, an annual self-assessment of 140 indicators is mandatory for all health facilities. This would indicate the level of compliance to standards regarding the physical requirements for facilities. PHC facilities use the ideal clinic indicators (DoH, 2016), which set standards to measure the quality of clinics and report on the gaps.

Health data management and indicators

In compliance with the prescripts of the NHA, the national health management information system (NHMIS) was established in 1996 to track health service delivery and health outcomes in the public sector, under supervision of the Health Information Task Team (HITT). In collaboration with stakeholders, the HITT publishes the National Indicator Data Set (NIDS), detailing the aspects for which information is gathered at all levels of the healthcare system.

In maternal and newborn care, both NIDS and CARMMA indicators exist. Information is also gathered through the evaluation of the effectiveness of health programmes, such as measures of maternal, newborn and child mortality. These indicators are briefly discussed in the following sections.

The monitoring of indicators (Department of Health)

The MNCWH and other directorates, in collaboration with the HITT, have adopted the following indicators for monitoring maternal and newborn quality of care and health outcomes:
- CARMMA indicators
- Obstetric and neonatal health facilities and levels of care
- Obstetric and neonatal signal functions:
  - Minimum signal functions for all facilities
  - Routine obstetric and neonatal signal functions
  - Signal functions for basic emergency care
  - Comprehensive or advanced signal functions.

CARMMA indicators

CARMMA focuses on the quality of maternal and newborn care and health outcomes. To this end, the following indicators and signal functions have been developed:
- Seven steps are indicated to assess the functionality of health facilities for neonatal care, focused on managers. The standard guidelines include three routine functions, seven basic emergency neonatal functions and two comprehensive emergency care functions that require competency from all healthcare staff.
- The level of care at which the facility functions, reflected in routine, basic and comprehensive care, is indicated.
- The availability and effectiveness of obstetric ambulances at district level is a critical aspect for quality improvement.

The indicators and signal functions are included on district health plans (DHPs) and monitored for effectiveness.

Obstetric and neonatal health facilities and levels of care

Obstetric and maternity care is functionally divided into levels of care, based on the type of services needed. There are two main types of essential obstetric clinics in South Africa, namely:
1. basic essential obstetric clinics (BEOCs) (SMI standard = four clinics per 500 000 of the population)
2. comprehensive essential obstetric clinics (CEOCs) (SMI standards = one clinic per 500 000 of the population).

Referral centres, district hospitals and specialised hospitals should be able to provide all the basic care according to the comprehensive signal functions, as indicated in the comprehensive care for mothers and babies guidelines for comprehensive emergency obstetric and neonatal care (CEmONC) (Pattinson et al, 2015)

The general standards for obstetric and neonatal health facilities are the following:
- Services to be available 24 hours a day, seven days a week
- A sufficient number or ratio of skilled providers, with a sufficient skills mix
- An effective referral system and functional communication for emergency transport
- Infrastructure with reliable water and electricity, heating and clean toilets.

Obstetric and neonatal signal functions

Signal functions are minimum life-saving interventions in obstetric health services that are globally recognised as factors that will make a difference to the quality of care and will prevent maternal and newborn deaths. Signal functions guide obstetric care for improved health outcomes for each level. All midwives need knowledge and skills to practise the signal functions routinely.

The *basic critical signal functions* that are applicable in all health centres, such as PHC clinics, MOUs and hospitals, are:
- the availability and skilled administration of magnesium sulphate as an intervention to manage severe hypertension and eclampsia
- the availability and skilled administration of oxytocin as an intervention in the management of postpartum haemorrhage (PPH).

The *routine signal functions* include the minimum signal functions detailed above and include standards for routine care for all mothers and babies, as detailed in Table 4.6.

Inclusive of the minimum and routine signal functions, all midwives should be competent at managing *basic emergency interventions* in facilities at any level of care. The signal functions for *basic emergency care* are:
- parenteral magnesium sulphate for pre-eclampsia and eclampsia
- assisted vaginal delivery
- parenteral antibiotics for maternal infection
- manual removal of the placenta in the case of retained placenta
- removal of retained products of conception through manual vacuum aspiration (MVA)
- parenteral oxytocic drugs for haemorrhage

Table 4.6

Routine obstetric and neonatal signal functions for all mothers and babies

Obstetric signal functions	Neonatal signal functions
Monitoring of labour using a partogram Washing hands and using gloves to prevent infections Active management of third stage of labour (AMTSL) HIV and TB screening and treatment	Thermal protection Immediate and exclusive breastfeeding for six months Prevention of infections (eyes and cord care) ART for PMTCT

▶ antibiotics for preterm or prolonged premature rupture of membranes (PROM) to prevent infection
▶ corticosteroids in preterm labour
▶ ventilation with bag and mask, for non-breathing babies
▶ KMC for preterm and very small or LBW babies
▶ alternative feeding in case of inability to breastfeed
▶ injectable antibiotics for neonatal sepsis.

Advanced procedures are indicated in the *comprehensive signal functions* (inclusive of the minimum, basic and basic emergency care). The comprehensive functions include advanced resuscitation, which can be performed at any level, and blood transfusion at all levels where births are conducted. Surgery, however, can only be done in district hospitals. Comprehensive care for all mothers and babies, in the form of CEmONC, includes:
▶ surgery and anaesthetics (Caesarean sections)
▶ blood transfusions
▶ intravenous fluid
▶ the safe administration of oxygen.

Health data management and monitoring and analysis

Data management is the key to identifying gaps in health service and problems with quality, as well as monitoring progress. Accurate data can be used to better plan healthcare and to indicate the effectiveness of healthcare and healthcare programmes.

Several monitoring systems have been developed in South Africa to measure quality and the effectiveness of programme implementation, interventions and clinical outcomes of mothers and newborns.

All managers and staff at all levels of the healthcare system have a responsibility to report accurately and timeously on the required indicators. The planning of care, staff and finances depend on accurate and reliable data.

The monitoring of indicators at provincial level

The provincial health departments take responsibility for data management, policy implementation and implementation of certain programmes in districts. Data collection regarding maternal deaths is a provincial function.

The National Committee on Confidential Enquiries into Maternal Deaths (NCCEMD)

The NCCEMD put systems in place to monitor maternal deaths using a confidential enquiry system. Information on maternal deaths is collected at provincial level in the maternal morbidity and mortality audit system (MaMMAS database) for fairly rapid analysis, which is reflected in annual interim reports and the tri-annual *Saving Mothers* reports (see Chapter 2). The *Saving Mothers 2011–2013* report (DoH, 2014) gives a summary of the causes of deaths, trends in maternal deaths and the progress in reducing maternal deaths in the country. The institutional maternal mortality ratio (iMMR) in the report refers to women who died in public healthcare facilities. The reports are published nationally.

Figure 4.3 on page 42 gives an overview of the number of maternal death cases reported since 1998. This is not a complete picture, because not all cases have been reported as yet.

One of the interventions suggested in the *Saving Mothers* reports to improve the quality of outcomes for mothers and babies is the mandatory up-skilling of all staff working in obstetrics through training on the ESMOE programme and regular practise of EOST drills, in order to maintain skills. ESMOE and EOST attendance are mandatory in order to maintain emergency care skills. This training is planned and documented in South Africa.

The monitoring of indicators at district level

Data management at district level occurs through the district health management information system (DHMIS). Information is gathered on a monthly basis and reports are generated on a quarterly basis.

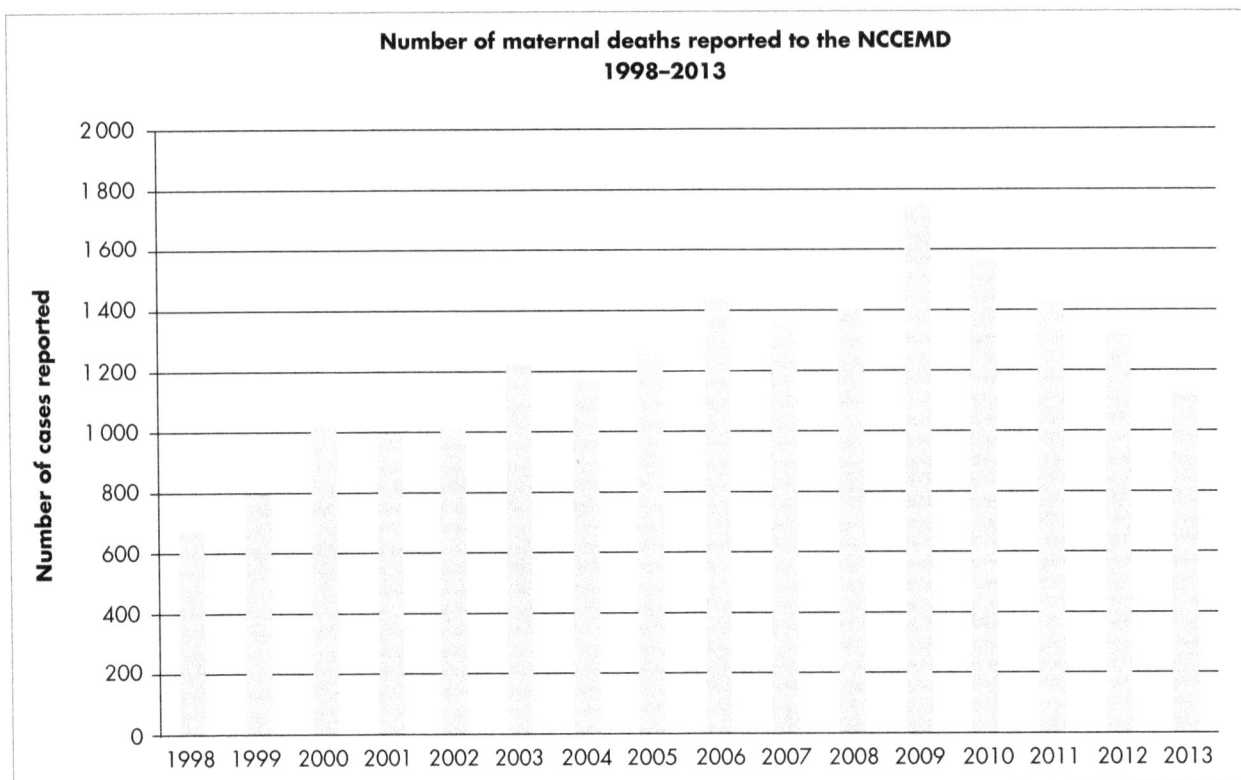

Figure 4.3 Number of maternal deaths reported 1998–2013 (collated from DoH, 2014: 3)

The DHB reports on maternal deaths per district through the DHMIS on an annual basis. The reliability of information depends on the quality of the data collected, captured and analysed. The essential principle of accurate record keeping by all staff becomes important to ensure accuracy of data.

The MNCWH dashboard

The MNCWH dashboard (UNICEF, 2013b) is used at district level to monitor the progress of maternal and child care against indicators on a real-time basis. This allows districts to monitor, report on and improve outcomes through action plans in DHPs. There are 25 selected indicators that can positively influence maternal morbidity and mortality, as identified by the district. The six indicators and targets most commonly used are the following:

1. The first visit during pregnancy (under 20 weeks), to make early contact with pregnant women for improved health outcomes
2. Antenatal client initiation on ART, aiming at 100 per cent counseling, testing and treatment of HIV in pregnant women

3. Deliveries in facilities for girls under 18, in order to monitor the effectiveness of prevention of pregnancy for teenagers
4. Delivery by Caesarean section to monitor appropriate procedures where needed, in line with national and international norms for safety
5. Maternal mortality in facility only, counting those deaths that happened in facilities (to monitor norms and standards of practice)
6. Maternal postnatal visits at six weeks, to monitor maternal and infant well-being in view of HIV/AIDS.

The PPIP

The PPIP is a database and tool to assist in the management of perinatal and maternal deaths at district level (also see Chapter 2). It allows the district to own the data and present them in graphs. The number of cases, as well as causes and avoidable factors, are identified and submitted by various facilities. This allows for real-time auditing and analysis and provides a quick response, which enables planning for action. Information can be presented at perinatal reviews. This consolidated information forms part of the *Saving Babies* reports (see, for example, Pattinson & Rhoda, 2014).

The Child Healthcare Problem Identification Programme

The ChildPIP is a mortality audit tool for children that has been in use since 2004. It currently reports on 200 hospitals in all nine provinces, with a focus on the five leading causes of mortality in children under 5 years of age (pneumonia, diarrhea, HIV, tuberculosis and meningitis) (Pattinson & Rhoda, 2014.)

Maternal and perinatal reviews

Maternal and perinatal review committees must be established and be functional at facility and district level, following standard guidelines.

Activity

Attend a perinatal review meeting and write a report on the standards set for these meetings.

4.6   Conclusion

The acceleration of programmes and interventions to reduce maternal and child mortality in South Africa depend on the local context, provinces and districts, and may differ between metros, urban and rural healthcare districts.

Nurses and midwives should maintain their competencies through continuous education. They should be flexible and be able to adjust, adapt and re-skill in times of transformation of the healthcare system. Competency also includes knowing the healthcare system and following guidelines effectively.

Section Two

The female reproductive system

The female reproductive organs

5.1   Introduction

This chapter explains the anatomical structure and function of the female reproductive organs. These are divided into the external and internal structures, as listed in Table 5.1.

Table 5.1

Structures found in the female reproductive system

External	Internal
Vulva (pudenda)	Vagina
Mons pubis	Uterus
Clitoris	Fallopian tubes
Labia majora	Ovaries
Labia minora	Supporting structures of female pelvis
Vestibule	
Urethral meatus	Bony pelvis
Skene's ducts	Pelvic floor
Bartholin's glands	Accessory breast tissue and milk ducts
Perineum	
Nipples	

Normal reproductive anatomy can be affected by:

▶ age
▶ genetic make-up
▶ birth or congenital defects
▶ malnutrition
▶ disease (eg TB, polio)
▶ trauma (eg a pelvic fracture)
▶ hormonal abnormalities
▶ previous births.

5.2   The external female genitalia

The external female reproductive organs are shown in Figure 5.1 on page 48. The vulva (also known as the pudenda) consists of all the structures externally visible, from the pubis to the perineum. It includes the mons pubis, clitoris, labia majora, labia minora, vestibule, urethral meatus, Skene's ducts, Bartholin's glands and perineum.

The mons pubis (also known as the mons veneris) is the fatty cushion over the pubic bone. It protects the pubic bone. After puberty it is covered with pubic hair.

The clitoris is a small erectile body beneath the mons pubis. It has an abundant blood and nerve supply. It is comparable to the male penis and becomes erect during sexual arousal.

The labia majora are the two folds of adipose tissue that conceal the underlying structures in a nullipara. In multiparous women, the labia may remain open. In menopause, they may shrink. The outer surface is covered with pubic hair and the inner surface is smooth. The labia majora are homologous to the scrotum in the male.

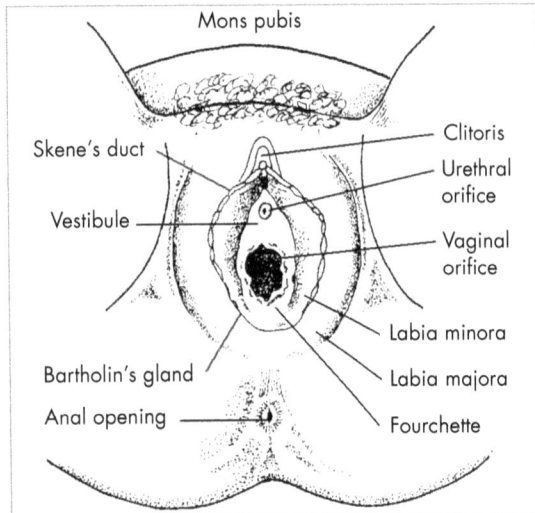

Figure 5.1 The structure of the female genitalia

The labia minora are two thin, hairless folds that lie between the labia majora. They are richly supplied with blood vessels and nerves. At the anterior they converge to form the frenulum of the clitoris and at the posterior they form the fourchette.

The vestibule is an almond-shaped area bordered by the labia minora. It stretches from the fourchette posteriorly to the clitoris anteriorly. The structures that open into the vestibule are as follows:

- *The urethral meatus of the urinary tract:* The opening is about 1.5 cm below the clitoris, and is sometimes difficult to find in multiparous women.
- *Two Skene's ducts (one on each side):* These ducts secrete mucus and are often infected in cases of gonorrhoea.
- *The vaginal introitus, or orifice:* The opening to the vagina occupies the posterior two-thirds of the vestibule. Before puberty, the opening may be partially hidden by a membrane known as the hymen. This membrane is usually ruptured during initial sexual intercourse, but can also be torn during strenuous physical exercise or by the use of vaginal tampons during menstruation. Further tearing takes place during the delivery of a child and the remaining tags of skin and fibrous tissue are known as carunculae myrtiformes.
- *Bartholin's glands (two):* These are situated on either side of the vaginal introitus. They are pea-sized, compound racemose (clustered) glands, and are situated posterior-laterally in the vestibule, embedded deep in the labia

majora and the bulbocavernosus muscle. These glands have a lubricating function, especially during sexual intercourse. They open into the vestibule on either side of the vaginal introitus through the Bartholin's ducts.

Bartholin's gland infection

A Bartholin's gland might become infected and form an abscess. This may be caused by a gonococcal infection. A Bartholin's duct could also be damaged by a badly performed or incorrectly positioned episiotomy.

The perineum, sometimes referred to as the obstetric perineum, is the small area of muscle and fascia between the vaginal opening and the anus. This area is often traumatised in childbirth. These layers of muscle and skin may tear or may have to be surgically incised during delivery. Perineal tears during delivery may also involve the anal sphincter (a third-degree tear).

The external female genitalia are highly vascular and are supplied and drained by branches of the internal pudendal vessels (from the internal iliac vessels). The external pudendal artery (a branch of the femoral artery) also supplies the vulva. Lymphatic drainage takes place via the sacral nodes, the internal iliac nodes and the inguinal nodes. This is a very sensitive area, richly supplied by branches of the pudendal nerve (sacral 2, 3 and 4). The posterior cutaneous nerve (sacral 1, 2 and 3), together with the genitofemoral nerve (lumbar 1 and 2) and the ilioinguinal nerve (lumbar 1), also supply the structures of the external genitalia.

5.3 The internal female reproductive organs

The structures that make up the internal genitalia are the vagina, the uterus (including the cervix), the uterine tubes and the ovaries, as shown in Figure 5.2. These organs are all contained within the true pelvis in the non-gravid (not pregnant) state.

The vagina

The vagina is a muscular tube that connects the vestibule with the uterus. It has three functions:

1. It is the excretory duct for menstrual flow.
2. It is the organ that receives the penis during sexual intercourse.
3. It is the birth canal.

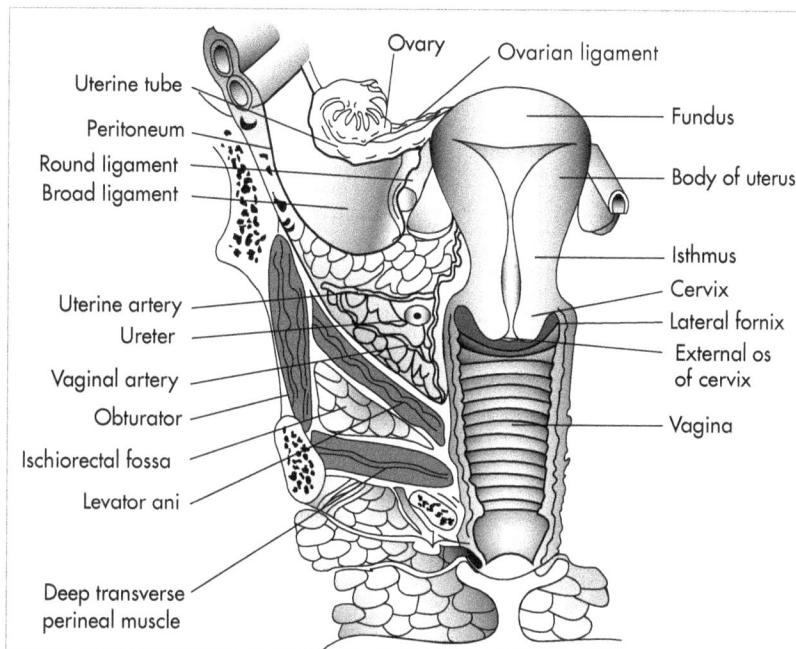

Figure 5.2 The internal female genitalia

The walls of the vagina are folded, with rugae (like a concertina), which allows the vagina to stretch during birth. The vagina is lined with stratified squamous epithelium, very similar to skin, but without glands. Under the influence of oestrogen, the squamous cells of the vagina lay down large stores of glycogen, which nourish the lactobacilli (Doderlein's bacillus) normally inhabiting the vagina. These bacilli produce lactic acid, which maintains the vaginal pH between 4.0 and 5.5. This acidic medium helps to reduce vaginal infections. Prior to puberty and after menopause, with reduced ovarian function, the pH of the vagina is less acidic and vaginal infections are more common.

The cervix opens into the posterior part of the upper vagina. The upper portion of the vagina is called the fornix, and it is divided into anterior, posterior and two lateral portions.

The vagina is a highly vascular organ and the blood vessels are full of turns and twists to allow for the stretching that is necessary during pregnancy and labour. Any trauma to the vagina during labour usually heals rapidly because of the generous blood supply. The main blood supply to the vagina is from the vaginal arteries and from the descending branches of the uterine arteries (branches of the internal iliac arteries) (see Figure 5.2). Lesser supplies are from the arteries of the bladder, the rectum and the internal pudendal arteries. An extensive network of veins accompanies these arteries. Varicose veins may affect the vaginal area.

The vagina is sensitive to stretching, but not to touch. It is supplied by sympathetic and parasympathetic nerve fibres.

Bacterial vaginosis (BV)

BV is a common vaginal infection that occurs during the female reproductive phase. It is caused by the excessive growth of bacteria.

White or gray vaginal discharge, which often smells like fish, is a common symptom of BV. Itching does not usually occur. The risk of infection with other sexually transmitted infections (STIs), including HIV, is approximately doubled when a woman is infected with BV. Pregnant women with BV also run a higher risk of early delivery.

BV is not an STI. It is caused by an imbalance of the bacteria that are found naturally in the vagina. New or multiple sex partners, douching, intrauterine contraceptive devices (IUCDs) and antibiotics are all risk factors.

Based on the symptoms, a diagnosis may be confirmed by a test of the vaginal discharge. If the vaginal pH is higher than normal and if bacteria are present in large numbers, BV will be diagnosed.

BV is treated with an antibiotic, such as clindamycin or metronidazole. These medications may also be used in the second or third trimesters of pregnancy. (See Chapter 49.)

Measurements of the uterus and the Fallopian tubes

The anterior view showing
the areas and measurements

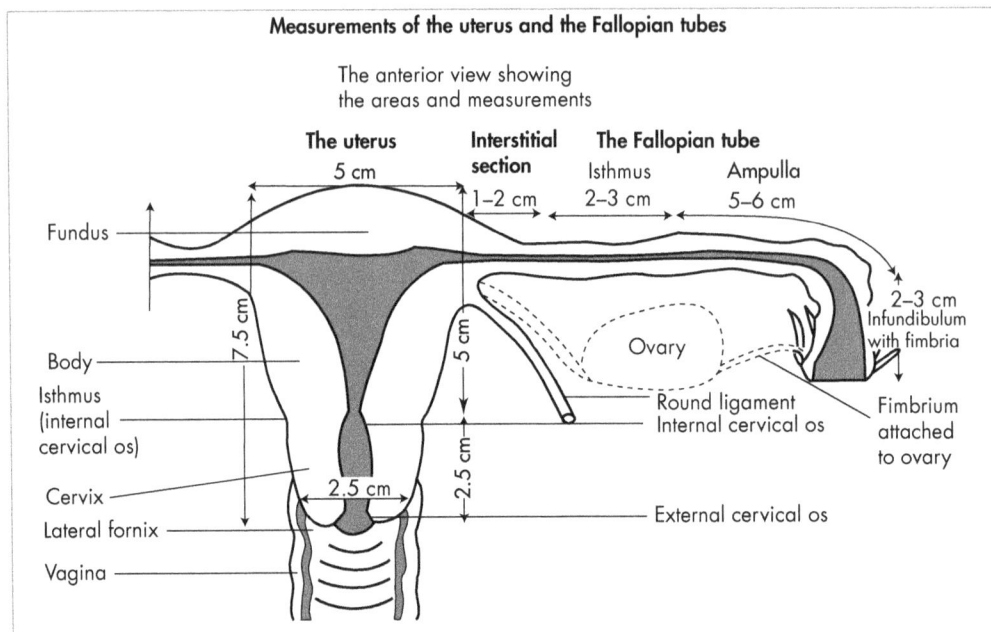

Figure 5.3 The size of the uterus

The uterus

The uterus is hollow and pear-shaped, and in its non-gravid state is approximately 7.5 cm long, 5 cm wide (at its widest point) and 2.5 cm thick, as shown in Figure 5.3. It is made up of a body and a neck, or cervix, which are joined at a constricted area, the isthmus. The cervix protrudes into the vagina and is sealed off with a thick mucus plug (operculum) during pregnancy.

The wide, rounded, upper portion of the uterine body is called the fundus. The fundus is the muscular part of the uterus. The uterus is functionally divided into the upper and lower segment in pregnancy. The fundus represents the upper segment and the cervix the lower segment. The isthmus divides the two segments. During pregnancy, the isthmus becomes larger and softer and Hegar's sign (in early pregnancy) is the softening that can be felt during vaginal examination. When pregnant, the uterus is referred to as gravid.

Immediately below the fundus, on either side of the body, the Fallopian tubes arise at the cornua (horns) of the uterus. The uterine cavity is continuous with the lumen of the uterine tubes.

The position of the uterus

The uterus is a pelvic organ in the cavity of the true pelvis, behind and above the bladder and in front of the rectum, as shown in Figure 5.4. In the normal non-gravid state, it leans forward in a position of anteversion. If it bends backwards

upon itself, it is in a position of anteflexion. The uterus is maintained in this position by several ligaments. The ones at the level of the cervix are the most important; these include the uterosacral, pubocervical, broad, round and ovarian ligaments (see Figure 5.4, Figure 5.6 on page 52 and Figure 5.7 on page 53).

The layers of the uterus

The uterus is composed of three layers, namely:
1. the endometrium
2. the myometrium
3. the perimetrium.

The endometrium

The endometrium is made up of three layers. The two most superficial layers are known as the functional layers, because they are shed during menstruation. The three layers of the endometrium are the following:
1. *The compact layer* lines the uterine cavity and is made up of columnar epithelial tissue.
2. *The spongy layer* consists of connective tissue (stroma) interspersed with glands that respond to the influence of oestrogen and progesterone by becoming more secretory. The thickness and the secretions of this layer of the endometrium depend upon the stage of the menstrual cycle. If the fertilised ovum does not implant, this layer and the compact layer are shed in menstruation.

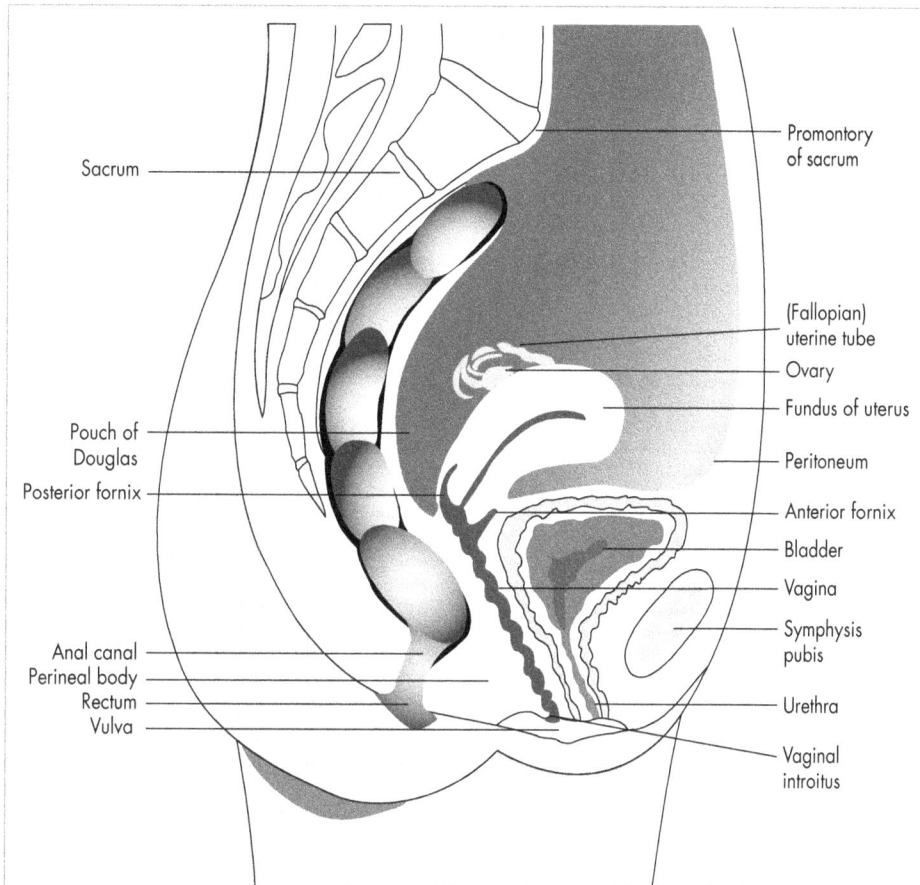

Figure 5.4 The position of the uterus and other reproductive organs

3. *The basal layer* also consists of connective tissue and glands, but it is not shed during menstruation, as it forms the basis for the regeneration of the two superficial layers of the endometrium after menstruation has taken place. Oestrogen acts on the cells of this basal layer to encourage regeneration. (See the menstrual cycle in Chapter 6 and colour illustration C1 on page 69.) If the basal endometrium is damaged, a woman cannot fall pregnant again. This is called Asherman's syndrome.

The decidua

In the gravid (pregnant) state, the endometrium is called the decidua. Under the influence of oestrogens and progesterone, it greatly increases in thickness and produces heavy secretions to receive and support the fertilised ovum, which is called a zygote.

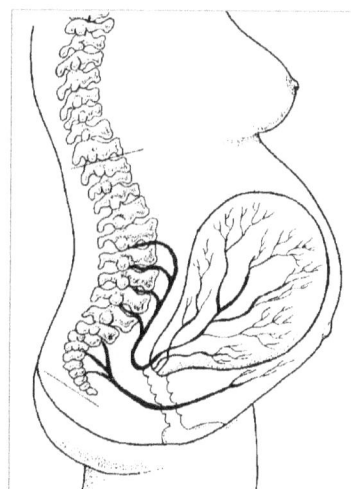

Figure 5.5 The uterine nerve supply

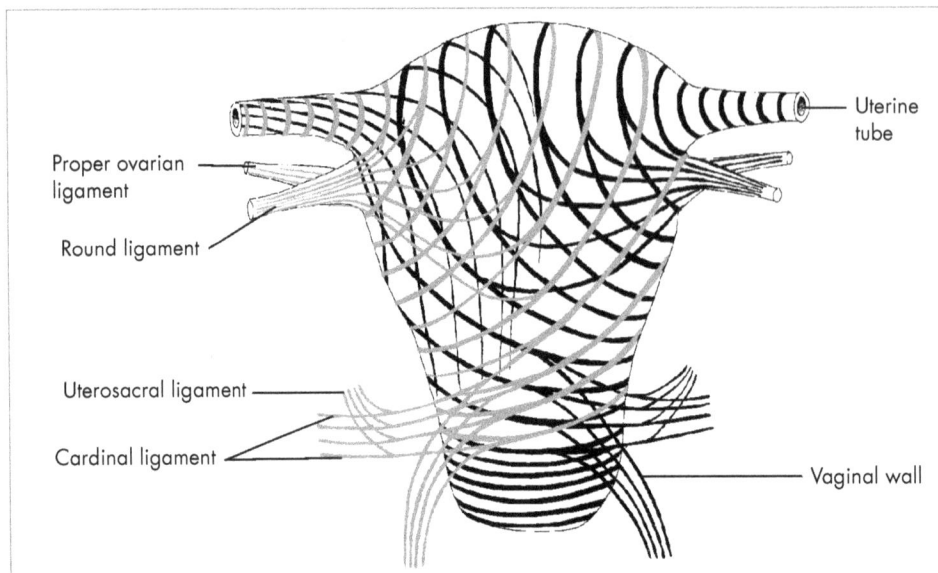

Figure 5.6 A schematic representation of the uterine musculature and ligaments

The myometrium

The myometrium is the thick, middle layer of the uterus. The myometrium is made up of three layers of muscle:

1. An inner layer of *circular muscle fibres* maintain the shape of the uterine cavity.
2. A middle layer of *criss-crossing fibres* enclose the numerous blood vessels supplying the walls of the uterus. The function of these fibres is to control bleeding from these vessels by acting as living ligatures after the detachment of the placenta in the third stage of labour.
3. An outer layer of *longitudinal muscle fibres* extend from the fundus of the uterus to the external cervical os, but are four times more plentiful in the fundus. New muscle fibres are developed in pregnancy to make the uterus a powerful muscular organ.

The contraction of these muscle fibres during labour causes the fetus (and/or other contents of the uterus) to be expelled.

Myomata

Myomata are growths in the myometrium common in women 30 years and older with high oestrogen levels. If present during pregnancy, they become large and vascular, causing complications that may cause placental abruption, malpresentation of the fetus, complications of birth and the risk of postpartum haemorrhage (PPH).

The perimetrium: The outer covering of the uterus

This is a layer of peritoneum that covers the body of the uterus and also divides the pelvic cavity from the abdominal cavity above. Anteriorly, it is reflected forward over the bladder, forming the uterovesical pouch, and posteriorly it is reflected upward over the rectum, forming the uterorectal pouch (of Douglas). On either side of the uterus, this layer of peritoneum covers the uterine tubes (and the ovaries) and is then attached to the sides of the pelvis to form the broad ligament/s (see Figure 5.7).

The cervix

The cervix, or lower third of the uterus, is cylindrical and is 2.5 cm in diameter and 2.5 cm long. The walls are 1.25 cm thick and surround a central canal, called the cervical canal. This canal is approximately 2.5 cm long and is constricted at either end, where it opens into the uterine cavity at the internal cervical os and into the vagina at the external cervical os. In pregnancy, the internal os becomes part of the uterine cavity.

The layers of the cervix differ slightly from those of the body of the uterus in the following ways:

▶ The inner layer or lining of the cervical canal is thrown into folds and is made up of ciliated columnar epithelium, interspersed with deep compound racemose glands, which secrete an alkaline mucus. The alkalinity of this mucus, which leaks into the posterior fornix of the vagina, affords protection to sperm deposited into the vagina during intercourse. (The acid medium of the vagina, while protecting the vagina from infection, is harmful to sperm.)

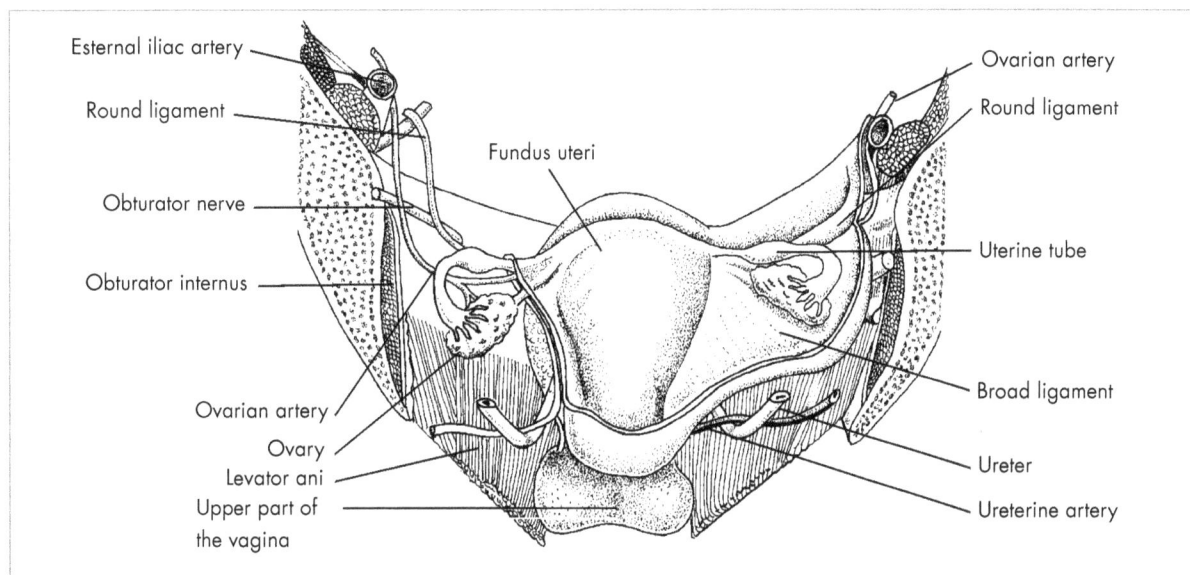

Figure 5.7 Ligaments supporting the uterus (posterior view)

▶ The alkaline mucus of the cervix, together with the cilia, which have an upward sweeping effect, helps the sperm move from the vagina into the uterine cavity.

During pregnancy, this mucus becomes thick and tenacious, forming a cervical plug, the operculum. This plug seals off the uterine cavity from the vagina and helps to protect the contents of the uterus from ascending infections.

The external cervical os is a small round opening. In a nullipara it is approximately 0.5 cm in diameter and is called the primip os. However, after vaginal birth it is an oval opening of 2 cm or more, is known as a multip os and is never completely closed again.

Cervical incompetence
Cervical incompetence describes a situation in which the cervix does not close and a woman cannot maintain a pregnancy. This may cause loss of pregnancies and needs medical intervention. Cervical incompetence may occur due to trauma at birth, but is usually idiopathic (spontaneous or due to unknown causes).

The Fallopian tubes

The Fallopian tubes (also called uterine tubes, oviducts or salpinges) stretch from the superior portion of the uterus to the ovaries and are approximately 10 cm long. Sperm enter the tubes from within the uterus and meet with the ovum that has been drawn in by the fimbria of the tubes, where fertilisation takes place. The cilia (small hairs) in the tube move the fertilised ovum towards the uterus via peristaltic movement. If the cilia are damaged by infections, the ovum may get stuck in the tube, where it then implants (an ectopic pregnancy). The tube may rupture when the ovum develops.

The ovaries

The ovaries lie on either side of the uterus in the true pelvis and are attached to the broad ligament. Each one is about the size and shape of an unshelled almond, approximately 3 cm long, 2 cm wide and 1 cm thick and greyish-white in colour.

The ovaries appear to lie outside the fold of peritoneum known as the broad ligament (see Figure 5.7), but they are attached to it on their anterior surfaces by a fold of the peritoneum known as the mesovarium. They are supported medially by the ovarian ligaments and laterally by the infundibulopelvic ligament.

The structure of the ovary and ovarian follicle

The ovary has a complex structure, with an inner medulla (middle) and an outer cortex (covering):

▶ The *medulla* is composed mainly of connective tissue, which forms the attachments for the ovarian and infundibulopelvic ligaments, which contain blood, lymph vessels and nerves.

The *cortex*, which is the functional part of the ovary, consists of theca cells (specialised connective tissue) interspersed with primordial and developing ovarian follicles, which contain the primary oocytes. The outer layer of the cortex of the ovary is made up of germinal epithelium, which is continuous with the mesovarium and is therefore probably a modified form of peritoneum.

The follicles are responsible for the gradual development of the primary oocytes, which will mature and become known as secondary oocytes and finally as ova (eggs). There are between 100 000 to 200 000 primordial follicles present in each ovary of a female child at birth. Under the influence of pituitary and ovarian hormones, these oocytes gradually develop and mature. It is only at puberty that these ovarian (Graafian) follicles begin to reach maturity, when one mature follicle will burst open approximately every 14th day of the 28-day menstrual cycle to expel a mature ovum into the peritoneal cavity. The follicles, which in the embryonic stage are solid structures of granulosa cells, gradually become cystic, with fluid forming between the ovum and the granulosa cells. The surrounding connective tissue develops into the theca (see Figure 5.8), encircling the follicle.

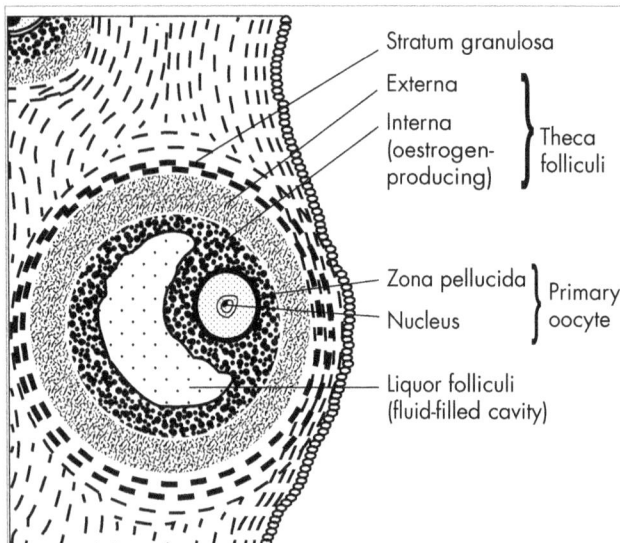

Figure 5.8 An ovarian follicle reaching maturity

The theca is divided into two functional layers:
1. The *theca externa*, or outer layer, is a highly vascular, connective tissue layer that becomes the capsule of the follicle.
2. The *theca interna*, or inner layer of cells, develops into epithelioid-like cells that are responsible for the secretion of the female hormone oestrogen, as are the granulosa cells.

Also see Chapter 6 for more details on menstruation.

Blood vessels

The blood supply to the ovaries is from the ovarian arteries, one on either side, which are direct branches of the descending aorta. The blood supply to the ovaries is augmented by the anastomosis of the uterine arteries with the ovarian arteries. These become enlarged in pregnancy. The venous drainage is via the ovarian veins, which drain into the inferior vena cava on the right side and into the renal vein on the left side.

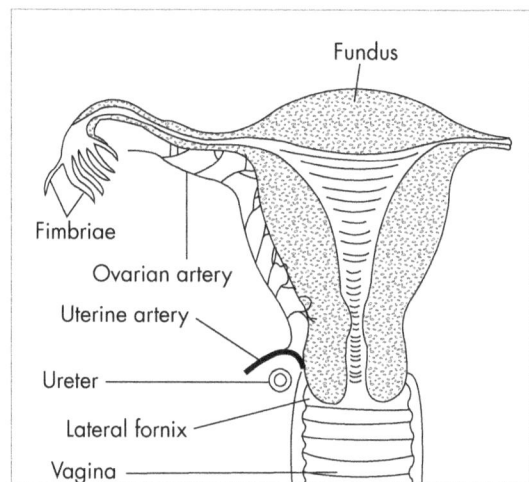

Figure 5.9 The uterine blood supply

Lymphatic drainage

This takes place via the para-aortic and inguinal nodes to the lumbar glands.

The nerve supply

The nerve supply (see also Figure 5.5 on page 51) is autonomic, with both motor and sensory, parasympathetic and sympathetic nerves accompanying the ovarian vessels from the ovarian plexus.

5.4   Congenital abnormalities of the female organs

In the female embryo, the two Mullerian ducts fuse to form the uterus. Anomalies occur when the fusion is incomplete or incorrect.

Some women are born with a congenital anomaly of the uterus, cervix, vagina or hymen. This means that these organs have developed differently than in most women, but may still be effective in fulfilling their primary functions, namely menstruation, vaginal intercourse and carrying a pregnancy.

Class U0: Normal uterus

Class U1: Dysmorphic uterus

Class U2: Septate uterus

Class U3: Bicorporeal uterus

Class U4: Hemi uterus

With rudimentary cavity

Without rudimentary cativity

Class U5: Aplastic uterus

Class U6: Unclassified cases

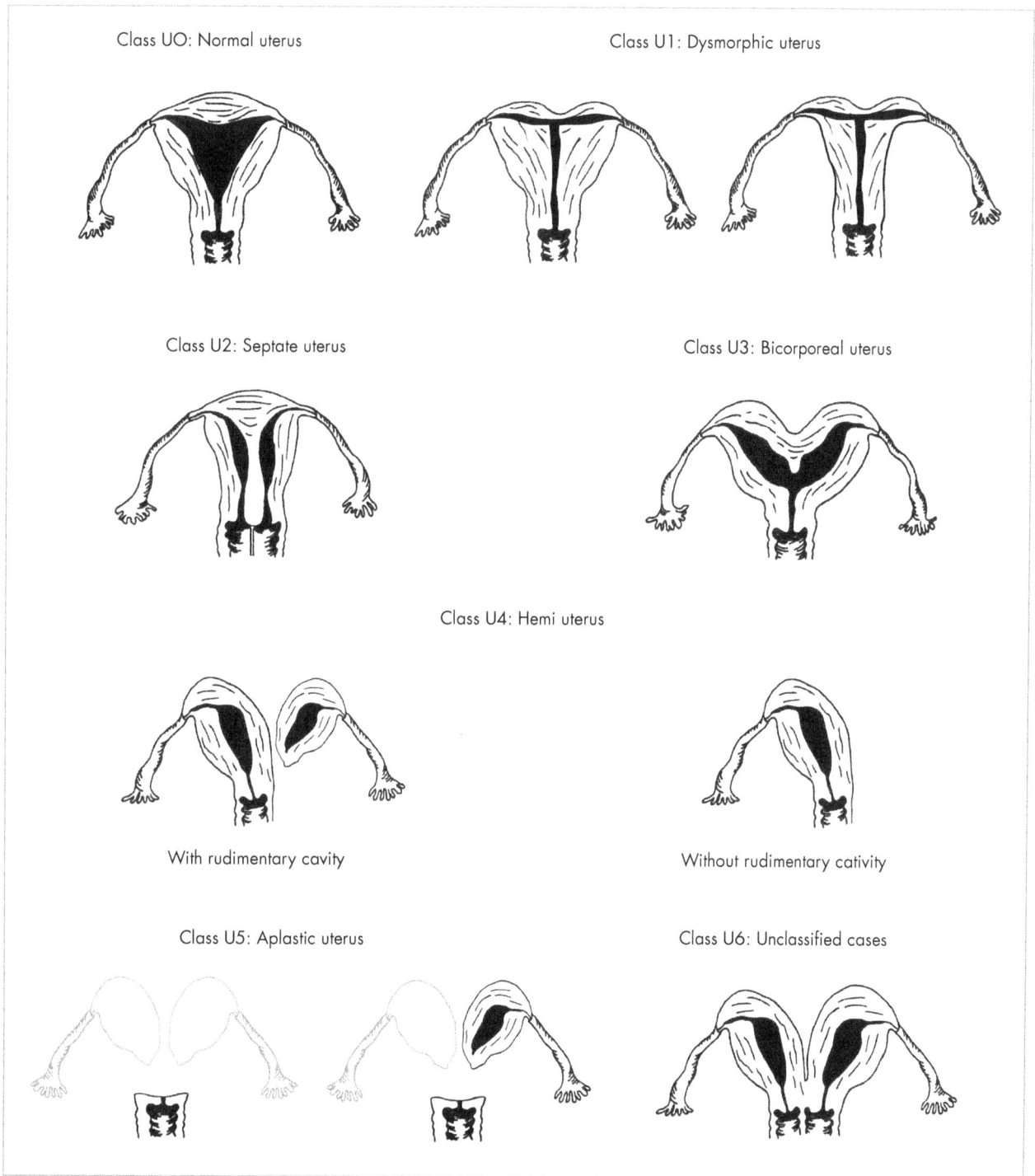

Figure 5.10 Congenitial abnormalities of the uterus

A woman or girl may not realise that she has an anomaly of the reproductive organs unless she has symptoms or undergoes imaging (such as an ultrasound) or an examination where it is discovered. Symptoms include not menstruating, abdominal pain with or without bleeding, pain or difficulty inserting a tampon, pain with intercourse or recurrent miscarriages, infertility, preterm labour or abnormal positions of the baby during pregnancy.

To diagnose a congenital anomaly of the uterus, cervix, vagina or hymen, a physical examination, an MRI or ultrasound, hysterosalpingogram (HSG) or laparoscopy may be indicated.

Hormonal abnormalities also exist, but in these cases the reproductive organs may be normal. Patients with uterine abnormalities may have associated renal abnormalities, including unilateral renal agenesis.

The classification of congenital malformations of the female reproductive system (see Figure 5.10) by the American Society of Reproductive Medicine was revised in 2013, based on the following agreed principles (Grimbizis et al, 2013):

- All anomalies are categorised based on the anatomy of the organ.
- The main classes of deviations of the uterus are of embryological origin.
- Subclasses indicate variations of degrees of deformity.
- Cervical and vaginal anomalies are classified in independent supplementary subclasses and are not included here.

Anomalies of the uterus are as follows (Grimbizis et al, 2013):

- *U0 – Normal uterus*
- *U1 – Dysmorphic, T-shaped or infantile forms of the uterus:* The shape of the uterus is abnormal or too small.

- *U2 – Septate uterus (partial or incomplete):* The two Mullerian ducts have fused, but the partition between them is still present, splitting the uterus into two parts. With a complete septum, the vagina, cervix and the uterus can also be completely divided. A uterine septum is the most common malformation that causes miscarriages. It is diagnosed using ultrasound or MRI. A uterine septum can be surgically corrected.
- *U3 – Bicorporeal (partial, complete or bicorporeal septate):* This occurs when the upper part of the Mullerian system that forms the uterus fails to fuse, partially or completely, with or without a septum, for example a bicornuate uterus.
- *U4 – Hemi uterus:* Only once side of the uterus was formed by one Mullerian duct, with or without a cavity.
- *U5 – Aplastic:* The uterus is underdeveloped, with or without a rudimentary cavity.
- *U6 – Unclassified:* The uterus may be absent and the vagina underdeveloped. Women with this condition have primary amenorrhea. In uterus didelphys, there are two uteruses, which may include one or two cervixes and vaginas.

5.5   Conclusion

In this chapter, the internal and external female reproductive organs were described. The vulva (external female reproductive organs) as well as the vagina, uterus, cervix, Fallopian tubes and ovaries were discussed in detail to illustrate their structure and function. Finally, congenital abnormalities of the female reproductive organs were briefly explained.

6

The menstrual cycle and hormonal control

LEARNING OBJECTIVES
On completion of this chapter, you must be able to:
▶ identify and describe the physiology and process of menstruation
▶ identify and describe the different hormones involved in menstruation and conception.

KNOWLEDGE ASSUMED TO BE IN PLACE
The endocrine system of the human body, with particular reference to the female hormones and the menstrual cycle

KEYWORDS
oestrogen • progesterone • gonadotrophin • human placental lactogen (HPL) • somatotrophin • prolactin • prostaglandins • luteinising hormone (LH) • follicle-stimulating hormone (FSH) • gonadotrophin-releasing hormone (GnRH)

6.1 Introduction

To be a midwife, one must have a working knowledge of the anatomy and physiology involved in pregnancy and childbirth. This chapter explains the function of the female reproductive hormonal system, hormonal control of menstruation and the hormones involved in the maintenance of pregnancy and lactation.

6.2 The female reproductive cycle

The female reproductive cycle consists of two cycles that take place simultaneously, namely:
1. *the ovarian cycle*, during which ovulation occurs
2. *the menstrual cycle*, during which menstruation occurs.

The female reproductive cycle is necessary to prepare the oocyte (egg) for fertilisation by the sperm as well as to prepare the uterus for implantation of the fertilised oocyte. If fertilisation does not occur, the unfertilised oocyte, as well as the endometrium (inner lining of the uterus), will be shed and expulsed by the uterus in the form of blood. The cycle then starts over again.

6.3 Female reproductive hormones

Reproductive (sex) hormones are chemical compounds that are responsible for female characteristics and the development of the female organs for reproduction. The primary hormones of the female reproductive system are follicle-stimulating hormone (FSH) and luteinising hormone (LH) (from the anterior pituitary), oxytocin (from the posterior pituitary), oestrogen and progesterone (from the ovaries). The reproductive hormones are controlled by the hypothalamic–pituitary–gonad axis, as illustrated in Figure 6.1 on page 58.

Figure 6.1 on the next page and colour illustration C1 on page 69 explain the cycle of hormones involved in the menstrual cycle:
▶ The *hypothalamus* secretes gonadotrophin-releasing hormone (GnRH) to the anterior pituitary gland.
▶ The *anterior pituitary gland* is then stimulated to secrete LH and FSH. The anterior pituitary contains five types of endocrine cells. One type is the gonadotropes, which secrete FSH and LH into the bloodstream. FSH and LH are glycoproteins that stimulate the granulosa cells of the Graafian follicle to secrete oestrogen and progesterone. LH also stimulates the production of inhibin A and B. As the levels of FSH and LH increase, they stimulate

the maturation of ovarian ova. These two hormones are responsible for the release of the mature ovum and the subsequent production of oestrogen and progesterone to regulate the ovarian cycle and the menstrual cycle.

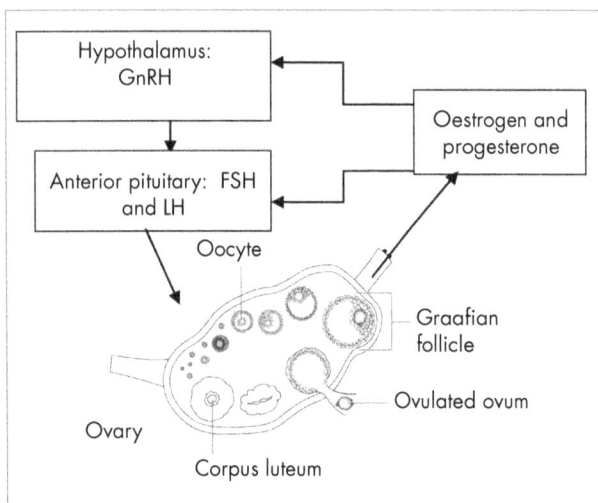

Figure 6.1 Hormones involved in the menstrual cycle

Only two hormones are secreted from the posterior pituitary gland: antidiuretic hormone and oxytocin. The last-mentioned is responsible for stimulating contractions in labour and plays a role in lactation.

The steroid hormones, androgens, oestrogens and progesterone are produced by the gonads and adrenals.

Cholesterol plays a role in the development of steroid hormones. Although most of the steroid hormones are produced from cholesterol in the gonads and adrenals, the placenta also produces progesterone and pregnenolone. Steroid levels vary throughout the reproductive cycle and in pregnancy.

Menstruation and pregnancy are controlled by the hormonal cycle. Failure to conceive and reproduce can be due to a range of causes, including nutritional and hormonal problems – particularly in teenagers – and malnutrition or anorexia nervosa.

In pregnancy and labour, severe hypovolaemia in postpartum haemorrhage (PPH) may cause hypoxia of the pituitary gland, resulting in failure to produce the hormones needed for lactation and menstruation. This may in turn result in failure to produce milk and an inability to fall pregnant again (Sheehan's syndrome).

Table 6.1

Female hormones and the menstrual cycle

Organ/ system	Actions of oestrogen	Actions of progesterone	Actions of gonadotrophins (GnRH)
Uterus	Stimulates proliferation of endometrium Increases cervical mucus (ferning and spinnbarkeit) Promotes uterine growth in pregnancy Increases myometrial response	Promotes secretory phase Makes mucus permeable for sperm, loss of ferning in mucus Promotes coiling of the uterine arteries Effect reaches a peak one week after ovulation Menstruation when no implantation	None
Fallopian tubes	Increases contractility	Decreases contractility	None
Vagina	Causes cornification of epithelium Maintains optimal pH of 3.5–4.2	Changes epithelium to intermediate and basal cell	None
Mammary glands	Promotes ductal system glands, nipples, alveolar and fatty tissue Increases prolactin in pregnancy	Develops lobules and alveoli during the menstrual cycle in preparation for lactation if conception occurred Causes breast swelling due to oedema before menstruation	None

continued

Organ/ system	Actions of oestrogen	Actions of progesterone	Actions of gonadotrophins
Ovaries	Releases ova Produces oestrogen	Unsure	FSH stimulates the ovarian follicle Promotes oestrogen production and secretion of LH, which stimulates the growth of the Graafian follicle and aids the corpus luteum Promotes progesterone
Skin	Diminishes sebaceous activity Increases water content of the skin	Increases sebaceous activity	Indirect
Cardiovascular system	Increases blood flow, angiotensin factor V and prothrombin	Causes vasodilatation and decreases contractility	Indirect
Secondary sexual characteristics	Causes female contours, fat deposits and hair distribution	Involved in breast development	Indirect
Thermogenic activity	None	Increases basal temperature by 0.4–0.6 °C after ovulation Deposits glucose in endometrium as nutrient for ovum	Indirect
Metabolism	Promotes sodium and water re-absorption from kidney tubules Affects calcium metabolism and bone growth	Progesterone has important effects on carbohydrate, lipid and protein metabolism It antagonises the effects of insulin on glucose metabolism in adipose tissue and skeletal	Indirect

Oestrogens

The human body forms two types of oestrogen: oestradiol and oestrone. Oestriol is an end product of both, and is of low functional value. Oestrogen is mainly synthesised by the theca interna of the corpus luteum in the follicular phase of the menstrual cycle and later from the placenta. A small portion comes from the adrenals (which is also the case in males). The steroid 17α-hydroxyprogesterone is important in the synthesis of oestrogens. Oestradiol is the main functional hormone. (See also colour illustration C1, page 69, on the menstrual cycle.)

Oestrogen is involved in the regulation and concentration of plasma proteins such as angiotensin II and T4. Oestrogen promotes protein synthesis for cell development. It also sensitises the receptors for progesterone and determines the effectiveness of the function of progesterone that will follow in the second phase of menstruation and/or pregnancy.

Progesterone

Progesterone is the hormone that maintains pregnancy; it is also called the pregnancy hormone. It is secreted from the Graafian follicle in small amounts in the follicular phase. The placenta secretes large amounts of progesterone and the adrenals secrete a small amount. The effect of progesterone is less marked in the body because it is only present at certain times. The minor disturbances of pregnancy are related to the effects of progesterone on vasodilatation, vascularity and the relaxation of smooth muscles in the body in pregnancy. The actions of progesterone are listed in Table 6.1.

Other hormones

Androgens are secreted in low concentrations from the adrenals and play a role in female reproduction. The chemical structure of androgens (testosterone) is similar to that of progesterone.

59

The onset of menarche

The first occurrence of cyclic bleeding in the young girl is called menarche and in many cultures signifies the transition to womanhood. In some cultures it is celebrated with festivals, while in others it is regarded as an inconvenience (Johnston-Robledo & Chrisler, 2011).

The mean age of menarche varies between populations and may be as young as 8 years. The average age of menarche is 12.7 years. Failure to menstruate by the age of 16 should be investigated. Factors that can delay the onset of menstruation are malnutrition (especially anorexia nervosa or obesity), stress, strenuous physical activity, ill health or congenital abnormalities of the female organs (see Figure 5.10 on page 55).

The onset of menarche is related to an increase in GnRH, which in turn increases LH levels. Initially, only oestrogen is secreted and the cycles are anovular and irregular. Generally, within two years the 28-day pattern will be established and ovulation starts.

The box below details a system described by Prof James Tanner in 1970 to classify the physical development of primary and secondary sex characteristics.

Tanner's stages of progression from childhood to maturity (Marshall & Tanner, 1970)

Stage 1 (pre-puberty):
- The vaginal mucosa is thin, red and dry.
- Breasts are undeveloped.
- No pubic hair is present.

Stage 2 (10–11 years):
- The breasts bud.
- The labia majora become more vascular.
- The vaginal mucosa becomes more moist, thicker and pink.
- The uterine fundus enlarges.
- The hips widen and body fat redistributes.
- A height spurt begins.

Stage 3 (11–12 years):
- The breasts enlarge.
- Pubic hair appears.
- The labia minora enlarge.
- The vaginal length increases, the mucosa thickens and a white discharge appears.
- The uterus enlarges and the Fallopian tubes increase in diameter.
- The sebaceous glands are activated, as well as sweat glands.
- Rapid growth takes place, with a peak in height.

continued

Stage 4 (12–13 years):
- The breasts enlarge and the areolas form.
- Pubic hair covers the mons veneris pubis and perineum.
- The vagina and uterus enlarge.
- Menarche starts, and linear growth decelerates.

Stage 5 (13–15 years):
- The breasts and genitals reach adult proportions.
- Pubic hair grows on thighs.
- Linear growth ceases.

6.4 The menstrual cycle

Menstruation (menses) is cyclic uterine bleeding under the influence of hormonal changes. It occurs when the ovum is not fertilised (about 14 days after ovulation in a 28-day cycle). Shedding of the lining of the uterus takes place, causing blood to exit via the vagina. This process lasts between five to seven days. (See colour illustration C1 on page 69.)

After menstruation, the lining of the uterus begins to thicken again in preparation for the next potential implantation of a fertilised egg. The period where the uterine lining is most hospitable for implantation is called the fertile window; it begins five days before ovulation and is about a week long. If an oocyte is not fertilised, the uterine lining will break down and the cycle begins again.

Women often do not know their menstrual cycle patterns accurately, due to the use of contraception or ignorance about the natural functions of their bodies. Once a woman is in a sexually active relationship, or experiences infertility problems, she usually becomes more aware, conscious and focused on how her body functions.

Although the average normal menstrual cycle is 28.1 days, cycles as short as 15 or as long as 45 days are reported and are normal for women with different hormonal profiles. Menstrual flow is normally four days long, with the heaviest flow on day two, with a blood loss ranging from 50–150 ml. Iron loss varies between 0.4–1 mg/day (12 mg/cycle).

Phases of the menstrual cycle

(Also see colour illustration C1 on page 69.)
1. The *follicular proliferation phase* is the oestrogen-dominant phase, with development of the Graafian follicle and oocyte and endometrium. Cycle length variations occur.
2. *Ovulation* takes place when the ovum is released.
3. The *luteal secretory phase* is a progesterone-dominant phase maintaining the endometrium for conception. The duration of the luteal phase is 14 days from ovulation.
4. Finally, menstruation or pregnancy occurs.

The follicular proliferation phase

Hormones of the endocrine system are responsible for the development and maturation of the ovarian follicle and the ovum in the ovary for ovulation and for the preparation of the female body for conception and pregnancy. Fertilisation and pregnancy are only possible when an ovarian follicle has been brought to maturation and when ovulation has taken place.

FSH is secreted by the anterior pituitary gland and the levels begin to rise in the last few days of the previous menstrual cycle. FSH is highest and most important during the first week of the follicular phase.

When FSH levels rise, five to seven ovarian follicles (the Graafian follicles) are prepared for ovulation. These follicles compete with each other for dominance. The so-called dominant follicle is selected seven days before ovulation. Two or three days before LH levels begin to increase, usually by day seven of the cycle, one (or occasionally two) of the recruited follicles emerges as dominant.

Throughout the entire follicular phase, rising oestrogen levels in the blood stimulate growth of the endometrium and myometrium of the uterus. Crypts in the cervix are also stimulated to produce fertile cervical mucus that reduces the acidity of the vagina, creating a more hospitable environment for sperm. The characteristic texture of the cervical mucus will guide sperm through the cervix and to the Fallopian tubes for fertilisation. In addition, the basal body temperature may fall slightly under the influence of high oestrogen levels.

On average, the follicular phase lasts about 13–14 days. Of the three phases, this phase varies the most in length. It tends to become shorter near menopause. This phase ends when the level of LH increases dramatically (surges). The surge results in release of the egg (oocyte).

Ovulation

High oestrogen levels increase LH levels 12–24 hours before ovulation (usually around day 12–13 of a 28-day cycle). LH stimulates the dominant follicle to bulge from the surface of the ovary. The Graafian follicle ruptures and discharges the secondary oocyte into the pelvic cavity, where the fimbria guide it into the uterine tube.

Mittleschmerz (abdominal pain) may be experienced by some women during ovulation and light bleeding may occur. The pain may last for a few minutes to a few hours. It is usually felt on the same side as the ovary that released the egg. The pain may precede or follow the rupture of the follicle and may not occur in all cycles.

The surge in LH can be detected by measuring the level of this hormone in urine. This measurement, and a raised body temperature, can be used to determine when a woman is fertile.

Fertilisation is more likely when sperm are present in the reproductive tract before the egg is released. Most pregnancies occur when intercourse occurs within three days before ovulation.

Egg release does not alternate between the two ovaries and appears to be random. If one ovary is removed, the remaining ovary releases an egg every month.

The luteal phase

This phase begins on the 15th day and lasts till the end of the cycle. Progesterone dominates the luteal phase. The following events occur during this phase:

1. The Graafian follicle released during the ovulation phase stays in the Fallopian tube for 24 hours.
2. If a sperm does not fertilise the follicle during that time, the cells of the ruptured follicle change to the corpus luteum (an irregular yellow structure).
3. The corpus luteum produces oestrogen, relaxin, inhibin and progesterone for approximately two weeks to develop the endometrium of the uterus.
4. If fertilisation occurs during this period, the corpus luteum will continue to produce the necessary hormones until the placenta can take over this role. During this period the cervical mucus becomes sticky and thick under the influence of progesterone.
5. Progesterone causes the body temperature to increase slightly during the luteal phase and to remain elevated until a menstrual period begins. This increase in temperature can be used to estimate whether ovulation has occurred.
6. During most of the luteal phase, oestrogen levels remain high to stimulate the endometrium to thicken.
7. The increase in oestrogen and progesterone levels causes milk ducts in the breasts to dilate. As a result, the breasts may swell and become tender.
8. If fertilisation does not occur, the corpus luteum degenerates 14 days after ovulation. The corpus luteum disintegrates and becomes the corpus albicans.
9. Hormone levels decrease and the hypothalamus produces GnRH to stimulate the production of FSH. The ovarian cycle starts again.

Menstruation

Menstruation is the shedding of the endometrium (the lining of the uterus) accompanied by bleeding. The menstrual cycle begins with menstrual bleeding (menstruation), which marks the first day of the follicular phase.

Bleeding occurs after oestrogen and progesterone levels decrease at the end of the previous cycle. This decrease causes arterial vasoconstriction and haematoma, resulting in the endometrium breaking down and shedding. At the same time, FSH levels increase slightly, stimulating the development of several follicles in the ovaries.

Menstrual bleeding lasts three to seven days, averaging five days. Blood loss during a cycle usually ranges from 50 to 150 ml.

6.5   Hormones in pregnancy

Pregnancy is an anabolic state and a range of complex processes and hormones are involved in maintaining pregnancy, supporting the growth of tissue and the fetus, and preparing for lactation.

Hormones of the anterior pituitary

The pituitary gland enlarges by at least 50 per cent during pregnancy and increases its production of all hormones, particularly the following:

▶ *Somatotrophin* (a growth hormone) promotes protein synthesis, gluconeogenesis and muscle resistance to insulin. It increases lipolysis.

▶ *Corticotrophin* controls the glucocorticoid formation in the adrenals.

▶ *Thyrotrophin* controls the absorption of iodine and the functions of the thyroid. The size of the thyroid gland increases in pregnancy.

▶ *Prolactin* plays a fundamental role in the production of milk. There is a low level of activity in pregnancy that is accelerated when the placental hormones drop after birth.

Hormones of the posterior pituitary: Oxytocin and relaxin

Oxytocin is normally produced by the paraventricular nucleus of the hypothalamus and released by the posterior pituitary. It is released into the bloodstream as a hormone in response to stretching of the cervix and is required for contraction of the uterus during labour. It is also released by stimulation of the nipples during breastfeeding. It helps with birth, bonding with the baby, and milk production.

Oxytocin may be used as a medication to induce contraction of the uterus, to accelerate labour and to stop bleeding following delivery. For this purpose, it is given either by injection into a muscle or into a vein.

The placenta breaks down oxytocin in order to prevent the uterus from contracting in pregnancy. It is therefore not possible to induce a woman with oxytocin if the uterus is not

ready for birth. Progesterone inhibits the action of oxytocin, while oestrogens have a tendency to increase the degree of uterine contractility.

In the female, relaxin is produced by the corpus luteum of the ovary, in both pregnant and non-pregnant females. It rises to a peak within approximately 14 days of ovulation and then declines in the absence of pregnancy, resulting in menstruation. It is also produced by the breasts and, during pregnancy, by the placenta, chorion and decidua.

During the first trimester of pregnancy, levels rise and additional relaxin is produced by the decidua. Peak levels of relaxin is reached during the 14 weeks of the first trimester and at delivery. It is known to mediate the haemodynamic changes that occur during pregnancy, such as increased cardiac output, increased renal blood flow and increased arterial compliance. It also relaxes other pelvic ligaments. It is believed to soften the pubic symphysis.

In males, relaxin enhances motility of sperm in semen.

Hormones of the placenta

The placenta is a very important endocrine organ, producing many hormones that affect the status of pregnancy and the maternal physiology. The placenta secretes both steroid hormones and protein hormones. The protein hormones include human chorionic gonadotropin (hCG) and human chorionic somatomammotropin (HCS), both of which have actions similar to those of some anterior pituitary hormones. The placental hormones hCG and HCS thus duplicate the actions of four anterior pituitary hormones.

Human chorionic gonadotrophin

This glycoprotein is similar to LH. The main function of this hormone is to prevent the degeneration of the corpus luteum, to continue the secretion of progesterone and oestrogens, and to maintain the endometrium after the implantation of the zygote.

As the embryo develops, maintenance of the endometrium is taken over by the placenta. The hormone hCG can first be measured in the maternal bloodstream eight to nine days after ovulation (shortly after implantation of the zygote). In general, the hCG level will double every two to three days in early pregnancy. Levels of hCG peak at about eight to ten weeks of pregnancy and then decline, remaining at lower levels for the rest of the pregnancy.

Pregnancies destined to miscarry and ectopic (tubal) pregnancies tend to show lower levels of hCG eventually, but often have normal levels initially.

Both blood and urine contain hCG. Home-based tests for pregnancy are based on the presence of this hormone in urine.

Human placental lactogen

Human placental lactogen (HPL, also called HCS) is structurally similar to the human growth hormone. Its main function is to regulate glucose availability for the fetus. The hormone is secreted by the cytotropic cells of the outer layers of the chorionic villi of the placenta from about the fifth week of pregnancy. It has a general metabolic action, with specific nutritional implications for both the mother and the fetus, particularly with regard to glucose and fat metabolism.

HPL is found in the maternal bloodstream and has been used to measure the efficiency of the placenta during pregnancy. If levels of HPL are low in early pregnancy, there is a risk of miscarriage and if they are low in later pregnancy, the growth of the fetus is at risk.

Oestrogens and progesterone

During pregnancy, the placenta synthesises oestrogens and progesterone. There is a relationship between the hormones in maternal urine and the size of the placenta and fetus. Oestradiol is the main hormone synthesised. Part of the development of the hormone takes place in the fetal adrenals, after which it is altered in the placenta and transferred to the mother. The placenta has an enzyme system that can synthesise oestrogens from cholesterol and steroids. The levels of the hormone in the mother and fetus are unequal. The placenta will not let oestrogens pass freely to the fetus. Progesterone concentration is also regulated by the placenta and the fetus.

Prostaglandins

Prostaglandins are present and synthesised in all human tissue. The different types are PGE1, PGE2 and PGF-2-alpha. These substances are biologically active when synthesised in tissue. Stretching of the cervix or local infections in the cervix or amnion can cause a release of prostaglandins that may cause the onset of labour.

6.6   Conclusion

The endocrine regulation of hormones in female reproduction is complex. The midwife needs to have a basic knowledge of the hormones that influence the health of the woman and the growing fetus during reproduction, pregnancy and lactation.

Colour illustrations

List of colour illustrations

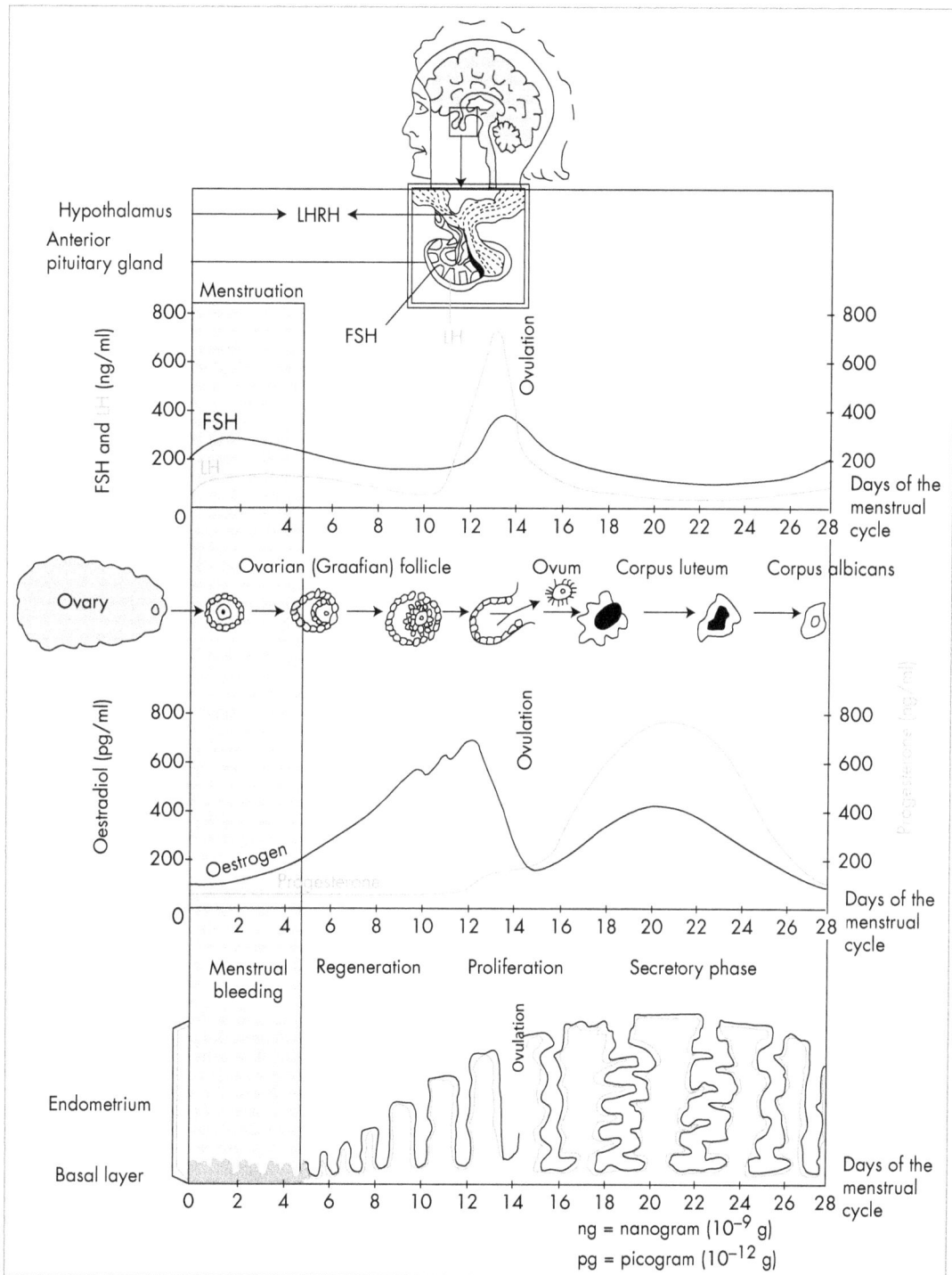

Figure C1 The menstrual cycle

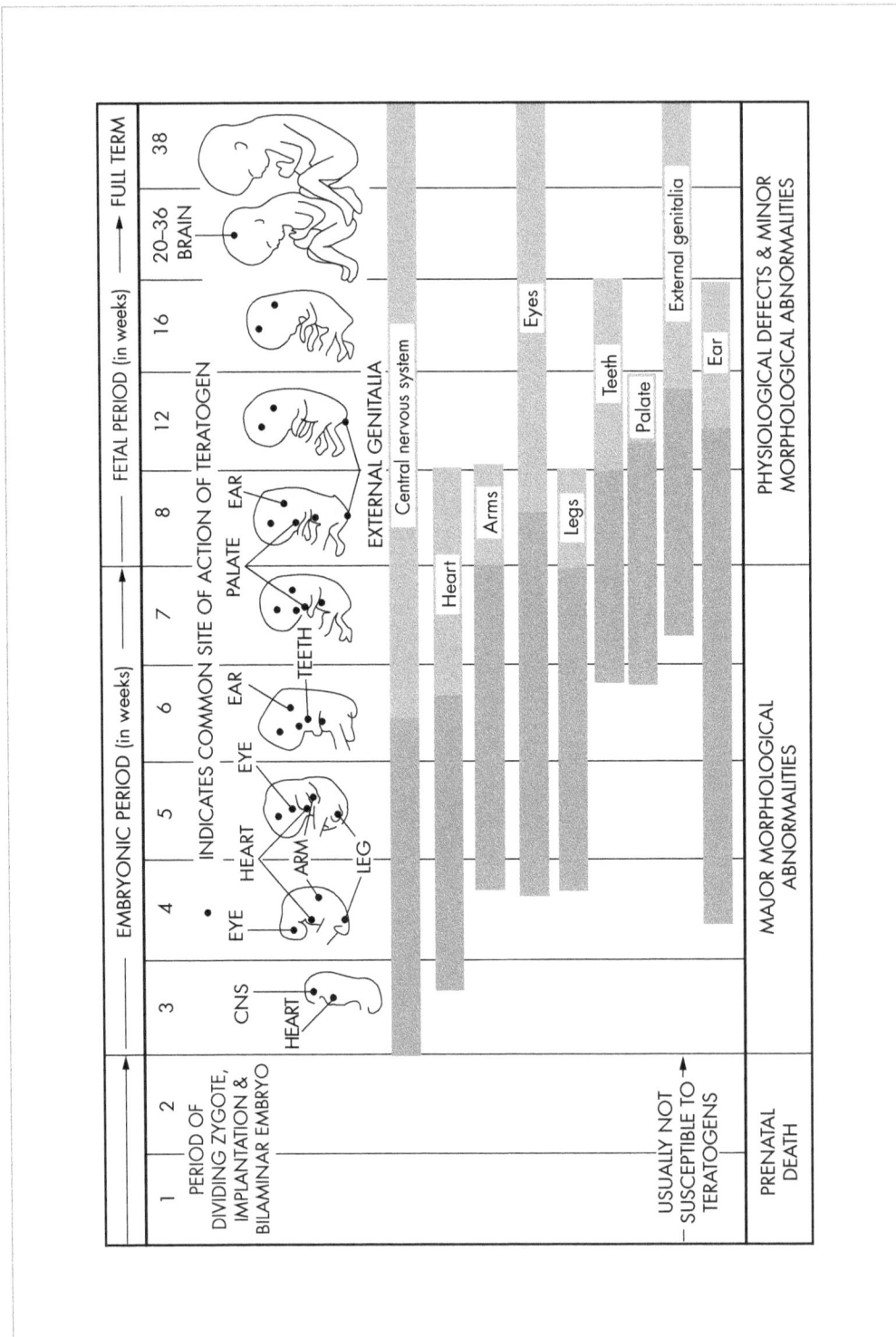

Figure C2 Organogenesis and fetal development

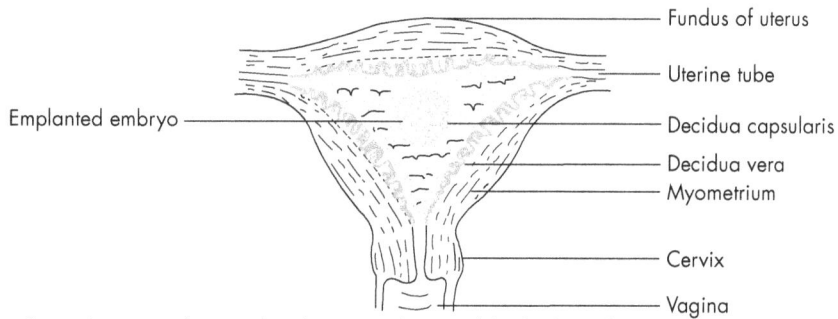

Figure C3 A gravid uterus showing the changing relations of the fetal membranes to the decidua

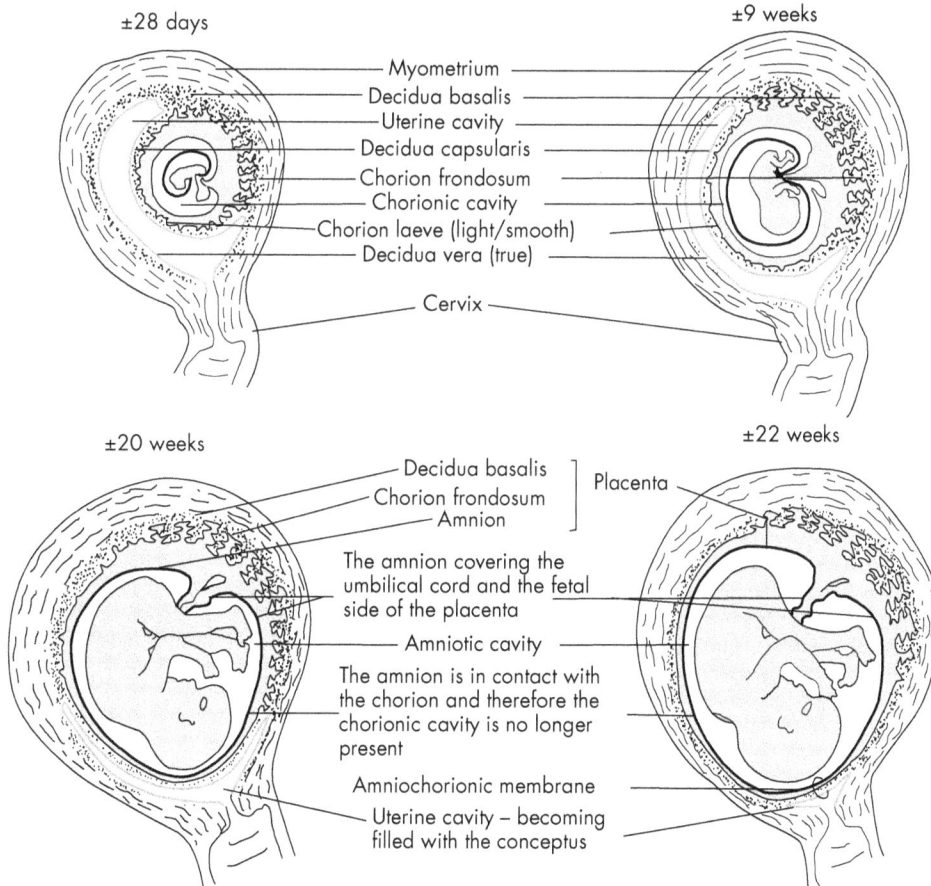

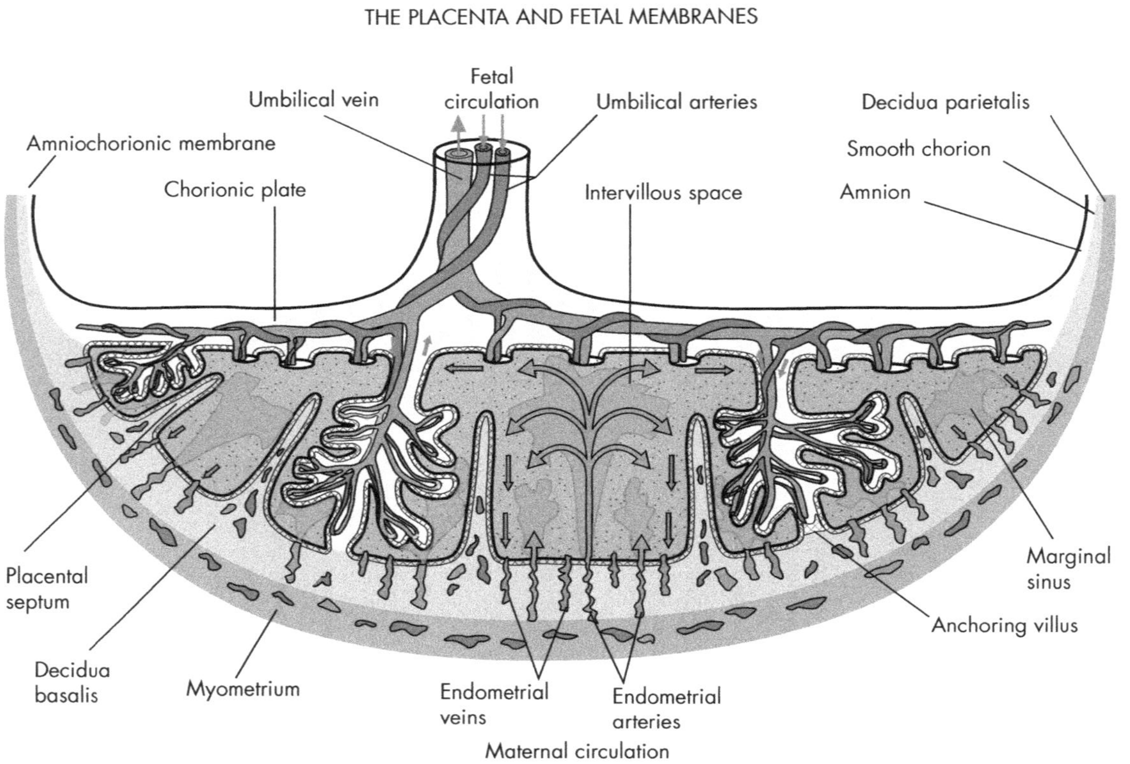

THE PLACENTA AND FETAL MEMBRANES

Fetal circulation

Umbilical arteries

Intervillous space

Umbilical vein

Amniochorionic membrane

Chorionic plate

Decidua parietalis

Smooth chorion

Amnion

Marginal sinus

Anchoring villus

Endometrial arteries

Endometrial veins

Maternal circulation

Myometrium

Placental septum

Decidua basalis

Schematic drawing of a section through a full-term placenta, showing (1) the relation of the villous chorion (fetal placenta) to the decidua basalis (maternal placenta), (2) the fetal placental circulation and (3) the maternal placental circulation. Maternal blood flows into the intervillous spaces in funnel-shaped spurts, and exchanges occur with the fetal blood as the maternal blood flows around the villi. The inflowing arterial blood pushes venous blood out into the endometrial veins, which are scattered over the entire surface of the decidua basalis. Note that the umbilical arteries carry deoxygenated fetal blood (shown in blue) to the placenta and that the umbilical vein carries oxygenated blood (shown in red) to the fetus. Note that the cotyledons are separated from each other by decidual septa of the maternal portion of the placenta. Each cotyledon consists of two or more main stem villi and their many branches. In this drawing only one main stem villus is shown in each cotyledon, but the stumps of those that have been removed are indicated (based on Ramsey, 1965).

Figure C4 Placental circulation at term

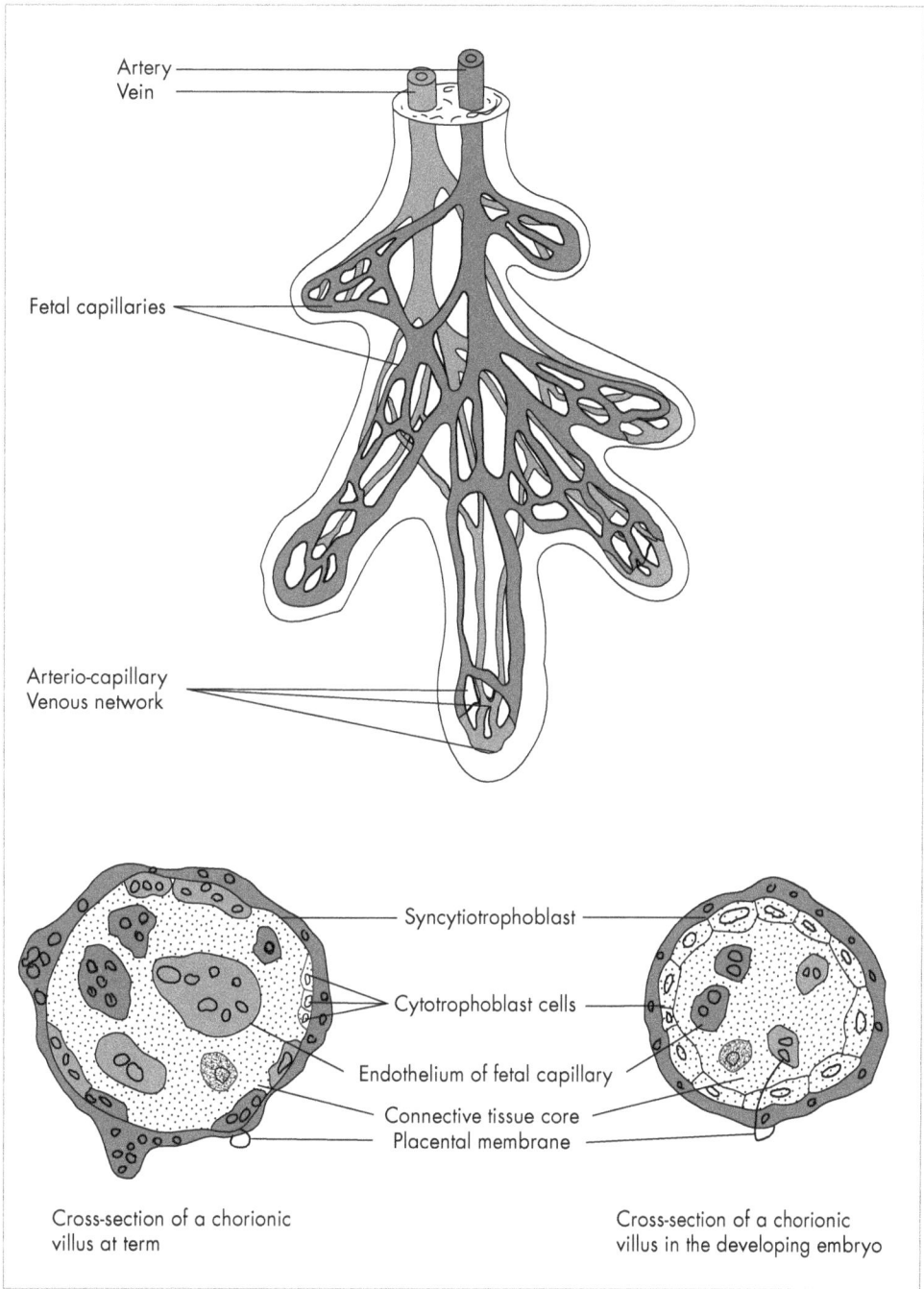

Figure C5 Chorionic villi at term

Artery
Vein

Fetal capillaries

Arterio-capillary
Venous network

Syncytiotrophoblast

Cytotrophoblast cells

Endothelium of fetal capillary

Connective tissue core
Placental membrane

Cross-section of a chorionic
villus at term

Cross-section of a chorionic
villus in the developing embryo

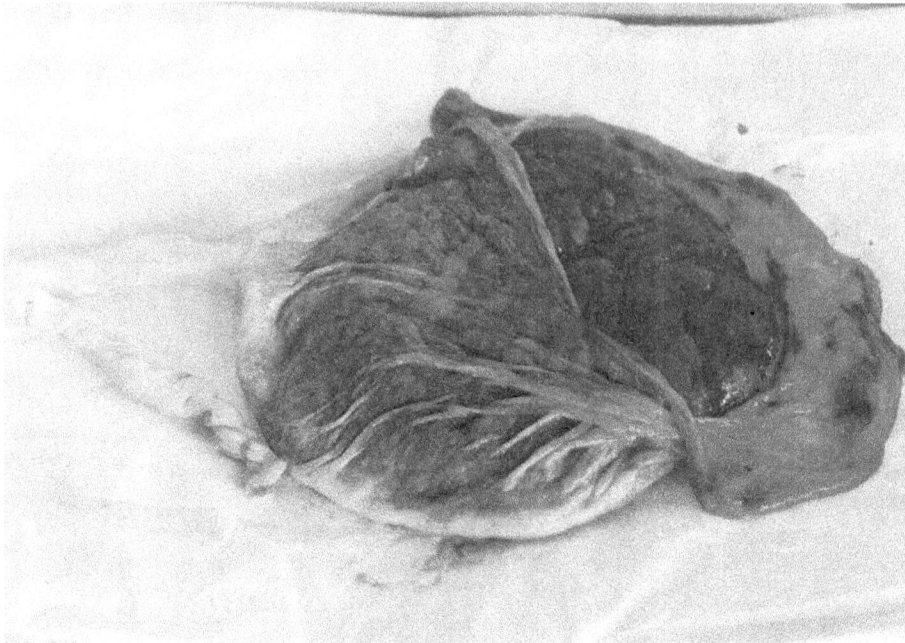

a. Maternal surface

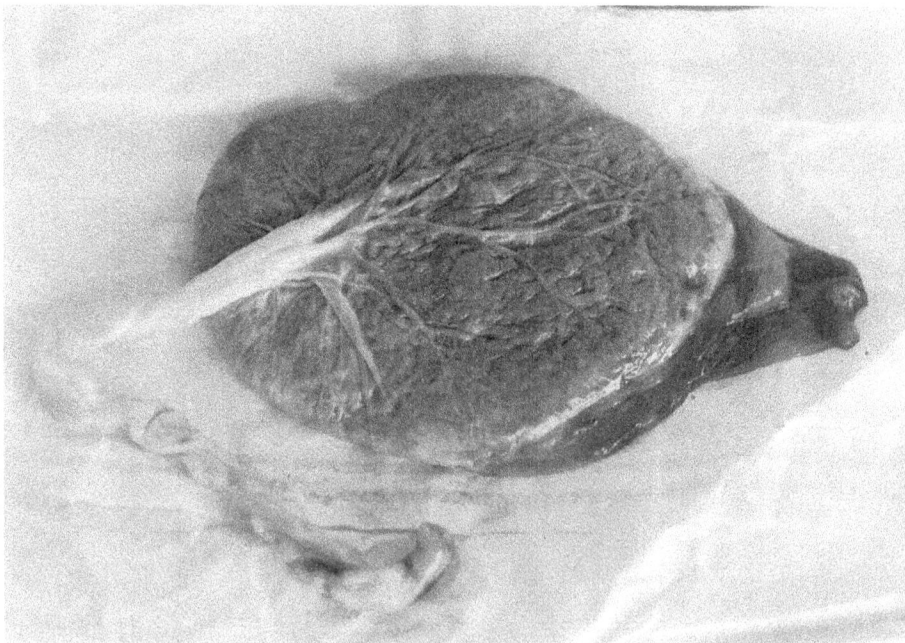

b. Fetal surface

Figure C6 Normal placenta

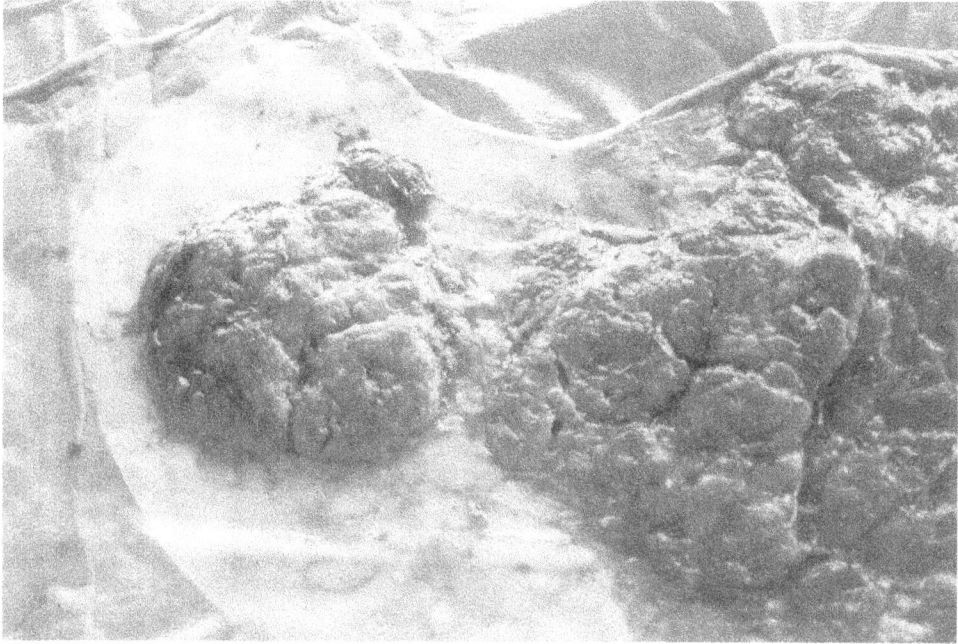

a. Maternal surface

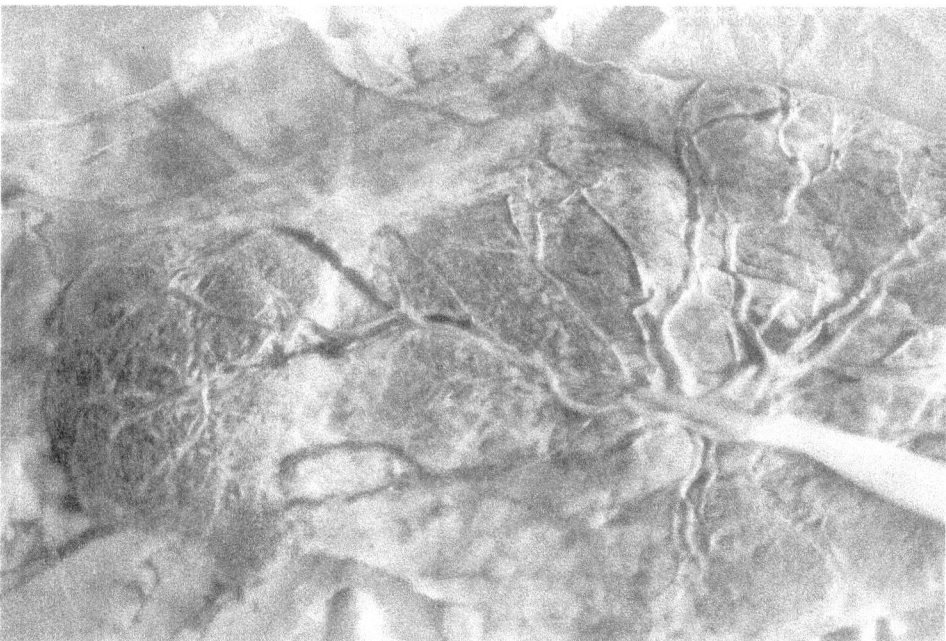

b. Fetal surface

Figure C7 Placenta succenturiate

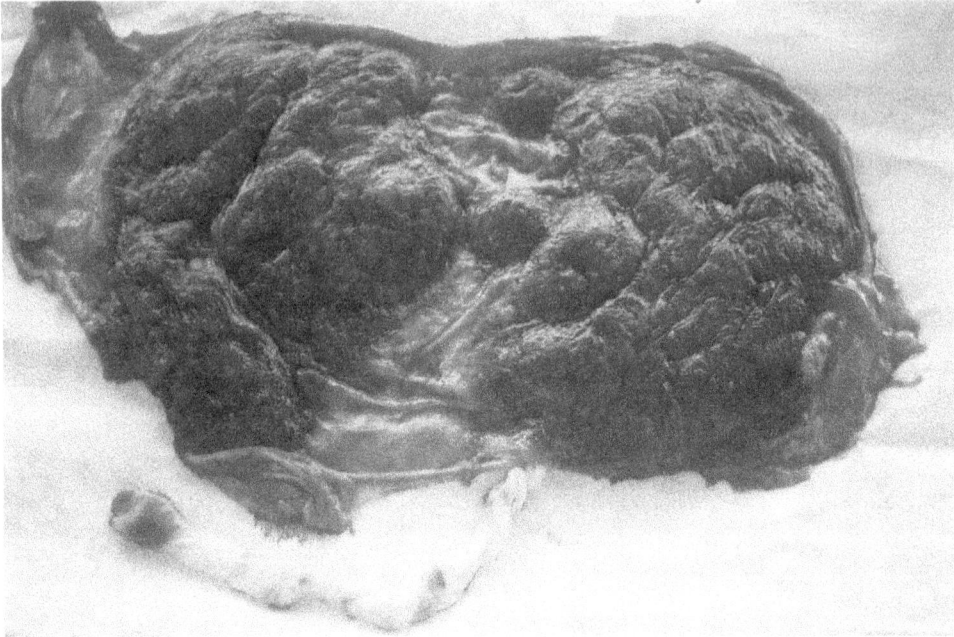

a. Maternal surface

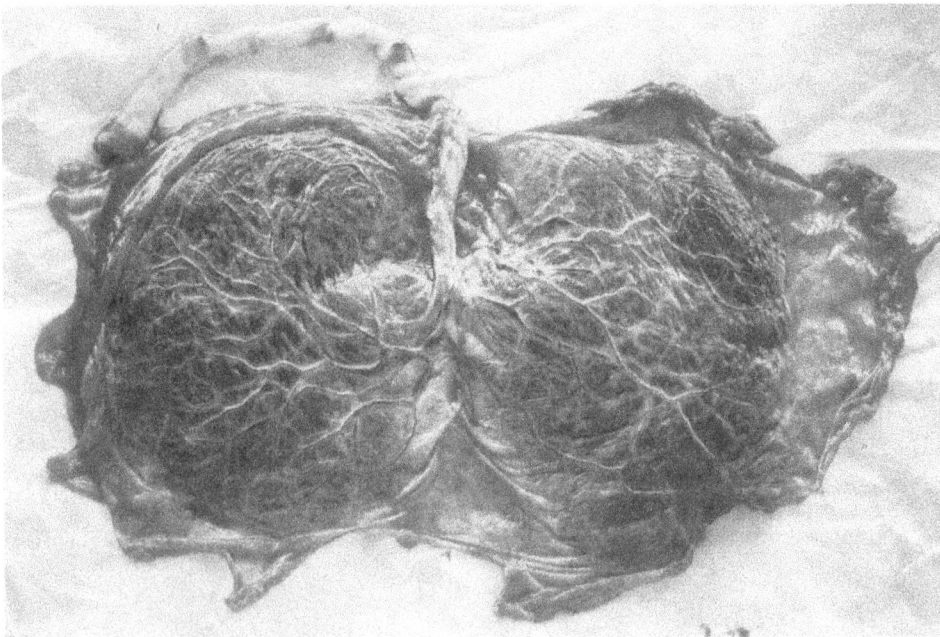

b. Fetal surface

Figure C8 Placenta bipartite or tripartite [1]

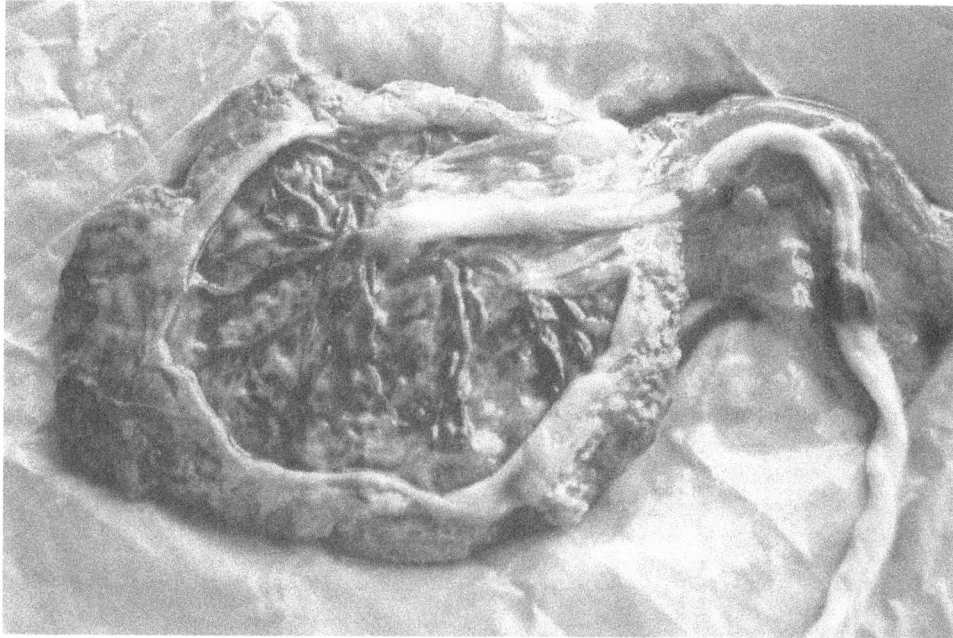

Figure C9 Placenta circumvallata

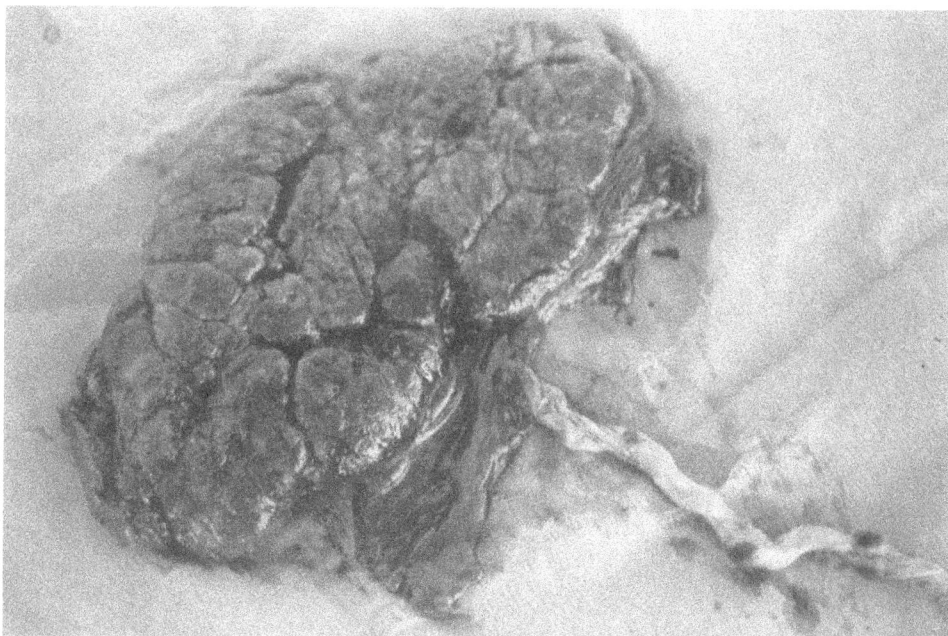

Figure C10 Battledore implantation of the cord

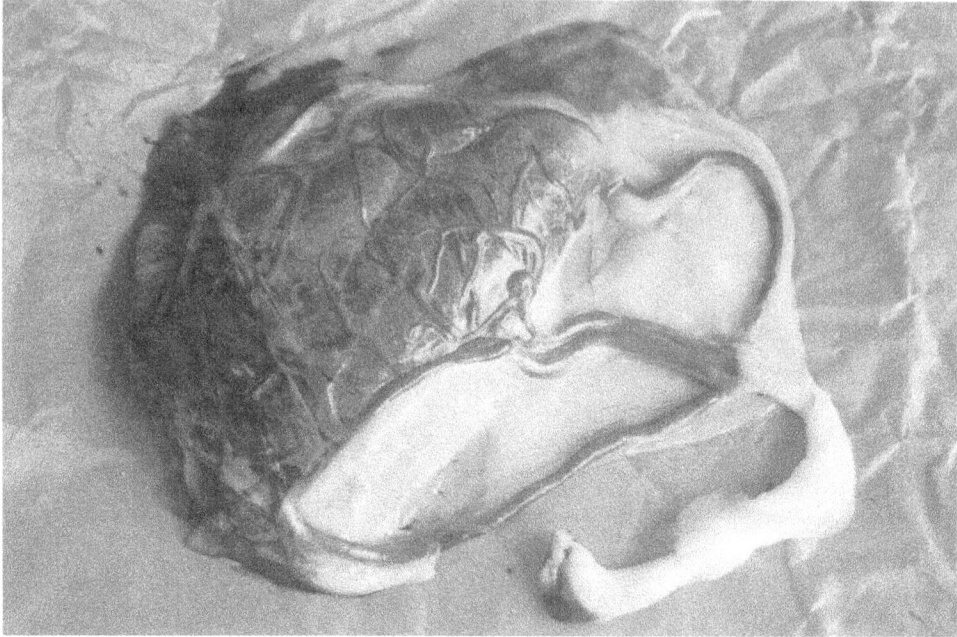

a. Velamentous placenta

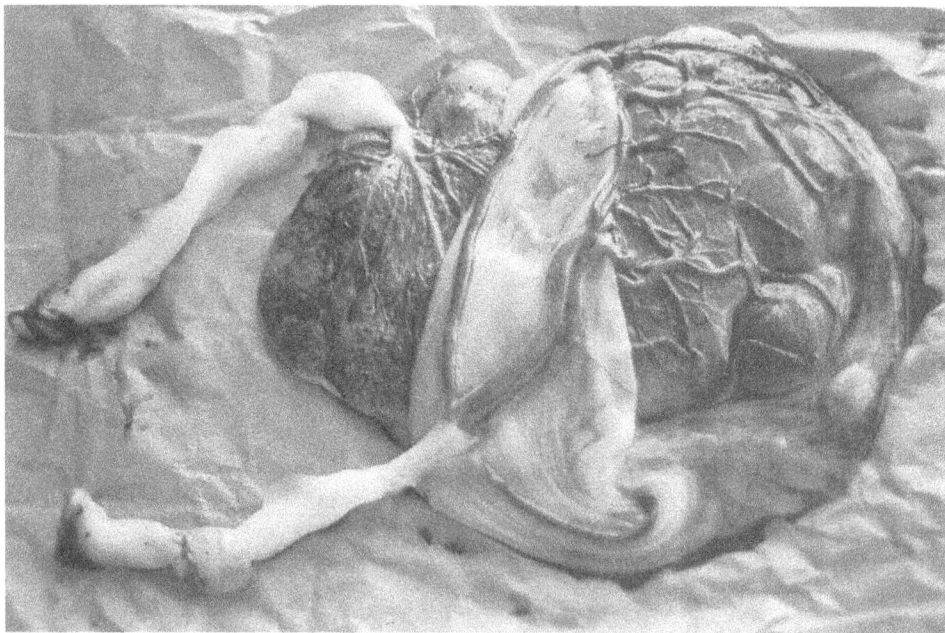

b. Velamentous and twin placenta

Figure C11 Placenta velamentosa

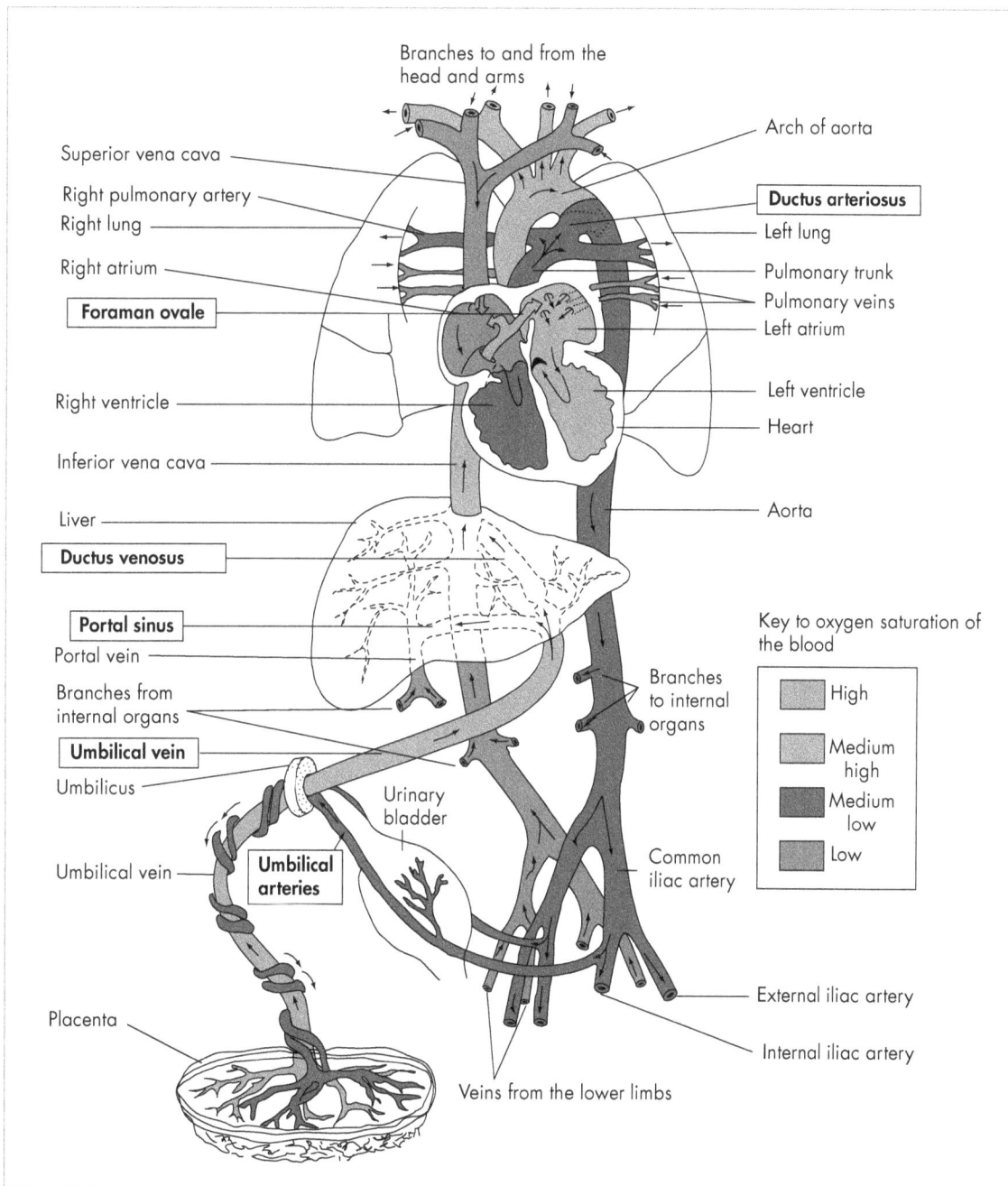

Figure C12 Fetal circulation

Branches to and from the head and arms

Arch of aorta

Superior vena cava

Ductus arteriosus

Right pulmonary artery

Right lung

Left lung

Right atrium

Pulmonary trunk

Pulmonary veins

Foraman ovale

Left atrium

Right ventricle

Left ventricle

Heart

Inferior vena cava

Aorta

Liver

Ductus venosus

Portal sinus

Portal vein

Branches to internal organs

Branches from internal organs

Umbilical vein

Umbilicus

Urinary bladder

Key to oxygen saturation of the blood

High

Medium high

Medium low

Low

Umbilical vein

Umbilical arteries

Common iliac artery

Placenta

External iliac artery

Internal iliac artery

Veins from the lower limbs

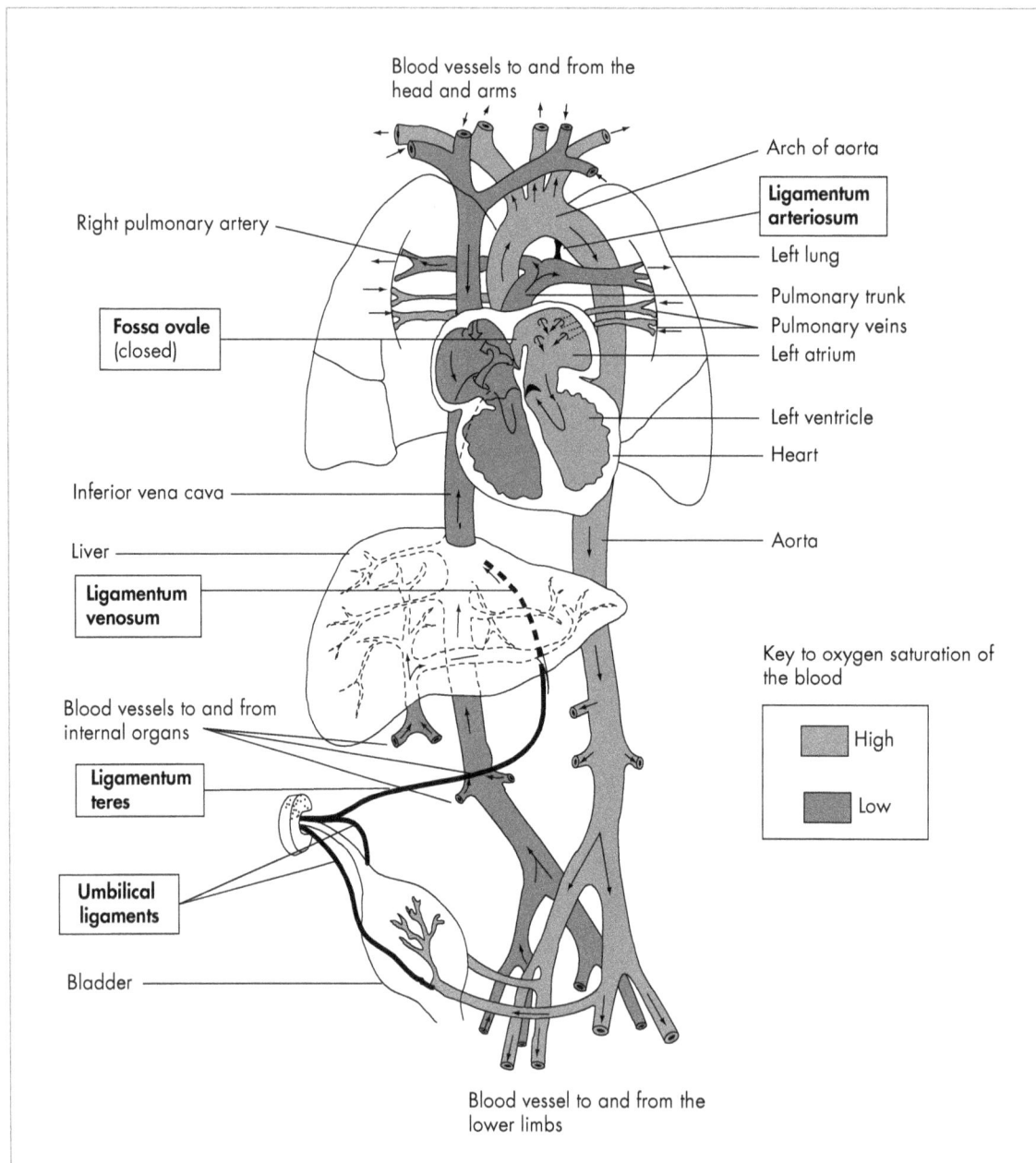

Figure C13 The (adult) general circulation of the blood, showing changes which take place at birth

Genetics, gametogenesis, fertilisation, placental development and embryology

LEARNING OBJECTIVES

On completion of this chapter, you must be able to:
- identify the national priorities for genetic disease management of newborns in South Africa
- explain the physiology of fertilisation, placental development and the stages of development of the embryo and fetus
- explain the anatomy of the placenta and membranes
- explain fetal circulation, changes at birth and how these apply to practice.

KNOWLEDGE ASSUMED TO BE IN PLACE

Basic anatomy and physiology
Terminology used in reproductive health

KEYWORDS

gametogenesis • fertilisation • placenta • embryology • genetics • stem cells • zygote • embryo • fetus • crown–rump length • gestational sac volume

7.1 Introduction

This chapter first gives an overview of genetics and discusses managing genetic defects and disorders in South Africa. Then the chapter explains normal cell division, namely mitosis and meiosis. Gametogenesis and the gametes are discussed. Conception and fertilisation are explained. The chapter then covers the development of the zygote, embryo and fetus. The placenta and membranes are discussed, including abnormalities of the placenta and umbilical cord.

7.2 Genetics

Genetics is the branch of biology concerned with the study of heredity (the transmission of characteristics from parents to their offspring) and the variation or genetic differences observed between living things.

Although most physical and other characteristics of humans are genetically determined, there are factors that may influence the expression of these aspects in life, starting from the day of conception. Even before conception, certain factors contribute, shape and influence the unique characteristics and well-being of a person; these factors include environmental influences and the parents' level of nutrition, exercise, education, background (social, cultural and family) and general well-being.

Human chromosomes and DNA

All living organisms are made up of cells. The human body is made up of billions of cells that have the same basic design. Each cell has a nucleus that carries chromosomes that contain deoxyribonucleic acid (DNA), the genetic material of the cell. DNA is shaped like a helix consisting of repeating nucleotide units attached to each other by base pairing (see Figure 7.1 on the next page).

Human somatic cells (cells of the body) have 46 chromosomes (23 pairs) in the nucleus and are said to be diploid (double), whereas the gametes (sex cells) have half that number (23 chromosomes) and are said to be haploid (single). Figure 7.2 on page 83 gives the karyotype (the number and visual appearance of chromosomes) of human genes.

Genetic abnormalities

All cells have enzymes that maintain and regulate the replication of DNA. Mistakes occur when the genetic code is altered; this is called a spontaneous mutation and can cause abnormal development. There are many environmental factors that may contribute to mutations, such as background radiation, pollutants and smoking.

Twenty per cent of pregnancies end in miscarriage, of which about 50 per cent is due to chromosomal defects. Genetic accidents are not restricted to one gene and can include the whole chromosome. Less than 1 per cent of children are born with a severe congenital abnormality globally. The data for South Africa are incomplete (Lebese, Aldous & Malherbe, 2016).

Heritable genetic disorders occur when mutations affect the gonads and these conditions are then passed on to offspring in ways that are governed by the laws of genetics. Families can be counselled about the risk of transmitting genetic diseases.

Not all genetic disorders are heritable. Screening is available in South Africa for some genetic disorders and birth defects.

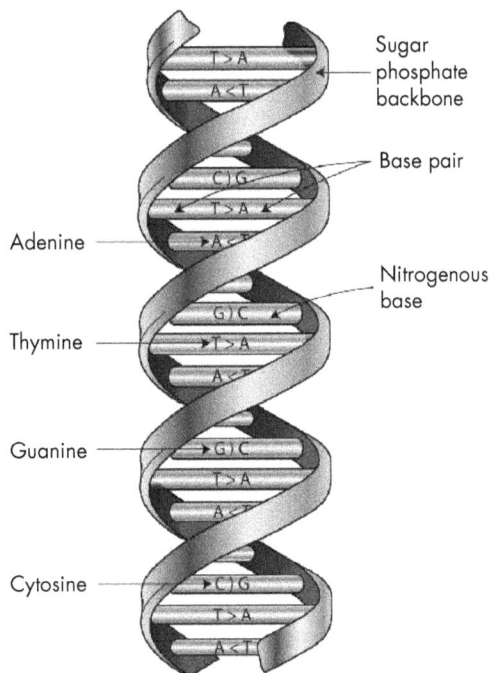

Figure 7.1 A DNA helix showing nucleic acid within the helix

Labels: Sugar phosphate backbone · Base pair · Nitrogenous base · Adenine · Thymine · Guanine · Cytosine

The Human Genome Project

The Human Genome Project (NHGRI, 2015), completed in 2013, was a collaboration between scientists from many countries. The aim was to map a complete and accurate sequence (blueprint) of the three billion chemical pairs of human DNA (20 000–25 000 genes), store this information in a database, develop related technology and address associated social, ethical and legal issues. The total genetic information of every human cell is now known.

continued

As researchers learn more about the functions of genes and proteins, this knowledge will have a major impact on the fields of medicine, biotechnology and the life sciences. However, a large portion of human DNA is now considered as non-coding (with unknown functions) and thus seen as 'junk'.

New developments and advances in genetics

Stem cells are the basic, undifferentiated cells present during the development of life. They have the potential to develop into any kind of cell, which may lead to cures for genetic diseases in the future. Stem cells are used in various forms of therapy.

Two different types of stem cells can be collected during childbirth: amniotic stem cells and umbilical cord blood stem cells. Amniotic stem cells collected from amniotic fluid during pregnancy are systematically examined and abnormalities and inherited conditions can be diagnosed. There are 2 000 conditions that can be identified at present. Umbilical cord blood stem cells can be stored in stem cell banks.

In 1997, a team of scientists in Edinburgh created an identical copy of an adult sheep from a stem cell (cloning). Her mother was therefore her identical sister.

Cloning could give scientists the ability to create organs for those who are awaiting organ donation. However, there are many ethical issues around this science. In South Africa, the Department of Health (DoH) has published guidelines in this regard, entitled *Human Genetic Policy Guidelines for the Management and Prevention of Genetic Disorders, Birth Defects and Disabilities* (DoH, nd[b]).

Genetic tests currently available in South Africa

There are 3 000 defects that have been catalogued. More than 2 000 tests have been developed to diagnose genetic defects. Genetic testing can be done on blood, hair, saliva, skin and amniotic fluid.

Antenatal testing includes:
▶ cordocentesis (fetal blood or placental tissue sampling in early pregnancy)
▶ chorionic villus sampling (CVS) – fetal blood or placental tissue sampling in early pregnancy (12 weeks)
▶ amniocentesis (testing of the amniotic fluid; 16–20 weeks)
▶ serum alpha-fetoprotein (16 weeks)
▶ fluorescent *in situ* hybridisation (FISH) test (20 weeks) during CVS or amniocentesis.

Postnatal testing includes a routine newborn test, which can be done from a heel prick.

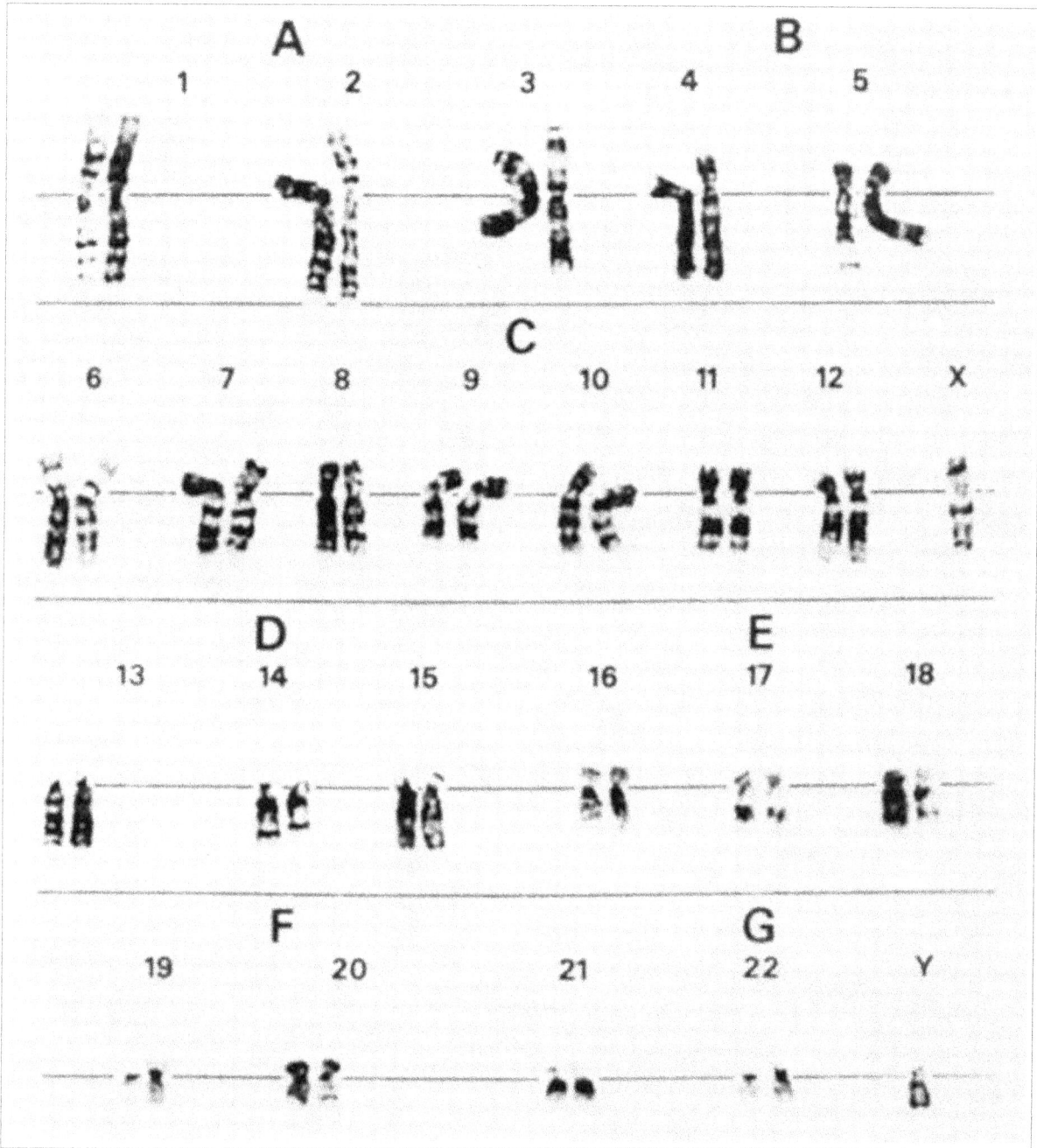

Figure 7.2 A human karyotype (Harrison, 2008)

Genetic services priorities in South Africa

The following congenital conditions (also see Chapter 45) are the priorities for genetic services in South Africa:

▶ Down's syndrome
▶ Neural tube defects
▶ Fetal alcohol syndrome (FAS)
▶ Albinism
▶ Cleft lip and palate
▶ Club feet (talipes equinovaris)
▶ Congenital infections from toxoplasmosis, other infections, rubella, cytomegalovirus and herpes (TORCH).

Table 7.1 gives some detail on how genetic disorders are to be managed in South Africa through primary, secondary and tertiary prevention. Primary prevention aims at preventing first occurrences of specific genetic disorders and birth defects. Conditions most amenable to primary prevention are birth defects caused by environmental factors that can be removed or neutralised, and non-hereditary genetic disorders such as chromosomal abnormalities, in which the association with advanced maternal age offers a basis for prevention. Secondary prevention aims at the prenatal identification of women at increased risk for having a child with a genetic disorder or birth defect. It also offers the option of termination of pregnancy.

Table 7.1

Strategies for the management of genetic defects and disorders in South Africa

Primary prevention	Secondary prevention	Tertiary prevention
Public efforts to improve health, nutrition, education and self-reliance, particularly of women	Identification of pregnant women at risk	Anticipatory guidance (eg prevention of obesity in Down's syndrome)
Avoidance of unintended pregnancies and achievement of proper birth spacing through access to contraception and family planning	Identification of pregnant women aged 35 years or more	Proper intervention to avert complications (eg laminectomy to alleviate spinal cord compression in achondroplasia)
Improved access to, and quality of, prenatal care and genetic counselling	Identification of pregnant women exposed to teratogens, eg alcohol, recreational drugs, infections (eg rubella, syphilis), medicines (eg phenytoin) or chemicals	Rehabilitation of disabilities (eg speech therapy, hearing aids in loss of hearing, physical therapy in neuromuscular diseases)
Improved quality of birth care	Ultrasound evaluation for all pregnant women to detect fetal defects	Psychosocial support for affected individuals and their families (an essential, albeit commonly neglected component of care relating to genetic disorders and birth defects)
Control of possible occupational risks	Amniocentesis or chorionic villus biopsy in appropriately selected pregnancies (eg previous chromosomal abnormality)	
Peri-conceptual supplementation of folic acid to women of reproductive age to reduce the risk of neural tube defects and perhaps other congenital defects	Termination of pregnancy for serious genetic disorders or birth defects	
Encouraging women to procreate at the ideal reproductive ages (20–35 years) to reduce the risk of chromosomal abnormalities		
Avoidance of teratogens (eg alcohol, recreational drugs, and certain chemicals and infectious agents) during pregnancy		

7.3 Cell division: Mitosis and meiosis

When a cell divides, the division results in two daughter cells, which are identical in every way to the parent cell. These daughter cells in turn become parent cells and each one divides into two more identical daughter cells. The original cell has now become four identical cells. These four cells continue to divide and each time produce two identical daughter cells, bringing the total to eight, then 16, then 32, then 64, and so on. Therefore, cell division results in a multiplication (reproduction) of cells. There are two types of cell division: mitosis and meiosis.

Mitosis

The nuclear division of somatic cells, resulting in diploid cells, is called mitosis (see Figure 7.3 on the next page).

As previously mentioned, in the nucleus of each cell in the human body there are 46 chromosomes (23 pairs). The similar chromosomes are said to be homologous chromosomes. These 23 pairs of chromosomes are made up of 22 pairs of autosomes and one pair of sex chromosomes. The autosomes determine the general characteristics of an individual, while the sex chromosomes determine the gender.

In each cell, the two chromosomes making up a homologous pair of autosomes are similar to each other in appearance (the same karyotype). However, the female chromosome is large and is known as the X chromosome, while the male chromosome is small and is known as the Y chromosome. Females have two X chromosomes, and males have an X and a Y chromosome.

During mitosis, the chromosomes, which are contained within the cell nucleus, divide in a way that ensures that identical chromosomal (genetic) material from the parent cell is duplicated and given to each of the daughter cells.

Mitosis is continuous, but it is usually divided into the following four stages, illustrated in Figure 7.3, to make the process easier to understand:

1. *Prophase:*

   Early: The chromosomes shorten and thicken and are seen as double strands in the cell, called *chromatids*. The genetic material of the cell forms long, thin chromatin threads.

   Late: The chromosomes divide to form two centrioles, which move to the opposite ends of the cell. In summary, a chromatin network is seen as chromosomes made up of two chromatids attached by a centromere (the point of attachment of the two chromatids).

2. *Metaphase:* Chromosomes are arranged at the equator (middle) of the cell.

3. *Anaphase:*

   Early: The spindle fibres shorten, pulling the chromatids to either end of the cell.

   Late: The cell membrane starts to constrict, leaving spindles at either end. In summary, chromatids move to the polar regions of the spindle and the chromatids split at the centromere. One chromatid of each chromosome moves to the opposite pole.

4. *Telophase:* Two daughter cells are formed, each identical to the parent. Each cell has one half of a chromosome (chromatid) that corresponds to an identical half in the other daughter cell. A nuclear membrane forms around the chromatids, making up the nucleus.

Between cell division there is a resting stage where no division occurs and the chromosomes are not easily seen. This stage is called interphase.

Meiosis

The nuclear division of sex cells, resulting in haploid cells, is called meiosis (see Figure 7.3). In the process of meiosis, the number of chromosomes in the parent cell (the diploid number in the human is 46) is reduced by half in the daughter cells (the haploid number in the human is 23).

The process of meiosis takes place in two steps, each step having a prometaphase, a metaphase, an anaphase and a telophase stage, as in mitosis. For the sake of convenience, the stages in the first step are referred to as meiosis I and the stages in the second step as meiosis II.

Meiosis I can be understood as happening in the following phases:

1. *Prometaphase I:* The chromosomes become coiled and a spindle forms. Homologous chromosomes join together to form bivalents. Crossing over occurs, with exchange of genetic material. The nuclear membrane disintegrates in this phase.

2. *Metaphase I:* The chromatids line up at the equator of the cell and the spindle fibres attach to the centromeres.

3. *Anaphase I:* Homologous pairs of chromosomes separate out and one member of each pair moves to the opposite pole of the cell.

4. *Telophase I:* The spindle fibre is broken down. The chromosomes uncoil and the cytoplasm begins to divide, which results in the formation of two cells. Each cell has only half the genetic make-up of the original cell because it has only one chromosome from each homologous pair. This means that another division is needed, because each cell contains two identical sister chromatids.

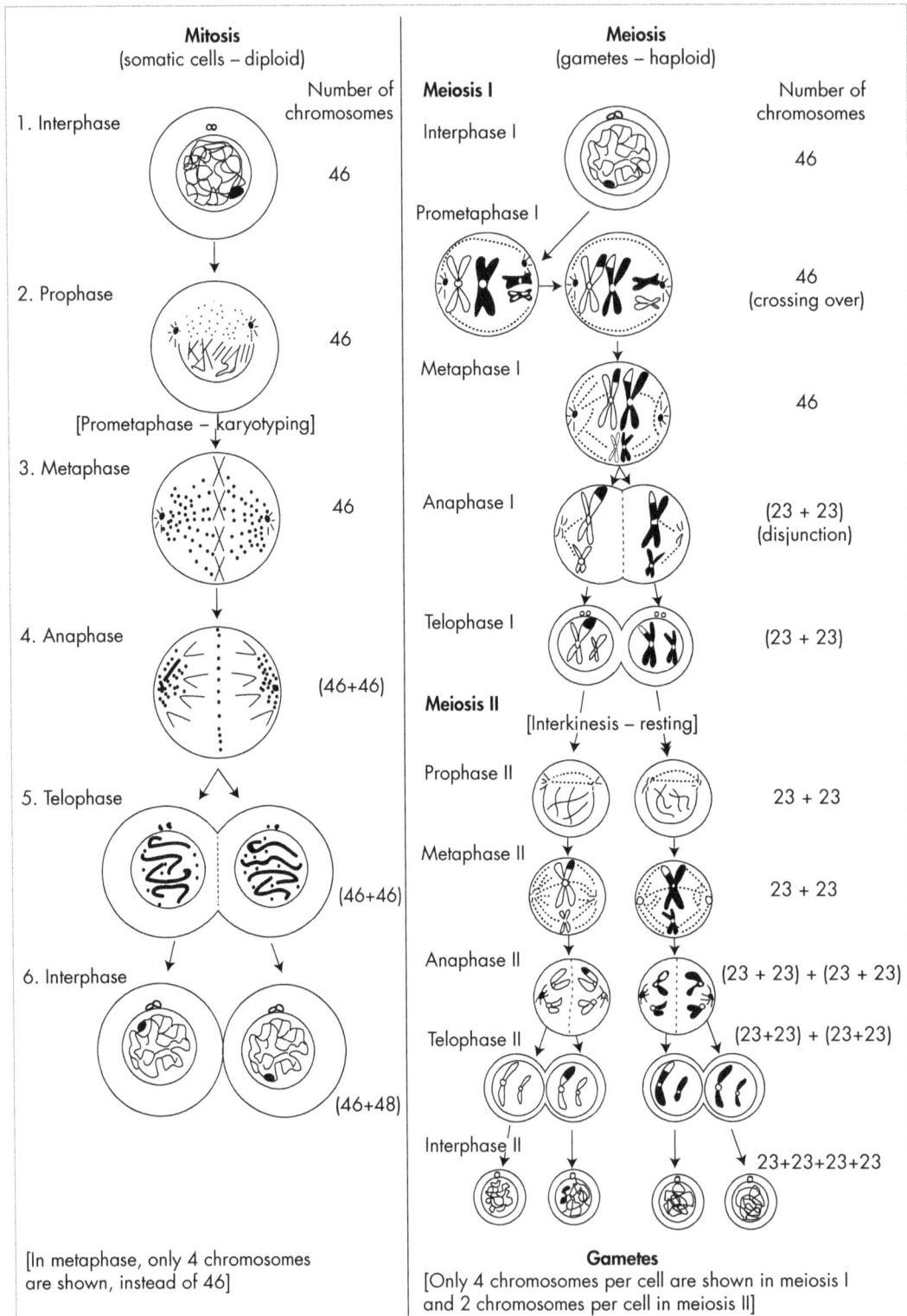

Figure 7.3 Mitosis and meiosis

The next division is called meiosis II and consists of the following phases:

1. *Prophase II:* Spindle fibres form in each of the two cells. The chromosomes re-form from the chromatin, but they are still made up of sister chromatids.
2. *Metaphase II:* Spindle fibres attach to the centromeres and the chromosomes align themselves along the equator of the cell.
3. *Anaphase II:* The centromere of each chromosome splits and the sister chromatids separate and move to opposite poles. The sister chromatids are now called chromosomes.
4. *Telophase II:* The chromosomes move to each pole, the nuclei re-form, the spindle breaks down, the cytoplasm is divided and two new cells form.

Fetal abnormalities due to chromosomal defects

It is during the processes of meiosis and mitosis that chromosomal defects can occur, resulting in fetal abnormalities. These chromosomal aberrations cause severe congenital abnormalities, most of which are not compatible with life. One of the abnormalities that is compatible with life – and one of the most commonly seen – is Trisomy 21 (Down's syndrome). Figure 7.4 shows the difference between abnormal and normal meiotic division in cells.

7.4 Gametogenesis and gametes

Gametogenesis

Meiosis produces mature gametes through the process of gametogenesis, the process by which the gametes – sperm and ova – are produced by the testes and ovaries. There are two types of gametogenesis: spermatogenesis and oogenesis.

1. *Spermatogenesis* is the process by which sperm are produced in the male sex cells. This takes place in the testes. Primary spermatocytes with 46 chromosomes divide to form two secondary spermatocytes, each with 23 chromosomes. These secondary spermatocytes divide to form a total of four spermatids, each with 23 daughter chromosomes. The spermatids eventually differentiate into spermatozoa (sperm). Meiosis in males always results in the production of four sperm.

   After the first meiotic division, both the secondary spermatocytes will be haploid; one of the secondary spermatocytes will have an X chromosome and the other will have a Y chromosome. After the second meiotic division, there will be four haploid spermatids; two of these spermatids will have an X chromosome and two will have a Y chromosome.

2. *Oogenesis* takes place in the ovaries to produce the egg. The primary oocyte in the ovary has 46 chromosomes and divides by meiosis to produce two cells that each have 23 chromosomes. One of these cells is called the secondary oocyte and the other is the polar body. The secondary oocyte receives almost all the cytoplasm. The polar body may disintegrate or it may divide again. The secondary oocyte begins meiosis II and then stops at metaphase. Meiosis in females produces only one egg and three polar bodies.

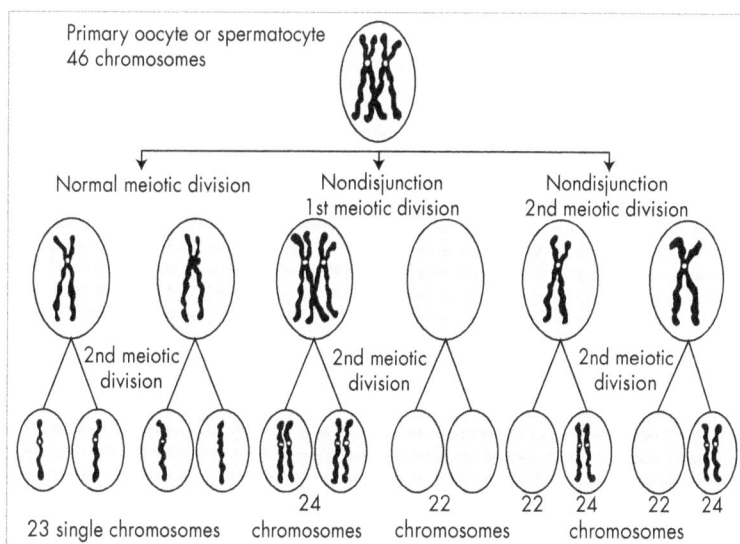

Figure 7.4 Normal and abnormal meiotic division

The structure of the mature ovum

The ovum consists of a central nucleus, surrounded by yellowish cytoplasm known as the vitellus, as shown in Figure 7.5. The vitellus is in turn surrounded by a space called the perivitelline space. The polar bodies, produced during the process of maturation of the oocyte during meiosis, are discarded into this space.

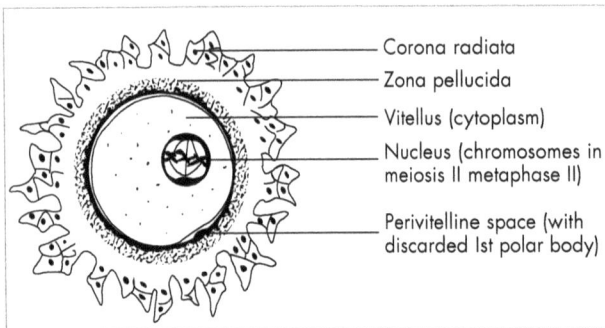

Figure 7.5 The human ovum, after ovulation but before fertilisation

The outer margin of the perivitelline space, formed by a thick membrane made from an opaque jelly-like substance, is called the zona pellucida, which acts as a protective shield around the ovum. The zona pellucida is encircled by granulosa cells of the ovarian follicle, which have clumped together and appear to radiate outward from the zona pellucida. This formation of granulosa cells, known as the corona radiata, gives the ovum

the appearance of a tiny, hairy ball. After ovulation the ovum is just barely visible to the naked eye, with a diameter of 100–150 microns.

As was discussed in Chapter 6, the ovum is expelled from the ruptured ovarian follicle and is propelled by the fimbriae lining the Fallopian tubes into the ampulla of the tube. After ovulation, the ovum must be fertilised within the first 12–24 hours. After this time, it begins to degenerate. Finally, if it is not fertilised, it disintegrates.

7.5 The male reproductive organs and sperm transport

The spermatozoa are produced in the testes, which are two oval-shaped organs suspended in the scrotum by the spermatic cords. The scrotum is a loose pouch of pigmented skin divided into two compartments. It is situated in the perineal area, behind the penis and in front of the anus, and is homologous with the labia majora in the female.

Each testis is made up of about 900 coiled seminiferous tubules, each about three-quarters of a metre long. Sperm are formed from the germinal epithelial cells called spermatogonia in the walls of these seminiferous tubules.

The seminiferous tubules lead into the epididymis, another coiled tube within each testis, which is about 6 m long. The sperm take several days to pass through the epididymis, during which time they undergo final maturation and become motile.

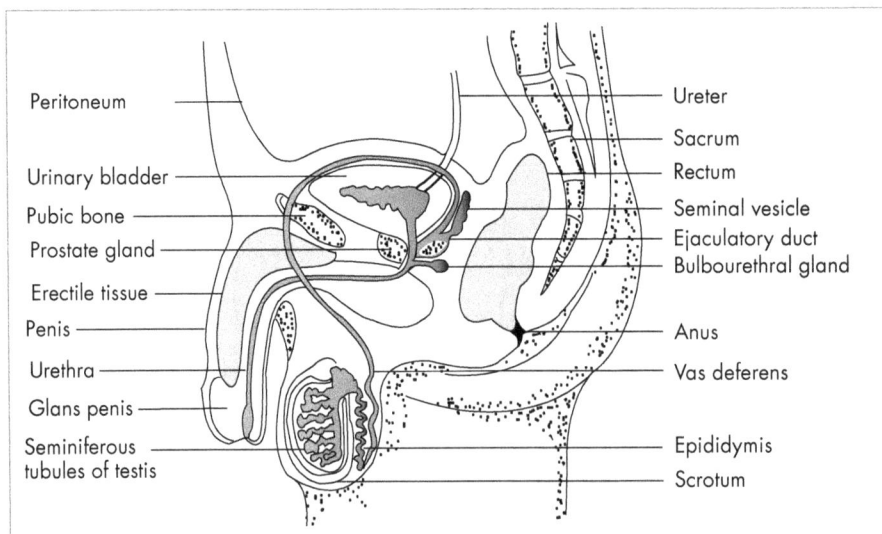

Figure 7.6 The male reproductive organs

The epididymis leads into the vas deferens, which is a long straight tube that leaves the scrotum and passes through the inguinal canal on either side of the pelvis and into the abdominal cavity. The vas deferens then curves over the bladder on either side, down the posterior surface of the bladder and back into the pelvis, where it joins with the duct of the corresponding seminal vesicle to form the ejaculatory duct. Most sperm are stored in the vas deferens and the ampulla of the vas deferens and can maintain their fertility for several months.

The ejaculatory ducts are two short ducts that pass through the prostate gland and then enter the urethra, which is a tube leading from the bladder, through the penis, to the outside of the body via the external urethral sphincter at the glans penis.

The testes, the epididymides, the vasa deferentia and the ejaculatory ducts are all paired – that is, they are situated on both sides of the body. Only the urethra is a single tube. It conducts both urine from the bladder and the fluid containing the sperm from the ejaculatory ducts, which leave the body via the penis.

The sperm together with the fluid in which they are suspended are called semen. This thick, white fluid is continuously secreted by the seminal vesicles, the prostate gland and the bulbourethral glands. Prostaglandins are also present in semen. On sexual stimulation, the penis becomes erect. On further stimulation, there is an emission of more fluid from the seminal vesicles, the prostate gland and the bulbourethral glands into the urethra. Finally, ejaculation occurs.

The structure of the spermatozoon

Sperm, as shown in Figure 7.7, have a tiny, pear-shaped head, which is about 5–7 microns long and contains the nucleus, which contains the chromosomes. The acrosome covers the front of the nucleus and contains hydrolytic enzymes, mainly hyaluronidase, and proteolytic enzymes, which disperse the cells of the corona radiata and dissolve the zona pellucida when the sperm penetrates an ovum at fertilisation.

The neck of the sperm is the constricted area between the head and the tail. In human sperm, a significant amount of cytoplasm often remains around the neck region. The tail is divided into a middle piece, a principal piece and an end piece. The middle piece, which is separated from the head by the neck, is about the same length as the head. Mitochondria are concentrated in the midpiece and generate the energy required for the flagellar movement of the sperm. The principal piece, which constitutes most of the tail, is made up of longitudinal fibrils, which are responsible for the motility of the sperm. The short end piece is merely the tapered end of the tail.

Male hormones

Androgens: Testosterone

The male hormones, called androgens, are produced by the interstitial cells, called Leydig cells, in the seminiferous tubules of the testes. The main androgen is testosterone. It is responsible for establishing male features in the embryo from the sixth week of development. It also stimulates the descent of the testes into the scrotum before birth.

When the male is about 10 years of age, the hypothalamus matures and begins to secrete hormones, which allow the anterior pituitary gland to secrete the gonadotrophic hormones – follicle-stimulating hormone (FSH) and luteinising hormone (LH) – as in the female. FSH stimulates the development of the seminiferous tubules and is thought to promote spermatogenesis. LH stimulates the Leydig cells to secrete testosterone.

Testosterone also promotes growth in the adolescent male, increasing the synthesis of proteins and the metabolic rate. It is responsible for the development of the primary sexual structures and for all the secondary sexual characteristics, namely facial, pubic and axillary hair, the deepening of the voice and the development of muscle. Testosterone is also responsible for the activity of sebaceous glands in the skin.

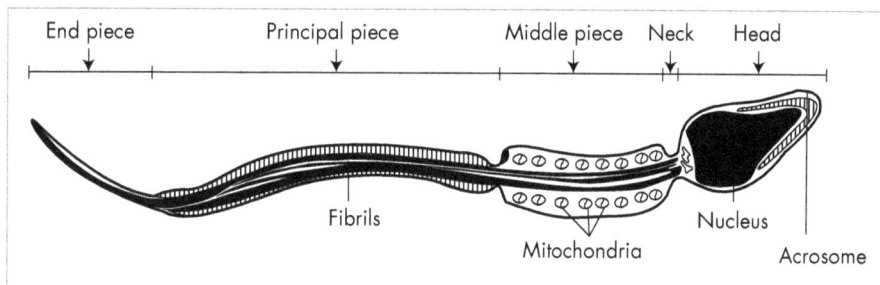

Figure 7.7 A human spermatozoon

Oestrogens

There are small amounts of the female hormones, the oestrogens, in the male. These hormones are thought to be secreted by specialised cells, the Sefton cells, which are interspersed with the germinal epithelium and the Leydig cells in the walls of the seminiferous tubules.

The Sefton cells provide a special environment in which the germinal cells can develop and they play a special role in converting the spermatocytes into spermatozoa. These cells also secrete other hormones necessary in the process of spermatogenesis, one of which is inhibin.

7.6   Conception and fertilisation

Conception refers to the process of joining the male and female elements. Fertilisation is the first phase in this process. Fertilisation usually takes place in the ampulla of the Fallopian tubes, soon after the ovum enters the tube (read more about ovulation in Chapter 6).

About three million sperm are deposited in the vagina, but only a few survive longer than 24 hours in the female genital tract. Most are destroyed by the lactic acid in the vagina, and many do not manage to negotiate the cervix, the uterus and the uterine tubes. Of the relatively few (1 000–3 000) that enter the tube containing the ovum waiting to be fertilised, only one will actually fertilise the ovum.

The sperm propel themselves forward by lashing movements of their tails. When a sperm meets the ovum, it must first penetrate a barrier formed by the corona radiata and the zona pellucida. At this point, the sperm become capacitated, a process whereby the outer membrane of the acrosome is broken down and the hydrolytic and proteolytic enzymes are made available (activated). Many sperm attempt to enter the ovum. The combined enzymes produced by all these sperm appear to be necessary for breaking down the barrier so that one sperm can penetrate into the cytoplasm (vitellus) of the ovum, as shown in Figure 7.8.

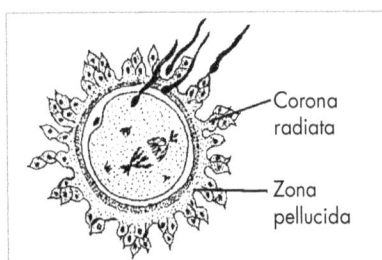

Figure 7.8 Fertilisation of the ovum

Once a sperm enters the ovum, the barrier of the zona pellucida reforms, so that no more sperm can penetrate. The head of the sperm enlarges rapidly to form the male pronucleus, and the tail degenerates. The ovum now completes the second meiotic division, forming the female pronucleus and expelling the second polar body into the perivitelline space.

The male and female pronuclei fuse on contact and lose their nuclear membranes. The 23 chromosomes from each nucleus fuse to form a new diploid cell, containing 46 chromosomes (23 pairs), which will be the beginnings of a unique human being. This fertilised ovum is known as the zygote.

As the sex chromosome from the ovum is always an X chromosome, the zygote will always have one X chromosome. The sex of the baby therefore depends upon which sex chromosome is contained within the nucleus of the fertilising sperm, which means that the male determines the gender of the baby.

The new cell, the zygote, then prepares itself for the first cleavage division in the process of mitosis, which will be discussed in the next section.

Birth ratio of male to female

There is a 50 per cent chance that a new zygote will be male (YX) or female (XX). More boys are conceived than girls, because sperm carrying the Y chromosome have a competitive advantage. There are 100 girls born for every 105 boys, but more boys than girls die before birth (Rojas-Burke, 2010).

7.7   Embryology

Embryology is the science of the development of the zygote, the embryo and the fetus in utero.

Terminology

The following terms are used when describing the development in utero from fertilisation to delivery:

▶ *Zygote:* This is the name given to the developing ovum during the period from fertilisation to the 21st day (the end of the third week).

▶ *Embryo.* This term covers the period from the 22nd to the 56th day after fertilisation (from the beginning of the fourth week to the end of the eighth week, ie five weeks). This period is best expressed in days, because the changes from fertilisation to the end of the embryonic period are so complex.

▶ *Fetus:* This term covers the period from the beginning of the ninth week after fertilisation to term. After the embryonic period, the fetal age is expressed in weeks.

The duration of pregnancy and the estimated date of delivery

Pregnancy in humans is 40 weeks, nine months or 280 days. It normally ranges between 37 and 42 weeks (259–294 days). The period of gestation in the human is divided into three trimesters (each a period of three months or approximately 13 weeks), which are known as the first, the second and the third trimesters.

The estimated date of delivery (EDD) is calculated as approximately 266 days after fertilisation. However, in order to have a recognisable landmark, the first day of the last normal menstrual period is used in obstetrics. Therefore, as fertilisation usually takes place within 24 hours of ovulation and ovulation takes place about 14 days after the onset of menstruation, 14 days are added to the 266 days, making the estimated date of delivery approximately 280 days after the onset of the last normal menstrual period.

When calculating the EDD in months, seven days are added to the date of the first day of the last normal menstrual period and then nine months are added (see chapters 1, 15 and 17). This is in accordance with Naegele's rule, which states: Add seven days to the first day of the last normal menstrual period, and then either subtract three months or add nine months (Baskett & Nagele, 2000).

Whether estimated in days, weeks or months, the periods of gestation given above are all approximate lengths of gestation and are merely guidelines.

The zygote: Cleavage, implantation and development

As mentioned, the term 'zygote' is applicable to the period from fertilisation up to the 21st day after fertilisation.

Because fertilisation usually takes place within 24 hours of ovulation, fertilisation and ovulation are practically interchangeable in expressing the age and development of the zygote.

The zygote now starts to divide by the process of mitosis into two identical daughter cells, then four, then eight, and so on (see Figure 7.9). This mitotic division of the zygote is known as cleavage and the daughter cells are known as blastomeres. The progress of the zygote, first along the Fallopian tube (see Figure 7.9) and then in the uterine cavity, is described using the days following fertilisation.

Days 1–5: Cleavage and entry into the uterine cavity

On the third day following fertilisation, a cluster of about 16 blastomeres form a solid ball, called the morula, as shown in Figure 7.10 on the next page. The cells increase in number as the morula passes from the Fallopian tube into the uterine cavity.

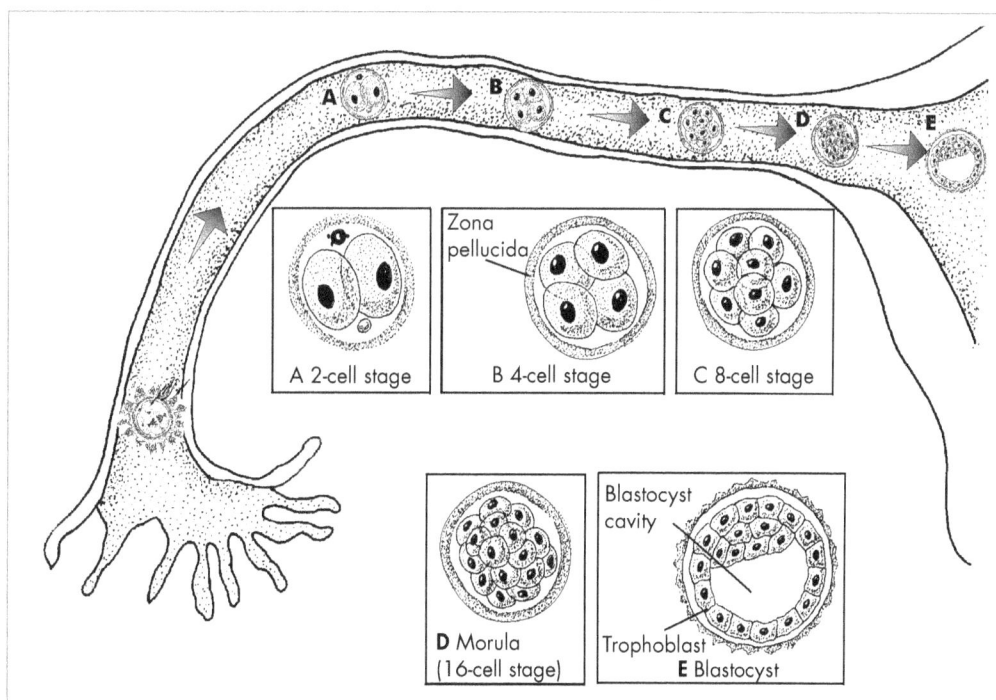

Figure 7.9 The transport of the developing ovum along the Fallopian tube: Day 1–5

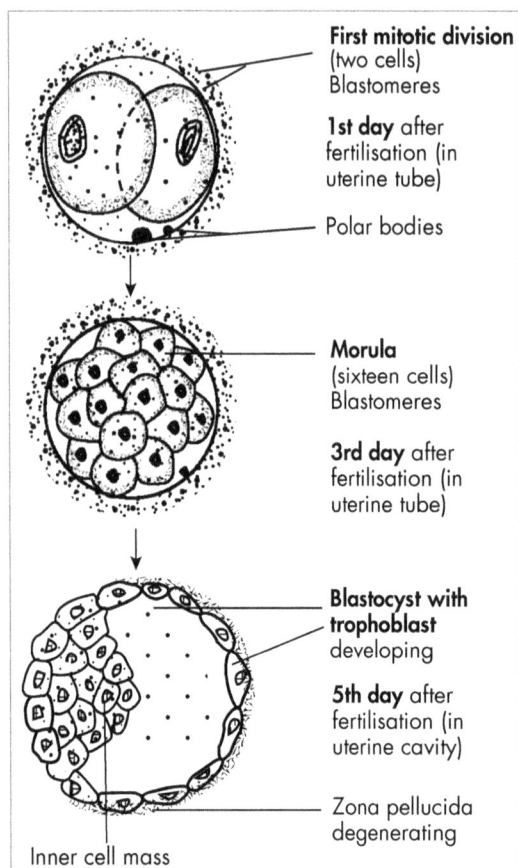

First mitotic division
(two cells)
Blastomeres

1st day after
fertilisation (in
uterine tube)

Polar bodies

Morula
(sixteen cells)
Blastomeres

3rd day after
fertilisation (in
uterine tube)

**Blastocyst with
trophoblast**
developing

5th day after
fertilisation (in
uterine cavity)

Zona pellucida
degenerating

Inner cell mass

Figure 7.10 Cleavage of the zygote

By the fourth day, fluid from the uterine cavity has penetrated the morula and formed a fluid-filled cavity (cyst), pushing the inner cell mass to one side. This changes the morula into a blastocyst, as shown in Figure 7.10. The inner cell mass will eventually become the embryo.

On the fourth and fifth days, the blastocyst remains free in the uterine cavity, receiving nourishment from the uterine secretions.

Days 6–7: Implantation of the embryo

From about the fifth day, the zona pellucida starts to degenerate and the blastocyst attaches to the uterine wall.

On about the sixth day, the outer cells of the blastocyst become highly specialised. They are now called trophoblastic cells. These cells secrete proteolytic enzymes that digest and liquefy the cells of the inner lining of the uterine endometrium, known during pregnancy as the compact layer of the decidua.

By the end of the seventh day, the blastocyst is superficially implanted into the lining of the decidua. In this way, the blastocyst is eventually able to embed itself into the spongy layer of the decidua and to acquire nourishment from the decidual cells. In order to achieve this, the trophoblastic cells develop into two distinct layers, which are together known as the trophoblast or syncytiotrophoblast, as shown in Figure 7.11. The embryo will implant into the endometrium about four days after reaching the uterus, about seven days after ovulation (in a normal 21-day cycle). The implantation takes about 24 hours and is facilitated through a protolithic enzyme excreted from the trophoblast cells.

The two layers making up the trophoblast or syncytiotrophoblast are:

1. *an outer syncytiotrophoblast layer* made up of syncytial cells which continue to secrete proteolytic enzymes and thereby continue to invade the decidua and nourish the blastocyst
2. *an inner cytotrophoblast or Langhan's layer* made up of cytotrophic cells, closely attached to the outer syncytial layer.

These two layers of cells therefore form the outer membrane of the trophoblast.

Implantation bleed
When the syncytiotrophoblast erodes the maternal decidua and blood vessels, the woman may present with slight vaginal bleeding. This may be perceived as an early and lighter-than-usual menstrual period, as the woman would not yet be aware of the pregnancy. This implantation bleed can cause difficulties with the EDD if the woman uses it as her last menstrual period (LMP). The actual date of delivery could, therefore, be about three weeks earlier than estimated.

Normal and abnormal implantation sites

The normal sites for implantation of the zygote are the posterior, anterior or lateral walls of the uterus, just below the entry to the Fallopian tube, roughly in the centre of the uterus.

Any implantation site other than the uterine cavity is abnormal and will give rise to an ectopic pregnancy. The following are some examples of abnormal implantation sites:

▶ Implantation in a *Fallopian tube* results in a tubal pregnancy, where the zygote implants anywhere along the length of the tube. The zygote will develop and grow and eventually become too large to be accommodated in the lumen of the tube. This will cause the tube to rupture, resulting in a ruptured (tubal) ectopic pregnancy and the death of the embryo. This is a very serious condition, causing severe pain and extensive intra-abdominal bleeding. Without emergency surgical intervention, it can result in the death of the woman. This pregnancy mostly does not progress past the first trimester.

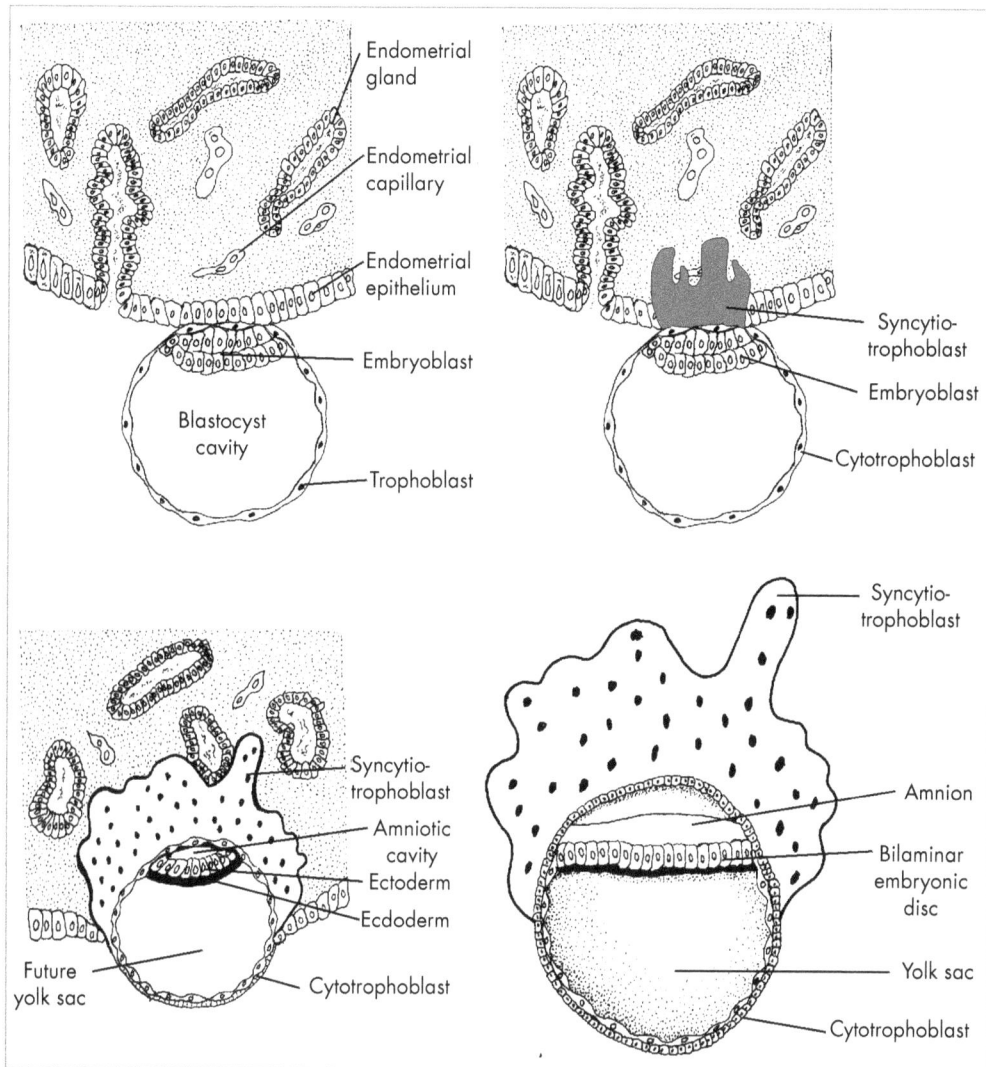

Figure 7.11 Stages of implantation of the blastocyst: Day 6–7

▶ Implantation in the *abdominal or peritoneal cavity* is called an extra-uterine or abdominal pregnancy. It is a very rare condition, with implantation in the ovarian tissue or in the mesentery, or in any organ, even the liver. Implantation in these tissues could result in the fetus surviving to term, but it usually results in early fetal death and fetal abnormalities. Sometimes, extensive damage to vital structures results in severe maternal intra-abdominal haemorrhage. Unless delivered by abdominal incision, the fetus would eventually die in the abdominal cavity due to a lack of nourishment, as it would not be able to be expelled by the uterus at term. The maternal system would eventually lay down calcium in the body of this dead fetus, resulting in a lithopedian or calcified fetus. Pauline Sellers once nursed an elderly woman who complained that she had had a large lump in her abdomen for a great many years. During a laparotomy it was found to be a large, probably full-term, lithopedian fetus. The placenta in this case cannot be removed due to the risk of haemorrhage and is left *in situ* to be reabsorbed.

▶ Implantation in the *lower uterine segment or the cervical canal* may result in a placenta praevia, which may cause severe bleeding from a detached placenta during late pregnancy and during labour. In addition, because of the dearth of criss-cross muscle fibres in the cervix, it may also lead to severe postpartum haemorrhage (PPH).

93

The development of the decidua

Changes occur in the secretory endometrium of the uterus during pregnancy, which then becomes known as the decidua (see colour illustration C3 on page 71). The decidua is made up of three layers:

1. The *basal layer* is the same as the basal layer of the endometrium in the non-pregnant state. It is not shed at menstruation and is the basis from which the new endometrium is regenerated each month; it is a permanent, regenerative layer.

2. The *spongy layer* is the broad band of connective tissue (stroma), interspersed with glands, which is regenerated from the basal layer under the influence of oestrogens and which then proliferates under the influence of progesterone. It is called the spongy layer because it is like a sponge in texture; the cells are loosely knitted together, with large spaces (lacunae) in-between the groups of cells. This layer is secreted under the influence of progesterone when the ovum is fertilised and the trophoblast is formed. During pregnancy, it becomes highly vascular and secretory in order to provide the blastocyst with nourishment. The penetrating trophoblastic villi, with their syncytial layer containing proteolytic enzymes, erode through the maternal blood vessels in the spongy layer of the decidua, causing the spaces between the villi to fill with maternal blood (see Figure 7.25 on page 111). These are then known as the intervillous spaces. These trophoblastic villi later become known as chorionic villi (chorion frondosum) and will eventually develop into the placenta.

3. The *compact layer* is the first layer that the ovum encounters when it enters the uterine cavity, as this layer is continuous with the lining of the uterine tubes. It consists of an outer layer of columnar epithelial cells, which forms the lining of the uterine cavity and keeps the cells of the spongy layer in place, together with an inner, thicker layer of connective tissue (stroma). These superficial stromal cells are swollen and enlarged and as a result are tightly packed together or compacted.

Situated on the basal layer, between the basal and spongy layers, is a specialised layer known as the 'postage-stamp' layer, or the fibrinous layer of nitabuch. This collagen layer becomes highly specialised and forms a barrier to the invading trophoblastic cells, preventing them from penetrating the basal layer of the decidua and into the myometrium. However, perforations in this layer allow the undamaged maternal spiral arteries and veins, supplying and draining the decidua, to pass through. Detachment of the placenta at this zone allows a uniform separation of the placenta from the decidua in the third stage of labour, hence the name 'postage-stamp' layer.

Should this layer not develop sufficiently, allowing some or most of the villi of the chorion frondosum to invade the basal layer of the decidua and even to extend into the myometrium, the placenta would become a morbidly adherent placenta. The result of this would be that a part or the whole of the placenta would not be able to separate from the uterine wall in the third stage of labour and would be retained within the uterus. This is known as either a partial or total placenta accreta.

The mature placenta and membranes are discussed later in this chapter, on pages 106–113.

Days 7–14: Embedding and development

The embedding and development of the zygote (blastocyst and trophoblast) occurs from day 7 to 14 after fertilisation, as shown in Figure 7.12. The cells of this inner layer begin to secrete human chorionic gonadotrophin (hCG), which is very similar to the LH of the pituitary gland.

Human chorionic gonadotrophin

The hormone hCG forms the basis of laboratory tests (of urine and blood) for the diagnosis of pregnancy.

In the non-gravid state, the corpus luteum in the ovary would start to degenerate by approximately the eighth day after ovulation, causing progesterone and oestrogen levels to start to fall. About 14 days after ovulation, the endometrium, which would no longer be sustained by these hormones, would slough away and be expelled and the unfertilised ovum would be expelled with it.

However, in pregnancy, hCG, with its LH-like action, is able to act on the corpus luteum and cause it to continue secreting progesterone and oestrogens. As a result, the following occurs:

1   The corpus luteum increases greatly in size.
2   More and more progesterone and oestrogens are secreted.
3   The endometrium grows larger and more vascular.
4   Greater invasion of the decidua by the syncytial layer of the trophoblast occurs.
5   The inner cell mass and, consequently, the developing embryo has all the nourishment that it requires to grow and develop.

On about the eighth to ninth day after fertilisation, the secretion of hCG can first be measured in the maternal blood. The rate of secretion rises rapidly and reaches a maximum at about seven to nine weeks after fertilisation, after which it decreases fairly rapidly to a much lower level by the sixteenth to twentieth week after fertilisation.

continued

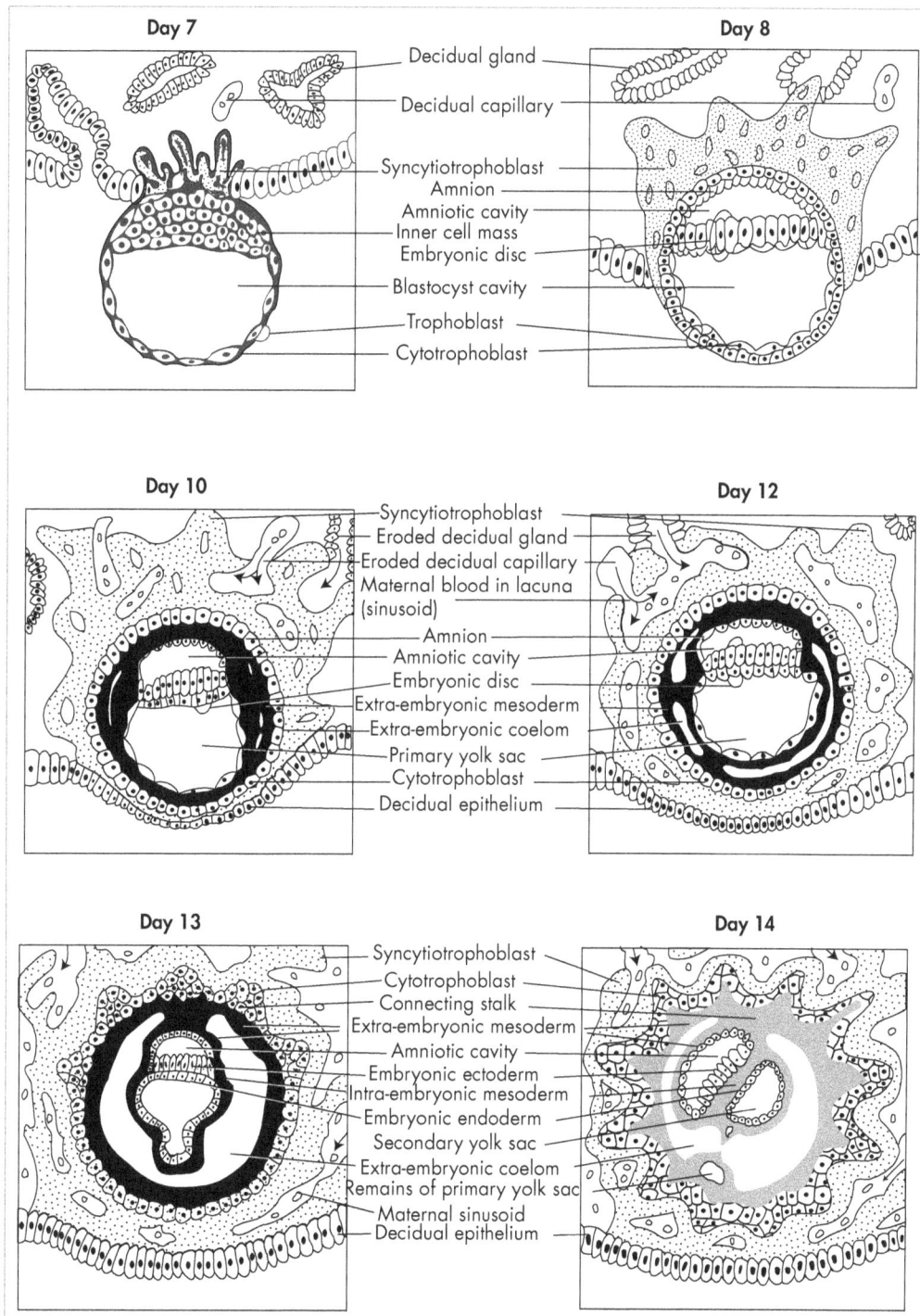

Figure 7.12 Embedding and development of the zygote (blastocyst and trophoblast) from the 7th to the 14th day

This low level is then maintained throughout pregnancy. Should the urine and blood levels of hCG remain high or even increase after 10–16 weeks of gestation, a hydatidiform mole (gestational trophoblastic disease) would be suspected. The diagnosis would be confirmed by an ultrasonic scan. Alternatively, multiple pregnancy would be a possibility.

With its LH-like effect, hCG stimulates the testes in a male fetus to begin producing small amounts of testosterone and thus causes the development of the male sex organs of the fetus *in utero.*

From about the 11th to the 13th day after fertilisation, the cells of the cytotrophic layer have greatly proliferated, pushing the syncytial layer outwards in finger-like processes or primary chorionic villi, which invade the decidua. The trophoblastic tissue therefore mingles extensively with maternal tissue, then known as secondary chorionic villi. Mesoblast cells also separate the trophoblast, which surrounds the zygote, from the inner cell mass.

These outer mesoblast cells are called the *extra-embryonic mesoderm.* By the end of the 21st day or the third week after fertilisation, they will have developed into fetal capillaries, as shown in Figure 7.13.

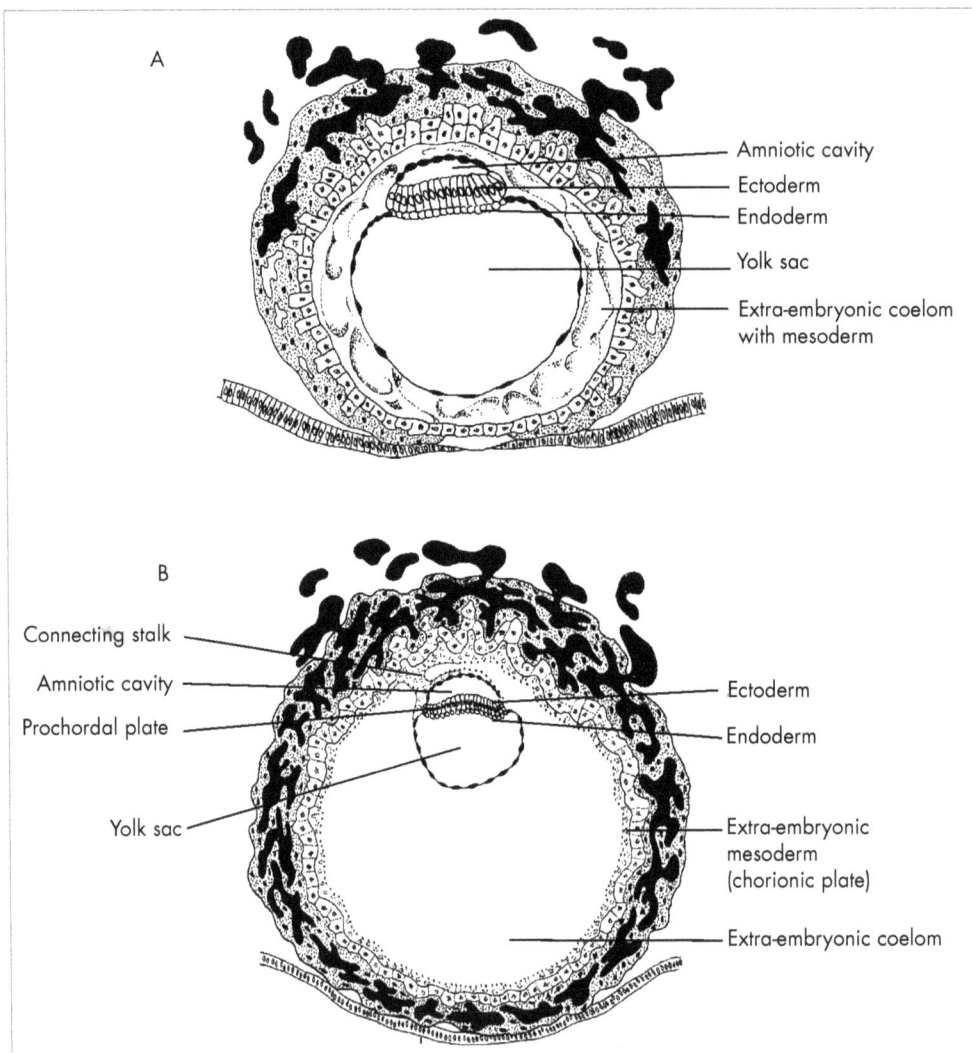

Figure 7.13 Development of the extra-embryonic mesoderm (A) and (B) coelom: Day 11–13

Once the fetal capillaries have been formed, the secondary chorionic villi become known as (tertiary) chorionic villi. These (tertiary) chorionic villi, together with the maternal decidua, will eventually form the placenta. The three layers making up the walls of the secondary chorionic villi are:

1. the *syncytiotrophoblast* (the syncytial layer), which is the outer layer
2. the *cytotrophoblast* (the cytotropic layer), which is the middle layer
3. the *mesoblast* (the mesenchymal core), which is the inner core.

By the 11th to the 13th day, changes have occurred in the inner cell mass of the blastocyst, as shown in Figure 7.14. Mesoblast cells have also formed within the inner cell mass. These will become the mesoderm at the centre of the embryonic plate, which, together with the ectoderm and the endoderm, will develop into the embryo.

The amniotic sac

The amniotic sac, which is a narrow, slit-like space lined with ectoderm cells, develops between the inner cell mass and the outer trophoblast layers, forming the beginning of the *amniotic cavity or sac* (see Figure 7.13).

The inner cell mass

The inner cell mass differentiates into an embryonic disc. This is made up of three layers (germ layers) as follows:

1. *The ectoderm:* Where the inner cell mass is closest to the trophoblast and on the side where the amniotic cavity has developed, there is a row of cells known as the ectoderm. This row of cells is continuous with the ectoderm cells which line the amniotic sac (see Figure 7.13).
2. *The mesoderm:* At the central part of the embryonic disc is the mesoderm. The row of mesoderm cells is continuous with the mesoblast cells within the chorionic villi, which later develop into the fetal blood vessels.
3. *The endoderm:* Lining the side of the mesoderm closest to the blastocyst cavity is a row of cells known as the endoderm. These cells are continuous with the cells lining the yolk sac.

The yolk sac

The cavity of the blastocyst has now developed into the yolk sac, which is lined with endoderm cells, as shown in Figure 7.13. The zygote has now differentiated into two distinct parts, namely:

1. the *outer trophoblast*, which is invading the maternal decidua and will eventually form the placenta and the chorionic membrane (the chorion), responsible for the nourishment and well-being of first the embryo and then the fetus

2. the *inner cell mass*, which will develop into the embryo and then the fetus. This will also form the amniotic membrane (the amnion) and will become filled with fluid called liquor amnii. The umbilical cord, which links the fetus to the placenta, will develop from the (connecting) body stalk.

By the 12th day, spaces have started to form within the extra-embryonic mesoderm. By the 14h day, the primary yolk sac has divided into two, and the remaining (secondary) yolk sac is much smaller. The extra-embryonic coelom has greatly enlarged and now surrounds the inner cell mass, except at the connecting or body stalk. The primary chorionic villi will have been established. This is the time at which the menstrual period would normally have taken place.

Days 15–21: Development of the zygote

The third week of embryonic life, which is the period immediately following the first missed menstrual period, is a time of rapid growth.

The trophoblast

The primary chorionic villi progress to secondary villi and then, when blood vessels have formed in these villi, to tertiary chorionic villi (see Figure 7.14). These vessels become connected to vessels developing in the embryonic heart via vessels in the connecting body stalk. By the 21st day, embryonic blood has started to circulate through the capillaries in the chorionic villi, and now carry nourishment from the maternal blood to the developing embryo and return waste products to the maternal circulation.

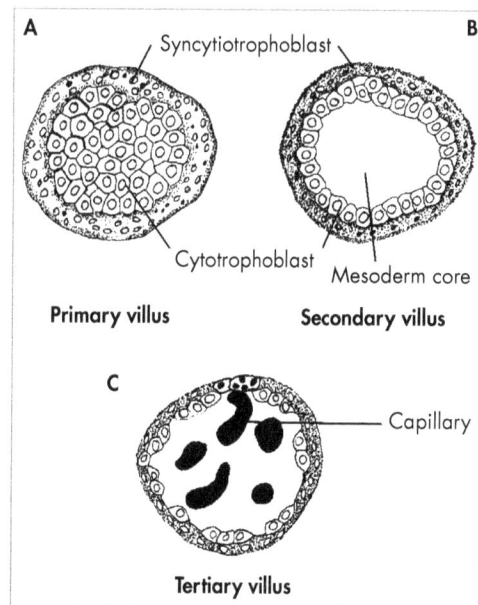

Figure 7.14 Structure of the villi: Day 15–21

The inner cell mass

The embryonic disc develops and changes from a flat disc to become pear-shaped and then elongated. The cranial area expands while the caudal area elongates. A fold or groove (the neural plate) develops longitudinally down the centre of the ectoderm and the mesoderm. This neural plate folds around on itself and by the end of the third week, the edges of the neural plate meet and fuse in the centre of the embryo.

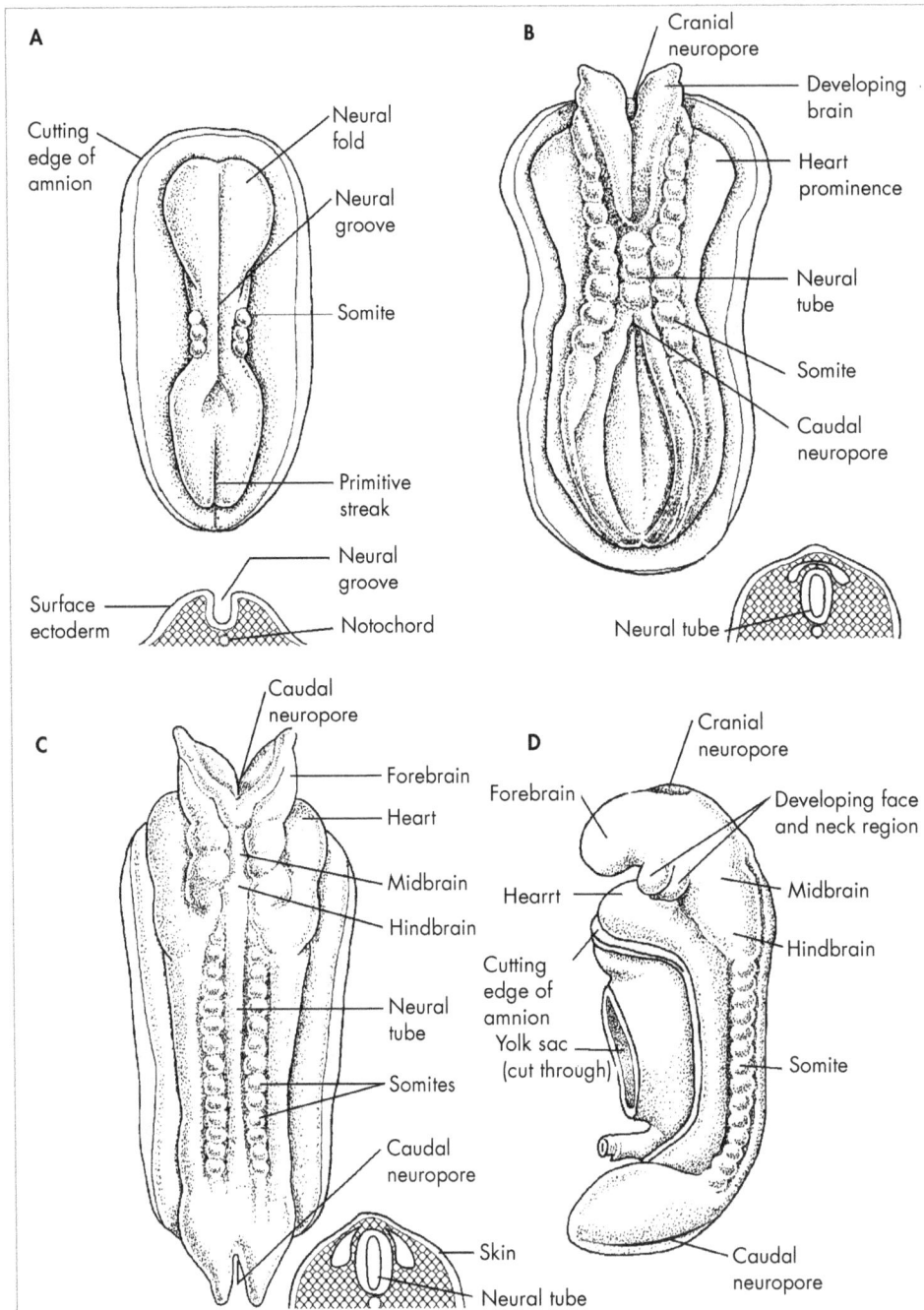

Figure 7.15 Development of the neural tube: Day 15–21

By the 21st day, the primitive cardiovascular and neural tubes have formed. The neural tube, as shown in Figure 7.15, is the precursor of the brain and the nervous system, together with the tissues covering and protecting the brain and spinal cord. Any disturbance during this process can result in severe abnormalities of the brain and spinal cord, such as anencephaly.

The intra-embryonic coelom or embryonic body cavities now appear as isolated intra-embryonic coelomic spaces within the intra-embryonic mesoderm. These spaces will later coalesce to form the heart and the pericardial cavity, the pleural cavities and the peritoneal cavity.

By the 21st day, a primitive cardiovascular system is established within the embryonic form and the yolk sac (see Figure 7.15).

The amniotic sac surrounds the embryonic form and begins to extend towards the yolk sac, which it will also ultimately surround.

Derivatives of the embryo and germ layers

The three germ layers that have been formed by the end of the third week give rise to all the tissues and organs in the embryo (see Figure 7.16). The main body systems are outlined as follows:

▶ The *ectoderm* gives rise to the nervous system, the brain, spinal cord, eyes, nose, hypophysis gland, epidermis, nails and enamel of the teeth, subcutaneous glands and the mammary glands, and the medulla of the adrenal glands.

▶ The *mesoderm* gives rise to the skeletal system, bone, cartilage and connective tissue, muscle tissue (striated and smooth), cardiovascular and lymphatic systems, heart, lungs, blood and lymph vessels, blood cells, spleen, urogenital system, kidneys and gonads (but not the bladder), the serous membranes lining the body cavities and the cortex of the adrenal gland.

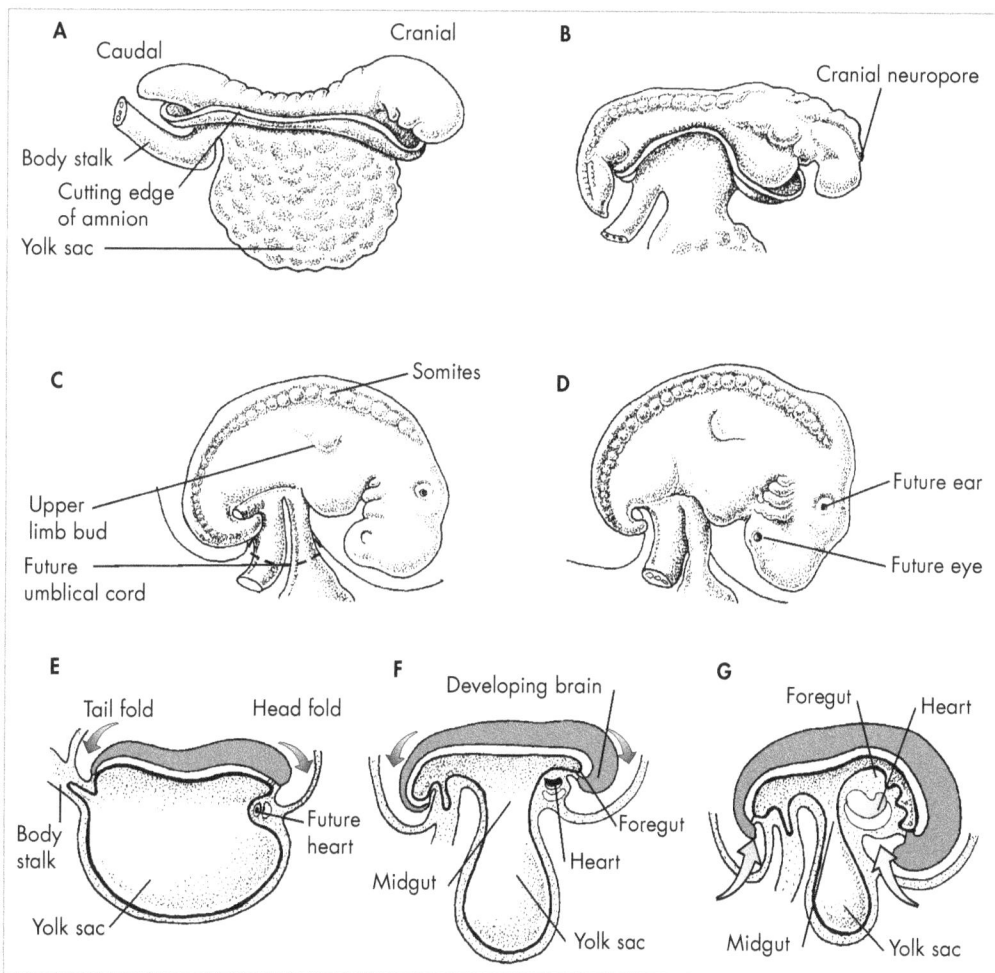

Figure 7.16 The folding of the embryo: Differentiation of tissue and organs by day 21

▶ The *endoderm* gives rise to the epithelial lining of the gastrointestinal (GI) tract, the respiratory tract, liver, pancreas, gallbladder, thyroid, parathyroid, thymus glands and urinary system.

The embryo: Days 22–56

The development of the embryo covers a period of five weeks, from the beginning of the fourth week to the end of the eighth week after fertilisation.

Until the sixth week, the size of the gestation sac is measured with ultrasound to confirm pregnancy. The gestational sac volume (GSV) is measured in millilitres (ml) (see Table 7.2 on page 103). Once the fetus is identified in the sac from the sixth week of gestation, the crown–rump length (CRL) is measured. This is the most accurate means of determining gestational age (GA) until the twentieth week. A viable pregnancy can be identified from the fifth week and is associated with the beating of a fetal heart (see Table 7.2).

This is an extremely important period of development in the human, and is called organogenesis. All the main organ systems have started to develop by the end of the fifth week and are differentiated into specific organs. The shape of the embryo gradually changes as these developments take place (see colour illustration C2 on page 70).

If the embryo is exposed to certain toxic agents during the period of organogenesis, it can lead to developmental anomalies, which will cause major congenital abnormalities. These agents are referred to as *teratogenic agents* and can include irradiation, cytotoxic agents, viruses, alcohol, many medications (drugs), as well as air, water and food pollutants. An agent that prevents cell reproduction is called an *antimitotic agent*, for example the medication thalidomide, which prevented the limb buds from developing into arms and legs in certain embryos.

While the systemic developments are taking place, the embryo takes on the fetal form and position in the uterus, as shown in Figure 7.17. The flat, straight, embryonic disc folds both longitudinally and transversely. This results in a cylindrical body form which curves, making the two ends (the head and the tail) approach each other so that the embryonic form then resembles the letter C. The curled embryonic form remains joined to the trophoblast by the connecting or body stalk, which is attached to the open end of the C and which will become the umbilical cord. The yolk sac is incorporated into the embryonic form at the open end of the C. This uncurved portion will gradually be enclosed to form the anterior abdominal wall.

Gradually, the amniotic sac completely surrounds and encloses the embryo. The amniotic membrane covers the umbilical cord and is continuous with the fetal skin at the umbilicus, as shown in Figure 7.18.

The umbilical cord (previously the body or connecting stalk) is attached into the centre of the developing placenta (chorion frondosum). The fetal side of the placenta is also covered with amniotic membrane.

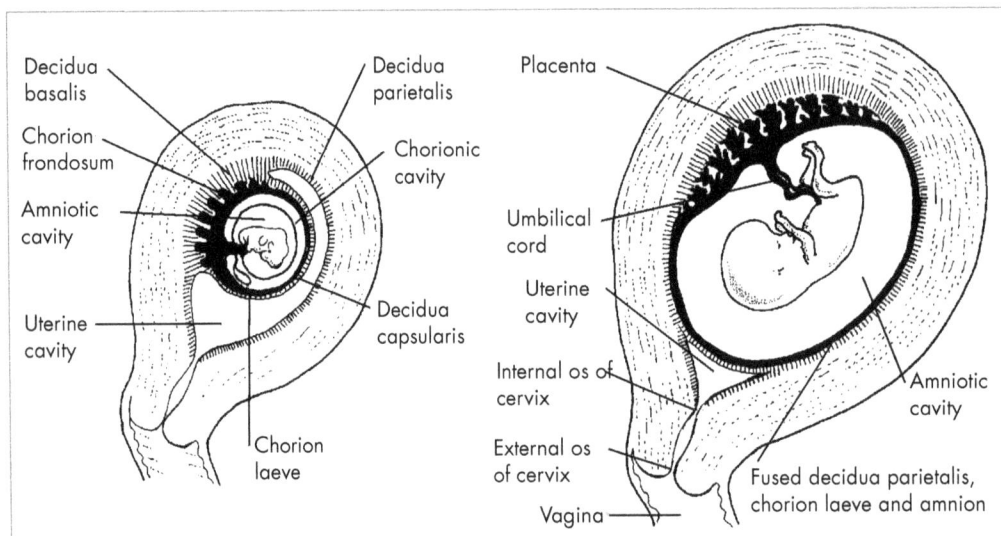

Figure 7.17 Formation of the chorion: The embryo takes on fetal form by days 22–56

Fundus of uterus

Myometrium

Decidua vera

Amniotic cavity

Decidua capsularis

Chorionic cavity

Uterine cavity

Decidua basalis

Chorionic villi

Amnion

Embryo

Yolk sac

Internal cervical os

Cervical canal

External cervical os

Vagina

±24 DAYS

±30 DAYS

Chorionic villi

Amnion growing outwards towards the chorion

Embryo

Connecting stalk

Yolk sac

Amniotic cavity

Chorionic cavity

±9 WEEKS

±20 WEEKS

Placenta

Amniotic cavity filled with liquor amnii

Amnion

Yolk sac within umbilical cord

The amnion covering the umbilical cord

Chorionic cavity

Chorion laeve (smooth chorion)

The amnion has taken up the chorionic cavity and the amnion has adhered to the chorion to form the fetal sac.

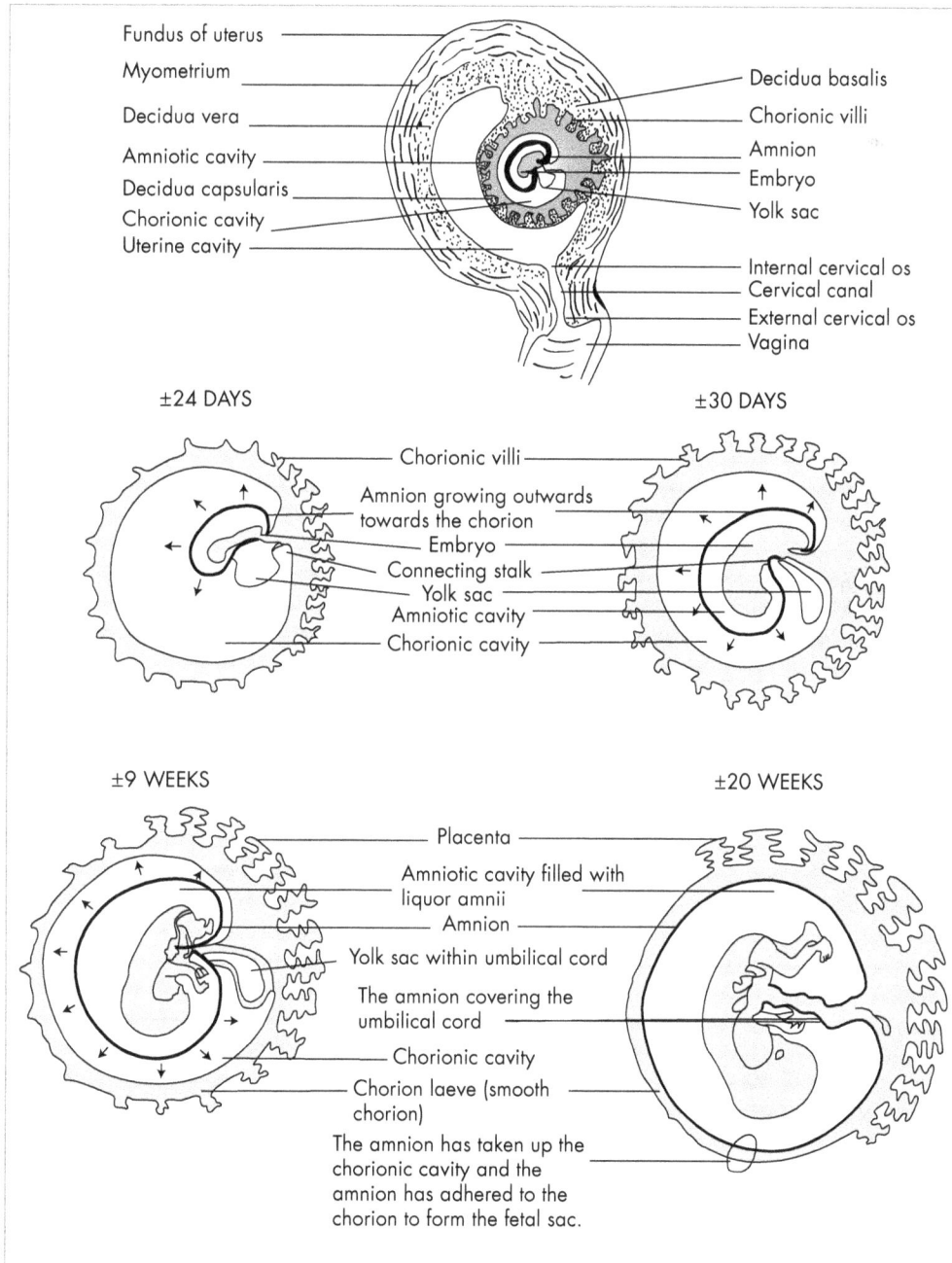

Figure 7.18 Sagittal section of a gravid uterus showing how the amnion covers the umbilical cord and how the fetal sac develops: Day 22–56

In Figure 7.19 on the next page, the age of the embryo is shown in terms of days after fertilisation. The actual length is shown on the left of each drawing and the measurement is shown as a dotted line on each drawing (GL = greatest length; CR = crown–rump; CH = crown–heel). Figure 7.20 on page 104 illustrates the development of the fingers.

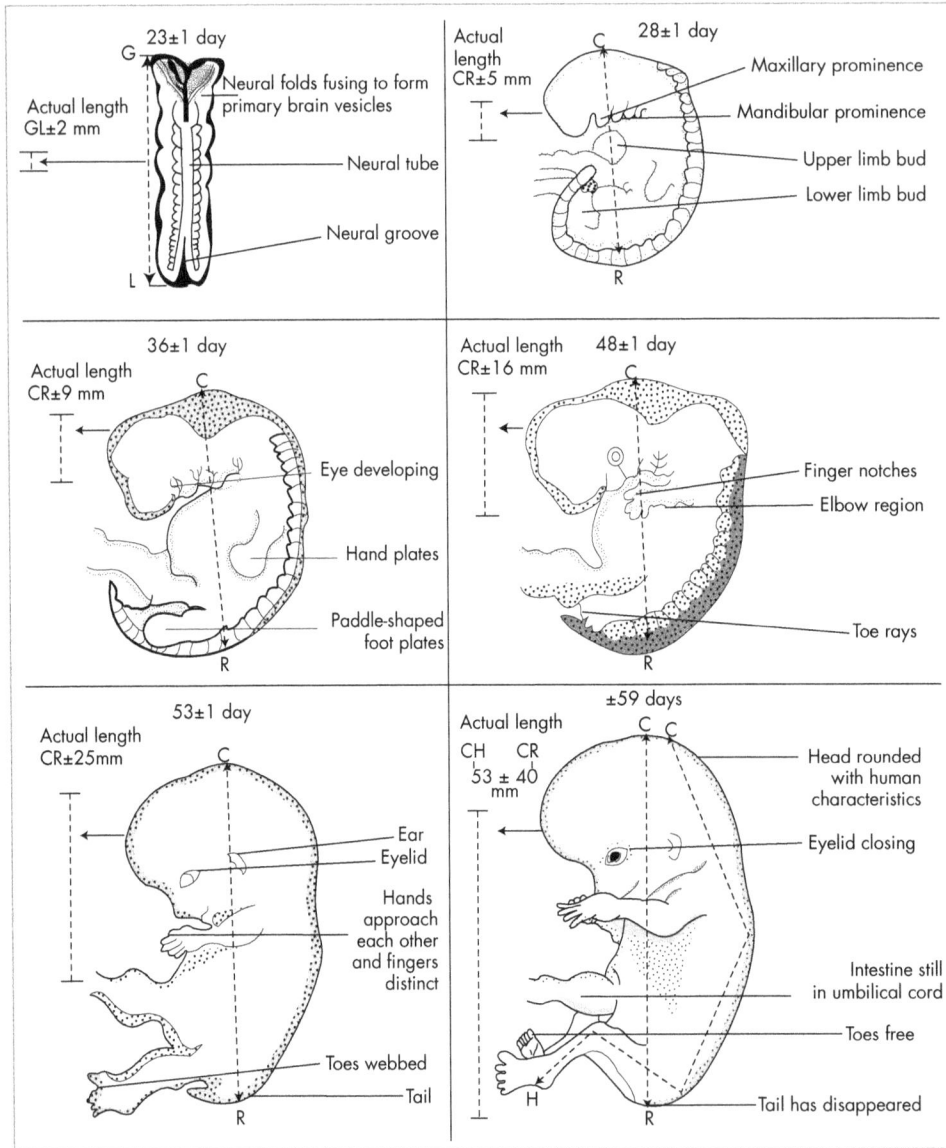

Figure 7.19 Development of the embryo from 23 to 59 days

The development and growth of the embryo and the changes that occur happen systematically and at specific times under normal circumstances. This facilitates the estimation of the stages of development in the embryo, as shown in Table 7.2.

Table 7.2

Early development of the embryo (Chudleigh & Pearce, 1995: 293)

Age: weeks	Age: days	GSV: ml	CRL: mm	Main characteristics
3 weeks	20–21	0.2		Neural groove present and neural tube forming
	22–23			Embryo slightly curved
	24–25			Embryo curving further; optic vesicles formed
	26–27			Upper limb buds and heart prominence appear
4 weeks	28–30	1.0	Fetus not noted	Embryo is C-shaped; upper limb buds flipper-like; lower limb buds and tail present
	31–32			Upper limb buds paddle-shaped
5 weeks	33–36	4.5		**Primitive heart beating**
	37–40			Foot plates formed; hand plates formed; lower limbs paddle-shaped
6 weeks	41–43	5.9	4	Finger rays appear; trunk straightening
	44–46		6	Toe rays and elbow region visible; eyelids forming; nipples and finger notches visible
	47–48		8	Limbs extend ventrally; trunk longer and straighter
7 weeks	49–51	17.8	10	Fingers distinct but webbed; toe notches seen
	52–53		12	Hands and feet approach each other; fingers distinct and longer; toes webbed
	54–55		14	Toes free and longer; eyelids and ears distinct
8 weeks	56	22.4	16	Head more rounded, with human characteristics; tail has disappeared; bulge still present in umbilical cord due to herniation of intestines; sex not yet distinguishable

The size and stage of embryo development are of use in estimating the age of an embryo that is aborted. However, an embryo of less than six weeks is very rarely seen, as it is minute and often not noticed in the blood clot.

The fetal heart beat

The cardiovascular system is the first system to function in the embryo. The primitive heart is contracting by the 22nd day and the formation of the heart is essentially complete by the 42nd day (the sixth week after fertilisation).

The gestational sac within the uterus of the pregnant woman can be seen on an ultrasound scan from four to five weeks after fertilisation (that is, six to seven weeks from the first day of the LMP). The embryo's heart can be seen beating by the seventh week.

The fetus: Growth and development

The fetal period is taken from the beginning of the ninth week after fertilisation to term (the end of the thirty-eighth week), or from the beginning of the eleventh week to the end of the fortieth week, after the first day of the LMP.

By the beginning of the ninth week after fertilisation, the human embryo has developed into a recognisable human being and most of the body structures have already started to develop (see Figure 7.19). The fetal period is mainly concerned with the differentiation and growth of tissues and organs that have already appeared. For this reason, the fetus is far less vulnerable than the embryo to the harmful and deforming effects of teratogenic agents.

5 weeks

Upper limb bud

Hand plate

A

B

6 weeks

Developing digits

Notches between developing digits

Elbow

C

D

8 weeks

Webbing between fingers

Fingers separated

E

F

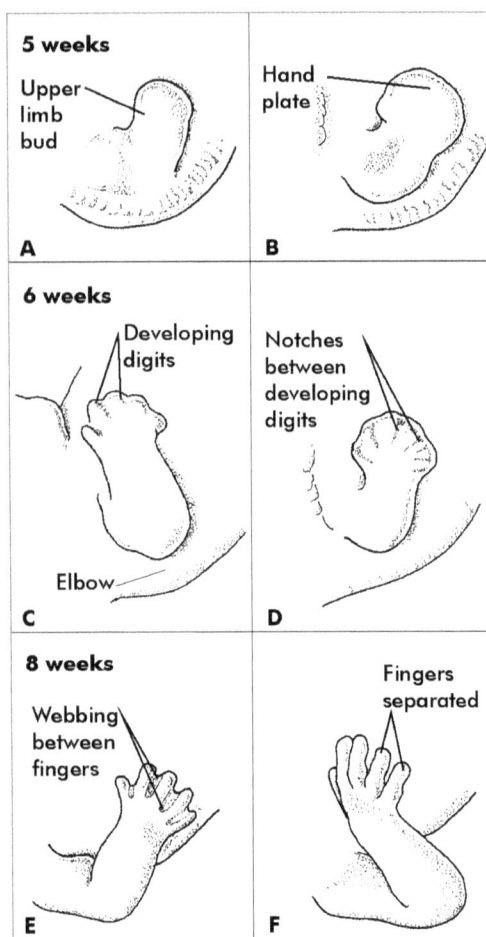

Figure 7.20 Development of upper limbs and digits by 5 to 8 weeks

The transition from the embryonic to the fetal form is gradual, although the rate of body growth of the fetus is remarkable, especially between the ninth and sixteenth weeks. There is also a significant gain in weight by the fetus in the third trimester, especially during the final month in utero.

Different fetuses will grow at different rates, blurring the findings of GA determined by ultrasound. A range of normal parameters are compared to determine fetal growth and development (such as biparietal measurements, femur length and abdominal circumference, as in Table 7.3). After the twentieth week of pregnancy, the fetal growth parameters have a two-week variance until the thirtieth week and a three-week variance until the fortieth week. The implication is that clinical estimations can differ by two to three weeks from the real GA. Even ultrasound, if not done before 20 weeks, carries a risk of error depending on the skills of the professional. Therefore, term is the fortieth week from the first day of the LMP and at term the average newborn baby is 500 mm (50 cm) long and weighs 3 400 g (3.4 kg).

Urinating, swallowing, hiccuping and peristalsis are all normal in the fetus. Defecating, however, is not normal and may indicate periods of hypoxia, bringing about relaxation of the anal sphincter.

Breathing movements of the lungs are present so that the lungs are able to exhale and inhale when the baby is born. The lungs are inflated with fluid derived from the lungs and from the amniotic membrane at term; this fluid has to be expelled at birth before it can be replaced by air.

Table 7.3 shows the mass, biparietal diameter (BPD) and characteristics of the fetus at different stages.

Table 7.3

The growth and development of the fetus after nine weeks (Chudleigh & Pierce, 1995: 294)

Age: weeks	BPD: mm	Average mass: gr	Characteristics
9		2	Eyelids closing or closed; head rounded
10		4	Intestine in abdomen; fingernails appearing; ossification centres have developed in most bones; urine is now excreted into the liquor amnii which is swallowed by the fetus
12	20	14	Sex distinguishable; neck well defined; the nasal septum and palate have fused
14	28	110	Head erect; lower limbs well developed
16	36	200	Ears stand out from head
18	40	320	Vernix caseosa present; toenails appearing; fetal movements present, which can be felt by the mother as quickening; the fetal heart can be heard on auscultation

continued

Age: weeks	BPD: mm	Average mass: gr	Characteristics
20	48	460	Lanugo (body hair) visible; brown fat starts to form for heat production
22	54	630	Skin wrinkled and red; brain development occurring
24	60	820	Fingernails developed; body is lean; traces of surfactant present in lungs and respiration is now possible
26	64	1 000	Eyes partially open; eyelashes present; slight breathing movements present
According to South African guidelines, the fetus is now viable.			
28	70	1 300	Eyes open; hair on head plentiful; skin slightly wrinkled
30	74	1 700	Toenails developed; body filling out; testes descending (if male); pupillary light reflex is present
32	80	2 100	Fingernails reach fingertips; skin pink and smooth
36	88	2 900	Body plump; lanugo almost absent; toenails reach toe tips; limbs flexed; grasp is firm; the circumference of the head and abdomen almost the same
38	92	3 400	Prominent chest; breasts protrude; if male, testes in scrotum or palpable in inguinal canals; fingernails extend beyond fingertips; ossification has progressed, especially at the ends of long bones
The fetus is at term.			

Figure 7.21 shows the growth of the fetus's head during pregnancy.

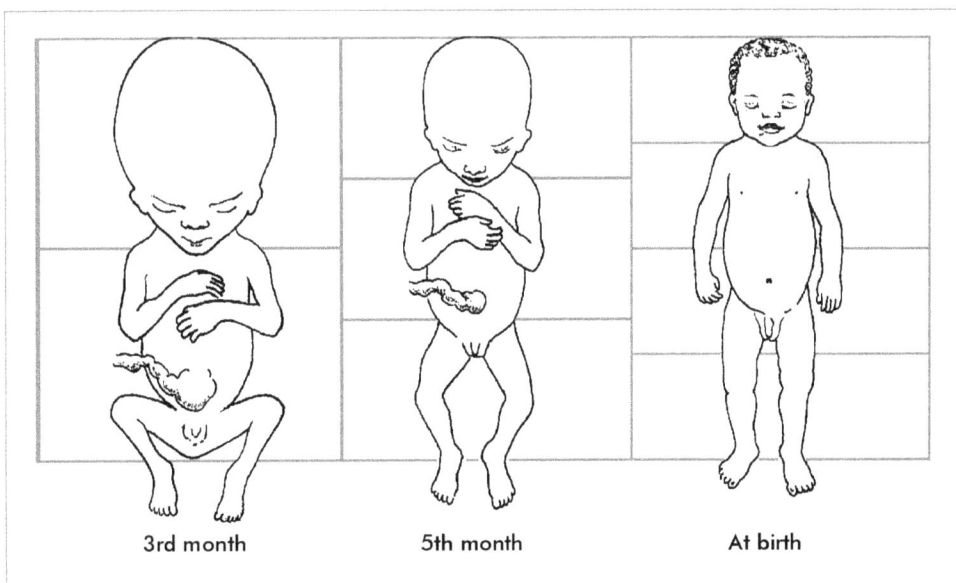

3rd month   5th month   At birth

Figure 7.21 Proportional growth of the head in pregnancy

Factors causing impaired fetal growth

The factors mainly responsible for fetal growth impairment are either directly acquired through the mother or are caused by an inefficient placenta, which is usually due to certain maternal conditions. Fetal causes are usually genetic. At birth, babies with growth retardation are small for gestational age (SGA).

A summary of the causes of growth restriction are as follows:

▶ Placental insufficiency or impaired uteroplacental blood flow causes growth restriction.
▶ Maternal conditions such as hypertension, hyperpyrexia, chronic infections and cardiac disease prevent the placenta from efficiently transmitting nutrients from the mother to the fetus.
▶ Genetic factors and chromosomal aberrations, such as Down's syndrome, achondroplasia and dwarfism cause babies to be SGA at birth.
▶ Smoking is known to affect the growth rate of the fetus because of its effect upon placental growth. The condition is worsened if the mother's diet is deficient.
▶ Alcohol and drug/substance addiction can cause growth impairment, congenital abnormalities and addiction in the newborn.
▶ Infections of the mother, for example viruses such as rubella and some other pathogens such as *Treponema pallidum*, can pass through the placental membrane and adversely affect fetal growth.
▶ With a multiple pregnancy, there is an increased nutritional burden on the mother for each additional fetus and the placenta and babies are smaller in size than a singleton.
▶ Maternal malnutrition plays an important role; if the mother is lacking in certain necessary nutrients, the fetus will also be deprived.
▶ Prolonged pregnancy is considered a factor in fetal demise. It is widely believed that the placenta ages progressively towards the end of pregnancy. Thus, the longer the pregnancy lasts after term, the greater the placental degeneration. This increases the risk of fetal hypoxia, together with intrauterine growth restriction (IUGR) and even fetal death.

The umbilical cord

The umbilical cord, attached to the fetus at the umbilicus, is the link between the fetus and the placenta. The other end of the umbilical cord is inserted into the centre of the placenta, which is attached to the decidua of the uterine wall.

The connecting or body stalk, which joins the inner cell mass to the trophoblast, develops into the umbilical cord, as explained in the development of the zygote (see Figure 7.18 on page 101). The body stalk consists of mesoderm cells, which develop into fetal blood vessels contained within the umbilical cord. These blood vessels transport nutrient-enriched fetal blood from the chorionic villi in the placenta along the umbilical cord to the fetal heart and then return the nutrient-depleted fetal blood back to the placenta for replenishment.

The blood vessels in the umbilical cord include (see colour illustration C4 on page 72):

▶ *one umbilical vein:* a thin-walled, wide-bored blood vessel which carries 85 per cent oxygenated blood from the placenta to the fetus
▶ *two umbilical arteries:* thick-walled blood vessels with a narrower bore that carry de-oxygenated blood (only 50 per cent oxygenated) from the fetus to the placenta.

The vein and the two arteries divide and narrow in the placenta until they become capillaries. They then anastomose, creating unbroken circulation from the fetal heart through the placenta and back to the fetal heart.

The arteries are usually wound loosely around the vein, along the length of the cord, and the vessels are surrounded by a jelly-like substance called Wharton's jelly, which protects and supports the vessels. Wharton's jelly sometimes forms lumps, which are known as false knots (see Figure 7.27 on page 116). Figure 7.22 shows the umbilical arteries and vein.

The outer sheath or covering of the umbilical cord is developed from the ectoderm cells of the amniotic membrane. At the placental end of the cord, the outer sheath is continuous with the amnion covering the fetal side of the placenta. At the umbilicus, the outer covering of the umbilical cord is continuous with the skin of the fetus.

At birth, the average diameter of the cord is 10–15 mm (1–1.5 cm) and the average length of the cord is 550–600 mm (55–60 cm). The cord should be inspected at birth to ensure that all three blood vessels are present, as the absence of an artery is often associated with a congenital abnormality. Very rarely, four umbilical vessels (two arteries and two veins) are present.

The membranes

The amnion and chorion

The amnion is also known as the amniotic membrane. The small cavity that appears in the ectoderm cells between the embedding trophoblast and the inner cell mass at the end of the first week after fertilisation is the beginning of the amniotic cavity or sac.

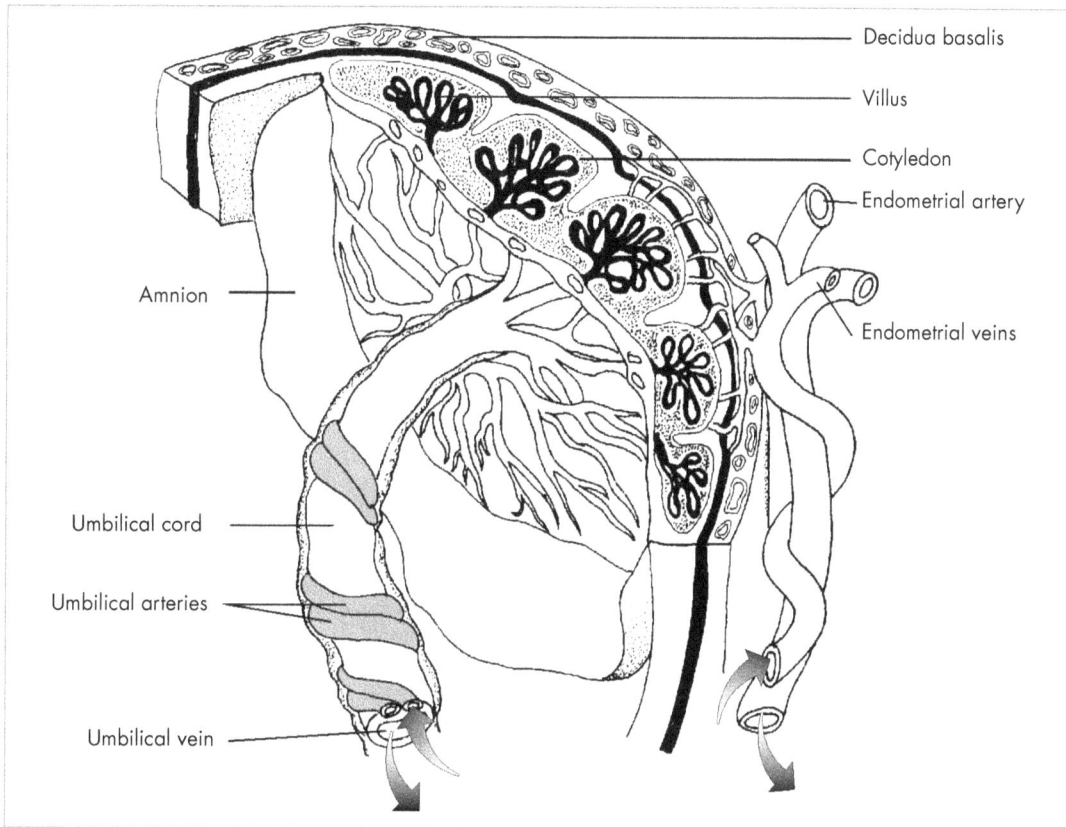

Figure 7.22 The umbilical cord

The membrane encompassing this cavity or sac, which is formed from these ectoderm cells, is known as the amnion. The sac becomes filled with fluid which is derived from the maternal blood and which diffuses through the trophoblastic cells. This fluid is known as the amniotic fluid or the liquor amnii.

The amniotic sac increases in size until it completely surrounds the embryo, which then floats freely in the amniotic fluid. As the amniotic sac swells in the chorionic cavity, the amnion envelops the umbilical cord, forming its outer covering. The amnion also comes into contact with the fetal side of the placenta and with the chorionic membrane (the chorion) and so completely fills the chorionic cavity by the twentieth week after fertilisation.

Where the amnion comes into contact with the chorion, they adhere. However, after the delivery of the placenta and membranes, these two membranes can be separated from each other, up to the insertion of the cord into the placenta.

The amnion (near the fetus) and the outer chorion (near the decidua) (the amniochorionic membrane) form the fetal sac (see colour illustration C3 on page 71).

The fully developed amnion is translucent and smooth and is a relatively tough membrane. This membrane usually ruptures at birth, allowing liquor amnii to escape. Should it not rupture and should the baby be born with the amnion over his or her head, it could suffocate the baby. This is known as being born with a caul. (According to legend, this caul is supposed to indicate magical or divining properties, and it is greatly prized in certain cultures.)

The chorion is opaque and is easily torn, whereas the amnion is tough. The chorion lies on the side of the uterus. If a piece of amnion or chorion remains in the uterus after birth, it can cause massive bleeding.

Amniotic liquor

The fluid that fills the amniotic sack is also known as the amniotic fluid or liquor amnii. It is normally a clear, pale, straw-coloured, alkaline fluid (pH 7.2).

The origin of the amniotic fluid is not clearly understood, but it is thought to be formed mainly by fluid diffusing through the chorionic and amniotic membranes from the maternal blood in the decidua of the uterus. Some fluid is also thought to diffuse through the umbilical cord.

The fetus passes urine into the liquor. The fetus also swallows the liquor, which is then absorbed from the fetal intestines, passed into the fetal circulation and so back to the placenta and the maternal circulation. Half the volume of fluid contained within the amniotic sac is exchanged every 90 minutes, or the whole volume every three hours. The amount of liquor in the amniotic sac increases at a rate which is fairly predictable, and is approximately as follows:

▶ 10 weeks: about 35 ml
▶ 10–20 weeks: a rapid increase in volume to about 300 ml
▶ 20–30 weeks: doubling to about 600 ml
▶ 30–38 weeks: a slow increase slowly to about 1 000 ml
▶ after 38 weeks: a decrease to about 600 ml at term (40 weeks).

Two abnormal conditions related to the volume of amniotic fluid are the following:

1. *Polyhydramnios* refers to too much liquor, or more than 1 500 ml. Polyhydramnios is often associated with abnormal conditions such as multiple pregnancy, or where the fetus cannot swallow, for instance a fetus with anencephaly or with oesophageal atresia (see chapters 24 and 45).
2. *Oligohydramnios* refers to too little liquor, or less than 300 ml. Oligohydramnios is usually associated with conditions where the fetus cannot pass urine, such as congenital absence of the kidneys or urethral blockage. It is often associated with IUGR due to placental insufficiency. There is also a marked reduction of amniotic fluid in prolonged pregnancies and, of course, in circumstances where the membranes have ruptured and the liquor has drained out (see Chapter 23).

The composition of the amniotic fluid

Amniotic fluid is similar to that of extracellular fluid. It is composed of:

▶ 98 per cent water
▶ 2 per cent solids, made up of:
  • electrolytes
  • proteins and derivatives: creatinine, urea, uric acid and all the known enzymes that exist in the human body
  • glucose
  • fats, lipids (phospholipids and cholesterol)
  • hormones: hCG, human placental lactogen (HPL), oestrogens and progesterone, prolactin
  • pigments: bilirubin in early pregnancy and in premature newborns, which disappears as the fetal liver matures after 30 weeks

• exfoliated matter from the amnion and fetus: hair, vernix, cells from the skin, mouth and urinary tract, etc
▶ prostaglandin, levels of which increase abruptly during labour.

The functions of the amniotic fluid

During pregnancy, amniotic fluid acts mainly to form a buffer between the fetus and the uterus to permit symmetrical growth of the embryo by equalising pressures and to prevent the amnion from adhering to the embryo and later the fetus. It also cushions the fetus from impacts to the maternal abdomen and maintains the fetus at a constant temperature. The fluid allows the fetus to move freely for the development of muscles. Together with the intact amnion, it protects the fetus from infection.

During labour, the amniotic fluid equalises the compression on the fetus caused by uterine contractions and prevents excessive diminution of the placental site and consequent hypoxia of the fetus when the membranes rupture. The fluid flushes the birth canal, and so helps to reduce the likelihood of the fetus becoming infected during birth.

The amniotic fluid is swallowed by the fetus and forms meconium in the colon. The fetus also breathes the fluid into the lungs and the lungs develop. When the fluid is diminished or lost, hypoplastic (under-developed lungs) may be present.

The placenta and fetoplacental unit

The placenta is the connecting link between the fetus and the mother. It is a circular or disc-shaped organ, with the chorionic membrane extending outwards from its edges to form a sac. The umbilical cord is attached to the centre of the fetal side of the placenta. The chorionic sac and the fetal side of the placenta are lined with the amniotic membrane, which is filled with amniotic fluid in which the fetus floats.

The fetus, placenta, umbilical cord, membranes and liquor are together referred to as the fetoplacental unit. The fetus can be seen as a true parasite, living within and deriving all its nourishment from and through the mother. Regular growth will take place and the fetus will thrive until term. Then, at birth, it should present as a normal newborn baby.

All the nourishment that the fetus derives from the mother is obtained through the placenta, which permits an exchange of nutrients from the maternal bloodstream through the placental membrane and into the fetal bloodstream. In this way, the maternal blood and the fetal blood do not come into contact with each other at all, unless there is an abnormal breakdown in the placental membrane. The mother and the fetus each have their own separate blood circulations and can have different blood groups. Figure 7.23 shows details of the placental circulation.

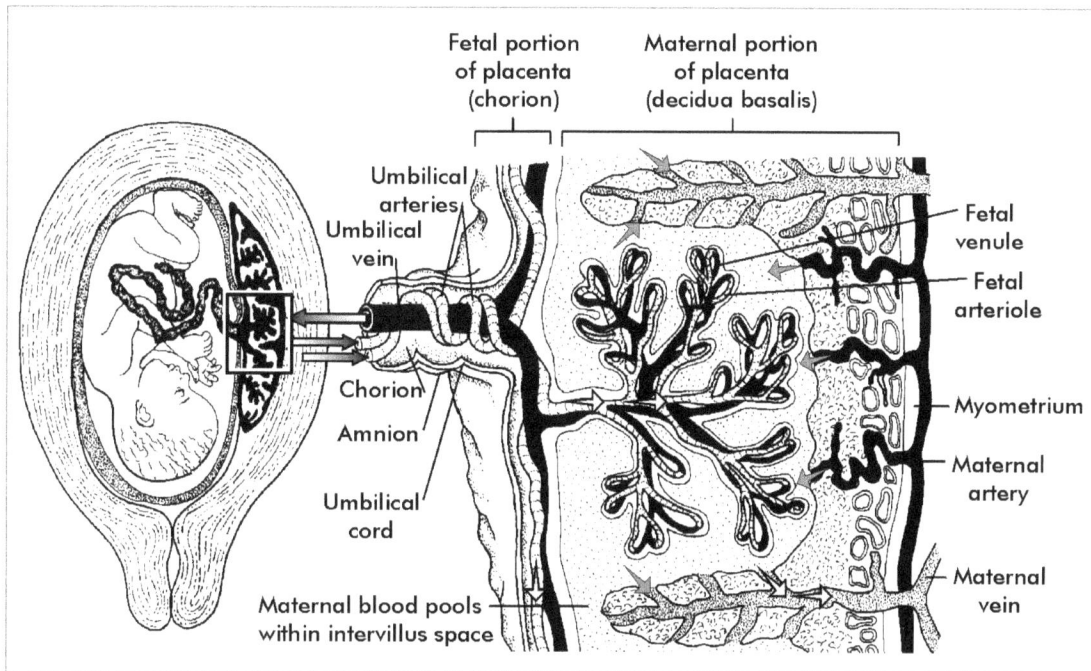

Figure 7.23 The placental circulation

Should the placenta not be as efficient as it is meant to be, the fetus will not receive all the necessary nourishment. This could also occur if the mother's intake of nourishment is insufficient or if the mother has an abnormal condition, preventing the nourishment from either reaching the placenta or penetrating the placental membrane.

The development of the placenta

The placenta and its chorionic membrane (the chorion) are continuous with one another and develop from the outer trophoblast layers of the zygote, which are the precursors of the chorionic villi. The primary chorionic villi develop towards the end of the second week after fertilisation, and as they grow, they become known as secondary chorionic. By the end of the third week they have become fully developed (tertiary) chorionic, as shown in Figure 7.24 on the next page. As explained in the development of the zygote, the outer syncytial layer of these villi produces a proteolytic enzyme, which has the ability to erode the maternal decidua and blood vessels.

When the zygote or embryo implants itself, the uterine endometrium changes to become the decidua that is divided into three regions or areas:

1. The *decidua basalis* (see Figure 7.17 on page 100) is that part of the decidua into which the trophoblast first embeds

and which lies under or is at the base of the zygote. The decidua basalis, together with the chorion frondosum, will eventually develop into the placenta.

2. The *decidua capsularis* (see Figure 7.17 on page 100 and Figure 7.18 on page 101) is that part of the decidua that grows over or encapsulates the zygote. As the embryo develops and grows inside the trophoblast, the decidua capsularis, which encircles the trophoblast, is stretched outwards into the uterine cavity. This stretching thins out the decidua capsularis and also the chorion laeve (smooth chorion) within it, forming two membranes, which gradually come into contact with the remaining decidua of the uterine cavity, the decidua vera.

3. The *decidua vera* or true decidua is that part of the uterine decidua that is not affected during the initial implanting of the trophoblast. However, as the conceptus grows and pushes the decidua capsularis and chorion laeve outwards, these eventually come into contact with the decidua vera. By 12 weeks the uterine cavity is completely filled.

The decidua capsularis and the decidua vera then fuse and the decidua capsularis disappears. The chorion laeve, made up of atrophied chorionic villi, remains and becomes the chorionic membrane or the chorion (see Figure 7.18 on page 101).

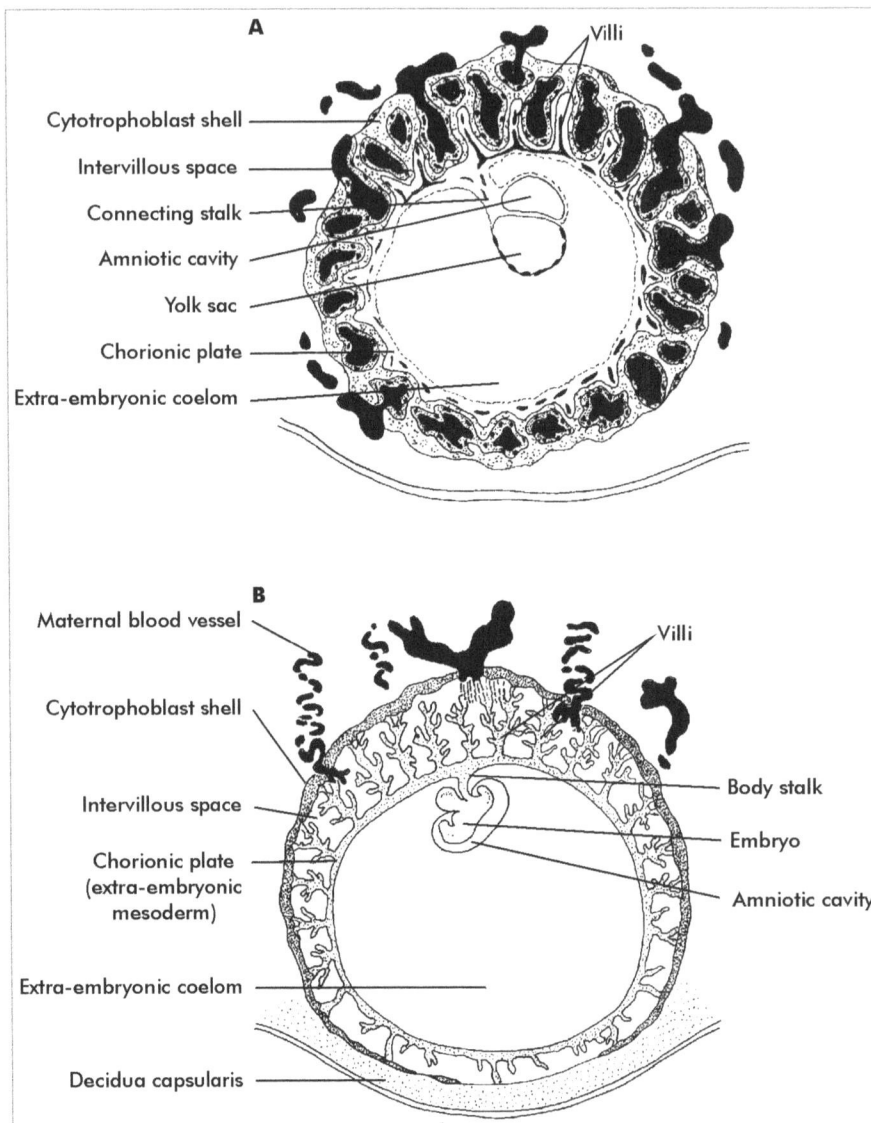

Figure 7.24 Radial appearance of villi

As the chorionic villi encroach into the maternal decidua, those villi that are situated in the decidua basalis are well nourished. They enlarge, branch out extensively and increase in size (see colour illustration C5 on page 73). This area of prolific growth of the chorionic villi is known as the chorion frondosum (leafy chorion) and this becomes the fetal portion of the placenta. The actual decidua basalis into which this chorion frondosum embeds itself becomes the maternal portion of the placenta. This maternal side of the placenta is divided into lobules or cotyledons by deep furrows or sulci.

The chorionic villi embedded in the decidua capsularis, on the other hand, are not well nourished. These villi shrink and atrophy, leaving a bare area, which is known as the chorion laeve (light chorion) and which becomes the chorionic membrane or the chorion.

When the decidua is eroded, some of the villi attach themselves firmly to the connective tissue of the decidua. These are known as anchoring villi. Most of the villi, however, are not attached to the maternal decidua; the ends of these villi are free-floating.

When the maternal arterioles are eroded, the maternal blood spurts into the spaces between the chorionic villi, the intervillous spaces (see Figure 7.25), and the free-floating villi are bathed in maternal blood, allowing an exchange of materials through the placental membrane. These open maternal blood vessels are known as the *maternal blood sinuses* (see Figure 7.23 on page 109).

The blood in the intervillous spaces, besides containing oxygen and nutrients from the maternal circulation, also contains fetal waste products, which are absorbed into the maternal circulation via the eroded maternal venules. The circulation in these intervillous spaces is slow and sluggish, allowing a free exchange of nutrients and gases by the processes of osmosis and diffusion through the placental membrane. A small percentage of these substances is actively transported through the placental membrane by enzymatic reaction and also by pinocytosis (similar to phagocytosis) (see Figure 7.23).

Placental functions and activities

All the functions and activities of the placenta are not yet fully understood, but a normal, functioning placenta is essential for fetal metabolism and well-being (see Figure 7.23).

The placenta as barrier

The membranes of the trophoblasts in the placenta form a barrier between the fetus and the uterus. The placenta thus is a barrier against harmful agents, especially in the first trimester. However, it is not as effective as was previously thought, and many substances are able to pass from the mother's bloodstream through the membrane into the fetal blood.

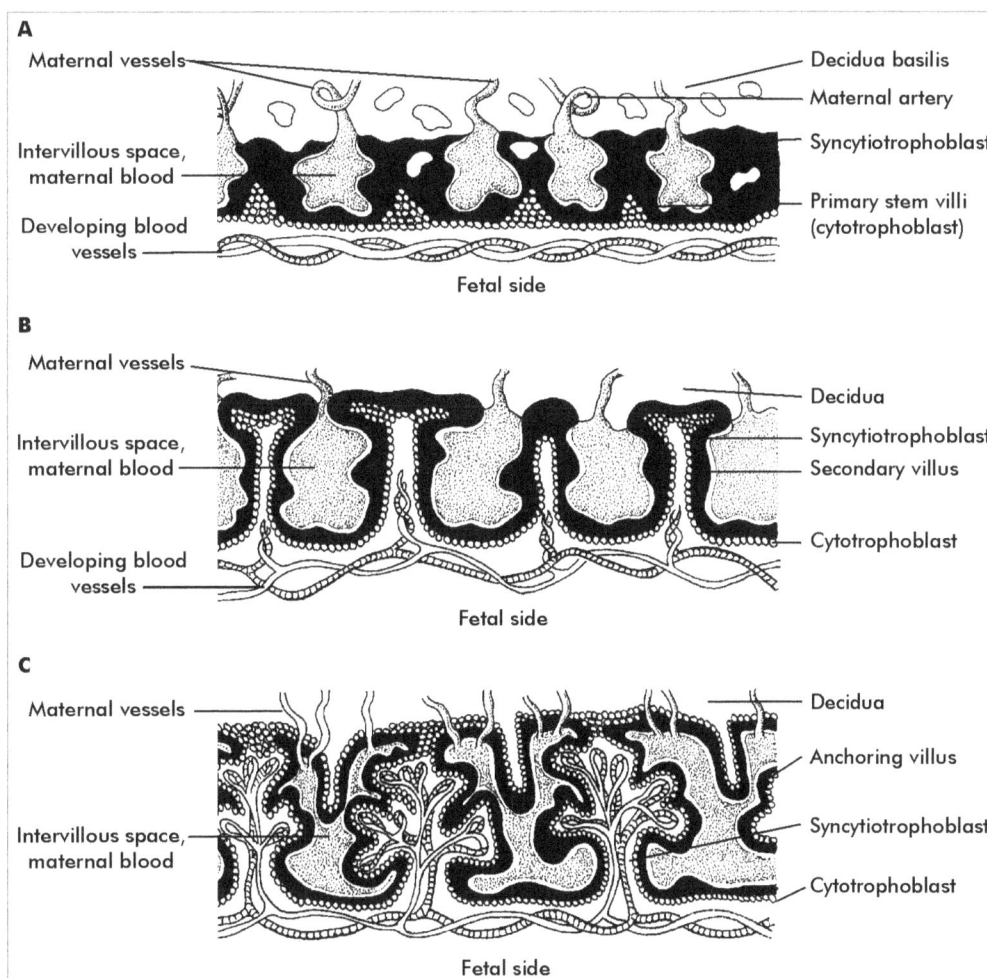

Figure 7.25 The development of intervillous spaces

From the third to about the twentieth week, the trophoblasts consist of four layers (Figure 7.12 on page 95), namely:
1. the *syncytiotrophoblast*, an outer layer of syncytial cells
2. the *cytotrophoblast*, the second layer of cytotropic cells
3. *mesoblast cells* or a connective tissue core, surrounding the fetal capillaries
4. the *endothelium* of each fetal capillary.

After the twentieth week, however, the trophoblasts may only consist of two or three layers, as the outer layers (the syncytiotrophoblast and the cytotrophoblast) become progressively thinner. These membranes separate the fetus from the uterus. Maternal and fetal blood never mixes.

Maternal and fetal erythrocytes are too large to pass through this membrane. It is thought, however, that a few fetal blood cells do escape into the maternal blood. They are instantly destroyed before antigens are made against them. During an abortion or in other instances when the chorionic villi are damaged, this barrier can be broken. Fortunately, many bacteria are too large to penetrate this membrane.

The placenta and hypertension in pregnancy

Evidence confirms that the infiltration of the trophoblast into the decidua, normally after 20 weeks of gestation, if deficient or partial is linked to the likely development of pregnancy-induced hypertension (PIH) (Lain & Roberts, 2002).

Towards the end of pregnancy, as the placenta begins to age, the surfaces of the villi are covered with fibrinoid material, which may decrease the permeability of the membrane (see Chapter 23).

Certain substances of larger molecular size are prohibited from passing through to the fetus; this is known as the *placental barrier*. The efficiency of the barrier depends upon the permeability of the placental membrane at a given time and on the size of the molecules present at that time.

The substances that do pass through the placental barrier may not all be of benefit to the fetus, and some may even cause fetal abnormalities. These substances include:
- *gases:* oxygen, carbon dioxide, carbon monoxide
- *nutrients:* water, glucose, amino acids, vitamins and mineral salts
- *hormones:* thyroxin, conjugated steroids, testosterone, some synthetic progestins
- *electrolytes:* these pass freely through the membrane, which means that intravenous electrolytes given to the mother will affect the water and electrolyte status of the fetus

- *antibodies:* IgG gamma globulins reach the fetus and provide passive immunity. However, a woman who is Rh factor negative and whose fetus is Rh positive will produce antibodies to the fetus's Rh factor, which can cause breakdown of fetal red blood cells
- *medications:* most medications pass through the membrane and some can adversely affect the embryo and later the fetus. In early pregnancy, the development of the embryo can be affected, for example, by thalidomide. Certain sedatives given during labour, for example morphine and barbiturates, can cause depressed respiration of the newborn baby
- *alcohol and narcotics*
- *infectious agents:* these can pass through the placental membrane, particularly viruses that are extremely small, for example the herpes and rubella viruses. *Treponema pallidum*, which causes syphilis, is able to penetrate the placental membrane after the first trimester
- *waste products:* of fetal metabolism, such as urea.

Respiration

The placenta acts as the respiratory organ for the fetus. Oxygen is transferred through the placental membrane from the mother's blood in the intervillous spaces to the fetal blood and circulation. This is essential for the development, growth and survival of the fetus. As a result of this anabolism (building-up process) and catabolism (breaking-down process), carbon dioxide levels in the fetal blood rise. The carbon dioxide is then transported by the fetal circulation back to the placenta and transferred across the placental membrane into the maternal blood circulation. It is then exhaled via the maternal lungs.

Nutrition

Nutrients necessary for normal fetal development, growth and survival, such as glucose, amino acids, vitamins and mineral salts, are transferred from the mother across the placental membrane to the fetus.

Excretion

Waste products, such as creatinine, urea, uric acid and bilirubin, which form as a result of the metabolism taking place in the fetal body, are transferred from the fetal bloodstream across the placental membrane to the mother's blood circulation for excretion.

Endocrine

The placenta is a temporary endocrine organ. The hormones produced by the placenta are essential for the maintenance of pregnancy and are responsible for the preparation of the maternal body for pregnancy, labour and feeding the newborn baby. The major hormones produced by the placenta are:

▶ hCG
▶ oestrogens
▶ progesterone
▶ HPL.

Enzyme function

The placenta contains a wide variety of body enzymes, most of which represent the range of structural and metabolic enzymes also found in all body cells. Some of the enzymes play an important role in the synthesis of proteins and steroids. Enzymes that are specifically produced in the trophoblast of the placenta are heat-stable alkaline phosphatases (HSAP), responsible for the active transport at membrane level in a variety of tissue, and cystine aminopeptidase (CAP), referred to as oxytocinase, which breaks down natural oxytocin (Chard & Klopper, 1982).

The placenta at term

After the birth of the newborn, the placenta and membranes are delivered. It is essential that the placenta and membranes are examined carefully to ensure that they look healthy and normal, and that no part of either the placenta or membranes has remained behind in the uterus. Should any of these be retained, the uterus would not be able to contract properly and postpartum bleeding could occur. This retained tissue would also make the patient more susceptible to infection.

The midwife must be able to recognise a normal placenta at term and must be able to identify what abnormalities can occur and what to observe the patient for. (See also colour illustration C4 on page 72.)

As mentioned, the umbilical cord connects the fetus with the placenta. It is covered with amnion and is usually inserted into the centre of the fetal surface of the placenta (colour illustration C6 on page 74). The length of the umbilical cord is about 55 cm. The average thickness of the cord is about 1.5 cm. It has three blood vessels. There should be one large, thin-walled vein and two smaller, thick-walled arteries. Wharton's jelly can be seen surrounding the vessels.

A normal placenta is shaped like a disc, with an almost even thickness throughout. The diameter is about 200 mm (20 cm). The central thickness is about 25 mm (2.5 cm). It has a mass of approximately one-sixth of the baby's mass, averaging 500 g. It has two surfaces, which are called the maternal and the fetal surfaces:

1. *The maternal surface* (colour illustration C6a on page 74) is composed of the decidua basalis and has thousands of chorionic villi containing fetal blood, which are embedded in the decidua basalis. The presence of maternal blood in the intervillous spaces gives it its deep red or purple colour. The maternal surface is divided into 16–20 lobules or cotyledons, which are separated by deep grooves or sulci.
2. *The fetal surface* (colour illustration C6b on page 74) faces the fetus during pregnancy and has the umbilical cord inserted into it. It is covered with the amniotic membrane (the amnion), which gives it a smooth, shiny appearance. The amnion can be stripped away from the fetal surface up to the insertion of the cord. Fetal blood vessels can be seen radiating from the insertion of the umbilical cord out towards the edges of the placenta. These blood vessels are branches of the umbilical vein and the two umbilical arteries. As they branch, they dip into the placental tissue and become smaller as they approach the placental edge.

The two membranes attached to the placenta are the chorion and the amnion. The amnion is the membrane on the fetus's side and the chorion is on the maternal side. The clinical significance of these two membranes is that the chorion tears easily, which means that pieces of the chorion can remain behind in the uterus.

7.8 Abnormalities of the placenta, membranes and cord

From time to time, certain placental, membrane and cord abnormalities are found. Some of these abnormalities are of significance because they pose a danger to the mother or the fetus. An abnormal placenta may also be an indication of an abnormal maternal or fetal condition.

Abnormalities of the placenta

Placenta succenturiate

An accessory lobe of placental tissue has developed separately from the placenta and there are fetal blood vessels running off the edge of the placenta, through the chorion, to and from the succenturiate lobe (see colour illustration C7 on page 75). This is a relatively common abnormality, where a group of chorionic villi which should have atrophied and become part of the chorion laeve have instead been nourished and have grown and hypertrophied.

This abnormality poses a danger, because this lobe may be retained in the uterus after the delivery of the placenta and could cause severe PPH and infection.

On inspection, a second hole may be noticed in the chorion, and after the amnion has been stripped from the chorion and from the fetal side of the placenta, blood vessels can be seen running off the edge of the placenta, through the chorion and ending at the hole.

If signs of a placenta succenturiate are found, they should be recorded and reported to a doctor immediately.

Placenta bipartite or tripartite

This is a very rare condition, in which the placenta has developed as two or even three separate lobes (see colour illustration C8 on page 76). The blood vessels from the separate lobes unite at one umbilical cord. Remember that in a multiple pregnancy, there will be a separate cord for each baby.

Placenta circumvallata

In this abnormality, the chorion (and sometimes the amnion as well) has folded back upon itself around the edge of the placenta, before continuing over the edge of the placenta to form the fetal sac (see colour illustration C9 on page 77).

This fold may be firmly attached to the placenta, or the examiner may be able to run a finger around the placenta, under the fold. The danger of this abnormality is that the chorion, or part of it, can become detached from the edge of the placenta and can be retained in the uterus.

Hydatidiform mole (gestational trophoblastic disease)

This is a developmental abnormality of the trophoblast that may occur in the first trimester if there is a vesicular change in the chorionic villi. The chorionic villi become swollen and cystic, like small grapes, and proliferate greatly. No fetal blood vessels develop in these cysts. Consequently, the zygote is not nourished, dies and is absorbed. The pregnancy usually ends in a spontaneous abortion or miscarriage before 20 weeks of pregnancy. In rare cases, the medical practitioner may induce the process to remove the products of conception and may perform a curettage even after a spontaneous miscarriage. If products remain, cancer may develop.

Placental infarcts

True infarcts of the placenta are areas of necrosis where the chorionic villi have been damaged, usually due to vasospasm of the maternal circulation, and the areas around these villi have become calcified. This makes the affected parts of the placenta incompetent. If severe, it causes placental insufficiency. The placenta is usually small and thin and instead of the usual deep red colour, large parts of the placenta have a whitish, anaemic appearance.

Perivillous fibrin deposits may be found in the placenta due to haemodynamic turbulence within the intervillous spaces. These tend to occur in a placenta with a particularly good maternal uteroplacental blood flow and this is part of the normal progressive functioning (ageing) of the placenta.

On the maternal surface, they are seen as tiny, light-greyish, 'gritty' deposits, while on the fetal surface they appear as small, white patches.

The placenta may present with a bruised, hollowed-out area, after the removal of a very dark red blood clot. This indicates that there had been an earlier retroplacental bleed, which could have been caused by either placental abruption or placenta praevia.

Placental colour

A large, pale placenta may indicate that the mother has diabetes mellitus. On the other hand, a large, pale, watery placenta can be an indication of hydrops fetalis due to Rh isoimmunisation, some pathological condition of the fetal kidneys or pituitary gland, or maternal syphilis.

A meconium-stained (yellow) placenta and cord is caused by meconium being passed in utero, for example in IUGR due to a period or periods of fetal hypoxia. Yellow staining can also be due to high levels of bilirubin in the liquor amnii caused by Rh isoimmunisation.

Placenta accreta, increta and percreta

This is a condition where the trophoblastic villi have penetrated through the basal layer of the decidua and become attached to the myometrial cells (placenta accreta). In some instances, the villi have penetrated the myometrial cells (placenta increta) or have even penetrated through to the serosal surface of the uterus (placenta percreta). This condition will usually result in retention of the placenta and will necessitate surgical intervention.

Haemangiomata of the placenta

This is the only common non-trophoblastic tumour of the placenta and occurs in about 1 per cent of all placentae (Fox, 1966). Haemangiomas are usually small and single, but may occasionally be large or multiple. The vast majority are not visible on external examination, but uncommonly large haemangiomas are most frequently seen as bulging protuberances on the fetal surface of the placenta. Occasionally, they are found on the maternal surface, where they may replace an entire lobe, or in the membranes, where they may be attached to the placenta by a vascular pedicle. Most haemangiomata are of no clinical importance, but those measuring more than 5 cm in diameter may be associated with maternal or fetal complications such as polyhydramnios, fetal hypoxia, IUGR and even intrauterine death (IUD).

Placenta venestra

In this condition, almost the entire chorionic membrane is covered with thin, but functioning, placental tissue. The thickness of the placental tissue is in inverse proportion to its area.

This means that almost the entire decidual lining will be expelled with the placenta after delivery and could therefore result in PPH.

Placenta in multiple pregnancy

Figure 7.26 gives the variations of the placenta and membranes in multiple pregnancies, with differentiation between monozygotic and dizygotic twins. (Also see Chapter 24.)

Abnormalities of the cord
Battledore insertion of the cord

If the cord is not inserted into the centre of the placenta but is inserted to one side, it is termed a lateral insertion. However, should the cord be inserted at the very edge of the placenta, it is called a battledore insertion, because it resembles the racquet used in the ancient game of battledore and badminton (see colour illustration C10 on page 77).

Placenta velamentosa

If the cord is inserted into the membranes instead of into the fetal surface of the placenta, it is known as a velamentous insertion of the cord (see colour illustration C11 on page 78). In this type of placenta, the vessels branch from the insertion of the cord and then run through the chorion to and from the placenta. This can be dangerous to the fetus during labour, as these vessels may lie over the cervical os and therefore in front of the presenting part of the fetus. This is termed a vasa praevia (vessels in front).

Vasa praevia

With a placenta velamentosa and the fetal blood vessels from the umbilical cord lying in front of the presenting part during labour, the danger is that as the membranes rupture, these vessels may also be torn or severed. This is a very rare condition but should it occur, it would cause a loss of fetal blood.

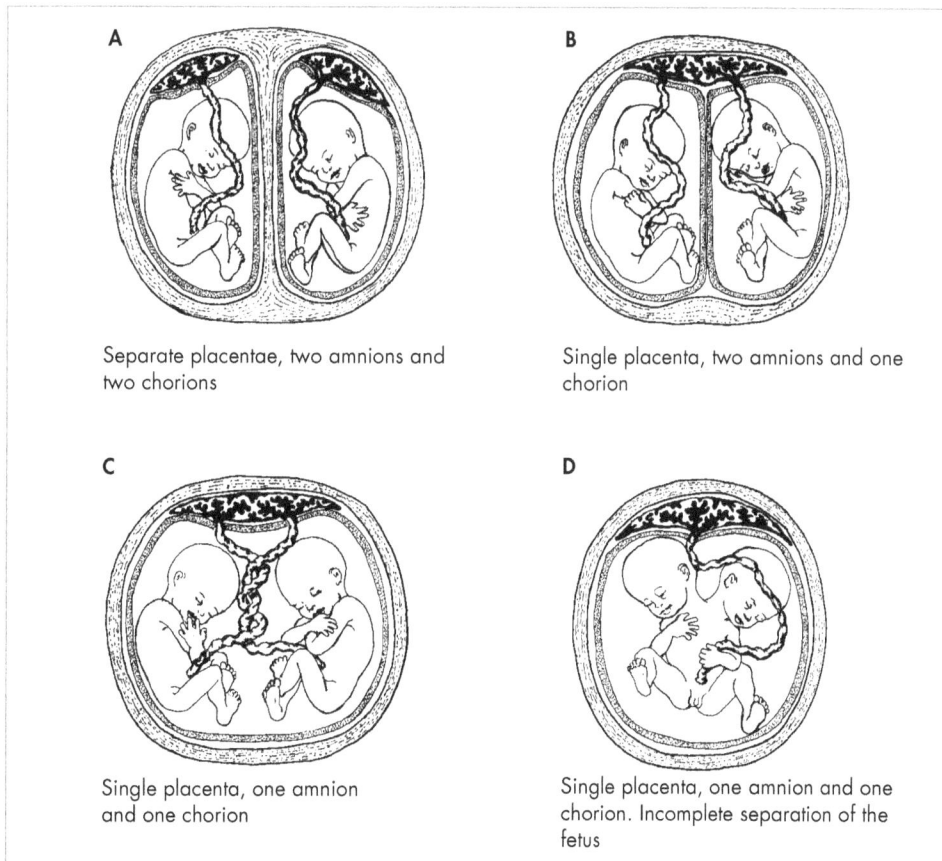

A
Separate placentae, two amnions and two chorions

B
Single placenta, two amnions and one chorion

C
Single placenta, one amnion and one chorion

D
Single placenta, one amnion and one chorion. Incomplete separation of the fetus

Figure 7.26 Multiple pregnancy

Amniotic bands

Owing to a lack of amniotic fluid, the fetus may come into contact with the amniotic membrane. The membrane may then become attached to and form a band of amnion around a limb. This can result in badly deformed limbs and may even result in the amputation of a fetal hand, foot or whole limb.

A short cord

A short cord is any cord less than 400 mm, but it could be as short as 200 mm. The dangers of a short cord include the following:

▶ It could delay or even prevent the descent of the fetus during labour.
▶ There could be early separation of the placenta, causing fetal anoxia.
▶ The cord may snap, which could result in fetal anoxia, loss of fetal blood and a retained placenta.

A normal or long cord that is wound around the fetus, leaving only a short free end, would present the same dangers as a short cord.

A very long cord

Cords of 1 500 mm have been recorded. Long cords may become wound around any part of the fetus and may even be wound two or three times around the neck of the fetus at birth. Should the cord be wound tightly around some part of the fetus, this could cause a reduced blood flow to the distal tissues, resulting in underdevelopment. It might even stop the blood flow, causing a limb to wither, or even fetal death if the cord is wrapped tightly around the neck or body of the fetus.

True knots in the cord

A true knot, as shown in Figure 7.27, is caused by the fetus passing through a loop of cord and forming a knot. This is most likely to occur with a long cord and during the period of gestation when there is a greater ratio of amniotic fluid to fetus, from 16 to 24 weeks. The danger is that during the delivery, the knot could be drawn tight as the fetus descends, causing anoxia and even fetal death.

7.9   Fetal circulation

The dynamic circulatory differences *in utero* and changes of the newborn after birth (from *in utero* to normal circulation) must be fully understood in order to be able to understand the dynamics of the fetal circulation as the basis for obstetric practice.

In utero, the fetal lungs and GI system do not function, because the fetus obtains the oxygen and nutrients necessary for development and growth from the maternal circulation. The waste products of metabolism pass back into the placenta to the maternal circulatory system for disposal (see colour illustration C12 on page 79).

As a result of these differences, certain modifications are found in the fetal blood circulation that are normally temporary and become redundant after birth (see colour illustration C13 on page 80).

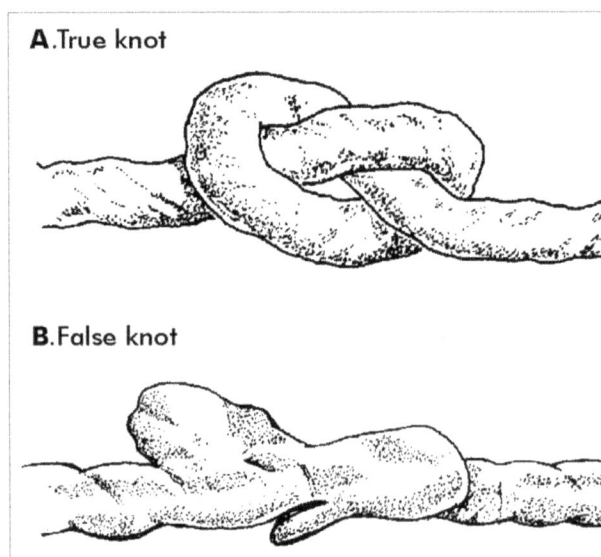

Figure 7.27 A true knot and false knot

Fetal haemoglobin

The Hb of a fetus *in utero* is uniquely adapted to support the growing and developing fetus, as the lungs are not functional and the fetus is dependent on the mother for oxygen through the placenta.

The diffusion of oxygen from the mother's blood through the placental membrane and into the fetal blood occurs in almost exactly the same osmotic process as oxygen diffusion through the pulmonary membrane. The dissolved oxygen in the maternal sinuses passes into the fetal blood because of the oxygen pressure gradient difference between the maternal and the fetal blood. Under normal circumstances, at term the partial pressure of oxygen (PO_2), which reflects the amount of oxygen dissolved in the blood, is about 50 mmHg in the healthy maternal placental sinuses, while it is about 30 mmHg in the fetal blood in the umbilical vein after oxygenation. This makes an average PO_2 difference of 20 mmHg between the maternal and fetal blood. The low PO_2 of only 30 mmHg in the oxygenated fetal blood would not supply the fetus with sufficient oxygen under ordinary circumstances.

The fetus exists in a relatively hypoxic environment. However, the reason why the fetal blood is able to transport almost as much oxygen to the fetal tissues as the mother's blood is able to transport to her own tissues is the greater percentage of Hb in the fetus. Fetal Hb carries more oxygen than normal Hb in red blood cells. Fetal Hb can carry as much as 20–30 per cent more than the maternal Hb. The Hb concentration of the fetal blood is about 50 per cent higher than that of the maternal blood. The Hb levels of a newborn is higher than those of an adult, at between 14 g/dl and 24 g/dl.

The Bohr shift, which allows Hb to transport more oxygen where there is a low partial pressure of carbon dioxide (PCO_2), is effective because large amounts of carbon dioxide in the fetal blood are diffused through the placental membrane into the maternal blood, causing a greatly lowered PCO_2 in the fetal blood. In addition, the loss of carbon dioxide makes the fetal blood more alkaline and the increase of carbon dioxide in the maternal blood makes the maternal blood more acidic. These changes force more oxygen from the maternal blood and at the same time enhance the oxygen in the fetal blood. This causes a Bohr shift in the opposite direction, which in effect results in a double Bohr effect.

This mechanism enables the fetus to receive an adequate amount of oxygen despite the fact that the fetal blood leaving the placenta has a PO_2 of only 30 mmHg. This gives an oxygen concentration of 85 per cent in the blood in the umbilical vein, which is transported to the fetus.

The temporary structures of the fetal circulation

There are various temporary functional structures that allow fetal circulation, bypassing the lungs. These are the ductus venosus, the two umbilical arteries, and the two cardiac shunts, the ductus arteriosus and the foramen ovale (see colour illustration C12 on page 79).

The ductus venosus

The ductus venosus is a connection between two veins. In the fetus it is the temporary connection between the umbilical vein and the inferior vena cava. This vessel is a continuation of the umbilical vein and transports 85 per cent oxygenated blood from the placenta to the fetus.

As the umbilical vein passes into the fetal abdomen, it branches off to the liver to supply the right lobe of the liver (the liver is a very important and large organ in the fetus). Through the umbilical vein the ductus venosus then joins the inferior vena cava just above the level of the fetal umbilicus.

De-oxygenated blood is transported from the fetal pelvis and lower limbs through the ascending inferior vena cava and is then mixed with the oxygenated blood from the umbilical vein and the placenta. This mixed blood is transported to the right atrium in the heart. From here, a small portion will flow to the right ventricle and supply the uninflated lungs through the pulmonary artery. The blood volume and pressure in the right side of the heart is then greater than the blood volume and pressure in the left atrium, causing a right-to-left shunt of blood from the right to the left atrium.

The foramen ovale

There are several structures in the body called 'foramen ovale', meaning 'oval window'. These are openings that connect structures, such as the opening at the base of the skull. In the fetus and newborn, the temporary structural opening in the septum between the right and left atria of the heart is called the foramen ovale of the heart. It allows oxygenated blood to flow from the right atrium to the left during intrauterine life. The foramen ovale is formed with a valve or flap (the septum primum) on the left side of the septum. As the pressure is greatest on the right side of the heart during fetal development, the pressure of the blood against the valve in the right atrium causes the foramen ovale to remain open and so allows the blood to flow through into the left atrium.

As the fetal lungs are not functioning, the blood bypasses the lungs. Most of the blood from the umbilical vein and the inferior vena cava passes directly from the right atrium into the left atrium (right-to-left shunt) through the foramen ovale.

The blood that flows through the foramen ovale into the left atrium is mixed blood. The blood flows from the left atrium to the left ventricle and to the aorta.

The ductus arteriosus

A ductus arteriosus is a connection from an artery to another artery. In the fetus, this is a temporary connection between the pulmonary artery and the aorta.

The blood from the left ventricle is pumped into the aorta. The reasonably well-oxygenated blood is mainly directed to the heart, the head and the upper parts of the fetus through the aorta. De-oxygenated blood from the head and upper parts and the lungs are transported through the ductus arteriosus to the aorta. This mixed blood then flows to the internal organs and lower extremities via the descending aorta and iliac arteries and its branches, the umbilical arteries. The blood is now only 50 per cent oxygenated.

The umbilical arteries

The umbilical arteries are branches of the internal iliac arteries, returning de-oxygenated blood (containing only 50 per cent oxygen) from the fetus back to the placenta for re-oxygenation. As these blood vessels enter the umbilical cord, they become known as the umbilical arteries.

Dynamics of the fetal circulation

The fetal blood circulation is reversed in terms of oxygenation. Blood that is transported from the placenta to the fetus through the umbilical vein is oxygenated and is functionally arterial blood, while blood returning through the umbilical arteries to the placenta is de-oxygenated blood – functionally, venous blood. This will change after birth.

The fetal circulation gives preference to the fetal brain and heart muscle.

The fetal and maternal blood never mix directly, and gas exchange takes place in the placenta through diffusion in the intervillous spaces separated by the cell layers of the placental villi.

Fetal circulation changes at and after birth

With birth, certain changes must occur to allow and establish extrauterine life (see colour illustration C12 on page 79) namely:
- the switching off of the placental circulation by the cutting of the cord or separation of the placenta
- the commencement of the working of the fetal lungs for respiration and gas exchange
- the closure of the two cardiac shunts.

The causes of and the order in which these immediate functional and permanent anatomical changes take place to allow for extrauterine life are not yet fully understood, but they occur in the following way:
- With the cutting of the umbilical cord, the low resistance of the placenta disappears and blood circulation to the placenta is prohibited. Placental circulation is stopped.
- When the baby starts to breathe, the lungs expand and this uncoils the pulmonary capillaries when blood flows through the pulmonary artery to the lungs. As blood is drawn into these pulmonary capillaries, it is oxygenated and returned to the left atrium via the now expanded four pulmonary veins. These changes increase the pressure in the left atrium and decrease pressure in the right atrium.

- There is a left-to-right pressure and blood volume shift that cause the closure of the foramen ovale. This is a functional closure of the foramen ovale at birth. In most individuals, the anatomical permanent closure of the foramen ovale occurs within months after birth, but in 25 per cent of adults, the foramen ovale does not fully close. Patency of the foramen ovale is referred to as a shunt or patent foramen ovale (PFO). The vast majority of cases do not require treatment. When the foramen ovale closes anatomically, scar tissue remains between the atria, termed the fossa ovalis.
- The oxygen tension in the blood rises and prostaglandins are released, which cause contractions of the smooth muscle in the wall of the ductus arteriosus between the aorta and the pulmonal artery. The closure becomes permanent by the end of two months, and a ligament is formed, called the ligamentum arteriosum. Should the ductus arteriosus not close, this would cause a condition called persistent or patent ductus arteriosus (PDA). PDA and non-closure of the foramen ovale have been attributed to factors such as:
  - neonatal hypoxic incidents
  - maternal infections (PDA is the most common heart defect in congenital rubella)
  - the possible effect of medications given to the mother.
- When the umbilical cord ceases to pulsate, when it is severed or when the placenta separates, no blood enters the umbilical vein and ductus venosus, which further reduces the pressure on the right side of the heart. The ductus venosus closes through muscle constriction soon after birth, but permanent anatomical closure takes weeks or months, with the proliferation of endothelial and fibrous tissues. It becomes the ligamentum teres hepatis.
- The umbilical arteries also constrict, atrophy and form the umbilical ligaments.

7.10   Conclusion

This chapter gave an overview of the basic development of the zygote, embryo, fetus, decidua, placenta and membranes. The fetal circulation was also discussed, as well as changes in the fetal circulation that occur at birth. Common pathologies that occur during development, and which midwives need to consider in practice, were discussed. Further in-depth reading and study needs to be undertaken in order to gain a thorough knowledge of the anatomy and physiology of pregnancy, as the body of scientific knowledge is constantly growing.

The three Ps of labour: Passage, passenger and powers

LEARNING OBJECTIVES
On completion of this chapter, you must be able to:
▶ explain the three Ps of labour (passage, passenger and powers)
▶ explain the integrated processes for normal labour
▶ describe and explain normal pelvic anatomy
▶ describe the fetal skull, its landmarks and functions in labour
▶ describe measurements of importance in childbirth
▶ identify and describe the essential soft tissue structures important in childbirth
▶ identify and describe the path that the fetus negotiates during normal birth
▶ describe normal uterine function in pregnancy and labour.

KNOWLEDGE ASSUMED TO BE IN PLACE
Basic anatomy and physiology of the reproductive system, the pelvis and muscles

KEYWORDS
obstetric pelvis • pelvic floor • perineal body • fetal skull • uterine action • levator ani • occipitoposterior (OP)

8.1   Introduction

The three Ps of labour summarise the three critical role players in birth: passage, powers and passenger. The passage includes the bony pelvis and the soft tissue of the pelvic floor, the passenger is the fetus and the powers include the uterus as the birthing organ. When these three Ps are within normal parameters, the birth can be expected to proceed uneventfully. In reality, each birth has unpredictable outcomes. The fetus needs to negotiate the bony pelvis and soft tissue of the pelvic floor to be born through various movements, called mechanisms. The working of the uterus is influenced by the 'fit' between these two factors.

This chapter explains the three Ps of labour by describing the anatomy of the bony pelvis and the muscles of the pelvic floor and the perineum, the fetal skull and normal uterine action.

8.2   The passage: The bony pelvis

Note: The pelvis is best studied with a model of a gynaecoid pelvis and a baby.

The bones of the pelvis are joined to form the pelvic canal, through which the fetus must pass during birth. The shape and the size of this canal, which depend upon the shape and size of the pelvic bones, determine whether a fetus of average size and shape will be able to negotiate it. The female-shaped bony pelvis is called a gynaecoid pelvis (see Figure 8.1 on the next page) and has specific characteristics that make it suitable for childbirth.

The four pelvic girdle bones that make up the pelvis are:
1. the two innominate bones, each made up of three fused bones, namely the ilium, the ischium and the pubic bones
2. the sacrum, made up of five fused vertebrae
3. the coccyx, made up of three to five fused rudimentary vertebrae.

The pelvis supports the internal organs, such as the intestines, liver and kidneys in the false pelvis and provides an entry for the openings of the rectum and bladder. Organs that are situated in the true pelvis are the uterus and bladder. In pregnancy, the uterus becomes an abdominal organ and the bladder is also pulled up in the abdomen. After pregnancy, the uterus returns to its normal position within six weeks. The pelvic girdle carries the internal organs and the gravid uterus in pregnancy.

The pelvic inlet or brim
(superior view)

Posterior

False pelvis

Iliac crest
Ala of sacrum
Sacral promontory
Sacroiliac joint
Sacrococcygeal joint
Iliopectineal line
Anterior superior iliac spine

Iliopectineal eminence

Pubic crest
Symphysis pubis

Transverse±13 cm
Antero-posterior ±11 cm

True   pelvis

Anterior

[All oblique diameters measure 12 cm]

The pelvic outlet
(inferior view)

Anterior

Symphysis pubis

Inferior ramus of ischium

Acetabulum

Anterior superior iliac spine

Antero-posterior ±11.5 cm

Transverse±11 cm

Ischial tuberosity

Sacrotuberous ligament
Promontory of sacrum
Iliac crest
Coccyx
Sacrococcygeal joint
Sacrum

Posterior

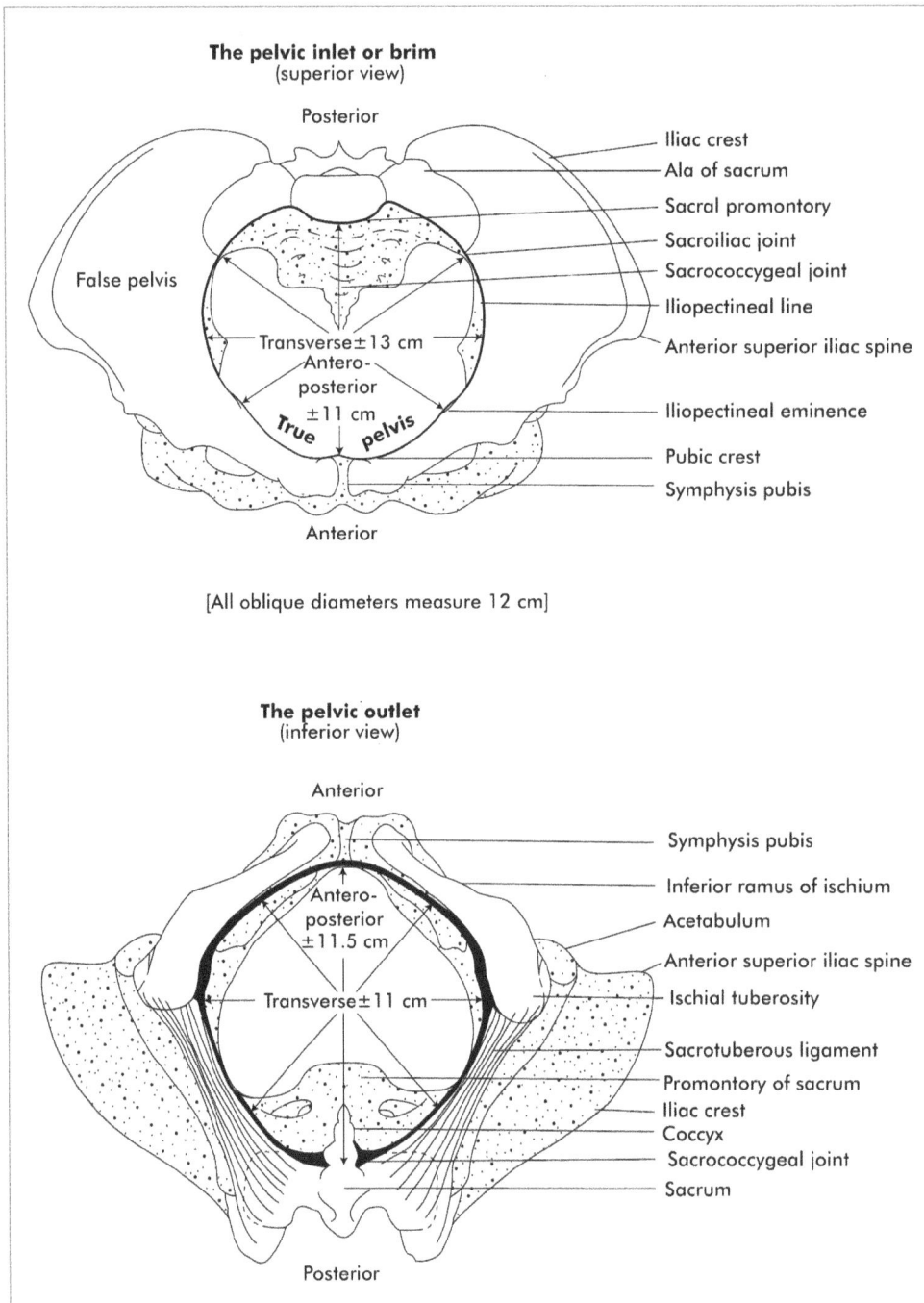

Figure 8.1 The female-shaped or gynaecoid pelvis

The innominate bones

There are two innominate bones, each made up of three bones that fuse completely during puberty or early adulthood. The three bones are the ilium, the ischium and the pubis, as shown in Figure 8.2. These three bones all meet on the outer aspect, in the acetabulum of the innominate bone, and on the inner aspect and in the lateral walls of the mid-cavity of the true pelvis.

The ilium

The ilium, called the innominate, is the strong, heavy superior bone of the pelvis.

The upper portion of the ilium forms the large flared-out part of the pelvis, known as the false pelvis. The posterior border articulates with the ala of the sacrum at the sacroiliac joint to form the girdle of the pelvis. The upper curved border is called the iliac crest, which ends posteriorly in the posterior-superior iliac spine and anteriorly in the anterior-superior iliac spine.

The lower portion of the ilium, which forms the upper part of the true pelvis, meets the inferior border of the ischium posteriorly and the pubic bone anteriorly.

At the junction of the upper and lower portions of the ilium there is a ridge, which forms the lateral division between the false and the true pelvis, called the iliopectineal line. This iliopectineal line also forms the lateral borders of the brim or inlet to the cavity of the true pelvis.

The ischium

This is the lowest part of the innominate bones. The thickened, lower border of this bone is known as the ischial tuberosity. In a sitting position, the full mass of the body is carried on these bones. They also form part of the outlet to the pelvic cavity.

A thin arm, the inferior ramus of the ischium, projects forwards and upwards from the tuberosity and meets and joins with the inferior rami of the pubic bones to form the pubic arch. In an average gynaecoid pelvis, the arch should form an angle of 90 degrees. Superiorly, the ischium widens and joins the ilium in the posterior portion of the acetabulum.

Directly above the tuberosity on the posterior border, a small spine projects posterior-laterally into the pelvic cavity, separating the greater sciatic notch from the lesser sciatic notch, called the ischial spine. This is an important landmark in the pelvis in childbirth.

The pubis or pubic bone

This bone consists of a body and two arms, the superior and the inferior pubic rami. The bodies of the two pubic bones meet anteriorly, to form the joint known as the symphysis pubis.

The upper or superior ramus forms the pubic crest and joins the lower anterior border of the ilium in the acetabulum. The lower or inferior rami, on either side, together make up the pubic arch, which also forms part of the outlet to the pelvic cavity. Where the two arms of the pubic bone meet the ischium inferiorly and the ilium superiorly, they form an oval-shaped window or hole in the anterior pelvic wall, known as the obturator foramen.

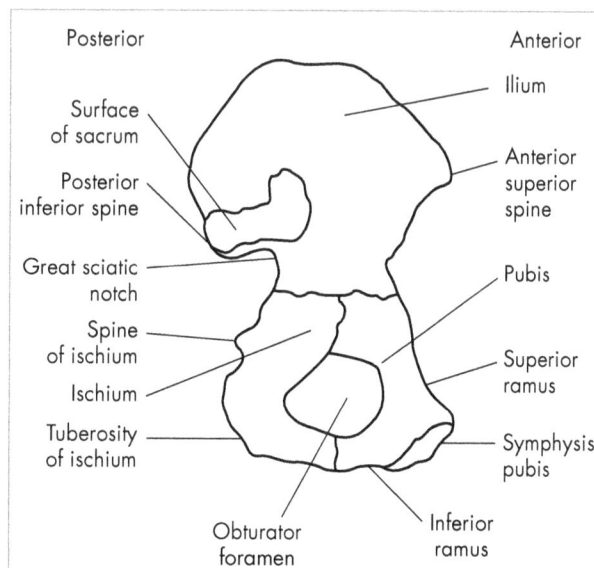

Figure 8.2 The innominate bones

The symphysis pubis

This is a cartilaginous joint. It is formed anteriorly where the two pubic bones join and is strengthened by fibrous tissue. There is a pad of cartilage between the bodies of the two pubic bones. As a result of hormone action, this joint may widen spontaneously during late pregnancy, giving rise to movement of the joint and pain on walking.

The sacrum

This is a strong, heavy bone, which forms the posterior part of the pelvis and articulates on either side with the ilium at the sacroiliac joints. The full weight of the body is taken on this bone and transferred via the sacroiliac joints to the acetabula and so to the legs. The forces generated by the legs and trunk converge on this strong bone.

The sacrum is made up of five fused vertebrae and is a wedge-shaped triangular bone. The wide end of the wedge is directed upwards, where it articulates with the fifth (last) lumbar vertebra and where the anterior border forms the promontory of the sacrum. The narrow end of the wedge is directed downwards and backwards and its inferior border articulates with the upper end of the coccyx.

As the sacrum is an extension of the vertebral column, it has a central canal containing nerves. Posteriorly, on either side of the short spinous processes, is a row of inter-vertebral foramina through which the sacral and coccygeal nerves pass. The main branch of the sacral plexus is the sciatic nerve, which is the largest nerve in the body. At the inferior end of the canal, there is an opening known as the hiatus, through which the filum terminale passes and is inserted into the coccyx.

The sacrum in the female pelvis is shorter than the sacrum in the male pelvis. It is wider and is well curved. This curvature is called 'the hollow of the sacrum'. It normally measures 15 cm in a normal gynaecoid pelvis and is suited for birth.

The coccyx

This is a small, wedge-shaped bone, consisting of three to five fused rudimentary vertebrae. It is situated at the end of the vertebral column. The wide edge of the wedge articulates with the lower end of the sacrum. The coccyx serves as the origin for important muscles of the pelvic floor and the hip.

The pelvic joints

The joints of the pelvis are very strong and the ligaments strengthening these joints are partly cartilaginous and partly fibrous. Normally, there is very little movement in these joints, but in the pregnant state, hormones cause softening and stretching of the ligaments, allowing some movement or 'give' in the pelvic joints.

Women often experience back pain, especially in late pregnancy, as a result of this joint laxity, which may also be carried over into the first few weeks after delivery. Women should be careful about posture and lifting objects during pregnancy.

If there is a minor degree of disproportion in size between a mother's pelvis and the head of the fetus (cephalopelvic disproportion, or CPD), the degree of give in the pelvis can be a factor contributing to a successful birth. The woman's position during labour influences the fetal–pelvic relation.

The sacroiliac joints and ligaments

The joints between the sacrum and the ilium are the strongest joints in the body. The joint formed between the articulation of the ilium and the sacrum on either side of the pelvis are called the right and left sacroiliac joints.

The sacrococcygeal joint

This joint is formed where the sacrum and the coccyx articulate and is much looser than the other joints of the pelvis. This enables the coccyx to bend backwards, allowing the fetal head to negotiate the outlet of the pelvic canal. Where there has been a previous fracture of the coccyx, or if the joint has become immobilised (the coccyx fused to the sacrum), there may be difficulty during the birth of the fetal head. The woman may also experience pain after delivery, especially when sitting.

The lumbosacral joint

The lumbosacral joint lies at the posterior aspect of the pelvis, between the fifth lumbar vertebra and the sacrum. Exceptionally strong ligaments strengthen this joint, but because of the backward inclination of the sacrum, considerable strain also occurs here during pregnancy. Occasionally, the fifth lumbar vertebra projects forwards and downwards, reducing the pelvic brim area.

The pelvic ligaments

Besides the ligaments that strengthen the pelvic joints, there are two additional ligaments of the pelvis that are important in childbirth:

1. The *sacrospinous ligament* runs from the lower sacrum and the coccyx to the ischial spine, and encloses the lower border of the greater sciatic notch. The sacrospinous ligament is covered by the coccygeus muscle of the pelvic floor.
2. The *sacrotuberous ligament* encloses the lesser sciatic notch and runs from the lower sacrum and the coccyx to the ischial tuberosity.

Together with the lower sacrum and the coccyx, these two ligaments form the posterior aspect of the pelvic outlet. Thus, the pelvic outlet is only partially encompassed by bone, unlike the pelvic inlet, which is totally encompassed by bone.

The birth canal

The word 'pelvis' is derived from the Latin word for basin, referring to its shape. It is also known as the hip girdle. There are four types of pelvis, as described in Table 8.1 on the next page, namely the gynaecoid, android, anthropoid and platypelloid pelvis. The classification of the pelvis for birth is based on its anatomical form and shape.

The gynaecoid or female pelvis is adapted for birth. Other pelvic shapes may complicate birth because of unfavourable diameters. The midwife therefore needs to know the favourable types and measurements in order to identify the types of pelvis that are less suitable and will complicate birth. Because the pelvis cannot be measured directly, signs and symptoms of pelvic disproportion may provide an indirect method of measuring the pelvis.

The gynaecoid pelvis is divided in two parts: the false pelvis and true pelvis. They are separated by a ridge, called the linea terminalis, as shown in Figure 8.3. The false pelvis is above the line and of little obstetrical interest. The true pelvis is extremely important in obstetrics, as this is the passage through which the fetus has to pass during labour (the process of birth).

In normal labour (when the head presents), the fetal head (skull) is the first part of the fetus to negotiate this passage. First, it has to enter the narrowest part of the inlet of the pelvis. Secondly, the fetus has to pass through the narrowest part of the curved cavity of the pelvis and, finally, it has to emerge from the narrowest part of the outlet. The fetus makes very specific moves to pass through this channel (see Chapter 25) and can get stuck at any point.

In obstetrics, therefore, three different planes or zones of the pelvis are described: the pelvic brim or inlet, the pelvic cavity or midpelvis and the pelvic outlet. In the typical or normal gynaecoid pelvis, these areas or zones have average dimensions, as shown in figures 8.4 and 8.5 (on page 125). Table 8.1 gives details of these areas in the four types of pelvis.

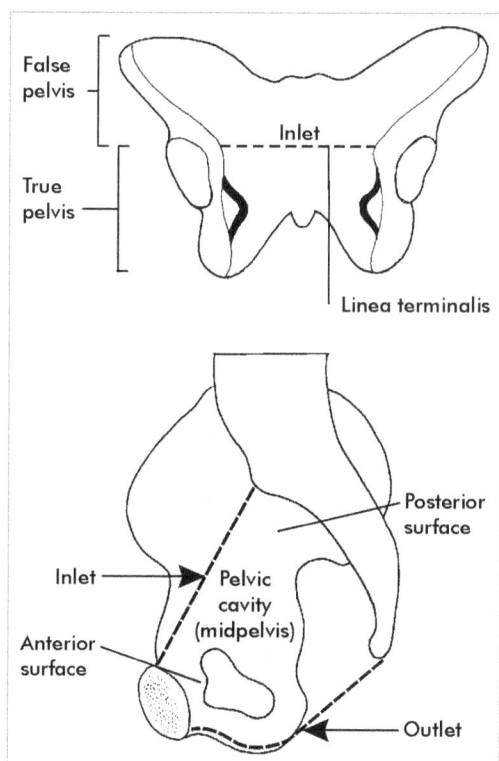

Figure 8.3 The anterior and sagittal view of the pelvic plane

The gynaecoid pelvis

In the gynaecoid pelvis, the brim is almost round, except for the posterior intrusion of the promontory of the sacrum. It is not possible to measure the pelvic inlet satisfactorily in a human without ultrasound, X-rays, CT or MRI scans.

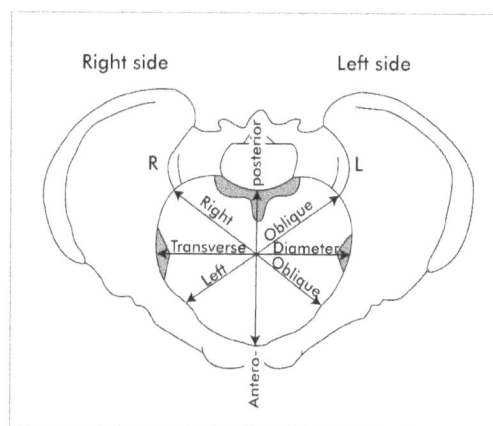

Figure 8.4 Diagram showing the diameters of the pelvic brim and from where they are measured

Table 8.1

Classical description of pelvic shapes

Type	Female-shaped (gynaecoid)	Male-shaped (android)	Ape-shaped (anthropoid)	Flat (platypelloid)
	This is the best type of pelvis for birth. 50 % of women have this type of pelvis	This type is the least favourable for birth	Labour does not usually present problems, but a direct occipitoposterior (OP) or occipitoanterior (OA) may occur	This type of pelvis has a kidney-shaped brim
Inlet	Rounded, oval brim anteroposterior (AP) diameter: 12 cm Transverse: 12.5 cm Non-prominent sacral promontory	Heart-shaped Narrowed AP diameter Short and heavily built women are more inclined to have an android pelvis	Oval-shaped Large AP diameter Reduced transverse diameters Women with this type of pelvis tend to be tall with narrow shoulders	Sacrum displaced forward or flat with a narrow cavity Narrowed AP diameter
Midpelvis	Shallow with straight side walls Non-prominent ischial spines 10 cm Concave sacrum Movable coccyx Sacrospinous ligament admits two fingers (4 cm)	Contracted midpelvis Prominent spines Sacrum straight and long Reduced interspinous diameter	Slightly narrowed intestinal diameters	Shallow pelvis
Outlet	Suprapubic arch 90 degrees (admits two fingers) Coccyx is movable Intertuberous diameter: 10 cm	Android outlet Narrowed subpubic arch	Intertuborous diameter is reduced	The diameter of the outlet is increased, except for AP diameter
Effect on labour	If the fetus is of average size and in the right position, labour should be normal	OP positions are more common Face and brow presentation If the ischial spines are prominent, this will prevent complete internal rotation of the head, resulting in deep transverse arrest Poor progress Obstructed labour Delayed second stage Fetal and pelvic floor trauma	Labour normally presents without difficulty Posterior positions may remain in persistent OP (POP) Prolonged first and second stage Higher incidence of obstetric interventions	High head slow to engage Prolonged and obstructed labour Increased face and brow presentations Once the head has passed the brim, no problems are expected in an average-sized baby

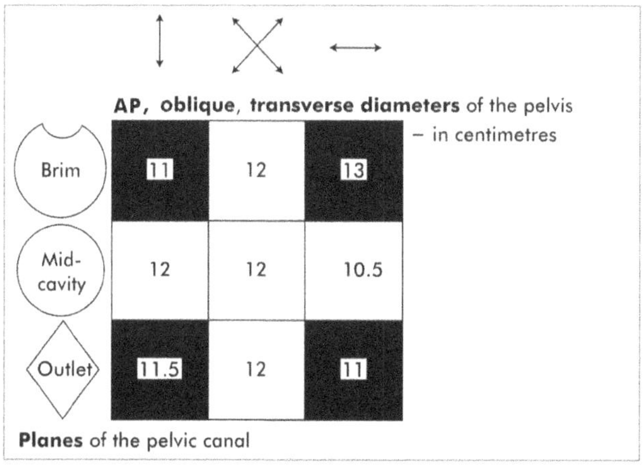

Figure 8.5 The measures of the gynaecoid pelvis

Other pelvic variations include those caused by dietary deficiencies (of vitamin D), resulting in a rachitic pelvis that was deformed in early childhood. This must be suspected if a woman's legs are bowed and spinal deformity occurs. A Caesarean section is indicated in severe contraction of the pelvis. Trauma to the pelvis (fractures or congenital dislocation of the hips) may impact the shape and size of the pelvis due to callus formation.

The gynaecoid bony pelvis, with its normal measurements, is well suited for labour and if the fetus is of average size and in the correct position, birth is uneventful or considered normal. It is the task of the midwife or medical practitioner to identify abnormalities in pregnancy and labour early and to refer the woman for appropriate care. Approximately 20 per cent of births will be complicated.

When the typical gynaecoid pelvis is described, certain specific characteristics and measurements are essential basic knowledge for midwives. This content should be studied with a model of the pelvis so that the specific landmarks can be identified (also see figures 8.4 and 8.5 and Figure 8.7 on page 127). The five landmarks and approximate measurements of each area of the pelvis, discussed in the following sections, are:

1. the pelvic brim, or inlet (see Figure 8.4)
2. the pelvic cavity, or midpelvis (see Figure 8.5)
3. the pelvic outlet (see Figure 8.5)
4. pelvic inclination (see figures 8.3 and 8.7)
5. the axis of the birth canal (see the curve of Carus in Figure 8.7).

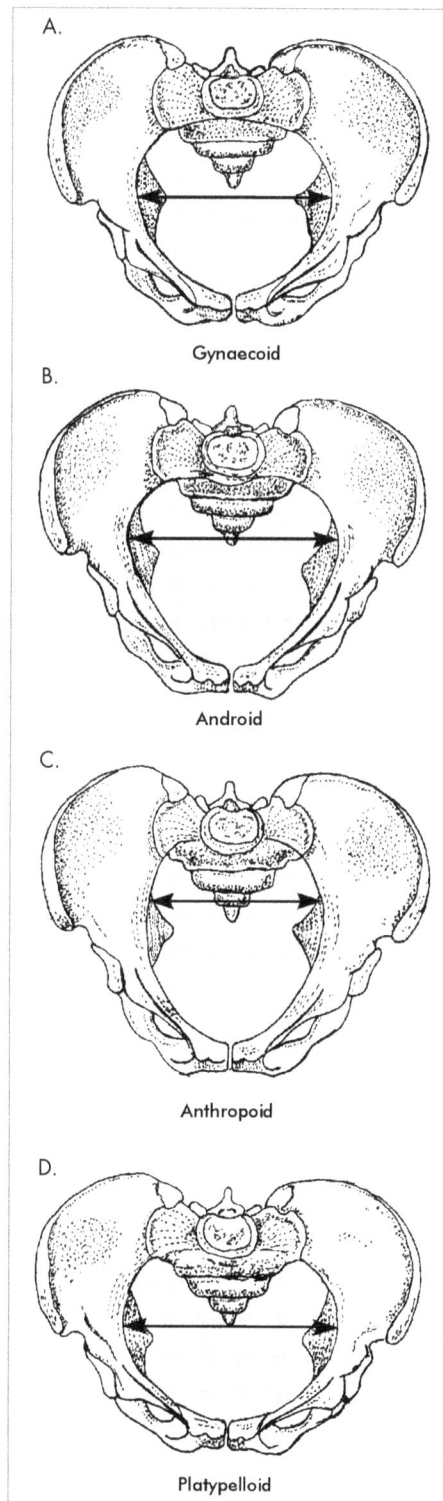

Figure 8.6 Classification of pelvises for birth

The pelvic brim or inlet

This area is particularly significant in childbirth, because if the fetal head cannot pass through the pelvic brim, labour becomes obstructed and complicated. If the largest presenting diameters of the fetal skull do pass through the pelvic brim, the fetal head is said to be engaged.

The size of this area is difficult to assess, because it is internal and all the landmarks cannot be felt on vaginal examination. The borders of the inlet are:

▶ posteriorly, the promontory of the sacrum, the alae (wings) of the sacrum and the sacroiliac joints
▶ laterally, the iliopectineal lines on either side of the pelvis and the iliopectineal eminences where the iliac bones meet the superior rami of the pubic bones
▶ anteriorly, the pubic crests on each pubic bone and the symphysis pubis.

The diagonal conjugate refers to the distance assessed (using vaginal examination) from the subpubic arch towards the sacral promontory. A measurement of 12.5 cm is considered adequate.

The true or anatomical conjugate is between 11 and 13 cm. The obstetric (true) conjugate is the narrowest point of the pelvic inlet and is measured from the back portion of the pubis to the sacral promontory. This can be determined by subtracting 1.5 cm from the diagonal conjugate (about 10 cm).

The pelvic cavity, or midpelvis

This area is between the inlet and the outlet of the pelvis. The pubic arch, ischial spines and tip of the sacrum form the borders of the midpelvis.

Because the sacrum has a concave curve from above, looking downwards, and because the pelvic cavity has a short anterior wall, the pelvic canal is curved anteriorly (see the curve or axis of the pelvic canal in Figure 8.7).

In a transverse section, the pelvic cavity is almost round and therefore all the measurements are approximately the same. The most important and narrowest diameter of the midpelvis is between the ischial spines, and is called the bi-spinous diameter. This measures between 10 and 10.5 cm.

The ischial spines are used as a landmark in labour to determine progress by determining the relationship of the fetal skull or breech with the spines.

The pelvic outlet

The outlet to the pelvis is diamond-shaped. The landmarks of the pelvic outlet are:

▶ posteriorly, the coccyx and the sacrotuberous ligaments, 4–5 cm

▶ laterally, the ischial tuberosities (transverse diameter: 11 cm)
▶ anteriorly, the pubic arch 90 degrees (AP diameter from subpubic arch to sacrococcygeal joint: 11.5 cm).

Even if the fetus has already negotiated the pelvic inlet and midpelvis, a narrowed, funnel-like outlet may be too small for birth.

Only the last two diameters can be measured directly with the hand. Prominence of the ischial spines is noted and if the subpubic arch does not admit two fingers with ease, it is considered suspicious.

Pelvic inclination

This is the relationship of the pelvic inlet to the maternal spine, allowing the fetus to enter the pelvis, as shown in Figure 8.7. The pelvic inclination is influenced by which position a woman is in.

In the standing position, the inlet makes a 55 degree angle with the horizontal. The anterior-superior iliac spine and pubis are on the same level when the woman is standing. In the supine position, the inlet is 25 degrees below the horizontal. The supine position is not considered to be natural or the best for birth and can complicate the birth process. The Better Birth Initiative (Smith et al, 2004) advocates that women should be allowed to adopt the position they find most comfortable during birth (as long as it does not compromise the fetus).

The axis of the birth canal

Theoretically, this is the path followed by the centre of the fetal head as it descends through the birth canal during labour, known as the curve of Carus, as shown in Figure 8.7. It is C-shaped and makes a 90 degree curve. The anterior border measures 5 cm and the posterior border is 15 cm. The fetus makes the necessary movements, which include curling up (flexion), stretching (extension) or turning (rotation) to negotiate the canal.

Important measurements of the pelvis
The three most important pelvic measurements are:
1 the obstetric or true conjugate of the pelvic inlet (AP diameter 10 cm)
2 the interspinous diameter of the midpelvis (10–10.5 cm between the ischial spines)
3 the AP diameter from the subpubic arch to the sacrococcygeal joint (11.5 cm). If the pubic arch is less than 90 degrees, this may be less.

Median sections of the female pelvis showing the pelvic planes and pelvic inclinations

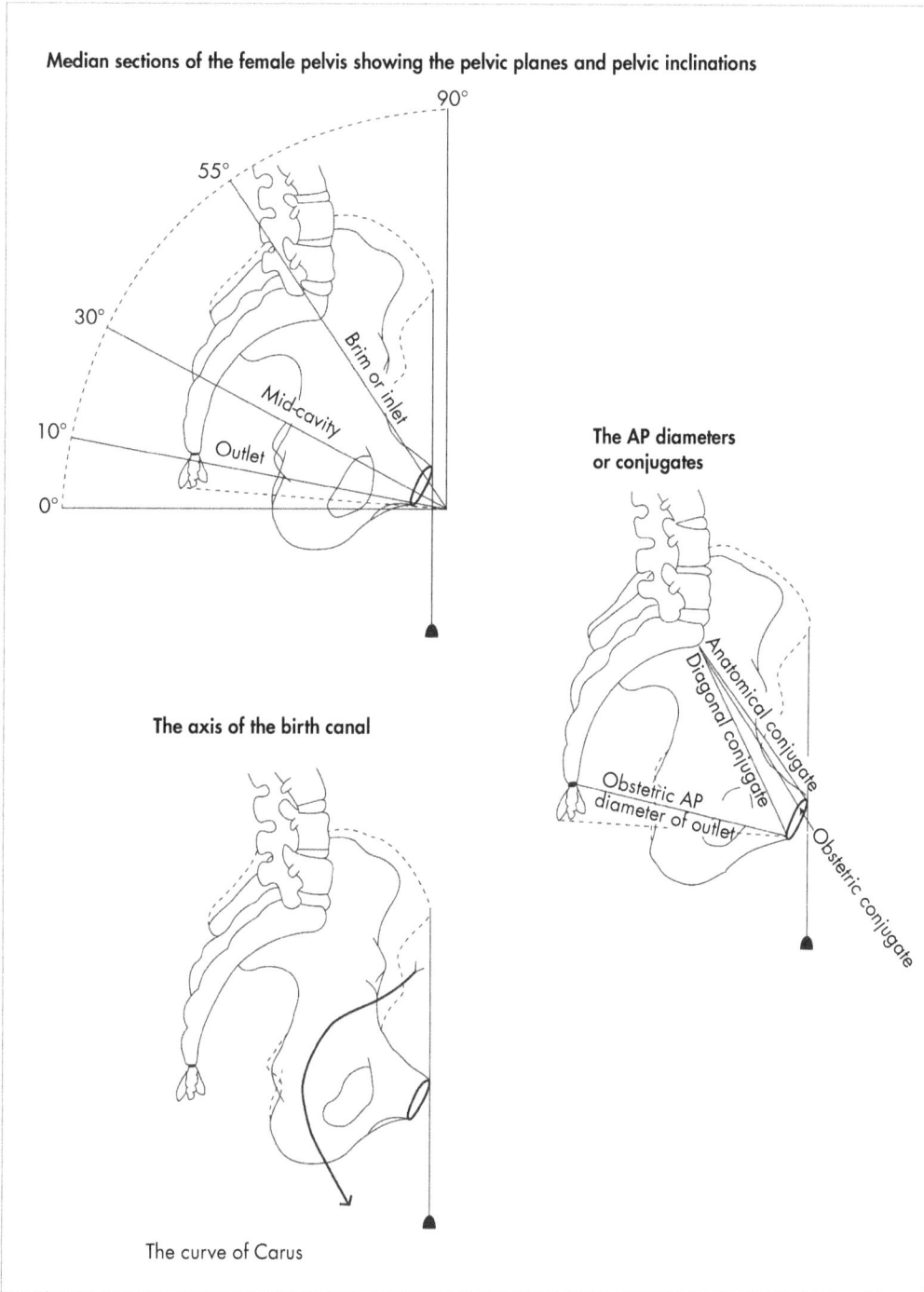

90°

55°

30°

10°

0°

Brim or inlet

Mid-cavity

Outlet

The AP diameters
or conjugates

Anatomical conjugate

Diagonal conjugate

Obstetric conjugate

Obstetric AP
diameter of outlet

The axis of the birth canal

The curve of Carus

Figure 8.7 Median sections of the female pelvis

8.3 The passage: The pelvic floor

The pelvic floor consists of soft tissues within the bony pelvis. These tissues enclose the outlet to the pelvis and are part of the birth canal. The functions of the pelvic floor are, first, to keep the pelvic and abdominal contents (including the gravid uterus) in place and, secondly, to contain the urethra, the vagina and the anus in position to connect the pelvic organs (the bladder, uterus and the rectum) with the external world.

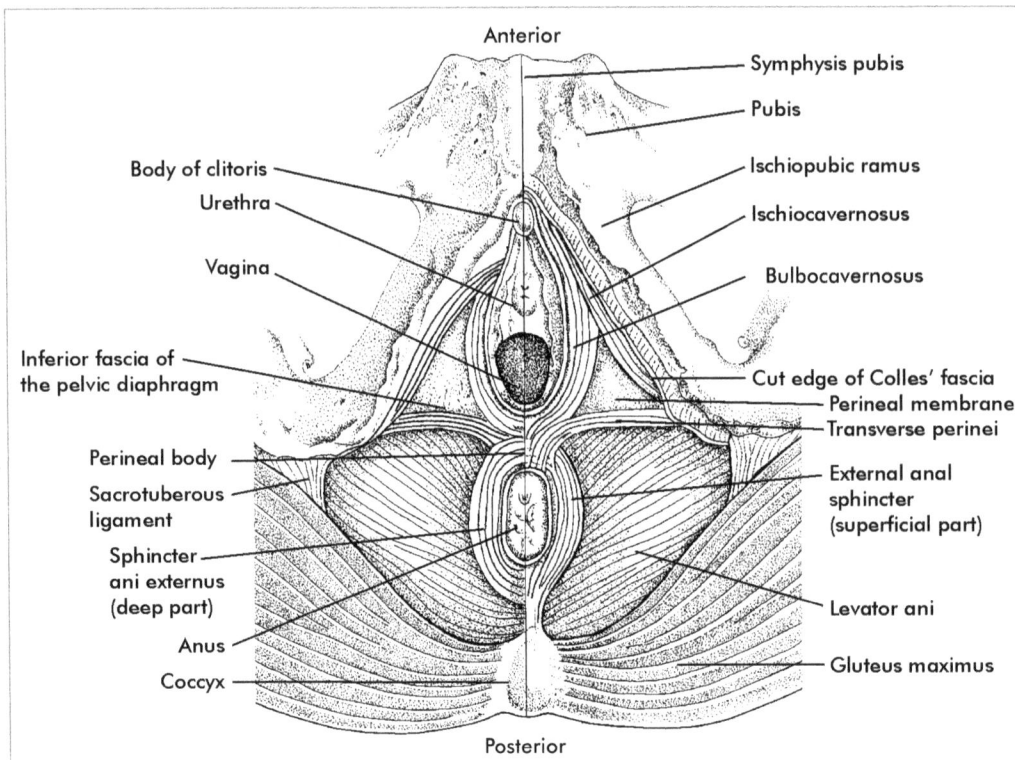

Figure 8.8 The pelvic floor: Inferior view

The pelvic floor consists of three layers or levels of muscle, which are covered by connective and adipose tissue and by skin on the outer body surface, as summarised in Table 8.2.

Table 8.2

Structures of the pelvic floor

Deep layer	Middle layer	Superficial layer
The levator ani · Ischiococcygeus Iliococcygeus Pubococcygeus Puborectalis Pubovaginalis	The deep transverse perineal	The bulbocavernosus The ischiocavernosus The superficial transverse perineal The anal sphincter
The vagina, rectum and urethra pass through the structures. Damage to the pelvic floor in birth can cause prolapse and fistulas.		These are the structures of the perineum that may be involved in trauma during birth or when cutting an episiotomy.

The deep muscle layer of the pelvic floor

The deep layer of muscles of the pelvic floor (levator ani) are highly specialised. They are attached to the inner circle of the pelvis at the front and sides and are inserted into the sacrum and the coccyx posteriorly. The muscles on either side are constructed in such a way that they slope downwards and forwards, and meet and decussate (the interlacing or crossing over of fellow parts) in the midline, to form a gutter or sling.

The formation of this downwards and forwards sloping gutter is of great significance during the birth process, because whichever part of the fetus meets the pelvic floor first is directed in a downwards and forwards direction, enabling it to follow the axis of the pelvis or curve of Carus through the pelvic canal. It is these muscles that move the fetus through the pelvic canal in the mechanism of labour.

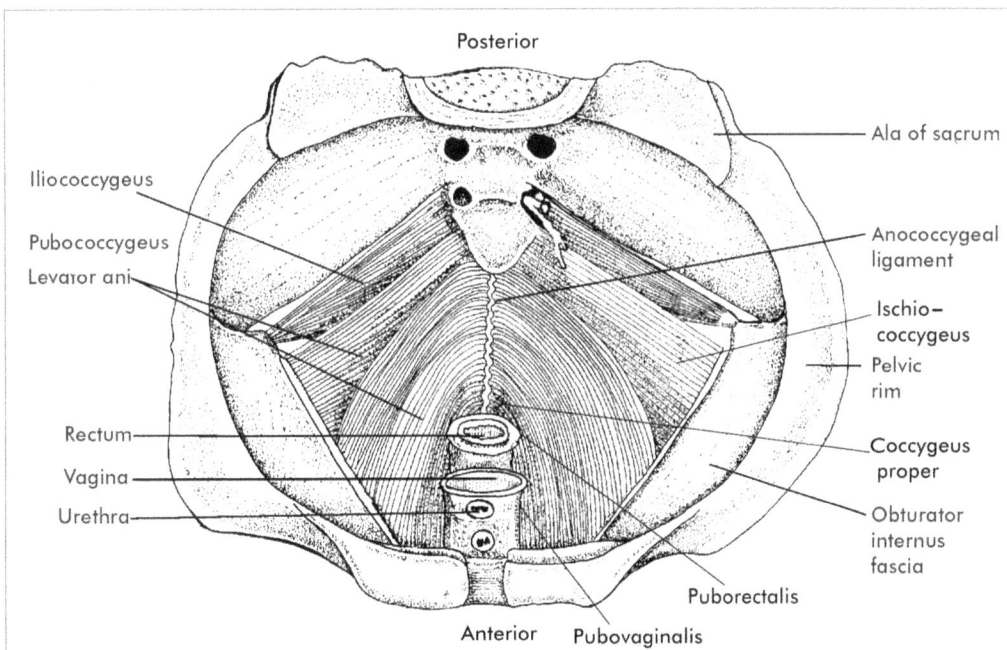

Figure 8.9 The pelvic floor: Superior view

The levator ani muscles maintain constant tone (except during voiding, defecation and the Valsalva manoeuvre) and are made up of the iliococcygeus and the pubococcygeus, as shown in Figure 8.9. These are highly specialised muscles that work like a sling around the vagina and rectum, giving passage to the anal canal, the lower third of the vagina and urethra. The pubococcygeus is divided into the puborectalis (rectum), pubovaginalis (vagina) and pubococcygeus proper. The white line of fascia is a ring of connective tissue that is formed where the muscles implant.

The ischiococcygeus and coccygeus muscles originate from the rami of the ischium, the white facia and the ischial spines. They cover the sacrospinal ligament on each side and are inserted in the coccyx and lower sacrum.

Kegel exercises

Kegel exercises are a set of exercises designed to strengthen and give voluntary control over the pubococcygeus muscles. Doing these is the best way to avoid postpartum complications. Performing Kegel exercises daily will ensure that the pelvic floor muscles are strong and in good shape. These are the same muscles used to stop urine flow. The exercises prevent or improve the stress incontinence that some women experience after childbirth.

In some cases, the muscles that support the uterus become so weak that the uterus sags down into the vaginal opening, a condition called uterine prolapse. In another condition, called cystocele, the bladder falls down into the vaginal opening. These conditions need surgical repair.

The middle layer of the pelvic floor

The strong perineal body lies below the levator ani muscles, making up the posterior portion of the urogenital triangle (diaphragm). This body is triangular and is made up of several muscles. The female perineal body is a mass of interlocking muscular, fascial and fibrous components lying between the vagina and the anorectum. The perineal body is also an integral attachment point for components of the urinary and fecal continence mechanisms, which are commonly damaged during vaginal childbirth. Injuries to the perineal body are caused by spontaneous tears or an episiotomy. They may need surgical intervention and may have serious consequences for the woman's health.

Activity

Visit http://www.fistulacare.org/pages/index.php and learn about the fistula project and the results of insufficient care in childbirth. Thousands of repairs have been done in eight North African countries, which have improved the lives of these women after birth.

The superficial area between the vestibule and the anal sphincter is known as the perineum (the structures commonly involved in tears and episiotomy incision).

The deep perineal muscles are distal to the coccygeus muscles. The origin of the deep transverse perineal muscles is the inferior ramus of the ischium on either side of the pelvis. They meet and intersect in the midline, where they fix to the central tendon. In the female, a portion of these muscles is specialised to form the constrictor vaginae, which acts to compress the vaginal orifice and greater vestibular glands. The deep transverse perinea are not usually involved in the episiotomy incision, but may suffer damage in birth as part of the perineal body.

The perineal body, including the adipose tissue and skin of the perineum, is the area most susceptible to injury and tears during the delivery of the baby (see the box on the next page). This is also the area that is incised when an episiotomy is performed. At the perineum, the pelvic outlet is divided into anterior and posterior sections by the transverse perineal muscles. The anterior portion is known as the urogenital triangle (diaphragm), while the posterior portion is known as the anal triangle. The spaces within these triangles are filled with adipose tissue.

The superficial layer of the pelvic floor (perineum)

The superficial area of the pelvic outlet, from the symphysis pubis anteriorly to the sacrum and coccyx posteriorly, is like a sling and is enclosed and strengthened by pairs of muscles interspersed with adipose tissue. The muscles meet and decussate at the midpoint, surrounding the urethra to form the urethral sphincter. They also surround the vagina and meet and decussate between the vagina and the anus at the perineum, forming the base of the strong perineal body. Behind the anus, they meet in the anococcygeal body, after surrounding the anus and forming the anal sphincter. See Figure 8.9.

The following muscles are found in the perineum:
- The *ischiocavernosus muscles* arise from the ischial tuberosities of the pelvis and pass upwards and inwards

along the pubic arch, to be inserted into the crura of the clitoris. In the female, they have a less functional role.

▶ The *superficial bulbocavernosus and deep transverse perineal muscles* arise from the inner surfaces of the ischial tuberosities and are inserted in the central tendon of the perineum, where they meet and decussate. These are usually not injured or involved in a midline episiotomy. However, the anatomic structures involved in a mediolateral episiotomy include the vaginal epithelium, transverse perineal muscle, bulbocavernosus muscle and perineal skin.

▶ The muscle fibres forming *the anal sphincter* are a continuation of the bulbocavernosus muscle. They arise in the perineum, surround the anus, form the anal sphincter and are inserted into the anococcygeal ligament.

A third-degree tear of the perineum is a tear that extends right through the perineum into the muscle fibres on the anterior border of the anal sphincter and can even extend into the rectal mucosa.

Perineal tears or episiotomies

The structures of the perineum involved in a perineal tear or episiotomy are:

▶ an outer layer of skin, which also forms the fourchette anteriorly
▶ the bulbocavernosus muscles
▶ the transverse perineal muscles (superficial and deep) – the perineal body.

8.4　The passenger

The fetus is the passenger, which has to negotiate the maternal passages in order to be born. The course of labour, therefore, will be influenced by several factors concerning the passenger, such as:

▶ the number of fetuses
▶ the gestational age (GA)
▶ the position of the fetus in the uterus
▶ the size of the fetus and its relation to the pelvis.

Approximately 95 per cent of all labour starts with the head of the fetus presenting over the pelvic brim, which means that most babies are born head first. The fetal head is relatively large compared with the body. It consists of a bony box (a skull) that is different from the adult skull and that contains the fetus's delicate brain.

Once the head is born, the body usually follows without any problem. (The exception to this is a large baby, with large, wide shoulders. In this case the shoulders can become caught up at the pelvic brim during delivery. Sometimes the mothers of these babies have diabetes mellitus.)

The head is the least compressible part of the fetus and whether it is delivered first or last (as in a breech presentation), it is the most difficult stage of the delivery. The fetal head and its contents can be damaged as the head is squeezed through the bony pelvis and any damage to the fetal brain may be permanent. The trauma to which the fetal head is subjected during the birth process can cause the death of the fetus, or – if the child should survive – it can result in cerebral damage with intellectual disability and/or spasticity.

All these facts indicate that the fetal head is the most important part of the fetus during labour.

The fetal skull

A fetal skull of normal shape and average dimensions is able to pass through an average gynaecoid pelvis with the minimum amount of difficulty if the presentation is a normal, well-flexed (chin on the chest) vertex presentation. In a well-flexed position, the head of a normal fetus of 37 weeks or more presents the best diameters for vaginal birth. In this case the head is like a round ball and the small diameters presented pass through the smallest pelvic diameters with ease.

However, if the presentation of the fetal head should be other than a normal, well-flexed vertex presentation, then larger diameters will present. This may cause difficulties when the head attempts to enter the pelvic brim, during its passage through the pelvic cavity and/or in negotiating the outlet. In this case the effect of a round ball has been lost. It is therefore important to know the diameters of the fetal head.

The anatomy of the fetal skull

There are certain areas and landmarks on the fetal head that are identifiable on abdominal palpation and on vaginal examination, and which enable the midwife to identify and estimate the size, presentation, position and state of flexion of the fetal head. It is necessary, therefore, for a midwife to know the bones, sutures and fontanelles, as well as the areas, landmarks and dimensions of the fetal skull.

Regions of the fetal skull

The skull can be divided into three main regions: the base of the skull, the face and the vault or cranium:

1. The *base of the skull* is the bony area surrounding the opening known as the foramen magnum. These bones are firmly united in order to protect the vital centres in the medulla.
2. The *face* extends from the root of the nose to the junction of the chin with the neck. The bones of the face are small and are also firmly united.

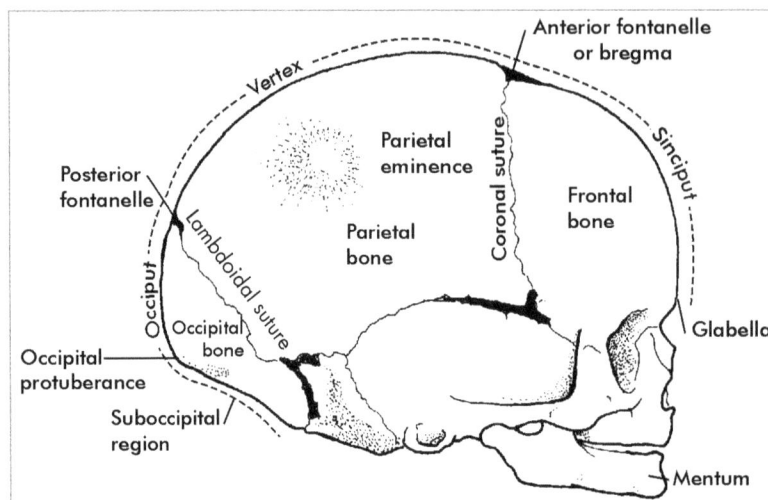

Figure 8.10 Bones, regions and landmarks of the fetal skull

3. The *vault* or *cranium* is the greater, upper, dome-shaped part of the skull that extends above the face in front to the base of the skull posteriorly and includes the temporal sutures laterally, as shown in Figure 8.10. The bones of the vault are formed from membrane and not cartilage. The intramembranous ossification of these bones starts by the tenth week of intrauterine life. The ossification begins at the centre of each skull bone and, as development takes place, spreads slowly outwards towards the periphery. At term, the ossification is not quite complete, leaving a thin line of membrane between each skull bone, which is called a suture. Where three or four sutures meet, a membranous area exists, which is known as a fontanelle. The sutures are very useful for identifying the position of the fetal head during labour, as they can easily be felt on vaginal examination.

At term, the skull bones are thin, especially at the edges, and are fairly pliable. The sutures allow these bones to overlap or 'override' when the head is compressed, thereby decreasing the dimensions of the presenting diameters. This overriding of the skull bones is known as moulding (as shown in Figure 8.15 on page 137 and discussed in that section), and this allows the head to pass through the pelvic canal more easily. However, if the bones are too soft (as with preterm infants) or if too much moulding takes place during labour (as with a contracted pelvis), then the contents of the skull are compressed and brain damage can occur.

The bones of the fetal skull

As shown in figures 8.10 and 8.11, the cranial bones (from the front of the fetal skull to the back) are:
▶ two halves of the frontal bone
▶ two parietal bones
▶ one occipital bone.

The sutures of the fetal skull

As shown in figures 8.10 and 8.11, the sutures are the following:
▶ The *frontal suture* (also called the metopic suture), which bisects the frontal bones down the centre of the forehead (sinciput), is a forward extension of the sagittal suture.
▶ The *sagittal suture*, which lies between the parietal bones and runs in an AP direction, divides the skull into left and right halves.
▶ The *coronal sutures* separate the frontal bones from the parietal bones. These two sutures run almost at right angles to the sagittal suture and the frontal suture, bisecting these sutures and thereby forming the anterior fontanelle.
▶ The *lambdoidal sutures* join centrally to form one long suture and divide the two parietal bones from the occipital bone. These sutures run transversely across the posterior end of the sagittal suture, thereby forming the posterior fontanelle.
▶ The *temporal sutures* lie on either side of the skull, between the temporal bones laterally and the frontal and parietal bones above. At the point where the coronal suture meets the temporal suture on either side of the skull, there is a small temporal fontanelle (the temple). It is between these points that the bitemporal diameter is measured.

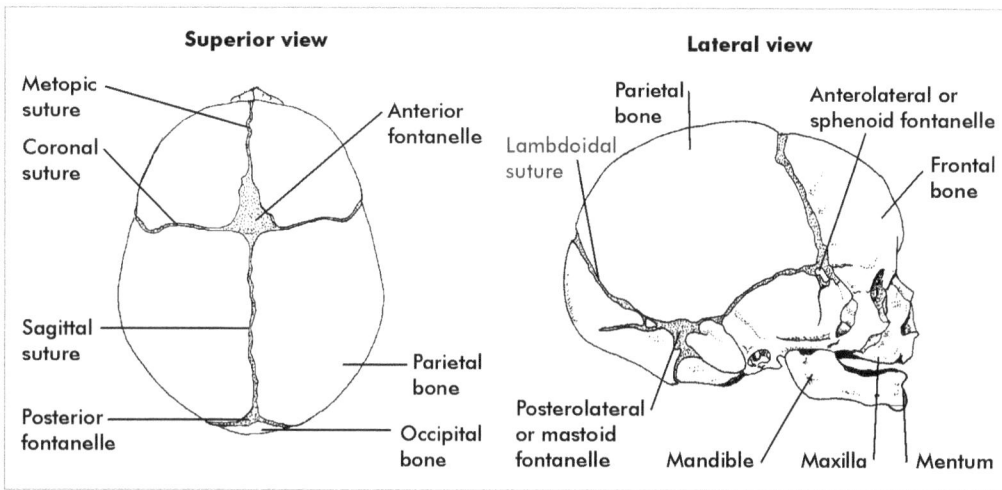

Figure 8.11 Regions of the skull

The two important fontanelles

The two important fontanelles that lie at the junction of the sutures (see Figure 8.11) are as follows:

1. The *anterior fontanelle,* or *bregma,* is diamond-shaped because it is formed by the junction of four sutures: the frontal, the sagittal and the two coronal sutures. It is situated centrally or at a midpoint on the top of the fetal skull, where the frontal and parietal bones meet.
2. The *posterior fontanelle,* or *lambda,* is triangular because it is formed by the junction of three sutures: the sagittal and the lambdoidal sutures. It is situated centrally, on the posterior aspect of the fetal skull, where the parietal bones meet the occipital bone.

Anatomical landmarks of the fetal skull

Taking a lateral view of the fetal skull and working from the point where the chin meets the neck anteriorly, continuing over the face and over the vault of the skull to the nape of the neck posteriorly, the following areas and landmarks are identified (see Figure 8.10 and Figure 8.12 on the next page):

- The *submental area* is the area below the chin. It extends to the angle where the chin meets the neck.
- The areas between the submental area and the vertex are:
  - the mentum
  - the face
  - the root of the nose
  - the orbital ridges above the eye sockets
  - the glabella, which is the elevated area between the orbital ridges

- the sinciput (the brow or forehead), which is the area bounded anteriorly by the glabella and orbital ridges and posteriorly by the bregma and coronal sutures.
- The *vertex* is the top of the cranium and is the lowest area on the fetal skull to enter the pelvic brim in a vertex presentation. The vertex is bounded by the coronal sutures and bregma anteriorly, by the lambdoidal sutures and lambda posteriorly and by the parietal eminences laterally.
- The *parietal eminences* are thickened and raised areas in the centre of each parietal bone, where the greatest amount of ossification has taken place. The diameter between these eminences is the widest part of the skull, and therefore the largest transverse diameter, called the biparietal diameter (BPD).
- The *occiput* is the area at the back of the head, which is formed by the occipital bone. It is posterior and below the lambdoidal sutures and the posterior fontanelle. The suboccipital area is the area below the occipital protuberance (the thick, raised area in the centre of the occipital bone). The suboccipital area extends from the occipital protuberance to the nape of the neck.

Measurements of the fetal skull

The diameter of the portion of the fetal skull that lies over the pelvic brim, and which attempts to enter the pelvic brim during pregnancy and labour, is of great importance. This is because the smallest diameters of an average-sized fetal skull will enter the brim of a gynaecoid pelvis with the least amount of difficulty, while the largest diameter of an average-sized fetal skull is too large to enter the pelvic brim, which means that the head could become obstructed.

133

A midwife should know the measurements of the fetal skull and the reasons why these are important. These measurements, as in Figure 8.12, are approximate for an average-sized fetal skull and are indicated between two landmarks on the skull:

1. The transverse diameters: The BPD of 9.5 cm is measured between the two parietal eminences. The bitemporal diameter of 8.2 cm is measured between the junctions of the corona and temporal sutures on either side of the skull (between the temples).

2. The AP diameters: These diameters and their application in cephalic presentations (presentations of the fetal head) are as follows:

   ▶ The suboccipitobregmatic diameter of 9.5 cm is measured from below the occipital protuberance to the centre of the anterior fontanelle. This is the diameter (together with the BPD of 9.5 cm) that presents in a well-flexed vertex presentation (round ball). As all the diameters in this presentation are small and also equal, the presenting part is an almost perfect circle, which fits well onto the circle of the internal cervical os. This creates an even pressure all around the cervix and brings about an even dilatation of the cervix during labour.

   ▶ The suboccipitofrontal diameter of 10 cm is measured from below the occipital protuberance to the centre of the sinciput. This is the diameter (together with the BPD) that presents a slightly deflexed vertex presentation, usually with the occiput lying posteriorly in relation to the pelvis.

   ▶ The occipitofrontal diameter of 11.5 cm is measured from the occipital protuberance to the glabella. This large diameter (together with the BPD) presents in a deflexed vertex presentation, also known as the 'military attitude', where the spine is straight, the head erect on the spine and the occiput lies posteriorly in the pelvis. This presentation often develops into a POP position. In this presentation, the wide diameter will also distend the vulva at birth.

   ▶ The submentobregmatic diameter of 9.5 cm is measured from the angle of the chin with the neck to the centre of the anterior fontanelle. This diameter (together with the bitemporal diameter of 8.2 cm) presents in a fully extended face presentation. Although this diameter is smaller than the suboccipitobregmatic diameter, it is not circular and therefore does not exert an even pressure on the cervix. In addition, although these diameters may negotiate the pelvic brim, the wide BPD, which still has to enter the pelvic brim, may become caught up as the face descends into the pelvic cavity.

▶ The submentovertical diameter of 11.5 cm is measured from the angle of the chin with the neck to the highest point on the vertex (about midway between the anterior and posterior fontanelles). This diameter (together with the bitemporal diameter) presents in an incompletely extended face presentation, particularly common in a mentoposterior position. This wide diameter also distends the vulva during the birth of a face presentation.

▶ The mentovertical diameter of 13.5 cm is measured from the tip of the chin, or mentum, to a point on the vertex that is just above the posterior fontanelle. This diameter is the largest on the fetal head. This extremely large diameter presents in a brow presentation. It is larger than any of the diameters of a gynaecoid pelvis and would usually become obstructed should it attempt to negotiate the pelvic brim.

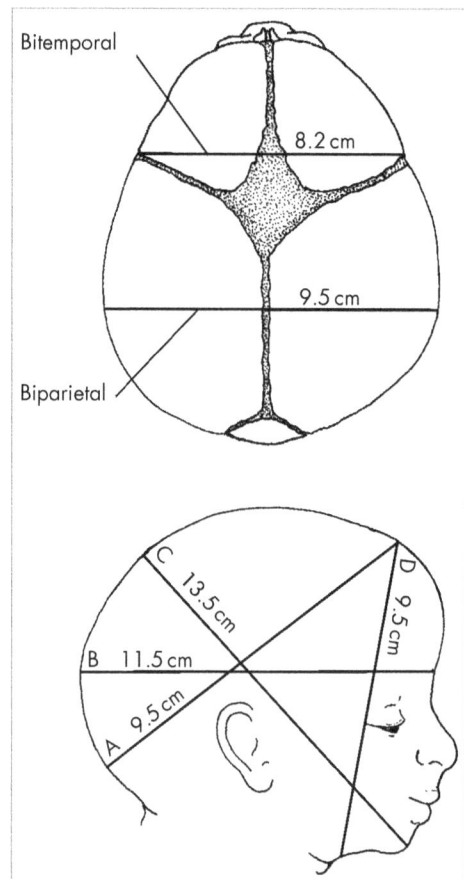

Figure 8.12 Measurements of the fetal skull: A = suboccipitobregmatic diameter; B = occipitofrontal diameter; C = mentovertical diameter; D = submentobregmatic diameter

Measurements of the fetal head in labour

The diameters of the fetal head can only be inferred in labour unless they are measured by ultrasound, CT scan or X-rays. Signs of malpresentation include poor contractions during labour, poor application of the presenting part on the cervix and failure of the presenting part to engage and descend. In addition, the midwife will have difficulty feeling the sutures and fontanelles on vaginal examination.

The Ferguson reflex

A well-fitting presenting part on the cervix releases local prostaglandins and stimulates the uterus to contract well. This is called the Ferguson reflex. Where it is absent, uterine contractions may be weak or abnormal.

Movements of the fetal head (attitude)

The fetal head is capable of a wide range of movements and can also rotate 90 degrees on the neck to either side of the body. The following movements are considered important:
▶ *Flexion:* The head is completely flexed, so that the chin of the fetus is in contact with the chest.
▶ *Extension:* The head is completely extended, so that the occiput is in contact with the fetal back.
▶ *Deflexion:* This is neither flexion nor extension, but somewhere between the two. The fetal back is straight, with the head erect. This is known as the 'military attitude'.

Engagement of the fetal head

Engagement of the fetal head has taken place when the widest presenting diameter, the BPD, has passed through the brim or inlet of the pelvis. This is applicable to the delivery of the head of any fetus, whether the presentation is a vertex presentation or not, or however large or small the fetal head may be.

The engagement of the fetal head is the most important facet in the delivery of the baby, because unless the BPD is able to pass through the pelvic brim, vaginal delivery cannot take place. See also Figure 8.13.

Clinical assessment of engagement

A clinical assessment of the engagement of the fetal head can be made through:
▶ *abdominal palpation,* where the part of the fetal head palpable above the pelvic inlet is calculated as fifths above the pelvic inlet
▶ *vaginal examination,* where with a normal vertex presentation and a normal pelvis, the fetal head can be felt at or near the level of the ischial spines. Figure 8.13 illustrates the relationship of the fetal head with the ischial spines. If the presenting part is felt at the spines, it is at 0. If the head is above the spines, it is potentially −1 to −5 cm above the spines and it is difficult to feel it clinically. If the head moves past the spines, it can be measured at 1 to 5 cm below the spines and is more easy to determine.

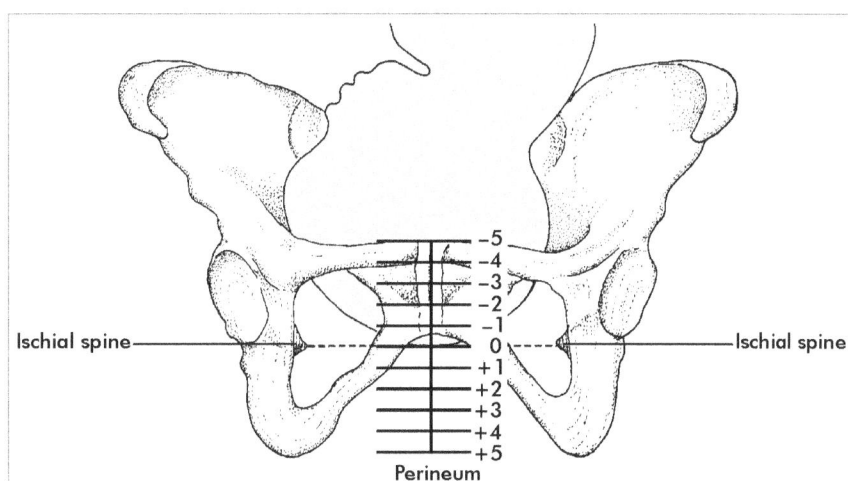

Figure 8.13 Stations of the presenting part in the pelvis

Synclitism and asynclitism

Synclitism exists when the fetal head is aligned with the spine and the sagittal suture line divides the pelvic cavity in two equal parts, regardless of the position of the head. On vaginal examination, the sagittal suture line will be felt in the middle and the applications may be good. Synclitism will provide a better 'fit' or application on the cervix.

Asynclitism, as shown in Figure 8.14, occurs when the pelvis is wide and the fetal head tilts on the shoulders and is mal-aligned. The suture line is off-centre and an ear can be felt on vaginal examination, with poor application. This may influence application of the presenting part on the cervix.

With posterior asynclitism (Litzmann's obliquity), the ear can be felt posteriorly. With anterior asynclitism (Naegele's obliquity), the ear can be felt anteriorly.

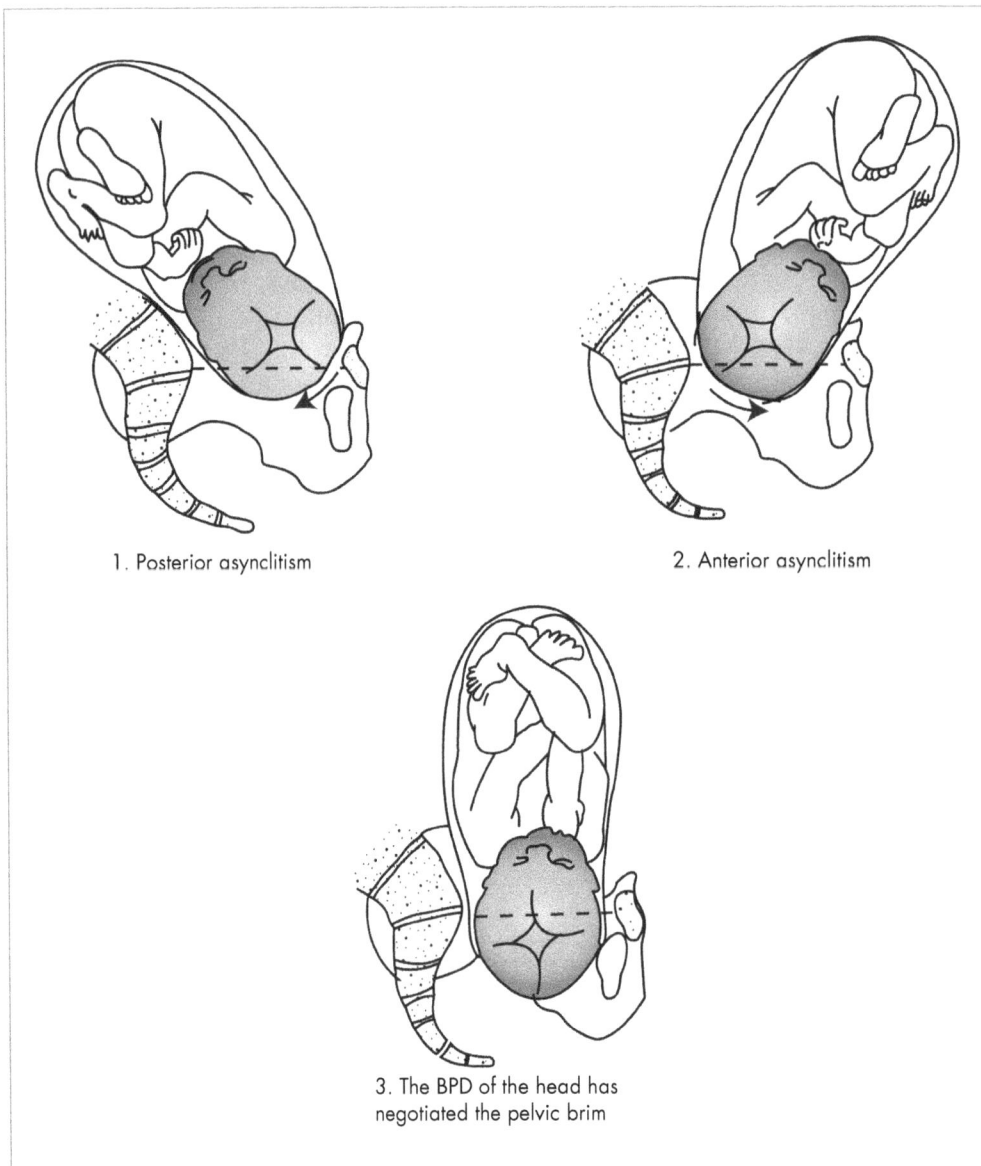

1. Posterior asynclitism

2. Anterior asynclitism

3. The BPD of the head has negotiated the pelvic brim

Figure 8.14 Asynclitism

Moulding of the fetal skull

Moulding, as shown in Figure 8.15, is the change in shape of the fetal head during its passage through the birth canal due to prolonged compression on the presenting diameters of the head as the head is forced through the bony pelvic canal.

While the presenting diameters are reduced, the diameters at right angles to the presenting diameters are increased. This means that in normal labour, with the average amount of force exerted by the uterine contractions, the actual area of the cranium is not altered. Where the space is diminished in one direction, it is increased in another direction.

Moulding is of the greatest value in the progress of labour, as it allows the widest presenting diameters of the fetal head to enter the pelvic brim (become engaged) and to negotiate the pelvic canal.

Moulding should be a slow process, occurring as the head passes into and through the pelvis. No damage of any consequence is caused to the brain of the baby as long as the moulding is not excessive. However, damage can occur:

▶ with prolonged labour due to CPD
▶ in a preterm baby, due to large sutures and soft skull bones
▶ in the after-coming head of a breech presentation or assisted delivery
▶ in a difficult or traumatic forceps delivery or vacuum extraction.

In the above-mentioned situations, the danger is tearing of the falx cerebri or tentorium cerebellum and the adjoining blood vessels in the brain due to sudden compression and decompression.

The change in shape of the fetal skull (see Figure 8.15) depends primarily upon the state of flexion or extension of the fetal head. This, in turn, determines which will be the largest presenting diameter. When this diameter is diminished, the head increases in size at right angles to this largest presenting diameter. For example, in a well-flexed vertex presentation, the largest presenting diameter is the suboccipitobregmatic diameter of 9.5 cm. Therefore the diameter which will be increased with moulding is the mentovertical diameter (which is at right angles to the suboccipitobregmatic diameter), causing the vertex to become extended outwards.

This change in the shape of the fetal head is possible because the sutures between the bones allow the edges of the bones to override one another and because the bone edges are thin and pliable. The parietal bones usually override the occipital bone posteriorly and the frontal bones anteriorly.

In a normal vertex presentation, the occiput lies over the cervical os and is therefore subjected to the greatest amount of pressure early in labour. This causes the edges of the occipital bone to slip under the edges of the parietal bones. One of the parietal bones then overrides the other parietal bone.

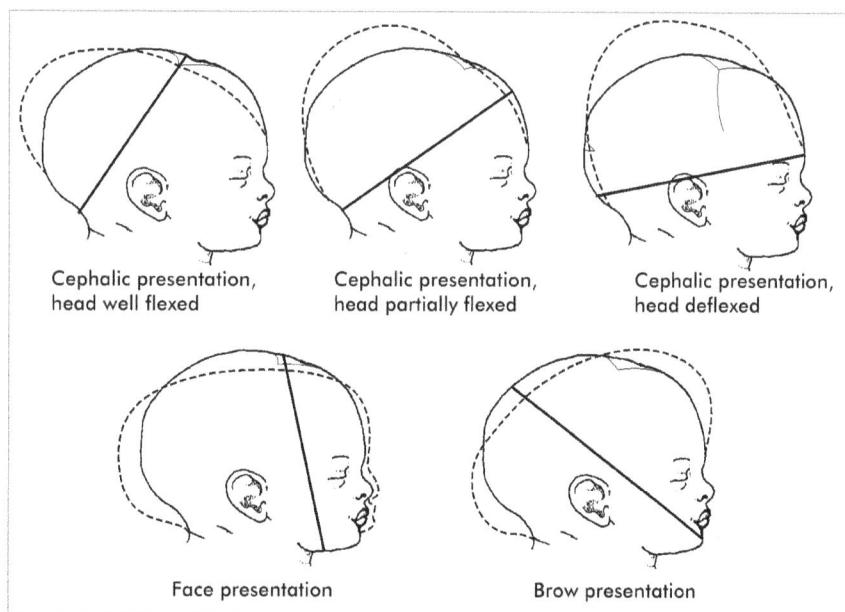

Cephalic presentation, head well flexed

Cephalic presentation, head partially flexed

Cephalic presentation, head deflexed

Face presentation

Brow presentation

Figure 8.15 Moulding of the fetal skull. The moulding is indicated with a dotted line as it would appear in different presentations

The posterior parietal bone is subjected to the most pressure during labour by the sacral promontory, and it is usually the edge of this bone that slips under the edge of the anterior parietal bone.

Caput succedaneum and cephalohaematoma

Caput succedaneum is a neonatal condition involving a serosanguinous, subcutaneous, extraperiosteal fluid collection with poorly defined margins. It is caused by the pressure of the presenting part of the scalp against the dilating cervix (tourniquet effect of the cervix) during delivery.

The position of the scalp over the cervical ring changes as the head negotiates the pelvic canal and therefore the site of this swelling is extended accordingly. A caput is present on the heads of all babies born as vertex deliveries. It starts to reduce in size soon after birth and disappears within 12–24 hours. If, however, the labour has been prolonged and difficult, the caput will be excessive and may persist for up to 36 hours.

Where labour has been prolonged and difficult, a subaponeurotic haemorrhage may occur, where bleeding takes place into the scalp, or a *cephalohaematoma* may develop, where bleeding takes place under the periosteum of one or more of the skull bones. (See Chapter 41.)

8.5   The powers: Uterine contractions

The uterine contractions are the primary powers in childbirth. The muscle fibres in the uterus hypertrophy. At term, the uterus is the largest and strongest muscle in the body. The uterine muscle (middle-layer myometrium) is very vascular and any myoma present will grow large in pregnancy and turn pink due to the vascular supply. This will return to normal size (degenerate) after birth and very seldom interferes with birth.

The muscle fibres of the uterus are specialised and can contract and retract. This means that during contraction the muscle becomes shorter and maintains this length while relaxing again instead of returning to its original length, as shown in Figure 8.16. As a result, the interior space in the uterus becomes smaller and the baby is pushed out. The uterine muscle fibres are arranged in a longitudinal, circular and diagonal way. The blood vessels that pass through these interlocking muscle layers are constricted when the uterus contracts, and bleeding is controlled. During labour the blood supply to the fetus is also constricted when the contraction reaches a particular peak.

A contraction is a motion of the uterus and part of the process of childbirth. Contractions, and labour in general, occur when the hormone oxytocin is released into the body. Oxytocin may be released because of the following:

- *Mechanical means:* The increased pressure and volume of the uterus may signal the start of birth (polyhydramnios and multiple pregnancy).
- *Endocrine action:* An increased number of oestrogen receptors prepare the uterus for oxytocin. The decreased function of the placenta and decreased hormones may signal the release of oxytocin.
- The membrane potential of the uterine muscle (with tubular cells called myocytes, which need large amounts of adenosine triphosphate, or ATP, in both the attachment and release phases) is increased through increased ATP. Prostaglandins are released when the fetal head engages and are involved in the stimulation of contractions and stretching the cervix in preparation for birth. The uterine action is improved through these two processes.
- *Neurogenic action:* The Ferguson reflex occurs when the lower segment of the uterus is stretched, causing a reflective contraction in the upper segment (see the box on page 135 on the Ferguson reflex).

A well-fitting presenting part is associated with good uterine contractions. Induction of labour can be stimulated in late pregnancy if the cervix admits two fingers (4 cm) with a 'stretch and sweep'. The fingers are placed in the cervix and the cervix is stretched. The membranes are then separated from the lower segment by moving the fingers once clockwise between the cervix and the membranes. This releases prostaglandins and may start labour. It is because of this that vaginal examinations are avoided in premature labour, as they may stimulate contractions.

Prior to actual labour, women may experience Braxton-Hicks contractions. These are pre-labour contractions less than 30 seconds in duration. They are irregular, with one or two in 10 minutes, and measure less than 40 mmHg in intrauterine pressure. Braxton-Hicks contractions prepare the cervix and may be involved in the 'ripening' of the cervix for labour. They are also associated with false labour, where contractions are present but the cervix is not dilating.

Under the influence of oxytocin, the contractions become regular and stronger or more intense. Labour starts, a process which is characterised by the presence of the mucus or 'show', changes of the cervix and the descent of the fetal head in a normal vertex presentation.

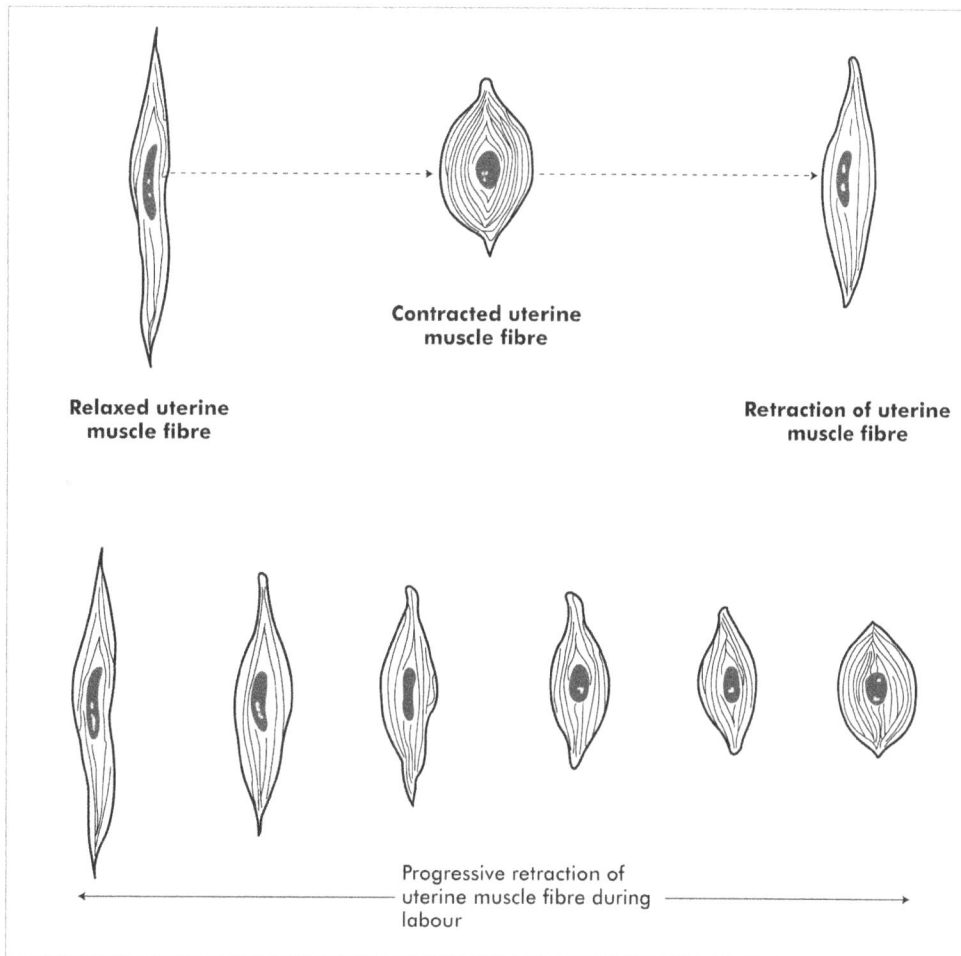

Figure 8.16 Contraction and retraction of the uterine muscle during pregnancy (Braxton-Hicks contractions) and during labour

Terminology

The following terms are important to understand in relation to the uterine action:

▶ *Contraction* is the spontaneous contraction of the uterine muscle, measured in Montevideo units (MVUs).

▶ *Retraction* is the ability of the uterine muscle to relax and become shorter with each contraction. This diminishes the uterine cavity and pushes the fetus out.

▶ *Tone* is the basic pressure in the uterus. The normal tone is 8–12 mmHg. The uterus will be at rest between contractions. Increased basal tone can interfere with placental and fetal blood flow.

▶ *Amplitude* (quantitative assessment) is also referred to as the intensity or 'strength' of a contraction. This can be accurately measured with intrauterine monitors but can also be observed manually or with external monitors.

▶ *Frequency* (qualitative assessment) is the number of contractions in 10 minutes. Clinically, two to three contractions per 10 minutes are required for labour. Scientifically, a total value of 200 mmHg (MVU) (the sum total of all the contractions in 10 minutes) is reached in 90 per cent of women who deliver normally.

▶ *Duration* is the time from the beginning to the end of a contraction. The observation of the duration of a contraction is observed as 'pain' by the patient and there will be a difference between the woman's perception and the midwife's findings on abdominal palpation of the contraction.

139

▶ The *physiological retraction ring* is the physiological border between the upper and lower segment. As labour progresses, the upper segment of the uterus becomes shorter and thicker and the lower segment stretches and becomes longer.

▶ *Effacement* is the changes in the cervix whereby it becomes shorter and is taken up into the uterine cavity to become part of the lower segment of the uterus during the descent of the presenting part. Effacement starts in late pregnancy, when the cervix ripens and the head engages in the pelvis and pushes on the cervix.

▶ *Dilatation* is the opening of the cervical os due to the descent of the presenting part. It is measured in centimetres. Full dilatation is 10 cm.

▶ *Effective contractions.* True labour is characteristised by contractions that will cause the descent of the presenting part and progress in the effacement and dilatation of the cervix. Labour reaches a stage where birth is irreversible.

Assessment of uterine function

In spontaneous labour, regular and frequent contractions indicate true, established and effective labour. Descent of the presenting part and cervical changes will result.

When labour starts, the uterus contracts regularly, and a point is reached where labour is irreversible. Although there are variations in uterus action among women, in 90 per cent of cases the uterus functions in a predictable pattern (see Figure 8.18 on page 142). This has been determined scientifically.

'Normal' uterine contractions in established labour have a specific pattern, strength and number, which can be assessed to determine abnormalities or deviations (see Chapter 31).

Quantitative assessment

As shown in Figure 8.17, a true quantitative assessment of uterine actions can only be done by an intrauterine pressure device. The pressure of the contraction is measured in MVUs. When there is no contraction, the resting tone (pressure) of the uterus is 8–12 mmHG. At the peak of a contraction, the pressure increases to 60–75 mmHg. A sum total of 200 mmHg in 10 minutes is required.

Clinical assessment of contractions is done manually by the midwife: She feels with her finger tips on the fundus of the uterus. A contraction is measured in seconds. This is an indirect estimation of contractions.

The effect of the contractions on the course and progress of labour is the measure of true labour and depends on all the Ps of labour.

Qualitative assessment

The number of contractions in 10 minutes can be observed manually or with an external toco transducer. The midwife can assess contractions manually on the abdomen by placing her finger tips on the fundus of the uterus for a period of 10 minutes every hour.

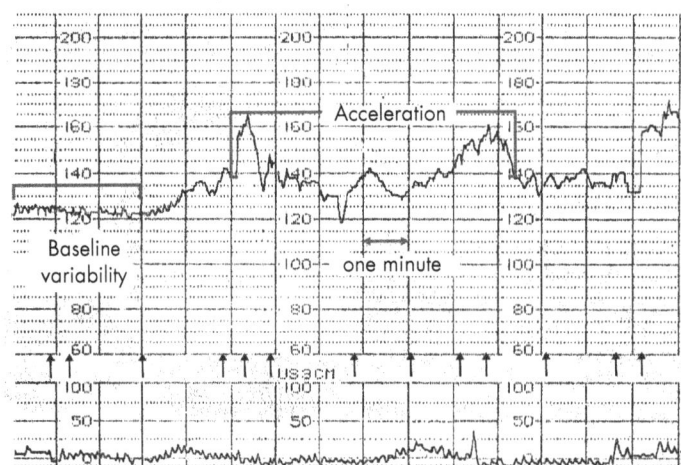

Figure 8.17 Schematic presentation of uterine contractions

The number (frequency) and duration (strength) of contractions in the 10-minute period are reported, for example three contractions of 45 seconds each. The contractions are considered weak, mild or strong based on the duration as 30 seconds, 45 seconds or 60 seconds respectively, and the strength or intensity.

Electronic monitoring of uterine action is useful, but cannot replace the midwife's direct observation of labour. It is a supportive tool, but can lead to inaccuracy and artefacts.

Women generally experience a contraction when the intrauterine pressure exceeds 30 mmHg. This creates a difference of 20 seconds between the woman's experience and the midwife's observation. Midwives need to be aware of this difference and rely not only on the woman's report. If a woman reports 'pain' before the midwife observes a contraction or after the contraction has gone, it may indicate abnormal uterine action.

Characteristics of normal uterine function

The physiology of labour depends on the relationship between the passage, passenger and powers. When the fetus is in a favourable position and the presenting part 'fits' well on the cervix, the pressure of the presenting part stimulates normal contractions.

Although the science of normal uterine action is described here, the midwife must always be aware of individual differences and other factors that affect labour. The midwife should be able to distinguish the normal from the abnormal.

Uterine actions are thus always considered in terms of the position of the fetus, the application and descent of the presenting part and the progress of dilatation. A well-flexed anterior vertex position that presents with a BDP of 9.5 cm and a suboccipitobregmatic diameter of 9.5 cm is ideal for labour if the baby is of average size and a well-fitting presenting part stretches the lower segment. The Ferguson reflex will kick in and labour should progress with good contractions.

Uterine tonus, dominance and polarity

Normal uterine contractions are characterised by a normal resting tone between contractions, fundal dominance (contractions starting in the fundus), polarity (the uterus contracting as a unit) and two to three contractions of 45–60 seconds in 10 minutes:

▶ *Uterine tonus:* There is always pressure in the uterus, even when in a state of rest. The resting tone of the uterus is 8–12 mmHg. When the uterus contracts, the pressure increases and reaches a peak (see Figure 8.17 and Figure 8.18 on the next page). During a contraction, the pressure on the fetal head measures up to 200 mmHg. In the

second stage of labour, the peak is 80 mmHg or more. An increase in the basic resting tone above 12 mmHg is suspect and needs attention; it may indicate a silent abruption. Hypertonic contractions indicate overstimulation of the uterus by medication in the induction of labour (IOL) (see Chapter 31). Hypertonic contractions during labour when an induction or augmentation was *not* performed may indicate obstructive labour.

▶ *Fundal dominance:* This indicates that the contractions start in the upper segment in the pacemakers of the fundus and spreads over the uterus 2 cm per second to the other pacemakers until the uterus contracts as one unit. This is called the contraction wave (see Figure 8.18 on the next page). If the contraction starts in the lower segment, there will be poor progress.

▶ *Polarity (or synchronised/symmetrical uterine action):* Effective uterine action occurs when the uterus contracts as a unit. This means that there is fundal dominance and that the contractual wave spreads over the uterus and both sides contract together. Apolarity means that some of uterine muscles contract independently. This can be referred to as a colicky uterus.

Does duration of pregnancy vary by ethnic group?

Research (Patel et al, 2004) provides evidence that the length of human gestation differs amongst ethnic groups in a heterogeneous maternity population. Black and Asian women may have shorter pregnancies than Caucasian women. The discrepancy in gestational length could be associated with earlier fetal maturation. To accurately predict estimated date of delivery (EDD), maternal factors may need consideration.

Pathophysiology of labour: Obstructed labour/Bandl's ring

When the uterus contracts, the upper segment contracts and retracts with each contraction. This means that the upper segment becomes shorter and thicker and pushes the fetus into the lower segment of the uterus. The lower segment becomes longer and thinner. If the fetus is obstructed by the pelvis, the process will continue until the upper segment reaches its maximum contractile ability and cannot contract any further. The upper segment is now a thick spastic bundle of muscle, and the lower segment is overstretched, long and thin. The fetus is jammed in the pelvis and labour is arrested. The difference between the two segments can be seen and felt on the abdomen and is called Bandl's ring. This is also known as the pathological retraction ring.

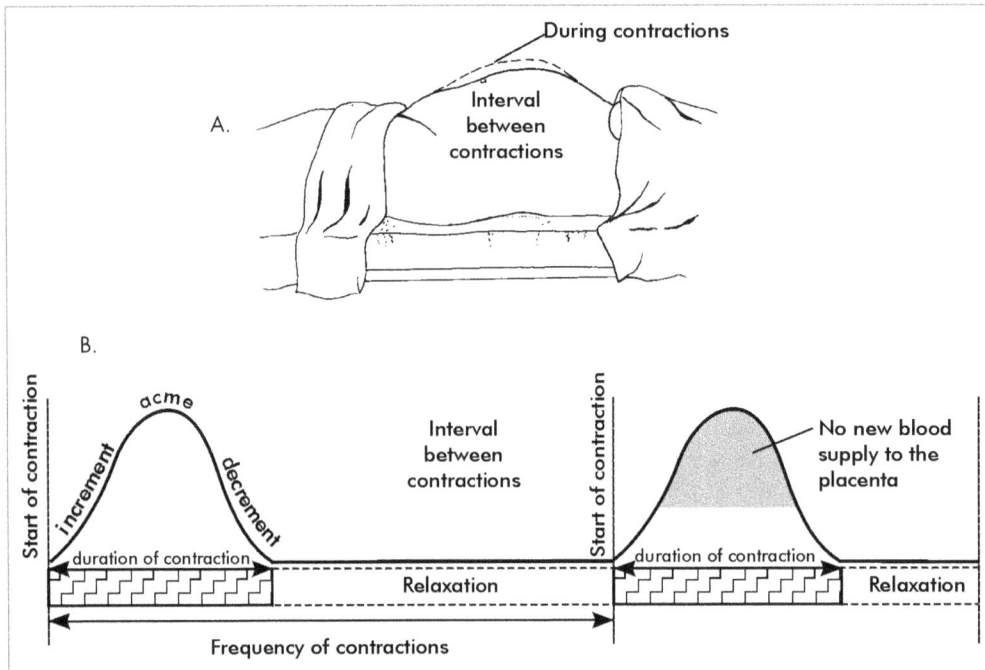

Figure 8.18 Uterine contractions: A = Changing of abdominal contours before and during the contraction; B = Wavelike pattern of contractions

A constriction ring can also occur, where a circular segment of the myometrium goes into spasm and constricts over the fetus, causing a delay in birth.

Obstructed labour is an important cause of maternal and fetal death and morbidity. The following are possible complications in different situations:

▶ *Complications for multiparae:* When there is obstruction of labour and the uterus has reached its maximum contractility, labour cannot proceed and can result in a ruptured uterus in multigravidae.

▶ *Complications for primigravidae:* When obstructed labour develops in a primigravida, the uterus tends to be less likely to tear because it is a first pregnancy. As a result, the woman will present with prolonged labour and the contractions will gradually disappear as the uterus reaches maximum contractility (with the development of Bandl's ring). Obstetric shock will develop, which may lead to abruption placenta and related complications for the baby and mother. If the baby is delivered by Caesarean section, postpartum haemorrhage (PPH) and death may occur. Abnormal uterine action is explained in Chapter 31.

Causes of obstructed labour

The most common cause of obstructed labour is CPD and malpresentations, pelvic abnormalities and large fetal size, or soft tissue dystocia (also see Chapter 31). Risk factors include:

▶ a large or pendulous abdomen
▶ a small woman
▶ a large fetus
▶ a ballotable fetal head when labour commences, with poor application of the presenting part
▶ excessive and early formation of caput and moulding in labour
▶ strong contractions that become progressively hypertonic and then gradually disappear
▶ prolonged labour, which leads to maternal and fetal exhaustion.

Prevention and intervention

The midwife is tasked with identifying women at risk for obstructed birth in the antenatal period already. If this is not done, the use of the partogram is an essential tool to assist the midwife in determining when a birth starts to exceed the normal expected progress in terms of time, the engagement and descent of the fetal head and the dilatation of the cervix. Standard care of good quality intrapartum can prevent a catastrophe. In the case of prolonged labour, the midwife refers the woman.

A rupture of the uterus is an emergency. Only a Caesarean section can correct this condition. Early identification and intervention are needed to prevent it. Obstructed labour and the development of Bandl's ring in a woman under observation by healthcare professionals indicate inexcusable negligence. A healthcare professional must be able to identify the problem in time and take the needed action, particularly by using the partogram correctly.

8.6 Conclusion

This chapter presented aspects of the three Ps of labour – the passage, the passenger and the powers – which are considered to be the three major factors in childbirth. An experienced midwife should know the normal from the abnormal. This starts with a thorough understanding of the normal.

9

Breastfeeding

LEARNING OBJECTIVES

On completion of this chapter, you must be able to:
- demonstrate knowledge of the anatomy and physiology of human lactation
- demonstrate an ability to apply your acquired knowledge in educating women in the antenatal and postpartum periods with regard to the production of breast milk
- demonstrate the ability to provide support on breastfeeding techniques
- demonstrate knowledge of the strategies for protection and promotion of breastfeeding
- identify advantages of and contraindications to breastfeeding.

KNOWLEDGE ASSUMED TO BE IN PLACE

Basic anatomy and physiology of the female breast

KEYWORDS

mammae • lactation • oxytocin • hypergalactia • galactorrhoea • agalactia • lactogenesis • galactopoiesis

9.1   Introduction

The importance of breastfeeding warrants a scientific view of evidence-based findings on breastfeeding and breast milk. To date, there is no true substitute for breast milk. Replacement feeding has been adapted to suit various special needs of infants, but can never be as good as the milk produced by a mother, which is tailor-made for the baby. However, breastfeeding is the mother's choice and she needs to be supported in whatever choice she makes. In places where breastfeeding is universal or the norm, this needs to be protected.

The midwife must have a thorough knowledge of the anatomy and physiology of the breast and other factors that may affect a woman's choice of feeding.

9.2   Protection and promotion of breastfeeding

The WHO and the United Nations Children's Fund (UNICEF) support and protect breastfeeding.

UNICEF's strategy for infant feeding

UNICEF's strategy for infant and young child feeding is based upon the Innocenti Declaration on the Protection, Promotion and Support of Breastfeeding. The Innocenti Declaration was adopted in 1990 and endorsed by the World Health Assembly (WHA) and UNICEF's Executive Board. The four Innocenti targets in the *Global Strategy for Infant and Young Child Feeding* adopted by the WHA in May 2002 include (WHO, 2003):

1 the appointment of a national breastfeeding coordinator of appropriate authority, and the establishment of a multi-sectoral national breastfeeding committee
2 ten steps to successful breastfeeding (the Baby-Friendly Hospital Initiative, or BFHI) practised in all maternity facilities
3 the global implementation of the International Code of Marketing of Breast-Milk Substitutes and subsequent relevant WHA resolutions in their entirety
4 the enactment of imaginative legislation protecting the breastfeeding rights of working women and the establishment of means for enforcement of maternity protection.

The lives of over 820 000 children under 5 years could be saved if all children 0–23 months old were optimally breastfed. Breastfeeding improves IQ and school attendance, and is associated with higher income in adult life (WHO, 2017). Breast milk alone is the ideal nourishment for infants for the first six months of life, because it contains all the nutrients, antibodies and hormones that an infant needs to thrive. It protects babies from diarrhoea and acute respiratory infections, stimulates their immune systems and responses to diseases, and aids the response to vaccination. (Also see Chapter 39.)

Breastfeeding also has many health and emotional benefits for the mother, including decreased blood loss postpartum, a delayed return to fertility and a decreased risk of cancer of the breast. Immediate postpartum breastfeeding helps the bonding between mother and child.

UNICEF's goal is that all women exclusively breastfeed for six months and continue breastfeeding, with complementary food, well into the second year and beyond. This requires support systems that will help women achieve this aim.

The midwife is the healthcare professional closest to the mother and infant in pregnancy, birth and the early and late neonatal periods. The midwife needs to guide the practice and promote breastfeeding within the framework of the UNICEF guidelines. Women should not be forced to breastfeed, but should be guided and supported to do so. In order to achieve this, midwives need a thorough understanding of the anatomy, physiology, sociology, psychology and pathology of breastfeeding.

South African Breastfeeding Week and policies related to breastfeeding

World Breastfeeding Week is celebrated every year on the anniversary of the Innocenti Declaration (1–7 August). The South African national Department of Health (DoH) supports this initiative.

After the Tshwane Declaration of Support for Breastfeeding was released in 2011, UNICEF and the WHO declared that South Africa is a country that actively promotes exclusive breastfeeding. The declaration ensures that South Africa will take active steps to include the promotion of breastfeeding in policy and legislation (also see Richter, 2016). The declaration includes guidelines for the development of human milk banks, the implementation of baby-friendly care (BFC) and kangaroo-mother-care (KMC). A decision was also taken that no formula feeds will be made available at public health facilities. All public hospitals strive to be accredited as part of the BFHI.

The *Infant and Young Child Feeding Policy* (DoH, 2013) gives guidelines for pregnant women and infants in South Africa.

9.3 Development and anatomy of the female breast

The breasts, known also as the mammary glands or mammae, exist in both sexes and are present as rudimentary glands at birth. In the male, they normally remain rudimentary throughout life, unless they are stimulated in some way by female hormones. The breasts are accessory glands of the female reproductive system.

In the female, the breasts are underdeveloped before puberty, but they undergo further development during and after puberty. During pregnancy, the breasts develop milk glands under the influence of oestrogen, and after giving birth, further development takes place to enable lactation.

The increased development of the glandular tissue of the breasts is stimulated by an increase in the female hormones at puberty, during pregnancy and lactation.

Breast development

During puberty, the breasts form two rounded eminences, one on either side of the anterior chest wall. They are situated within the superficial fascia of the chest wall. They are separated from the chest muscle, the pectoralis major, by the deep fascia and by a zone of loose areolar tissue, the sub-mammary space, which allows the breast some degree of movement on the deep fascia.

The shape and size of the breasts differ in each individual, as well as at different ages in each individual.

Just below the centre of each breast there is a small, cylindrical projection that is harder and darker in colour than the rest of the breast; this is known as the nipple or papilla. In the nulliparous woman, it usually lies at about the level of the fourth intercostal space.

The tissue of each breast extends vertically from about the second to the sixth rib, and horizontally from the side of the sternum to near the mid-axillary line. The tissue of the upper outer quadrant of each breast extends upwards and laterally towards the axilla, forming the tail, which may pass through the deep fascia and lie in close contact with the axillary lymph nodes.

In all mammals in early fetal life, a line of immature breasts extends from the axilla to the inguinal region on either side (embryologic mammary ridges). In humans, the majority of these breasts disappear, leaving only two. However, occasionally, some of these breasts and nipples persist. They are known as supernumerary or accessory breasts. They seldom rival the proper breasts in size and function and when only a nipple persists, it can be mistaken for a pigmented mole.

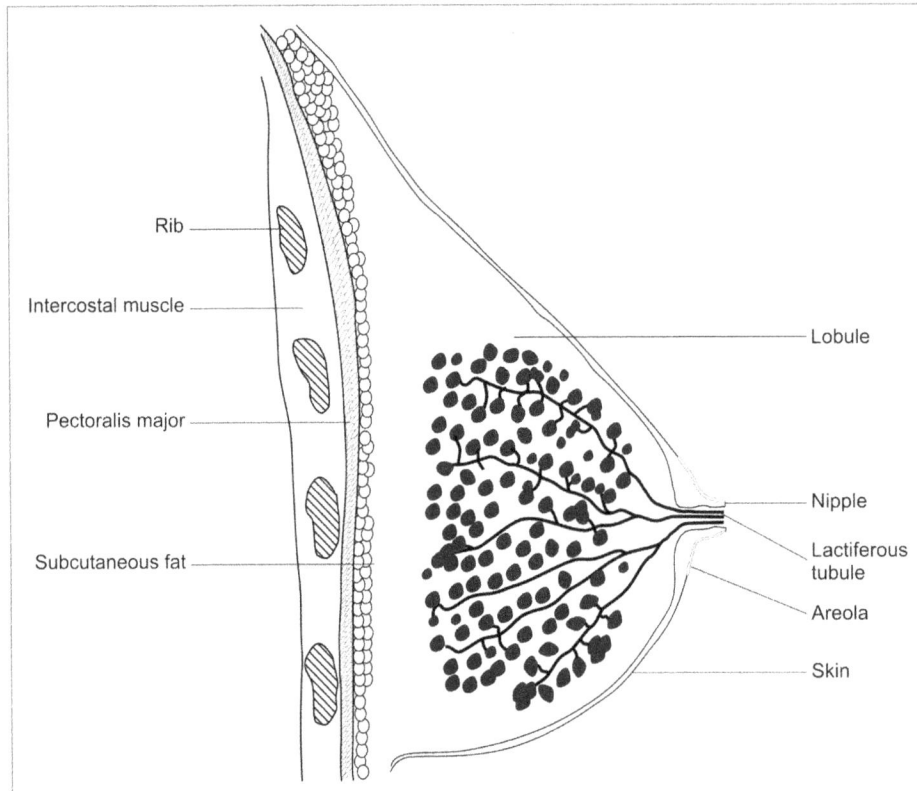

Figure 9.1 Sagittal view of the female breast

Some women have nipple lines down one or both sides of the chest and abdomen, and many of these rudimentary breasts also secrete milk in various quantities after delivery.

Anatomy of the female breast

The breast is made up of glandular tissue, fibrous tissue and adipose tissue, and is covered on the outside by skin. Figure 9.1 shows the structure of the female breast from the sagittal view.

The skin and areola of the breast

The breast is covered with skin and subcutaneous tissue, but at the centre of the breast, around the nipple, the covering consists of primary areolar tissue, which is a specialised form of skin. This areola is pigmented and because it contains more glands, it is less smooth than the skin covering the rest of the breast.

During pregnancy and lactation, this primary areola becomes even darker and more extensive and the areolar glands situated within it become larger and more active; this is then known as the secondary areola. Some of the glands in the areola are sebaceous glands, some a combination of sebaceous and sweat glands and some, Montgomery's glands, are small oil glands. The oily secretion from these glands provides a protective lubricant for the areola and nipple during lactation.

The subcutaneous tissue which encloses the breasts sends numerous septa into the breast to surround each lobe.

The adipose tissue

This forms the bulk of the breast tissue. The amount of adipose tissue present determines the size of the breast.

The fibrous tissue

The fascia on which the breast rests sends out extensions in the form of fibrous processes from the back of the breast forwards to the subcutaneous tissue underlying the skin and nipple, in order to give support to the breast. These processes are the suspensory ligaments of Cooper.

The glandular tissue of the breast

There are 15–20 lobes in each breast, which are made up of glandular tissue and ducts. Each lobe is made up of 30–40 tiny lobules, which are connected to ducts by loose connective tissue and by blood vessels.

Each lobule, when fully developed during pregnancy and in the puerperium, consists of a rounded cluster of 10–100 acini, also called alveoli, which produce milk. These alveoli open up into tiny ducts, which are the smallest ducts of the breast. These tiny ducts unite to form larger ducts draining each lobule and they in turn lead into still larger ducts, known as the lactiferous ducts, which drain each lobe. These ducts converge towards the areola, where they become slightly distended, forming the lactiferous sinuses, which will serve as reservoirs for milk during lactation. The lactiferous ducts then continue as narrow, straight ducts, which pass through the nipple and lead to tiny openings at the end of the nipple, as shown in Figure 9.2.

The nipple, which is composed of erectile tissue, is surrounded by smooth muscle fibres and nerve endings, which cause erection of the nipple.

The alveoli and tiny ducts are surrounded by neo-epithelial cells known as myoepithelial cells. The myofibrils of these cells contract under the hormonal stimulation of oxytocin, causing the 'let-down' of milk. When these myofibrils relax under sympathetic stimulation, the 'let-down reflex' is inhibited.

The blood supply to the breast

The arterial supply

Blood supply increases in pregnancy and lactation. Breast fullness and visible veins in the breasts are early signs of pregnancy. The following arteries supply the breast:

▶ *The internal mammary artery:* This artery branches from the first part of the subclavian artery above the sternal end of the clavicle. It descends into the thorax behind the cartilages of the upper six ribs, branching off to organs and tissues on the way. The anterior intercostal branches are distributed to the upper six intercostal spaces. These branches supply the intercostal mucles and send further branches through them to the pectoral muscles, the breast and the skin.

▶ *Branches from the axillary artery (external/lateral mammary branches):* The axillary artery is a continuation of the subclavian and begins at the outer border of the first rib. As it descends down the arm, it sends off branches, one of which follows the lateral border of the pectoralis minor to the side of the chest and is called the lateral thoracic artery.

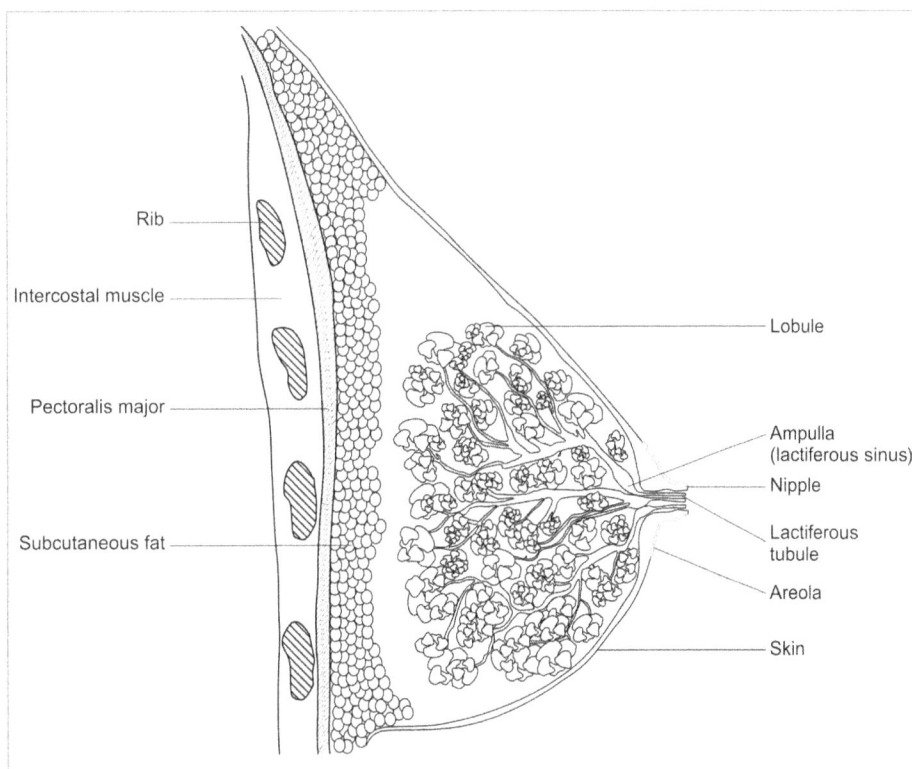

Figure 9.2 A sagittal section through a lactating breast and the anterior chest wall

In the female, the lateral thoracic artery is large and gives off lateral mammary branches, which wind around the lateral border of the pectoralis major to reach the breast.

▶ *Upper/posterior intercostal arteries:* The descending thoracic aorta branches out to the thorax. Arising from the back of the aorta are the posterior intercostal arteries. These are distributed to the intercostal spaces and send off mammary branches to the second, third and fourth spaces. During lactation, these arteries increase considerably in size.

The venous drainage

The *circulus venosus* is an anastamotic circle at the base of each nipple and it drains into the axillary vein and the internal thoracic vein. Both of these veins drain into the subclavian vein, which becomes the brachiocephalic vein and, finally, the superior vena cava.

Each mammary branch of the posterior intercostal artery is accompanied by a corresponding vein and nerve. There is more blood circulating in the breasts during pregnancy and lactation than in the non-gravid state.

The lymphatic drainage of the breast

The lymph vessels originate in a plexus (an interconnected network of lymph vessels) in the interlobular connective tissue and in the walls of the lactiferous ducts. This plexus communicates with a subcutaneous lymphatic plexus beneath the areola surrounding the nipple. The lymphatics of the two breasts communicate freely with one another.

The lymph drains to the following regional nodes:

▶ *The axillary glands in both axillae:* These are the pectoral lymph nodes, which commonly receive more than 75 per cent of the lymph from the breasts.
▶ *Glands in the anterior mediastinum:* These are the parasternal nodes, which drain the medial halves of the breasts.
▶ *Glands in the portal fissure of the liver.*

The nerve supply to the breast

The nerve supply to the nipple is good, but it is poor to the remainder of the breast. There is no voluntary central nerve supply to the breast and no parasympathetic nerve supply.

The nerve supply to the breast is from the autonomous system and made up of sympathetic fibres only:

▶ *Sensory (afferent) somatic fibres:* Impulses are transmitted from the nipples via the spinothalamic tracts to the hypothalamus and so to the pituitary gland. When the baby suckles on the breast, these fibres transmit impulses to the hypothalamus that are then transmitted from there

to the anterior pituitary gland to release the hormone prolactin into the bloodstream. At the same time, the posterior pituitary gland releases the hormone oxytocin into the bloodstream.

▶ *Motor (efferent) sympathetic fibres:* Impulses are transmitted from the brain via the thoracic prevertebral ganglia to the breast. These impulses cause a reflex erection of the nipple whilst the baby suckles. The same reaction occurs by tactile stimulation, but tactile stimulation by pressing the palm of the hand on the nipple can also cause reflex vasoconstriction of arterial blood supply and therefore relaxation of the myoepithelial cells, thereby causing inhibition of the milk flow (inhibition of the 'let-down reflex'). This also comes about as a result of pain, fear, worry, embarrassment or distaste. There is a close relationship between the nerve supply to the breast and hormonal influences on the breast.

9.4   The physiology of lactation

Terminology

The following are important concepts related to lactation that the midwife must know and understand in order to apply her knowledge in the care of breastfeeding women:

▶ *Lactogenesis* is the onset of milk secretions through a series of mammary epithelial cellular changes whereby alveolar cells are converted from a non-secretory state to a secretory state.
▶ *Galactopoiesis* requires prolactin for milk secretion and oxytocin that is critical for the milk let-down reflex in response to suckling.
▶ *Hypergalactia* refers to the overproduction of milk.
▶ *Galactorrhoea* is abnormal milk production.
▶ *Agalactia* indicates an inability to lactate.

Hormonal influences on the breast

During puberty, the influence of hormones on the breasts increases, and it persists until menopause. The breasts respond to cyclical variation in hormonal levels each month, corresponding to the menstrual cycle and also to alterations in hormonal levels during pregnancy and lactation.

The hormones that influence the breasts and the manner in which the breasts respond include oestrogens, progesterone, prolactin, oxytocin, human growth hormone (HGH), adrenal glucocorticoids (see Whirledge & Cidlowski, 2010), human placental lactogen (HPL), thyroxine, prolactin-inhibiting factor and insulin. They are detailed in the following sections and in the box on the next page.

Oestrogens and progesterone

These hormones are produced by the Graafian follicles and the corpus luteum of the ovary under the influence of the hypothalamus and anterior pituitary gland. They influence the breasts during and after puberty and are responsible for the development of these accessory (secondary) glands of the female reproductive system. During early pregnancy, the trophoblast produces human chorionic gonadotrophin (hCG), which stimulates the ovary to continue producing oestrogens and progesterone. Later, the placenta produces oestrogens and progesterone in large amounts. These hormones are responsible for the breast development that takes place during pregnancy and lactation.

From the onset of puberty and during pregnancy, oestrogen causes the duct system to grow and to branch, and also increases the quantity and the deposition of connective tissue and of fat in the breast. Oestrogen causes enlargement of the nipple and areola.

Progesterone acts upon the tissues already prepared by the oestrogens, causing proliferation of these tissues (it also causes premenstrual fullness and congestion of the breasts). During pregnancy, progesterone increases the secretory tissue and develops the secretory characteristics of the alveoli (acini) cells. Both oestrogens and progesterone have the specific effect of inhibiting the effects of prolactin and thereby inhibiting the actual secretion of milk during pregnancy.

Prolactin

This hormone is secreted by the anterior lobe of the pituitary gland. Unlike the other hormones, which are stimulated by the hypothalamus, prolactin production is inhibited by the hypothalamus. Prolactin is carried in the bloodstream during pregnancy. Together with the oestrogens, it increases the development of the duct system of the breasts and is responsible for the secretion of milk at the onset of lactation and during the maintenance of lactation.

The secretory effect of prolactin is inhibited by high levels of oestrogens and progesterone. This means that, although there are high levels of prolactin in the bloodstream towards the end of pregnancy, the secretory effects of prolactin are severely curtailed by the high levels of oestrogens and progesterone. A small amount of colostrum is, however, produced in the breasts towards the end of pregnancy. The sudden drop in oestrogens and progesterone with the delivery of the placenta at birth allows prolactin to assume its function of promoting milk production.

Hyperprolactinaemia can also be present in conditions of severe stress. If a woman suddenly develops engorged breasts or produces milk in pregnancy, this may be a sign of decreased placental function.

Oxytocin

This hormone is secreted by the posterior lobe of the pituitary gland under the influence of the hypothalamus. It is mainly stimulated by the baby suckling on the breast, but may also be stimulated by the mother just seeing or hearing her baby, or by an increase in temperature. Oxytocin is carried in the bloodstream to the breasts, where it causes the myoepithelial cells that surround the outer walls of the alveoli to contract, thereby causing milk to be expressed from the alveoli and into the duct system. At the same time, oxytocin is carried to the uterus, where it causes contraction of the uterine muscles and helps in the involution of the uterus.

Hormones affecting lactation	
HGH and adrenocorticotrophic hormone (ACTH)	Establishing and maintaining lactation. There is an intimate relationship between the hypothalamus and the anterior pituitary with respect to the secretion of ACTH and HGH. Both hormones play a role in lactogenesis
HPL	Has mild lactogenic properties and supports prolactin
Thyroxine	Important in the maintenance of lactation
Prolactin-inhibiting factor	Controls the secretion of prolactin
Insulin	Supports prolactin in milk synthesis

Lactogenesis

As mentioned, lactogenesis refers to both the initiation and production of milk by the breasts. The stages of milk production are colostrum, transitional milk and mature milk.

Colostrum is present during pregnancy and is the first food for the infant. It has a particular function. It is a thick, yellowish fluid with a specific gravity (SG) of 1 040 to 1 060. (The SG for mature milk is 1 030.) The yellow colour is due to high levels of beta carotene (vitamin A). Colostrum is unique and is rich in components, of which 50 per cent are unique to human colostrum (Godhia & Patel, 2013). Colostrum continues to be secreted for up to two weeks postpartum. Its benefits are as follows (Ballard & Morrow, 2013):

▶ It provides a continuation of the immunity that was available to the fetus via the placenta.

▶ It is rich in immunoglobulins, which protect an infant from viruses and infections.

▶ It is high in protein.

▶ It is high in fat-soluble vitamins and minerals.

▶ It contains high amounts of sodium, potassium, chloride and cholesterol to encourage the optimal development of a baby's heart, brain and central nervous system (CNS).

▶ It is a natural laxative that encourages the passage of meconium, which reduces the risk of jaundice in the baby.

The energy value of colostrum is 67 cal/100 ml (280 kJ), versus 75 cal/100 ml (313 kJ) in mature milk. The volume varies between first mothers and multigravidae and is about 2–10 ml per feed per day for the first three days. Sodium, potassium, chloride, fat, protein, fat-soluble vitamins and minerals are present in greater concentrations than in mature milk. The fats present in colostrum are directly excreted from the mother and are smaller than the fat globuli that will be synthesised in mature milk.

Transitional milk is produced between day seven to ten, for two weeks. The composition of milk changes gradually to mature milk.

Mature milk will be present after 14–21 days and looks watery rather than creamy, because of the high concentration of whey.

The volume of water as the main constituent of breast milk is depended on the concentration of glucose in breastmilk (Ballard & Morrow, 2013). Breast milk meets the requirements of the baby, and no added water is needed.

When hormones are released, lactation starts. It is maintained by the stimulation of the nipple and the emptying of the breast. Milk synthesis continues, but 80 per cent of milk production occurs during suckling. Milk production depends on suckling, which releases the hormones for milk production. The rate of milk synthesis is 11–58 ml per hour per breast.

Emptier breasts make milk faster than fuller ones. Regular emptying of the breasts is the main way to produce more milk. The 80/20 principle is applicable. Breasts will make 15–20 per cent more milk than the baby takes. If the baby drinks 80 per cent, the milk will fill up. If the baby takes less than 80 per cent, the breasts will make less. The rate at which milk is pumped out of the breast depends on how empty the breasts are at that stage.

Synthesis of human milk

The synthesis of human milk is unique. It makes a tremendous demand on the maternal system, with a marked change in the woman's metabolism. This includes a redistribution of blood, which causes cardiovascular changes in the mother, with increased blood flow to the breasts, gastrointestinal (GI) tract and liver, and an increased cardiac output. The increase in the metabolic rate places a burden on the thyroid gland. The thyroid is enlarged during lactation.

Breast milk changes during the course of a feed and throughout the day. It is secreted first as foremilk, which satisfies a baby's initial thirst. Hindmilk, which is secreted as the feeding progresses, is high in fat and calories to promote the growth and development of the baby.

Preterm milk differs markedly from full-term milk by offering premature babies longer access to colostrum, to higher levels of immunoglobulin A (IgA) and other anti-infective properties. Preterm milk also contains greater concentrations of triglycerides and long-chain fatty acids. It is 20 per cent higher in nitrogen (protein) than milk for term babies, to meet the growth needs of the small baby. These qualities offer the premature infant optimal nutrition for short-term energy needs as well as for long-term neurological and visual development. Preterm milk also offers the best protection from necrotising enterocolitis (NEC), an often fatal condition in premature babies.

The composition of breast milk is influenced by the mother's fluid and food intake. Human milk contains at least a hundred ingredients not found in any artificial infant milk. Milk is produced by apocrine (where the secretion contains part of the cell) and merocrine (where the cell remains an intact mechanism with minimal mitosis) metabolic processes, as shown in Figure 9.3.

Metabolic processes of the mammary gland	
Component in breastmilk	**Type of metabolic process used by the mammary gland**
Protein	Apocrine
Fat	Apocrine
Lactose	Merocrine
Ions	Diffusion and active transport
Water	Diffusion

Milk is synthesised in the alveolar cells of the acini. The epithelial cells of the milk gland contain stem cells and are highly specialised at the terminal duct. They are stimulated by HGH and insulin. Prolactin synergises the cells to start their activity and is mainly responsible for the synthesis of milk that takes place during suckling. The plasma levels of cortisol are also increased during suckling.

As shown in Figure 9.3, the secretory cells are cubical at the beginning of suckling. Because of increased water uptake, they change into cylindrical cells prior to milk secretion. The cell's nucleus is at the base of the cell and moves to the apex before

secretion. The cytoplasm is granular, but changes to striated as milk secretion begins. The enlarged cell, with its thickened apical membrane, becomes club-like and the tip pinches off, leaving the cell intact (apocrine). The portion containing fat, protein and a small amount of cytoplasm floats free. The baby will ingest a freshly secreted cell portion.

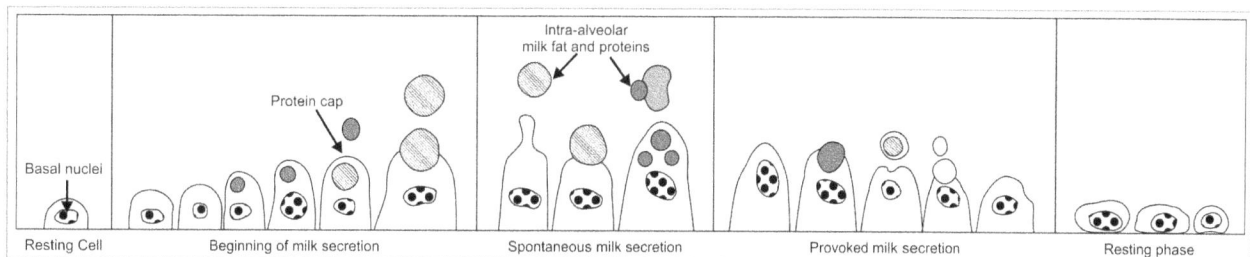

Figure 9.3 Synthesis of human milk at a cellular level

Properties of human milk

The following are unique characteristics of human milk:

▶ *Immunological properties:* Breast milk contains 4 000 cells – mainly leukocytes, which are high in colostrum – per millilitre. Breast milk also contains macrophages. These cells kill bacteria, fungi and viruses. The macrophages secrete lysozyme and lactoferrin, while the lymphocytes produce IgA and interferon. Neutrophils are also present. Lactoferrin coats and protects a baby's intestines. When combined with lysozyme, this has a direct antibiotic effect on bacteria such as *Escherichia coli* and staphylococci. Secretory IgA, along with other immunoglobulins, protect the ears, nose and throat, as well as the GI tract, against foreign viruses and bacteria. These antibodies are capable of altering their protective qualities to fight any allergens or pathogens that may be present. This action decreases an infant's chances of developing allergies, respiratory infections, otitis media and asthma (Stuebe, 2009).

▶ *Enzymes:* Some enzymes enter mother's milk from the maternal intercellular fluid and others are broken down in the mammary cells. These include xanthine oxidase, aldolase and alkaline phosphate. Lipase assists with fat metabolism. Other enzymes, such as amylase, do not seem to contribute to infant digestion.

▶ *Electrolytes, minerals and water:* Water and electrolytes (sodium, potassium, chloride, magnesium, calcium, phosphate and sulphate) cross the membrane in both directions. The water secretion in human milk depends on the availability of glucose. The sodium and potassium

levels are lower than in plasma, with a ratio of 1:3. Human milk has lower monovalent ions (sodium and potassium) and higher lactose content than the mother's plasma; this relationship distinguishes human milk from that of other species. Trace minerals, such as zinc, copper, selenium, manganese and iron, are low in human milk.

▶ *Glucose (carbohydrate) metabolism:* This is a key function in milk production and is the main source of energy. It is critical to the volume of milk produced. Lactose is derived from blood glucose and the process is regulated by progesterone. Lactose accounts for the majority of carbohydrates in human milk. The concentration is 6.8 g/100 ml versus 4.9 g/100 ml in cow's milk. It enhances calcium absorption and metabolises carbohydrates into galactose and glucose, which supply energy to an infant's rapidly growing brain. The largest portion of the carbohydrate is monosaccharide, with a low percentage of glucose. The enzyme to metabolise lactose is not present in preterm babies under 30 weeks and it disappears at the age of 3 years.

▶ *Fats:* The alveolar cells are able to synthesise short-chain fatty acids. Long-chain fatty acids come directly from the blood plasma of the mother. Prolactin stimulates the increase of enzymes to assist the capillaries with the production of fats. The fat droplets accumulate in the base of the cell and form larger drops that move to the apex. These are secreted by the apocrine process described in Figure 9.3. The fat droplets mainly contain polar lipids and phosphatidylcholine.

Human milk contains numerous long-chain fatty acids, including docosahexaenoic acid (DHA) and arachidonic acid (ARA) (Innis, Gilley & Werker, 2001). At least 167 different fats have been identified in human milk. These lipids are responsible for cell membrane integrity in the brain, retinas and other parts of a baby's body. If a mother's milk contains 20 per cent fat on the seventh day postpartum, breastfeeding will most probably be successful. A woman's food intake has a direct influence on the type of fat in her breast milk.

▶ *Protein (nitrogen):* This is produced by free amino acids in the cells. Protein is 75 per cent of the total nitrogen in human milk versus 95 per cent in cow's milk. Prolactin, insulin and cortisol are involved in protein synthesis. Casein, lactoglobulin A and B, glycoprotein and immunoglobulin are the main proteins synthesised by the ribosomes through apocrine secretion. Some proteins are secreted by merocrine actions. Casein has a specific amino acid composition: the methionine/cysteine ratio is close to 1:1 in human milk, similar to plants. Taurine (a sulphur-containing amino acid) is present in high concentrations in human milk. It is a neurotransmitter and it plays a role in bilirubin and bile conjugation. The ratio of casein to whey protein in humans is 1:5. Human milk is low in curd, due to the high whey content, and is easily digested. If expressed breast milk is left standing, the clear fluid seen is whey.

▶ *Vitamin content:* This is dependent on the nutrition and vitamin intake of the mother, and can be critically low if the mother is not well nourished. The vitamin content of mature milk is lower than colostrum for vitamin C, vitamin A, riboflavin, vitamin B6, thiamine and niacin. Vitamin D is present and B12 and folic acid abound. However, the baby needs to be exposed to sunlight to produce his or her own vitamin D. Vitamin content varies between foremilk and hindmilk in the same feed.

▶ *Nucleotides:* Expressed as nucleotide equivalents, the concentration in mother's milk varies between mothers and the period of location, and is 55–68μmol/ℓ. Nucleotides are important in protein synthesis and provide energy for biosynthesis. They play a role in anabolism and growth. Failure to thrive on breast milk, if all other factors are excluded, may be because of low nucleotides in the breast milk.

9.5 Breast milk advantages and reasons for avoidance

Advantages of breast milk

Evidence confirms the advantages and superiority of human milk. Babies who are breastfed have a decreased chance of developing:
▶ respiratory and ear infections
▶ allergies and atopic diseases
▶ asthma
▶ urinary tract infections (UTIs)
▶ diarrhoeal infections, gastrointestinal reflux and NEC
▶ bacterial meningitis
▶ sudden infant death syndrome (SIDS)
▶ juvenile rheumatoid arthritis
▶ childhood lymphomas such as Hodgkin's disease and leukaemia.

Discontinuation or avoidance of breast milk

There are certain medical reasons for not breastfeeding.

Agalactia (inability to breastfeed)

The significant inhibiting factors for breastfeeding include factors such as breast surgery, retained placenta, Sheehan's syndrome or pituitary shock, where a woman fails to lactate.

Suppression of breast milk

In some cases, breast milk production is suppressed by hormonal contraception. Breast milk can be suppressed if there is a risk of contamination of milk by bacteria or viruses (such as HIV), or by drugs or prescription medication that may affect the baby.

Replacement feeding and milk banks

If a mother cannot breastfeed an infant, replacement feeding may be an option. Infants can still get the benefit of breast milk through certified donor milk banks (DMBs).

DMBs exist in many centres, and provide a safe source breast milk for the low-birth-weight (LBW) and preterm infant.

Social factors

Rates of breastfeeding differ between cultures and socioeconomic groups. As more women work away from home, the demands of breastfeeding may be too high, and such women may opt for formula feeding as a more convenient feeding method. However, more affluent women in developed countries are beginning to opt for breastfeeding. In less developed countries it is the accepted practice.

Working women need support to breastfeed and policies around maternity leave will influence rates of breastfeeding. Women also need support in the form of breastfeeding consultants to help them to continue to breastfeed.

Breastfeeding rates

In South Africa, the goal for exclusive breastfeeding (EBF) (1–6 months) is 50 per cent by 2030. In 2015, the EBF rate for infants up to the age of six months was 12 per cent (Sibiza et al, 2015).

Psychological factors

Motherhood and breastfeeding are learned behaviour. If young women are not exposed to breastfeeding when they grow up and do not see it in the community, they may find it more difficult than anticipated, even if they have positive attitudes towards it. Psychological factors that play a role include a woman's relationship with her own mother, her relationship with the father of the baby and whether or not the pregnancy was planned and wanted.

Psychological factors in breastfeeding

Research shows that the duration of breastfeeding is associated more with psychological than with socioeconomic factors. Psychological factors include an optimistic outlook, feeling comfortable with breastfeeding, faith in breast milk as a food, expectations of breastfeeding, anxiety and the planned duration of breastfeeding.

The baby may pick up cues from the mother, and may refuse the breast if he or she does not feel contained. Factors that affect successful feeding include the attitudes of doctors, midwives and other healthcare professionals during pregnancy and birth, and the level of support received. BFC improves breastfeeding support.

Contamination of breast milk

Breast milk reflects the contamination found in the environment. It is therefore monitored throughout the world to determine the level of toxins in the environment (contamination of water, food, pesticides and air). For example, pesticides such as DDT may be present in human milk.

9.6 Conclusion

Successful breastfeeding is dependent on a range of complex sociodemographic, economic, political, psychological, anatomical, physiological and personal factors. Midwives must support each individual mother within the personal and social framework that exists for her.

Section Three

Psychosocial and cultural aspects of childbirth

Psychosocial and cultural issues of pregnancy and childbirth

10.1 Introduction

This chapter reflects on the psychosocial aspects of society, cultural beliefs around childbirth, as well as the cultural differences relating to childbirth in a multicultural, post-apartheid society in the process of transformation. As indicated in Chapter 1, the influence of the colonial period resulted in the modification of patterns of behaviour and practices that had existed over ages. (For example, women used to give birth in the squatting or standing position, but today most women give birth in the supine position, ie lying down.) Women in South Africa, according to Chalmers (1990), embraced Western medicine alongside traditional practices, which played a part in the transformation of the care of women in South Africa. The country has also been in a constant process of political and socioeconomic transformation since the end of the apartheid period in 1994. This has an influence on healthcare practices.

This chapter also touches on social and cultural aspects of pregnancy and birth, such as fertility, unwanted pregnancies, teenage pregnancy and responses to pregnancy and the newborn by family members.

The supportive vs non-supportive care model is mentioned as best practice example. The unique behaviour of the newborn is explained in an attempt to alert midwives to aspects that they must be familiar with in order to educate mothers and fathers about the newborn's behaviour.

10.2 South African society

South Africa is a multicultural society – often referred to as the 'rainbow nation' – where several groups reside as traditional indigenous people. They represent four main ethnic groups, and there are 11 different official languages in the country.

The South African population is diverse and according to the 2011 census, 79 per cent are African, 8.9 per cent white, 8.9 per cent coloured, 2.5 per cent Indian and 0.5 per cent of unknown ethnic origin. The African population is divided into the Nguni (Zulu, Xhosa, Ndebele and Swazi groups), Sotho-Tswana (southern, northern and western), Tsonga and Venda. A group of Khoisan (the oldest indigenous people) still live in South Africa. White South Africans include white people who have been born and raised in South Africa over

10–12 generations and those of European descent that have migrated here. There is also a significant number of Chinese people in South Africa.

Migration

Post-apartheid South Africa has experienced an influx of people from Africa (Meny-Gilbert & Chiumia, 2016). There are two categories of migrants, namely international visitors (those who do not stay more than 12 months) and migrants (those who change their residence for a period of at least 12 months). Research in 2016 indicated that people migrating to South Africa mainly come from Zimbabwe, Mozambique, Lesotho, Malawi, the UK, Swaziland, the DRC, Namibia and Nigeria (Meny-Gilbert & Chiumia, 2016). The presence of migrants of various cultures, whether their presence here is known to South African authorities or not, impacts on healthcare delivery and increases the complexity of the cultural diversity in South African society.

The current multicultural South African population is diverse in terms of culture, language, ethnic groups, socioeconomic status, rural or urban residency, politics and expectations for the future. Healthcare delivery in this context requires a cross-cultural approach, which falls into the domain of sociology.

10.3 Key concepts in sociology and cultural competency

To be able to consider sociological changes in societal living and in healthcare, an understanding of the key sociological concepts is needed.

In healthcare, it is particularly important to know and understand diverse societal values, beliefs and traditional practices, particularly when working in communities and especially in rural areas. While South African communities are in social transition and have adapted to different lifestyles and habits, many people still ascribe to beliefs and 'ways of being' that are rooted in tradition. Healthcare professionals also hold different traditional views and may still subscribe to traditional practices that may or may not contradict evidence-based health information and influence the care they offer. A brief review of the definitions of culture and society, manifestations of culture in society and societal transition are presented in the following sections to orientate students to sociological thinking.

Definitions

Various sociologists define 'culture' as the cumulative deposit of knowledge, experiences, beliefs, values, attitudes, religions, time periods, roles, spatial relations, concepts of life and death, understanding of the universe, material objects and possessions acquired by a group of people over the course of generations through individual or group efforts. People are what they learn, but are also able to change later in life and adapt to new ideas and practices (Li & Karakowsky, 2001). Culture is thus also dynamic.

Sociologists define 'society' as people who interact in such a way as to share a common culture. Society is seen as a social organism. Several definitions sum up society as an ever-changing, complex system or web of social relationships.

Manifestations of culture in society

Cultural diversity expresses itself in various ways. Diverse cultural groups think, feel and act differently in society. The following section explains concepts characteristic of culture.

Symbolism

Symbolism is the most superficial expression of deep-core cultural values and is expressed in aspects such as language, attire, decorations and rituals:

- *Language* is a symbolic expression using words, gestures, pictures or objects that carry a particular meaning, which is mainly understood by those who share a particular culture. Old symbols may disappear and can easily be replaced by new ones, or may be copied between cultures. This is why symbols represent the outermost layer of a culture.
- *Role models, examples or heroes* are the models – real or fictional, past or present – that are valued and prized in a society.
- *Rituals* are socially essential collective activities (eg ways of greeting, paying respect or social ceremonies) used for specific purposes.
- *Values* are the broad, often unconscious core aspects of a society that form the basis of all practices, indicating preferences in terms of judgements such as good or evil, right or wrong, natural or unnatural. Values are indirectly observed from the way people act under different circumstances.

Key concepts in cultural competency

Culture is complex and dynamic in nature. Cultural competency is a new field in nursing care which supports healthcare professionals to be competent in working with a culturally diverse population. The following concepts are important in understanding cultural competency:

- *Diversity* includes aspects of race, colour, ethnicity, origin and immigration status. It also includes religion, age, gender, sexual orientation, ability/disability, economic status, education, occupation, spirituality, marital status and residence in an urban versus rural a community.

▶ *Discrimination* occurs when one person or group acts based on prejudice and denies others their fundamental rights, treating them differently based on diversity. Discrimination results in disrespect, marginalisation and the disregard of the rights and privileges of others who are different.

▶ *Cultural awareness* is when people become knowledgeable of their own thoughts and feelings and how these can affect others.

▶ *Cultural imposition* occurs when one cultural view is applied to all.

▶ *Cultural sensitivity* is indicated by the use of neutral language (verbal and non-verbal) to avoid interpretations that may offend others.

▶ *Acculturation* occurs when the cultural attributes of another culture are adopted when groups come in contact, leading to new cultural variations. This can also be referred to as social transition.

Social transition

Culture is dynamic, and constantly changing and shifting. Social change refers to an alteration in the social order of society. It may include changes in the nature of society, social institutions, behaviours and relationships.

In South Africa, the Constitution (1996) provides the basis for the development of a healthy society where all cultures can co-exist.

The Bill of Rights

The Constitution of the Republic of South Africa, 1996, and its Bill of Rights are progressive and lay the foundation for an open society. The Constitution reaffirms South Africa's determination to build a healthy society based on equality, law and democracy. It upholds:
▶ non-racialism and non-sexism
▶ supremacy of the law and Constitution
▶ democracy, free and fair elections, accountability, responsiveness and openness.

10.4   Transcultural nursing

Since 2002, several models and frameworks have been developed to support the practice of working with diverse cultures (see Table 10.1 on the next page). The principles of transcultural nursing are implied in the South African Nursing Pledge (see the box below), as well as in the Batho Pele principles.

Definition

Transcultural nursing is defined as the 'how to' of professional nursing interactions, taking into account the concept of cultural diversity (Leininger, 1991).

Professional conduct

The South African Nursing Pledge for professional nurses and midwives expresses the intention that professional nurses and midwives must behave and conduct care in a neutral manner. In the current social environment, this demands transcultural caring skills.

The Batho Pele policy ('putting people first') provides the framework for putting the needs of other people before one's own in healthcare services (DPSA, nd). The 11 standards of the Batho Pele documents are well known and are available from www.dpsa.gov.za/documents/Abridged%20BP%20 programme%20July2014.pdf.

The South African Nursing Pledge (SANC, 2016)

I solemnly pledge myself to the service of humanity and will endeavour to practise my profession with conscience and with dignity.

I will maintain, by all the means in my power, the honour and noble tradition of my profession.

The total health of my patients will be my first consideration.

I will hold in confidence all personal matters coming to my knowledge.

I will not permit consideration of religion, nationality, race or social standing to intervene between my duty and my patient.

I will maintain the utmost respect for human life.

I make these promises solemnly, freely and upon my honour.

Transcultural competency and care

When nurses learn transcultural competency, it increases the quality of care to the population they care for (Murphy, 2006).

The principles of transcultural care

Transcultural nursing requires that nurses:
▶ understand the diverse health perspectives, worldviews and understandings of the meaning of life held by the societies they seek to serve

Table 10.1

Nursing models for culturally competent care (AACN, 2008)

Theory and models	Description	Comparison of the models' concepts, assumptions and frameworks
Campinha-Bacote (2009): The Bacote model of cultural competence	This model sees institutions and organisations as having an intrinsic motivation to engage with cultural competence within differences in cultural awareness, knowledge, skills, cultural encounters and desire.	Cultural awareness Cultural knowledge Cultural skills Cultural encounters Cultural desire
Giger and Davidhizar (2002): The transcultural assessment model	This model sees people as unique beings influenced by culture, ethnicity and religion within six areas of diversity.	The model identifies six areas of diversity: 1. Communication 2. Space 3. Social orientation 4. Time 5. Environmental control 6. Biological variation
Leininger (2006): Cultural care, diversity and universality theory or the transcultural nursing model	This model acknowledges similarities and differences in culture and gives guidelines for culturally congruent action for care with principles of transcultural care.	The principles of transcultural care are the following: • Care is essential to healing and cure. • Every culture has indigenous care knowledge and practices which vary transculturally. • Values, beliefs and practices are influenced by the worldview, language and philosophy of a culture. • Cultural conflict develops when care fails to be fairly congruent with the recipient's values and beliefs, leading to non-compliance. • Within the model, nurses can adopt culturally congruent actions: cultural preservation, maintaining current patterns of care, cultural accommodation and negotiation, and cultural restructuring of beliefs.
Purnell (2002): The model of transcultural healthcare	Four levels have been developed for the practitioner to move through to achieve cultural competency in healthcare: 1. Unconscious incompetence 2. Conscious incompetence 3. Conscious competence 4. Unconscious competence.	The model as a whole contains various macro-aspects, namely global society, commerce, economy and technology that shapes worldviews. All healthcare providers in any practice setting can use the model, which makes it especially desirable in today's team-oriented healthcare environment. The micro-aspects consist of 12 domains, namely heritage, communication, family roles, workforce issues, ecology, high-risk behaviours, nutrition, pregnancy and birth, death rituals, spirituality, healthcare practices and practitioners. Each domain contains concepts common to culture. It is used to give insight into a person's cultural needs.
Spector (2009): The health tradition model	Spector refers to three theories to explain healthcare in transition and has developed a 'heritage' assessment tool to indicate to what degree a person or family adheres to traditions.	Spector refers to Zitzow and Estes's heritage consistency theory (1981) and Giger and Davidhizar's model for health tradition (2002) to observe how people adapt their lifestyles from a tribal culture to embrace new values.

- use cultural knowledge to understand health behaviour and refer to the views and knowledge of the society, while interpreting how these differ from their own knowledge and viewpoints (Murphy, 2006)
- respect the fact that all cultures are not alike and that each person is unique.

Cultural competency

Cultural competency is a combination of culturally congruent behaviour, practices, attitudes and policies that allows nurses to work effectively in cross- or multicultural situations.

Culturally competent nurses consciously address the cultural assumptions that affect nurse–patient exchanges. They make allowances and have compassion for cultural preferences if these are not harmful. They strive to increase their knowledge and cultural sensitivity (Leininger, 1991).

Assumptions of transcultural care

Transcultural care is the broadest holistic perspective for care in nursing, because it includes the perspective of the culture it serves. It accepts that every human culture has folk remedies, professional knowledge and care practices that vary and can be useful if explored. These practices could be beneficial and may enhance well-being and the satisfaction of the community being cared for.

The care of women and their families must be appropriate to the individual or group and take into account cultural and religious beliefs. Many traditional practices are wholesome and useful, but some traditional practices have been found to be harmful.

Harmful traditional practices for women and children

Several practices related to reproduction, pregnancy and birth that are potentially harmful to women and children have been identified.

In 1979, the UN Commission on Human Rights (UNCHR) appointed a special rapporteur on violence against women. Harmful traditional practices identified were categorised in 1994. These include (UN, 1994):
- female genital mutilation (FGM)
- son preference: Girls are weaned from the breast sooner than boys
- female infanticide
- early marriage and dowries

continued

- early pregnancy: Young girls are expected to have children as soon as they reach puberty
- nutritional taboos: Most pregnant women in developing countries have a lower food intake than the average for males, as most societies in Africa have taboos on food intake during pregnancy
- superstitions: The belief that certain animal parts or plants can cause harm to the baby
- traditional substances: The use of herbal mixtures and magic is common in pregnancy in Africa. Some are beneficial (see Chapter 52), while others are lethal, particularly when taken in high concentrations.

A further harmful traditional practice is the use of fundal pressure in obstructed labour to try to force the baby out. Some birth attendants perform surgical procedures to extract the fetus, cutting the labia and vagina. This is called the 'Gishiri cut'. Sometimes, obstructed labour is blamed on marital infidelity and the woman is coerced to confess to such. In cases of obstructed labour, a mortality rate of 37 per cent is associated with these practices (Walker-Smith & Murch, 1999: 713).

The WHO supports traditional practices that enhance health. In 1994, Resolution WHA 47.10 against harmful practices was adopted.

10.5 Social and cultural aspects of reproduction

Sexuality, reproduction and childbirth are highly emotional, psychological and social phenomena, with deep cultural and religious roots. Even communities and women who have embraced Western lifestyles may still maintain traditional habits and practices around reproduction and childbirth. Selected beliefs, habits and practices are briefly discussed in the following sections.

Common views on reproduction and childbirth

Fertility, sexuality and reproduction are deeply embedded in the worldviews, cultural and religious views and practices of communities. Individuals and societies may develop and adopt different views as knowledge and science increase and when they are exposed to different experiences, but they often return to traditional practices. In South Africa, women hold on to traditional beliefs and practices while at the same time adopting Western healthcare practices and medicine, and accepting contraception and hospital healthcare for birth. The following sections briefly discuss aspects of societies' beliefs and practices in terms of fertility, sexuality and reproduction.

Fertility

It is generally accepted that fertility is a sign of prosperity and health. For women, fertility refers to the ability to bear children and also to the number of children a woman is able to give birth to. The pregnancy of a man's partner or wife confirms the man's fertility, as does the number of children he has fathered.

Views on fertility are culturally influenced and directed, and also influenced by religious beliefs. Young people are educated and guided by cultural principles regarding having children and socialised into desired patterns of cultural behaviour. For example, through cultural pressure, young women are often encouraged to fall pregnant to show their fertility. It is seen as a duty they have to fulfil. Becoming a mother is seen as a rite of passage to a higher status in society and is often viewed as a sign of riches and future prospects.

Women in rural areas have a higher fertility rate (number of children) because they still lead lives following traditional practices. In urban areas, women often have access to higher levels of education and have careers. Young women in rural areas often have higher ambitions for education and career development. The result is that women often delay pregnancy or space their children, which leads to fewer children.

Across all religions, infertility is seen as punishment for wrong-doing (Sewpaul, 1999). Interference in fertility through contraception and the use of technology to assist those with fertility problems are rejected by many traditional and religious beliefs, and spiritual guidance and traditional medicine are often used to cure infertility.

Access and encouragement to use contraception will influence fertility prospects. Males often have traditional views on contraception and discourage their partners from taking contraceptive precautions. In South Africa, having a child is still seen as important by society.

Sexuality and gender roles

Sexuality and gender identity are part of a person's identity and are also culturally influenced.

Traditionally, sexuality is considered as natural and the consequence of pregnancy is also seen as natural and even desired as an essential step of transition to womanhood by women in most societies. Pregnancy and childbirth are viewed as positive events in most societies, although cultural differences still exist.

Gender roles are culturally prescribed, but are also changing as more women are educated, become career-driven and gain control over their fertility through contraception. Same-sex relations are protected in the South African Constitution, but are often still frowned upon and rejected by cultures and religious groups.

Practices to initiate young people into their gender roles differ across societies. These practices are also influenced by cultural development through education and information in the social media era. The initiation process and rituals carried out are expressed in song, dance, through masks, various tests/ordeals, tattooing, and other events. This gives symbolic expression and verifies the individual's transition to a new role and function. The expression of the practice varies across societies; some focus on bravery and toughness, others on spiritual aspects or practical education (Davis, 2011).

Rites of passage are still important rituals in African culture. The aim is to prepare young men and women for their responsibilities in the community and to give them a clear understanding of these responsibilities. Rites of passage enshrine sexual and gender identity as well as roles and responsibilities (Davis, 2011).

Reproduction

Normally, pregnancy is viewed as a sign of growth, cohabitation and prosperity. However, there is a global awareness that uncontrolled reproduction is not sustainable and that the world may run out of space and resources. This awareness has led to a shift in reproductive behaviour through the use of contraception in Western societies, which has caused a change in demographics. Many countries now have a negative population growth, particularly in Europe (Haub, 2012). A fertility rate of two children per woman is needed to maintain a constant population (UN, 2015). Fertility control through contraception is an acceptable practice promoted or even enforced in many societies.

The box on the next page details an example of a case of involuntary reproduction control, enforced in China from 1979 to 2015 through a Chinese national policy called the Chinese one-child policy.

In 2012, the United Nations Population Fund (UNFPA) projected that the region with the largest population growth by 2015 would be Africa (Haub, 2012). In 2014, the UNFPA emphasised the need to improve reproductive healthcare and contraception in order to reduce poverty in the face of continued rapid population growth. Reproductive healthcare and the acceptance of this care by communities irrespective of cultural and religious beliefs are of importance.

The use of contraception in Africa is still low and the maternal and perinatal mortality rate is high. Many countries in Africa view contraception as immoral (Lipka, 2014).

The Chinese one-child policy

Because of a rapidly growing population (790 million in 1979), Chinese leader Deng Xiaoping introduced the one-child policy for the ethnic minority Han Chinese in 1979. Between 1979 and 2010, 400 million births were estimated to have been affected, and the population in 2010 was 1 339 million. The policy was enforced by a penalty called a 'social child-raising fee' or 'family planning fine'. Both men and women had to pay the fine. In this case, like in many other societies, male children are still preferred and societal rules may influence family planning decisions. The consequence of the one-child policy was that male children were allowed to live, while girl children were allowed to die. This led to an unnatural sex ratio at birth. The policy distorted the natural population ratios and will lead to an estimated 30 million more men than women by 2020, leading to social instability and courtship-motivated emigration. The policy was changed in 2015 to a two-child policy (Eberstat, 2015).

In African cultures, the birth of a child calls for celebration. Each infant is believed to come from the spirit world with important information, bringing unique talents and gifts – indeed, a unique purpose, mission, message or project – to offer the community.

Traditionally, the name of a child reflects his or her life purpose. Whenever the name is called, it also serves as a powerful reminder of the individual's life work and his or her mission. The family and community, through consultation with elders and/or diviners, determine the mission of the infant in order to successfully guide him or her along a life path.

Most other cultures also have rites and rituals regarding the birth of a child, which are expressed in different ways.

Today, many societies experience a tension between traditional beliefs and the demands of a modern lifestyle, women's rights and reproductive health choices. The cultural expectation that young women should prove their fertility still exists and the passage to womanhood, as defined culturally through pregnancy and childbirth, is still highly prized. This often leads those who fail to fall pregnant to resort to abducting a baby. Because of this cultural pressure, young women engage in sexual behaviour early and fall pregnant either intentionally or unintentionally.

Teenage pregnancy, unintended pregnancies and child brides

Teenage pregnancy

Teenage pregnancy is a global phenomenon. However, the response of individuals and communities to pregnancy in this age group will differ between societies and will depend on demographic and socioeconomic status. This issue is also closely linked to the status of the girl child in a community and the empowerment of women to make their own reproductive choices.

Pregnancy will impact on the ability of the teenage girl to complete her education and become economically independent. It may also lead to risky behaviour, such as opting for an unsafe abortion. The lack of support for teenage mothers is also a concern.

In 2013, there were 99 000 teenage pregnancies in South Africa (Willen, 2013). According to findings by UNICEF, in 2009 the teenage pregnancy rate in SA differed between population groups as follows: 71/1 000 for black African people, 60/1 000 for coloured people, 22/1 000 for Indians and 14/1 000 for white people (UNICEF, HSRC & DoE, 2009).

In rural areas, women may fall pregnant at a younger age, even if they are unmarried. This may be intentional and form part of cultural practices. It is not unusual for women to have children while awaiting *lobola*. The traditional practice in Africa of *lobola*, or 'bride price', has become modernised in recent times, with exchanges of cash and payments by credit card; this is also embraced by the church.

Unintended or unwanted pregnancy

Unintended pregnancies are pregnancies that are unplanned and often unwanted. In some cultures, an unintended pregnancy is shameful and will be hidden from the community; the baby may be given up for adoption. In African culture, generally, unintended pregnancies are accepted and babies are seldom given up for adoption; rather, they remain in the family. In rural communities, this practice has remained unchanged.

If the unintended pregnancy is also an unwanted or teenage pregnancy, it may lead to abuse or an illegal abortion. Traditionally, abortion on demand is not an acceptable practice in African culture and centres for abortion are not well supported. Since the Choice on Termination of Pregnancy Act 92 of 1996 came into effect, abortion services have become more accessible in urban areas. (This Act is discussed in Chapter 48.) In all cultures, if legal options are not available, women seek and use illegal abortions to remedy unwanted pregnancy.

There are also regular reports of abandoned newborn babies, some dead and some alive. In certain circumstances a young woman may hide her pregnancy and abandon the baby after birth. It is commonly cited that around 3 500 babies were abandoned in South Africa annually.

Child brides

Marriage before the age of 18 is a fundamental violation of human rights (UNICEF, 2017). Child marriage among girls is most common in South Asia and sub-Saharan Africa, and the 10 countries with the highest rates are found in these two regions (UNICEF, 2013a). To raise awareness, UN Women declared an International Day of the Girl Child, celebrated since 2012, to underline the severity of the problems around the status of young women globally. Between 2011 and 2020, more than 140 million girls will become child brides, according to the United Nations Population Fund (UNFPA) (UNICEF, 2013b).

The practice of child marriage exists in many parts of the world. In Africa, girls may be symbolically 'promised in marriage' at a young age and then 'married off' to a man when they reach puberty. A report by UNICEF (2005) gave a statistical overview of child marriages in the world in 2005. In 2013, the report *Ending Child Marriage* was published (UNICEF, 2013a). The UNFPA has declared child marriage to be a human rights violation (UNICEF, 2017). The legal minimum age of marriage in South Africa is 18 years for boys and girls, according to Section 26(1) of the Marriage Act 25 of 1961, read with sections 17 and 18(3)(c)(i) of the Children's Act 38 of 2005. (Mahery & Proudlock, 2011)

In South Africa, *ukuthwala* is the practice of abducting girls or women and forcing them into marriage (DoJ & CD, 2017), a practice which still continues. This practice is discouraged and contravenes human rights.

10.6 Psychological responses to pregnancy, birth and parenthood

The range of responses to pregnancy, birth and parenthood share certain similarities across different societies and can be explained scientifically. Psychologists, anthropologists, sociologists and other professionals in the medical field have examined and described these processes and responses. A person's early experiences, expectations, mental status and culture are some factors that may influence his or her experience of and responses towards pregnancy, childbirth and parenthood. The following sections briefly investigate these aspects and responses. The first task is for the woman, the father of the child and the community to accept the pregnancy.

Maternal responses to pregnancy

Some pregnancies are planned; others are not. However, not all unplanned pregnancies are rejected by the woman and not all planned pregnancies are greeted with enthusiasm. Much depends on the circumstances of conception, the woman's current family situation, her marital or relationship happiness, her reasons for wanting or not wanting a baby, the timing of her pregnancy and her cultural context. While it is easy to accept that the news of an unplanned baby may cause shock, it is less easy to understand that planned babies may also arouse negative or ambiguous reactions.

Women who are obliged by tradition to have children may not find joy in it and see it only as a task they have to fulfil. On the other hand, career women in particular may experience conflict between wanting a baby and not wanting to jeopardise their professional lives. Women therefore respond to a pregnancy within the given context.

A woman's response may also be influenced by culture. For example, in some traditional African cultures, women are not allowed to talk about the pregnancy, the symptoms they experience or the date of conception out of fear of 'bewitching' or 'bad luck'.

A woman can experience various adaptations in pregnancy, as detailed in the following section.

Psychological adaptations to pregnancy

Maternal responses can vary between happiness, anxiety, uncertainty and denial. Psychological patterns of adaptation include the following:
- *First trimester:* The woman focuses on herself to try to understand the pregnancy and may experience minor symptoms as a form of 'disease' (see Chapter 20).
- *Second trimester:* When the woman feels the baby move, the pregnancy becomes a reality and her focus moves to the baby. She fantasises and daydreams about the baby and withdraws from her husband and other children. By now she accepts the pregnancy, if she had not done so previously. She becomes closer to her mother or other older female relatives who serve as mother figures for support and re-evaluates her husband as a partner.
- *Third trimester:* 'Nesting' occurs, to prepare for the baby. The woman fears the delivery, does not sleep well and wants the birth to be over. Ambivalent feelings come and go and emotional lability is common.

Common feelings experienced in pregnancy

Anxiety

Some level of anxiety during pregnancy is normal. Anxiety levels may be elevated in the early months of pregnancy, partly due to the initial adjustment to being pregnant and partly in reaction to physical discomfort experienced, such as nausea and tiredness. However, anxiety is usually lowered during the middle trimester and rises again as the expected time of birth approaches. In this later stage in particular, anxiety may be accompanied by nightmares.

While psychological upheaval may be readily expected in a first pregnancy, it is interesting to note that anxiety frequently appears to be even greater with second and subsequent pregnancies. It is possible that the experience of pregnancy and parenthood leads to an increased knowledge and understanding of the possible dangers as well as the commitments of pregnancy and parenthood. Greater awareness with later pregnancies leads to a more realistic and less romantic view of parenthood.

Fear

Fear is a universal reaction during pregnancy, and includes fear of miscarriage or abnormality, of dying in labour or of the baby dying, of hospitals and doctors, of the mother's illnesses affecting the baby and of pain. Many of these fears are not expressed, particularly in the case of African women, who are not traditionally allowed to talk about the baby and their fears. However, if the woman can express her fears, this may help her to deal with them and to understand exactly what it is that she fears. Women (and their husbands or partners) should be encouraged to talk about their concerns in an environment that allows frank and open discussion; this will take time, but may well lead to an easier adjustment to the pregnancy and parenthood.

Another major concern during pregnancy is fear of intercourse. A woman may be concerned not only about the effects of sexual intercourse during pregnancy, but also about losing her attractiveness. Sexual activity during pregnancy for most couples is a matter of personal desire. Unless there are medical reasons for abstaining (such as a history of miscarriage), couples should be encouraged to approach sex during pregnancy as an added dimension to their sexual lives – offering opportunities for exploration and adventure, as physical changes in the woman's body demand alterations in sexual behaviour.

One common concern is that the man's penis may hurt the baby in some way during intercourse. This fear can often be dispelled by examining pictures of the anatomy of the baby in utero. Talking about the fear often helps. Sometimes, this fear can make a husband or partner less willing to engage in sexual intercourse during pregnancy, and acknowledging the concern may help to explain this behaviour. If unexpressed, the woman may interpret her partner's reluctance as a response to

her possible loss of attractiveness or may even imagine that he is being unfaithful. Long-term misunderstandings may well be prevented by discussing sexuality within a professional setting.

Emotional lability

One common reaction during pregnancy is mood swings or emotional lability. Hostility or irritability frequently occur. Some women become dependent and insecure, even if they are normally assertive and independent. Increased emotionality may well be particularly influenced by hormonal changes. Nausea and tiredness in the early months and a cumbersome feeling in the last trimester may easily contribute to feelings of being emotionally 'down'.

Many women become increasingly introspective as the pregnancy progresses. Less involvement in the outside world may be nature's way of ensuring that the woman avoids situations that may be hazardous for herself and her baby. She becomes, in effect, an 'incubator', concerned with monitoring the safety of her baby.

The middle trimester of pregnancy is usually the most comfortable and may well be the period which gives rise to the feeling of 'radiance' often experienced during pregnancy. This period also corresponds with the time at which life is first felt, a pleasurable experience. It is possible that in this middle period, the woman is most receptive to guidance and advice on motherhood.

The father's response to the pregnancy and birth

Chapter 11 contains a discussion on the role and value of the father in pregnancy and birth. Traditional views on the family and the role of the father differ across cultures. Traditionally, men were not involved in pregnancy and birth. This has changed and in urban areas African men tend to be more inclined to attend the birth when it takes place in private birth centres and selected public institutions.

Siblings' responses to the pregnancy and birth

If there are siblings or other children, they require special care during their mother's pregnancy. All children need preparation for the forthcoming baby, but the nature and method of instruction will differ depending on the age of the siblings and cultural beliefs and practices. It is particularly important to reassure each child that he or she is loved and wanted and that the coming child will not replace him or her in the parents' affections.

While giving time and attention to siblings is possible during pregnancy, this becomes more difficult after the baby is born. Parents need to foresee this challenge and spend time during pregnancy planning possible means of overcoming this problem after delivery. Often, solutions will entail involving the father more actively in the care of older children. In the traditional extended family, siblings are easily managed by a 'gogo' (grandmother) or family member.

If siblings are much older than the new baby, the mother's pregnancy offers a wonderful opportunity for the siblings to learn about pregnancy and parenthood.

Grandparents' responses to the pregnancy and birth

The woman's own mother, in particular, may assume an important role during and after pregnancy. In some African cultures, the mother-in-law is prominent and has decision-making powers. Pregnant women often experience an increased feeling of dependence. This frequently presents as a need to be mothered, which may be strongest after the baby is born. It is understandable that at a time of personal challenge as well as threat, a woman should have a predominant need for security and care from someone she trusts. In this case, and depending on the traditional roles they are fulfilling, grandparents should be included in some of the couple's preparations for parenthood.

Friends' responses to the pregnancy and birth

Pregnancy may make the prospective parents realise the value of friends. Friends in similar positions – pregnant or with young children – provide a marvellous opportunity for learning about babies and baby care and these friendships should be cultivated. This is of particular value in African cultures, where the loss of the extended or traditional family means that many women no longer learn about pregnancy, birth and parenting at home.

Friends, however, do sometimes make comments or relate stories (especially horror stories) about others' experiences in pregnancy or during birth. These are often anxiety-provoking and may arouse fears in mothers-to-be. A pregnant woman will welcome opportunities to discuss these stories or comments with a midwife. Horror stories or challenges experienced by others may also alert the woman to possible future scenarios and may prepare her with a coping mechanism should she experience such a situation.

Birth experiences

The sacredness of birth is culturally defined. Birth is a family experience and highly revered, touching all the family members. Birth has the potential to be a critical spiritual experience and is the transition to motherhood.

Birth has become medicalised in most healthcare settings. Under the influence of 'modern' healthcare practices, birth care has become less personal and the place for birth has been moved from the home and community to a medical healthcare setting, where the mother's and baby's lives can be saved if necessary. This medicalised environment is often unsupportive in terms of warmth, care and love. In the Western model, traditional practices are often not honoured.

In South Africa, out-of-hospital births are discouraged. In 2003, only 6.6 per cent of women in South Africa birthed at home; in 4.7 per cent of births the carer was not known (DoH, 2003: 125). It is the policy of the Department of Health (DoH) that women in South Africa give birth in a clinic or hospital. Women who give birth in the public sector often do not have the privilege of being allowed the presence of a significant person during birth. This leaves them isolated and alone, without the comfort, encouragement and support of a significant person. In some institutions, a doula (often a volunteer but trained lay worker) may be available to be with the woman. In most private institutions, the father of the baby or a family member is allowed to be part of the birth.

In African cultures, there is still an emphasis on birth as a natural process and women are traditionally supported by older, wise women during out-of-hospital births. This may lead to women remaining at home and only coming to hospital when problems arise. In rural areas, women stay at home as long as possible and come to the hospital only to deliver, often too late. In these cases, babies are born before they reach the hospital, which puts the mother and baby at risk. Often, young African women living in urban areas prefer to go home to rural areas to give birth within the cultural environment and support of the family.

In South Africa, there is a perception that care in some public institutions during pregnancy and birth is sub-standard, as reported by Jewkes, Abraham and Mvo (1998) and reflected by Rosman (in Penn-Kekana & Blaauw, 2004: 20). Penn-Kekana and Blaauw (2004) indicated that 84.5 per cent of women reported that no companion was allowed during birth. This issue of quality in the healthcare system may have a negative effect in that women who need medical assistance may not receive quality care during pregnancy and birth.

There are several deep-rooted traditional practices that are in conflict with current obstetric practices, such as the following:

▶ *The position of the mother during birth:* The dorsal position (on the back, or supine) is not a natural position to give birth. In traditional practices, women used to give birth while squatting or standing up.

- *The management of pain relief:* Rosman (in Penn-Kekana & Blaauw, 2004: 20) indicated that, in 2004, 83.2 per cent of women in the public sector were not offered pain relief in labour in South Africa. This may be due to traditional practices in which it is thought that a woman must be strong and endure labour to become a mother.
- *The presence of a significant person:* Traditionally, women were supported by a family member or wise woman.
- *The care of the placenta:* Traditionally, the placenta was buried in the ground, but today the placenta is destroyed by the hospital. However, the mother is allowed to take the placenta or other products of conception home, according to cultural beliefs and as arranged according to local policy.

Supportive versus unsupportive care environments during birth

To compensate for the loss of supportive practices, a philosophy of *humane care*, which describes a supportive and non-supportive environment, has been developed.

Women-centred or *humane care* (also referred to as compassionate care) is now the hallmark of midwifery globally. This represents an effort to restore the sacredness of birth. It requires that the midwifery philosophy and model of care be instituted. The midwifery model of care consists of the three Cs, as explained in the box below. This model of care is considered to be supportive and gives one-to-one care and education to a mother and baby. Several natural birth units exist in South Africa in the private sector that give one-to-one care.

The three Cs of the midwifery model of care

- *Continuity of carer:* One person or a team cares for the woman.
- *Choice:* The woman has a choice over where she delivers and who is present during the delivery.
- *Control:* The woman is given control to negotiate changes and foster a positive birth experience in terms of pain management, position, persons present, bonding and breastfeeding.

Responses in the postnatal period

The postnatal period is important for the mother in terms of recovery, but the first 1 000 days are viewed as critical for the well-being of the baby. This relates to the time *in utero* and the first two years after birth. The mother needs to be supported in this period (Thurow & Hansen, 2016). The presence of a partner, family and the community makes it possible for the woman to be successful.

There are also different types of family, and families have evolved. The traditional roles of the extended family are in many cases no longer applicable. The nuclear family, consisting of a working mother and father, needs the assistance of a larger family or a helper. Families headed by single women are common, leaving the mother and children vulnerable.

The intensity of care that needs to be given to the baby requires one or both of the parents in a supportive environment of family and friends. Several aspects may impact on the woman's adaptation in the postnatal period, as discussed in the sections that follow.

Maternal adaptation after birth

The postnatal period is critical. It is also the period of emotional transition to motherhood. (Lothian, 2008)

Studies indicate that becoming a mother is a journey that includes physical, social and psychological changes and challenges (Javadifar et al, 2013). This may affect a woman's psychological wellness and her personal and family life. Although the period after birth is a time of contentment and wonder, it is also stressful, with a lack of sleep. This may endanger the mother's mental health and her ability to adjust to her new role. The loss of independence, loneliness, lack of time and potential loss of a professional livelihood may alter her identity and is part of her journey.

Traditionally, after birth, African women were separated from the community and cared for in a special hut. They were supported after birth by a trusted older woman, mother or mother-in-law until the cord of the baby had separated. Thereafter, the woman was allowed into the community. Currently, women give birth in clinics and are expected to return home from the hospital within three to six days after birth, often using public transport.

A woman's adaptation to motherhood has been described by researchers such as Rubin (in Jordan et al, 2013). Kiehl and White (2003) found that if a mother identifies with the motherhood role in the antenatal period, she is likely to experience more satisfaction after birth. Mercer (2004) gave evidence that the mother, through commitment and involvement, redefines herself in her new role.

The maternal role attainment theory (Mercer, 2016) lists four stages of acquisition:

1. The *anticipatory stage* is a period of psychological and social adaptation to the maternal role. In this stage, learned expectations and fantasies about the role exist.
2. The *formal stage* includes the assumptions of the maternal role and birth. The mother in this stage is guided by others in the social network for decision making.

3. The *informal stage* allows the mother to establish her own independent methods of mothering, separate from the social system, that work for her and the child.

4. The *personal stage* is the joy of motherhood, with harmony, confidence and competence in the maternal role.

Several factors affect adaptation after the birth of a baby and each woman will adapt at her own pace. Midwives who observe and support women must consider the following factors:

▶ *First impressions:* Reactions immediately after birth can vary widely, from excitement to dejection, and even rejection of the infant. Chapters 11 and 12 explain the complex process of bonding between mother and baby and father and baby. Separation of mother and child is discouraged and should only happen in case of life-threatening conditions.

▶ *The first hour after birth:* Most maternity units allow parents to spend some time together, as a family, during the first few hours after birth. This is a special time when mother, father and baby can enjoy the excitement of the birth. This recent change in maternity hospital policy is to be applauded and encouraged, as it allows time for couples to re-live the experience of birth. Although tired, many women have heightened alertness and energy after birth. This is the time to bond with the baby and begin breastfeeding within the first hour.

Changes in healthcare practices allow mothers to be discharged within 24 hours in the case of a vaginal birth and three to four days after a Caesarean section. However, the mother may not have the needed support at home. Often, young mothers have to leave employment and go back to rural areas to be close to their family and support structure. Alternatively, they may leave the baby with an extended family member, such as the grandmother, and return to work.

Postnatal 'blues'

The first few days or weeks after the birth is often a time of emotional lability. This, however, is not the same as postpartum depression, which is potentially a serious mental illness. The 'baby blues' can generally be dealt with by supportive healthcare professionals, relatives and friends. The cause is not clear, but it may be hormonal, or simply a response to a complete change in lifestyle. Some specific factors that may contribute to the onset of the 'baby blues' are the following:

▶ *The birth experience:* A disappointing birth experience may have an emotional effect on the mother.

▶ *Relief after a momentous event:* As with any major, long-anticipated event, there is often a feeling of disappointment after the birth is over, particularly if the mother's expectations were not met.

▶ *Feelings of responsibility for the newborn:* The sense of responsibility and the enormous undertaking of parenthood may contribute to weepiness.

▶ *The baby's behaviour:* For example, a crying baby can precipitate feelings of inadequacy, and consequently weepiness in the new mother.

Working mothers

In South Africa, women are entitled to 60 days maternity leave. The Basic Conditions of Employment Act 75 of 1997 (as amended in 2014) allows for three days' family responsibility leave in a 12-month cycle after four months' service.

The mother's return to work requires the woman to either take the baby to a caregiver or hire a caregiver to look after the baby at home. Many women will leave their babies with family members in rural areas. In this case, the mother may only see the baby over weekends or during holidays, which can be stressful and disturbs the mother–child attachment. Women are not always in the type of stable relationship that could assist with a smooth adaptation to motherhood and may need to return to work as soon as possible. The earlier the mother returns to work, the more pressure is experienced in the adjustment to parenthood. Women need to be supported in their role as mother for the benefit of the development of the child.

Breastfeeding

Traditionally, African women practised prolonged breastfeeding. Today, young women in social transition often leave the baby with a caregiver, and prolonged breastfeeding has therefore declined in this African population group. The poorest and richest women in all cultures have a high rate of prolonged breastfeeding. The rate is unacceptably low in South Africa, putting children at risk.

Parenting the newborn

Several issues become important in the early months of parenthood; some of these relate to the mother, some to the family and some to the new baby. Regardless of cultural preferences, the well-being of the baby depends on the care and love received after birth. Separation from the mother may have lifelong effects on the baby. In terms of survival, the first 1 000 days (the time *in utero* and the first two years of life) are considered critical.

Learning to know and care for the baby is a normal developmental task for parents. Being in the caring environment of an extended family or community may be supportive. In some cases, postnatal support groups are available to support young mothers after birth and assist them in the transition to motherhood. Broader reading on the subjects of child development, child rearing and fathering could benefit any midwife who works with parents.

The Brazelton Neonatal Behaviour Assessment Scale

Midwives are encouraged to study the Brazelton Neonatal Behaviour Assessment Scale (BNBAS), developed by T Berry Brazelton (Lundqvist & Sabel, 1999). The BNBAS suggests that newborns are well equipped for social interaction and that they have the capacity to influence others around them. Babies are not passive; instead, they will encourage or discourage caretaking activities. The development of parental love is not without feedback from the baby. The absence of feedback from the baby, associated with separation, may impair the development of parental love.

The first task of the parent is to become aware of the unique behavioural responses of his or her baby. Brazelton showed that normal babies will differ in activity (state of consciousness), feeding patterns, sleeping patterns and responsiveness to the environment. These differences in sleep-and-waking patterns are present in all normal newborns and parents are encouraged not to compare babies, but to learn about the unique qualities of their own baby and adapt care to suit the baby's needs.

States of consciousness

The state of consciousness of the newborn fluctuates between light and deep sleep, lethargy and irritability. This can be divided into:

- *two sleep states:* deep and light sleep
- *four waking phases:* drowsiness, quiet alert, active alert and crying.

The quiet alert stage is the optimal state of arousal. During this phase, the newborn is:

- focused on external stimuli
- performing active manipulation of the outside world
- able to co-ordinate eye movements
- smiling (later in infancy)
- vocalising
- watching his or her parents' faces and responding.

Each state of consciousness has its own characteristics. The states are explained in greater detail in Table 10.2.

Table 10.2

Sleep and wake cycles

Phases	Body movements	Eye movements	Facial movements	Breathing	Level of response
Deep sleep	Body action: Still	None	None Sucking at intervals	Smooth and regular	Threshold high Intense stimuli required to wake up
Light sleep	Twitches, with occasional body movements	Rapid eye movement (REM) sleep, with fluttering eyelids Eyes closed	Smiles briefly Makes fussy sounds	Irregular	More responsive to external stimuli May stay in light sleep, return to deep sleep or wake up
Awake/ drowsy	Smooth movements Mild startle response	Open or closed eyes Dull, glazed appearance	Some movement Face appears still	Irregular	Reacts to sensory stimuli Delayed responses when stimulated
Quiet alert	Minimum	Bright and wide eyes	Bright, attentive, responsive	Regular	Attentive to environment Focuses attention on any stimuli Optimum state of arousal
Active alert	A great deal of activity and fuss	Open eyes Less bright	Facial movements not bright	Irregular	Increasing sensitivity to disturbing stimuli
Crying	Movements accompanied by colour change	Tightly closed or open	Grimacing	Irregular	Extreme response to unpleasant internal or external stimuli

Factors that influence the state of consciousness are the following:

▶ *Gestational age (GA):* The maturity of the central nervous system (CNS) of the newborn will affect behaviour. In a premature baby, for example, the whole body will respond to stimuli, while a mature infant will react to stimuli in a more specific way, for example by withdrawing only a foot.

▶ *Time of day:* A baby has one period of eight hours sleep in 24 hours. When in deep sleep, it is difficult to wake a baby up.

▶ *Time of the last feed:* Babies have small stomachs and if a baby is being fed with breast milk, the stomach empties within two hours. Therefore, some babies wake up within two hours and ask for another feed.

▶ *Stimuli and environmental events:* Bright lights, noise, tension in the environment (for example a hospital) or tension in the mother can affect the baby.

▶ *Medication, anaesthesia and analgesia given to the mother:* This will affect the newborn up to the fifth day after birth and may inhibit responses.

Teaching parents about the psychology and abilities of the baby and the sleep–wake cycle empowers the parents and reduces stress in the care of the newborn. Ante- and postnatal support and information are powerful support strategies.

10.7   Conclusion

Cultural views and traditions that have developed over the course of time influence how the next generation is received and socialised. In many societies, women are still oppressed. The empowerment and rights of women and girls as seen through the global lens are issues that have been placed on the global agenda. The reproductive choices of women and their childbirth and child-raising practices are often dictated by societal influences. In reproductive healthcare, many women are moving away from cultural practices to embrace modern Western practices. However, some traditional practices remain. Midwives can support women within their belief systems (as long as such practices are not harmful) through developing transcultural care competencies and integrating these into their practice in a structured way. Most women in South Africa currently give birth in healthcare facilities and as such the midwife is in a position to support women during childbirth.

The 'normal' psychological and social experiences observed and documented in childbirth are universal, but are often suppressed and denied when strong traditions prevail. The common responses of the mother, father and others have been highlighted in this chapter. Considering that South Africa is a country in the process of social transition, culturally competent healthcare professionals are those who are able to offer technical care of high quality while honoring the traditional and cultural beliefs of the women and children they assist.

Pregnancy and childbirth: The father's experiences

LEARNING OBJECTIVES

On completion of this chapter, you must be able to:
▶ explain the potential positive and negative responses of fathers to pregnancy
▶ explain the five phases of adaptation to fatherhood
▶ explain aspects of father–child bonding
▶ explain the role and function of midwives in promoting the father's involvement in childbirth.

KNOWLEDGE ASSUMED TO BE IN PLACE

Social groups, interaction and family structure and dynamics
Normal pregnancy and birth processes

KEYWORDS

father–infant bonding • father involvement • father deprivation • Couvade syndrome

11.1 Introduction

Pregnancy is a time when a couple may develop a different relationship with one another. It is a normal developmental phase, but also a transitional phase that may make some members of the family feel unbalanced; it therefore requires emotional, behavioural and physical adjustments. Each pregnancy is unique and will challenge the couple and individual members of the family to adapt. Men and women experience and respond differently to pregnancy and birth.

In this chapter the adaptations to fatherhood are considered. Midwives are encouraged to learn more about fathers in their cultural environment, to improve and develop best practice for the care of fathers in pregnancy and labour.

11.2 Fatherhood and childbirth

The transition to fatherhood demands a role adaptation in all cultures. Although this is a normal developmental phase, it is also a period of change and stress.

The level of stress a father will experience during the role transition is determined by the motivation for the pregnancy, his expected role (influenced by culture) and his ability to make changes and adapt to the demands of the new role.

The motivation for the pregnancy

Ambivalent feelings about pregnancy are normal in men and levels of ambivalence may be related to the motivations for the pregnancy. The reasons for pregnancy are divided into:
▶ *rational reasons:* being ready for a family; natural development
▶ *subconscious reasons:* cultural and family demands and expectations, or wanting an heir
▶ *conscious reasons:* trying to save the relationship, or to keep a woman in the relationship.

How fathers adapt to their changed role

A man who has fathered a baby may not necessarily be interested in the pregnancy. He may choose not to be involved in the pregnancy or even reject it. If a man accepts the pregnancy, the role of father makes emotional and other adaptational demands on him and challenges him, even if it is not a first pregnancy. How a new or first-time father adapts to fatherhood and his ability to adjust to the changes brought about by pregnancy and birth may depend on many factors. For instance, the father is required to examine his role, with particular reference to his role as provider and the financial implications around having a child or another child.

The man's own childhood experiences and interaction with his father (or lack thereof) will influence his perception of being a father. This may create anxiety about his ability to be a father. The potentially positive and negative adaptations to fatherhood are as detailed in the following sections.

Positive adaptations

Physical changes may include:
▶ weight gain
▶ the need to grow a beard or moustache
▶ the need to shave a beard or moustache if he has one.

These signs and symptoms can be exaggerated by Couvade syndrome, in which the man experiences the same symptoms as the woman in pregnancy, for example nausea, vomiting and birth pains when the woman is in labour.

Negative adaptations

Minor defective behavioural changes on the part of the father may include:
▶ nausea and vomiting
▶ headaches
▶ irritability
▶ looking up old friends
▶ staying away from home
▶ anxiety
▶ depression.

Psychological adaptations

These may include:
▶ a change in affection shown
▶ changed sexual patterns
▶ a loss of interest in the relationship.

More serious defective behaviour patterns

The development of fatherhood can have a profound influence on a man's mental health and well-being. He may start to abuse alcohol and develop negative responses if unresolved issues or the demands of the role are too overpowering or if he does not have the skills to adapt to the demands of the new role. Although not enough research has been done on men, Condon, Boyce and Corkindale (2004) found that 'pregnancy, rather than the postnatal period, would appear to be the most stressful period for men undergoing the transition to parenthood'. Xu, Sullivan and Homer (2016) found that during the seventeenth or eighteenth weeks of pregnancy, 3 per cent of surveyed fathers reported high levels of 'psychological distress'. Fishbein (1981) found that in 2 per cent of cases where men were admitted for mental health disorders, the root cause was pregnancy. Mental disorders among fathers significantly impacted on the co-occurence of mental disorders among mothers.

Serious defective responses to pregnancy among men include:
▶ alcoholism
▶ theft
▶ becoming unemployed
▶ absconding from work.

11.3   The five phases of adaptation to fatherhood

There are five phases of normal adaptation to fatherhood that have been observed and described. These are briefly presented in the sections that follow.

Phase 1: Acceptance of the pregnancy

The first and most important adaptation for the father is to accept the pregnancy. Without this, it may be difficult for the woman to adapt positively. Negative feelings on the part of the father may affect the woman's feelings of self-worth. She may feel that the father is rejecting her and the child, which may affect her bond with the child. This may lead to rejection of the pregnancy by the mother, resulting in termination of the pregnancy or abortion, preterm birth or intrauterine growth restriction (IUGR) or even abandoning the baby after birth.

For the father, acceptance of the pregnancy is the first step to the development of fatherhood. It indicates his commitment to becoming a father.

Phase 2: Awareness of the mother's emotional and physical changes during pregnancy

It is of fundamental importance for the future role of the father that he becomes aware of the mother's physical and emotional changes throughout pregnancy. His emotional and physical involvement will determine his preparedness for fatherhood. Positive adaptations will influence his experience. If the father is involved with the mother and her experiences of the pregnancy, the baby will become real to him and not just exist in his mind. This involvement will reduce his level of anxiety.

In addition, the mother needs the father's presence and involvement in order to experience the pregnancy positively and to develop her role as mother. When the father shows an interest in the pregnancy and is actively involved, positive and supportive, the mother feels loved and cared for. It enhances her ability to accept the baby and make positive emotional investments in the baby, which will influence the development of the fetus. Stress in women, caused by any stressor, has been shown to have a negative effect on the fetus (O'Connor et al, 2002).

The relationship

The relationship between the father and the mother is vital and has a dynamic effect on the development of parenthood. There is a positive correlation between the couple's relationship and the progress and outcome of pregnancy.

This is also a period where couples re-evaluate their relationship. Women who are secure in their relationships are more able to make positive investments in the pregnancy and the baby. They experience pregnancy more positively and are more self-confident, which in turn improves their partner's self-confidence and self-image. A problematic relationship uses all the woman's emotional resources and she cannot plan effectively for the future. This may lead to depression.

The relationship also has an effect on the father's well-being and, possibly, mental health. Condon, Boyce and Corkindale (2004) found that 'men appeared to be ill-prepared for the impact of parenthood on their lives, especially in terms of the sexual relationship'. Sexual intercourse is a concern during pregnancy. Men may avoid it because they are afraid of hurting the baby or the woman. An open discussion between the couple and the midwife or other healthcare professional may set the man's mind at rest.

Emotional support

The man's main task is to provide emotional support to the woman during pregnancy and the birth.

In the first trimester, the experiential gap that exists between the man and woman is due to the lack of physical involvement of the father in the experience of pregnancy. This may cause tension in the father and he may find it difficult to support the woman. This often leads to the emotional withdrawal of the man from the situation so that he can work through his ambivalent feelings. The father may adapt to his new role and minimise his stress by escaping from the situation through reassuming sport activities, starting a new hobby, working longer hours or engaging in other behaviour to find emotional support from others (Hangsleben, 1983). Women often go to their own mothers, sisters or close family members for emotional support in this period.

It is essential that the father's inner conflicts about fatherhood be resolved so that a satisfactory role division can be developed. This will ensure that his partner's pregnancy is a healthy developmental phase for him. Midwives need to be aware of the father's role and needs during the pregnancy and should involve him in the care of the mother and baby by using structured evidence-based guidelines.

In the mid-trimester, the woman may shift her emotional needs away from her mother and sisters to her partner. The man may experience feelings of unease due to this increased emotional demand. The mid-trimester is the period where the physical changes of pregnancy are obvious. The father can feel the baby moving and the fetal heart is audible. The baby therefore becomes a reality to him. If he attends an ultrasound procedure and sees the baby, it can cause a strong emotional response and enhance the adaptation. Generally, the father now becomes involved, which leads to him becoming more involved in developmental tasks and activities of pregnancy. He may show 'nesting' behaviour, which includes preparation for the baby's arrival and future. This involvement is characterised by the redefinition of his role and the acceptance of the emotional impact of the pregnancy through the collaborative planning of a constructive role.

The father's involvement

The father shows his involvement by taking responsibility for:
- childcare activities
- attending antenatal classes and speaking to the caregiver
- raising the income of the family
- improving or enlarging the home
- providing things for the baby.

The financial burden and responsibilities of fatherhood are important factors that can cause tension. Fathers often work harder and longer hours to plan for the future. Pregnant women are sometimes required to stop working by their partners, with a resultant loss of income, which may increase financial stress.

Phase 3: Anticipating the birth

In the last trimester, the father generally experiences intense anxiety in terms of his partner and baby, the potential problems and the risks of death. He may question his own ability to assist his partner in birth due to his lack of experience. If he has had previous experience of birth, this may influence him positively or negatively. Daydreaming and fantasies are common during this period and are a form of role-play in which the father plans what to do, for example when 'the waters break', when he has to take his partner to the hospital, how to deal with the appearance of the baby, and how he will act and behave towards the baby.

His experience and involvement at this point may become so intense that he develops Couvade syndrome, where he experiences all the physical symptoms of pregnancy and birth. This is seen as a positive psychological adaptation for the father.

The fears and anxiety of the father may be increased by:
- the strange environment of the hospital
- the attitude of healthcare professionals

▶ the quality of care provided for the woman and baby
▶ uncertainty about how he should act and behave
▶ uncertainty about what he is allowed to do
▶ fear of what will happen if the caregiver is not present
▶ uncertainty about what to do about the pain that will be experienced by his partner during the birth.

An unprepared father's fears and anxieties can be transferred to the mother, making her delivery more difficult. The father's self-confidence can be improved by developing realistic goals and anticipating problems that the couple need to solve rationally beforehand. The healthcare professional can help the father develop clear goals to reduce his fears and support him and his efforts.

Phase 4: Involvement in labour

The experience of labour has an enormous impact on the father, independently of his experience of pregnancy. The birth of the baby is a special crisis period and his tension levels may be very high. The father generally has two main fears during birth. These are:
▶ that the mother may die
▶ that the baby may be abnormal.

The mere presence of the father at birth does not necessarily indicate his involvement. Ideally, and if culturally appropriate, the role of the father during birth is that of an active participant giving emotional support to his partner while she is in labour. If the father is sympathetic and actively involved and is emotionally supportive, the mother tends to rely on him for her emotional needs; medical personnel and caregivers then become technical helpers and assistants.

All fathers need support, help and guidance during labour. No pressure should be placed on the father during this time. The father needs to be supported and should be encouraged to be part of the process by supporting the mother through care-giving activities. The degree and level of support provided to him may also influence his level of participation with the birth process. Healthcare professionals and institutions are tasked with creating a supportive environment that includes and responds to the needs of the father if he is present at the birth. The presence of a competent midwife and the quality of care provided to the woman during the birth are strong supportive factors for him. The midwife should inform and guide the father by encouraging him, reminding him to eat and drink, showing him what to do – for example how to rub the mother's back or make her comfortable – and keep him informed of the progress. The father remains the emotional supporter of the mother, and this role will place a high demand on him during labour.

The father's presence during labour seems to have a positive influence on labour in the following ways:
▶ The labour process is shortened, because the woman is more relaxed.
▶ The woman's pain perception is influenced and less pain relief is required. Women tend to request and use fewer painkillers as a result of the help and support and physical presence of the father.

A shared experience of birth can influence the future of the relationship, foster father–child bonding, increase the father's self-confidence and encourage him to be more involved in caring for the mother and baby. Fathers who share birth experiences have more positive perceptions if the mother had a positive birth experience. A difficult delivery, on the other hand, may leave him with negative impressions and a delayed or negative response to the child.

Note that in some cultures (for instance in the Jewish and Muslim cultures), the presence of the father during birth is a cultural taboo. However, this does not mean that these fathers are less interested in the pregnancy and birth than other fathers. In these cultures, women accompany the mother during birth. In the social transition to modern patterns of living, it has become a more common phenomenon to make provision for and allow fathers to attend the birth.

Phase 5: The father and the postnatal period

The postnatal period in itself is a period of crisis for the father. The pregnancy and the baby are no longer a fantasy, but are real, and the father is challenged by the reality of events and the direct demands of fatherhood. Directly after birth, the father may compare the baby with his expectations and images from his dreams and imagination. He also needs to come to terms with the gender of the baby. His response to and acceptance of the baby's gender will influence the mother's responses.

Furthermore, the father must work through the stress of the birth and resolve this, particularly if the birth did not go the way it was anticipated. If the baby is premature, sick or abnormal it may cause an enormous amount of emotional strain and disappointment. The father may not be able to support the woman until he has resolved his own stress, emotional loss, grief and disappointment. Specific interventions and support are needed from health professionals in such a case, as described in Chapter 13.

The postnatal period requires the father to develop further skills in order to take care of the baby, for example to change nappies, bath and feed the baby. Women have special emotional needs and require reassurance and encouragement in the postnatal period, particularly in relation to breastfeeding.

The postnatal period, whether for the first or a later child, is unique and it makes special social, emotional and caregiving demands on the father and mother, which require a role change. These role changes depend on:
- the antenatal adaptations in men
- the father's experience of the birth
- the opportunity the father has had to develop skills
- the support and guidance available from family and caregivers.

Father–infant bonding

During this stage, the father ideally also develops a bond with his infant. Father–infant bonding has been proven to be just as strong as maternal–infant bonding, or stronger; babies seem to prefer their mothers to their fathers only when they are hungry (Gay, 1981).

Father–infant bonding starts in the antenatal period, but develops after birth and is strongly influenced by the development of fatherhood through the five phases described in this section. Fathers who assist their partners during labour develop special feelings towards their babies that are visible and permanent. Fatherly involvement through these phases, if positive, creates a strong and lasting bond between the father and the infant.

Fathers are generally not passive observers of their babies, but display the same bonding responses as mothers and actively seek involvement with their babies. Early contact with the child is the moment the father has been anticipating for nine months and it is the first opportunity to make physical contact. Fathers have been seen to respond to their babies within five minutes after birth by touching them. This early postnatal contact with the father will enhance the bonding and the father will develop strong connections with the infant. Fathers that had early contact with their babies talk more to the children and touch them more often.

The type of delivery and degree of father–infant bonding result in and contribute to continued and intensified involvement with the mother and child by the father taking over some of the childcare activities, such as feeding the baby.

The effect of the father on the infant

The father's role in the development of the child is fundamental, dynamic and active. Researchers have found that children need both a mother and a father to realise their talents to the maximum (Brazelton, 1983).

The presence of a father who is positively involved with the infant will have a positive influence on the child's development.

Interaction with both the father and the mother is thus considered essential for the development of the child. Research found that fathers and mothers influence child development in unique ways and that the absence of a father has a specific negative influence on the development of the child. Boys are more affected than girls when a father is absent.

There is a difference in childcare activities between mothers and fathers. Mothers tend to be more caring and less verbal with babies, while fathers tend to be more verbal and engage the child in physical activities and play. Directly after birth, the father's activities are more passive – holding, carrying and transporting the baby – but they soon change and become more focused on playing.

In addition, the baby is not a passive recipient of care from the father; instead, a two-way relationship develops. The baby shows great interest in the father by responding to his voice, or following him with the eyes when he leaves.

The absence of a father in a child's life is called *father deprivation* (or absence). This affects the child in a unique way that differs from maternal deprivation. The effect of the separation will depend on the age of the child and the duration of the separation. Father deprivation can also happen when the father is present, but is ineffective emotionally or unstable.

There are two particular areas where the child is most affected by the father:
1. *Socialising:* Father–infant bonding lays the foundation for the future social milieu and affects the socialisation of the child positively. Studies have shown that in children with a good father–infant bonding experience, there is less separation anxiety when not with the mother. The father's contact with the infant is the infant's first contact with the world. Children with good father–infant bonding are more curious and explorative in terms of their environment. They respond more positively towards strangers and during complex stimuli. The positive effect of socialisation also enhances the cognitive development of the child.
2. *Cognitive and motor development:* Children with good father–infant bonding have more advanced motor development and are more secure in exploring new situations. Fathers tend to be more tolerant than mothers to explorative behaviour.

11.4 The role of the midwife in promoting paternal involvement

Midwives, when caring for women in pregnancy and labour, are also involved with the family, significant people and the father of the baby. As such, midwives need to invite these categories of significant persons into the care of women and educate or guide them on what to expect.

The midwife is tasked with and should acquire the knowledge and skills to manage the involvement of the father during the process of pregnancy and birth. It has become common practice globally to facilitate greater involvement of the father during pregnancy and birth. In practice, however, there are challenges that need to be addressed, such as encouraging the father to attend antenatal visits and training as well as the birth, and actively involving the father in postnatal care activities such as bathing the baby.

Activity

Consult the following source for insight into the complexity of fatherhood in the traditional South African context:
Richter, L. 2006 *BABA: Men and fatherhood in South Africa*. Cape Town: HSRC Press.

Guidelines for involving fathers in childbirth

In South Africa, childbirth has been accessible to fathers in the private health sector for more than 40 years. In the public sector there is a definite intention to allow the father access to his partner during childbirth, but certain prerequisites need to be met for successful practice, such as the principles of privacy and control. This is a good intention and speaks to the ideal situation, but a policy change is required. Such practices need to take place within a structured programme that follows strict guidelines and considers the following principles:

▶ Wards should have a written policy and guidelines on how to involve fathers during pregnancy, birth and the postnatal period.

▶ Specific culturally sensitive guidelines are required to manage the father during pregnancy and birth, such as knowledge of cultural and religious taboos.

▶ Midwives need focused education and training on:
  • the assessment, implementation and evaluation of the father's involvement during all the phases of pregnancy and the birth
  • measures to support the father
  • practical considerations relating to the environment to protect the father and others in the unit by ensuring privacy, giving the father time to rest, reminding him to eat and making sure there is a toilet that he can use
  • legal implications, which include the understanding that the man may not legally be the father of the baby, or that he may take a photo and put in a claim for damages in case of emergency
  • safety considerations in case the man faints or becomes intoxicated or violent.

11.5   Conclusion

The support of the employer, management and the midwife is required to create an enabling environment that accommodates the father's support and involvement in childbirth, with consideration of the cultural variations and social stressors of poverty, family disintegration and violence against women that are present in South African society. Remember that education is a powerful tool to help families during the cycle of childbirth.

It is also essential to develop best practice policies, procedures and a physical environment that will allow for the participation of the father during pregnancy and labour.

The mother–infant relationship, 'good-enough mothering' and perinatal loss

LEARNING OBJECTIVES

On completion of this chapter, you must be able to:
- explain the principles and processes of mother–infant bonding and attachment
- explain the concept of maternal containment and 'good-enough mothering'
- explain factors that impact on the maternal–infant relationship
- explain potential short- and long-term effects of mother–infant separation on the infant
- explain the midwife's role in the observation and promotion of the mother–infant relationship.
- assist and manage the loss of a baby, using evidence-based standards, guidelines and protocols.

KNOWLEDGE ASSUMED TO BE IN PLACE

Basic knowledge of psychology, and cultural and religious diversity
Normal child development and attachment theory
Theories of 'good-enough mothering' and deprivation

KEYWORDS

baby • infant • good-enough mothering • maternal–infant bonding • attachment • deprivation • battering • Kübler-Ross • loss • grief

12.1   Introduction

The relationship between a mother and her newborn baby is dynamic. The relationship that starts during pregnancy and the birth process is sub-conscious and abstract (a psychosocial conscious process), but when the baby is born, a process called *bonding* begins, which is now concrete and real.

Mother–infant bonding refers to the emotional bond and relationship that develops between the mother and baby. Maternal–infant bonding is expressed in maternal physical and verbal behaviour that can be observed. Attachment is the process of establishing the bond. This is not automatic and is dependent on a variety of factors, including the social and physical environment, the healthcare environment, the birth experience, feelings of well-being after birth and the support

structures that are in place. The early experience of an infant from the time of birth is contained in the process of bonding and attachment, and may have long-term psychological and social consequences for the development and well-being of the infant and child.

This chapter will look at the factors that affect bonding and attachment, and the effects on the baby. The attributes of maternal containment or 'good-enough mothering' will be discussed. These terms are used to describe the basic (emotional and social) conditions that must be in place for the baby/infant to experience normal psychosocial development in a safe environment.

Maternal instinct is not necessarily universally displayed in all mothers. 'Mothering' is considered to be learned behaviour, with strong cultural roots and influence. Midwives are close to the mother in this sensitive period and are well positioned to identify problems, facilitate bonding, and educate and support mothers to be 'good-enough mothers' in this complex and on-going process of care of the baby, infant or child. The first 1 000 days are important, starting from intrauterine life to the days, weeks and months of the first two years of life, which lay a foundation for the well-being and future of the child.

12.2 Motherhood and baby/infant health

Motherhood is fundamental to the future physical and mental health of a population and must be considered when planning the provision of maternal healthcare.

Child care and human rights

The human rights approach to healthcare has influenced the way in which healthcare has developed, and increasing attention has been given to the rights of children through the work of the United Nations Children's Fund (UNICEF), the Millennium Development Goals (MDGs) (UN, 2006) and Sustainable Development Goals (SDGs) (UN, 2015).

The Children's Act 38 of 2005 (CA) promotes the protection, development, well-being and rights of the child. It addresses single parenthood and/or a family that has reached a point of severe breakdown and is unable to stay together as a unit, as well as instances where abuse and neglect are evident. The CA sets out principles relating to the care and protection of children and defines parental responsibilities and rights.

MDGs 4 and 5 were concerned with aspects related to motherhood that impact on child health. UNICEF (2015) stresses the need for children to get the best start in life. Parents who struggle to raise a child under less than favourable conditions experience intense family stress. This effect may start before and during pregnancy and exist in early childhood, when mothers are often separated from their children.

UNICEF plays a pivotal role in strengthening the training and education of midwives and developing the skills and competencies of midwives. The aim is to improve professional development for better maternal and newborn outcomes.

Effective mothering

Ideally, the biological mother should be the primary caretaker of the baby. In all societies, effective mothering requires a stable, supportive environment. To this end, childbirth preparation and positive parenthood are initiatives that are valuable resources in technologically sophisticated (usually urban) environments to prepare parents for the care they need to give.

Preparation for parenthood in traditional populations is often quite different and governed by tradition. The transitional development of large portions of South African society from rural to urban living has disturbed traditional patterns and may affect a women's physical and mental well-being in pregnancy, which in turn can affect mothering patterns and practices. Innovative support systems are needed to protect children under these circumstances.

If the biological mother is not available or is unable to care for the baby, it is possible for substitute mothers or alternative carers to meet all the baby's physical needs through the provision of emotional, age-appropriate cognitive stimulation and care to ensure the basic development of the child.

Single-parent families are also a concern, not only because single mothers are more likely to struggle, but because it is assumed that good mothering requires the financial and emotional support of a partner or a community.

12.3 Mother–infant bonding

The bond between a mother and her infant is not automatic nor instinctive. 'Mothering' involves a mother getting to know her baby practically through interactions with her baby, and each mother adapts at her own pace. Each baby, from each separate pregnancy, places specific and unique developmental demands on the mother. Not all pregnancies are planned or wanted, which may affect the bonding process and behaviour. Even in wanted pregnancies, depending on the timing of the pregnancy, women may bond differently to their babies.

A range of factors can affect the mother's experience of and thoughts on the baby and delay mother–infant bonding. The mother may feel threatened on a variety of levels in pregnancy and after birth, for example by:

▶ the physical changes to her body
▶ changes to her relationships
▶ challenges in terms of her financial commitments
▶ changes to study opportunities and/or future goals
▶ the loss of her independence.

Bonding may already be strong during the pregnancy, but it generally only really takes hold after birth when the mother and baby interact – through eye contact, skin-to-skin contact, body warmth and movements. Depending on cultural beliefs – for example, some cultures avoid eye contact or are not overly verbal – most women seek contact with their babies within six hours after birth, but sometimes bonding happens over a longer time. Mothers may need to consolidate and reflect on the experience of birth and come to grips with their expectations of the baby. There appears to be a sequence of behaviour involved in bonding, as explained in the box that follows.

Typical bonding behaviour
Typical bonding behaviour and responses of the mother include the following: ▶ *Touching:* The mother looks at the baby at first and then naturally displays touching behaviour that follows a natural sequence. The mother touches the baby using her finger tips, beginning at the baby's extremities and moving towards the trunk, often using stroking movements. When the palm of the mother's hand meets the baby's trunk, the sequence is complete. The mother then lifts the baby up to her face for eye-to-eye contact. ▶ *Verbalising:* The mother asks questions or compares the baby to other members of the family, eg 'She looks like …'. A typical positive response is when a mother makes a statement such as 'This is the most beautiful baby I have ever seen', indicating her perceptions and expression of love. The mother speaks to the baby in a high-pitched voice. Speaking to the baby and not about the baby is a positive bonding activity.

Factors influencing mother–infant bonding

Motherhood is a normal developmental phase and each pregnancy and birth is a unique experience that affects the mother's mental well-being and ability to be a mother, even on a subconscious level. Several factors influence the bonding process and the mother's ability to mindfully respond to the baby's anxieties and give comfort – also referred to as 'maternal containment'. Factors that may influence maternal–child bonding include:

▶ the motivation for the pregnancy
▶ the woman's experiences and relationship with her own mother
▶ poverty, or the financial support available
▶ support from the community or environment
▶ support from healthcare professionals and healthcare practices
▶ problems experienced in pregnancy and birth
▶ the mental health of the mother.

The motivation for the pregnancy may determine the mother's attitude towards the baby. If the father accepts the pregnancy, the mother is likely to be more positive towards the baby. If the mother views the pregnancy as her social duty or a duty towards her husband, she may be less invested in the pregnancy and less responsive to the baby after birth. She may even abandon the

baby. On the other hand, if she has the support of the father of the baby, financial security and family support, this will assist her to focus on her newborn.

When a woman is pregnant or becomes a mother, she tends to reflect back on her own experiences of being mothered. If this was negative, or if she experienced insecurity, rejection, discomfort or abuse from her primary caregiver, her ability to be a mother may be severely affected and she may even repeat this behaviour with her own baby. The developmental tasks of mothering are therefore influenced by experiences and the relationship the woman had with her own mother, as well as the environment in which she grew up. This will include experiences with and examples of baby care she has learned from her environment. Although the maternal instinct is natural, mothering is also learned behaviour. Evidence shows that these patterns are unconsciously repeated through generations. The way the mother has resolved these stages in her own childhood may distort her view of her child and create anxiety that will influence and affect her ability to be an effective mother.

The availability of healthcare, the attitude of staff and the level of information and support provided during pregnancy and birth may have an influence on the mother's response to her baby. Important aspects in healthcare include the practices followed during birth, in creating a bonding environment (eg care, information and support) and in allowing for early breastfeeding. This is even more important when the baby is not well or the mother and baby are separated. In case of a separation, staff can assist by trying to overcome the separation and finding ways to keep contact. They can keep the mother informed and find ways to bring the mother and infant together. This may play an important role in initiating bonding behaviour.

It is normal for women to experience ambivalent feelings towards the baby in pregnancy and after birth. Women fantasise about their babies. Most pregnant mothers have dreams or nightmares in late pregnancy about their inability to care for the baby (such as starving the baby or forgetting the baby in a car or shopping centre). They also feel fear and anxiety about the actual process of giving birth.

Depending on the underlying fantasies and fears in pregnancy, birth itself may be experienced as a joy, a wonder, a relief, a loss, a trauma or a discovery. It is probably a mixture of all of these, regardless of the mother's cultural beliefs. The actual events of the birth also make a significant contribution, in terms of the quality of the experience, for parents and their babies. The degree of anxiety and discomfort or comfort experienced, the availability of technological interventions, the nature of the birth environment and the amount of stress, danger or confidence experienced all play a part. The external reality of these events may be beautiful or harsh, but the meaning and extent to which they are felt to be pleasurable, distressing, manageable or unbearable will be intimately related to the internal psychological disposition of all concerned.

Often, the exhilaration and relief of a safe delivery may be followed by a period of depression and disappointment. Sometimes, a period of 'mourning' may even occur, as the mother mourns the loss of the baby from her womb to become a separate being, now born. The mother may become passive and demand to be cared for, thus neglecting the baby's needs.

The birth of the baby can also bring about feelings related to unmet emotional needs in the mother and/or the father. For instance, the parent's own neediness may be so overwhelming that the baby's emotional or physical needs are neglected.

After birth, some women verbalise feelings of distance, unreality, or not knowing the child. Indifference to the child is not uncommon. On the other hand, women with mental health disorders may express behaviour inconsistent 'with maternal bonding, such as ignoring the baby, not feeding the baby and making negative comments about the baby – for instance, calling the baby 'it'.

Midwifery practice in early bonding

It has become standard practice to advocate for putting the baby to the breast within an hour after birth and to avoid the separation of mother and baby as far as possible. This is a very important part of the bonding process, because after birth, the mother is focused and psychologically open (due to hormonal effects) and wants to interact with the infant. Even if the mother is separated from the infant at birth, midwives need to facilitate contact within 24 hours. (It should be noted that best practice guidelines require mothers and babies be together 24 hours a day through rooming-in in birthing units.)

The midwife plays an important role in helping the mother to recover from the birth and facilitates the first crucial moments in the physical presence of her baby. Midwives should observe the bonding process and be sensitive to a mother's particular circumstances. Once the initial sequence of bonding has taken place (during the first hour after birth), the baby should be ready for breastfeeding; evidence-based best practice in maternal and 'baby-friendly' care (BFC) requires this.

For most babies, the primary caregiver or 'need satisfier' is the biological mother – the source of food, protection, warmth, stimulation and affection. If a baby does not want to latch to the breast, it may be due to delayed or interrupted bonding. It is a good idea to take the mother through the process of skin-to-skin contact and eye contact and encourage her to talk to the baby in the face-to-face position. This encourages breastfeeding.

The bond, or attachment, that a mother forms with her baby begins during pregnancy, possibly when she first feels movement within her body. It is a gradually unfolding relationship that blossoms with the baby's birth. The first minutes, 24 hours and days after birth have special significance. Certain events, or mental illness, may disturb early attachment and possibly have adverse effects on the later mother–child relationship.

Signs of potential faulty, failed or delayed attachment include the woman saying that she did not want the pregnancy or the child, not being happy with the gender of the baby, not wanting to look after the baby, complaining about the baby, and calling the baby 'it' instead of by name (if named). Clues would be failing to feed the baby, refusing breastfeeding or bottle feeding and not wanting the baby in the room. Kangaroo-mother-care (KMC) is one way to promote bonding, particularly when mothers and babies are separated for periods due to complications of pregnancy and birth.

The quality of the mother–child relationship is based on the mother's own psychological resources, which can be strengthened by a supportive environment, or weakened by a lack of support. Her relationship with the baby will either grow well or become troubled, which could have lifelong consequences for the child.

Maternal containment or good-enough mothering

Ideally, the biological mother should be the primary caregiver, because of the biological and emotional bond assumed between the mother and infant. Mothering is interactive and has a direct influence on the baby. The baby is not a passive participant and gives the mother clues as to its needs. The mother should be able to identify, interpret and respond to the baby's clues and needs. After birth, the mother–infant unit is still seen as one. The baby is totally dependent on the mother. The concepts explained in the following sections express dimensions of mothering.

Maternal containment

'Containment' is a concept and psychoanalytic theory that was developed by Bion (in Finlay, 2015) and Cartwright et al (2010). It refers to the intent and action to keep something harmful under control or within limits. Containment is embedded in mothering and starts with maternal–infant bonding (Salomonsson, 2014) and the mother's desire to keep the baby comfortable and safe.

If maternal–infant bonding is adequate, the mother is able to read and interpret the baby's needs and respond adequately to them. This is called maternal containment. It refers to the psychological component of the relationship whereby the mother is able to understand what the infant wants and respond appropriately to the baby's inner life. It also refers to the mother's response to the demands the infant places on her from this inner life in order to create comfort and alleviate anxieties. The term 'containment' refers to what happens when the mother receives, processes, absorbs and responds to the demands the baby makes on her (Salomonsson, 2014). It deals with the mother's ability to create a safe emotional space for the baby to grow and develop by being able to hear, understand and interpret the baby's needs and clues.

Good-enough mothering

Maternal containment is needed for good-enough mothering. This term refers to a set of known conditions that are needed for the normal development of babies, infants and children, provided either by the biological mother or a substitute mother. Where there is maternal containment, the baby feels safe and cared for and secure attachment behaviour develops. Good-enough mothering also suggests that an absent mother or the presence of an 'ineffective mother' with mental health problems may have a negative effect on the growth and development of the infant. Good-enough mothering implies that a substitute mother who is able to act according to the known conditions for normal development and comfort may be able to create the safe environment needed by a baby or infant.

Babies and infants are vulnerable and depend on the mother not only for survival but also for their developmental needs, as explained in the maternal containment models. The mother's failure to meet the individual emotional needs of the infant has long-term consequences for the child's psychological, emotional and cognitive development. If the mother is uneasy or troubled, she may not be able to interpret and respond to the baby's or infant's clues and may fail to respond appropriately, leaving the baby's or infant's needs unmet. This will have adverse consequences for the baby's development, particularly if the mother is severely depressed. If the mother is preoccupied with concerns about other members of the family, with work or outside interests, her depression, illnesses, absences, or even her death, are transformed into experiences of rejection and desertion for the baby, infant or child.

If a baby or infant experiences fluctuation between aggressiveness, love and understanding in the mother's care during the developmental phases, this may have an adverse effect on his or her development and sense of security. Frustration, discomfort and pain (also seen as persecution) enter into the baby's feelings about the mother and the world, because in the first few months the mother or primary caregiver represents the whole of the external world. Therefore, both good and bad comes from the mother, and this leads to an ambivalent attitude towards the mother and the world, even under the best possible conditions.

The infant reacts to persecutory impulses of an unfavourable environment with anxiety, predisposing the child in later life to behavioural disorders, learning disabilities and personality disorders. These include antisocial behaviour, drug and alcohol abuse, insecurity, low self-esteem, eating disorders and depression, as well as an inability to form lasting and meaningful relationships.

Substitute mothering

Maternal–infant bonding, containment and good-enough mothering may be absent in cases where mothers are not able to take care of the needs of their babies because of their own physical or social problems, or mental health status. Women with a history of abandoning their children or who were abused themselves are at risk of becoming abusive mothers. The demands of the care of the baby may revive in the mother her own childhood conflicts and experiences. If these where stressful, it may cause a crisis in her own perception of and adaptation to her new role as a mother.

If a biological mother is sick or absent, a foster or substitute mother who meets the needs of the infant can provide good-enough care. This is confirmed by many cases of adopted children growing up to be well-adjusted adults.

Attachment and separation

Spontaneous parental attachment behaviour becomes the known world of the baby or infant, where the baby's needs are met and where he or she finds comfort. There is consensus that a major developmental shift occurs in babies at around seven months after birth. They become able to experience themselves and their mothers as whole persons, separate from one another. This is a normal developmental phase and needs to be recognised and managed.

The baby will now be able to maintain an internal relationship to the mother in his or her mind while she is externally absent. It is this internal relationship that allows secure attachment behaviour and for the baby to develop a sense of his or her own person and the mother. A child should have a secure base and be able to return to that safe haven while exploring the world (see the box on the next page). This process starts from the moment the baby is born: The mother makes eye contact and even if the baby looks away, the mother is there waiting when the baby looks back.

Maternal deprivation

Maternal deprivation is the absence of a consistent caregiver for the critical first two years of life.

Bowlby's maternal deprivation theory (McLeod, 2007) found that babies who stayed close to their mothers survived to have children of their own. The continuous care of one single figure for the first year of life is essential for the baby to form an attachment with one person that will result in a secure base for the infant to explore the world.

The short-term separation of a baby or infant from this caregiving figure causes distress. Continuous interruption or brokenness of this attachment in the critical two-year period will cause irreversible long-term consequences associated with maternal deprivation.

The circle of security
The circle of security (the parent's attention to the infant's needs) is a process whereby the parent creates an environment where the child can explore, by moving or looking away from the parent (FSU, 2016). The parent remains present while the infant ventures away. The infant asks the parent to allow him or her (ie watch me, delight in me, enjoy with me and help me). When the infant experiences discomfort, he or she realises the need for the parent and comes back to the safety of the parent's hands and arms (ie protect me, comfort me and help me to organise my emotions).   The following are guidelines for parents: ▶ Always be big, strong, wise and kind.   ▶ If possible, always follow the child's need.   ▶ Whenever needed, take charge.

When an infant experiences lack of maternal containment, the infant feels physical discomfort, pain and emotional distress, which are powerful and negatively charged experiences. This forces the infant to rely primarily on his or her own resources and to withdraw emotionally, become apathetic, not interested in the world and avoid eye contact. Children in whom this deficiency is severe seem to grow up lacking the conviction that distress can be tolerated. Deprivation thus refers to a lack of the experiences or resources in life considered basic for physical, emotional and social development. This absence of experience leads to protest, despair and detachment in the baby or infant.

Children who experience maternal deprivation may develop insecure or disorganised attachment behaviour and suffer a loss that influences cognitive and social behaviour

or causes a 'failure to thrive'. The long-term consequences of maternal deprivation include delinquency, reduced intelligence, increased aggression, depression and affectionless psychopathy or anti-social behaviour (McLeod, 2007).

A mother suffering from depression in the first year of a baby's life, if untreated and unsupported, may have the same effect on the baby's development as an absent mother.

Battering

Despite all the joys and pleasures of a wanted pregnancy, the new mother may also feel, for the first time, unexpected fears and anxieties that are not part of the playful interaction of mother and baby. She may experience a core of loneliness that she is unaccustomed to. The most devoted mother can experience times of intense loneliness with her baby and symptoms of mental illness (postnatal depression [PND] and anxiety) may contribute to uncontrolled emotions. Other elements that may lead to battering include a mother's personal experiences or history of being battered herself, the stress of being a single or teenage mother, or severe family breakdown.

Many parents have felt intense rage and an impulse to smack a baby at a time of stress. Assistance is needed in the form of family or friends taking over the care of the baby to relieve the tension between mother and child. If mothers are unsupported, it may result in unintended battering. Midwives and healthcare professionals are by law obliged to report cases where babies are neglected or where emotional or physical abuse is suspected, observed or reported. Alerting features that should prompt the midwife or health professional to suspect child maltreatment include (NICE, 2009):

▶ persistently harmful parent– or carer–child interactions (emotional abuse, shouting at the infant in public)

▶ persistent emotional unavailability and unresponsiveness from the parent or carer towards a child, in particular towards an infant (emotional neglect, leaving the child alone or punishing the infant by ignoring him or her).

12.4 The psychosocial role of the midwife in maternal and newborn care

Psychological aspects of care are an important competency and part of the standards of midwifery practice. Midwives and ward-based outreach teams (WBOTs) in primary healthcare (PHC) need to understand the emotional, cognitive and psychosexual development of the baby, and should guide the mother, parents or primary caregivers in stimulating these skills. In addition, the midwife should make helpful observations in diagnosing problem areas in the mother–child relationship. Midwives are also required by the CA to identify and report cases where a child may be in danger.

Observations during mother–infant interactions

The following are observation guidelines the midwife can use to identify positive or negative parental interactions:

▶ *Preparation:* How did the mother prepare for the arrival of the baby?

▶ *Bonding behaviour:* Did bonding occur? What was the initial response of mother and baby after birth? What were the mother's verbal responses (eg cooing, soft and friendly, or harsh and impatient)? Does she make and keep eye contact?

▶ *Aspects of care:* How does the mother respond to the baby's physical needs (temperature of the room, appropriateness of clothing, need for nappy changing, sleep and feeding)?

▶ *Holding:* Does the mother keep the baby in her mind by holding and containing the baby? Does the mother respond to the baby's needs for comfort and warmth? How does the baby respond – what is the baby's expression? How long does the mother leave the baby in the push chair or cot unattended?

▶ *Handling:* How does the mother pick up and hold the baby? Does the mother handle the baby in a caring and safe way? What are the baby's responses to being changed or handled? How does the mother speak to the baby?

▶ *Safety:* What does the mother think about safety issues in general? Is her attitude appropriate for the baby's age and stage of development?

▶ *Feeding:* Can the mother recognise that the baby is hungry and respond appropriately? How does she hold and speak to the baby while feeding? How does she cope with challenging situations such as a dirty nappy, vomiting and wriggling distress? What feeling does this encounter evoke in the midwife?

▶ *Play:* Does the mother adapt to the baby's mood, playing appropriately and in a friendly, caring way, following cues from the baby? Can she recognise when the baby is tired?

▶ *Comforting and settling to sleep:* Does the mother recognise whether or not the baby needs to sleep? Does she respond appropriately? Does she talk to the baby when putting him or her to sleep? Is she happy to get rid of the baby or does she give loving and caring instructions to others when leaving the baby with them? How does she negotiate a break for herself and does she ask for help?

▶ *Relationships:* Does she protect the baby from her own feelings of upset, anger or sadness and the effect of these feelings on the baby? How do mother and father work

as a couple, with the family and the healthcare staff – are they forming a positive relationship? Is there consistency of mood and response?

Midwives need to empower themselves by self-development and a process of life-long learning. This will enable them, in turn, to educate mothers and to ensure that their supervision and care of the mother–infant dyad contribute to positive experiences of motherhood.

12.5 Perinatal loss and grief

There are several causes and forms of grief that a woman may experience in motherhood. The healthcare professional needs to manage grieving and bereavement through following best practice, grief processes or models of counselling and care (Flenady et al, 2014; Kersting & Wagner, 2012). If this is neglected, the grief can stay unresolved for a lifetime. Different forms of loss are briefly mentioned in the sections that follow.

Forms of perinatal loss

Infertility

Women who use artificial means to fall pregnant are generally offered professional counselling; however, women who fail to conceive go through a process of grief and are often highly stressed.

Early pregnancy loss

A spontaneous abortion, ectopic pregnancy or termination of an abnormal fetus may result in the grief of acute loss. This grief may not be recognised by society, as the event is considered an abortion.

The loss of a pregnancy through choice of termination may bring early feelings of relief, and grief is often suppressed. This may have long-term effects on the mental health of women who choose termination of pregnancy (TOP), and counselling is not always available at TOP clinics in the public healthcare sector. A systematic review of literature did not find evidence that women have long-term mental health problems after abortion on demand; the review found that only a minority of women experienced sadness, grief, regret and depression (Charles et al, 2008).

Intrauterine death or stillbirth

The loss of a baby *in utero* (IUD) is usually a period of intense grief and pain. The events that follow the diagnosis may worsen the problem. The choice of delivery, the choice of burial and going home to a room that had been prepared to receive a baby can cause great distress.

The experience of stillbirth may be even worse. When a woman is in labour, expecting to deliver a healthy baby, and the baby dies during labour, the psychological impact on the mother, father and staff is acute. This woman may be at risk for post-traumatic stress disorder (PTSD). In these cases the delivery is often an emergency procedure, without time for preparation. In the case of twin or multiple pregnancies, the woman may lose one baby *in utero* or may have to choose to terminate one baby to save another. This can cause enormous tension and grief.

Physical or mental disability

The parents of a baby who is sick and physically or mentally disabled will grieve for the loss of a normal baby. Parents often experience conflict around this event. They may also fear that the baby may die or have long-term health problems and subsequent attachment with the baby may be affected. In addition, parents often experience conflict around such a traumatic event, while costs and the time spent caring for the

baby can be overwhelming and may add to feelings of stress, guilt and hopelessness.

Giving up a baby for adoption; surrogacy

The decision to give a baby up for adoption may be a relief for a woman who cannot care for the baby. Some women experience intense grief, while others can let go easily.

Surrogate mothers will carry a baby for another couple and sign an agreement to let the baby go after birth.

The experience of loss and grief

Although the stages of grieving are similar, people differ in the way that they experience loss and grief and how they express this experience. These differences depend on an individual's personality, gender and culture. Elizabeth Kübler-Ross (1969) observed and described typical behaviour associated with loss and grief regardless of age, culture or gender. This behaviour includes denial, anger, bargaining, depression and acceptance. The time a person takes to move through these phases differs.

PROCEDURE   Caring for bereaved parents

Principles
The care of a family that has experienced perinatal loss requires skill and maturity. It takes time to guide a woman and her family through this traumatic experience. Several principles need to be considered when caring for a woman after a perinatal loss. It is also important to have a written policy in the unit on how to manage perinatal loss, birth defects and stillbirths.

Breaking the news
One of the main signs of IUD is that the baby is not moving. A woman may suspect or know that something is not right and come for advice. The midwife must always be honest and involve the woman and her family in the process. If possible, a medical doctor needs to make or confirm the diagnosis. An ultrasound is usually sufficient, and it also allows the parents to see that the fetal heartbeat is absent.

A skilled midwife needs to be appointed to take care of the family after news of a perinatal loss. The following are guidelines for managing this part of the process:
- After the loss of a baby, a woman should never be placed in a ward with other women who have babies.
- Early discharge is only recommended if the woman does not need medical care.
- In cases of IUD a vaginal birth – if possible – is better than a Caesarean section.
- The woman needs to be allowed time to express her fears and needs. The midwife should be standing by (not actively involved, but present and observant) and available for support. The physical presence of a midwife can be supportive to the woman, but her space should not be invaded.
- Communicate information clearly, as people in shock do not take in messages well. Give time for questions and answer them honestly, using therapeutic verbal and non-verbal communication skills (see Chapter 3). Empathetic listening and quiet reflection are helpful.
- Assistance can be sought from other professionals such as social workers, psychiatric nurses, psychologists and psychiatrists if the risk factors warrant this.
- Consider genetic counselling if required. In most cases, the cause of the death is not obvious, but parents tend to want a reason to help them understand. If there is an obvious cause of death, point it out.

continued

▶ Observe and respect cultural wishes and practices. Groups such as Hindus, Muslims, Christians, Jews and African groups all have different ways of dealing with grief and practise different rituals. For example, Jewish and Muslim parents need to have the body prepared by a priest and buried before the sun sets. Ask the mother and family what they prefer and assist them, as long as it is within the law. A baby that was viable (28 weeks) cannot be removed from a clinic or hospital without a death certificate. Only the police can give permission for a body to be transported by the family rather than by a registered undertaker.

▶ Explain the need for a birth certificate and a death certificate as well as other legal requirements to the parents. The authorities must be informed of the baby's birth through the completion of the official notification of birth, accompanied by a death certificate. If the baby was viable, it has to be buried or cremated by a registered institution. Parents of a fetus of less than 1 000 g may also agree to incineration. Formal processes and hospital protocols should be followed in a sensitive way, with two people present.

▶ One of the most important aspects when dealing with grief is to allow the parents to experience the event. Allow the parents and family to see and to hold the baby. This process should never be forced. Parents must be told that they have a right to see and hold their child and that there will be an opportunity to do so in the next 48 hours or before the baby is taken to the undertakers. Initially, parents may be shocked, surprised or confused. They may at first refuse, but eventually most people want to see and hold the baby, even if the baby is severally malformed or macerated.

Creating memories
It should be the hospital's policy to create reminders of a lost child to assist the family in the grieving process.

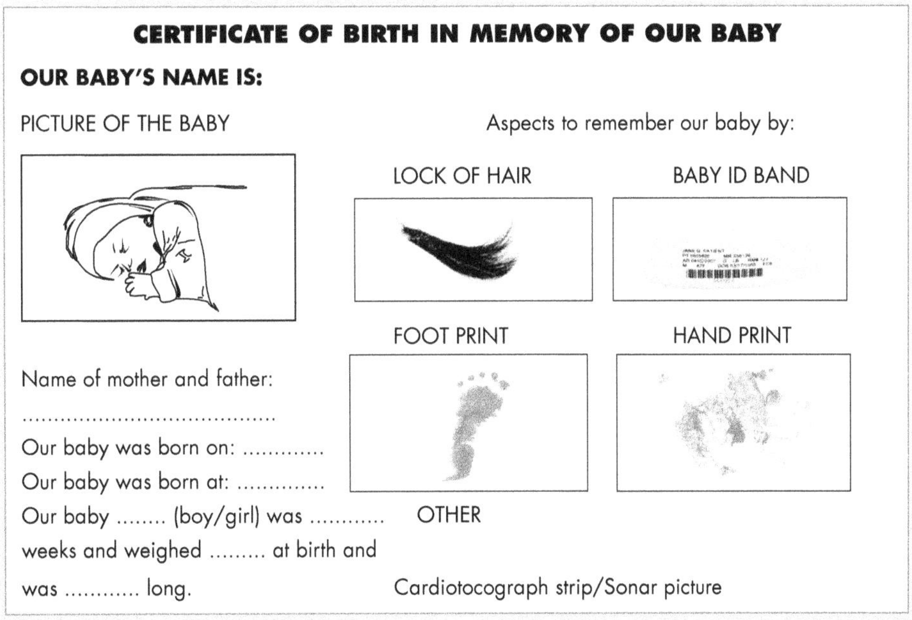

Figure 12A Creating reminders

With the parents' permission, the following can be done:
▶ Take a photo of the baby or allow the parents to take a photo. (This is valuable, as memories fade fast and it is not possible to hold on to a brief moment.)
▶ Make a footprint or handprint.
▶ Give the baby a name (if culturally appropriate).
▶ Create a name tag with the full details of the date, time, the baby's mass, the baby's length and so on.
▶ Cut off a piece of hair and put it in a booklet for deceased babies.

continued

Most institutions have a specific booklet in which the information and evidence can be collated before it is given to the parents. This is most helpful in the grieving process.

Following up

It is important to prepare the mother and family for the aftermath of the event. Often, women want to talk about the experience, yet family and friends avoid it. This leads to emotional discomfort and a breakdown in communication. One way to assist parents is to refer them to services that support women who have lost a child or other services in the community. (For example, The Compassionate Friends assist parents after the loss of a child. Find out more by visiting www.compassionatefriends.co.za.)

It is important not to forget about physical care for the wound, the breasts and Hb. In addition, family planning and all the normal postnatal care should not be neglected.

12.6　Conclusion

The midwife should be able to assess the mother and her needs for information, her expectation of the pregnancy and baby, her relationship with a significant person and available family support. The the nature of the relationship between the mother and infant, including verbal interaction, emotional sensitivity and physical care of the infant, should also be assessed at every point of contact. It is important to discuss any concerns that a mother may have about her relationship with her baby and to provide information and treatment. Education about parenting and guided assistance before, during and after birth can make all the difference to the mother's actions and understanding of her role and function in caring for her baby.

It is essential to recognise that a woman with a mental health problem may experience difficulties with the mother–baby relationship; the midwife should consider further intervention or referral to improve the problem. Nursing care plans should include not only physical and obstetric indicators but also mental health and psychosocial aspects of the mother and child (see Chapter 13). Skills need to be developed to allow respect and space for the mother to vent feelings and express anxieties while maintaining professional boundaries.

Women with special health needs

LEARNING OBJECTIVES

On completion of this chapter, you must be able to:

▶ assess a woman's mental health status in pregnancy and act according to the risk factors

▶ demonstrate the necessary knowledge and skills to assess and monitor mental health in women during pregnancy and after birth and make decisions regarding treatment, give appropriate advice or refer women

▶ demonstrate basic knowledge of the management of female genital mutilation (FGM)

▶ manage women who are in situations of violence according to national and international guidelines.

KNOWLEDGE ASSUMED TO BE IN PLACE

Basic knowledge of psychology, and cultural and religious diversity
Basic knowledge of mental health and mental illness

KEYWORDS

depression • anxiety • psychosis • psychotropic medication • mental health • female genital mutilation (FGM) • gender-based violence

13.1 Introduction

This chapter will consider the special health needs associated with mental health, social habits, behaviour pathology and violence against women during pregnancy and childbirth. Pregnancy and birth are a period of stress even though this a normal transitional development phase. Even when pregnancy and birth are normal and uneventful, it can affect a person's mental health.

13.2 Mental health disorders in pregnancy

Midwives play an important role in mental healthcare promotion and care, as pregnancy is considered as a life stressor event (AIS, 2017), even when the pregnancy is uneventful. One approach to mental health assessment is the mental status examination (MSE), as stipulated in the primary healthcare (PHC) screening tool detailed in the *Ideal Clinic Manual* (component 16, element 110) (DoH, 2016). A number of other assessment scales are available, such as the Edinburgh Postnatal Depression Scale (EPDS), patient health questionnaire (PHQ-9) or the 7-item Generalized Anxiety Disorder Scale (GAD-7), which can also be downloaded from the internet. Because of the fear of stigmatisation, it is important to know that women might be unwilling or reluctant to admit to mental health problems and midwives need to show empathy and non-judgemental respect at all times. In addition, midwives need to have referral routes and options to refer women for specialised care when needed.

Mental health conditions may first manifest in pregnancy because of the increased physical, hormonal, emotional, social and mental stress. These conditions include anxiety, depression and bipolar mood disorders. Women who are particularly vulnerable are those with a history of mental health problems, those who are diagnosed and under treatment and the intellectually disabled. A mother's ability to take care of her baby may be affected by these conditions. Some of the more serious existing conditions are schizophrenia, panic disorders, psychosis, addictions and eating disorders such as anorexia. Obsessive compulsive disorders tend to worsen in pregnancy. A traumatic birth experience may also lead to post-traumatic stress disorder (PTSD).

Rahman et al (2013) state: 'There is growing evidence that, in low- and middle-income (LAMI) countries, the negative effects of maternal mental disorders on the growth and development of infants and young children are independent of the influence of poverty, malnutrition and chronic social adversity.' Instead, these negative effects are rooted in the mental health of the mother and the mother–child interaction on a day-to-day basis. The authors further state: 'In low-income settings, maternal depression has been linked directly to low birth weight and undernutrition in the first year of life, as well as to higher rates of diarrhoeal diseases, incomplete immunization and poor cognitive development in young children' (Rahman et al, 2013). Interventions expressly designed to improve maternal mental health have been found to have a positive impact on infant health and development.

Depression

Depression may already be present during pregnancy, but often only presents in the postnatal period as postnatal depression (PND). The actual prevalence of PND is unclear, with rates varying between 0.5 and 60 per cent (Abdollahi et al, 2011). Symptoms include insomnia, irritability, tearfulness, poor concentration, poor appetite and restlessness, being overemotional, an inability to stop crying, forgetfulness, emotional reserve, antisocial behaviour, tension, disorientation, anxiety, overdependence and suicidal thoughts. A useful tool for the identification of PND is the EPDS.

Puerperal psychosis

Puerperal psychosis is a very serious condition and occurs in one to two cases per 1 000 live births (Harlow et al, 2007; Kendell, Chalmers & Platz, 1987). Puerperal psychosis presents within days of the birth and is characterised by insomnia, suspicion, abnormal behaviour, neglect or overprotection of the baby and loss of a sense of reality. Women with puerperal psychosis may harm their babies and infanticide is a risk, although rare. This catastrophic outcome can be prevented by early recognition and intervention.

13.3 Mental health status assessment

Risk indicators for mental illness

Pregnancy or life stressors may be a trigger for a mental condition in a woman with a predisposition for such a condition, especially if she is unsupported during pregnancy and her life stressors are too high. Risk factors include:

- a previous history of depression or other mental health conditions
- lack of support from her partner
- pregnancy complications
- the loss of her own mother when she was a child
- an accumulation of misfortunes such as bereavement, post-traumatic stress, job loss, housing and money problems.

In the assessment of a woman during history taking in pregnancy, midwives must also take note of the risk factors for mental disorders and refer the woman for psychological care if necessary.

Mental health assessment

An assessment of the mother's mental health status is needed in the ante- and postnatal periods or in high-risk situations such as indicated in the preceding section. The WHO indicates that, worldwide, 10 per cent of pregnant women and 13 per cent of women who have just given birth experience a mental disorder; in developing countries, 20 per cent of women are affected (WHO, 2008). The WHO's comprehensive mental health action plan for 2013–2020 was adopted by the 66th World Health Assembly (WHA) in 2013 (WHO, 2013).

A systematic review of the epidemiology of maternal depression in low- and middle-income countries found that

a non-psychotic depressive episode of mild to major severity is one of the major contributors of pregnancy-related morbidity and mortality and it is an enormous unrecognised and untreated burden (antepartum or post partum) with negative health-related behaviours and adverse outcomes, including psychological and developmental disturbances in infants, children, and adolescents. (Gelaye et al, 2016)

The disorder may be so severe that the mother commits suicide or harms the baby. All women are at risk for one year after birth, but poverty, migration, extreme stress, violence, conflict situations, natural disasters and a low level of social support increase the risks.

Mental healthcare should be integrated into maternal and child care. However, a skilled professional in mental healthcare or psychiatric nursing is needed to do an effective assessment with appropriate actions. Figure 13.1 represents an algorithm for mental health problems in pregnancy and the postnatal period.

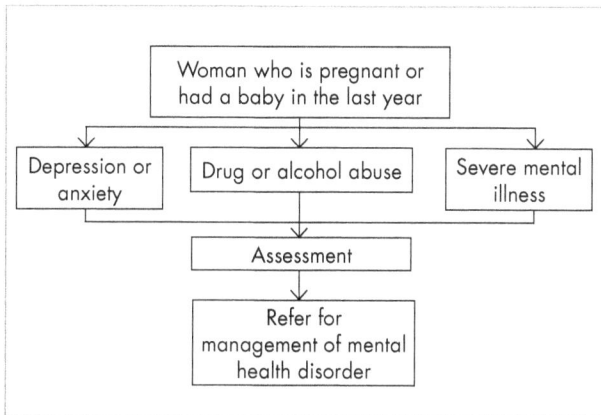

Figure 13.1 Algorithm for the identification of mental health problems (NICE, 2011)

Observations for mental health

The acronym POPSAMSS (see Table 13.1 on the next page) guides observations that are needed for mental health assessment in midwifery (Uys & Middleton, 2013):

▶ *P: Psychiatric history.* History of mental illness; family history of mental illness; on psychiatric treatment; under supervision of the psychiatrist and obstetrician

▶ *O: Obstetric history.* Obstetric risks; traumatic births; perinatal deaths or Caesarean sections

▶ *P: Partner relationship.* Single; stable relationship; conflict in relationship; nature of conflict; mechanisms to resolve conflict

▶ *S: Support network.* Material resources; social resources; perception of resources

▶ *A: Attitude.* Quality, intensity and duration of response to unborn child; attitude towards feeding and child care (mother–child relationship); attitude towards staff, family and friends

▶ *M: Mental status.* Table 13.1 on the next page gives a guideline for aspects to consider during pregnancy and after birth to assess women's mental health

▶ *S: Self-concept.* Personality strengths; perceptions; beliefs (false or true); skills in negotiation; use of resources

▶ *S: Suicide ideation.* History of attempts; expression of intent (direct or indirect); method planned; risk to the baby.

Activity: Using POPSAMSS

Use the steps outlined above (the POPSAMSS guideline) to review the aspects to observe in a woman's history for signs of mental illness or family history of mental health. Then apply it to the scenario below and suggest appropriate actions:

> Miss Zebra started crying (after birth in the clinic), saying that she feels hopeless and guilty that she cannot be a good mother to her baby. She says she will not be able to cope on her own and is so tired. She has no energy because she is nauseous and has not been eating for days. She has been on Fluoxetine for a long time, but she stopped taking that because it made her feel sick during pregnancy. She is worried about the HIV and sometimes she feels that she is better off dead, but she also wants to be a mother for her baby.

1 How would you describe Miss Zebra's mood?
2 What are the psychosocial implications and risks of this situation to the mother and the baby?
3 What short-term interventions can you implement to support Miss Zebra?

13.4 Treatment of mental illness in pregnancy and after birth

The primary goals of the treatment of psychiatric disorders in pregnancy are to maintain mental stability while minimising the risk to the mother and fetus, and to develop support systems and a plan for management of the baby and its needs post-delivery. In some cases, symptom control is the main aim. The mental well-being of a mother may warrant the termination of a pregnancy and is permitted under the Choice on Termination of Pregnancy Act 92 of 1996.

Psychotropic medication use during pregnancy and the postnatal period

Before starting any treatment, discuss the changing risk–benefit ratio for psychotropic medication and the likely benefits of psychological interventions, such as cognitive behavioural therapy, psychotherapy, relaxation, meditation and mindfulness. Should the woman prefer to continue or stop psychotropic medication and/or psychological interventions, the midwife has a duty to ensure that the woman is supported and that she is referred to a specialist mental health professional to prescribe the lowest effective dose. Ensure that she knows about any associated risks to herself, the fetus or baby when stopping or starting psychotropic medication.

Table 13.1

Adapted POPSAMSS mental health status assessment guide (NICE, 2003; Uys & Middleton, 2013)

MSE	Aspects of mental functioning	Risk to the mother	Risk to the baby	Referral or intervention (up or down)
General appearance	Grooming Restlessness Sleep patterns Eating habits	Exclude socioeconomic aspects Self-respect Self-awareness Disinterest	Neglect: inattention to basic physical needs	Recording and reporting of observations Refer to ward-based outreach teams (WBOTs)
Affect (mood)	Mood swings Depression Anxiety Flat affect	PND Depression (suicide) Generalised anxiety Bipolar mood disorder	Bonding difficulties Insecure attachment Flat facial expression Less eye contact or smiles	Psychiatric evaluation and interventions Psychotropic medication
Thoughts and thought patterns Perception	Coherent Delusional Suspicious Bizarre Hallucinations	Puerperal psychosis Risk of harm to self False and unrealistic beliefs Conflict in relationship with others	Risk of harm to the baby Anxious baby Incorrect interpretation of care or needs and signals from baby	Emergency: Admission and observation (Mental Health Care Act 17 of 2002)
Cognition Judgement Orientation Insight	Awareness of condition Confused, disorientated	Neglect of wound care and appointments Relapse Non-compliance with medication/treatment Unaware of risks to self	Neglect, not in touch with baby's needs Abuse and false recollection of incidents	Health professionals Interventions Psychotropic medication
Speech	Slurred Rapid Yelling Incoherent Pressured Mute	Manic, excited Impulsive spending and inappropriate behaviour Aggression	Neglect Emotional abuse Shouting No eye contact Sleep disturbances	Interventions Health professionals and home care
Psychomotor behaviour	Stiff Shaky Bizarre Ritualistic Hyperactive Uncoordinated	Injury to self Obsessive-compulsive behaviour Discomfort and shame	Holding and handling Feeding of baby Risk of injury when holding and handling the baby (also during feeds)	Interventions: cognitive behavioural therapy Health professionals

If a pregnant woman has taken psychotropic medication with known teratogenic risks at any time in the first trimester, do the following:

▶ Advise the woman on the common stressor and factors that can put her mental health at risk during and after pregnancy.

▶ Advise the woman of the risk to the fetus of using medication for mental health during pregnancy.

▶ Confirm the pregnancy as soon as possible.

▶ Explain that stopping or switching the medication after pregnancy is confirmed may not remove the risk of fetal malformations.

▶ Offer screening for fetal abnormalities and counselling about continuing the pregnancy.

▶ Seek advice from a specialist and explain the need for additional monitoring.

If a pregnant woman has a mental health problem that requires medication, it is essential that the medication does not put the fetus at risk. It is therefore important to refer the woman for specialised care to ensure safety. Some medication is unsafe to use during pregnancy, as discussed in the box below.

Alert: Psychotropic medication safety

Valproate is prescribed as a treatment for epilepsy and bipolar disorder. It was introduced in 1974, and there have always been warnings about the risk of birth defects. In recent years the risks to unborn babies have been better understood, leading to further warnings. A woman who takes valproate during pregnancy runs a 1-in-10 chance of having a baby with a birth defect, such as:

▶ spina bifida

▶ facial and skull malformations (including cleft lip and palate)

▶ malformations of the limbs

▶ malformations of organs such as the heart, kidney, urinary tract and sexual organs.

The long-term negative effects of valproate are not known, but can include:

▶ a delay in the baby learning to walk and talk

▶ a lower intelligence compared to children the same age

▶ poor speech and language skills

▶ poor memory and learning problems.

Children exposed to valproate *in utero* are more likely to suffer from autism or autistic spectrum disorders.

continued

Some evidence suggests that these children may be more at risk of developing attention deficit hyperactivity disorder (ADHD).

Valproate should not be used in women or girls of childbearing age, women who are planning a pregnancy or women who are pregnant, unless other treatments are ineffective or not tolerated and the woman is monitored (Drugs.com, 2017). Women or girls of childbearing potential must use effective contraception during treatment.

A woman who is on valproate should not stop taking the medication without consulting her doctor. The healthcare profession must carefully weigh the benefits that valproate treatment may bring against the risks. If there is no treatment option other than valproate, women of childbearing age should use effective contraception. The treatment of women on valproate must be reviewed regularly.

(Source: MHRA, 2016)

General information and advice

The following general advice and information should be noted by professional midwives:

▶ Provide culturally relevant information on mental health problems.

▶ Consider referring a woman to a secondary mental health service for preconception counselling if she has a past or present history of mental illness.

▶ Discuss treatment and prevention options and any concerns the woman has about pregnancy or the fetus/baby.

▶ If a woman needs to stop some psychotropic medication in order to breastfeed, discuss the benefits and potential risks.

▶ Seek more detailed advice from specialist mental health professionals about the possible risks that mental health problems pose to the mother and baby.

▶ Assess and agree to the level of contact and support needed and monitor the woman regularly for symptoms throughout pregnancy and the first few weeks after birth.

Table 13.2 on the next page lists the assessments and observations required for specific mental disorders, the appropriate psychological interventions or medication, and the associated risks.

Table 13.2

Mental health disorders, psychotropic medication and associated risks (NICE, 2016)

Disorder	Assessment/observations	Medication or high-intensity psychological interventions	Risks to mother or fetus/baby
Depression or PND	Assess suicide risk Patient health questionnaire (PHQ-9) Ask well-being questions (WHO5 well-being index): 1. During the past month, have you been bothered by feeling down, depressed or hopeless? 2. During the past month, have you often been bothered by having little interest or pleasure in doing things? Use the EPDS for assessment of risk Conduct repeat and follow-up checks	Refer to mental health professionals Seek advice High-intensity psychological interventions (cognitive behavioural therapy), counselling and psychotherapy or in combination with medication, ie: • tricyclic antidepressant (TCA) • selective serotonin reuptake inhibitor (SSRI) or (serotonin-) noradrenaline reuptake inhibitor ([S]NRI) • electroconvulsive therapy for severe depression (rare) or a manic episode when physical health or fetus is at risk	Assess the risk of breastfeeding Assess the safety of drugs (there is a known risk of fetal cardiac abnormalities and persistent pulmonary hypertension in the newborn) Assess risks associated with changing or stopping a previously effective medication Assess neonatal adaptation syndrome in the baby (paroxetine and venlafaxine)
Anxiety and obsessive compulsive disorder	GAD questions: 1. Over the last two weeks, how often have you been bothered by feeling nervous, anxious or on edge? 2. Over the last two weeks, how often have you been bothered by not being able to stop or control worrying?	Psychological interventions Do not prescribe or gradually stop benzodiazepine **Exception:** short-term treatment for anxiety and agitation	Seek advice on use of medication or gradually withdraw in breastfeeding when mother or infant at risk. If addicted, withdrawal symptoms may occur
Severe mental illness: Postpartum psychosis	See MSE Find out if there is any history of severe mental illness (family, past or present mental illness) Exclude neurocognitive complications of HIV/AIDS Observe risk of harm to mother and/or baby	Refer to mental health professional and emergency admission (within four hours) Antipsychotic medication: Rapid tranquillisation (short-term management for disturbed or violent behaviour) Dietician: diet and weight control Do not offer depot (long-acting injections) If stable on antipsychotics and pregnant and likely to relapse without medication, rather continue, but observe, support and advise	Gestational diabetes Weight gain Measure prolactin levels on planning of pregnancy and after conception Prevent injury to self or baby but do not restrain or seclude the mother

continued

Disorder	Assessment/observations	Medication or high-intensity psychological interventions	Risks to mother or fetus/baby
Epilepsy and bipolar mood disorder	A health professional assessment includes EEG, PHQ-9 depression test and/or the WHO5 on emotional well-being	Psychological interventions of choice Cognitive behavioural therapy and couples therapy Anticonvulsants: Do not offer valproate or lithium, or stop gradually – measure lithium levels Avoid carbamazepine If on lamotrigine: check levels	Birth/developmental defects Lithium: Stop, monitor and explain risk of relapse when stopped If pregnant on lithium: Monitor the levels Risks: fetal heart problems Toxicity in breast milk
Alcohol, drug addiction and other psychosocial problems during pregnancy and the postnatal period	If suspected, take a history, test and assess as follows: • Family, physical well-being (weight, smoking, nutrition, activity) • Past/present mental health and treatment • Attitude towards pregnancy • Mother–baby relationship • Living conditions: support or isolation, responsibilities towards other children • Domestic violence and child abuse	Brief interventions or refer to substance misuse services Assisted withdrawal or detoxification programmes Collaboration with support and multidisciplinary services Referral to outreach and WBOTs Regular supervision and observation	Measure adherence and monitor risk to baby (neonatal assessment) Observe for fetal alcohol syndrome (FAS), intimate partner violence, child maltreatment Physical complications of the newborn, ie liver, heart, gastric and other

13.5 Gender-based violence

Gender-based violence occurs across the social spectrum. Evidence suggests that this type of violence is preventable, since it may result from community, cultural and other external factors. Gender-based violence is a public health concern and a violation of human rights. Women often experience violence from intimate partners and this is often linked to sexual issues.

International Day for the Elimination of Violence Against Women

In 1993, the UN adopted the Declaration on the Elimination of Violence Against Women. In 1994, a special rapporteur was appointed to investigate causes and consequences of violence against women. In December 1999, the General Assembly of the UN adopted Resolution 54/134, proclaiming 25 November to be the International Day for the Elimination of Violence Against Women (see http://www.un.org/en/events/endviolenceday/).

continued

The first global report on violence and health was released by the WHO on 3 October 2002, recognising violence as a global health problem (WHO, 2002). This gave violence against women a public face and created a mandate to:

▶ collect information from governments, agencies and non-government organisations (NGOs) and respond to it
▶ recommend measures to be implemented
▶ work closely with the UN High Commission on Human Rights (OHCHR).

Scope of the problem

At the Fourth World Conference on Women in Beijing in September 1995, it was recognised that two of the 12 critical areas identified as obstacles in the advancement of equality, development and peace of women in society include violence (UN, nd). The 2005 WHO multi-country study on women's health and violence against women in 10 low- and middle-income countries found that in rural Tanzania, Peru and Bangladesh, of women aged between 15–49, the first sexual encounter of 17–30 per cent of these was forced (WHO, 2016). The information in the box below gives a general overview of the global problem. It is difficult to get accurate statistics in South Africa due to unreported cases.

Gender-based violence: Statistics

▶ Globally, 35 per cent of women (one in every three) has been beaten.

▶ In 30 per cent of cases, the abuser is a family member.

▶ In 38 per cent of murders of women, the male intimate partner is guilty.

▶ In Gauteng, one in every six women that dies is killed by an intimate partner.

▶ South Africa has a high incidence of rape of babies and children (13 800 child victims per year).

▶ In South Africa, someone is raped or sexually abused every 24 seconds.

(Sources: WHO, 2016; The Tembisan, 2015; Givengain. com, 2017)

Types of violence

Violence in adult life is often part of a cycle – people who have experienced a violent upbringing or come from a violent society or community have learnt patterns of violent behaviour that they may repeat in their own relationships, families and communities.

The following are all forms of violence: rape, child trafficking for sex, exploitation of female labour and migrant workers, forced prostitution, human trafficking, forced pornography and cultural practices such as female genital mutilation (FGM). Further forms of violence include:

▶ family violence associated with traditions and economic issues

▶ sexual assault and harassment within a marriage

▶ dowry-related violence and early marriage

▶ custodial violence against women.

The state and government can also commit acts of violence through the detention, torture and of refugees or displaced women by police and the armed forces. Breaking the cycle of violence requires an intensive effort along with programmes put in place by trained psychologists, psychiatrists or other professionals.

FGM is a form of violence against women. According to UNICEF (2016), there are more than 200 million women and girls alive who have undergone FGM, in 30 different countries. At the beginning of the new millennium, Rao et al (2000: 135) noted that the amount of women and girls who have undergone FGM and who are living in North America and Western Europe is increasing. They relate that a man from Mali was convicted in France for the death of his baby girl, who died from an infection related to FGM. They also mention that Canada granted refugee status to a Nigerian woman, based on her fear of persecution for not performing FGM on her own daughter. As Rao et al (2000: 135) note, many governments across the world have engaged in educational campaigns to teach people about the adverse health effects of FGM.

The South African population does not practice FGM, but, just as in Europe and North America, a growing number of female immigrants and refugees from Africa and the East use services in the public and private health sector. South African midwives are not trained to deal with FGM. This aspect should be added to the curriculum so that midwives are able to appropriately and respectfully manage women who have undergone FGM. The activity below deals with important guidelines for the management of FGM.

Activity: Read up on FGM

The WHO has developed policy guidelines for nurses and midwives on the prevention and management of health complications, which can be found at http://apps.who. int/iris/bitstream/10665/66858/1/WHO_FCH_ GWH_01.5.pdf.

Also see the WHO's factsheet on FGM at http:// www.who.int/mediacentre/factsheets/fs241/en/.

The role of healthcare workers

Women face the highest risk of domestic violence and abuse. The Domestic Violence Act 116 of 1998 (as amended) offers women and children in South Africa protection against all forms of violence. The underlying characteristics predisposing a person to violence are identifiable.

Injured women are often seen in maternity units, as violence frequently occurs during pregnancy. Women who suffer physical violence during pregnancy are three times more likely to die from future physical abuse. Clinics need to have a policy and a protocol for recognising abuse, providing counselling, doing referrals and following up to prevent future deaths. Midwives can intervene in the cycle of violence by helping women to understand their options and to take appropriate action. Parenting classes, conflict management and social programmes can assist in combating violence in the family and community.

If healthcare professionals are to help others to resolve issues around violence, they should consider their own beliefs and experiences of violence. Training and education are important steps in developing knowledge and the skills to manage violence. Midwives will frequently come across women who have experienced violence during pregnancy and birth. In general, healthcare professionals can create awareness, educate and empower the community and help to change beliefs and attitudes. It is important not to ignore violence when it is encountered. Midwives can be guided by the following principles:

▶ Avoid indifference or judgemental reactions.
▶ Learn to ask questions in an empathetic, supportive and respectful manner.
▶ Give the care required, such as medical care or family planning.
▶ Offer counselling and refer the woman to a support group.
▶ Give the woman options that can empower her.
▶ Document events and injuries.
▶ Reach out to men to inform and support them.

At community, governmental and national level, actions include the development of national legislation, providing legal aid and counselling, creating shelters and rehabilitation centres. Pornography and violence in the media should be eliminated. Through educational programmes, the non-stereotyping of women and behaviour modification skills can be fostered.

13.6   Substance abuse and dependence

There is an acknowledged link between mental health disorders and the use of substances. Most of these substances place either the mother or the fetus at risk. After birth, the risk to the baby continues (Forray, 2016). The degree of risk may depend on the type of substance being used, as the degree of placental permeability depends on the chemical properties and molecular weight of the drug and whether it is used alone or in combination with other drugs.

Commonly used drugs are alcohol, cocaine, crack, dagga, amphetamines, barbiturates, hallucinogens, heroin, caffeine and nicotine. Dagga (or marijuana) contains 400 complex chemicals and interferes with the production of hormones that are critical for sexual and reproductive development. Drugs used during pregnancy are often found in the same concentration in the baby and may cause respiratory and cardiovascular suppression in the baby. Drugs such as LSD are also teratogenic.

A comprehensive team approach is needed for safe outcomes for mother and baby. The midwife's task involves the evaluation of medical, socioeconomic and legal aspects, and is aimed at the early identification of cases that are at risk. Fetal surveillance during pregnancy is important, as the fetus is affected and at risk. The baby should be delivered in a maternity unit with a neonatal unit attached (a Level 3 facility).

Alcohol in pregnancy

Alcohol use and abuse during pregnancy is common. As there are no determined safe levels of alcohol intake during conception and pregnancy, current advice is that women should not drink alcohol when pregnant. FAS, which is particularly common in the Western Cape, is a preventable condition. Babies of women who do not usually drink but consume a lot of alcohol at certain times, for example Christmas or New Year, or who consume alcohol in early pregnancy not knowing that they are pregnant, are also at risk of being born with FAS. Midwives need to educate women on the adverse effects of alcohol in pregnancy. (Also see Chapter 51.)

The potential effects of alcohol

Alcohol may have the following potential effects on the fetus:

▶ Two or more drinks per day: Intrauterine growth restriction (IUGR), decreased placental weight, immature motor activity/tone, poor sucking, increased risk of stillbirth
▶ Four or more drinks per day: Structural brain abnormalities
▶ Six or more drinks per day: FAS
▶ Mental retardation is the single most serious problem associated with alcohol use in pregnancy. Although babies do not always present with full-blown FAS, other effects may be present that will affect the child for life.

Screening tool for alcohol abuse

A very simple tool that can be used to screen for alcoholism or substance abuse is the CAGE questionnaire. It consists of four questions, from which the acronym CAGE is created. It focuses on Cutting Down, Annoyance by Criticism, Guilty Feelings and Eye Opener:

1   Have you ever felt you ought to CUT DOWN on your drinking?
2   Have people ANNOYED you by criticising your drinking?

continued

---

3   Have you ever felt GUILTY about your drinking?
4   Have you ever had a drink first thing in the morning to steady your nerves or get rid of a hangover (EYE OPENER)?

Scoring: Two 'yes' answers indicates probable alcoholism.
(Source: Ewing, 1984; O'Brien, 2008)

Nicotine and smoking

When smoking a cigarette, the blood levels of nicotine peak at 14–41 ng/ml, depending on the way in which the person smokes. Depth and length of inhalation will affect nicotine blood levels. Nicotine is reabsorbed by the fetus, with an increase in fetal heart rate (FHR). Nicotine is also secreted in breast milk for a period of seven to eight hours after smoking the last cigarette.

The most common effect of regular smoking on the fetus is IUGR, with an average reduction of 200 g in the mass of a smoker's baby. The relationship is dose-dependent; more cigarettes means a greater reduction in growth. Smoking 11 or more cigarettes per day increases the risk of spontaneous abortion by 16.7 per cent (OSG, 2004). The greatest risk of damage to the fetus is during the first trimester, but the effects are most potent in the last trimester, when the central nervous system (CNS) develops.

Midwives need to encourage pregnant women to stop smoking by utilising effective cessation-of-smoking programmes that do not include the use of nicotine patches. Positive changes such as improved fetal mass and improved placental function occur when a woman stops smoking during pregnancy. Positive outcomes include a lower risk of respiratory distress and sudden infant death syndrome (SIDS).

Effects of nicotine in pregnancy

The number of women smokers is rising and has in some areas exceeded the numbers of male smokers. Most smokers start between the ages of 14 to 19 years and 10 per cent of teenagers in South Africa are smokers (Mashita et al, 2011). A written health warning on all cigarette products in South Africa alerts the population to the dangers of smoking in pregnancy.

13.7   Conclusion

Pregnancy and birth are emotionally charged events. Women who are already compromised through a history of mental health disorders, substance dependence or violence need to receive care that suits their needs. The failure to provide appropriate care can have far-reaching consequences for the mother and baby, the family and the community.

Section Four

Pregnancy

The physiology of pregnancy

14.1   Introduction

Dynamic changes take place in the body of a pregnant woman to maintain the pregnancy and accommodate the growing fetus, nourish the fetus during the periods of development and growth, and provide the woman with energy for the delivery and lactation. These changes take place throughout pregnancy and are caused by the action of hormones from the trophoblast.

The woman's whole body is affected by the pregnancy and her endocrine balance and metabolism are also changed. These changes are responsible for the signs and symptoms (clinical features) of pregnancy and form the basis for the diagnosis of pregnancy. Because these changes occur in a predictable pattern throughout a normal pregnancy, they can be used as a guide for formulating a programme of antenatal care. In this way, abnormalities occurring during the pregnancy can be detected and treated early.

Although most of the changes are reversible, when the woman's body returns to a non-pregnant state, some anatomical changes (such as stretch marks and cervical changes) are permanent and will be noticed by clinicians as indications of previous pregnancies.

14.2   The endocrine system

The physical and physiological changes of pregnancy are based on the endocrinological factors unique to hormones produced during pregnancy, as explained in Chapter 6.

14.3   The reproductive organs

Physiologically, it is the reproductive organs that are predominantly affected by pregnancy.

The uterus

The uterus is the organ that undergoes major changes in pregnancy, as it contains and nourishes the fetus and gives birth to the baby at term.

Functions of the body of the uterus and the cervix

The uterus consists of a body and a cervix (neck), as described in Chapter 7. During pregnancy, the body of the uterus must relax and form new muscle fibres in order to grow to be the largest muscle in the body by term. The cervix remains closed and becomes part of the uterine cavity in order to maintain the pregnancy.

The size of the uterus

There is a huge increase in size, weight and volume of the uterus during pregnancy. The approximate increases from the non-gravid state to those at term are as follows:
▶ Increase in size: from 7.5 × 5 × 2.5 cm to 30 × 23 × 20 cm
▶ Increase in weight: from 50–60 g to 900–1 000 g
▶ Increase in volume: from 6 ml to 5 000 ml (holding capacity of the cavity).

At eight weeks, the uterus can easily be felt on bimanual vaginal examination and is the size of a grapefruit. The uterus is palpable above the symphysis pubis after 12 weeks. In the first 20 weeks of pregnancy, the increase in size is due mainly to an increase in the number of muscle fibres (muscular hyperplasia) and the size of the muscle fibres (muscular hypertrophy). The uterus continues to grow and can be visibly observed or palpated and measured (see Chapter 17).

The body of the uterus

The uterus is functionally divided in pregnancy into the upper and lower uterine segments, as explained in Chapter 5 (see Figure 14.1).

During normal pregnancy, the uterus is functionally changed in the upper and lower segments. (The upper segment includes the fundus and isthmus). Normally, the blastocyst implants in the upper segment and develops into the fetus, cord and the placenta.

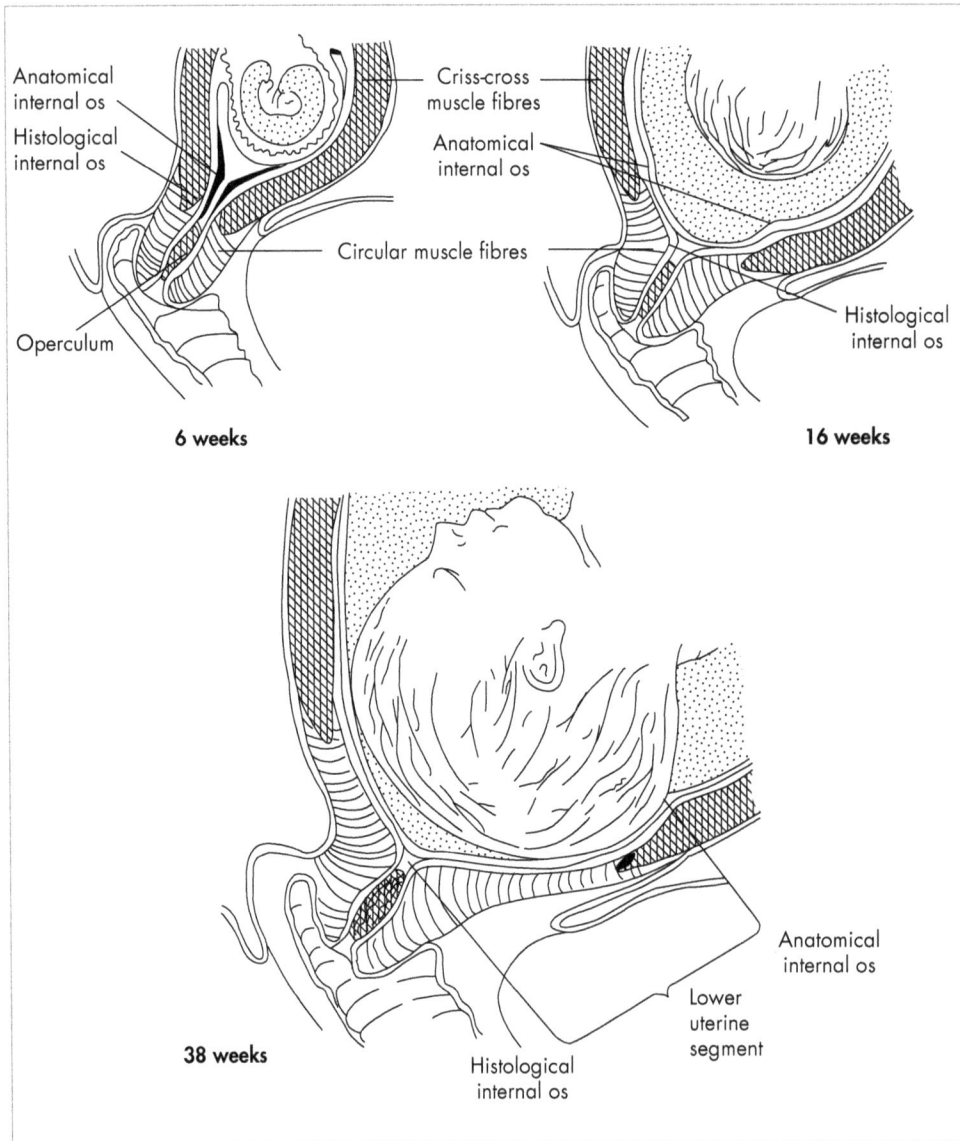

Figure 14.1 Formation of the upper and lower segments of the uterus (redrawn from Lewellyn-Jones, 1982)

The lower segment is the lower part, between the isthmus and the cervix, which softens and lengthens in early pregnancy. The softening of the cervix and isthmus forms the basis for Hegar's sign of pregnancy, as explained in Chapter 15. After the first trimester, as the fetal sac begins to fill the uterine cavity, the elongated isthmus is gradually drawn up. This forms the lower uterine segment, which starts to develop from three weeks of pregnancy and is only fully developed by 30 weeks. The lower segment is less vascular, with fewer muscle fibres. A lower-segment Caesarean section is therefore preferred, but is difficult to perform before 32 weeks.

Braxton-Hicks contractions

The uterine muscles contract throughout pregnancy. These contractions are known as Braxton-Hicks contractions, as shown in Figure 14.2. These painless contractions assist with the formation of the lower uterine segment and play a role in the blood circulation in the uterus.

In early pregnancy, the contractions are mild and irregular and although they remain painless, they increase in frequency and intensity as the pregnancy nears term. Before 30 weeks' gestation, the intrauterine pressure remains below 5 mmHg. After 30 weeks, the intrauterine pressure may rise intermittently to about 12 mmHg, which is still below the pain threshold of 25 mmHg.

The stronger contractions are now thought to be brought about by the progressive release of prostaglandins, derived from the uterine decidua towards the latter part of pregnancy and by the fact that the uterine muscles become increasingly sensitive to oxytocin as labour approaches. (Nipple stimulation during pregnancy will release oxytocin, which then stimulates the uterus to contract.)

Contractions prepare the uterus for labour. Once the contractions are regular, increasing in intensity and not more than 20 minutes apart, labour may start. Labour is only positively diagnosed when it has been determined that the cervix is starting to dilate (see Chapter 25).

Position of the uterus

The non-pregnant uterus is a pelvic organ in anteversion and anteflexion (see Figure 5.4 on page 51). In pregnancy, it becomes an abdominal organ and at 12 weeks the uterus can be felt above the pelvis. The uterus moves up in the abdomen and displaces the abdominal organs as it does so.

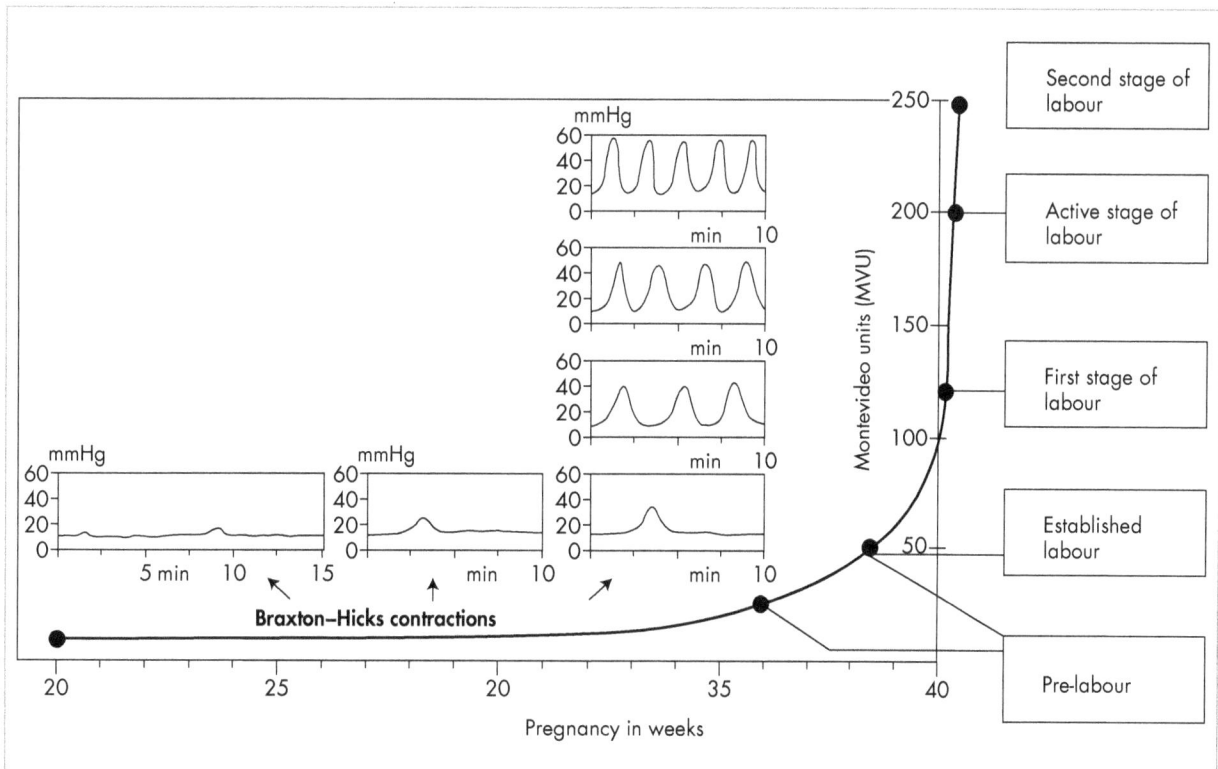

Figure 14.2 Schematic presentation of uterine activity in pregnancy and birth (adapted from Llewellyn-Jones, 1992)

The round ligaments grow longer and become soft. At 20 weeks, the uterus is dextroverted, turning to the right side to lift from the aorta and inferior vena cava. This places pressure on the right ureter and it is this side that is most prone to pyelonephritis.

These changes of the uterus can be measured between 20 and 35 weeks to determine the gestational age (GA) (by means of the symphysis fundal [SF] measure). Every 1 cm equals one week.

An abnormal position of the uterus, such as retroversion or retroflexion, multiple pregnancy and polyhydramnios will influence these measurements. A grand multipara may also have an over-stretched uterus and ligaments, which can cause the uterus to take any position.

The growing uterus displaces the abdominal organs, which may cause misleading signs and symptoms of disease in abdominal organs, for example an appendix that lies in an abnormal position.

False labour

When the presenting part engages and the lower segment is stretched, contractions can become quite intense and frequent in the last two weeks of pregnancy. Some pain may be experienced, especially by anxious women and by primigravidae who have not previously been in labour. This may result in what is called false labour, which can lead to further anxiety. The woman and her family should be reassured and the signs of true labour should be made clear to them. It is important that they be advised to wait for the start of true labour. False labour is distinguished from true labour by lack of 'show' and the absence of changes of the cervix. If the membranes rupture prematurely, care is different and specific (see Chapter 32).

The cervix

In pregnancy, the cervix changes its consistency and becomes soft. It will also change position, particularly in primigravidae, and maintain a relatively constant length of about 2.5 cm. Due to the increased vascular supply to the uterus, the cervix changes from pink to a dark purplish colour – this change is diagnostic of pregnancy. The cells of the cervix also change during pregnancy, and a Pap smear can only be done until 28 weeks and again at six weeks postpartum.

The cervix remains posterior during the first two trimesters and remains firm until the end of the first trimester. In the second trimester, the cervix widens and softens and there is a marked proliferation of cervical mucosa glands, resulting in increased glandular activity. The mucus secreted at this time is thick and viscid and forms a mucus plug, which occludes the cervical canal. This plug, known as the operculum, acts as a barrier against ascending infection.

The softening process is accentuated as the pregnancy reaches term and labour approaches. This is known as *ripening of the cervix*. The cervical position may change to anterior, indicating readiness for labour (see the Bishop score in Table 34.1 on page 539). In the latter weeks of pregnancy, the cervical canal becomes partly effaced or taken up into the lower uterine segment, also as a result of Braxton-Hicks contractions. The ripening of the cervix and the effacement of the cervical canal prepare the cervix for labour and make it favourable for dilatation (see chapters 24, 25 and 34).

Cervical changes can be used to predict the success of induction of labour (IOL) using the Bishop score and will also predict the progress of labour. A posterior, closed cervix when labour starts can predict a long labour in a primigravida.

The blood supply to the uterus

The volume of blood to and from the uterus increases with uterine growth and the tortuous blood vessels straighten out. The uterine blood flow at term ranges from 500 ml to 700 ml per minute. This greatly increased blood supply to the uterus is vital for fetal development, growth and well-being.

During systole, the blood at the placental site is forced from the endometrial arteries under pressure, causing it to spurt into the intervillous spaces and against the chorionic plate. The streams of blood being forced against the chorionic plate are dispersed like fountains, thereby allowing the blood to circulate around the chorionic villi, which are floating freely in the maternal blood. The velocity of the blood flow slows and this allows for the transfer of nutrients and the exchange of oxygen and carbon dioxide to and from the fetus across the placental membrane. Thereafter, the blood drains away via the endometrial veins during diastole. This procedure is repeated with the following systole.

In labour, the blood supply can be cut off in hypertonic uterine contractions.

The vagina

The muscle fibres of the vagina hypertrophy during pregnancy and there is softening of the connective tissue, causing the vagina to develop a larger lumen and increasing the stretching ability of the vaginal walls. The vagina becomes very vascular and assumes a dark purplish colour.

Owing to the influence of extra oestrogens in pregnancy, the mucosa becomes thicker and there is a larger amount of glycogen in the squamous cells. This leads to an increased desquamation of the superficial vaginal mucosal cells and consequently to an increased vaginal discharge. The pH of the vagina changes in pregnancy as a result of hormonal changes, predisposing the woman to vaginal infections. The increased vaginal discharge may become infected with pathogens such as bacteria, fungi (*Candida albicans*) or parasites (*Trichomonas vaginalis*) (see Chapter 49). The resultant vaginitis can be troublesome during pregnancy.

The vulva

During pregnancy there is an increased vascularity of the vulva, resulting in a darker colour. Varicosities of the vulval veins may occur.

The Fallopian tubes

The uterine tubes, together with the broad and round ligaments, hypertrophy and become more vascular and pliable. As the uterus grows and becomes an abdominal organ, the Fallopian tubes are also lifted out of the pelvis.

The ovaries

The blood supply to the ovaries is increased. The ovaries are drawn up into the abdominal cavity with the uterus and uterine tubes. At term, the ovaries are situated posteriorly in the abdomen, just below the costal margins.

During the first 12 weeks of pregnancy, under the influence of human chorionic gonadotrophin (hCG), the corpus luteum increases in size to almost 20 mm in diameter. However, from the third month (second trimester), there is a regression of the corpus luteum as the placenta starts to take over the function of producing oestrogens and progesterone.

14.4 The breasts

The breasts undergo extensive changes during pregnancy in order to be prepared for the nourishment of the infant at birth. Breast changes are often the first signs of pregnancy that a woman notices, and are as follows:

▶ At three to four weeks, there is a prickling and tingling sensation. The duct and alveolar systems of the breasts enlarge under the influence of oestrogen and progesterone respectively.
▶ From six weeks, the breasts gradually increase in size. On examination, the breast tissue changes from being soft and smooth to having a tense, nodular feel.
▶ There is an increased vascularity of the breasts from about eight weeks, which can be seen under the skin as a network of subcutaneous veins. This vascularity increases until, near term, the veins have ramified over the whole anterior aspect of the thorax.
▶ By the twelfth week, the nipples have enlarged and become more prominent. Together with the primary areola, which has become raised and moist, the nipples

have become more pigmented to a brownish colour. The darker the woman's complexion, the darker the pigmentation becomes.
▶ By the twelfth week, the modified sebaceous glands in the primary areola enlarge and become more prominent. They are known as Montgomery's follicles or tubercles. Their secretions keep the areola and nipple soft and pliable during pregnancy and lactation.
▶ By the sixteenth week, the areola has extended over a larger area of the breasts, and becomes known as the secondary areola. This is more noticeable in brunettes and dark-skinned women.
▶ From about the sixteenth week, colostrum can be expressed from the nipples. This colostrum will only change to milk on about the third day after the birth of the baby. The milk supplied by a woman's breasts provides exactly the correct form of nourishment for her baby, no matter at what period of gestation the baby may be born.

14.5 The skin

High hormonal levels cause an increase in pigmentation of the skin during pregnancy. This is more pronounced in brunettes and dark-skinned women and can be noticed on the breasts, the abdomen, the vulva and the face. When present on the face, this pigmentation is called chloasma or the *mask of pregnancy*. It usually occurs on the cheeks and forehead.

The linea alba, a thin white line extending from the symphysis pubis to the umbilicus, may darken appreciably. It then becomes known as the linea nigra (black line).

Increased pigmentation of the skin gradually fades after pregnancy.

The high levels of circulating hormones and the rapid stretching of the skin of the abdomen, thighs and breasts are probably responsible for small pinkish-brown streaks or scars that develop in these areas. They are known as *striae gravidarum* and may become quite dark in multigravid brunettes and dark-skinned women. These striae gravidarum, or 'stretch marks', fade after the pregnancy and later appear as silvery streaks on a white skin or as shiny dark streaks on a dark skin.

14.6 Other body systems

The cardiovascular system

The cardiovascular system is hyperdynamic in pregnancy. The changes to the cardiovascular system are reversible and are mediated by circulating hormones and the demands of the enlarged vascular bed. In most pregnancies, these effects

203

do not compromise the mother. However, if the mother has underlying health problems, she or the fetus may be compromised.

Changes include modification of the blood volume, plasma volume, red blood cell (RBC) volume and cardiac output. Anatomically, the heart is displaced upwards by the enlarged uterus and moves into a more horizontal position. The heart is slightly enlarged.

The heart

Pregnancy places a high demand on the heart:

▶ *Cardiac output:* This increases by 30–50 per cent by eight weeks and continues increasing steadily until the third trimester, due to the increase in blood volume and venous return. Most of the increased output is managed by an increase in the stroke volume (the amount of blood ejected per beat). In late pregnancy, cardiac output is affected by the woman's physical position. Twins and triplets affect cardiac output more than singleton pregnancies.

▶ *Heart rate:* The normal range for heart rate in pregnancy varies by 20–60 beats. Both heart rate and venous return are increased in pregnancy – the increase in heart rate is about 10–20 beats. Extra systolic beats are normal in pregnancy. In women with small hearts, the rate can be increased to 90 or 100 beats per minute; smaller women also have difficulty dealing with cardiovascular changes in pregnancy.

Blood pressure

In early pregnancy, BP, especially diastolic pressure, decreases by 10–15 mmHg due to the enlarged vascular bed and a drop in peripheral resistance. Both parity and age have an effect on BP: increased parity is associated with a decrease in diastolic pressure, and increased age with an increase in diastolic pressure. From 20 weeks, BP gradually increases. The woman's position (standing or sitting) is associated with a gradual drop in diastolic BP in pregnancy until the third trimester, which means that the woman's BP must always be measured when she is in the same position.

Systemic vascular resistance

The increased blood volume, together with vasodilatation, causes a decreased vascular resistance in peripheral vessels. In late pregnancy, the gravid uterus may contribute to poor venous return, which may cause distension of the veins and oedema of the legs, vulva and anal canal; varicose veins and haemorrhoids are quite a common problem.

Supine hypotensive syndrome

This syndrome is caused by the pressure of the enlarged uterus on the dilated inferior vena cava when the pregnant woman lies on her back. The uterus blocks the return of blood to the heart and results in the patient feeling faint and becoming pale and sweaty. The woman's BP may be low or even unrecordable. This can also have an adverse effect on the fetus because of a reduction in the oxygen supply to the placenta. This condition is managed by turning the woman onto her side to alleviate the obstruction of the blood flow to the heart by the uterus. Pregnant women should never lie in the supine position; instead, they must always lie on the left side.

Distribution of blood flow

The greatest proportion of the increased blood flow goes to the uterus, to nourish the enlarging uterus and its contents. At term, the blood flow to the uterus is 500–700 ml/min, which is 10–20 per cent of the cardiac output. There is also increased blood flow to the lungs, the skin and mucous membranes, and particularly to the kidneys.

The uterine spiral arteries undergo marked changes in pregnancy. They become completely dilated and are not responsive to the stimulation of the autonomic nervous system.

Total blood volume

One of the major changes in pregnancy involves changes in the cardiovascular system. The total blood volume (TBV) increases by about 1 500 ml (30 per cent) to supply the enlarging uterus and the placenta (hydraemia of pregnancy). From the sixth to about the thirty-fourth week of pregnancy, there is a rapid increase in plasma volume, which reaches about 3 800 ml, about 30–50 per cent more than in the non-gravid state. There is a direct correlation between the increase in blood volume and the weight of the fetus. This hypervolaemia of pregnancy is substantially greater in twin (65 per cent) and multiple pregnancies (more than 65 per cent), placing a greater demand on the cardiovascular system. There is increased total body water and increased plasma renin, both of which cause intracellular fluid retention and an increased cardiovascular distensibility. Body fluid distribution changes and in the supine position blood accumulates in the legs, which may cause swelling in the feet and varicosities. There is a slow plasma volume increase in women with pre-eclampsia.

Red blood cells

RBC volume increases slowly from approximately 10 weeks and continues to increase throughout pregnancy. Since there is only an 18 per cent increase in RBC volume (200–450 ml) compared to the 30–50 per cent increase in TBV, the concentrations of Hb and serum albumin and other proteins are lower than in the non-pregnant state. This lowered Hb concentration (haemodilution) is known as the physiological anaemia of pregnancy, reflected in lower haematocrit and Hb levels. This peaks at the period when blood volume is at its highest, at 30–32 weeks. Hb therefore drops by 2 g/dl in pregnancy, reaching its lowest level when plasma volume peaks at 32 weeks. The lowest acceptable Hb in the third trimester is 10.5 g/dl. The mean haematocrit is 33.8 per cent.

Lowered serum albumin levels may contribute to oedema. The expanded blood volume also leads to lowered concentrations of the water-soluble vitamins. On the other hand, serum levels of the fat-soluble vitamins and lipid factions, such as cholesterol, triglycerides and free fatty acids, are elevated.

White blood cells

In early pregnancy the total white blood cell (WBC) count increases slightly. The total WBC count is 4.8–10.8 × 109/ℓ. Changes are minimal.

Platelets

There is a slight decrease in a platelets in pregnancy. The acceptable range for platelets in pregnancy is 130–400 × 109/ℓ. Moderate to severe thrombocytopaenia is present in 5 per cent of healthy women (Parnas et al, 2006). The HELLP syndrome (haemolytic anaemia, elevated liver enzymes, low platelet count) is associated with dangerously low levels of platelets. (This syndrome is described in Chapter 21.)

Plasma components

Protein requirements increase dramatically in pregnancy, as it is required to build new tissue, the placenta and the fetus. There is a resultant tendency for serum protein to drop by 10–14 per cent, a contributing factor in oedema in pregnancy. Total protein, albumin and gamma globulin levels fall in the first trimester and then rise slowly to term. Beta globulin and fibrinogen fractions rise by 50–80 per cent, causing a fourfold increase in the erythrocyte sedimentation rate (which cannot be used as a diagnostic measure during pregnancy). Alterations in plasma protein affect the pharmacokinetics of substances such as calcium and other drugs. Note that the dosages of some drugs may need to be altered during pregnancy.

Serum iron decreases in the plasma. The stored quantity of iron is withdrawn for maternal and fetal use. The greatest drop in iron values is between 12 to 25 weeks, when the number of RBCs increase.

There is an increase of 40–60 per cent in serum lipids, especially cholesterol – the oestrogen and progesterone precursor – and phospholipids, a major component of cell membranes.

Coagulation factors

Pregnancy is an acquired hypercoagulable state, resulting in an increased risk of thrombosis and coagulopathies such as disseminated intravascular coagulation (DIC). There is an increase in coagulation components, such as fibrinogen and factors VII, VIII, IX and X, and a decrease in the anticoagulation components – the fibrinolytic system.

The hypercoagulable state of pregnancy is further magnified during labour. This protects the woman against excessive blood loss, providing rapid haemostasis after delivery of the placenta. These changes in the cardiovascular system increase the risk of superficial thrombophlebitis and also deep vein thrombosis (DVT) during pregnancy and in the puerperium. If a woman already suffers from a weak heart, the cardiovascular changes in pregnancy can result in HELLP syndrome and DIC.

The immune system and defence mechanisms

Defence mechanisms consist of immunological and non-immunological factors. Non-immunological factors include the skin, mucosal barriers, digestive enzymes, pH, temperature, proteins, enzymes, lysozymes, transferrin and interferon.

The immune system and defences are altered in the pregnant woman. Pregnancy requires that the mother achieve a balance between tolerating the products of conception and maintaining normal defences against microorganisms.

Serum levels of immunoglobulin G (IgG) fall as pregnancy progresses, except in intrauterine death (IUD) and intrauterine growth restriction (IUGR). IgA and IgM decrease or remain stable in pregnancy. IgE changes are minimal and IgD increases to term. Pregnancy zone protein (PZP) appears to inhibit inflammatory processes. This is a glycoprotein produced by the mother and is found in phagocytosis near the decidua trophoblast. Pregnancy-associated plasma proteins (PAPPs) are produced by the syncytiotrophoblasts and have an inflammatory regulating function. Altered levels of PAPPs have been associated with complications in pre-eclampsia and diabetes and are increased in multiple pregnancies.

The respiratory system

Biomechanical factors

Changes in respiration in pregnancy include a relaxation of the muscles in the thorax, which broadens the ribcage by about 6 cm. This increases the air volume by 50 per cent per minute. The increased intra-abdominal pressure pushes the diaphragm up and breathing becomes diaphragmatic.

During pregnancy, breathing remains diaphragmatic, but due to pressure from the enlarged uterus, the movement of the diaphragm is reduced. To counteract this, pregnant women breathe more deeply (due to the effect of progesterone on the respiratory centre), thereby increasing the tidal volume.

Biochemical factors

There is greater mixing of gases during pregnancy, and an increased oxygen consumption of 20 per cent occurs at term. The effect of progesterone in dilating the pulmonary vasculature and the increased blood volume cause an engorgement of the pulmonary vessels, which can clearly be seen on chest X-rays taken during pregnancy.

Pregnant women are in a state of compensatory respiratory alkalosis.

The results of these changes are an increased oxygen tension (PaO_2) and a decreased carbon dioxide tension ($PaCO_2$). These are both beneficial to the fetus; the raised PaO_2 causes more oxygen to be transferred across the placental membrane to the fetus, and the lower $PaCO_2$ helps the fetus to dispose of carbon dioxide across the placenta to the maternal circulation.

Clinical implications

Dyspnoea may be experienced by some pregnant women. This may be due to pulmonary capillary engorgement combined with the pressure from the enlarged uterus.

Upper capillary engorgement may result from progesterone causing swelling of the nasopharynx, larynx, trachea and bronchi. This may be uncomfortable, with an increase in inflammation and nose bleeds.

Pregnant women may be more prone to upper respiratory infections and viral pneumonia.

Asthma is the most common respiratory problem in pregnancy (0.4 to 1.3 per cent) (Duque, Reche & López-Serrano, 2002). It may improve, remain the same or worsen in pregnancy.

The renal system

The kidneys are critical in the maintenance of body homeostasis. Structural and functional alterations in pregnancy affect the normal function of the renal system. Pregnancy is characterised by sodium retention and increased extracellular volume, both of which alter renal functioning. Normal parameters and values for renal function are altered in pregnancy.

A number of changes affect the urinary tract during pregnancy:

▶ The kidneys enlarge by 1 cm and renal volume increases by 30 per cent. This is partly due to the increase in vascularity and partly due to the effect of progesterone, as relaxation of the smooth muscle leads to dilatation of the renal pelvis and the ureters.

▶ Pregnancy is characterised by physiological hydroureter and hydronephrosis, with marked dilatation of the renal pelvis as early as the seventh week.

▶ Progesterone causes dilatation of the ureters, which may result in kinking in the middle portion because of loose support in this region.

▶ The bladder muscle also becomes relaxed as a result of the effect of progesterone. This, together with the dilatation of the renal pelvis and the ureters, can lead to stasis of urine. The result of these changes is an increased risk of urinary tract infection (UTI).

▶ With the growth of the uterus, the bladder is pulled up and also becomes an abdominal organ. However, the neck of the bladder is pushed forwards against the symphysis pubis. In late pregnancy, the enlarged uterus can compress the ureters at the pelvic brim, which causes a reduced flow of urine.

▶ At 20 weeks, dextroversion of the uterus affects the right kidney, with an increased risk of pyelonephritis in the right side.

▶ Because of the increased blood volume, there is an increase in renal blood flow and the glomerular filtration rate until, by the sixteenth week of pregnancy, they have increased by 40–50 per cent, which is then maintained throughout pregnancy. This results in increased urine production by the kidneys and causes frequent micturition, particularly in early pregnancy.

▶ Although blood flow and glomerular filtration rate are higher, tubular reabsorption remains unaltered. As a result, the capacity of the tubular cells to reabsorb certain substances is exceeded, and there is an increased clearance of certain substances, particularly sugar, amino acids, folic acid, water-soluble vitamins, iodine and waste products such as urea, uric acid and creatinine. This accounts for the frequency of glycosuria found during pregnancy (lowered renal threshold).

▶ Protein in the urine may be due to contamination caused by vaginal discharge. Consistent and increased proteinuria needs investigation. Protein in the urine after 20 weeks of pregnancy is of diagnostic value for pre-eclampsia.

▶ The increased glomerular filtration rate could also lead to the excessive loss of sodium and chloride, but there is a compensatory mechanism that causes increased reabsorption of sodium and chloride from the renal tubules and so preserves maternal electrolyte homeostasis. This is a consequence of increased production of steroid hormones by the placenta and the adrenal cortex during pregnancy.

The alimentary system

The gastrointestinal (GI) and hepatic systems are altered to accommodate essential maternal and fetal nutritional demands in pregnancy.

The gastrointestinal system

During pregnancy, changes in the GI tract may affect the food intake and nutrition of the mother. Early in pregnancy, hormonal changes result in loss of appetite, nausea and vomiting ('morning sickness') and, consequently, reduced food intake. This period is followed by increased appetite, thirst, changes in taste, food aversions, cravings and pica. Food intake increases by 15–20 per cent in early pregnancy. The alteration in insulin and glucagon levels, combined with oestrogen and progesterone, influences food intake.

The high levels of progesterone needed to relax the smooth muscle of the uterus also relax the smooth muscles of the GI tract. This leads to decreased motility and longer transit time throughout the GI tract. This is an advantage in the upper GI tract, as absorption of nutrients is increased. In the large intestine, however, increased water absorption and reduced motility may give rise to constipation.

Indigestion may result from relaxation of the oesophageal sphincter and pressure on the stomach from the growing fetus. In late pregnancy, pressure of the uterus on the GI tract makes consuming large meals difficult. Small, frequent meals are required at this stage.

Pregnancy does not demineralise teeth. Fetal calcium is withdrawn from maternal body stores. Gingivitis and tooth decay during pregnancy are caused by hormones in the saliva. Gingivitis occurs in 30–100 per cent of women. The gums become highly vascular, oedematous and hyperplastic. Bleeding while tooth brushing is more common in pregnancy.

Saliva becomes more acidic in pregnancy. Saliva does not increase in pregnancy, but some women may experience ptyalism, which is excessive salivation of up to 1 ℓ per day. The cause is unknown.

The liver

The enlarged uterus displaces the liver superiorly and posteriorly. The liver's production of protein, bilirubin and enzymes is altered. Spider angiomata and palmar erythema (found in liver conditions) due to high oestrogen levels are common in pregnancy. These appear after two to five months and disappear after pregnancy.

Weight gain in pregnancy will be discussed in Chapter 51.

The neuromuscular and sensory systems

The effects of the changes of pregnancy on the sensory system are well documented. Discomfort is common in pregnancy and birth and is considered a normal part of the process.

In pregnancy, ocular changes include oedema of the cornea in late pregnancy – a thickening of the cornea that may change refraction – and a slight fall in intraocular pressure. Women with contact lenses may find they cannot wear them anymore due to the changed shape of the eye ball. These changes are dependent on hormonal changes and BP changes. The composition of tears also changes slightly.

Otolaryngeal changes are associated with fluid dynamics and increased vascularity. Nasal congestion and stuffiness and increased snoring and sleep disorders are more common. The sense of smell may be altered.

Pregnant women may also complain of ear stuffiness that is not relieved by swallowing, and there may be a transient mild hearing loss and vertigo.

Sleep patterns are altered. Insomnia, dreams and nightmares are common in the third trimester. Hormonal changes decrease REM (rapid eye movement) sleep and increase non-REM sleep. Pregnancy-associated sleep disorders have been described. (Read more about common minor disorders of pregnancy in Chapter 20.)

The musculoskeletal system

Pregnancy is characterised by changes in posture and gait. External rotation of the femurs cause a 'waddling' gait to compensate for the redistribution of body mass. The symphysis pubis may widen by 10 cm. Lower limb pain may develop due to increased load on the lateral side of the foot, and many women need to wear a bigger size shoe. The risk of ligament injury increases in pregnancy and muscle cramps are common in the third trimester and at night. Compensatory lordosis develops due to the shift in the centre of gravity.

Diastasis of the rectus abdominus may occur and if this persists in the postnatal period, it may need to be corrected surgically.

Calcium balance remains normal during pregnancy if the diet contains adequate dairy products. The bones, therefore, are unchanged in normal pregnancy. These changes may give rise to discomfort and backache in advanced pregnancy.

14.7 General metabolism

'Metabolism' comes from the Greek word meaning 'change'. The principles of human metabolism include the maintenance of plasma glucose and an optimal supply of protein for enzyme function and muscular mobility. Excess protein is stored as fat; nitrogen is excreted in the urine.

Metabolic changes

The basal metabolic rate (BMR) increases by an average of 15 per cent during pregnancy. However, this varies among women because of differences in pre-pregnant nutritional status.

The thyroid enlarges in pregnancy and high levels of hormones are synthesised and metabolised in the system. This increase is due to the increase in the amount of metabolically active tissue of the fetus, placenta and mother, the higher level of effort required from the mother (for example cardiovascular and respiratory work) and tissue synthesis.

The metabolism of macronutrients (carbohydrates, proteins and fat) is adapted to shift nutrients to the fetus for growth, to meet the increased needs of the mother during pregnancy and to build up maternal stores needed by the mother during lactation.

In a well-nourished woman, the fetus accounts for 25 per cent of her weight gain, while in an undernourished woman, the fetus accounts for 60 per cent of her weight gain. Nutrition and weight gain are explained in Chapter 51.

Carbohydrate metabolism

The most marked changes occur in carbohydrate metabolism. This promotes the storage of energy as fat for later use in gestation and during lactation.

The fetus is dependent on the mother for glucose and this is actively transported across the placenta. Human placental lactogen (HPL), progesterone and cortisol are involved in the maintenance of glucose.

Glucose production remains sensitive to insulin and increases by 15–30 per cent in pregnancy. Blood glucose levels in a pregnant woman are 10–20 per cent lower than in a non-pregnant woman, so there is a tendency towards hypoglycaemia and ketosis.

In early pregnancy, insulin secretion increases, leading to 'accelerated starvation'. Accelerated starvation is a drop in blood glucose and metabolic processes to counteract the effects of hypoglycaemia. The mother compensates by breaking down fat for energy. This draining of glucose and amino acids by the fetus may lead to increased maternal appetite. Dieting and carbohydrate restriction in pregnancy are dangerous for the mother and the baby.

The 'diabetogenic' state of pregnancy is caused by increased resistance to insulin. This means that blood sugar does not drop when insulin is excreted. This is a protective measure to make sure that glucose is available for the fetus even when the mother is fasting. This effect is mainly present in the second and third trimester.

Protein metabolism

Decreased serum protein and amino acid levels are found in pregnancy. During the first half of pregnancy, maternal protein storage increases, with a retention of 1.3 g/day (nitrogen). Most is transferred to the fetus, but some is stored. In the second half of pregnancy, protein utilisation is more economical, with less urinary excretion.

Lipid metabolism

Marked alterations in lipid metabolism occur in pregnancy. Triglycerides increase by 40 per cent by 18 weeks and 250 per cent by term. Phospholipids and cholesterol also increase.

Maternal fat stores are most prominent between 10 and 30 weeks, before the peak of fetal demand. In the third trimester, fat is broken down into free fatty acids and glycerol, associated with the fetal demand for increased glucose and amino acids.

Calcium metabolism

Maternal serum levels fall progressively after fertilisation by an average of 1–1.5 mg/dl, with the lowest levels between 28 weeks and term. Calcium absorption doubles in pregnancy, with storage to meet the later demands of the fetus. Bone mass is not normally lost in pregnancy.

14.8   Thermoregulation

The amount of heat produced in pregnancy increases by 30–35 per cent, with an increased tolerance for cooler temperatures and an intolerance for heat. Peripheral vasodilatation is increased four to seven times, with increased activity of sweat glands. The mother's temperature increases by 0.5° C. The fetus cannot control its temperature independently of the mother. The fetus's temperature must be higher than the mother's for heat to move from the fetus to the mother. High maternal temperature can affect the fetus, causing hypoxia, altered haemodynamic teratogenesis and preterm birth.

14.9   Thyroid function

Serum thyroglobulin increases in the first trimester but is most marked in late pregnancy, with an associated enlargement of the thyroid. The degree of hyperplasia depends on iodine intake. Nausea and vomiting in pregnancy are associated with altered thyroid function.

Untreated hyperthyroidism will complicate pregnancy. Women with hypothyroidism have a high incidence of infertility and spontaneous abortion. The fetal thyroid is not dependent on the mother for development but the neurological development of the fetus in the first trimester may be affected.

14.10 Conclusion

The anatomical and physiological changes of pregnancy are complex, and changes in the mother take place in order to favour fetal development. However, the well-being of the mother is important. Antenatal care and education involve the assessment of maternal and fetal well-being.

15

The signs, symptoms and diagnosis of pregnancy

LEARNING OBJECTIVES

On completion of this chapter, you must be able to:
▶ identify the signs and symptoms of pregnancy
▶ use a scientific process to diagnose pregnancy
▶ select and use diagnostic tests to confirm pregnancy.

KNOWLEDGE ASSUMED TO BE IN PLACE

The anatomical and physiological changes of pregnancy

KEYWORDS

Hegar's sign • human chorionic gonadotrophin (hCG) • amenorrhoea • quickening • Osiander's sign • Jacquemier's/Chadwick's sign

15.1 Introduction

The diagnosis of pregnancy is important. Midwives use a variety of strategies to gather information in order to make conclusions or diagnoses. The accurate determination of pregnancy can influence the progress of the care and interventions that follow.

15.2 The diagnosis of pregnancy

The diagnosis of pregnancy is based on:
▶ symptoms experienced by the woman
▶ physical signs found on examination
▶ special investigations.

The signs and symptoms are based on the physiological changes that take place in a pregnant woman's body. These changes are influenced by the effects of human chorionic gonadotrophin (hCG), which is secreted into the woman's bloodstream when the trophoblast embeds and later by the hormones produced by the placenta. These effects, together with the development and growth of the products of conception (the embryo – which later becomes the fetus – the placenta, the membranes and the liquor amnii), give rise to the signs and symptoms of pregnancy (see chapters 6, 7 and 14).

Although there are many signs and symptoms of pregnancy, only a few of these are diagnostic. Most of these diagnostic signs are only present after 20 weeks of pregnancy. However, with the development of modern technology and the use of ultrasonography in obstetrics, it is possible to obtain a conclusive diagnosis of pregnancy as early as the seventh week from the first day of the last menstrual period (LMP), when the fetal heart can be seen beating (see Chapter 7).

Most women suspect that they are pregnant and either visit the antenatal clinic, their doctor or a midwife to confirm the diagnosis. Women living in remote areas may not be able to visit a clinic or be seen by a midwife or a doctor; they may have to rely on the traditional signs and symptoms of pregnancy. These include the cessation of menstruation, enlargement and pigmentation of the breasts, the presence of colostrum, the presence of chloasma and food cravings. However, all of these can be found in non-pregnant women as well. Pregnancy in these circumstances is usually confirmed at between four and six months (12–24 weeks).

Subjective signs and symptoms of pregnancy

Each of the signs and symptoms discussed in the following sections is subjective and nonspecific and could sometimes be caused by conditions unrelated to pregnancy.

Amenorrhoea

Pregnancy is the most common cause of cessation of menstruation in young women.

However, amenorrhoea may also occur in times of emotional stress and change of environment, in some endocrine disorders or in anaemia. After the use of the contraceptive pill, a period of amenorrhoea may occur and women should be informed of this. Poor nutrition may cause amenorrhoea. Young women with anorexia nervosa do not menstruate.

On the other hand, scanty vaginal bleeds sometimes occur during pregnancy. More frequently, however, a small vaginal bleed may take place during the time of implantation of the zygote. It is therefore important when estimating the gestational period to ask the woman if her last period was of normal amount and duration.

Breast changes

From three to four weeks, signs and symptoms such as tingling of the breasts and breast heaviness and enlargement may be the first indications of pregnancy. However, these features may also be experienced by non-pregnant women, particularly immediately prior to menstruation, due to high hormonal levels.

Morning sickness

More than 50 per cent of pregnant women experience nausea and vomiting between the fourth and the fourteenth week after the beginning of the LMP. This usually occurs in the morning, but may continue throughout the day. The cause is thought to be due to the high blood levels of hCG and oestrogens (see Chapter 20).

Should the vomiting persist after 14 weeks or if there is excessive vomiting, then it would no longer be considered normal.

Bladder irritability

Frequency of micturition without any signs of infection such as burning or pain often occurs in early pregnancy, particularly between the eighth and fourteenth weeks. This is due to the increased blood volume, which causes increased renal blood flow and glomerular filtration rates with an increase in urine production, together with pressure from the enlarging uterus on the bladder (see Chapter 14).

Quickening

The fetal movements the pregnant woman notices are called *quickening*. It is recognised as early as 16 weeks by multigravidae and at about 18–20 weeks in primigravidae.

Temperature elevation

When fertilisation and implantation have taken place, a woman's temperature is elevated.

In some instances, the woman is advised to take her temperature regularly throughout a normal menstrual cycle to establish her basal temperature, which usually rises at ovulation and then gradually returns to normal about 10 days after ovulation. If in subsequent cycles the woman's temperature remains elevated after ovulation, there is a strong likelihood of her being pregnant. This method is a particularly useful guide to pregnancy when a woman comes off the contraceptive pill.

It has also been observed that from the fourth week of pregnancy, the skin temperature over the breasts is about 0.7 °C higher than the temperature of the skin over the sternum, probably because of the increased vascularity of the breasts. This can be detected by a sensitive infra-red thermometer. However, an elevated temperature could be due to almost any infection, and this is not a reliable indicator of pregnancy.

Changes in body shape

A woman may report that her clothes do not fit, and her abdomen feels full.

Objective signs of pregnancy

Objective signs are more reliable than the subjective signs and symptoms, but could still be caused by conditions other than pregnancy.

Skin changes

Pigmentation of the skin often occurs during pregnancy and chloasma is usually noticeable from the sixteenth week (see Chapter 14). The linea alba changes to the linea nigra on the midline of the abdomen. The nipples may darken and the secondary areola appears.

Breast changes

From eight to 12 weeks, subcutaneous veins become noticeable and there is an increase in the size and pigmentation of the nipple and areola, and Montgomery's follicles/tubercles appear. From 16 weeks, colostrum can be expressed.

Changes in the pelvic organs

These signs are demonstrated during vaginal examination. All pregnant women, including those being attended by a professional midwife or attending an antenatal clinic, should be referred to and seen by a doctor at least once during pregnancy. The doctor will usually perform a vaginal examination to exclude any abnormalities. If the visit takes place early in the pregnancy, the following signs would help to confirm the pregnancy:

▶ *Hegar's sign:* At six to 12 weeks the embryo still only occupies the upper part of the uterus and the isthmus has softened and elongated. On bimanual examination, with two fingers of one hand in the vagina and the fingers of the other hand pressing downwards and backwards on the anterior abdominal wall, the fingers of both hands feel as though they meet because of the soft, elongated isthmus, which is in contrast to the rounded, full, upper segment above and to the much harder cervix below.

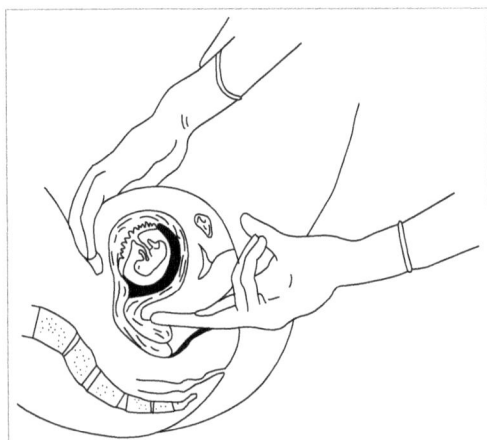

Figure 15.1 Hegar's sign

▶ *Jacquemier's/Chadwick's sign:* From the eighth week, there is a dark purplish discolouration of the mucous membranes of the cervix, vagina and vulva, which is caused by increased blood volume causing congestion of these tissues. The vagina is warm and blue and the cervix is soft.

▶ *Osiander's sign:* From the eighth week, increased pulsation is felt in the lateral fornices of the vagina, due to the increase in vascularity.

▶ *Uterine enlargement:* On vaginal examination, the uterus is the size of a grapefruit at about eight weeks. This is a very accurate diagnostic sign, because in the early stages of pregnancy, uterine size does not vary much between women. From the eighth week, the uterus increases in size and becomes more globular in shape. From about the twelfth week the fundus can be palpated abdominally, just above the symphysis pubis, and with the gradual increase in size, the uterus becomes an abdominal organ. From the twelfth week the cervix begins to soften. This 'ripening' process continues gradually until, at term, the cervix is ready or 'favourable' for dilatation. From 16 weeks, the uterus becomes more ovoid in shape.

▶ *Abdominal enlargement:* From the twelfth week, as the uterus grows and becomes an abdominal organ, the height of the fundus rises and the abdomen enlarges.

▶ *The uterine souffle:* From the sixteenth week a soft blowing sound that synchronises with the pregnant woman's pulse (normally about 80 beats per minute) can be heard on auscultation. It is the sound of the maternal blood coursing through the enlarged uterine vessels. It must not be confused with the sound of the fetal heart, which is a much more definite and rapid double-beat (normally about 140 beats per minute).

▶ *Braxton-Hicks contractions:* From the twentieth week these painless contractions are present.

15.3   Diagnostic procedures

The basis for all pregnancy tests is the presence of hCG. During the first 60 days of a singleton pregnancy, the hCG level doubles every two days. There is a relationship between the level of hCG and the gestational age (GA). Urine is used in most of these tests. However, maternal blood is used in the sensitive serum assays, which are the latest tests available.

Biological tests for pregnancy

Urine tests

These immunological tests are the most frequently used, because they are 99 per cent reliable and easy to use. They are available in kit form and contain reagents that are added to a woman's urine.

The objective of these tests is to detect hCG in the urine. At least 25 different tests are available. The modern immunometric assay, which can be used one week after the missed menstrual period, is used for these tests.

The urine specimen used for testing should be 25 ml of the first early-morning midstream specimen, which should be as free as possible from any contamination, particularly blood and protein.

Risks of the hCG urine test

Either a false positive or negative pregnancy test is possible. A false positive would indicate a pregnancy, even though there is none. A false negative result can occur if the test is done earlier than 14 days after the LMP. The test should then be repeated after at least a seven-day interval, when the hCG levels in the urine have increased. A false negative pregnancy result may also be obtained if the urine is contaminated with protein, which may coat the particles carrying the immunological reagent. In this case, the test should also be repeated as described above.

Urine and reagents used straight from the refrigerator may result in delayed agglutination.

Conditions such as hydatidiform mole and choriocarcinoma will give a strong positive pregnancy reaction due to high levels of hCG in the urine. A positive pregnancy test eight days after the first missed period indicates that the woman is probably pregnant. However, if the woman denies the possibility of pregnancy, the test should be repeated after seven days.

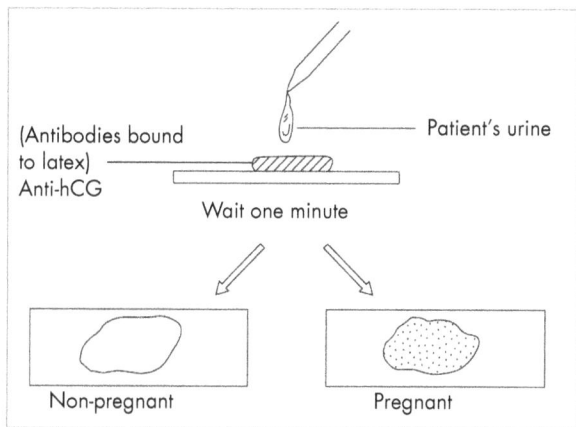

Figure 15.2 Immunological test for pregnancy

Sensitive serum assays (blood tests)

This blood test is similar to that of the urine test and also detects hCG. These tests are much more sensitive than urine tests but require a specialised laboratory. Very reliable results are possible, even before the first missed period, and the results can be read within 15 minutes if the equipment is available.

These tests can also be used for conditions such as ectopic pregnancy and threatened, missed and tubal abortion. Quantitative tests which give the exact amount of hCG in the blood may also be performed.

Potential sources of positive hCG results

This is the most sensitive of all the pregnancy tests and uses the beta-subunit of hCG. Very low levels of hCG can be detected, which means that pregnancy can be detected several days after conception. This test includes immunoradiometric assays, enzyme-linked immunosorbent assays, fluoroimmunoassays, phantom hCG and pituitary hCG.

15.4 Conclusive diagnostic signs

The following signs give conclusive proof of pregnancy. However, those signs that are not dependent upon modern electronic technology can usually only be demonstrated after 20 weeks of pregnancy.

Fetal heartbeat

The fetal heartbeat can be detected in the following ways:
- *Auscultation:* With the use of Pinard's stethoscope, an experienced examiner can hear the fetal heartbeat from 20 weeks after the LMP.
- *Ultrasonic devices:* These machines use ultrasound to detect and 'hear' the sound of the fetal heartbeat. The fetal heartbeat can be detected by ultrasound as early as six to seven weeks. Detection with other devices and doctors' stethoscopes or fetal stethoscopes is only 100 per cent reliable from about 15–20 weeks after the LMP if the information of cessation of menstruation is accurately identified by the woman. Often, women are unsure.
- *Electrocardiotocograph:* Using the electrocardiotocograph machine and an abdominal (fetal) transducer, the fetal heart can be detected from about 15 weeks.

Quickening and fetal parts

On abdominal palpation, the fetal parts can be felt from about 28–30 weeks of pregnancy and the lie and presentation can be defined in most instances.

Fetal movement

Quickening is the first sensations, often described as 'gas' or 'butterflies', that the woman has of the fetus. In first pregnancies, it is identified from about 20 weeks, but in follow-up pregnancies women may identify it from 15–16 weeks. Fetal movements can usually be felt on abdominal palpation by 22 weeks after the LMP.

Ultrasonic evidence

The fetal sac can be outlined using ultrasound from five weeks, and the heart can be seen beating by seven weeks after the LMP in 95 per cent of cases.

X-ray evidence

The fetal skeleton can be demonstrated by 15 weeks of pregnancy. However, because of the danger of radiation, this method is only used where there are indications of fetal death. No alternative methods are available to determine the fetal position, the presence of a suspected multiple pregnancy or fetal abnormality.

Signs of previous pregnancies/deliveries

For personal reasons, a woman may sometimes not admit to a previous pregnancy. There are signs, however, which give some indication that a woman may have had a previous pregnancy. This knowledge may be useful to the labour ward staff, because if a woman has had a previous vaginal delivery, both the first and second stages of subsequent labours are shorter than those of the first labour.

The following signs are not positive, but together with the woman's attitude, they may suggest the probability of a previous pregnancy:

- The breasts may be flabby with prominent nipples and persistent pigmentation of the areola.
- The abdomen muscles may be stretched, the skin loose and silver (old) striae gravidarum may be seen.
- The fetal parts are often easier to palpate than in a primigravida.
- The vulval pigmentation may have persisted with gaping of the labia and the vaginal introitus. The hymen may be torn and replaced by small tags (carunculae myrtiformes), and scarring of the perineum from an episiotomy or tear may be present.
- The vagina may be lax and roomy, or there may be signs of a cystocele or rectocele.
- The cervix usually provides the most conclusive sign. On speculum examination, the external cervical os is seen as a transverse slit, which easily admits at least one finger. In a nullipara, the cervical os has a small, round opening.
- There may be scars from a Ceasarean section.

Pseudocyesis

Pseudocyesis is a false or phantom pregnancy and is often the result of an intense desire for a child. This may cause stimulation of the hypothalamus, with the release of gonadotrophic hormones. Sometimes this intense desire may be associated with a deep-seated fear of pregnancy or of parenthood.

Many of the signs and symptoms of pregnancy are demonstrated, such as amenorrhoea, fullness of the breasts together with the secretion of fluid from the nipples and an enlarged abdomen (usually due to flatus). Examination and tests, however, fail to reveal any positive signs. Today, ultrasound can diagnose false pregnancy earlier. The husband or partner should be present if possible.

These women and their partners should be referred for psychological counselling, both to cope with the experience and to determine and – if possible – remedy the cause of the condition.

15.5   Conclusion

The diagnosis of pregnancy and the correct management of pregnancy, as well as the signs and symptoms have been discussed in this chapter.

Correlation between theory and practice in the diagnosis of pregnancy is of utmost importance to minimise medico-legal risks, especially with regard to record keeping.

Evidence-based antenatal care

16.1 Introduction

The science of midwifery practice evolved over time and guidelines for clinical midwifery competencies have been stipulated for the 21st century. This includes the Basic Antenatal Care (BANC) guidelines, which are used to ensure minimal standards of care for women during pregnancy. The guidelines are based on a system of recording basic care that reflects the quality factors for maternal care determined for the specific context. This chapter discusses antenatal care in terms of safe motherhood strategies, evidence-based care, the WHO's model for low-risk pregnancies and the BANC programme's guidelines.

The BANC programme was adapted from the focused antenatal model of care approach (FANC) and was rolled out as a quality improvement strategy in antenatal care in South Africa by the end of 2008 (Patience, Sibiya & Gwele, 2016). The WHO (2016) suggested new guidelines for innovative, evidence-based antenatal care to improve quality and make pregnancy a positive experience. This recommendation advocates for a standard of maternal and fetal assessment that includes nutrition and psychosocial aspects, and counselling for intimate partner violence. In South Africa the adjusted programme is referred to as BANC Plus, adjusting the number of antenatal visits from four to eight, starting no later than 20

weeks. Nine standard operating procedures and eight protocols guide the new BANC Plus application.

This chapter considers general national and international initiatives to improve antenatal care, including BANC and BANC Plus.

16.2 Safe motherhood strategies

The Safe Motherhood Initiative (SMI), which started in 1987, is a global programme aimed at improving the quality of care by the multiple care providers who are involved in care during pregnancy, birth and the postpartum period. This multi-professional approach forms part of a global effort to reduce maternal and perinatal mortality. The midwife is integral to this approach, as midwives are the main caregivers for women in childbirth.

The SMI is about avoiding not only death but also morbidity; it strives to improve the quality of healthcare for improved health outcomes for mothers and babies. This includes the physical, mental and social well-being of the childbearing woman before, during and after childbirth, to facilitate the birth of a healthy baby who will be able to thrive and grow into a healthy child. This approach is in keeping with the constitution of the WHO, that defined health in the broader sense as 'a state of complete physical, mental and social wellbeing and not merely the absence of disease or infirmity' (WHO, 2017a).

Many of the factors that lead to maternal death are not always identifiable. A more realistic approach to the provision of pregnancy care is to provide a woman with the necessary care and services to help her stay on the road to health and to keep a close watch over her health status. This is referred to as BANC and BANC Plus, which is focused on risk identification particular to the South African healthcare system and is part of the primary care approach to maternity care.

The SMI sees the midwife as the preferred primary caregiver for women and families in childbirth. Strategies for improving care for mothers and babies before, during and after pregnancy are summarised in Table 16.1. Several principles and values underpin the safe delivery of care to women and children. These are briefly explained in the box on this page.

The aspects presented in Table 16.1 have been addressed through the *Saving Mothers* (DoH, 2014) and *Saving Babies*

(Pattinson & Rhoda, 2014) report recommendations for South Africa (see Chapter 4), the *National Core Standards for Health Establishments in South Africa* (DoH, 2011) and the *Ideal Clinic Manual* (DoH, 2016).

Values and principles of perinatal care

Care for a normal pregnancy and birth should involve the woman during decision making and should be:
- de-medicalised
- based on the use of appropriate technology
- regionalised
- evidence-based
- multidisciplinary
- holistic
- family-centred
- culturally appropriate.

Table 16.1

Safe motherhood strategies

Factors	Strategies
Infrastructural or environmental	Ensure access to safe water. Provide appropriate systems of support that address the socioeconomic and psychological needs of women and their families. Provide infrastructure with readily available emergency obstetric care. Provide a clean environment for the birth.
Organisational	Provide access to appropriate maternity care. Refer to specialist care when needed. Provide easy access to family planning services.
Norms and standards of care	Screen women for complications. Educate and inform women about their pregnancy and birth and about warning signs of emergencies so that they know what to expect and can participate in their own care. Set protocols (guidelines to be followed) for dealing with major problems. Provide tetanus immunisation after delivery (where tetanus is a problem locally).
Norms and standards of staff	Ensure the availability of a skilled birth attendant (a skilled midwife with life-giving skills is the primary care provider for most deliveries). Provide a basic education programme for midwives, which balances academic credibility with clinical excellence. Provide a continuing professional development (CPD) programme for all healthcare professionals, which combines clinical excellence with academic credibility.

Birth as a normal physiological process

The focus of care for women and newborns acknowledges childbirth as a normal physiological process. There is a global move to de-medicalise birth. De-medicalisation should be aimed at considering pregnancy as a physiological event rather than a disease, and birth and the newborn should not be regarded as a problem, nor should the woman be considered a 'patient'. However, an uncritical approach to de-medicalisation should be avoided. In order to achieve safe de-medicalisation, skilled attendance should be ensured during pregnancy, at birth and after birth, for each birth, at each level of care. Healthcare systems are challenged to adopt this approach while increasing the quality of care and reducing maternal and perinatal mortality. Bearing this in mind, the quality of education for midwives and the effective correlation of theory to practice cannot be overemphasised.

Technology and childbirth

The use of technology in healthcare is important. It saves time and can provide accurate findings that influence care. In the developing world, appropriate technologies are defined as methods, procedures, techniques and equipment that are scientifically valid, adapted to local needs and acceptable both to those who use them and to those for whom they are used, and which can be maintained and used by the community with resources the community can afford.

The incorporation of appropriate technology in maternal care is essential in order to improve care. Great advances have been made particularly to support care in rural areas and in primary healthcare (PHC), where medical care and expensive equipment may not be cost-effective. One example is the training of healthcare workers in the skills and techniques of Helping Babies Breathe (HBB) (described in Chapter 46) for the effective resuscitation of the newborn using room air.

Accessibility of care

Making healthcare accessible for all is another challenge. Effective and safe maternal and perinatal care should be available at each level of care in an integrated network between primary (minimal), secondary (intermediary) and tertiary (intensive) levels of care. This will ensure that regionalisation of perinatal care takes the place of the previously centralised, out-of-date and non-functional system.

Culturally sensitive care

Culturally sensitive care incorporates and respects all acceptable traditional practices of care – after they have been tested for safety and efficacy. Each intervention in new initiatives should be evaluated in the national context for its impact on cultural attitudes and an effort should be made to facilitate its acceptance through information and discussion.

Civil society collaboration

Women's participation in decision making, the implementation of initiatives and advocacy should be enhanced and encouraged in South Africa. Midwives need to partner with women to give care that will satisfy the community. The South African Civil Society for Women's, Adolescents' and Children's Health (SACSoWACH) was launched in Kalafong hospital in 2015 to raise public awareness regarding issues in reproductive health to improve quality of care and health outcomes.

16.3 Evidence-based healthcare

Common practices, professional skills, protocols and policies should be based on scientific evidence and regularly updated. Care should be able to satisfy the physical, emotional and psychosocial needs of mothers, newborns, fathers and families in a holistic way. Care and interventions therefore have to be centred on the information, motivation and participation of the whole family and local community.

Evidence-based care requires healthcare professionals to investigate their practice and constantly ask the following questions:
▶ What am I doing?
▶ Why am I doing it?
▶ Does the practice achieve its aim?
▶ Is there evidence of better or more effective ways of achieving this aim?

It is clear that some practices in healthcare are not supported by evidence of efficacy. Many actions or interventions are now being carefully re-assessed. As a result, many healthcare practices have been shown to be unnecessary, wasteful of resources and, frequently, harmful. Midwives need to:
▶ use a process of practising evidence-based practice (EBP)
▶ know where to find the best evidence
▶ understand what is meant by the terms 'sensitivity', 'specificity' and 'randomised controlled trial'
▶ be able to critically appraise research
▶ appreciate that care should be evidence-based and individually tailored.

EBP has been defined by Sackett (2000) as the integration of best research evidence with *clinical expertise and patient values and preference*.

217

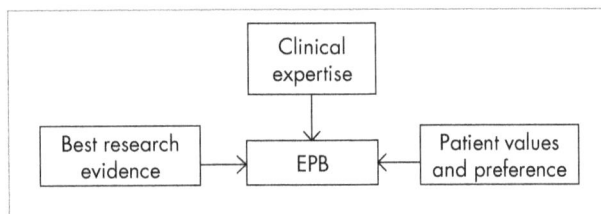

Figure 16.1 Evidence-based practice (Sackett, 2000)

Best research evidence is described as 'that which is clinically relevant'. The evidence may be obtained from basic sciences, but is usually from patient-centred clinical research addressing the following questions:

▶ What are the accuracy and precision of the diagnostic tests (including clinical examination) used?

▶ What is the power of the prognostic markers? Is the evidence about prognosis valid? If valid, how important is it for the patient? (Is the prognosis valid over time and how precise is it?)

Clinical expertise is defined as the ability to:

▶ use clinical skills and experience to identify each patient's health state accurately

▶ diagnose the individual risks and benefits of any potential intervention for that person

▶ identify the patient's values and expectations.

Patient values are identified as the unique preferences, concerns and expectations each patient brings to a clinical encounter and which must be integrated into clinical decisions.

The scientific process of care

Midwives should use a scientific process to assess, diagnose and treat women in childbirth. The scientific process of care follows a specific pathway, namely:

1. the gathering of information
2. the analysis and interpretation of the information
3. reaching conclusions through special examinations
4. the plan and execution of care
5. the evaluation of care.

Each parameter in the abovementioned process is equally important. This assessment and care is comprehensive and includes all the woman's healthcare needs: physical, psychological and social. It is a dynamic and ongoing process.

Without an attitude of 'caring', effective practice will not meet the required levels of quality and satisfaction, and can be harmful. A scientific method and a caring attitude allow for control of care and permit self-correction. This attitude guides practice, makes care measurable and fosters accountability,

quality and satisfaction for the carer and pregnant woman. In addition, problem solving is an essential part of scientific reasoning and distinguishes professionals from other workers.

Antenatal psychological and mental health assessment

Antenatal and maternal healthcare are expanded beyond technical care, which focuses mainly on physical health. The mental and psychological health of women and families should also be assessed. As antenatal psychological problems may be associated with unfavourable healthcare outcomes, the midwife should consider psychological health evaluation. Issues of great concern to the woman, her family or the caregiver usually indicate a need for additional support or services. If concerns are identified, for example in mental health, follow-up and/or referral should be considered (see Chapter 13).

Nutrition

Nutrition remains one of the critical aspects to ensure a positive outcome for mothers and newborns. Nutritional aspects are referred to throughout this book and particularly in Chapter 51.

16.4   Principles of antenatal care

Antenatal care should start when pregnancy is diagnosed. In South Africa, the target is to start antenatal care no later than 20 weeks. If a woman visits a clinic early on in her pregnancy, the information gathered will be more accurate, which means that interventions can take place to identify factors associated with adverse outcomes for mother and fetus. Ultrasounds at 12 weeks and 20 weeks are able to identify most fetal abnormalities. The triple test at 16 weeks can screen for open neural tube abnormalities and Down's syndrome. Other conditions such as HIV, syphilis, multiple pregnancy and medical conditions can be identified early and the appropriate care can be instituted.

The following are some guidelines to be followed in providing antenatal care:

▶ The antenatal care provided has to be effective. When the woman is involved in planning and implementing her care, the effectiveness of antenatal care is enhanced. A holistic approach should be utilised. Early attendance to care as well as involving women and their families in the care can be realised when there is a trusting relationship between the woman and the healthcare professionals. This trusting relationship should be developed at the initial booking visit and sustained during the period of care.

▶ To facilitate establishing a trusting relationship, the healthcare professionals (midwives, medical personnel and ancillary staff) should display a welcoming and caring attitude and behaviour as well as professional interpersonal skills and competencies.

▶ A detailed history, particularly personal information, should be obtained. This must be done with respect, ensuring privacy and confidentiality.

▶ The *Guidelines for Maternity Care in South Africa* (DoH, 2015a) highlight the importance of dialogue and mutual respect between private caregivers and the public health sector in managing women during pregnancy and the process of childbirth.

▶ The nursing process can be used to guide provision of care. This involves assessing the woman's health needs, planning to meet her individual health needs, implementing the plan, evaluating the effect of the implemented actions and re-adjusting the plan where necessary. The attending healthcare professional must be able to recognise potential complications, including making timely referrals to the next level of care based on individualised healthcare needs utilising the holistic approach.

▶ Provide health education on topics related to pregnancy and childbirth (such as prophylaxis, personal hygiene, appropriate health-promoting behaviours during pregnancy such as a healthy lifestyle, the labour process and parenthood) to facilitate informed decision making. This information should include the available antenatal services, the services provided by other service providers as well as the higher levels of care that can be accessed in case of deviations from normal.

▶ Accurate, clear and comprehensive documentation of all information should be obtained, including nursing care plans and the implementation and evaluation of care. All documentation should be kept in the woman's file.

▶ The care should not only follow the process guidelines of the BANC programme, but also meet the clinical guidelines found in the *Guidelines for Maternity Care in South Africa* (DoH, 2015a). Care should adhere to the skilful competent caring of midwifery, considering the individual needs of women.

The WHO model for low-risk pregnancies: Antenatal visits

According to the WHO's new guidelines for antenatal care (WHO, 2016), the number of visits are increased to eight for low-risk pregnancies, and more for others, to ensure a positive pregnancy and reduce perinatal mortality. The WHO (2016) indicates that eight or more quality visits during pregnancy can reduce perinatal deaths by up to 8 per 1 000 births

when compared to four visits. In South Africa, the BANC Plus programme has extended antenatal visits to eight, for improved surveillance, early identification of problems and early intervention.

A low-risk pregnancy is one where:
▶ no risk factors are identified in the history or during the antenatal period
▶ there is only one fetus (a singleton pregnancy)
▶ the baby is in the vertex position
▶ the mother is not younger than 16 years or older than 37 years
▶ the mother does not have a medical condition such as HIV/AIDS, diabetes or hypertension.

The content of the antenatal care visits, based on the WHO model for low-risk pregnancies, includes (2016):
▶ an initial assessment to obtain baseline health information about the woman and her family as it relates to pregnancy and childbirth (medical history, surgical history, history of chronic illnesses, genetic disorders, obstetric and gynaecological)
▶ a clinical examination (head-to-toe and abdominal)
▶ screening tests based on geographical location to exclude:
  • malaria
  • tuberculosis
  • syphilis
  • HIV
▶ haematology – full blood count or Hb, blood group, Rh
▶ vital signs and measurements – BP, maternal weight and height
▶ immunisations and prophylaxis – tetanus toxoid to prevent neonatal tetanus, iron, folic acid, calcium and vitamin A supplementation (VAS).

The BANC quality programme and BANC Plus

The BANC programme was launched to standardise and improve the quality of antenatal care in order to lower maternal and perinatal death rates. The programme is focused on analysing and grouping women according to their risk factors, which facilitates caring for low-risk women and referring high-risk women. BANC uses the integrated PHC approach: the principles of good antenatal care that were put forward by the WHO and which have been adapted for South Africa.

The BANC Plus 2016 programme is an extension of the BANC of 2008–2014 and specifically focuses on quality improvement. It is based on the recommendations of the *Saving Mothers* (DoH, 2014) and *Saving Babies* reports (Pattinson & Rhoda, 2014), the Committee on Mortality and Morbidity in

Children under five (CoMMiC) and the National Perinatal Morbidity and Mortality Committee (NaPeMMCo).

The BANC programme trains healthcare professionals in antenatal care implementation by using training facilitators. Healthcare professionals are identified by PHC facility managers. The facility then receives a package containing:

▶ a manual to be used for training the trainers
▶ notes for the facility manager
▶ referral hospital notes
▶ a task book
▶ protocols and audit criteria
▶ a handbook
▶ the WHO's basic antenatal care guidelines
▶ protocols for the prevention of mother-to-child transmission (PMTCT) (of HIV)
▶ training posters.

Research on the effectiveness of BANC in South Africa

Several studies have investigated how effective the BANC programme has been in South Africa. Two studies useful to read are the following:

1 Snyman, JS, 2007. *Effectiveness of the Basic Antenatal Care package in primary health care clinics.* MCur thesis: Nelson Mandela University.

2 Patience, NTS, Sibiya, MN & Gwele, NS. 2016. 'Evidence of application of the Basic Antenatal Care principles of good care and guidelines in pregnant women's antenatal care records'. *African Journal of PHC and FM,* 8(2): 1016. https://www.ncbi.nlm.nih.gov/pmc/articles/PMC4913450/ (Accessed 3 August 2017).

The study by Patience et al (2016) identified evidence of incomplete application of the BANC principles of good care and guidelines in pregnant women's antenatal care records, which indicated that the BANC approach was not being successfully implemented. Recommendations made include policy development, institutional management and practice, nursing education and further research to assist in the successful implementation of the BANC approach in line with the guidelines and principles of good care.

Selection for BANC

At the first visit, pregnant women are divided into two groups according to pre-set criteria:

1. Those qualifying for the BANC programme
2. Those requiring a higher level of care, who are then referred for medical care.

The BANC objectives

The objectives of BANC are to (DoH, 2015a):

▶ save time
▶ improve the level of contact with pregnant women for the early identification of problems
▶ reduce workload through focused planning and intervention
▶ improve the chances of a good outcome of pregnancy through a structural standardised programme that lends itself to auditing the quality of care rendered.

Priority considerations in the BANC programme

Table 16.2 indicates the conditions that are screened as priority in the BANC programme. These are conditions which can be detected and treated in pregnancy.

Table 16.2

Priority conditions in the BANC programme

Maternal	**Fetal**
Anaemia	Poor fetal growth
Hypertension and pre-eclampsia	Post-maturity
	Congenital syphilis
Medical conditions: diabetes mellitus, epilepsy, cardiac conditions	Congenital abnormalities
	Twins
HIV	Abnormal lie
Chronic TB	Rh incompatibility
Urinary tract infections (UTI)	
Vaginitis and sexually transmitted infections (STIs)	
Malnutrition	

Staff skills

Appropriately trained nurse-midwives and midwives are required to have the knowledge and skills to deliver effective quality of care in the PHC context. Effective intervention follows the clinical process of:

▶ checking the antenatal card
▶ looking, listening and feeling (assessing)
▶ recording findings
▶ classifying the findings
▶ treating, advising or referring.

Standards

Various factors are checked at each visit, namely:

▶ iron and calcium supplementation

▶ nutritional advice
▶ warning signs appropriate for the gestational age (GA) and risk profile
▶ the birth plan
▶ transport arrangements
▶ the complete checklist
▶ the date for a follow-up appointment.

Protocols

The BANC programme requires close collaboration between referral hospitals and clinics. There are protocols for antenatal care to be signed and agreed upon between clinics and referral hospitals, including improved communication between levels of care. These should be updated regularly and signed by all parties.

The protocols are designed locally to suit a local context. They address a problem, offer preventive measures, show screening criteria and procedures and provide evidence-based treatment and intervention.

Treatment regimens

In the original BANC programme, there is a hierarchy of treatment regimens:
▶ Policy guidelines are developed by the Department of Health (DoH).
▶ Management guidelines are developed by evidence-based principles and research (WHO).
▶ Institutional protocols use these guidelines to add details suitable to the area and context.

The BANC Plus has revised clinical protocols and standard operating procedures to improve the quality of care, satisfaction and outcomes, including an increase in the number of visits.

Clinical programmes
There are several programmes for care in PHC that a midwife needs to be able to implement, such as newborn care charts, Integrated Management of Childhood Illnesses (IMCI), Integrated Chronic Disease Management (ICDM) and PMTCT of HIV. District clinical specialist teams (DCSTs) have been appointed with a view to strengthening maternal and child care and are involved in the monitoring and support of districts and clinics.

The BANC programme has a checklist that needs to be completed, which will guide and direct decisions. The first clinical checklist and follow-up checklists are designed to focus on specific conditions with specific protocols to manage the women, based on the results.

Auditing

Auditing of care is used within the BANC programme to determine and improve quality of care. With the assistance of the DCSTs, all facilities conduct regular auditing, not only of BANC but also of partograms and mortality and morbidity reviews, to improve health outcomes.

Activity
Attend a maternal or perinatal mortality and morbidity meeting in your district and write a report.

Referrals

The following referrals are indicated by the BANC programme:
▶ Routine referral to a medical practitioner
▶ Non-acute referral
▶ Referral to a social worker
▶ Referral for food supplementation.

Implementation of the BANC and BANC Plus programmes

The implementation of the BANC and BANC Plus programmes will improve the quality of antenatal care, especially at PHC level. The success of these programmes relies on the availability and accessibility of its services, policies, guidelines and protocols, the type of communication about the programme, the incorporation of PHC services and the training and in-service education, support and direction that midwives receive.

Facilities implementing the programme must undergo a process of change. Guidelines and policies should also be available for successful implementation of the programme.

16.5   Standards, protocols and regimens

The *Guidelines for Maternity Care in South Africa* (DoH, 2015a, and as these are updated) guide the principles of care at district level. All institutions and clinicians involved in maternity care use these guidelines to develop and implement protocols and regimens to improve care. Generic protocols and guidelines are printed on posters and should be visible in all clinics and clinical areas.

Guidelines and protocols are evidence-based and are reviewed. These include training in the Essential Steps in the Management of Obstetric Emergencies (ESMOE) and essential obstetric care (Emergency Obstetric Simulation Training, or EOST). Midwives' skills and competencies are updated and they receive a certificate of competency for effective practice.

Besides these maternity guidelines, midwives should develop protocols for 'caring'. The particular hallmark of midwifery is 'being with women' and 'caring' in pregnancy and birth and the postnatal period. Caring is the domain of the midwife and extends beyond technical care. Specific guidelines for caring should be reflected in protocols of caring (see Chapter 3).

The value of records

Records are scientific tools used to assist the healthcare professional to gather and interpret information during pregnancy and to communicate the findings to the rest of the team for decision making for best outcomes during pregnancy, birth and the postnatal period.

Record keeping calls for a systematic process of gathering and communication of information using a set record system (generic). It is part of a process of quality improvement and allows for an audit to measure the quality of care. The information gathered is only as good as the skills of the user. Complete records should be maintained at all times.

Maternity case records

The maternity case record (MCR) is started, completed and issued with the first visit. The woman keeps the record with her and produces it at any point of entry into the healthcare system. She is thus required to bring her record with her to any clinic visit for recording health information until birth. The MCR is used to relay information on the mother's health status to the next level of care during the antenatal period, referral, birth and the postnatal period. After birth, the MCR is used until after the six-week postnatal visit. During the antenatal and birth processes and after the woman has given birth, the antenatal records and birth records and partogram are audited for quality purposes.

The BANC programme includes structured tools to gather and store information for evidence-based assessment and evaluation of improved quality decision making and care.

Improving standards for healthcare establishments

The national DoH has implemented the six priorities in the *National Core Standards for Health Establishments in South Africa* (DoH, 2011) for improved quality of care delivery. The *Ideal Clinic Manual* version 16 (DoH, 2016) provides guidelines to improve the infrastructure of clinics. To meet standards, it has 10 components, 32 subcomponents and 186 elements, which are monitored.

16.6   Conclusion

This chapter discussed strategies for safe motherhood, with an emphasis on the role of the midwife as primary caregiver before, during and after birth. Next, the importance principles of evidence-based antenatal care was explored. The use of a structured approach and records guide the clinician and should not only make care focused, but also enhance communication between levels of care during the pregnancy and birth processes.

The chapter explained the principles of antenatal care based on the WHO's model for low-risk pregnancies and the BANC programme's guidelines. Finally, the importance of standards, protocols and regimens was emphasised. The BANC and BANC Plus programme are guides for practice, but they do not prevent the midwife from using her midwifery professional knowledge to add to the care and make conclusions and diagnosis beyond the scope of the programme. In fact, it is important to identify problems and refer these women.

Health screening and planning of care at the first antenatal visit

LEARNING OBJECTIVES

On completion of this chapter, you must be able to:
- take a complete health history and do a complete health screening in pregnancy
- use a scientific process to diagnose pregnancy
- select and use appropriate diagnostic tests to confirm pregnancy
- perform the needed physical examinations in pregnancy
- identify and perform special examinations in pregnancy
- identify and refer women to a higher level of care
- plot information correctly on a growth chart and keep accurate records
- use the Basic Antenatal Care (BANC) programme to classify maternal risk.

KNOWLEDGE ASSUMED TO BE IN PLACE

The anatomy of the female reproductive system, including the breast

The potential psychological, sociological and physiological effects of pregnancy on the woman and her family

The nursing process

Basic Antenatal Care (BANC) and auditing according to the *Guidelines for Maternity Care in South Africa* (DoH, 2015a), Chapter 4

KEYWORDS

human chorionic gonadotrophin (hCG) • amenorrhoea • quickening • pelvimetry • biometry • ultrasound

17.1 Introduction

Antenatal care is the care given to women during pregnancy, from the time of conception to the onset of true labour. With the first contact, the midwife takes a full history, performs a physical general examination, carries out tests of urine and blood and does an obstetric examination. It is essential to diagnose the pregnancy and identify risk factors. The midwife and pregnant woman then develop a plan of care based on the findings.

Antenatal preparation entails screening for physical, psychological and socioeconomic considerations in the planning of care. Pregnant women who are at risk for complications or those who present with complications during pregnancy or have pre-existing medical conditions are referred for medical care.

Antenatal care provides an opportunity for skilled healthcare professionals to promote healthy behaviours following childbirth, such as infant feeding options, early postnatal care and spacing of children.

17.2 Terminology and general obstetric status

Terms used in midwifery practice and the general obstetric status of a woman are explained in the boxes on the next page. A midwife needs to know the terminology used in obstetrics in order to summarise a woman's obstetric history. The ICD 10 classification of disease has categorised all conditions. The codes most often associated with the primary diagnosis in obstetrics and comorbidities are given in Annexure A. It is thus possible to categorise a woman according to the ICD 10 codes.

Terminology

▶ *Fetal viability.* In South Africa, a fetus is considered viable at 28 weeks of gestation (1 000 g). The WHO's definition of viability is 24 weeks or a weight of 500 g. Fetal viability is determined according to lung maturity or the ability to survive based on respiratory development and function.

▶ *Miscarriage.* A pregnancy that has terminated spontaneously before reaching fetal viability (24–26 weeks or a weight of 500 g) is termed a miscarriage.

▶ *Termination of pregnancy (TOP).* This is the number of pregnancies that were terminated by choice or due to maternal complications or fetal abnormalities, usually before fetal viability (24–26 weeks or 500 g), also expressed as abortions.

General obstetric status

▶ Gravidity refers to the number of times a woman has been pregnant.
  • A primigravida is a woman who is pregnant for the first time (gravida 1).
  • A multigravida is a woman who has had at least one previous pregnancy (gravida 2, 3 or more).

▶ Parity refers to the number of viable births (including fetuses born after fetal viability, whether alive or stillborn). Stillborn babies are counted if the mother gives birth after 28 weeks. The births are counted and not the number of babies or the status of the baby. This means that multiple pregnancies count as one birth.
  • A nullipara is a woman who has not carried a pregnancy to viability, referred to as para 0.
  • A primipara is a woman who has had one viable pregnancy, referred to as para 1.
  • A multipara is a woman who has given birth to two or more viable pregnancies, referred to as para 2, 3 or more.
  • A grande multipara is a woman who has had five or more viable pregnancies (para 5, 6 or more).

Determining obstetric status

Consider the following example:
▶ A woman who has had three previous pregnancies and is now pregnant for the fourth time will be grav 4.
▶ If only two of her previous pregnancies were viable (lasted 26 weeks or longer), she will be grav 4 para 2 (G4P2).

continued

▶ If one of her viable pregnancies produced twins (alive or stillborn) then she will still be grav 4 para 2 (G4P2).
▶ If the first viable pregnancy produced twins and the second viable pregnancy produced quadruplets, then she will still be grav 4 para 2 (G4P2).

17.3   The initial visit (booking visit)

Ideally, women of childbearing age should receive pre-conception care. This care will ensure that the woman is in an optimal state of health when she is pregnant to minimise health problems which can affect pregnancy.

The goal of the initial antenatal visit is to accurately diagnose the pregnancy and develop a treatment plan based on any early underlying conditions identified or the presence of factors that put the mother or fetus at risk, such as HIV. The initial antenatal visit is also intended to allow for preventive measures, such as prevention of congenital syphilis, anaemia and malaria (in certain geographical areas). These conditions are known to cause adverse outcomes (DoH, 2015a).

Women who come to an antenatal clinic for the first time after 20 weeks of gestation, when they experience problems or when they are already in labour are at risk. This limits the number of appropriate interventions that are available, for example in the case of Down's syndrome, open neural tube defects (NTDs) and structural abnormalities of the fetus, which could have been detected before 20 weeks of gestation. Early contact with healthcare services is therefore recommended.

An examination during the first trimester, if done before 20 weeks of gestation, provides a more accurate date of conception and therefore:
▶ a more accurate estimation of the delivery date
▶ more accurate baseline information (before change and adaptation in pregnancy) with which to observe and assess the progress of the pregnancy.

Standards of care for the first antenatal visit

These include the following:
▶ The staff (admission personnel, midwives, medical practitioners, etc) should have a welcoming attitude.
▶ Personal information should be obtained in an effective and confidential manner and prescribed records should be completed.
▶ A detailed history is taken and recorded on the antenatal card, which the woman is expected to carry and bring along when she reports for antenatal care, visits a doctor or reports for other health-related services, and the Basic Antenatal Care (BANC) records, which stay in the clinic.
▶ Baseline information is gathered using a standard process.

Health assessment

The health assessment includes a full history (see Table 17.1), an interpretation of the woman's obstetric status and a physical examination. The aim is to screen the woman to determine her well-being and identify any existing abnormalities or factors that may complicate pregnancy and birth. The history obtained provides baseline health information to be used to complement physical examinations during future antenatal care visits and also forms the basis for planning the level and content of care. Abnormalities can be detected early and treatment started immediately; these can then be evaluated and treated as the pregnancy progresses.

As mentioned, all information gathered (the assessment, examination and tests) and all care provided to the woman are recorded in the BANC records and on the antenatal record card.

Taking an antenatal history

Taking a history is an art and a competency needed in midwifery practice, as it requires effective and culturally sensitive communication skills. History taking is an extremely important aspect of antenatal care that must be mastered, because it is a screening procedure to identify factors that may be detrimental to the normal course of pregnancy and birth.

The BANC checklist, as presented in the *Guidelines for Maternity Care in South Africa* (DoH, 2015a), should be completed. These guidelines indicate factors that need further attention and reflect the actions that should be undertaken at each antenatal visit. Table 17.1 summarises the information that should be obtained during history taking at the first antenatal care visit.

Table 17.1

History to be obtained at the first antenatal visit

Component	Details
Personal information	Full name Full address (check accessibility to the health facility) Telephone number Date of birth Population group Occupation (in detail) Religious affiliation (if any) Husband or partner's full name, address, occupation, business address and contact telephone number Name, address and telephone number of closest relative Name of health facility Name of healthcare provider Personal preferences about the delivery process (Is there need for a support person or any preferred person to conduct the delivery?)
Social history	Level of education Financial situation and employment (The woman may have difficulty attending the clinic if she is employed) Support systems, including aftercare for mother and baby An age of less than 16 or more than 35 years is associated with higher maternal and neonatal morbidity and mortality Marital status: If the woman is unmarried, there is the possibility of less support. If she is married, is the husband employed and supportive? Residential address: If in a poor socioeconomic area, find out details such as overcrowding or poor sanitation and financial situation Distance to the clinic and means of transport: This plays a role in the accessibility of care and clinic visits Nutritional habits, food security and safe water: If employed, check opportunities for regular breaks for nutritional snacks Alcohol, drug or tobacco use or exposure to teratogenic substances

continued

Component	Details
Social history (continued)	If the woman is employed, maternity leave arrangements The nature of her work: Are there occupational health hazards, such as high temperatures, standing for long hours, or working with chemicals? Any cultural or religious affiliations that may affect the birth process (eg women from North Africa may have undergone female circumcision) Any other information that the woman believes to be of importance **Note:** Should the woman's social history reveal any problems, a social worker should be consulted.
Family history	**Note:** This is important in terms of possible genetic conditions. Include both families (the father's and mother's families). Any history of multiple pregnancy, particularly on the maternal side Family history of chronic medical conditions such as hypertension, diabetes, rheumatic fever, cardiac conditions, haematological (blood) disorders Any hereditary conditions such as Down's syndrome, haemophilia, muscular dystrophy, cystic fibrosis, phenylketonuria (PKU), albinism, Tay-Sachs disease (if Jewish), albinism, achondroplasia, dwarfism, giantism, talipes, deafness, blindness, cleft lip and palate, etc
Medical/ surgical	Significant past medical and surgical history Immunisations, such as rubella, hepatitis B and tetanus toxoid Childhood diseases Operative procedures such as abdominal or spinal surgery or surgery for varicose veins, etc Accidents, especially involving the spine, lower limbs or pelvis Any previous chronic conditions or abnormal conditions, such as poliomyelitis, rheumatic fever, hypertension, renal disease, cardiac disease, respiratory disease, diabetes mellitus, anaemia, malignancy, asthma, thrombosis, endocrine dysfunction, psychiatric disorders, sexually transmitted infections (STIs) Any medication, current or previous, such as cortisone, insulin or oral medication for diabetes, other hormones, anticoagulants and anti-epileptic therapy, etc Bleeding tendencies and previous blood transfusions Any abnormal symptoms which may affect the current pregnancy, maternal and fetal health
Current history	Pre-pregnant weight Any weight gain or weight loss within the past six months Blood group and Rh factor Current complaints, eg recurring urinary tract infections (UTIs) or vaginal infections
Gynaecological history	Age at menarche: If first menstrual period occurred after 16 years of age, consider congenital abnormalities Type of menstrual cycle, such as 28-day cycle, and whether regular or irregular Any history of menstrual problems such as dysmenorrhoea, periods of amenorrhoea, profuse menstruation Any vaginal discharge: Give the name if known or otherwise ask the woman to describe the consistency, colour and odour STIs such as gonorrhoea, syphilis, herpes 2, HIV Any previous surgery to the reproductive system, such as Caesarean sections or myomectomy, surgical repair of torn vagina and perineum, previous cone biopsy, Shirodkar stitch Contraceptive history: type of contraceptive used, the date of removal of an intrauterine contraceptive device (IUCD) or when contraceptive pills were last used

continued

Component	Details
Past obstetric history	History of infertility or subfertility, including any treatment Number of sexual partners (Are the women's children from the same father?) History of previous pregnancies: number of normal pregnancies (that continued to term and presented no serious problems) The dates and spacing of pregnancies Any abnormalities related to pregnancy, such as pre-eclampsia and eclampsia, early or late bleeding during pregnancy, intrauterine growth restriction (IUGR), polyhydramnios or oligohydramnios, etc History of previous labours: type of delivery and reason for interventions (forceps, Caesarean sections), abnormalities and complications, precipitate labours, prolonged labours, perineal tears or episiotomies, primary postpartum haemorrhage (PPH), fetal distress, pain relief methods or spinal/epidural anaesthetics Experience of labour (presence of significant person at birth) The history of previous postnatal periods (from the end of labour to six weeks): any abnormalities, such as sub-involution of the uterus, bleeding or secondary PPH, thrombosis Infections: general, of the perineum, the birth canal or the breasts History of breastfeeding and duration of breastfeeding or infant feeding Any psychological problems Number of viable children and their birth weights Birth weight of last baby: < 2 500 g or > 4 000 g Perinatal deaths, stillbirths (macerated or fresh) or neonatal loss, if any: age of infant deaths and cause of death Number of live children and their health (state any abnormal conditions they may have) Duration of pregnancy: preterm or post-term babies
Present obstetric history	The date of the first day of the last menstrual period (LMP): Was this period a normal period, in amount and length? The woman's attitude to this pregnancy: Was it a planned or unintended pregnancy? If not, explain. Has the pregnancy been normal and without complications? Has she been sleeping and eating well and doing antenatal exercises? Any common disorders such as feeling faint, nausea and vomiting, constipation, heartburn, itching of the skin or pruritis, varicose veins, haemorrhoids, backache (explain in detail) Any serious disorders, such as bleeding, excessive vomiting, severe headaches, high temperatures (explain in detail) Any infections, particularly viral rubella, cytomegalovirus (CMV), influenza, herpes, HIV Other: syphilis, toxoplasmosis, or any other treatment or exposure, particularly to X-rays, cytotoxic treatment or any accidents, any surgery or anaesthetics

Estimation of gestational age

The first day of the last normal period is used to determine the gestational age (GA). This is only valid if the woman is sure of her dates and where palpation of the uterus and symphysis fundal height (SFH) measurements are compatible with the given dates. GA must be calculated from the first day of the last normal menstruation period. However, most women are not sure of their dates. The longer the time between the LMP and the clinic visit, the more inaccurate this date becomes.

Calculation of estimated delivery date

Several methods can be used to calculate the estimated date of delivery (EDD):

▶ *The obstetric calendar* is easy to use. Once the LMP is determined, the EDD can be read on the next line.
▶ *The obstetric wheel,* as shown in Figure 17.1 on the next page, is also easy to use and gives both the EDD and the current GA based on the LMP. The EDD can also be determined by using Naegele's rule (see the box on the next page).

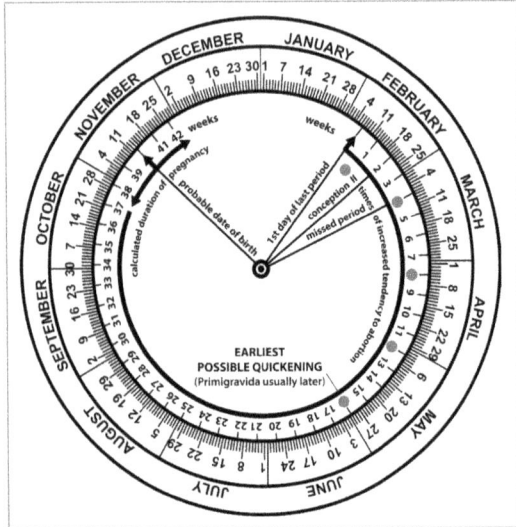

Figure 17.1 The obstetric wheel

The classic calculation of Naegele's rule

The duration of pregnancy in humans is nine lunar months or 37–40 weeks or 266 days (38 weeks). Forty weeks is nine months and six days calculated from the first day of the last normal menstrual period plus seven days (when implantation occurs) plus nine months or minus three months.

For example: A woman's LMP started on 10 April.
Add seven days: 10 + 7 = 17 April.
April is the fourth month. Add 9 months = January.
The EDD is 17 January.
Alternatively, three months can be deducted from the fourth month: 4 – 3 = 1 = 17 January.

After confirmation of pregnancy, the duration of the pregnancy is determined.

PROCEDURE The measurement of symphysis fundal height

Definition
Fundal height is generally defined as the distance from the pubic bone to the top of the uterus, measured in centimetres. Fundal height measurement is a tool for gauging fetal growth and gestational age; it is not an exact science.

The fundal height in centimetres correlates well with weeks of gestation (eg 26 cm correlates with 26 weeks' gestation) and serial measurements of a single pregnancy provide an indication of fetal growth and well-being during pregnancy.

Usefulness
A combination of the SFH measurement and an abdominal palpation and assessment by ultrasound scan provides a reasonably accurate GA estimate. However, the SFH measurement is of little value before 24 weeks and it is not reliable in late pregnancy (> 35 weeks). In early pregnancy, bimanual and abdominal palpation can be used, and after 29 weeks palpation of the fetal head is useful. Assessing GA by means of palpation requires skill and experience.

SFH measurement should be used:
▶ where technology is unavailable, such as in units with poor resources
▶ to identify high-risk factors such as polyhydramnios and multiple gestations
▶ to assess fetal growth and development during a single pregnancy
▶ for early identification of a small-for-gestational-age (SGA) baby, and subsequent referral of the woman to higher levels of care.

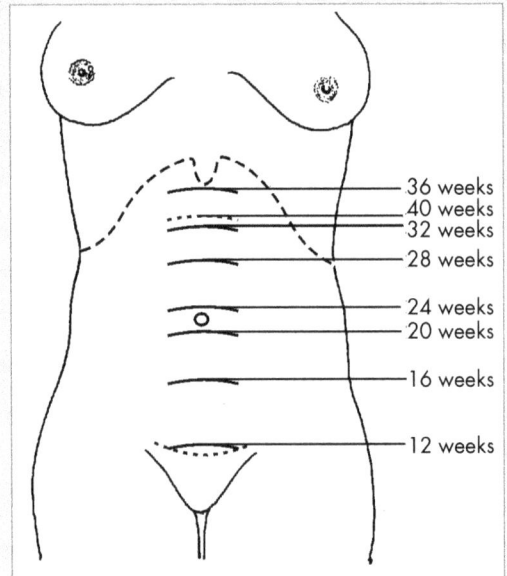

Figure 17A Duration of pregnancy according to estimated abdominal measurements

continued

Principles

The following principles should be followed during SFH measurement:

▶ A single SFH measurement is ineffective. Serial measurements are necessary for a more accurate assessment of fetal growth (see Figure 17A).

▶ Using a tape measure is simple and inexpensive.

▶ Measuring SFH does not replace abdominal palpation; rather, it supplements it.

▶ To be most accurate, the SFH measurement should be done by the same examiner at each assessment.

▶ The bladder should be emptied before the measurement is done.

▶ Maternal position (such as torso elevation and flexing of the legs) may influence the SFH measurement.

▶ If a woman is very tall, very short or obese, this will influence the accuracy of the findings of fundal height measurements.

▶ Maternal conditions (such as uterine fibroids or hydramnios) distort the uterine size and cause an inaccurate assessment of fetal size.

▶ For women weighing more than 100 kg, 1 cm is subtracted from the obtained measurement.

▶ Variations in fetal weight during the last trimester will decrease the accuracy of SFH measurement.

▶ A variation of +/− 2 cm is considered normal.

▶ A lag in the progression of fundal height may indicate IUGR.

▶ Early detection of IUGR can reduce the chance of perinatal death.

▶ A sudden fundal height increase may indicate the presence of twins or hydramnios.

▶ A measurement of 40 cm in a singleton pregnancy after 36 weeks may be an indication of a bigger-than-expected baby (increasing the risk for shoulder dystocia).

▶ The assessment should not be done through clothing.

▶ The measuring of SFH is not painful. Any tenderness should therefore be investigated.

▶ The expected fetal growth for a single pregnancy in a non-obese woman is 1 cm per week. A measurement of 26 cm, for example, will therefore indicate a pregnancy of 26 weeks.

▶ If the dates and uterine size differ by more than three weeks, accept the uterine size as the better parameter of duration. The dates are considered correct if the difference is less than four weeks (See Figure 17C on the next page).

Preparation

▶ The midwife ensures privacy and obtains informed consent.

▶ The midwife washes and warms her hands.

▶ The woman's bladder should be empty and her abdomen exposed.

▶ The woman should be in a supine position with her head and shoulders slightly elevated on a pillow, with arms at her side and the legs flexed. Flexing the legs relaxes the abdominal muscles.

▶ Use a non-stretch measuring tape for a more accurate assessment.

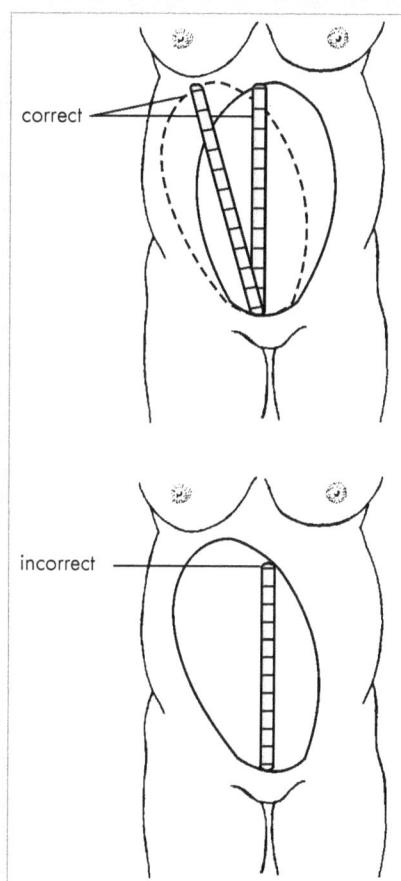

Figure 17B SFH measurement

Procedure

1 Gently place the dominant hand on the lower segment of the uterus.

2 Facing the woman, use the side of your non-dominant hand to palpate the uterus gently inwards towards the spine to locate the top of the fundus. For accurate measurement, one hand stabilises the uterus while the other hand locates the top of the fundus without pushing the uterine fundus downwards.

continued

3 Determine the position of the fundus in relation to the midline of the body. If it is not in the midline, locate it and assess the bladder for distension. (A full bladder causes an inaccurate assessment because it pushes the uterus aside.)

4 Determine the highest point of the fundus, even if it is not in the midline of the abdomen.

5 Retain an imaginary mark on the skin.

6 Secure the tape measure at the fundus with one hand.

7 Measure the SFH from the top of the symphysis pubis over the curvature of the abdomen to the imaginary mark on the fundus. The tape measure should stay in contact with the woman's skin.

8 Plot the measurement on the woman's antenatal card.

9 Correlate the SFH with the dates and the size of the uterus (see Figure 17C).

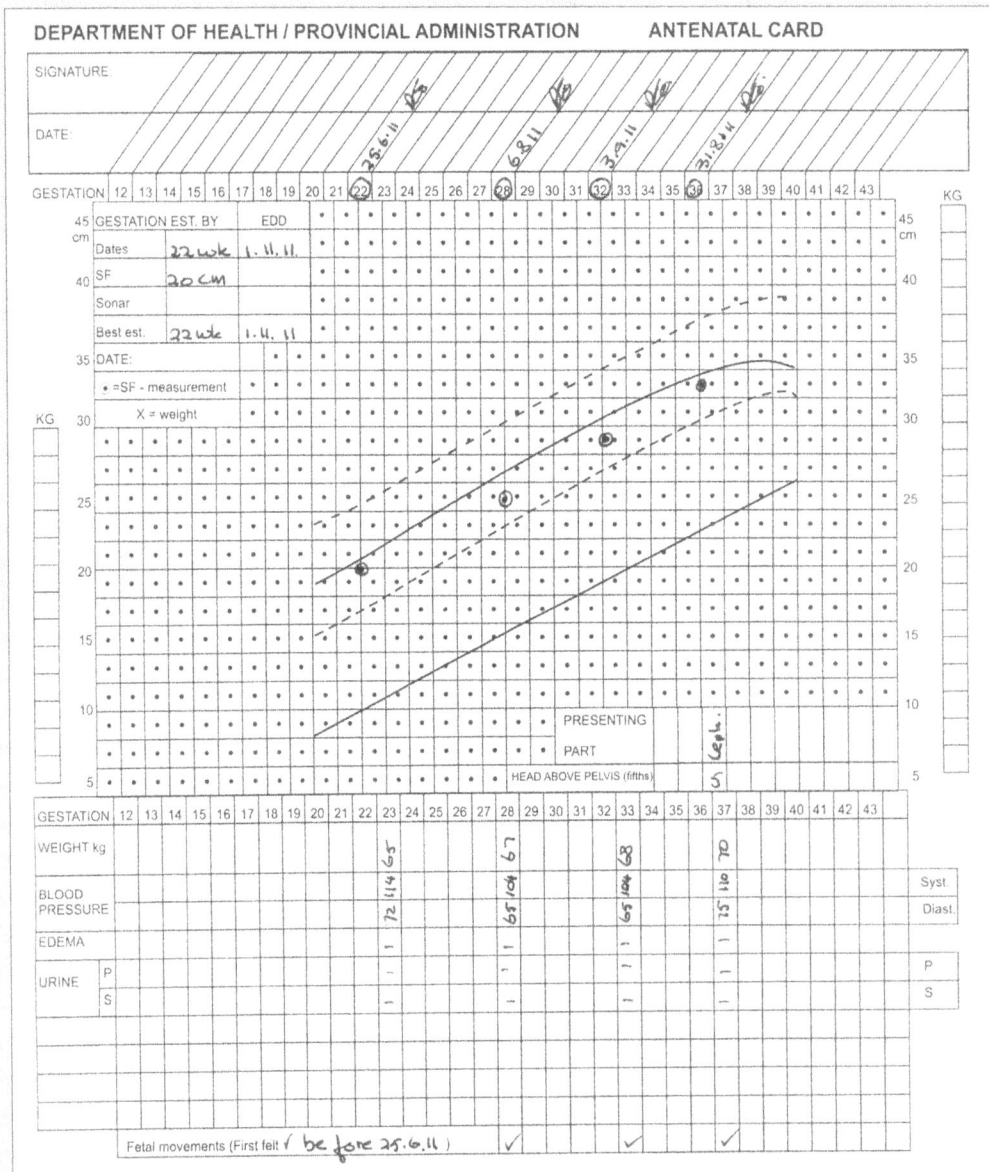

Figure 17C SFH graph and antenatal card for monitoring progress, of a woman with correct menstrual dates

continued

Interpretation

McDonald's rule for determining the length of gestation adds precision to the measurement of fundal height during the second and third trimester:

Height of fundus (cm) x 2 ÷ 7 = gestation in lunar months

Height of fundus (cm) x 8 ÷ 7 = gestation in weeks

A fundal height *below* the umbilicus indicates a pregnancy of less than 22 weeks. A fundal height *at the level of the umbilicus or higher indicates* a pregnancy of 22 weeks or more.

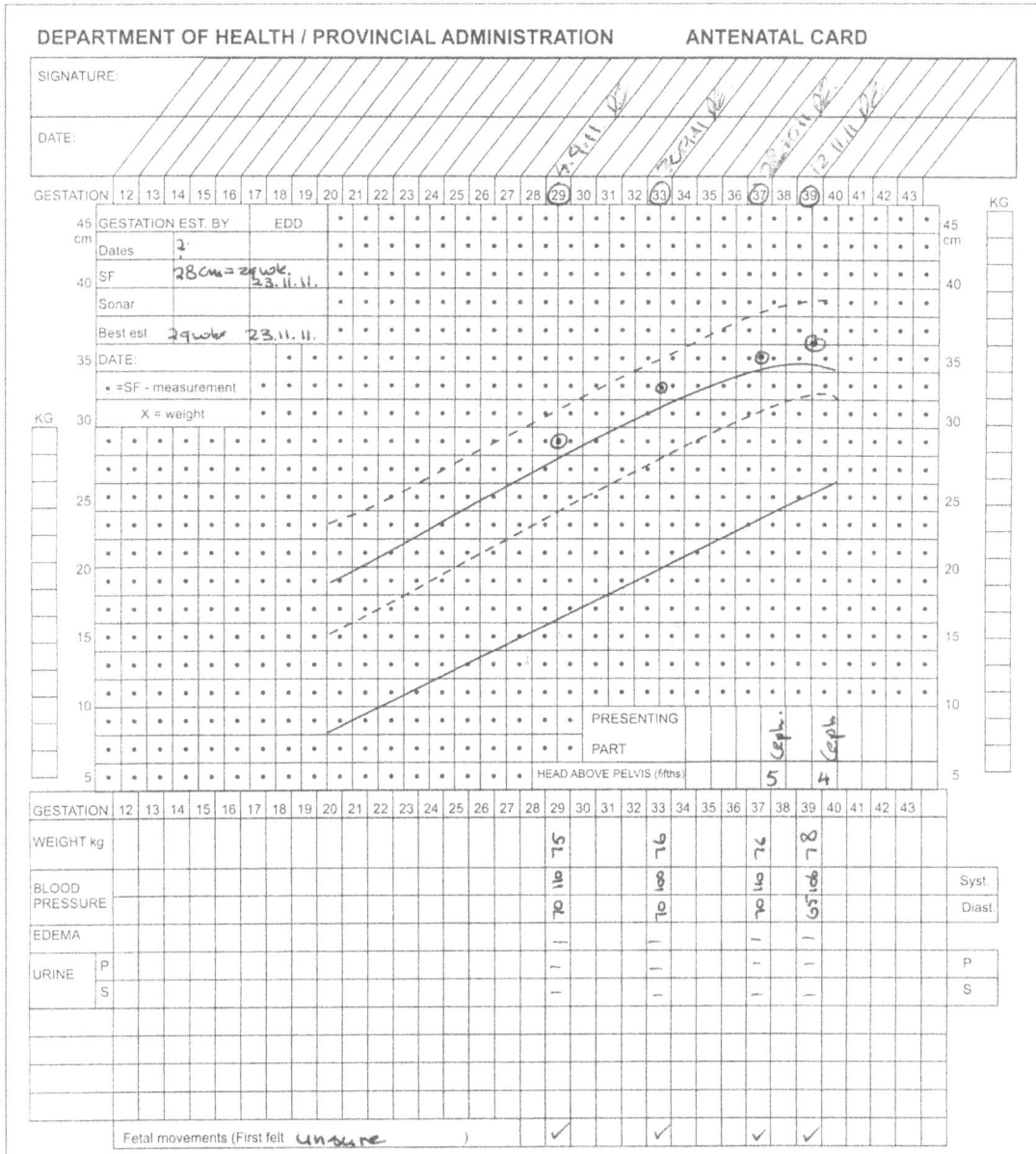

Figure 17D SFH graph and antenatal card for monitoring progress, of a woman whose menstrual dates are unknown

continued

The measured SFH is plotted in centimetres onto the 50th centile line on the SFH graph, providing the midwife with a graphic display of fetal growth. The SFH growth curve is compared with the duration of pregnancy, usually according to the estimated dates.

▶ The solid line on the SFH growth card represents the 50th percentile and the upper and lower dotted lines represent the 90th and 10th percentiles.

▶ With normal intrauterine growth, the SFH will be plotted between the 10th and the 90th percentile, allowing the corresponding GA to be read from the graph.

▶ Confirmation of the GA can be made by abdominal palpation and ultrasound.

▶ Refer the woman for further investigations if two successive or three separate measurements are below the 10th percentile or three measurements remain the same without necessarily crossing below the 10th percentile. The 10th percentile means that 10 per cent of fetuses fall above this line. If the measurement falls below the 10th percentile, the fetus may be growth restricted (see Figures 17C and 17D).

Abnormalities
Causes of an abnormal fundal height include:

▶ a high body mass index (BMI)
▶ a full bladder
▶ an especially tall and thin or short and heavy mother
▶ a multiple pregnancy
▶ abnormally slow growth due to placental insufficiency, resulting in IUGR

▶ rapid fetal growth due to maternal gestational diabetes
▶ oligo- or polyhydramnios
▶ too little or too much amniotic fluid
▶ uterine fibroids
▶ fetal malposition (breech, transverse)
▶ premature fetal descent.

Physical examination

The purpose of the physical examination must be carefully explained to the woman. The midwife should engage and communicate with the woman during the process of physical examination. This helps the woman relax and can provide the midwife with information about the woman's emotional state.

The examination is performed systematically, from head to toe, always maintaining privacy and respect for the woman's culture and beliefs. Table 17.3 on pages 234–237 provides a summary of the normal findings and possible deviations from normal. The main focus is on the general condition of the mother, including anaemia, malaria, hypertensive conditions, tuberculosis and varicosities. The well-being of the fetus is assessed through monitoring mid-upper-arm circumference (MUAC), abdominal measurements in centimetres (fundal height) and the fetal heart rate (FHR). The woman should also be educated on breast self-examination and instructed how to examine her breasts for lumps.

During the physical examination, the following aspects should be considered:

▶ *Maternal weight.* The weight of the woman allows the midwife to rule out obesity and abnormally low weight, both of which can have an adverse effect on the fetus. Obesity is associated with pregnancy-induced hypertension (PIH) and gestational diabetes mellitus. Abnormally low weight may contribute to IUGR,

resulting in the delivery of an SGA baby. The monitoring of maternal weight gain is no longer used in the public sector. The MUAC is now the standard assessment of nutrition in pregnancy. (This procedure is explained in the box on the next page.)

▶ *Blood pressure.* This provides baseline data to monitor the woman for PIH. Changes in the systolic pressure are usually minimal. BP reaches its lowest peak at 32 weeks' gestation, as a response to the relaxing effect of progesterone on the blood vessels. Normal BP ranges between 110/70 and 120/80 mmHg.

▶ *Urinalysis.* This is done at all antenatal visits to exclude bacteriuria, proteinuria, glucose and ketones. Bacteriuria is asymptomatic; if noted, the woman should be treated to prevent pyelonephritis, which might further complicate the pregnancy and lead to preterm labour. Proteinuria in the presence of oedema or raised BP may indicate pre-eclampsia (see Chapter 21).

▶ *General observations.* The woman's general response to pregnancy is noted, as some women may require emotional support. This is particularly likely in the case of a first pregnancy, if the current pregnancy is unintended or if there were adverse events in the previous pregnancy. Checking vital signs during the initial antenatal care visit provides an opportunity to document baseline observations. As the body adapts to pregnancy, it may contribute to some of the changes in baseline vital signs. Normal values for vital signs are presented in Table 17.3 on the next page.

▶ *Oedema.* The woman should not present with oedema of the lower limbs or any facial oedema. During subsequent visits, oedema should be checked. Mild oedema of the lower limbs is considered normal, while oedema that extends to the knees and facial oedema should be investigated. Physiological oedema of the lower limbs is more marked during the day due to gravity, as the woman spends most of the time walking or standing. This oedema subsides overnight as the woman sleeps (see Chapter 20).

▶ *Varicosities.* Some women experience varicosities during pregnancy, predisposing them to deep vein thrombosis (DVT). Varicosities may also occur on the vulva. Haemorrhoids are also common during pregnancy. Women should be examined for varicosities at every antenatal visit.

PROCEDURE Measuring mid-upper-arm circumference

Principles

MUAC is preferable to BMI, for the following reasons:

▶ Height does not need to be measured.
▶ Accurate scales are not required.
▶ The woman does not have to stand up straight.

▶ No calculation is needed.
▶ Unlike weight, MUAC does not normally increase significantly during pregnancy.

The MUAC is recorded in a number of African countries and gives useful information on nutritional status and pregnancy risk. It can easily be performed during the antenatal period or labour. As an indicator, MUAC measurement is preferred to pre-pregnant weight in pregnancy. All pregnant women are measured at the first antenatal visit, in the labour ward or postnatally to determine their nutritional status. The National Committee on Confidential Enquiries into Maternal Deaths (NCCEMD) (DoH, 2014) also included the MUAC in the national maternal death notification form.

Procedure

The MUAC should be measured immediately after checking the BP. If it is greater than 33 cm, a large cuff is used for the BP. Measure the MUAC at any gestational period, or during or after labour.

1 The arm should hang freely (elbow extended).
2 Measure the arm circumference on either the right or left arm, midway between the tip of the shoulder (acromion) and the tip of the elbow (olecranon). Use a soft tape measure.
3 Record the measurement to the nearest 1 mm.
4 Record the MUAC on the antenatal card or in the labour ward admission notes.

Interpretation and recording

Table 17.2

Interpreting the MUAC measurement

MUAC > 33 cm	MUAC ≤ 23 cm
Suggests obesity Is associated with an increased risk of pre-eclampsia and maternal diabetes Is associated with an increased risk of delivery of a larger-than-normal infant Indicates that BP measurement with a normal-sized adult cuff may be an overestimation	Suggests under-nutrition or a chronic wasting illness Is associated with delivery of a smaller-than-normal infant

On its own, an abnormal MUAC:
▶ is not a reason for more frequent antenatal visits
▶ is not a reason for referral to a higher level of care
▶ does not require special investigations, eg chest X-rays or glucose testing.

However, an abnormal MUAC requires vigilance to ensure good nutrition and the monitoring of fetal well-being.

The general assessment of a pregnant woman includes a physical and psychological assessment. The general appearance of the woman may be that of being aware, co-operative and communicative, or dull and unresponsive, calm or agitated and anxious, happy or depressed. These variations are taken note of and explored further to provide individualised care and support. Table 17.3 provides details of the possible normal findings and significant deviations from normal during pregnancy.

Table 17.3

The physical examination

System	Normal	Abnormal
General appearance	Healthy-looking Groomed Appearing stable with no signs of discomfort or distress	Untidiness and changes in mood may signify psychological conditions. Wasted, pale and appearing to be in distress: may be a result of anaemia, malaria, HIV infection or tuberculosis
Vital signs and measurements: BP, pulse, temperature and maternal weight	BP: 110/70 to 120/80 mmHg	A BP of 140/90 on three successive occasions prior to 20 weeks may indicate essential hypertension and after 24 weeks it may indicate PIH. Such an increase, if accompanied by proteinuria and marked ankle or pretibial oedema in the absence of other conditions such as renal disease, may signify pre-eclampsia.
	Pulse: 60–90 bpm	Marked tachycardia or bradycardia may signify infection or cardiac disease.
	Temperature: 36.2 °C to 37.5 °C	Hyperpyrexia may indicate infection.
	Weight: Expected to increase by 2 kg in the first 20 weeks' gestation and 500 g per week from 20 weeks till term.	Weight gain below the expected may contribute to IUGR, while weight gain above the expected may signify multiple pregnancy or a big baby in the absence of any pathological condition in the mother. Weight gain on its own may not be suggestive of nutritional deficiency. The measurement of the MUAC may therefore be very relevant as regards assessment of the woman's nutritional status.
Skin: the body, face, breasts and abdomen	Colour: The skin's natural colour is normally consistent with the woman's racial background. The condition and texture or feel of the skin should be smooth and elastic, with no or slight oedema (50 to 70 % of women have slight oedema in late pregnancy). No rashes or other lesions should be present. Linea nigra: Darkening of the secondary areola of the breasts and chloasma	Pallor (palms and nail beds): This may be natural, but can be due to anaemia or other blood disorders, or to inborn errors of metabolism such as PKU. Dark pigmentation, secondary areola and chloasma: This can be normal in pregnancy due to physiological changes. It may also be due to birthmarks or moles (naevi). Alternatively, it may be abnormal and a sign of neurological or immunological disorders. Jaundice: hepatitis or other conditions causing hyperbilirubinaemia

continued

System	Normal	Abnormal
Skin: the body, face, breasts and abdomen (continued)		Cyanosed or dusky: cardiac and respiratory conditions Roughness: hypothyroidism, malnutrition and vitamin deficiencies Inelasticity: dehydration, malnutrition, advancing age Oedema: pre-eclampsia, cardiac or renal disease Rashes or other lesions: infections, STIs, parasites Bruises or petechiae: trauma, bleeding tendencies
Head and hair	Size of head: appropriate for the size of the body Face: symmetrical Scalp: normal pattern, and neck allows smooth mobility The temporal artery is palpable without causing discomfort to the woman. The colour and texture of the hair is consistent with the woman's racial background and distributed normally.	Weakness of the facial muscles may indicate a cerebral vascular accident in the presence of pre-eclampsia. Abnormalities of mobility may indicate a muscular or nerve disorder. Oedema of the face may indicate pre-eclampsia in the absence of other pathology. Abnormalities of hair texture and distribution may be due to malnutrition or hypothyroidism. Alopecia: At times the loss of hair can be genetic.
Eyes	Generally bright, alert and clear White sclera Round, equal pupils that respond to light No swelling of the eyelids Pink conjunctivae	Deformities, strabismus, ptosis, lesions, sight impairment, nystagmus, discharges Pale conjunctivae may indicate anaemia. Yellow pigmentation of the sclera indicates jaundice; red sclera may indicate infection. Dilated or pinpoint pupils may indicate the use of drugs such as dagga or heroin, respectively. Oedema of the eyelids and surrounding areas may indicate pre-eclampsia, renal disease or other pathology.
Nose and sinuses	Unrestricted and silent nasal breathing Normal sinuses Nasal mucosa oedematous with or without nasal stuffiness due to the effect of oestrogen	Blocked nose Broken nose Rhinitis and discharge, bleeding or red nasal mucosa may indicate infection. Sinuses blocked, headaches, postnasal drip or cough and epistaxis
Mouth, teeth and tongue	Lips, gums, buccal mucosa, palate and pharynx are pink and free of lesions. Teeth are even and without dental caries; breath of normal odour. Tongue has full mobility in mouth, is pink, with papillae moderately rough.	Lips: oedema, lesions, pale, obvious deformities Gums: pale, lesions, bleeding Teeth: broken, dental caries Breath: offensive; other odours such as alcohol or dental decay (a throat swab can be taken if necessary) Tongue: a large or thick tongue may indicate hypothyroidism; may protrude from the oral cavity; speech difficulties; tongue-tied Buccal mucosa: pale, jaundiced, lesions Palate: cleft, which may cause speech difficulties Pharynx: enlarged, inflamed or septic tonsils; inflamed, ulcerated throat

continued

System	Normal	Abnormal
Neck and thyroid	Neck mobile, with good muscle tone and no stiffness Thyroid gland of normal size Carotid pulses palpable	Neck stiffness may indicate spinal or neurological conditions. Poor muscle tone may indicate muscular dystrophy. An enlarged thyroid may indicate hyperthyroidism. If the carotid pulse is diminished or absent, it may indicate cardiovascular disease. Rolls of fat may indicate obesity.
Shoulders, arms and hands	The shoulders, arms and hands are relaxed and flexing, with good muscle tone; neither fat nor thin. All the joints are of a normal size and mobile. The hands and all the fingers are present, with no extra digits. Radial pulses are good. Hands and fingers are the right colour for the woman's racial group, warm and slightly moist; nail beds pink and firm. MUAC ≤ 33 cm Pulse felt on both sides; regular and full.	Tension of muscles: lack of muscle tone Obesity or excessive thinness Very tight-fitting rings may indicate oedema and pre-eclampsia. Enlarged joints may indicate arthritis. Clubbing and cyanosis of fingertips may indicate cardiac or respiratory disease. Spoon-nails may indicate iron-deficiency anaemia. Chipped nails may indicate a mineral deficiency. Carpal tunnel syndrome MUAC > 33 cm raises potential risks for hypertension or gestational diabetes.
Chest, heart and lungs	Normally shaped, symmetrical chest Sternum and ribs not prominent Normal lung and heart sounds	A barrel or pigeon chest could indicate asthma, emphysema, chronic pulmonary or cardiac disease. Pulse irregular, skipping beats Abnormal lung and heart sounds or murmurs
Breasts	Skin smooth: in primigravidae, the breasts firm and supple; in multigravidae, the breasts less firm and old striae may be seen. The areola pigmented and veins are prominent from eight weeks. The nipples and Montgomery's follicles are enlarged by 12 weeks. Secondary areola appears and colostrum can be expressed from 16 weeks. The nipples are supple and prominent and do not retract when gently squeezed between the fingers, just behind the nipple.	Lumps and/or coarse 'orange-peel' appearance of skin of the breast may indicate carcinoma. Tender lumps, or areas of redness and heat may indicate infection. Nipples that are flat, depressed, inverted, bifid (cleft), or have any cracks or lesions Supernumerary or auxiliary breasts may be present.
Abdomen	Probable signs of pregnancy include linea nigra and striae gravidarum.	An unduly large abdomen may indicate a big baby or multiple pregnancy.
Legs	Good muscle tone Symmetrical legs Normal skin colour No lesions or varicose veins Joints of normal size and mobility Feet and toes normal and all the toes present (no extra digits)	Abnormalities/deformities of feet and toes may be due to congenital disorders or accidents. Very small feet may suggest a small pelvis. Oedema of feet and/or legs (pitting on digital pressure): If oedema is present, note how extensive it is. Extensive oedema accompanied by proteinuria or raised BP may indicate pre-eclampsia.

continued

System	Normal	Abnormal
Legs (continued)	Femoral pulses present No oedema	Varicose veins may indicate blood disorders.
Back	Normal spinal curves, with possible increased lumbar curve in late pregnancy and therefore often some backache	Spinal deformities eg kyphosis, abnormal curves; spina bifida Severe backache, especially in early pregnancy
External genitalia (vulva) and perineum	Covered with hair in an inverted triangular shape Normal appearance: no lumps or lesions Vulva moist, with normal secretions Perineum of normal length and thickness	Anatomical abnormalities may indicate congenital deformities, cystocele or rectocele or a prolapsed uterus. Rashes, lumps, warts or lesions may be due to infections, diabetes mellitus, abscesses, STIs or cancer. Abnormal vaginal discharges and offensive odours may indicate infections such as *Monilia*, *Trichomonas* or STIs such as gonorrhoea. A very wide or very thick, rigid perineum Perineal scars may indicate previous episiotomy or perineal tears. How much scar tissue is there; was the wound well sutured?
Buttocks and anal area	Normal appearance	Any abnormalities such as congenital deformities, bleeding or haemorrhoids, anal fissures, rectal prolapse Sacral pilonidal sinus Rashes, lumps, tenderness, excoriation, etc may be due to allergies, infections, abscesses, diarrhoea.

Abdominal examination

The process of abdominal examination includes inspection, palpation and auscultation (described in Chapter 18). Abdominal palpation is essential in all women. However, it can only be significant if the woman is 24 weeks and above or when fetal parts become palpable, particularly the head. Its purposes are to:

▶ confirm the signs of pregnancy
▶ estimate the period of gestation
▶ estimate the growth of the fetus
▶ identify the lie, presentation, position and engagement of the fetus
▶ identify any deviations from normal
▶ estimate the relationship between the fetus and the pelvis.

These findings are compared with all other information gathered in pregnancy.

Special examinations

In pregnancy, women undergo essential investigations as well as special screening tests for those who present with deviations from normal (in both the mother and the fetus). Ward tests or side-room tests are quick and inexpensive and do not require laboratories or specialised staff. These tests are used for screening and more accurate testing is done if a problem is suspected. The boxes below and on the next page list the essential or standard tests in pregnancy, as well as the special tests currently available in the public sector in South Africa.

Essential routine screening tests in pregnancy

Essential screening tests may be done as side-room tests or blood may be collected and sent to the laboratory.
Essential screening tests include the following:

▶ Pap smear: before 28 weeks or at six weeks postpartum
▶ Urinalysis for protein, sugar and ketones (each visit)

continued

- Hb level: This can be estimated using the portable haemoglobinometer or copper sulphate screening method. If within the normal range, this is repeated at about 32 weeks' gestation or 36 weeks' gestation in preparation for labour. If below 12 g/dl, it is repeated more frequently.
- A rapid plasma reagin (RPR) test for primary or secondary syphilis: If the RPR test is positive, this should be confirmed by the *Treponema pallidum* haemagglutination (TPHA) test, especially for false positive results from RPR and also for tertiary syphilis.
- ABO blood grouping
- Rh factor: If the woman is Rh negative, a medical practitioner is advised and blood is tested for the antibody titre, and repeated at specified intervals. The husband or partner's blood is also tested for Rh factor. Rh (D) blood group is done by using a rapid test.
- Hepatitis B antigen
- HIV serology using a rapid test kit.

Special screening tests in pregnancy

Special tests are carried out on a particular woman as indicated by the identified need based on health assessment findings. These tests include:
- the triple test for abnormalities at 16 weeks
- the fluorescent *in situ* hybridisation (FISH) test for selected abnormalities after 18 weeks
- ultrasound at 12 and 20 weeks to exclude fetal abnormalities
- rubella testing before 20 weeks, if exposed
- blood glucose screening, if indicated
- urine microscopy, culture and sensitivities (MC&S), in women with history of preterm labour and UTIs.

Vaginal and cervical investigations

Vaginal examinations are not routinely done in pregnancy, but it may be necessary for the medical practitioner or the midwife to take the following specimens for laboratory investigation:
- Pap smear (before 28 weeks)
- A high vaginal swab if there is an undiagnosed vaginal discharge.

Special assessments

If there are indications of specific problems, the woman may be referred for a higher level of care or specialised care. Special assessments may include any of the following:

- Nutritional assessment, if the MUAC is more than 33 cm or less than 23 cm (see Chapter 51).
- Mental health assessment, if there is a history of mental health problems or previous postnatal depression (PND) or psychosis (see Chapter 13).
- HIV counselling and testing; the latest maternal guidelines from the Department of Health (DoH, 2015a) require universal testing of pregnant women (see Chapter 50).
- Genetic counselling, if there is a history of congenital abnormalities or if the woman falls into a risk category.

The care plan

After the woman has been assessed, the care plan will be instituted, based on:
- the gestational period
- factors present that place the woman in a category that requires a higher level of care or specialised care.

Routine care

All pregnant women should receive basic iron and folic acid supplementation and tetanus toxoid immunisation. All other interventions will be planned according to the antenatal protocols for specific conditions. Women who are categorised for a higher level of care are referred for follow-up at that level. Women who are categorised as low risk are scheduled for BANC.

Low or high risk

The initial visit is aimed at the identification of risk factors in the woman's history, based on her current physical status or during basic screening. As mentioned, the BANC checklist should be used to assess and categorise women into one of two groups, namely (DoH, 2015a: 42):
1. those qualifying for the BANC programme
2. those requiring a higher level of care, who are then referred for medical care.

Danger signs

The woman should be educated on the danger signs of pregnancy. She should be instructed to immediately report to the clinic or hospital, or seek medical assistance, if she experiences:
- headaches
- blurred vision, seeing stars or dots
- abdominal pain (epigastric)
- a leaking of abdominal fluid
- vaginal bleeding
- reduced fetal movement (kick chart)

- contractions
- vomiting.

Self-care or health information

The woman should be given information on:
- nutrition and exercise
- hygiene and breast care (breast examination)
- medication (see Chapter 53)
- avoiding smoking, alcohol and over-the-counter medication and traditional medication.

17.4 Conclusion

This chapter explored health screening and planning, based on the first antenatal visit. The first antenatal visit should ideally be before 20 weeks, to allow for the early identification of potential risk and to allow time for intervention and development of a care plan for the pregnancy with the mother and family. Late contact with the mother puts the pregnancy and fetus at risk, even if the mother has four antenatal visits. All health services should have clear referral routes and support services for high-risk cases, even if there is outreach available through advanced midwifery or medical support.

18

Maternal obstetric care and fetal surveillance with emphasis on follow-up visits

LEARNING OBJECTIVES

On completion of this chapter, you must be able to:

▸ monitor the well-being of low-risk pregnant women
▸ give appropriate basic antenatal follow-up care in pregnancy
▸ make an accurate diagnosis on the progress of the pregnancy and fetal growth and well-being in order to act appropriately
▸ identify and refer women with risk factors to a higher level of care
▸ effectively observe the growth and development of the fetus (fetal surveillance) and refer appropriately
▸ plot information correctly on an antenatal chart and keep accurate records
▸ develop skills in fetal surveillance and the interpretation of findings.

KNOWLEDGE ASSUMED TO BE IN PLACE

The potential psychological, sociological and physiological effects of pregnancy on the woman and her family
The scientific nursing process
Basic Antenatal Care (BANC) and auditing according to Chapter 4 of the *Guidelines for Maternity Care in South Africa* (DoH, 2015a)

KEYWORDS

follow-up visits • low and high risks in pregnancy • fetal surveillance

18.1 Introduction

The first antenatal visit should ideally occur before 20 weeks of pregnancy. This will enable the midwife to diagnose the pregnancy, take a general and obstetric history, do a physical examination and carry out the needed routine, essential and special examinations to:

▸ identify risks
▸ ensure maternal well-being
▸ monitor fetal growth and development.

However, some women present for the first time in the second trimester or even at birth. In such cases, all the observations and tests described in Chapter 17 should still be performed.

Women whose antenatal care started before 20 weeks will return for follow-up care as indicated by the Basic Antenatal Care (BANC) protocols. This chapter describes the standard care during follow-up visits, including screening, clinical and obstetric assessment and clinical examinations, namely abdominal palpitation and pelvimetry. Lastly, various methods of fetal surveillance are discussed.

18.2 Classification and scheduling of antenatal care

As mentioned, antenatal care should preferably be commenced as soon as possible, but not later than 20 weeks of pregnancy. Women who qualify for BANC, or low-risk care, will be scheduled for a further minimum of eight visits, depending on the stage of the pregnancy (DoH, 2015a).

Women who do not qualify for BANC will be referred and a specific programme or plan will be developed for them, including the specific interventions and the number of visits needed. Such women will be observed by an advanced or specialist midwife, a medical practitioner, obstetrician or specialist, depending on the problem. If the fetus is not growing, is abnormal or at risk, the woman may be cared for by a perinatologist. In rural or outlying areas where obstetricians are not readily available, advanced midwives may give weekly care at high-risk clinics. Alternatively, a medical practitioner may provide care in conjunction with weekly outreach services. In severe cases – when the mother or baby is in danger – the woman would be transferred in an obstetric ambulance to the nearest appropriate level of care.

Care for BANC clients

The purpose of the follow-up visits for low-risk BANC clients is to provide appropriate care for the woman, to monitor fetal growth and development and to observe for danger signs.

Antenatal visit schedules

The WHO recommends a minimum of eight antenatal visits for a pregnant woman who started to attend antenatal care before 20 weeks. Should any risk factors be identified, the visits will be adapted as needed. If the woman did not attend antenatal care, she is considered to be 'unbooked' and care is then focused on all aspects from the first visit.

The following guidelines can be followed in scheduling antenatal visits:

▶ BANC consists of a schedule of a minimum of eight follow-up visits. This schedule is applicable to women with no known risk factors at that stage.
▶ If a woman had her first visit before 12 weeks, return visits should be scheduled for 20, 26, 30, 34, 36, 38 and 40 weeks.
▶ If a woman reports late for the first visit, the return visits are scheduled according to the findings of the gestational age (GA). If all the tests have been done, the woman may have to return sooner for a re-evaluation, or be notified to return should it be necessary.

Standard routine BANC during follow-up visits

The following tasks must be completed during the follow-up visit (DoH, 2015a: 43):

▶ Revisit the woman's history and take the history of any problems that the woman may have experienced since the last visit.
▶ Assess the woman's needs.
▶ Give antenatal advice on physical exercise.
▶ Discuss a provisional plan for delivery and emergency transport.

▶ Do a routine assessment, including:
  • basic vital data (maternal well-being)
  • urine test: evaluate the results from previous tests and repeat or follow-up tests, eg mid-stream urine for microscopy, culture and sensitivity (MC&S)
  • fetal surveillance to monitor the progress of growth and development.
▶ Monitor the continuation of oral supplementation and Hb levels.
▶ Do routine specific observations for the level of pregnancy and plot the results on the antenatal card.
▶ Complete the BANC checklist and institute the required actions.
▶ Give appropriate health education.

MOMConnect

In the public sector, women have the option of enrolling for a free service called Mobile Alliance for Maternal Action (MAMA) through the mobile health tool MOMConnect. This tool creates awareness of the health services available on the national database from the twenty-first week of pregnancy. Appropriate SMS messages are sent according to the stage of pregnancy. These messages continue for one year after birth.

Return care for women with risk factors

Return visits for women with risk factors are scheduled depending on their specific problems. This includes referral to a high-risk clinic, advanced midwife or medical practitioner. Risk factors that indicate the need for referral are listed in Table 18.1 on the next page. Alternatively, women may be admitted to a hospital or maternity waiting home, should such facilities be available in the district.

Maternity waiting homes

The South African government advocates for and supports maternity waiting homes – homes designed to cater for pregnant women with complications or high-risk pregnancies, or those who live far away from healthcare facilities. Once labour starts, the woman can easily be transferred to a maternity ward. Women who live far from birthing facilities and whose lives or babies may be in danger should have the opportunity to stay close to a facility where safe care is readily available. Each province or district is urged to create such facilities.

Table 18.1

Risk factors indicating the need for interventions (DoH, 2015a)

Obstetric history	Current pregnancy	Risk factors that arise during antenatal care
Previous stillbirth Previous neonatal death Previous low birth weight (LBW): < 2.5 kg Previous large baby: > 4.5 kg Previous pregnancy admission for hypertension or pre-eclampsia/eclampsia Previous Caesarean section Previous myomectomy Previous cone biopsy Previous cervical cerclage Previous Rh isoimmunisation	Diagnosed or suspected multiple pregnancy Age < 16 years Age ≥ 37 years Rh isoimmunisation Vaginal bleeding Pelvic mass General medical conditions Diabetes mellitus Cardiac disease Kidney disease	Anaemia that does not respond to iron tablets Uterus large for dates: > 90th percentile symphysis fundal height (SFH) Uterus small for dates: < 10th percentile SFH SFH decreasing below 10th percentile Breech or transverse lie at term Extensive vulval warts that may obstruct vaginal delivery Pregnancy beyond 41 weeks Abnormal glucose screening: glucose tolerance test (GTT) or random blood sugar Reduced fetal movements after 28 weeks

Risk factors requiring hospital delivery	
Obstetric history	**Current pregnancy**
Previous postpartum haemorrhage (PPH) Parity ≥ 5	Epilepsy Asthma (on medication) Active tuberculosis Known substance abuse, including alcohol Any severe medical condition

18.3 Routine care in BANC

The BANC programme highlights factors that should be prioritised during the four antenatal visits (DoH, 2015a: 44). Regulation 2488 (of 26 October 1990) of the South African Nursing Council (SANC) guides midwives on the conditions under which registered and enrolled midwives may carry out their profession. This serves as a standard of care against which they are accountable in practice.

HIV-positive women are referred for specialised care. The following aspects, which are discussed in the rest of the chapter, are included in the routine antenatal care of HIV-negative women:
▶ Screening
▶ Clinical and obstetric assessments, such as BP, hypertension, weight and SFH
▶ Clinical examinations, including:
  • abdominal palpitation and auscultation
  • pelvimetry
▶ Providing information to the woman
▶ Record keeping
▶ Fetal surveillance.

Activity

Compare the BANC checklist (Pattinson, 2007) with the SANC Regulation 2488 dated 26 October 1990. Chapter 1 of the BANC checklist and Regulations 4, 5, 6 and 10 of R2488 reflect on the professional duty of the midwife.

Screening

At the first visit, a history is taken (see Chapter 17) to determine if the woman is eligible for BANC or whether she should be classified as high risk and referred. At each follow-up visit, the midwife reviews the findings of the previous visits:
▶ Ensure that the estimated date of delivery (EDD) is calculated correctly. GA must be calculated from the first day of the last normal menstrual period or by carrying out early ultrasound before 20 weeks, which is more accurate. Note that the EDD estimation is only valid if the woman is sure of her dates, and where palpation of the uterus and

SFH measurements are compatible with the given dates (see figures 17C and 17D on pages 230 and 231).

▶ Be sure to revisit the tests done at the first visit for HIV, TB, anaemia, Rh factor and diabetes.

To revise, the tests that should be done at the first visit are the following:

▶ *HIV and TB:* Ensure that voluntary testing and counselling are done and make sure that the HIV test results are in the file. Screen for TB (current cough, fever, loss of weight, drenching night-sweats).

▶ *Anaemia:* Do an Hb test and ensure that the Hb has been tested after 20 weeks and repeated after 30 weeks. Respond appropriately to Hb of 10 mg/100 ml and lower.

▶ *Rh factor:* Perform a rapid Rh test and ensure that the Rh test is recorded.

▶ *Urine test (dipstix):* Urine is tested at each visit.
  • If protein is detected in the urine, it may indicate an infection. A midstream test is then required.
  • Glucose in urine during pregnancy is common and may be considered normal, but should be followed up.
  • If ketones are also present, it may indicate diabetes.
  • The cause of the presence of blood in urine needs clarification.

Also refer to figures 17C and 17D on pages 230 and 231.

Clinical and obstetric assessments

The following assessments need to be done at each follow-up visit:

▶ *Observation of BP:* Follow best practice guidelines for accuracy. The woman's BP should be evaluated against the GA and risks at each visit. The correct cuff size should be used and standard procedures followed, with the woman in the left lateral position to avoid the inferior vena cava syndrome (IVCS).

▶ *Hypertension:* Ask questions about possible headaches, visual disturbances (seeing stars) and pain in the upper quadrant of the stomach at each visit to detect risk for hypertension disease in pregnancy and related problems.

▶ *Observation of weight gain:* Women should gain 8–12 kg in pregnancy in general. Insufficient weight gain after 20 weeks of gestation needs further consideration. Women who are obese are at risk for miscalculations due to difficulty in taking accurate BP readings and abdominal palpations.

▶ *SFH:* Serial SFH measurements are done mainly to determine uterine size for intrauterine growth restriction (IUGR) and to do fetal surveillance. The

SFH measurements taken between 20 and 36 weeks and serial measures are plotted on a graph and must show constant growth of the uterus correlating with all other parameters, such as the last menstrual period (LMP), EDD and ultrasound done before 20 weeks. Excessive uterine growth may indicate multiple pregnancy or polyhydramnios. Conditions or deviations such as breech presentation after 34 weeks can be detected and should be referred.

Providing information

During each visit, give the woman clear and accurate information about the following aspects:

▶ Explain the results of the tests.

▶ Discuss future plans regarding the care needed and the number of visits preferred.

▶ Discuss plans regarding the delivery mode, place of birth and professional support as well as transport to a birth unit, clinic or hospital.

▶ Discuss plans for lactation and contraception after birth.

▶ Discuss danger signs in pregnancy. Explore all options for emergencies and record such.

▶ Clinic checklist: Determine a follow-up date according to the findings. If the pregnancy reaches 41 weeks, refer the woman to a high-risk clinic to be seen within one week.

▶ Refer to higher care as needed.

Record keeping

Record all information on the antenatal card or maternity case record (MCR) and give this to the woman to carry with her in case she needs to be hospitalised.

18.4 Clinical examinations

At each antenatal visit, abdominal palpation and pelvimetry are carried out.

Abdominal palpation

Abdominal examination is a clinical skill used by midwives or doctors to gather information on the number of fetuses *in utero*, the lie and presentation of the fetus, the amniotic fluid volume and fetal size and growth. The fetal parts are mainly palpable after 30 weeks of pregnancy. In the second trimester, the head and back can be palpable through the uterus, but the position is only determined in the third trimester. The following subsections discuss the basic knowledge that a midwife must master for effective practice.

The relationship between the fetus and pelvis

Midwives should be familiar with the terms used to describe the relationship of the fetus to the uterus and pelvis, such as lie, attitude, presentation, denominator, position, presenting part and engagement. This knowledge will enable the midwife to identify any deviations from the normal and take appropriate action.

Lie

The lie is the relationship of the long axis of the fetus (spine) to that of the long axis of the mother (spinal column). The lie may be longitudinal, transverse or oblique, with either the head or the breech occupying the lower pole of the uterus. If the head is in the lower pole, the lie is cephalic and if the lie is breech, it is podalic.

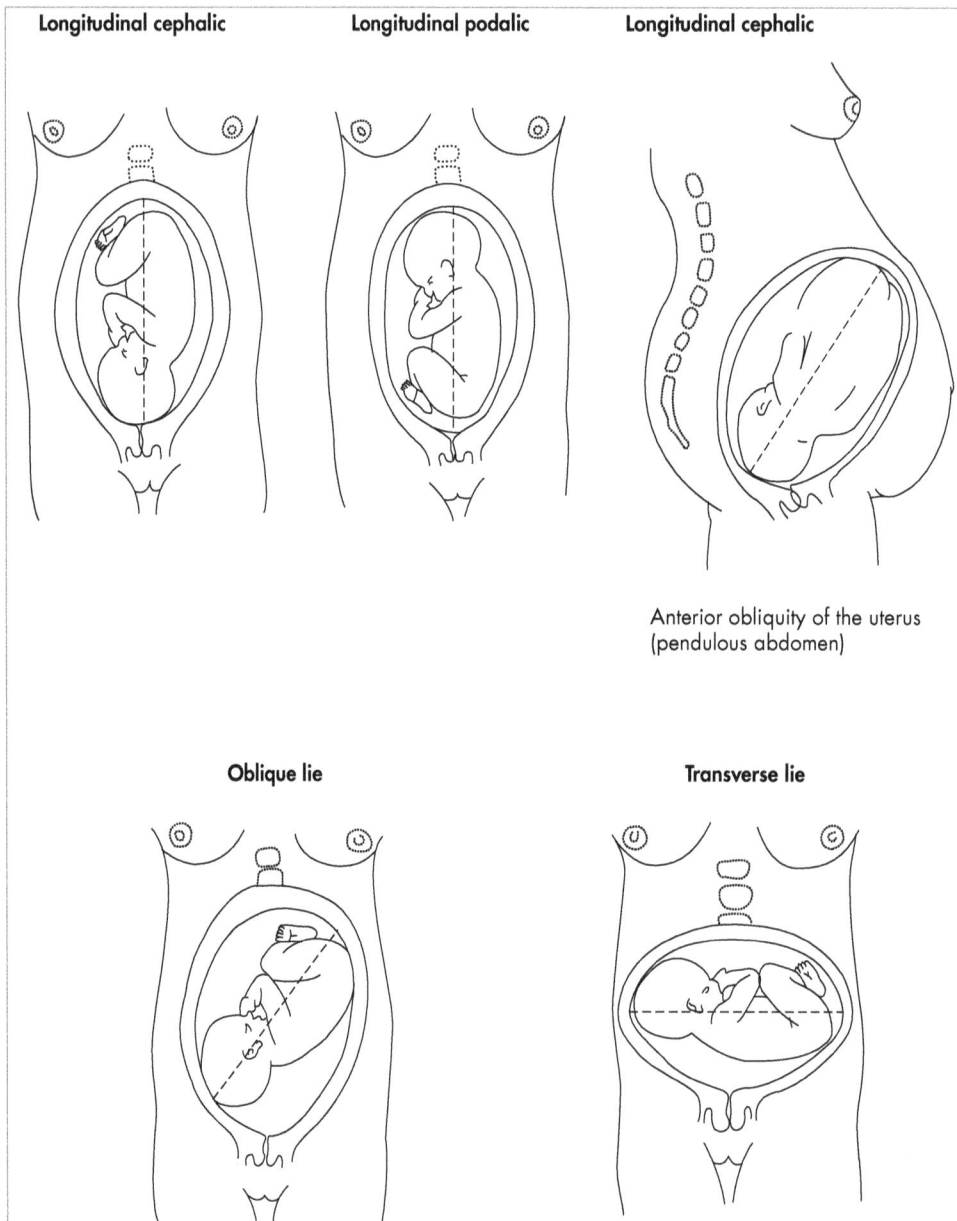

Figure 18.1 Variations in the lie of a fetus

In a transverse or an oblique lie, the long axis of the fetus (spinal column) lies across (either perpendicular to or at an oblique angle to) the maternal spinal column in the uterine cavity. A shoulder usually occupies the lower pole of the uterus and lies over the pelvic brim, but in rare instances an arm or some part of the trunk may present at the pelvic brim. A transverse lie is an extremely serious condition, because the fetus (unless very small) would be unable to pass through the pelvic canal and an obstructed labour would result.

In conditions such as grand multiparity, multiple pregnancy and polyhydramnios, where there is overstretching of the uterine muscles and a reduction in muscle tone, the uterus becomes round instead of ovoid and may not support the fetus in a longitudinal lie.

Attitude

The attitude of the fetus is the relationship of the fetal parts to one another – that is, the relationship of the fetal limbs and head to the fetal trunk. The attitude position is normally flexion, but can be deflexion or extension:

▶ *Flexion.* Normally, the fetus adopts the attitude of full flexion (fetal position). The fetus usually lies with its back curved slightly in a C-shape, so that the head is bent forward or flexed, with the chin on the chest, and the buttocks bent forward with the thighs flexed onto the abdomen. The lower legs are flexed onto the thighs and the arms are bent and flexed onto the chest. The diameters of the fetal head that present in flexion are the most favourable for passing through the pelvis.

The biparietal of 9.5 cm and the suboccipitobregmatic of 9.5 cm presenting in this case forms a round circle. This facilitates good application on the cervix with good contractions, referred to as the Ferguson reflex.

▶ *Deflexion.* In this attitude, the fetal back is straight, with the head deflexed and upright on the spine (also called the 'military attitude'). The limbs remain flexed on the fetal trunk. Larger diameters of the head will lie over the pelvic brim.

▶ *Extension.* The upper spine is curved backwards, with the head bent backwards so that the occiput approaches the spine. The face of the fetus lies at the opposite pole to the buttocks and in a cephalic presentation the face will engage at the pelvic brim. The limbs remain flexed on the fetal trunk.

Presentation

The presentation is (see Figure 18.3 on the next page) that part of the fetus that lies in the lower pole of the uterus and which presents at the pelvic brim. The presentation may be a vertex, breech, face, shoulder or brow presentation:

▶ *Vertex presentation.* The largest diameters of the head that present in a well-flexed vertex presentation are the suboccipito (with a bregmatic diameter of 9.5 cm) and, at right angles to and bisecting this diameter, the biparietal diameter (BPD) (which is also 9.5 cm). This means that the circumference of the part of the head that presents is round and symmetrical and that the largest diameters of the head are smaller than the narrowest diameters of the pelvic canal.

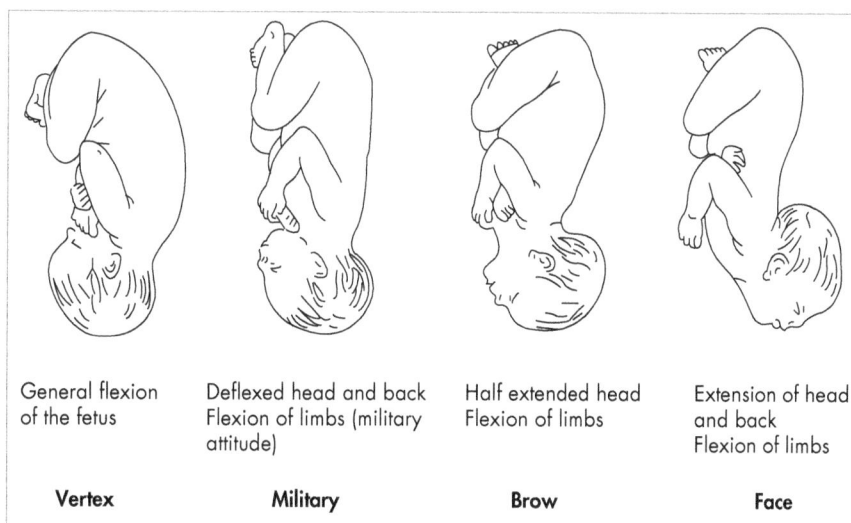

General flexion of the fetus	Deflexed head and back Flexion of limbs (military attitude)	Half extended head Flexion of limbs	Extension of head and back Flexion of limbs
Vertex	**Military**	**Brow**	**Face**

Figure 18.2 Attitude

A. Vertex presentation

B. Face presentation

C. Brow presentation

D. Complete breech

D₁ Frank breech

D₂ Footing breech

D₃ Kneeling breech

E. Shoulder presentation

F. Compound presentation

G. Cord presentation

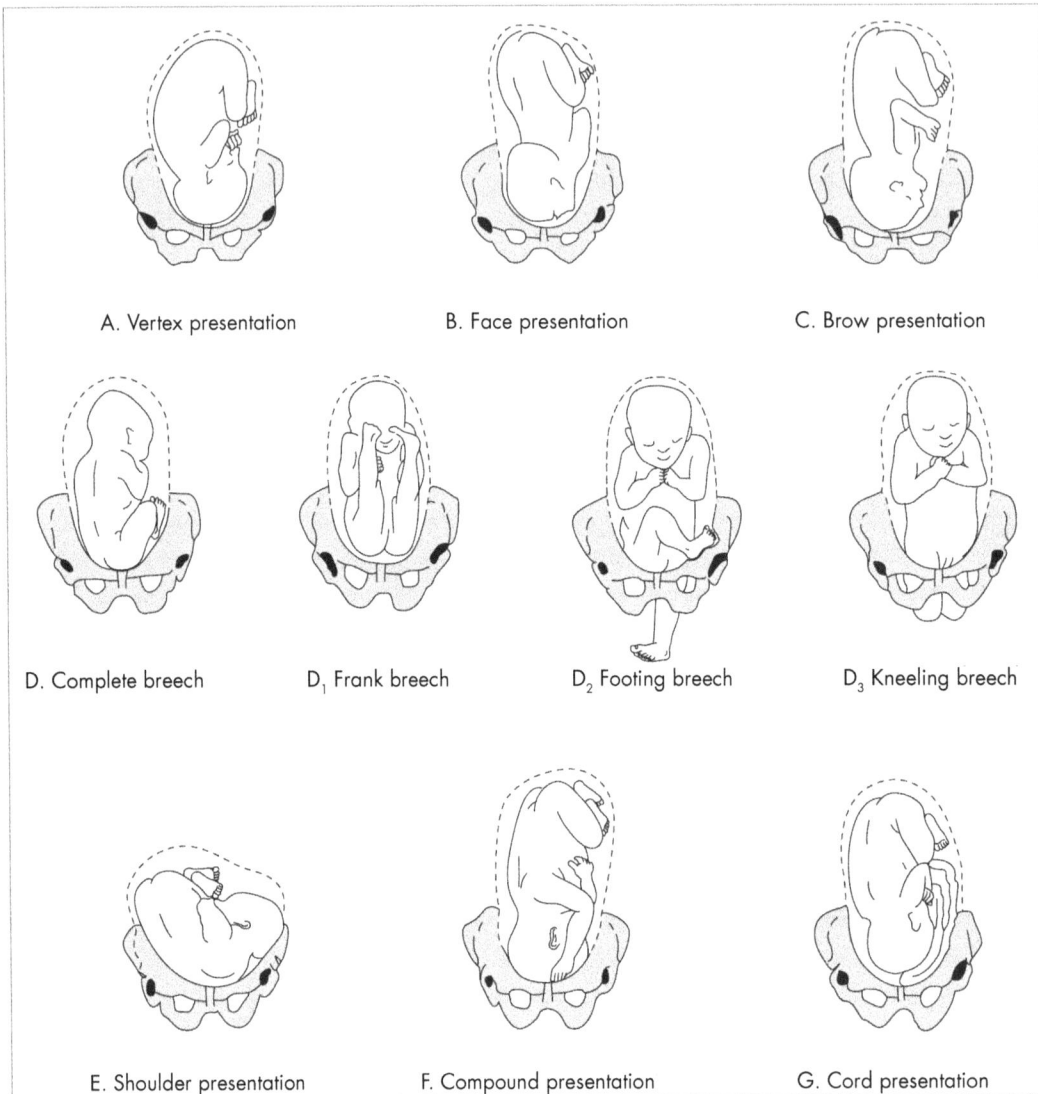

Figure 18.3 Variations in presentation of the fetus

▶ *Breech presentation.* When the lie is longitudinal and the buttocks of the fetus present at the pelvic brim, this is called a breech presentation. This type of presentation is often present between 26 and 34 weeks, because the small fetus is able to move freely in the plentiful liquor amnii and the uterine walls are as yet not able to confine the fetal form. The attitude of the fetus can be that of general flexion, with the buttocks and the feet presenting, or one or both legs may be extended at the knee. If both legs are extended, it is a frank breech and on abdominal palpation the fetal form would feel longer and thinner than normal for the gestational period. The extended legs would also cause splinting of the fetal body, possibly preventing it

from turning spontaneously or from being turned into a vertex presentation. A breech presentation in the second half of the third trimester is a serious condition; a breech delivery holds many potential hazards for the baby, and the woman must be seen by a medical practitioner. Breech presentation may be an indication of cephalopelvic disproportion (CPD). Very rarely, a foot or a knee may present, mainly in preterm birth; this is considered a complicating factor.

▶ *Face presentation.* In a face presentation, the lie is longitudinal and the presentation cephalic, but the attitude of the fetus is one of complete extension of the head and the face enters the pelvis. This rare presentation may deliver vaginally if the fetal chin is anterior (mentoanterior), as the diameters are similar to those in the vertex presentation. However, mentotransverse and mentoposterior presentations usually cause prolonged labour or obstructed labour. All face presentations must be referred immediately for medical intervention.

▶ *Brow presentation.* The brow presents at the pelvic brim when the head of the fetus is halfway between flexion and extension in a longitudinal lie of the cephalic type (military position). The diameter that attempts to enter the pelvic brim in a brow presentation is larger than any of the diameters in an average-sized pelvis and the fetal head may become caught up in the pelvic brim, causing obstructed labour. This presentation is usually only diagnosed when the woman is in advanced labour and the woman must be seen by a medical practitioner immediately.

▶ *Shoulder presentation.* The shoulder may present at the pelvic brim in a transverse lie. In this presentation the fetus is unable to negotiate the pelvic canal and the labour will become obstructed. As this is an extremely serious condition and the life of both the fetus and the mother are at risk, the woman must be referred immediately to a medical practitioner. Very rarely, a hand may present.

▶ *Compound presentation.* In a compound presentation, a prolapsed hand and/or foot may present together with the head, or a hand may present with the breech. This could be diagnosed on vaginal examination. There is a risk of cord presentation or prolapse.

The denominator

The denominator is that part (landmark) of the presentation that indicates the position of the presentation in relation to the pelvic brim and gives the position its name. This is the part that is felt first on vaginal examination. The occiput becomes the leading part in a normal vertex presentation and the mentum (chin) in a face presentation. Note the following:

▶ The occiput is the denominator in a cephalic presentation.
▶ The sacrum is the denominator in a breech presentation.
▶ The mentum is the denominator in a face presentation.
▶ The acromion process is the denominator in a shoulder presentation.

Position

The position of the fetus is indicated by the relationship of the denominator to six points or landmarks on the pelvic brim (see Figure 18.4 on the next page). The landmarks on the pelvic brim are:

▶ anteriorly: the left and right iliopectineal eminences
▶ laterally: the mid-point of the iliopectineal line on either side of the pelvis (the widest diameter of the brim in a gynaecoid pelvis)
▶ posteriorly: the left and right sacroiliac joints.

In a cephalic presentation with the occiput as the denominator, the position may be as indicated as in Table 18.2.

Table 18.2

Position in a cephalic presentation with occiput denominator

Landmark on pelvic brim	Description
Left occipitoanterior (LOA)	The occiput lies adjacent to the left iliopectineal eminence. The sagittal suture of the fetal skull will lie in the right oblique diameter of the pelvis, with the posterior fontanelle lying anteriorly and to the left of the pelvis and the anterior fontanelle lying posteriorly and to the right of the pelvis. The oblique diameters of the pelvis are always named from the posterior – that is, from the sacroiliac joint on the left or right of the pelvis, which corresponds to the woman's left or right hand.
Right occipitoanterior (ROA)	The occiput lies adjacent to the right iliopectineal eminence. The sagittal suture of the fetal skull will lie in the left oblique diameter of the pelvis, with the posterior fontanelle lying anteriorly and to the right of the pelvis and the anterior fontanelle lying posteriorly and to the left of the pelvis.
Left occipitoposterior (LOP)	The occiput lies adjacent to the left sacroiliac joint. The sagittal suture of the fetal skull will lie in the left oblique diameter of the pelvis, with the posterior fontanelle lying to the left and posteriorly, and the anterior fontanelle lying to the right and anteriorly in the pelvis.
Right occipitoposterior (ROP)	The occiput lies adjacent to the right sacroiliac joint. The sagittal suture of the fetal skull will lie in the right oblique diameter of the pelvis, with the posterior fontanelle lying to the right and posteriorly and the anterior fontanelle lying to the left and anteriorly in the pelvis.

± 7%	ROP		LOP	± 3%
± 25%	ROL		LOL	± 40%
± 10%	ROA		LOA	± 15%

Diagram of the six cephalic positions and their approximate frequency

Right occipitoposterior

Left occipitoposterior

Right occipitolateral (ROL)

Left occipitolateral (LOL)

Right occipitoanterior

Left occipitoanterior

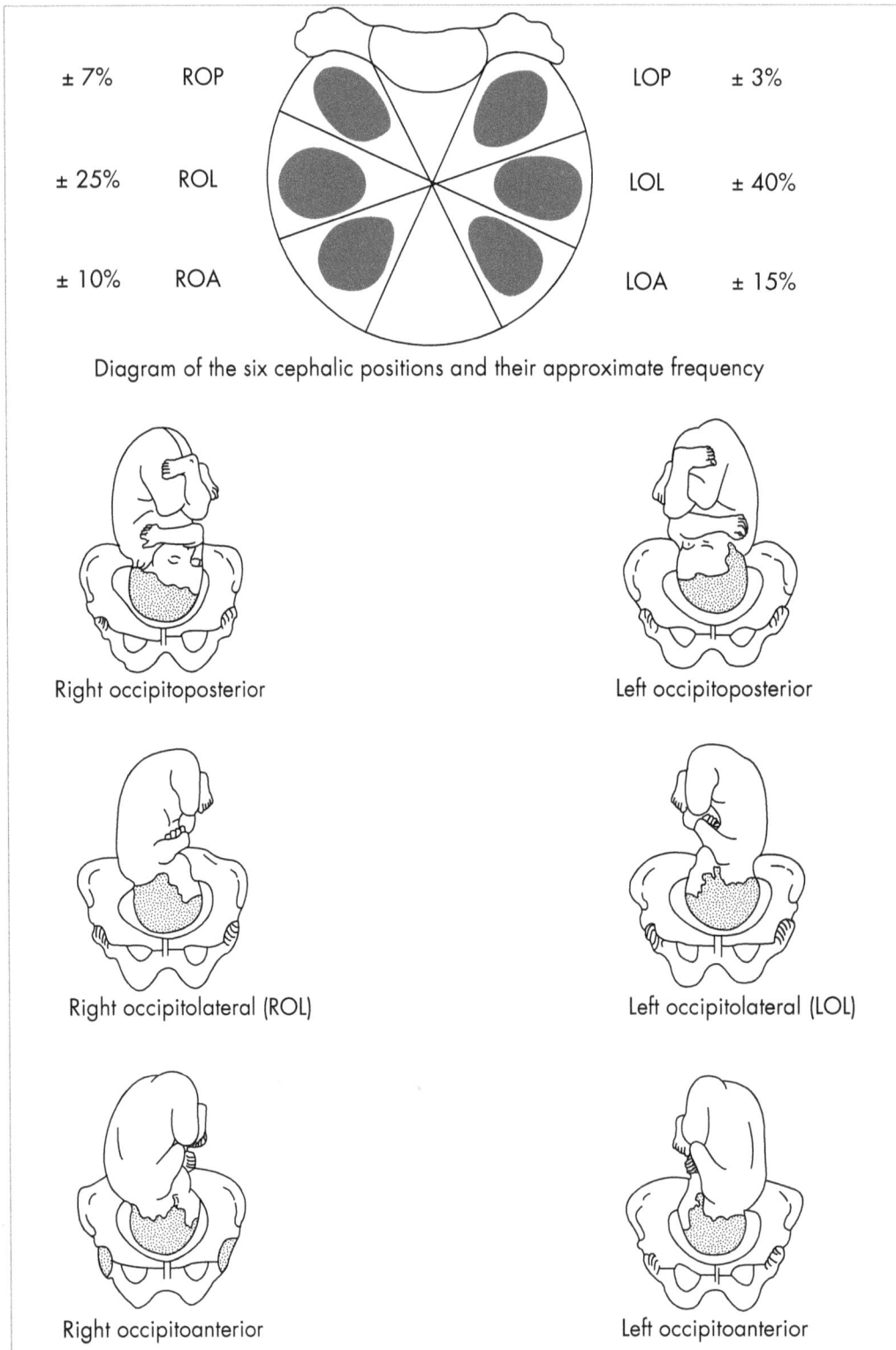

Figure 18.4 Six positions of the fetus in a cephalic presentation

The lateral and anterior positions occur more frequently in a cephalic presentation, because the curved fetal back is more easily accommodated against the concavity of the woman's abdomen than against the rigid spine. There is also more room in the lateral and anterior portions of a gynaecoid pelvis for the broad biparietal diameter of the fetal head.

The LOP is the least frequent position in cephalic presentations, as the descending colon takes up a large part of this area in the pelvic cavity. In a cephalic presentation, when the abdomen is palpated, the back of the fetus will be found on the same side of the abdomen as the denominator (the occiput). This will also apply in a breech presentation, but not in a face presentation.

Positions in breech and face presentations

In breech and face presentations, these positions will correspond to those of the cephalic presentation, with only the denominator changing. In breech and face presentations, the sacrum (S) and the mentum (M) respectively take the place of the occiput in the cephalic presentation:
- LSA and LMA correspond to LOA.
- RSA and RMA correspond to ROA.
- LSL and LML correspond to LOL.
- RSL and RML correspond to ROL.
- LSP and LMP correspond to LOP.
- RSP and RMP correspond to ROP.

The presenting part

The presenting part is that part of the presentation that lies over the cervical os during labour. It is therefore upon this portion of the presentation that the caput forms.

Descent of the presenting part

The amount of descent of the presenting part (fetal head or sacrum) into the mother's pelvis is assessed on abdominal examination and is calculated as fifths of the fetal head above the pelvic brim.

At 36 weeks, there is a slight descent of the fetus in the uterus, known as lightening. The descent of the fetal head within the uterus is brought about by increased pelvic vascularity, causing softening of the cervix, and by the taking up of the cervical canal due to the action of Braxton-Hicks contractions.

In multiparous women, who often have lax abdominal muscles that are unable to give good support to the uterus, the fundus of the uterus usually settles slightly forwards when the woman is standing and the abdomen becomes more prominent. In these women, the fetal head seldom engages in the pelvis before the onset of labour.

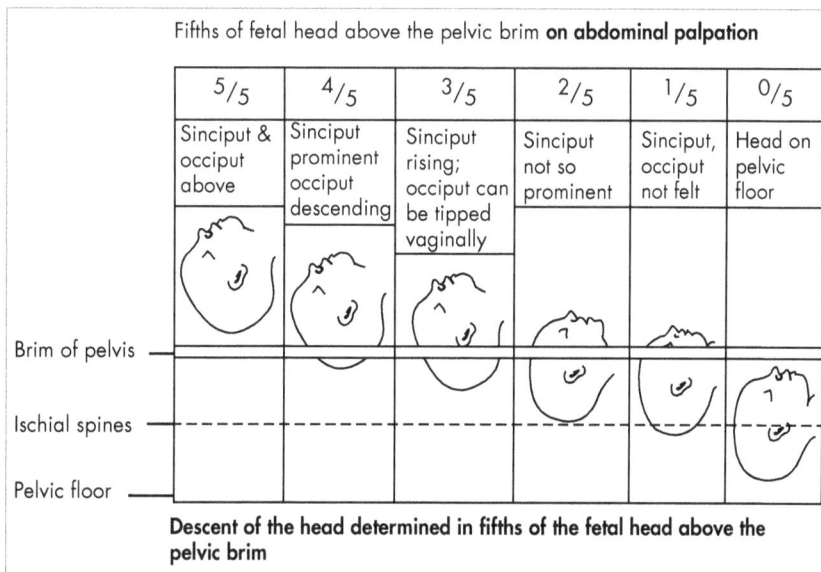

Fifths of fetal head above the pelvic brim **on abdominal palpation**					
$^5/_5$	$^4/_5$	$^3/_5$	$^2/_5$	$^1/_5$	$^0/_5$
Sinciput & occiput above	Sinciput prominent occiput descending	Sinciput rising; occiput can be tipped vaginally	Sinciput not so prominent	Sinciput, occiput not felt	Head on pelvic floor

Descent of the head determined in fifths of the fetal head above the pelvic brim

Figure 18.5 Engagement of the fetal head

Engagement of the presenting part

In a longitudinal lie of the cephalic presentation, engagement of the fetal head takes place when the largest presenting diameter *and* the BPD have passed through the brim of the pelvis. In a longitudinal lie, an engaged breech occurs when the bitrochanteric diameter has passed through the pelvic brim. However, this does not guarantee that the presenting diameters of the head, which comes after, will also be small enough to enter the pelvic brim.

Engagement of the fetal head is crucial to the delivery of the fetus, because unless these diameters have negotiated the pelvic brim, delivery cannot take place. The size of the fetal head (diameters), the presentation, the position, the moulding of the fetal head (with pliability and overriding of the fetal skull bones), together with the size of the pelvis, the degree of 'give' of the pelvic joints and the inclination of the pelvic brim, will all play a role in enabling the fetal head to engage. (See Chapter 8 for more on the fetal head, pelvic diameters and moulding.) Once engagement has taken place, delivery is usually possible, but there are instances where problems can still arise in the mid-cavity and the outlet of the pelvis.

Clinical significance of engagement

During abdominal palpation in the last few weeks of pregnancy, the midwife should check for engagement of the fetal head, especially in the primigravida or nullipara. If the head is not engaged, this should be recorded on the antenatal case notes.

Non-engagement of the fetal head at term is important in white and Asian primigravidae and could denote some CPD, with possible prolonged and difficult labour. In black women, however, it is not as significant, as a very much lower percentage of fetal heads are engaged before the onset of labour, possibly due to pelvis shape. Nevertheless, it should not be ignored.

Causes of non-engagement of the fetal head

It is important to know the different causes of non-engagement of the fetal head in order to be able to make a correct assessment during abdominal palpation. These include:

) an inaccurate calculation of EDD (the pregnancy is not as advanced as had been calculated)
) a full bladder (this may prevent the fetal head from entering the pelvis and therefore the bladder should be emptied before examination)
) large presenting diameters (a deflexed head, brow presentation, a large baby, hydrocephalus)
) a contracted pelvis
) polyhydramnios
) multiple pregnancy
) breech presentation or transverse or oblique lie
) placenta praevia
) tumours or abnormalities of the uterus, ovaries or pelvic structures
) a pendulous abdomen or anterior obliquity of the uterus
) unknown causes.

The station of the presenting part

The descent of the presenting part within the pelvis (on vaginal examination) and in relation to the ischial spines is known as the station of the presenting part (also see Chapter 8). Usually, the fetal head is engaged when the bony skull of the presenting part (not the caput succedaneum) has reached the level of the ischial spines at station 0.

The findings on abdominal palpation can be verified by vaginal examination. Vaginal examination is relevant when the woman is in labour, but it is not done routinely during the antenatal period.

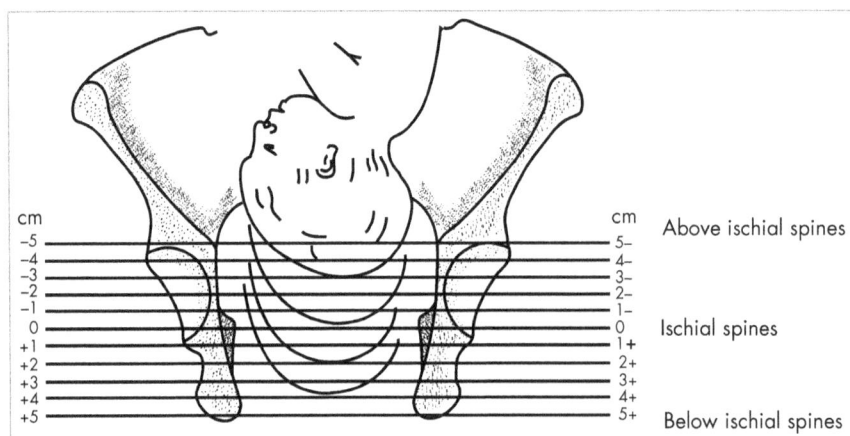

Figure 18.6 Stations of the presenting part on vaginal examination

PROCEDURE Abdominal examination

Abdominal examination includes inspection, palpation and auscultation.

Basic procedure and principles

▶ Always obtain informed consent before performing an abdominal palpation.
▶ Include the assistance of a chaperone or a translator during the procedure.
▶ Inform and reassure the woman during the procedure.
▶ Wash and warm your hands before the procedure.
▶ Advise the woman to empty her bladder.
▶ Position the woman as comfortably as possible on the examining bed at an adjusted angle of 30°. In later pregnancy, the patient should be positioned at a higher angle or in the left-lateral tilt position to avoid aortocaval compression.
▶ Expose the woman's abdomen, ideally from the lower chest (just below the breasts) to the symphysis pubis.
▶ Place a modesty sheet over the exposed area to maintain the woman's dignity.
▶ Right-handed healthcare professionals should stand on the woman's right-hand side, and vice versa.
▶ The procedure is done systematically, starting with inspection, followed by palpation and auscultation (see detailed notes in the rest of this box).
▶ Leopold's manoeuvres, which are a systematic way to determine the position of the fetus, describe the fundal grip, umbilical or lateral grip, Pawlick's and pelvic grips.
▶ Additional grips include the walking grip, moving the hands over the abdomen to feel for small parts, and the deep pelvic grip, similar to the pelvic grip.
▶ The presence of a fetal heart may confirm a pregnancy, but the absence of a fetal heart needs to be followed up with more investigations. Tumours and pseudo-pregnancies may occur.

Step 1: Inspection of the abdomen

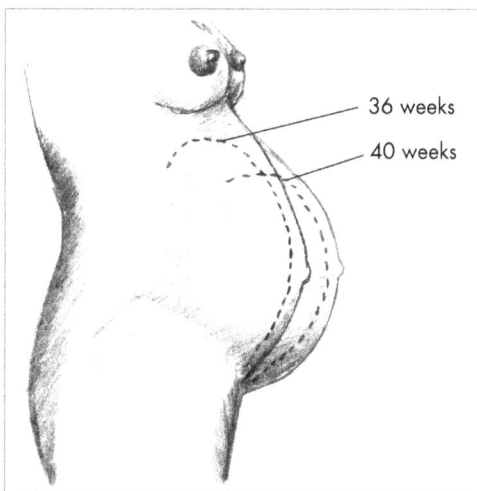

Figure 18A Size of fundus of the uterus

The shape and size of the uterus:
▶ The rounding and size of the uterus is normally visible at 12–14 weeks of gestation.
▶ The fundus of the uterus will reach the level of the umbilicus at around 20 weeks of gestation.
▶ The fundus of the uterus reaches maximum height at the level of the xiphisternum at 36 weeks.
▶ In a singleton pregnancy the uterus has a symmetrical, oval shape and a longitudinal lie.
▶ In a multiple pregnancy, or in the case of polyhydramnios, the shape of the uterus will be round.
▶ A 'flattened' (indented) lower abdomen suggests a vertex presentation with an occipitoposterior position (ROP or LOP).
▶ A suprapubic bulge suggests a full bladder or an OP position after 36 weeks.

continued

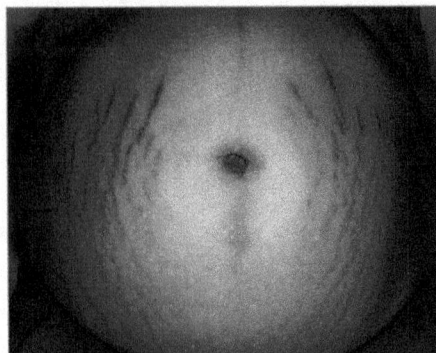

Figure 18B Striae gravidarum

Look for:
▶ any abdominal scars, such as laparoscopic and laparotomy scars, or scars due to physical abuse
▶ a Pfannenstiel scar (transverse, lower abdomen), which indicates a previous Caesarean section
▶ skin changes such as striae gravidarum (red and inflamed) or silvery grey skin on the lower abdomen, thighs and buttocks and the linea nigra (hyperpigmentation) of the midline linea alba
▶ fetal movements (visible after 24 weeks), which can be used as a way to confirm viability of the fetus
▶ a protruding umbilicus, which may indicate the possibility of an umbilical hernia
▶ a full bladder, which may be visible just beneath the umbilicus
▶ the presence of any rashes (determine the cause and document).

Step 2: Palpation

SFH measurement is done from 20 to 36 weeks. Measuring the fundal height is of little value before 20 weeks (when the fundus reaches the level of the umbilicus) and after more than 35 weeks' gestation. (The procedure for measuring the SFH is explained in Chapter 17, on pages 228–232.)

As the uterine ligaments and the pelvic viscera become more vascular and soften, and due to ripening of the cervix and partial effacement of the cervical canal, the presenting part descends and may even pass through the pelvic brim (inlet) into the pelvic cavity, causing the height of the fundus to drop. This is called lightening.

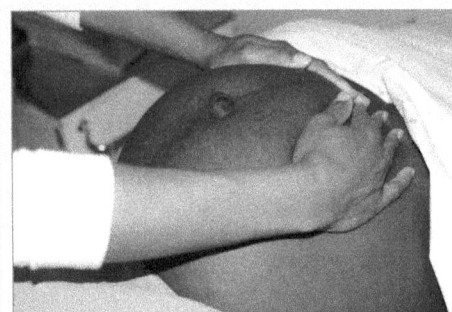

Figure 18C Bimanual fundal palpation (How many poles in the fundus?)

What is in the fundus? The fundal grip by means of Leopold's manoeuvres
▶ Facing the mother and using both hands, palpate the superior border of the fundus to determine the shape, size, consistency and mobility of the fetus in this part of the fundus.
▶ The fetal head is firm, hard and round and moves independently from the trunk.
▶ The breech feels softer and symmetrical. It moves with the trunk.
▶ Is there only one pole?

Alert: A bicornuate uterus or myoma can give a false indication of a second baby.

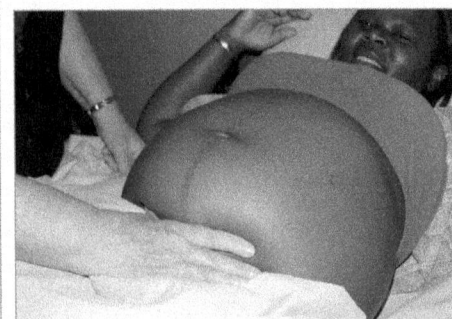

Figure 18D Pawlick's grip (What part of the fetus is presenting?)

What is in the pelvis? Pawlick's grip
▶ Use the right hand to feel which part is in the pelvis. Is it harder and ballotable?
▶ Is this part still above the symphysis or is it moving into the pelvis?
▶ The size of the presenting part may give an indication of GA.
▶ The head can really only be identified after 30–32 weeks.

continued

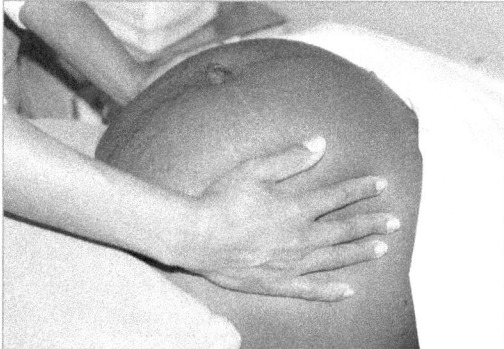

Figure 18E Lateral uterine palpation (Where are the back and the small parts?)

Where are the back and the small parts? Lateral grip: Using both hands

▶ Determine the location of the fetal back. Record whether it is on the right or left side of the maternal abdomen.

▶ Facing the mother and using both hands, palpate the mother's right side with the left hand and the mother's left side with the right hand.

▶ The fetal back feels firm and smooth. The side where the small parts are feels emptier.

▶ In a normal anterior position, the back may be near the umbilicus and the small parts may be lower, towards the back.

▶ In a posterior position, the back may be lower towards the back and the fetal parts may be felt all over the abdomen.

▶ Feel and estimate the amount of liquor: if there is an excessive amount of fluid, the uterus will be tense and it will be quite difficult to feel for fetal parts.

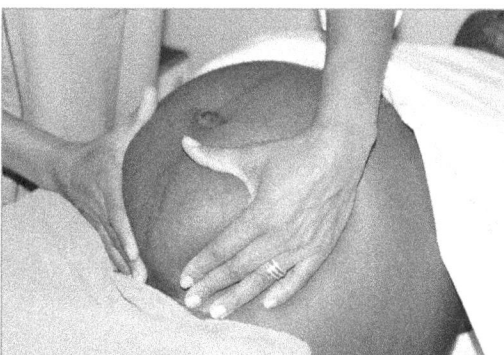

Figure 18F Deep pelvic palpation (level of engagement or descent)

Is the head engaged or deflected? (36 weeks): Deep pelvic grip

In late pregnancy, when palpation findings are unclear, do the following:

▶ Ask the woman to bend her knees and follow the fetal back with one of your hands. Facing the feet, attempt to locate the cephalic prominence or brow. This landmark will assist you in assessing the descent of the presenting part into the pelvis.

▶ Move the fingers of both hands down the sides of the uterus towards the symphysis pubis.

▶ If the fetal head is extended, the occiput is the first cephalic prominence felt and is located on the same side as the back.

▶ The position of the hands on the diagrams (to the left) indicate the potential findings in both scenarios.

▶ These findings may be confirmed with a vaginal examination.

▶ The final assessment relates to engagement of the fetal head, where the fetal head is divided into fifths.

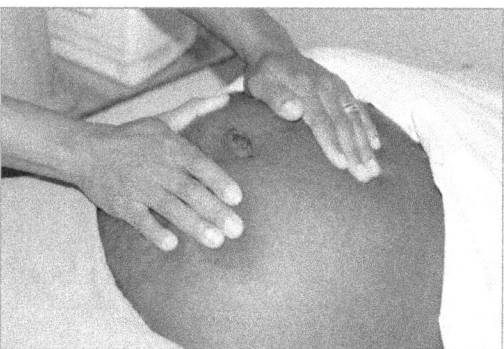

Figure 18G 'Walking' the fingertips over the abdomen (Where are the small parts?)

continued

Step 3: Auscultation

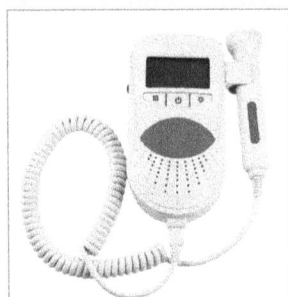

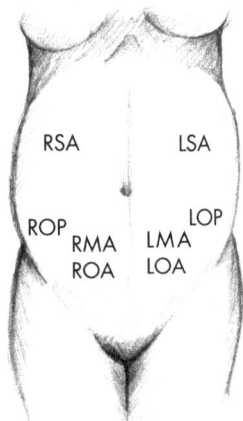

Figure 18H Auscultation positions

Labels in figure: RSA, LSA, ROP, LOP, RMA, LMA, ROA, LOA

Principles:
- The fetal heartbeat is a positive sign of pregnancy.
- Use a hand-held Doppler monitor, a Pinard stethoscope or an electronic fetal monitoring device to determine the fetal heart rate based on abdominal palpation findings.
- Take the fetal heartbeat while observing the maternal pulse for a full minute.
- The fetal heartbeat is rhythmical, regular and is influenced by many factors, such as the woman's sleep and wake cycle, fetal movements and uterine contractions. There may thus be periodic accelerations and decelerations that are within normal boundaries.
- A normal fetal heartbeat is 120–140 beats per minute (bpm) and has a double beat.
- In multiple pregnancies, both heartbeats should be taken simultaneously.

Anterior vertex positions:
- Place the Doppler transducer or the Pinard stethoscope over the identified back of the fetus in an OA position, usually between the symphysis pubis and the umbilicus.
- Feel simultaneously for the maternal radial pulse to distinguish between the two individuals.

Posterior vertex positions: The fetal heartbeat is heard over and around the umbilicus.

Breech positions: The fetal heart is heard above the umbilicus.

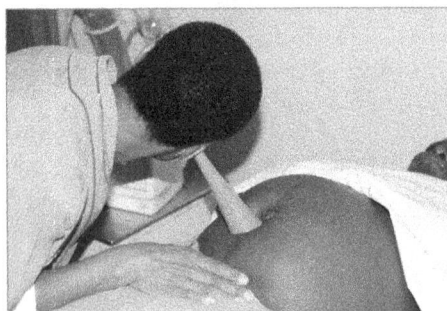

Figure 18I Auscultation of the fetal heartbeat using Pinard's stethoscope

Sounds
- The sound of the fetal heart is a clear, sharp, double beat. It should be distinguished from cord and placental sounds.
- A funic souffle is a high-pitched but muffled sound. It comes from the pulsating cord and is synchronised with the fetal heartbeat.
- The uterine souffle is a muffled sound that is heard strongly, but the beat corresponds with the maternal pulse. It is the sound of the uterine arteries and placental blood flow. If the placenta is implanted anteriorly in the uterus, it may hide the fetal heart. It is vital that the midwife only records factual and accurate fetal heartbeat data.

Recording and interpretation
- Document all findings on the maternal obstetric record and partogram.
- Report abnormal findings.

Pelvimetry for pelvic assessment

Pelvimetry is the examination of the size and shape of the pelvis to determine if a fetus can safely pass through the pelvis. Radiography in the form of X-ray and CAT scan pelvimetry is the most accurate way to assess the adequacy of the pelvis. Due to the risks to the baby, exceptional use of radiography is only allowed after 32 weeks of gestation. Ultrasonography can be used to estimate the size of the fetal head and the fetal weight.

Differences in pelvises affect the outcome of labour. A woman's pelvic inlet may be adequate, but there may be a narrowing in the midpelvis or outlet. If the pelvis is contracted in any way and/or if the fetus is over-sized, then difficulties must be anticipated and the woman should be referred to a medical practitioner as soon as possible. The fetal head may have difficulty negotiating the pelvic brim, and/or difficulties may occur in the pelvic cavity (midpelvis) and/or at the outlet.

An SFH of 40 cm or more may indicate a large infant; such a baby may well have difficulty negotiating an average-sized pelvis. On the other hand, a small baby may quite easily negotiate a slightly contracted pelvis.

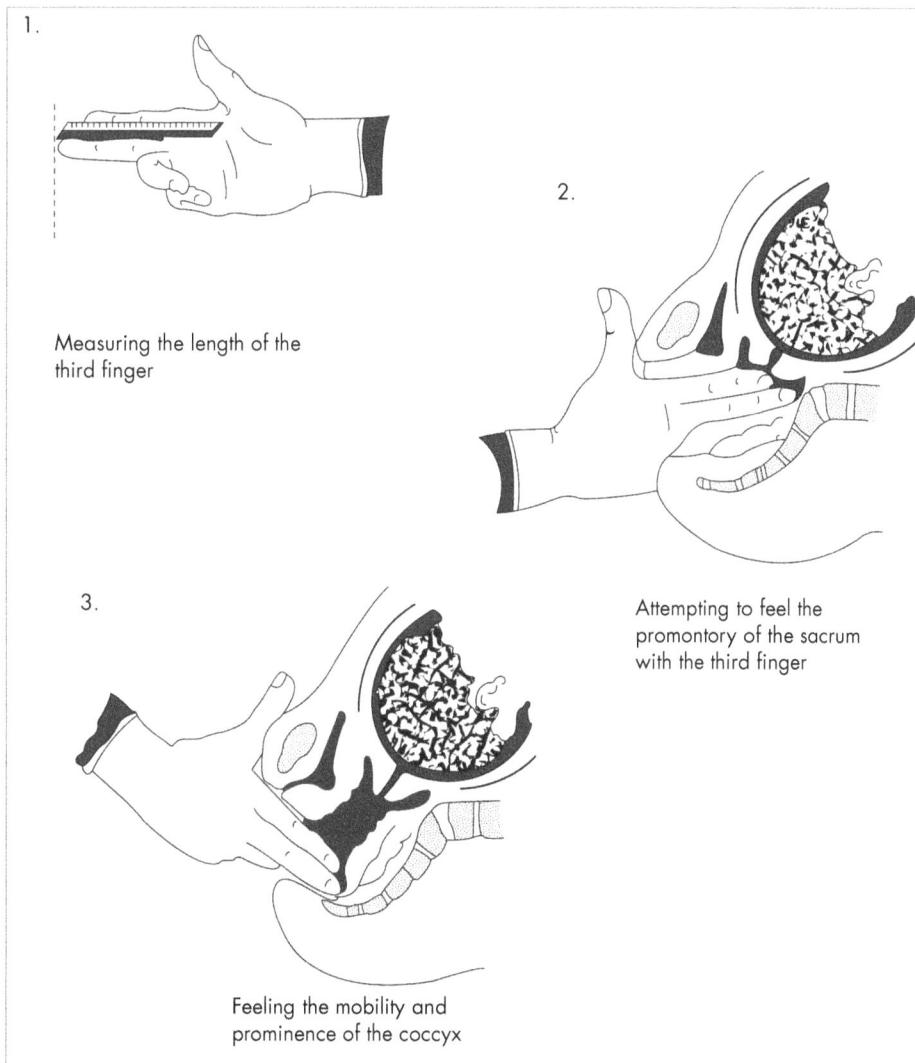

1. Measuring the length of the third finger

2. Attempting to feel the promontory of the sacrum with the third finger

3. Feeling the mobility and prominence of the coccyx

Figure 18.7 Clinical pelvic assessment

4.

a. Greater
   sciatic notch

b. Ischial
   spine

a. Measuring the
approximate size of the
greater sciatic notches

b. Noting the prominence of
the ischial spines

5.

Measuring the approximate
angle of the sub-pubic arch

6.

Measuring the approximate
width of the ischial
tuberosities

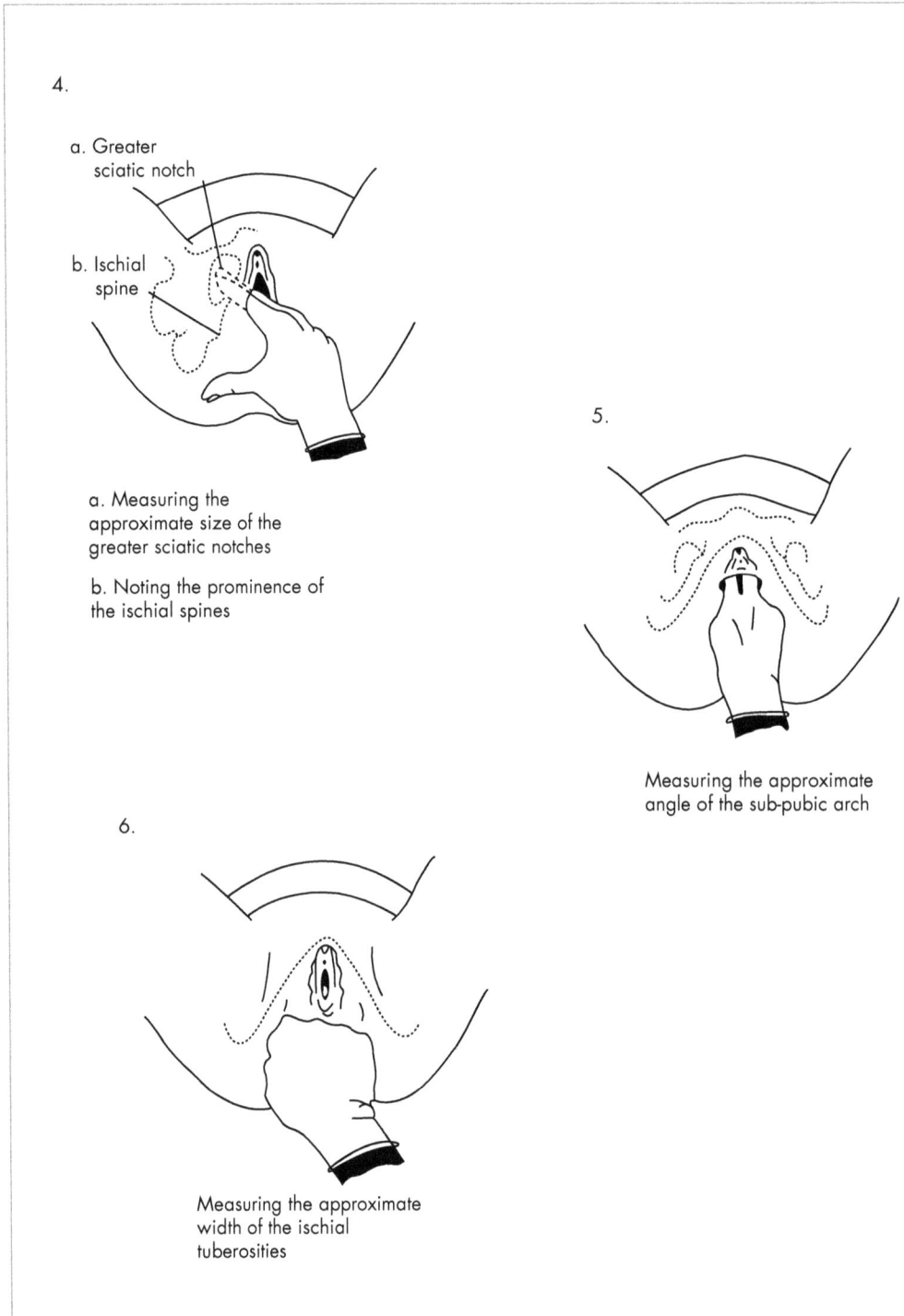

Figure 18.7 Clinical pelvic assessment (continued)

PROCEDURE	Clinical assessment of the pelvis

Definition
Clinical pelvimetry is the clinical assessment of a pelvis to determine if it is adequate for birth. This procedure is seldom used in pregnancy; it is normally used in labour. Although clinical pelvimetry is not used in many areas, it may be of use and midwives need to know the underlying principles of the obvious abnormalities that they may encounter.

Indications
▶ A primigravida after 36 weeks (SHF greater than 38 cm) (Note that the head may be engaged after 36 weeks in a primigravida.)
▶ Women who had previous prolonged labour or OP positions
▶ Vaginal birth after a Caesarean section (VBAC) for reasons other than CPD (not allowed in primary healthcare [PHC] clinics)

Preparation and principles
▶ The procedure is performed using an aseptic technique with gloves.
▶ Ensure maximum privacy.
▶ Explain the procedure to the woman and reassure her.
▶ The woman's bladder should be empty.
▶ The position of the patient is either lithotomy or a dorsal position with flexed legs and thighs.
▶ Perform abdominal palpation.
▶ You should know the measurements of your hand, as the hand becomes the tool for assessment. Knowledge of the normal measurements of the pelvis is important.

Procedure (Figure 18.7)
1 Gently introduce the index and middle finger into the vaginal orifice, first in a downward and backward direction and then in an upward and backward direction. The tip of the middle finger feels for the centre of the sacral promontory. The diagonal conjugate extends from the inferior margin of the symphysis pubis to the centre of the sacral promontory and should measure 12.5 cm (this cannot be determined during a normal examination). If the hand measurement is less than 12.5 cm, the sacral promontory should not have been reached in an average-sized pelvis. The obstetrical conjugate of the pelvic brim can be calculated by subtracting 1.5 cm from the diagonal conjugate, for example: 12.5 − 1.5 cm = 11 cm. The diagonal conjugate cannot be measured if the presenting part has entered the brim of the pelvis.
2 Gently run the tip of the middle finger down the curve of the sacrum. The sacrum should be smooth and broad (15 cm) and should have a rounded concave curve. It should not be long, narrow or straight, as this would indicate a narrowing of the pelvic cavity or canal.
3 Gently press the end of the coccyx. The coccyx should be slightly mobile and not prominent. It should not be fixed or projecting unduly into the anteroposterior (AP) diameter of the outlet of the pelvis, as this would indicate a narrowing of this diameter.
4 Fit two fingers on the ligament between the sacrum and the ischial spines on both sides of the sacrum. The greater sciatic arch on either side of the sacrum should admit at least two fingers on the ligament.
5 Move the fingers to the ischial spines. They should not be easily palpated. In other words, they should not be prominent in a normal gynaecoid pelvis. Prominent ischial spines can be the cause of delay or obstruction in the second stage of labour. Prominent ischial spines feel like the knuckles of a clenched fist. Non-prominent ischial spines feel like the knuckles of an open hand.
6 While slowly removing the fingers, estimate the width of the subpubic arch by turning the fingers horizontally and pressing them gently upwards, against the lower border of the arch. If the arch accommodates two fingers, it is estimated that the subpubic arch is about 90 degrees. If not, this may indicate a narrow arch.

continued

257

7   The distance between the tuberosities is an indication of the shape of the pelvis. The bituberous or intertuberous diameter should easily admit a fist. This is a rough measurement only. If the width of the hand at the knuckles is able to fit comfortably between the ischial tuberosities, the transverse diameter of the outlet is considered adequate. The average measurement is 10.5 cm.

Interpretation

▶ The sacral promotory should not be felt.
▶ Midpelvis: The sacrum should be curved and the coccyx moveable. The ligaments should allow two fingers and the spines should not be felt.
▶ Outlet: The subpubic arch should allow two fingers and the intertuberosities should easily allow a closed fist.

Actions

In the case of abnormal findings on performing pelvimetry, refer the woman to a medical practitioner.

Pelvic differences

In 1950, Evans and Steyn (Keller et al, 2003:15) found that pelvises of black women tend to be 20 per cent smaller than those of Caucasian women, thus explaining the higher rate of CPD and Caesarean sections in black women.

Other examinations

As part of routine care, the following should be done:
▶ *Breast examination.* At every visit, observe the breast and nipples and examine them for changes and lumps.
▶ *Legs.* Observe the feet and legs for oedema, varicose veins and tenderness that may indicate deep vein thrombosis.

18.5   Fetal surveillance

One of the aims of antenatal care is to monitor the well-being of the fetus *in utero*. The well-being of the fetus is linked to the well-being of the mother. Any disease (eg medical condition, cardiac condition, diabetes or thyroid problem) or infection (HIV and TB) of the mother will put the baby at risk.

The assessment of fetal well-being includes the risk factors of the mother (infections, Hb), gravidity, parity, age, previous pregnancies and births, previous perinatal deaths, the history of this pregnancy, the first day of the last normal menstrual period, the gestational period, when the baby's movements were first felt, maternal nutritional status, mid-upper-arm circumference (MUAC), mental and social status, and findings on abdominal palpation. The antenatal observations to monitor fetal growth is explained in Ch 17 and this chapter (see the procedure for measuring SFH and the antenatal card on pages 228–232).

The fetus and placenta function as the fetoplacental unit. At eight weeks, all major fetal organs are formed, the heart beats and the ovaries are formed in the female fetus. By 20 weeks, organogenesis is completed. The last structural change is the palate, which closes at 20 weeks. However, by 28 weeks, the lungs are not yet mature enough for independent functioning to sustain life, because of the lack of surfactant and the collapse of the lung alveoli on exhaling. The last trimester is a period of accelerated fetal growth. The fetus gains 200–250 g (or 10 per cent) per week – the same mass the baby will gain per week after birth. (See Chapter 7 for more on embryology.)

When only abdominal palpation is relied upon, observations and measurements of fetal growth and development are indirect and subject to misinterpretation and error. Maternal size and weight, the position of the placenta, the amount of amniotic fluid and the number and size of fetuses all play a role in the findings on palpation. Other aspects that may contribute to inaccuracies are late booking, inaccurate information regarding the LMP, inconsistent clinic attendance and change of staff.

Fetal surveillance includes serial measurements for the detection of deviations of fetal well-being against a variety of clinical parameters. These include maternal weight gain, uterine enlargement, SFH measurements between 20 and 36 weeks, the volume of amniotic fluid, fetal movements (kick chart) and feeling the fetal parts on abdominal palpation after 28 weeks.

Non-invasive measures include:
▶ SFH measures
▶ the Cardiff count-to-ten kick fetal movement count
▶ electronic fetal monitoring: non-stress test (NST) if not in labour
▶ ultrasound.

The measurement of the SFH is essential to determine if the fetus is growing. This requires accurate measurement and recording of the abdominal findings at five visits (see figures 17A on page 228 and 17C on page 230). In addition, the observation of fetal movements by the mother (discussed in the next subsection) is an easy way to ensure that the baby is well.

The interventions to support clinical findings include serial ultrasound assessments, biophysical profiling and Doppler studies. These are explained in the rest of this section.

Fetal movements

Fetal movements are reliable signs of fetal well-being and depend on subjective observation. Mothers are taught to observe fetal movements and to report on the movements with each visit.

The Cardiff count-to-ten kick fetal movement count

The kick count is a simple way of teaching mothers to observe the fetus in the third trimester. Babies usually move ten times in two hours. The mother is instructed to choose a time of day that the baby usually moves and to observe ten movements and write them down. A sharp deviation in patterns of movement or less than ten counts in 24 hours requires immediate attention. (See WHO 2016.)

The following instructions can be given to the mother (Crews, nd):

1 Choose a time during the day when the baby is normally active. (Most babies are active in the evenings.)

continued

Make sure that you will be able to pay attention to the baby during this time. Also make sure that you will be able to do the count the same time each day.

2 Count all the movements of your baby, including stretches, rolls, kicks and punches. Hiccups should not be counted. If the baby performs a flurry of movements, such as kicks, count it as one movement.

3 If within in an hour you have not felt any movements, lie down on your left side. Really concentrate on the baby.

4 When you have counted ten movements, record how long it took. Fill in the fetal movement chart.

In ten hours, the mother should feel at least ten movements. (Generally, she will feel ten movements in the first hour already.)

The mother should contact a healthcare professional if:

▶ less than ten movements are felt within 10 hours
▶ the movements steadily decrease from day to day
▶ the mother has lain down on her left side but still has not felt any movement after 90 minutes
▶ the mother is worried about the baby's activity levels for any reason. This may necessitate further tests.

PROCEDURE   Electronic fetal monitoring (non-stress test)

Definition

The NST is a non-invasive method to indirectly determine fetal well-being *in utero* using external electronic monitoring of the fetal heart rate (FHR) in the absence of uterine contractions.

Indications

The test is usually performed after 27 weeks if there is a suspicion of at-risk findings. The fetus is not sufficiently neurologically developed before this time to respond to the test protocols and the heart rate patterns of a preterm fetus after 27 weeks is tachycardic and flat.

Principles and preparation

▶ In the case of twins, both heart rates are monitored at the same time.
▶ The woman should have had something to eat or drink prior to the test.
▶ The woman should have an empty bladder.

Procedure

1 Explain the procedure to the woman and get her verbal consent.
2 Position the woman in the semi-Fowler's position or on her left side.
3 Make sure that both the transducer for the fetal heart and the probe for the uterine contractions are attached, in working order and a clear recording of the real event.
4 Explain to the woman that she needs to monitor the baby and report each time the baby moves by pressing a button that will make a mark on the tracing paper.
5 Make observations over 20 minutes and make sure everything is recorded well.

continued

6 Take the woman's BP during the test to exclude IVCS and record it. (The woman's BP must be stable throughout the test.)

7 Exclude the presence of contractions. An NST requires conditions of 'no stress'; thus, no contractions should be present. The presence of contractions must be eliminated by monitoring uterine activity.

8 Stay with the woman during the test.

Interpretation

During a normal non-stress period (ie no contractions for 20 to 40 minutes), the fetus will have at least two fetal movements. This will result in an acceleration of the FHR of 15 bpm above the baseline for 15 seconds (after 32 weeks) or 10 bpm for 10 seconds (before 32 weeks) in the absence of contractions. If this is not present, the woman must be admitted or referred. Findings can be categorised as:

▶ reactive or reassuring: two movements with acceleration in 20 minutes

▶ non-reactive, non-reassuring or suspect: no movements or movements with no acceleration in 20 minutes.

Actions

If there is an abnormal pattern or fetal movements with deceleration, the woman must be referred for medical care or a biophysical profile.

Recording and interpretation

The cardiotocograph (CTG) test, as shown in Figure 18J, is a legal document. It should be clearly marked with the woman's details. Findings and actions taken should be documented and filed.

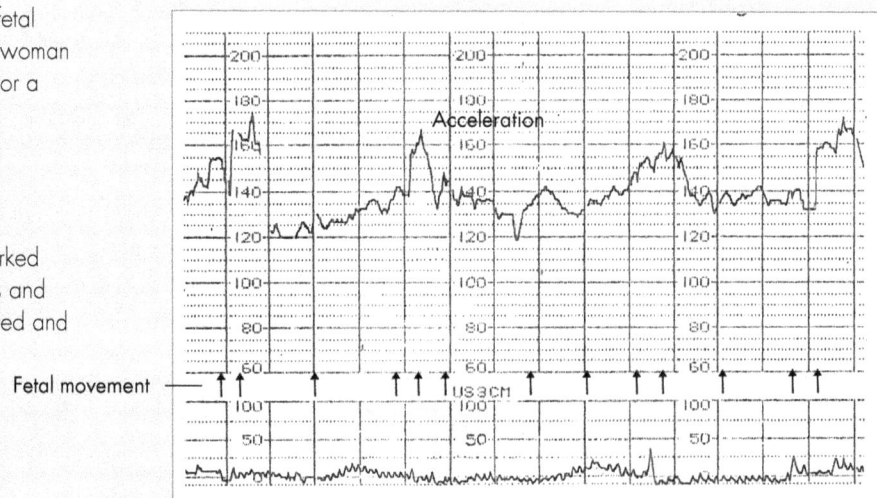

Figure 18J A CTG test

Ultrasound

Routine ultrasound in pregnancy has become common in South Africa. However, the availability of ultrasound in the public sector – and particularly in PHC – is problematic. Many clinics have been provided with ultrasound equipment and advanced midwives receive informal training to use it. There is also portable ultrasound equipment and some provinces have made these available.

Ultrasound functions through a transducer that produces sound waves that can penetrate liquid. The transducer is connected with the skin through contact gel. The sound waves penetrate the area of liquid in the womb and reflect back a real-time image of the structure of the fetus and its organs.

The frequency of ultrasound is 20 000 Hz (the human hearing range is 20–20 000 Hz).

Table 18.3 gives the indications for ultrasound in obstetrics. Two critical periods for ultrasound are at 12 weeks, to determine the position of the placenta and the number of fetuses present, and 20 weeks, when the palate closes and Down's syndrome can be detected.

The margin of error in interpreting ultrasound increases as the pregnancy progresses. In the third trimester, estimations can vary by a margin of three weeks if not compared with other parameters. GA estimations are more accurate when done before 20 weeks.

Table 18.3

Ultrasound findings in obstetrics

Period	Use of ultrasound	Observations made with ultrasound
First trimester: **Error margin =** **+ 1 week**	Diagnosis of pregnancy Duration of pregnancy Determination of threatening abortion Diagnosis of ectopic pregnancy Hydatidiform mole Ovarian mass Multiple pregnancy	Volume of amniotic sac at 9 days Crown–rump length (CRL) 3–5 days Femur length 6–9 days Fetal head 6–9 days Abortion Sac must be attached to the uterine wall with fetal heart heard Blighted ovum: 3 cm sac with no embryo Hydatidiform mole: snowlike appearance
Second trimester: **Error margin =** **+ 2 weeks**	Fetal abnormalities Fetal growth and development Cervical incompetence Position of the placenta	Serial measures are required Biparietal, after 34 weeks 1 mm/week femur length Abdominal circumference Mass 18 weeks: 95% of congenital abnormalities can be diagnosed Structural umbilical arteries Neural tube, anencephaly, hydrocephalic, spina bifida, encephalocele, microcephaly Palate and lip Heart, skeletal, gastrointestinal (GI) Urinary system, genitalia Tumours
Third trimester: **Error margin =** **+ 3 weeks**	Placental localisation and maturity Fetal position Amniotic fluid Biophysical profile	Placental maturity in four grades: 0 = homogenic 1 = proliferation on maternal side 2 = small spaces in placenta 3 = proliferation and calcification 4 = lobule appearance Level 4 + = lung maturity
Postpartum	Haematoma Neonatal complications Brain haemorrhage	Retained products of conception Haematoma Congenital abnormalities and fetal brain haemorrhage can be detected
Other	Cordocentesis, a genetic diagnostic test: Blood from the fetal umbilical cord is tested to detect fetal abnormalities Fetal Doppler studies Amniocentesis	Amniocentesis: localisation of placenta and cord Amniotic pool identified

Biophysical profiling

This is a non-invasive test that can only be performed by a skilled medical practitioner, sonographer or a midwife trained in sonography after 28 weeks of pregnancy. It is time-consuming and can easily take 45 minutes (excluding the NST). The clinician makes observations on the physical and functional aspects of the fetus *in utero*, namely fetal breathing, gross fetal body movements, fetal body tone and amniotic fluid volume. These are reflected in Table 18.4. A fetus with an abnormal biophysical profile will be referred for Doppler studies.

Table 18.4

Biophysical profiling

Biophysical profile	Rating	
Biophysical parameter	**Normal (2 points per variable)**	**Abnormal (0 points per variable)**
NST	Reactive pattern: at least two FHR accelerations of > 15 bpm and > 15 seconds in duration, associated with fetal movement in a 20-minute period	Non-reactive pattern: < two FHR accelerations of > 15 bpm and 15 seconds duration associated with fetal movement in 40 minutes
Fetal breathing movements	Present: At least one episode of fetal breathing of > 60 seconds within a 30-minute period	Absent: Absence of fetal breathing movements or the absence of an episode of fetal breathing of 60 seconds during a 30-minute period
Gross fetal body movements: The number of fetal movements is monitored over 30 minutes. Simultaneous limb and trunk movements are counted as a single movement.	At least three discrete episodes of fetal movement within a 30-minute period	Less than two movements in 30 minutes
Fetal body tone	Upper and lower extremities in full flexion Trunk in position of flexion and head flexed on chest At least one episode of extension of limb with return to position of flexion or extension of spine with return to flexion	Decreased: • Limbs in position of extension or partial flexion • Spine in extension • Fetal movement not followed by return to flexion • Fetal hand open
Volume of amniotic fluid	Fluid evident throughout the uterine cavity Largest pocket of fluid >1 cm in vertical diameter	Decreased: • Fluid absent in most areas of uterine cavity • Largest pocket of fluid measures <1 cm on vertical diameter
Interpretation: Total score Normal: 8–10 Equivocal: 4–6 Abnormal: 0–2		
Actions < 8: Refer if oligohydramnios is present. Refer: Doppler Immediate medical attention		

Doppler ultrasound

Doppler studies are done with ultrasound by a skilled sonographer or medical doctor. They consist of the observation of the umbilical artery and the rate of blood flow, which indicates if the blood flow from the placenta to the fetus is sufficient.

If the umbilical artery resistance is below the 95th centile, placental insufficiency is likely. When placental insufficiency is present, the diastolic BP to the fetus drops, which is shown by an increase in the resistance index in the umbilical artery to above the 95th centile. The implication is a malfunctioning placenta with a decreased blood flow to the fetus. The cerebral flow and venous ductus arteriosus can show the redistribution of blood to safeguard organs.

Doppler ultrasound is a highly sophisticated procedure done only by specialists. Fetuses with non-reassuring NSTs, biophysical and Doppler studies *in utero* are not likely to withstand the stress of labour. Intrauterine death (IUD) and fetal distress can be prevented if the cases at risk can be referred and the service is available.

The Modified Biophysical Profile (MBPP) uses the NST and the amniotic fluid index (AFI) only. The NST must be reactive and the amniotic pool must be greater than 5 cm (Preboth, 2000).

18.6   Conclusion

The assessment, diagnosis and treatment of women in pregnancy require that midwives be equipped with the relevant knowledge, skills and appropriate attitudes to provide quality basic antenatal care. While most women have uneventful pregnancies and births, a number of women will need intensive and specialised antenatal care. It is the task of the midwife to identify women with healthcare needs beyond the midwife's scope of practice and competency and to refer them for appropriate care.

19

Childbirth education and preparation

LEARNING OBJECTIVES

On completion of this chapter, you must be able to:

▶ explain evidence-based childbirth preparation
▶ demonstrate competency in individual and group education in pregnancy
▶ identify common problems relating to exercise in pregnancy
▶ explain the general and specific principles of exercise in pregnancy
▶ know the important information that a midwife needs to provide to a woman with regard to preparation for childbirth.

KNOWLEDGE ASSUMED TO BE IN PLACE

The physiological changes and common problems of pregnancy
Principles of health education
The ability to present a health talk

KEYWORDS

childbirth education • relaxation • doulas • significant person • health literacy

19.1　Introduction

The midwife has an important role to play in preparing the woman, her partner and family for childbirth and parenthood. The preparation focuses mainly on health promotion and how the woman can be assisted to maintain or improve her health and that of the fetus in preparation for labour, childbirth and parenthood, as well as promoting a healthy puerperium. This preparation, support and education should be extended to the father of the baby and, where possible, the family. Preparation and education should be culturally sensitive. The values and beliefs of the woman and her family related to pregnancy and childbirth must be respected.

19.2　Childbirth education as specialist care

Childbirth education can be provided to individuals, couples or a group of women or expectant parents. These classes provide an opportunity for parents to establish relationships and share experiences as well as the challenges they may face in bringing up their children. Childbirth education provides an opportunity for expectant parents to prepare for parenthood physically, mentally and emotionally. Expectant parents are empowered to make informed decisions about childbirth, care of the newborn and parenting practices that are likely to enhance attachment (bonding) relationships between them and their children.

In most cases, face-to-face and one-on-one health education is given during care. Group discussions, on the other hand, enable parents to understand their feelings and increase their confidence in their abilities. Principles of adult education should be applied in all these situations to facilitate understanding, cooperation and compliance with information learnt.

Preparation for health education

Childbirth education has become a speciality field in midwifery, and midwives can obtain a certificate in childbirth education. The International Childbirth Education Association (ICEA) has developed an accredited programme for childbirth educators to ensure that evidence-based information and care are given during pregnancy and birth. South Africa is associated with the ICEA through the Childbirth Educators' Resource Group (CBERG). Midwives and other professionals can join this group and complete a special programme in childbirth education.

Ideally, midwives who offer childbirth preparation, support and postnatal support services need to receive further training and education. The Department of Health (DoH), in collaboration with CBERG, has declared an annual national pregnancy education week in February. In addition, CBERG conducts annual workshops countrywide to educate pregnant women and educators. A magazine called *The Expectant Mothers' Guide for South Africa* provides information for health educators (see www.expectantmothersguide.co.za).

It is available at various retailers and contains the names of childbirth educators and other supportive services for pregnant women.

Activity
1 Obtain a copy of *The Expectant Mother's Guide for South Africa*, which has information about support groups in South Africa, at http://www.expectantmothersguide.co.za/about/.
2 Visit the ICEA's free online journal for childbirth educators, the *International Journal for Childbirth Education* (*IJCE*), at http://icea.org/about/icea-journal/ and learn about childbirth education.

Selected services and support groups available in South Africa	
Abortion	Marie Stopes Services South Africa: http://www.mariestopes.org.za/safe-abortion/
Adoption	Neo Birth Pregnancy Crisis Centre Adoption South Africa: https://government.cybo.com/ZA-biz/neo-birth-pregnancy-crisis-centre
AIDS	National HIV and AIDS helpline: 0800 012 322
Autism	Autism South Africa: http://aut2know.co.za/
Breastfeeding	Le Leche League: www.llli.org/southafrica.html
Cerebral palsy	The United Cerebral Palsy Association of South Africa (UCPA): http://ucpa.za.org/
Child welfare	Child Welfare South Africa: www.childwelfaresa.org.za
Cleft lip and palate	The Genetic Alliance: http://www.geneticalliance.org.za/
Cystic fibrosis	The South African Cystic Fibrosis Association (SACFA): www.sacfa.org.za
Deafness	The South African National Deaf Association (SANDA): www.sanda.org.za
Down's syndrome	Down Syndrome South Africa: www.downsyndrome.org.za
Genetic counselling	www.geneticcounselling.co.za
Haemophilia	The South African Haemophilia Foundation: http://www.haemophilia.org.za/
Marfan syndrome	South African Marfan Syndrome Organisation (SAMSO): http://www.heartnewslinks.com/directory/heart-groups/south-african-marfan-syndrome-organisation-samso
Multiple births	South African Multiple Birth Association (SAMBA): http://www.samultiplebirth.co.za/
Poison information centre	Poison information centre, Red Cross Children's Hospital 24 hours: 0861 555 777
Postnatal depression	Postnatal Depression Support Association South Africa (PNDSA): www.pndsa.org.za National helpline: 082 882 0072

19.3   Health education as the role of the midwife

Midwives who are not accredited childbirth educators still have an obligation to give health education to all the pregnant women they encounter at all levels of care. If possible, women should be referred to structured antenatal and parenting classes that are accredited and in line with the philosophy of the hospital or institution. Women who have initiated their own care should be supported and accommodated.

Types of childbirth education programmes

Institutions that do not offer childbirth classes but which provide care for women during pregnancy are obliged to develop and create supportive programmes for before and after birth. These programmes must be evidence-based and supportive and must meet the needs of women in the community. Supportive programmes can take many forms, such as:

▶ a structured programme for couples
▶ health literacy (a range of written pamphlets that help women to access all the forms of care available)
▶ call centres for postnatal support
▶ a group of midwives who supply breastfeeding support and care before, during and after birth
▶ online programmes (medical aid programmes and private clinics)
▶ special services (such as a 'stork nest' in private clinics).

Alternatively, women can use a private midwife who will provide one-on-one care.

Principles of education programmes

The following principles should be adhered to during the presentation of childbirth education, in order to ensure a supportive environment:

▶ *Standards.* When starting a childbirth preparation course, the midwife should try to give the highest standard of care at all times and should make sure that all the information provided is evidence-based, accurate and not conflicting. Women often complain of receiving conflicting advice from healthcare professionals. It is therefore important to have consensus in a given institution.
▶ *Confidentiality.* Women feel more secure when they work with small teams. The 'know your midwife' campaign, implemented in many healthcare systems, is geared to create conditions where midwives are allocated to specific women for support during their pregnancies. Whatever

the situation, the midwife must ensure confidentiality and listen to the concerns and problems voiced by the women and their partners and give appropriate care and advice.

▶ *Continuity of messages.* The independent childbirth educator should, where possible, make contact with all the healthcare professionals, midwives or medical practitioners involved so that the lines of communication remain open, and also to ensure continuity of care. If independent, the midwife should also have a good relationship with all the hospitals or clinics in the area and, where possible, give support before and during the delivery.
▶ *Cultural and individual needs.* The needs of the parents must be considered, bearing in mind their socioeconomic, cultural and religious backgrounds. Programmes should be carefully structured to meet individual needs as far as possible.
▶ *Evaluate the effectiveness of programmes.* The midwife should evaluate the woman's experiences of the programme at the end of each course.
▶ *Relevant and up-to-date information.* The midwife needs to stay well informed and use up-to-date information. The course content should be reassessed for relevance at regular intervals and changes should be made if necessary.

Doulas

Doulas are trained lay-people who support women in labour to relieve the burden of care on midwives and the healthcare system, and to make the birth environment more supportive for women. Some public institutions use trained doulas in South Africa.

19.4   Ante- and postnatal exercises

The value of physical exercise for the birth process and recovery after birth has been known since 1912. Grantly Dick-Read's theory on the fear, tension and pain cycle in childbirth (1959) focused on relaxation in childbirth. In the 1950s, psychoprophylaxis became popular in birth preparation and many methods were taught and used to prepare women for motherhood, including breathing and preparation for childbirth.

Today, psychoprophylactic and physical exercise preparations use a collaborative approach.

Each member of the multidisciplinary health team has a unique contribution to make towards preparation for childbirth. Physiotherapists and occupational therapists also provide help with physical exercises, as well as child and family relations and development.

Physical fitness and health can be promoted through safe stretching and muscle-toning exercises to prepare for the demands of pregnancy, labour, breastfeeding, handling the baby and parenthood. Exercise and relaxation programmes are designed to:

- help women to adjust physically and psychologically to the stresses of childbirth
- advise on physical activity
- adapt work and leisure
- gain or maintain fitness
- provide pelvic floor education
- prevent back problems
- teach relaxation and breathing
- teach a healthy body posture.

The midwife needs a thorough knowledge of the anatomy and physiology of pregnancy, the pelvis and the pelvic floor and the effects of pregnancy on the rectus abdomini, the levator ani and the perineum. The midwife should understand the effects of hormones on the endocrine and cardiovascular systems and the effects of the enlarged uterus on the lower extremities and back. The midwife should be able to help the woman to have a more comfortable pregnancy.

General principles and recommended exercises

It is clear that, due to the wide range of differences in women's bodies in pregnancy, universal antenatal exercises cannot be offered to all women. However, there are general principles to adhere to when antenatal exercises are considered:

- Women with a regular programme can continue with their usual exercise programme when pregnant, with certain adaptations.
- Women who do not already have a regular programme of exercise should do gentle exercise such as walking and swimming, which are safe in pregnancy.
- Women are encouraged to do exercises that will strengthen the back and upper arm muscles for post-delivery and the abdominal muscles.
- Gentle exercise will prevent constipation and help with improved sleep and rest.
- Women should avoid standing for long periods.
- Pelvic floor exercises (Kegel's exercises) should be linked to daily activities and done in any position.
- When doing exercises for the deep abdominal muscles, the back must not be arched. Instead, the knees must be kept together (Pilates).
- The transverse abdominis needs exercise.

- Women must practise pelvic rocking (as shown in Figure 19.2 on page 269).
- Women must use the correct technique for lying down, getting up, lifting and performing household tasks, as shown in Figure 19.1 on the next page.

The recommended exercises illustrated in Figure 19.2 are described in Table 19.1 on pages 270–272.

Risky exercises to be avoided

Women must be advised about the risks inherent in:

- sit-ups and double leg raises (straining the abdominal muscles with diastasis recti)
- jumping and riding or any exercises at high speed (risk of losing balance and falling)
- tennis, hockey, skiing and cycling (risk of losing balance and falling)
- any cardiovascular exercise that raises the core temperature (the fetus cannot cool down in the womb).

Relaxation and deep breathing

Several relaxation and breathing methods have been found to be helpful during pregnancy and birth. These include body massage, aromatherapy, imagery and suggestion, hypnosis and yoga. Women are often already using a method of their own choice and the midwife should support the woman's choice.

Women who do not have their own programme may be directed to accredited services where they can learn about relaxation techniques that will improve their feelings of well-being, reduce levels of stress and reduce anxiety and fear of labour. Men are often encouraged to attend antenatal relaxation classes as well.

Body massage and aromatherapy

Aromatherapy may enhance general well-being. The oils are used for massaging the woman or are inhaled by the woman, particularly during labour to ease labour pain. (See Chapter 52.) The doula, partner or midwife can rub the woman's back at the beginning of a contraction.

Imagery

The woman can be trained during the antenatal period to use imagery. At the beginning of a contraction, she is advised to reflect and concentrate on something that amuses her or which she likes very much, in order to divert her mind from the labour pain. The woman can be advised to listen to her favourite music or watch an amusing video.

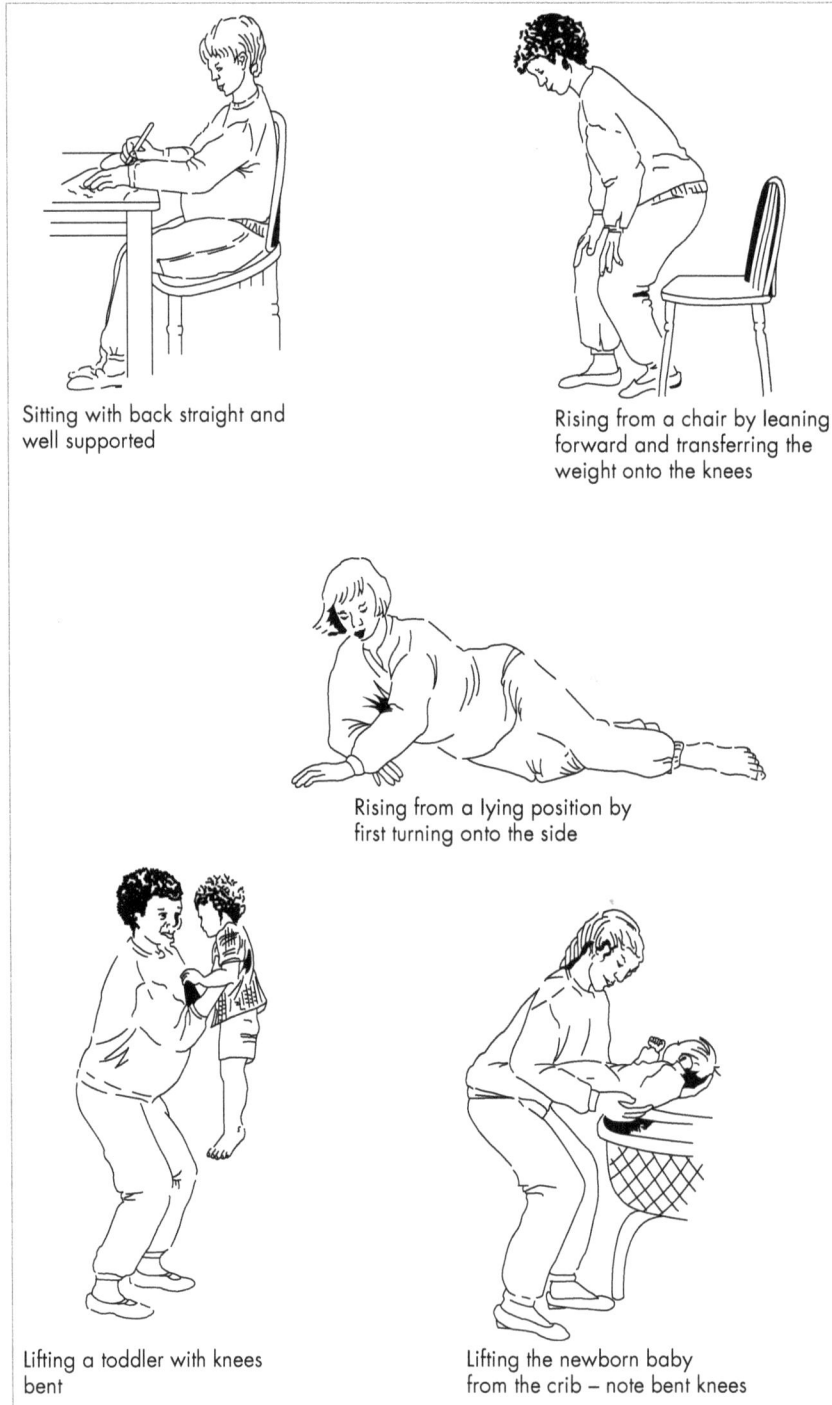

Sitting with back straight and
well supported

Rising from a chair by leaning
forward and transferring the
weight onto the knees

Rising from a lying position by
first turning onto the side

Lifting a toddler with knees
bent

Lifting the newborn baby
from the crib – note bent knees

Figure 19.1 Correct postural positions before and after delivery

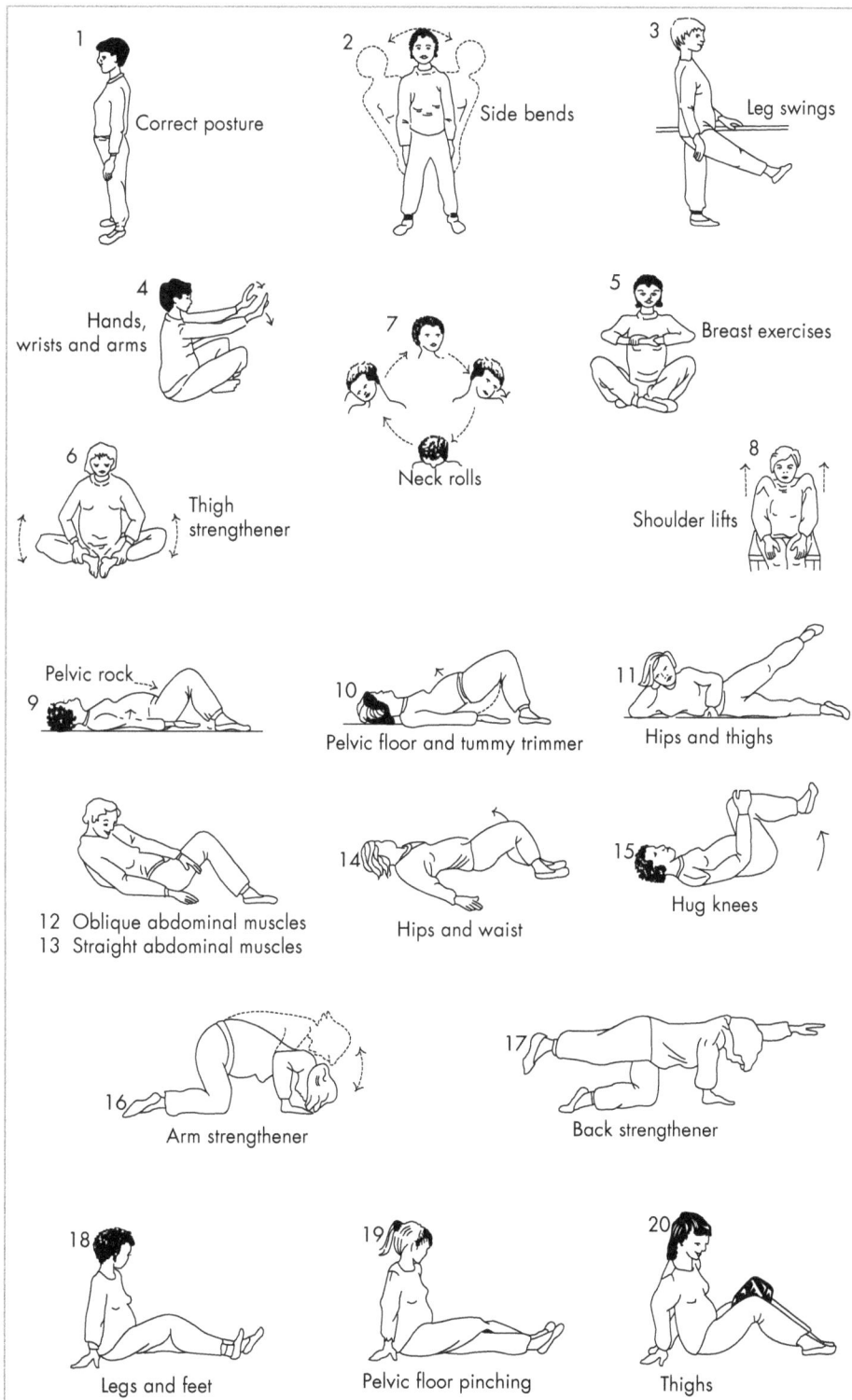

Figure 19.2 Recommended antenatal exercises

Table 19.1

Recommended antenatal exercises (as illustrated in Figure 19.2)

Exercises and starting position	Movement and instruction	Reason for exercise and muscles involved
1. Correct posture: Stand with feet comfortably apart.	Tuck the bottom in and under, pull the tummy in, keep the shoulders back but comfortably relaxed.	A supple, lengthened spine helps prevent many aches and pains that poor posture can cause. It also allows for maximum room for the baby and for the woman's breathing. Correct posture involves most of the main muscles of the body.
2. Side-bends: Stand with feet comfortably apart, legs straight, shoulders back and arms at sides (as in correct posture).	Bend sideways and reach down the side of the leg towards the knee. Be careful not to lean forward. Repeat five times each side.	For posture and beauty. Works muscles at the sides and front of waist.
3. Side leg swings: Stand in correct posture position, holding on lightly to the back of a chair (for balance).	Swing the leg gently and slowly forwards and back and across and out, away from the body. Repeat five times with each leg.	Improves circulation in hips and legs. Hip adductors are involved.
4. Hands, wrists and arms: Sit with legs crossed, back straight, arms stretched out straight in front.	Rotate the wrists, turning the hands in one direction and then the other. End off by flicking the fingers out. Repeat five times.	Stretches and strengthens biceps and triceps; loosens and warms up hands, fingers and wrists.
5. Breast exercise: Sit with legs crossed, back straight.	Raise the arms to just above shoulder height. Clasp each wrist with the opposite hand. Squeeze the wrists and push the skin towards the elbows. Contract and relax rhythmically. Repeat ten times.	Strengthens pectoral muscles and improves circulation to breasts.
6. Thigh strengthener (tailor sitting): Sit on the floor with the soles of the feet together.	Hold the ankles and bring the pelvis as close to the heels as possible. Keep the back straight. Press the thighs down gently towards the floor. Repeat five times.	Useful preparation for labour, as it loosens groins and hips and stretches the muscles of the inner thighs.
7. Neck rolls: This exercise may be done sitting or standing.	Bring the left ear to the left shoulder and roll the head around with the chin on the chest until the right ear is on the right shoulder. Lift the head across, left ear to left shoulder and back again. Then bring the right ear to the right shoulder. Roll the head around with chin on chest until the left ear and shoulder meet. Repeat twice. Do this exercise slowly and carefully.	Helps relieve stiff neck, headaches and tension. Note: Do not do this exercise if any pain is experienced.

continued

Exercises and starting position	Movement and instruction	Reason for exercise and muscles involved
8. Shoulder lifts: Sit with legs crossed, back straight.	Relax the arms and hands. Raise the shoulders to the ears, hold and relax. Repeat five times.	Releases tension in the shoulders and across the back of the neck.
9. Pelvic rock/tilt: Lie down on the back with the knees bent (crook lying) and the feet on the floor.	Breathe in, blow out, pull in the abdominal muscles and press the small of the back firmly onto the floor. Squeeze the buttock muscles together to tilt the bottom upwards. Hold for three counts. Relax and repeat five to ten times.	Mobilises the lumbar spine and prevents and relieves backache.
10. Pelvic uplift: Lie down on back with knees bent and the feet on the floor.	Do a pelvic tilt but continue to push the hips up off the floor until the back is in a straight line from shoulders to knees. Do not lift any higher, as this will over-arch the back. Repeat five times. Do not arch the back.	Strengthens thighs, pelvic floor, abdominal and buttock muscles.
11. Hips and thighs: Lie on the right side with the head resting on the right hand and the legs stretched out straight.	Keep the hip leaning forward and the abdominal muscles pulled in firmly. Lift the left leg straight up as high as is comfortable, hold for three counts and then lower. Repeat ten times with each leg.	Strengthens thighs and hips.
12. Oblique abdominal muscles: Lie on the back with the knees bent and the feet on the floor.	Keeping the back and shoulders relaxed, tilt the pelvis to flatten the hollow of the back. Pull in the abdominal muscles firmly and raise the head and shoulders, bringing the right hand towards the left knee. Hold for three counts. Lower back onto the floor. Repeat with left hand to right knee. Repeat alternating sides, five times each side, slowly and gently.	Strengthens oblique abdominal muscles. Note: Do not do this exercise if any pain is experienced.
13. Straight abdominal muscles: Lie on the back with the knees bent and the feet on the floor.	Do the procedure as for exercise number 12, but raise the head and shoulders, reaching both hands up to the knees. Hold for five counts. Lower and repeat five times.	Strengthens straight abdominal muscles. Note: Do not do this exercise if any pain is experienced.
14. Hips and waist: Lie on the back with the knees bent and the feet on the floor.	Keeping the shoulders flat on the floor and the knees together, rock the knees from side to side as far as they will go. Repeat five times.	Mobilises lumbar spine and sacroiliac joints. Relieves backache.
15. Hugging knees: Lie on the back with the knees bent and the feet on the floor.	Bring the knees onto the chest and hold with the hands (hug the knees to the chest). Feel the stretch in the back. Repeat five times. Addition: bring one leg up at a time, pulling the knee to the armpit around the side of the abdomen.	Stretches muscles of the back. Relieves pain in the sacroiliac joint.

continued

Exercises and starting position	Movement and instruction	Reason for exercise and muscles involved
16. Arm strengthener: Kneel on all fours. Keep the back well rounded.	Bend the elbows out to the sides and drop the body to the floor. Lift up slowly. Repeat five times.	Strengthens biceps and triceps.
17. Back strengthener: Kneel on all fours, with the weight evenly distributed.	Lift the left arm and right leg and stretch them away from the body. Stretch forwards with the fingers, and backwards with the heels. Keep the arm and leg parallel to the floor and in a straight line with the body. Look down at the floor. Repeat three times and then repeat with the other arm and leg.	Stretches and strengthens the lumbar area.
18. Legs and feet: Sit with the legs stretched out straight. Lean back on the hands.	Rotate the ankles in big circles, turning the feet in one direction and then the other. End by stretching and flexing the feet. Repeat ten times.	Improves and enhances circulation in legs and feet.
19. Pelvic floor pinching: Sit as in exercise 18.	Cross the ankles. Squeeze the thighs together as firmly as possible and hold for five counts. Hold the thigh squeeze and pinch and tuck the pelvic floor muscles (vaginal wall muscles) and hold for five counts. (Pinch as if holding back the flow or urine.) Keep pinching and end by squeezing the buttock muscles and the muscles surrounding the anus tightly for five counts. Relax all three areas. Repeat five times.	Tones inner thigh muscles and especially pelvic floor muscles. Do this exercise as often as possible during the day.
20. Thighs: Sit as in exercises 18 and 19, but bend the knees up slightly, feet on the floor.	Place a cushion between the knees, pull in the abdominal muscles firmly, pinch and tuck the pelvic floor muscles and then squeeze the knees together as tightly as possible. Hold for ten slow counts. Relax and repeat five times.	Tones inner thigh muscles and pelvic floor muscles. Note: Exercises 19 and 20 are essential to regain and maintain tone in these muscles, which are stretched during pregnancy and birth. Prolapse and stress incontinence will result from weak, poorly toned muscles.

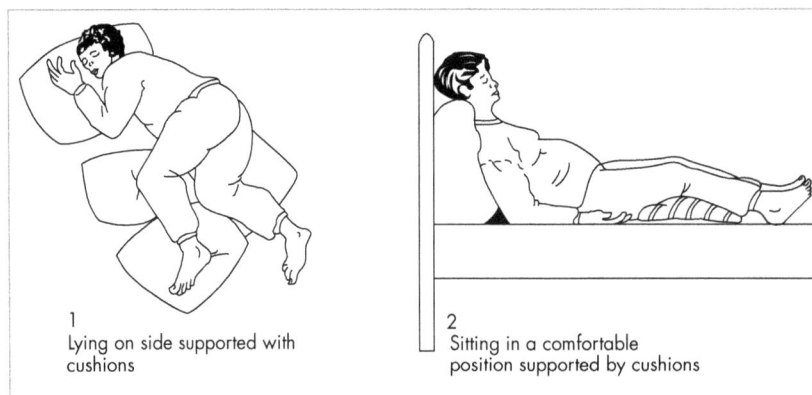

1
Lying on side supported with cushions

2
Sitting in a comfortable position supported by cushions

Figure 19.3 Positions for relaxation

Yoga

Imagery phrases can also be used in yoga classes. The woman will need to attend lessons with a yoga instructor in order to be able to utilise yoga in managing labour pain and the process of childbirth.

Relaxation exercises

The relaxation drill is basic training for women to learn so that they can concentrate on themselves and identify tension. This teaches the importance of self-awareness:

- The midwife must show the woman and her partner the different positions that can be used for the relaxation drill, as shown in Figure 19.3. The midwife should, if possible, have rugs or a mattress with pillows for each woman and partner during the class. If these cannot be supplied, then the couples should be asked to bring their own for each class.
- Soft, relaxing music may be played in the background.
- Lights can be dimmed where possible.
- The midwife should deliver instructions in a soft, low and pleasing voice. The midwife should try to talk slowly, with distinct pauses at appropriate places during the drill. Intervals of silence are important to enable the woman to continue to concentrate on body awareness and body rhythms.
- These positions (see Figure 19.3) are practised while lying on the floor during the classes, but must be adapted for each particular circumstance in the labour situation.

19.5   Common problems during pregnancy and childbirth

Lower back pain

More than 50 per cent of women experience lower back pain in pregnancy. This is caused by the effect of relaxin on the ligaments, combined with weight gain and postural changes during pregnancy. Multiparity and multiple pregnancies contribute to increased lordosis, which may contribute to lower back pain.

All pregnant women should be given advice on:

- wearing comfortable shoes with a low heel or no heel
- making sure that their posture is correct, with lordosis minimised (see Figure 19.2 on page 269)
- checking work surfaces and body mechanics
- contracting the abdominal muscles before changing position
- bending their knees and rolling on one side with knees together when getting up from a supine position (as shown in Figure 19.1 on page 268)

- avoiding lifting heavy things, including other children
- sleeping with a pillow under the waist to support the back
- sitting in a supportive chair.

Posterior back pain may develop due to pressure on the sacroiliac ligaments. Only 1 per cent of women will have true sciatica (Babycenter.com, 2017). Good posture is important for both the prevention and management of back pain. Women who experience backache due to pressure on the sacroiliac ligaments are advised to:

- sleep with a pillow between the legs
- wear a pelvic support girdle
- not sit with crossed legs
- always keep the knees and shoulders in line
- not twist the body
- use pillows to lift the baby to the breast if breastfeeding or to the bottle if bottle feeding
- bend their knees when lifting something.

Dysfunction of the symphysis pubis

Symphysis pubis dysfunction and discomfort occur in 1: 300 women (Wikipedia, 2017a). There is a 35 mm relaxation between the pubic bones in pregnancy. When the pubis is unstable, the gait is affected and the pain is worse when standing on one leg. A woman presenting with symptoms should be advised to:

- rest as much as possible
- avoid weight-bearing exercises, climbing stairs or squatting
- keep her knees together when getting out of bed
- deliver the baby in the side-lying position.

Pregnancy-associated osteoporosis

Pregnancy-associated osteoporosis is poorly recognised and can lead to fractures in pregnancy. Symptoms start in the third trimester and women usually present with pain of unknown origin that is exacerbated when they lift something up. Older women may be more affected than younger women. The condition can only be diagnosed by ultrasound and X-rays or bone-density measurements. Lactation may be contraindicated if the diagnosis is made.

Dysfunction of the pelvic floor

Pelvic floor dysfunction may include both antenatal and postnatal urinary incontinence (stress incontinence) and uterine prolapse. Urinary incontinence is a common problem, and occurs in 40–60 per cent of pregnancies. Supervised antenatal exercises improve this condition in 70 per cent of affected women and 66 per cent of women show improvement or are cured after eight weeks of intensive exercise (Bradshaw, 2003).

A woman suffering from a mild case of uterine prolapse after normal birth may benefit from pelvic floor exercises. However, surgery is needed for more severe cases.

Diastasis recti

Diastasis recti is a condition where the rectus abdominis muscles separate or herniate by more than 2.5 cm. The hernia can reach a size of 10 cm; the largest recorded hernia was 23 cm in late pregnancy (Bradshaw, 2003). There is a 66 per cent incidence in women who have constant backache.

The separation of the muscles is clearly visible on abdominal examination. When the woman is asked to lift her head in the supine position, two columns of muscle are visible on the side of the uterus. In severe cases the uterus and baby are felt very clearly, as the muscle is pulled away.

Women presenting with this condition are advised to:
- avoid curl-ups
- support the abdomen when sitting up from a lying position, by bending the legs and turning on the side first (see Figure 19.1 on page 268)
- always bend the legs when lying in the supine position and tilt to the side to relieve strain on the back and abdomen and to prevent inferior vena cava syndrome (IVCS).

A gap of 3–4 cm will resolve over a week postnatally; larger gaps may still be present at 12 weeks or until six months or may need surgical intervention.

19.6 Preparation for birth and parenthood

Women should be educated about what may happen in pregnancy, during labour and postnatally. The education programme should focus on the following aspects:
- *Pregnancy:* Common problems, nutrition, preparation of the breasts and nipples, prevention of stretch marks, signs of labour, when to go to the hospital, danger signs of pregnancy, kick chart, exercise, sleep, relaxation and labour drills, maternity leave, wearing a seatbelt, travelling by plane, going on holiday, having hair treatments and colouring, mouth hygiene, gingivitis and going to the dentist, emotional adjustments, and time and financial planning.
- *Birth preparation:* This deals with positions in labour, woman-friendly care, development of a birth plan, management of pain, choice of birth place, choice of birth method, choice of providers, the presence of the significant person of the woman's choice at the birth, the use of a doula, scenarios where complications may occur, maternal–child bonding and early breastfeeding, the role of healthcare professionals in labour and the costs of care.
- *Postnatal education:* This looks at the changed roles of the couple, the development of skills of baby care (eg fathers are taught to bath the baby). In many institutions, the father is given the opportunity to give the baby its first bath under supervision. Education should include instruction on breastfeeding and kangaroo-mother-care (KMC), abilities of the newborn, baby behaviour, crying, stools, jaundice, care of the cord and eyes, hygiene, immunisation, growth and development, introduction of solids, and safety aspects such as how to carry and transport the baby and where the baby should sleep.

Seatbelts
Both the American Academy of Family Physicians (AAFP) and the USA's National Highway Transportation Safety Administration (NHTSA) agree that pregnant women should always wear seatbelts.

Activity
1 Compile a programme that covers relevant topics.   2 Gather evidence-based information on each aspect and keep it in a file.   3 Design an information brochure.   4 Form a health education group and give a presentation on any topic of your choice to a class or a group of pregnant women.   5 Let the group of mothers evaluate the talk.

19.7 Breathing techniques

Women tend to be anxious about labour. It is important to teach the full range of breathing techniques that can be used at different times during labour, all of which help the labouring woman to relax, conserve energy, remain in control of her own body and work through the pain. This also helps to calm her and prevents her from becoming tense and afraid. When women have been taught that they can, with practice, have a high degree of control over their own bodies by concentrating on the breathing techniques, they will soon become confident in facing labour and will look forward to applying these techniques.

Methods of breathing in the first stage of labour

This technique is useful in various instances, namely:
- from the beginning to the end of each contraction, throughout the first stage of labour
- whenever an uncomfortable or anxiety-producing procedure is being done
- to overcome feelings of nausea.

The main principle behind this method of breathing is to keep the breathing rhythmic and controlled, which produces a calming effect and is ideal for the beginning and the end of each contraction. With this method, the woman will be able to achieve a high degree of relaxation and control instead of allowing the pain to envelop her. This helps the woman to 'ride out' each contraction.

The doula, husband or partner, significant person or midwife can play the role of 'birth coach', guiding and supporting the woman in labour.

Method

Breathing

Explain the following method for controlled, rhythmic breathing:
1. The woman places her hand on her abdomen. The hand must lift when she inhales. Abdominal breathing relieves the pressure on the uterus.
2. As soon as a contraction starts, the woman breathes in deeply through her nose, feeling the abdomen rise upwards. This is followed by a slow, deep exhalation through her mouth. It is important for the midwife to stress that each woman must find the depth and rhythm of breathing that is comfortable for her.
3. As each breath is released, the woman relaxes her entire body and tries to remain as relaxed as possible throughout the contraction.
4. As the contraction strengthens, the deep breathing may change to a shallower, lighter and slightly quicker rhythm of breathing; the midwife must stress the importance of the woman concentrating only on her breathing.

The sense of hearing

During a contraction, the woman listens to her breathing and thus keeps her sense of hearing under control.

The sense of sight

If the woman closes her eyes, she may retreat into a dark and pain-filled 'cocoon'. If she gazes around wildly, she may feel out of control and her fear and anxiety may increase. If,

however, she fixes her eyes on someone or on some object as the contraction starts, she should experience a better sense of control, enabling her to concentrate on her breathing.

The sense of touch

The woman should keep her hands relaxed and free. If she clutches onto someone or something else, such as a blanket or the sides of the bed, she will be tensing her whole body and this will increase the pain and also waste oxygen. Her hands can be used in the following ways:
- Effleurage is a French word describing a light type of massage, which can be done by the woman herself. She gently runs the tips of her fingers over her abdomen. She starts with both hands just above the pubic bone, using only the finger tips. She then runs her fingers up towards her sternum. She then parts her hands, and runs them around the uterus and down, to meet above the pubic bone. This roughly traces the shape of a butterfly. These actions sensitise the peripheral nerves below the skin surface and are very soothing (counter-stimulation). The woman can learn to do this to the rhythm of her breathing.
- The woman may find that having her hands at her sides and using her fingers to tap out the rhythm of her breathing is very helpful. She may also find that by holding her hands very lightly over her abdomen during a contraction, she can keep in touch with the rhythm of her breathing.

The sense of taste

Obviously, the sense of taste cannot be controlled, but here the midwife can give the woman advice on preventing her mouth from becoming dry during labour (with all the deep breathing). The woman should:
- move her tongue up and down, which will stimulate the secretion of saliva
- drink sips of iced water (which the birth partner can give her), suck ice or apply lip-ice to her lips at regular intervals to prevent her lips from drying and cracking.

The transitional and second stages of labour
Controlled breath-holding and pushing, bearing down

This technique is used in the second stage of labour with the urge to push or bear down. (For delivery positions, see management of the second stage of labour, in Chapter 28). The technique is as follows:
- The woman is advised to bear down when the contraction reaches its peak. The best position for labour is squatting.

The woman is allowed to assume a comfortable position during the second stage.

▶ When bearing down, her head is forward with her chin on her chest. Her mouth and eyes are closed. She pushes or bears down into her perineum, which is a similar action to that used for defecating.

▶ One or two long and sustained, strong pushes are given during the duration of the contraction, rather than frequent, ineffective pushes. This is known as the Valsalva manoeuvre.

▶ Between contractions, the woman lies back and relaxes, either on the cushions or against her husband or partner. However, she should remain in a sitting position if the delivery is to be undertaken in the dorsal position (modified dorsal position). She must conserve her energy as much as possible.

▶ If the woman delivers in this upright position, she will be able to see her baby emerge and possibly be involved with the final stage of delivery by placing her hands under the baby's armpits and delivering her baby onto her tummy. This can be a very exciting experience, but the woman should not feel guilty if she is feeling too tired and does not wish to do this, or if her medical practitioner does not allow her to.

Panting or fast light breathing

This technique is used during the period of transition from the first into the second stage of labour, to stop the woman from bearing down before the cervix is fully dilated, or during the second stage of labour when the baby's head is crowning.

1. The woman has to overcome the urge to push, in order to give the perineum time to stretch slowly to accommodate the baby's head. The midwife should stress the importance of this and explain that pushing when the baby's head is crowning can cause unnecessary tearing of the perineum.

2. Reassure the woman that she will be getting a tremendous amount of support and encouragement throughout the second stage and that she needs only to listen to any guidance given to her and do what is required of her.

3. The woman is taught to take a number of short, shallow breaths (similar to a dog panting), followed by a long exhalation after every five to ten pants, in order to prevent hyperventilation. For example: 'pant, pant, pant, pant, pant, blow'.

4. The women uses her chest and lungs to take short, shallow breaths. This type of breathing is not used for any length of time, but only to allow slow crowning and delivery of the head.

Hyperventilation

The signs of hyperventilation are dizziness, light-headedness, tingling sensations in the tips of fingers and/or lips and eventual fainting. Too much oxygen enters the system and carbon dioxide falls.

In order to prevent over-breathing or hyperventilation, the woman should be taught to recognise and report any early signs of hyperventilation. She should then be given or should ask for a paper bag, which she holds closely over her mouth and nose while she takes slow breaths in and out for a short period, until the dizziness passes.

In labour, holding the breath and bearing down causes a slight rise in the maternal partial pressure of carbon dioxide (PCO_2), as less carbon dioxide (CO_2) is exhaled. On the other hand, deep breathing during contractions has the opposite effect and causes PCO_2 levels to fall. This can result in symptoms of hyperventilation if the levels fall below 16–18 mmHg.

19.8 The ward visit

In most birth units, women are given an opportunity to visit the unit (during a ward round) to familiarise themselves with the place where they will give birth. This is often done by the childbirth educator once a month as a standard programme in the institution. Fathers are encouraged to come as well. Couples are allowed to ask as many questions as they want and are introduced to the ward's staff. A typical birth is explained and the delivery rooms, theatre and nursery or neonatal unit are shown and discussed. The philosophy and protocols of the unit (and the limitations) are explained as well as the mother- and baby-friendly principles and how these are applied in the particular unit.

Women are encouraged to develop a birth plan and discuss it with caregivers before or on admission. The birth plan should clearly indicate wishes such as choice of birth, pain relief, significant person to attend birth, feeding method, and any other wish or desire. The birth plan may include coping mechanisms for labour pain and anticipated birth experiences and birth outcomes.

The ward visit may help allay fears and uncertainties. Women are encouraged to book the bed, usually completing all the needed paperwork beforehand to avoid emergency situations when in labour. Women are instructed on what to bring to the hospital, where to keep emergency numbers for transport and what to do in case of an emergency. Women are usually instructed to come straight to the ward and not to go to admissions when in labour.

The woman is then taken through a series of exercises. The birth may be viewed on a video and the birth and the relaxation drill are done to prepare her for birth.

19.9   Conclusion

Childbirth education and preparation are important supportive processes. However, they need to be evidence-based and be carried out according to accepted norms and standards that are congruent with current practices, add value and are not conflicting. Midwives need to keep themselves updated on new developments, work well with others and evaluate the effectiveness of their actions.

20

Common minor disorders in pregnancy

LEARNING OBJECTIVES

On completion of this chapter, you must be able to:

▶ understand the physiology behind the minor disorders of pregnancy

▶ identify common minor disorders of pregnancy

▶ appreciate the scope of health promotion in managing minor disorders of pregnancy

▶ identify the role of the midwife in promoting the health of the pregnant woman during pregnancy

▶ demonstrate competency in evidence-based interventions for each condition

▶ explain the advice to give the pregnant woman for each condition.

KNOWLEDGE ASSUMED TO BE IN PLACE

The anatomical and physiological changes of pregnancy

The normal progress of pregnancy

KEYWORDS

nausea and vomiting • morning sickness (emesis gravidarum) • insomnia • human chorionic gonadotropin (hCG) • micturition • carpal tunnel syndrome • pruritis • heartburn

20.1 Introduction

The anatomical and physiological changes that take place during pregnancy were discussed in Chapter 14. It is largely due to these changes that some women experience discomfort. Certain conditions may interfere with the woman's diet and nutrition, and/or with her exercise and sleep, and may eventually undermine her general health. If these common (minor) disorders are not attended to promptly, they can become serious.

20.2 Identifying minor disorders during antenatal visits

While taking the history at each antenatal visit, the midwife should tactfully ask the woman if any of these conditions are troubling her. Some women are reticent about complaining of these very personal conditions. The woman may think the condition is not worth mentioning if it is not troubling her too much.

During the physical examination, the midwife may notice or pick up signs of some of these disorders. She should treat and/or give advice for each disorder. If the condition does not respond to the midwife's treatment, or if the condition has become serious, the woman should be referred to a medical practitioner.

20.3 Descriptions, causes and treatment

Fainting

Dizzy spells and/or fainting in early pregnancy can be worrying to the pregnant woman and her family. This condition arises early in pregnancy due to the likely drop in BP caused by the progesterone-induced general vasodilation of pregnancy, which has not yet been counterbalanced by the increase in blood volume. Fainting may occur when the woman has been standing for a while, especially in a hot, confined or crowded place. Wearing tight clothing, over-exertion, lack of sleep, excitement and shock may also be contributing factors.

Fainting may occur in late pregnancy as a result of pressure on the aorta and/or on the inferior vena cava by the enlarged uterus, particularly if the woman has been lying in the supine position for a while (supine hypotensive syndrome). Sudden changes in posture, such as moving swiftly from the recumbent to the upright position or standing for long periods, especially in hot weather, may contribute to fainting attacks.

Care and advice

If fainting occurs in early pregnancy, reassure the woman and her family that the condition usually resolves itself after the first trimester.

▶ *History:* Take a history to make sure that there are no serious problems. Pay specific attention to the woman's weight and daily intake of food in terms of energy as well as type of food.
▶ *Physical examination:* Take the woman's BP.
▶ *Special examination:* Check Hb and blood glucose.
▶ *Advice:* In the case of hypotension, refer the woman for medical attention. However, if no other conditions are identified, advise the woman to:
  • not stand for long periods, as the blood accumulates in the lower parts of the body and the diastolic BP drops
  • lie down at once (left lateral) if she starts to feel dizzy, or to sit down and put her head between her knees
  • avoid sitting or standing up quickly from a lying down position; the cardiovascular system cannot accommodate sudden changes
  • eat five small regular meals a day to boost glucose levels, as blood glucose may be low
  • turn onto her side and avoid lying in the supine position for more than 15 minutes at a time during the third trimester.

Nausea and vomiting (morning sickness/emesis gravidarum)

During weeks 4–14, most women experience some nausea and about 50 per cent of women will vomit. Nausea usually occurs immediately after rising in the morning, as does vomiting. When aggravated by other factors, such as a large meal, rich food or travel by car, boat or aeroplane, vomiting can occur during the day. Morning sickness is not considered to be serious and will usually have abated by the end of the first trimester.

The cause of nausea and vomiting in early pregnancy is not completely understood, but it is probably related to the increasing levels of oestrogen and/or high levels of human chorionic gonadotropin (hCG) in the bloodstream, which stimulates the chemoreceptor trigger zone in the brain and

initiates nausea and vomiting. However, over time the body becomes accustomed to the high levels of oestrogen and/ or hCG. It is thought that there are changes in the thyroid function as well. The altered carbohydrate metabolism, low blood sugar and the effects of the thyroid on the basal metabolic rate (BMR) cause changes in food preferences and may cause cravings.

If vomiting continues into the day and becomes excessive, preventing the woman from digesting and absorbing food, the condition is no longer normal and the woman should be referred to a medical practitioner. This is also the case if morning vomiting continues after the first trimester. Timely treatment can, in most instances, prevent the condition from deteriorating into hyperemesis gravidarum.

Excessive vomiting in early pregnancy may suggest a multiple pregnancy or hydatidiform mole (due to high hormonal levels). If no nausea or vomiting is experienced in early pregnancy, there is a raised chance of spontaneous abortion and preterm labour (due to low hormonal levels).

Care and advice

▶ *History:* Determine the extent, duration, time and periods when vomiting occurs. Also determine the presence or history of fever, headaches and abdominal pain.
▶ *Physical examination:* Observe signs of weight loss and dehydration.
▶ *Special examination:* Check urine specific gravity (SG) and ketones.
  • If there is no sign of dehydration or ketones, the woman is supported and advised.
  • If the woman cannot function or ketones are present; refer for medical attention.
▶ *Advice:*
  • Reassure the woman that morning sickness is transient and explain that the condition usually disappears after the first trimester.
  • Reorganise her daily nutritional programme and routine. Low glucose levels seem to aggravate the nausea and vomiting and are also not good for the fetus. Advise the woman to have a high-calorie drink (milk) before going to sleep and dry biscuits before getting out of bed in the morning.
  • The woman should have more frequent, smaller meals, with plenty of protein. She should not eat rich, fatty or spicy foods or large meals. She should eat the kind of food that best agrees with her condition and that she feels like, provided that she gets a balanced diet. Ginger can be an effective non-drug treatment for

nausea. Chamomile (for example chamomile tea) may relieve nausea for some women.

- If the woman already had a tendency to become nauseous and vomit when she felt worried or anxious before the pregnancy, the anxieties, fears and added responsibilities of pregnancy may aggravate her problem.
- The woman should not take over-the-counter (OTC) medication or self-medicate. A doctor may prescribe anti-emetic medication, of which meclozine appears to be the safest. Meclozine 25 mg is often combined with pyridoxine 50 mg, two tablets at night. Other antihistamine or anti-emetics such as promethazine may also be prescribed. These medications may cause drowsiness and the woman should be warned about this if she drives a car.
- If the woman is unable to tolerate any food, and if she has shown significant weight loss within a short period and/or if there are ketones in her urine, she will usually be admitted to hospital for observation and treatment.

Ptyalism (excessive salivation)

Some women experience excessive salivation, called ptyalism, during pregnancy. It usually occurs from the eighth week of gestation and may accompany heartburn. The saliva produced is tasteless, making it difficult for the woman to swallow the saliva. The condition may cause a lot of stress, particularly when in public places. The real cause is unknown.

Care and advice

No specific investigations are recommended. Listen to the woman attentively and display a great deal of sensitivity. Explain the physiology and offer psychological support. Advise the woman to eat oranges and chew gum if possible, as this may provide some relief.

Pica

Pica is a psycho-behavioural disorder characterised by the abnormal craving for non-food substances such as starch, clay (soil) or ice. The causes of pica are unknown, but there are a number of misconceptions about its causes such as psychological stress, dyspepsia, general hunger and a side effect of iron deficiency.

Pica may displace the intake of nutritious foods or interfere with nutrient absorption. There are various other potential complications, depending on the items consumed. These include lead poisoning, faecal impaction, parasitic infection, toxaemia, prematurity, perinatal mortality, low birth weight

(LBW) and anaemic infants. In addition, pica can cause iron deficiency anaemia.

Care and advice

Pica should be discouraged, as it increases the risk of nutritional inadequacies:

- When counselling the pregnant woman, determine what is ingested and why. Remain non-judgemental but stress the importance of an adequate diet, the use of iron supplements and the potential danger of pica.
- Educate the woman based on the type of craving. For example, if the woman is craving sand, educate her on the health problems which may occur as a result of consuming sand.
- If the substances taken are harmful to either the mother or fetus or both, refer the woman to a medical practitioner.

Breast tenderness

During pregnancy, the duct and alveolar systems of the breast enlarge under the influence of oestrogen and progesterone. Breast tingling and tenderness are some of the earliest symptoms of pregnancy. Later in pregnancy there is an increased vascularity, together with a general enlargement of the breasts, and the woman may experience tenderness and discomfort.

Care and advice

- *History:* Take a history of breast health, previous breastfeeding and care of breasts.
- *Physical examination:* Do a full examination of the breasts and nipples to feel for any lumps.
- *Special examinations:* No special examinations are required if all is normal. If a lump is present, an ultrasound may be needed.
- *Advice:* Reassure the woman and advise her:
  - that breast discomfort and enlargement are natural occurrences in preparation for breastfeeding
  - that she should buy and wear a good supportive brassiere
  - that the application of local warmth may help relieve tenderness of the nipples with breastfeeding
  - how to do self-assessment of the breasts.

Frequency of micturition

In early pregnancy the urine production by the kidneys increases, leading to frequency of micturition, particularly at night. The muscle-relaxing effect of progesterone causes stasis of urine within the urinary tract, which increases the risk of urinary tract infection (UTI). Pressure on the bladder from the enlarged uterus, particularly in late pregnancy when the presenting part enters the pelvis, may also lead to frequency of micturition and a retention of residual urine.

Care and advice

▶ *History:* Determine the pattern of the problem as well as any history of UTIs.
▶ *Physical examination:* Take the woman's temperature to exclude infection. Consider the possibility of multiple pregnancy or an abnormal position of the uterus. Palpate the abdomen.
▶ *Special tests:* Test the urine (clean-catch midstream specimen) for clarity, pH, protein and leukocytes.
▶ *Advice:* If no abnormality is present, advise the woman:
  • that her frequent micturition is caused by the uterus pressing on the bladder and that it should improve after 20 weeks
  • to reduce her intake of fluids in the evenings and before bedtime
  • not to stand for prolonged periods, particularly before bedtime, as the tissue fluids return to the vascular system when the woman lies down and this leads to nocturia
  • to empty her bladder regularly
  • that in later pregnancy, residual urine can be more easily voided if she leans forward during the final stage of passing urine.

Fatigue

The metabolic processes of pregnancy and the circulating hormones may interfere with sleep, causing fatigue in combination with relative hypoglycaemia. This is now seen as nature's way of ensuring that the woman slows down, both physically and mentally, in these early stages of pregnancy. It is sometimes known as the 'incubating' or 'nesting' phenomenon. During pregnancy, a woman needs more sleep than in her non-pregnant state and fatigue may also result from the cumulative effect of too little sleep. The effort of carrying around the increased weight of the enlarged uterus may also cause fatigue in late pregnancy.

Care and advice

▶ *History:* Determine the woman's daily activity and sleep pattern, including diet pattern and mental health status.
▶ *Physical examination:* Check the woman's physical condition, body and facial expression and emotional status.

▶ *Special examinations:* Complete the Edinburgh Postnatal Depression Scale (EPDS) – with the woman's permission – and check her Hb level to exclude anaemia.
▶ *Advice:* If no serious problems are identified, advise the woman:
  • that gentle exercise is needed daily
  • to attend an antenatal class and support group
  • to take rest and sleep periods during the day
  • to eat a balanced diet
  • to identify disturbances in her sleep
  • on which sleep positions are best
  • not to take OTC medication or self-medicate.

Headaches

Headaches are a fairly common complaint in early pregnancy and are probably due to the effects of oestrogen and progesterone on the circulatory system and in particular on the intracranial vascular system. They are very similar to premenstrual tension headaches and usually disappear after the first trimester. Occasionally the condition may persist throughout pregnancy.

Care and advice

▶ *History:* Take a neurological history of headaches and other problems.
▶ *Physical examination:* Take the woman's temperature and BP and check for oedema.
▶ *Special examinations:* Check urine for protein to exclude hypertension.
▶ *Advice:* If no serious problems are found, advise the woman:
  • that her headaches will pass after the first semester
  • that adequate rest, relaxation and, occasionally, paracetamol may relieve the headache
  • that if her headaches are severe or continue, she should see a medical practitioner
  • to take only prescribed medication.

Stuffy nose

A stuffy nose occurs as a result of increased blood supply to the nostrils due to the effect of oestrogen. In response, the nasal mucosa becomes congested and the woman continuously feels congested and blocked.

Care and advice

Advise the woman to:
▶ blow her nose gently
▶ avoid explosive sneezes

- use a humidifier, steam inhalation or normal saline nasal drops, which may help decongest the nose
- avoid decongestants
- breathe through the mouth while sleeping (and keep a glass of water nearby to prevent a dry mouth)
- sleep in the lateral position to minimise snoring
- seek medical attention if she is worried.

Epistaxis

Epistaxis is usually also due to the effects of oestrogen and progesterone on the circulatory system, causing engorgement of the blood vessels lining the nasal passages. Bleeding may be spontaneous or may be brought about by overheating or forceful nose-blowing. Frequent short bleeds with minimal blood loss are common and usually harmless; severe, short bleeds may indicate an underlying condition. If bleeding persists, it may contribute to anaemia.

Care and advice

- *History:* Determine risk factors, the occurrence of nasal stuffiness and the pattern of nose bleeding.
- *Physical examination:* Check for generalised oedema.
- *Special examination:* Check Hb.
- *Advice:* If no serious problems are found, advise the woman:
  - that nose bleeds are common during pregnancy
  - to pinch her nostrils hard while hanging her head over a basin – firm pressure for a few minutes should stop the bleeding
  - to use saline nose spray on a regular basis to keep the nasal mucosa soft
  - not to blow the nose hard or forcefully
  - that if her nose bleeds are recurrent or severe, she will be referred to a medical practitioner.

Varicose veins

The effects of oestrogen and progesterone on the circulatory system cause increased growth and dilatation of the veins which, together with the increased blood volume, are the main causes of varicose veins. The condition is further aggravated by the pressure of the enlarging uterus. If the woman has an inherited tendency to poor veins, coupled with long periods of standing, this can lead to incompetence of the veins in the legs.

Between 10 and 20 per cent of pregnant women suffer from varicose veins in the legs. The condition is also more common with an increase in parity and age. The woman may complain of tiredness and aching legs, which may become oedematous as the day progresses. At night, she often experiences cramps in her leg muscles. The veins may become distended and tortuous

and very unsightly. The varicose veins usually improve after the pregnancy, but it may take up to three months before the veins subside. However, the condition is aggravated by each subsequent pregnancy. Varicose veins of the vulva and vagina are less common.

The following complications – which may lead to thromboembolism – may occur:

- Haemorrhage and ulceration
- Thrombophlebitis (inflammation of the superficial veins of the leg, with thrombosis)
- Phlebothrombosis (deep vein thrombosis [DVT] of the leg).

Care and advice

- *History:* Identify women with risk factors, eg multiple pregnancy, polyhydramnios, previous thrombosis. Take a history of daily activities.
- *Physical examination:* Observe both legs and the vulva and consider haemorrhoids.
- *Special examinations:* Ultrasound should be done by a medical practitioner.
- *Advice:* Advise the woman:
  - to see a medical practitioner if she has a history of risk factors
  - that if her work requires her to sit or stand, she must not cross her legs or maintain the same position for more than half an hour
  - that she can continue to work after 32 weeks of pregnancy
  - to rest in the left lateral position
  - to do gentle exercises.
  - to rest with her legs and hips elevated for an hour at least twice a day
  - to wear supporting antithrombosis stockings (elastic stockings)
  - to avoid wearing garters and other tight garments around the legs.
- *Treatment and precautions:*
  - The surgical excision of incompetent veins may be necessary, but if possible this should be left until about three months after pregnancy.
  - During delivery, great care should be taken not to incise or tear vulval or vaginal varicosities, as they can bleed profusely.

Haemorrhoids

Haemorrhoids are varicose veins of the anal canal and are caused by the same factors as varicose veins in the legs or other areas. They can be internal and/or external. The condition is further aggravated during pregnancy by constipation, causing straining during defecation, and also by prolonged bearing down in the second stage of labour.

The complications of haemorrhoids are similar to those of varicose veins, although bleeding is more common and thrombosis is rare.

Care and advice

▶ *History:* Take a history of risk factors such as multiple pregnancy and constipation.
▶ *Physical examination:* Observe the haemorrhoids.
▶ *Special examinations:* If necessary, a rectal examination should be carried out by a medical practitioner.
▶ *Advice:* Advise the woman to:
   • eat a high-fibre diet, increase fluid intake and exercise more often to reduce the incidence of constipation and pain on defecation
   • prevent constipation and straining.
▶ *Treatment:*
   • The management of haemorrhoids is mainly directed towards preventing bleeding and relieving pain and discomfort.
   • Soothing ointments and suppositories may be ordered by the medical practitioner.
   • For prolapsed haemorrhoids, the woman should rest for about half an hour in the left lateral position with the foot of the bed raised. Then, after lubrication, the haemorrhoids may be gently replaced.
   • For bleeding, cold astringent packs can be applied to the area, using either hypertonic saline, magnesium sulphate or zinc sulphate solutions.
   • Haemorrhoids, like varicose veins, take up to three months to improve after delivery. Surgery is best left until then, if possible.

Heartburn and oesophageal reflux

Oesophageal reflux, which occurs in over 60 per cent of pregnant women, is the reflux or regurgitation of the gastric juices into the oesophagus or into the mouth, when it is commonly known as waterbrash. The effect of hormones in pregnancy, specifically progesterone, relaxes the oesophageal sphincter, resulting in incompetence of the cardiac sphincter (cardia). This, combined with the pressure on the stomach from the enlarging uterus, causes oesophageal reflux.

Women usually complain of heartburn, experienced as discomfort, burning or pain in the epigastrium, in the second and third trimesters of pregnancy. Although this is not a serious condition, it can be very distressing and is not easy to treat.

The acidic gastric juice causes irritation of the lower oesophagus and oesophagitis may occur. The condition is worse at night, when the woman is lying down, and may prevent restful sleep. Incompetence of the pyloric sphincter can result in bile being present in the gastric juice.

Care and advice

▶ *History:* Take a history of gastrointestinal (GI) problems and nutritional habits.
▶ *Physical examination:* Check the size of the abdomen.
▶ *Special examination:* No special examinations are required.
▶ *Advice:* The following may help to relieve the symptoms:
   • Small, fairly frequent meals should be taken, so that the stomach can empty easily.
   • The type of food is important. Meals should not consist of rich, fatty, oily, spicy or indigestible foods.
   • The last meal should not be taken after 6 pm or within three hours of going to sleep.
   • The woman may use an extra pillow when resting or sleeping.
   • The woman should stop smoking. If that is not possible, she should reduce the amount of cigarettes smoked and should not smoke after the last meal of the day.
   • If the acidic gastric juice is causing the problem, an antacid such as magnesium trisilicate or aluminium hydroxide may be prescribed by a medical practitioner.
▶ *Referral:* If the condition does not respond to the above advice and treatment, a medical practitioner may do further investigations. Refer the woman if the condition is continuous.

Constipation

Pregnant women tend to experience constipation, in the form of the infrequent emptying of the bowels, the passing of hard faecal matter or both. Constipation occurs due to the effect of progesterone, which acts on the smooth muscles of the GI system and causes relaxation of the smooth muscles of the bowel and small intestine. This relaxation effect contributes to reduced peristalsis, which in turn results in increased absorption of water from the gastric contents, causing constipation. Alternatively, it may result from pressure of the fetus on the intestines. Other contributory factors may include a decrease in physical activity and an inadequate intake of fluid and fibre. Constipation may also be a side effect of the consumption of iron supplements. If iron supplementation is a contributory factor, the woman may be advised to reduce the dosage or frequency of the supplement, if possible.

Care and advice

▶ *History:* Take a history of the woman's bowel action and diet patterns.

▶ *Physical examination:* Observe the woman's general appearance.

▶ *Special examinations:* No specific examinations are required.

▶ *Advice:* The woman should be advised:
  * that if she follows the advice given to her by the midwife at her antenatal visits, constipation should not be a problem
  * to eat foods high in roughage or fibre and low in carbohydrates or sugars
  * to eat regular, balanced meals
  * to eat high-bulk bran, which can be bought from health shops, and bran biscuits, wholewheat cereals and wholewheat bread
  * to drink plenty of fluids, particularly plain water, to help to keep the bowel contents soft and easier to evacuate
  * to do exercise, such as a short walk around the block, especially just before or just after breakfast
  * on bowel training, ie to use the toilet at specific times, such as after breakfast each morning
  * that aperients and laxatives are not recommended.

▶ *Referral:* If the constipation is not resolved within a few dasys, refer the woman to a medical practitioner.

Pruritis

Itching of the skin may be experienced during pregnancy, usually starting at the abdomen. This is caused by high levels of circulating oestrogen and the inability of the liver to metabolise the oestrogen, as well as the slight increase in circulating bilirubin. Itching of the skin of the abdomen and breasts may be caused by stretching or, if there is a generalised itching, it could be hormonal. Itching can also be caused by scabies, which the midwife should easily be able to recognise.

Pruritus vulvae may be hormonal, related to diabetes or due to vaginal and/or vulval infections such as *Candida albicans*, *Trichomonas vaginalis*, condylomata lata (syphilis) or condylomata acuminata (vulval warts).

In some instances, pruritus may be associated with a mild jaundice. Women with itching and jaundice must be referred to a medical practitioner.

Care and advice

▶ *History:* Check for any allergies.

▶ *Physical examination:* Observe for the type of rash and the distribution. Check for scabies.

▶ *Special examinations:* Check the urine for bilirubin.

▶ *Advice:* The woman should be advised:
  * on good hygiene, such as daily bathing, exercise, etc
  * on eating a balanced diet
  * not to wear clothing against the skin that could be irritating
  * to wear cotton rather than nylon underwear
  * to apply a soothing lotion such as calamine lotion.

▶ *Referral:* Itching may be related to a pathological condition such as jaundice. Persistent itching should therefore be referred to a medical practitioner for further investigations and treatment.

Oedema

Oedema of the feet and ankles is a common condition in late pregnancy, occurring in about 40 per cent of pregnant women. The increased blood volume, together with the distension of the veins and the added mechanical pressure of the enlarged uterus, may cause oedema of the feet, ankles, vulva and anus. Standing for prolonged periods aggravates the condition, but the swelling usually subsides after a good night's rest.

Care and advice

▶ *History:* Check the history for cardiac problems.

▶ *Physical examination:* Check the woman's BP and for generalised oedema.

▶ *Special examinations:* Check the Hb. Test the urine for protein.

▶ *Advice:* Reassure the woman and advise her:
  * not to stand for long periods, but to take frequent rests with her legs elevated
  * to elevate the foot of the bed; this will facilitate the return of fluid in the tissues of the legs to the general circulation
  * to see a medical practitioner if the oedema is troublesome or extends beyond the ankles
  * not to use diuretics
  * to see a medical practitioner if the oedema does not subside after a good night's rest, or if her fingers or face are swollen.

Leucorrhoea

Leucorrhoea is increased vaginal discharge during pregnancy. This occurs as a result of the high levels of oestrogen in pregnancy, which contributes to an increased shedding of superficial mucosal cells in the vagina. Leucorrhoea is a clear, whitish, non-offensive vaginal discharge. It indicates a normal physiological process in pregnancy.

Care and advice

Exclude any infection and explain the physiology behind the discharge to the woman. Then reassure the woman and inform her that this will resolve itself after the delivery of the baby. Educate the woman on:

▶ the physiological aspects
▶ good personal hygiene
▶ the use of cotton underwear, which is absorbent and non-irritant
▶ avoiding tights.

Carpal tunnel syndrome

About 28 per cent of pregnant women experience this condition, usually in the second or third trimester (O'Donnell, Elio & Day, 2010). It is associated with the hormonal changes of pregnancy, oedema and the compression of the median nerve, particularly in women presenting with gestational diabetes.

During pregnancy, some women may complain of numbness and tingling sensations ('pins and needles') in their hands and fingers. This can occur at any time of day, but is usually worse in the morning. It may become extremely painful and debilitating.

Swelling of the hands may cause carpal tunnel syndrome, where the nerves to the hand are compressed as they pass under the flexor retinaculum at the wrist. This results in severe pain in the hand and in muscle weakness, which may reduce the sensory and motor function. The condition usually resolves following childbirth.

Care and advice

No specific tests are recommended and the woman should be advised on how to make the symptoms better and reduce the pain and discomfort.

▶ *History:* Take a history of daily activities and nutrition.
▶ *Physical examination:* Observe for generalised oedema.
▶ *Special examinations:* No specific tests are recommended.
▶ *Advice:* Reassure the woman and provide the following information:
  • Studies have shown that resting the fingers, hand and wrist in a neutral position is the most effective way to reduce pressure in the carpal tunnel.
  • She should avoid repetitive work and take rests.
  • She should eat a low-salt diet.
▶ *Treatment and referral:*
  • Splinting may be a treatment in pregnancy.
  • An orthopaedic surgeon may inject cortisone in the wrist.
  • An operation to relieve the compression may be necessary.

Insomnia

Sleep and rest are essential during pregnancy, but there are many conditions, both psychological and physical, which may cause a disruption in sleep patterns. Insomnia usually occurs from 28 weeks of pregnancy until term. Many of the common disorders in pregnancy also tend to disturb or prevent sleep. Some of the contributory factors to insomnia include undue worry and anxiety about pregnancy-related issues, frequent micturition or difficulty in finding a comfortable position as a result of the pressure symptoms related to the gravid uterus.

Care and advice

▶ *History:* Observe the woman's sleeping patterns, fatigue levels and verbal responses.
▶ *Physical examination:* No specific examination required.
▶ *Special examinations:* No specific investigations recommended.
▶ *Advice:* The woman should be advised:
  • on the importance of a good, balanced diet
  • to get adequate amounts of exercise and rest
  • that sleeping disorders are common in late pregnancy
  • to avoid sleeping too often during the day (frequent naps)
  • to take a warm bath or a warm glass of milk before bedtime
  • to avoid caffeinated drinks
  • on how to adopt a comfortable position when sleeping, eg placing a pillow under the abdomen and another between the knees when lying in the lateral position.
▶ *Referral:* If the condition is severe, refer the woman to a medical practitioner.

Backache

Backache is a common complaint in late pregnancy. It is caused by the increased lumbar curve (lordosis) that occurs when the woman has to hold her shoulders back in order to counterbalance the enlarged uterus in front. Relaxin and progesterone cause a softening of the spinal and pelvic ligaments. This creates strain on the muscles of the back and results in backache and fatigue.

Lax abdominal muscles and a pendulous abdomen (anterior obliquity of the uterus) will further aggravate the condition.

Care and advice

▶ *History:* Take a history of skeletal events such as accidents and previous problems.
▶ *Physical examination:* Carry out abdominal palpation (see Chapter 18). Observe the size of the uterus and its effect on the body.

▶ *Special examinations:* No specific tests are recommended.
▶ *Advice:* The woman should be advised to:
  • rest frequently
  • not stand for long periods
  • not wear high-heeled shoes, as this will aggravate the condition
  • consider antenatal exercises (see Chapter 19)
  • maintain good body posture (see Chapter 19)
  • consider a supportive maternity corset.
▶ *Referral:*
  • If the backache is troublesome, refer the woman to a medical practitioner.
  • If necessary, refer the woman to a physiotherapist for help with body posture.

Muscle cramps

Muscle cramps affect about a third of all pregnant women. These occur in late pregnancy, especially at night, but are not usually troublesome more than three or four times in each pregnancy. Muscle cramps are associated with slowed venous return and decreased venous tone, attributed to the effect of progesterone on the blood vessels as well as nutritional deficiencies. Involuntary muscle contraction is also attributed to the build-up of lactic and pyruvic acid. In late pregnancy, the presenting part of the fetus can cause leg cramps when moving through the pelvis.

Care and advice

▶ *History:* Take a history of cramps and nutritional patterns.
▶ *Physical examination:* No specific observation is required.
▶ *Special examinations:* No specific investigations are recommended.
▶ *Advice:* The woman should be reassured and advised:
  • to rest frequently during the day
  • to flex the foot during a spasm, by pulling or pushing the toes up, and to massage the calf muscles gently
  • to consider calcium or magnesium supplementation if so advised by a midwife or medical practitioner; muscle cramps respond well to this treatment
  • to rest in the knee–chest position (see Figure 32A on page 504) to relieve pressure on the pelvic floor and nerves.

20.4   Conclusion

Some of the common minor disorders in pregnancy may contribute to maternal morbidity. The midwife must know about these disorders and the physiological factors surrounding them in order to mitigate their impact on the health of the woman. The midwife should also adopt a sensitive attitude to the woman who presents with a common minor disorder in order to provide appropriate care and timely referrals.

Medical and surgical conditions that complicate pregnancy

LEARNING OBJECTIVES

On completion of this chapter, you must be able to:
- ▶ recognise the medical and surgical conditions that complicate pregnancy
- ▶ demonstrate competence in preventing complications arising from medical conditions in pregnancy and birth
- ▶ demonstrate competence in the treatment and specific care of conditions that complicate pregnancy and birth.

KNOWLEDGE ASSUMED TO BE IN PLACE

The knowledge and ability to assess and care for low-risk pregnant women

KEYWORDS

pre-eclampsia • eclampsia • HELLP syndrome • peripartum cardiomyopathy (PPCM) • haemaglobinopathies in pregnancy • diabetes mellitis • epilepsy

21.1 Introduction

According to the *Saving Mothers* report (DoH, 2014), complications arise in about 20 per cent of pregnancies. The early identification of factors that indicate problems is essential. Early contact with the pregnant woman makes it possible to gather baseline information that will assist the midwife in identifying health problems in pregnancy, labour and the puerperium.

The age of the woman and the number of pregnancies (gravidity and parity) are factors that may lead to complications in pregnancy. In addition, pregnancy can be complicated by infections and medical or surgical conditions. This chapter will focus on the main causes of maternal mortality in South Africa and some other common problems.

Non-obstetrical medical or surgical problems, trauma or malignancies which can occur during pregnancy are not discussed in this chapter. HIV/AIDS is discussed in Chapter 50 and other infections are discussed in Chapter 49.

21.2 Obstetric risk assessment

Reducing maternal mortality depends on the healthcare system working effectively as a whole. No one single factor can be identified as the most important.

Midwives are specialists in low-risk birth and refer women with pregnancy-related complications to obstetricians and other specialists. The availability of medical practitioners has a significant influence on maternal mortality. In areas where medical practitioners are unavailable, midwives may be called on to practise outside their legal scope of practice.

New approaches to understanding risk provide a more liberal perspective on care during pregnancy. The traditional methods of classifying women as low risk, moderate risk and high risk have been shown to be an ineffective means of predicting complications in pregnancy, birth and the puerperium. Sanders (2003) found that labelling women as 'high risk' affects the psychological state of those women. According to Stahl and Hundley (2003), the way in which risks are documented and communicated needs revision. All women should be considered as having a normal pregnancy until there is clear evidence to the contrary.

No single instrument has so far proved effective (sensitive) in predicting outcomes in pregnancy and birth. The Safe Motherhood Initiative (SMI) moved from risk screening as a way to reduce maternal deaths to setting criteria for essential obstetric care (EOC) and other facilities, such as focusing on the quality of the environment. Table 21.1 details various factors of a woman's antenatal history that must be evaluated.

In South Africa, the development of norms and standards of the environment is particularly important. Therefore, guidelines for the referral of cases have been developed. However, the tenth interim maternal mortality report (Pattinson, Fawcus & Moodley, 2013) demonstrated that despite the tendency to refer high-risk cases to higher levels of care, maternal mortality remained unchanged, as women still died at different levels of the healthcare system under medical supervision.

A previous abnormal birth does not mean that a woman's next birth will also be abnormal. Equally, one normal birth is not necessarily followed by another normal birth. Complications can develop suddenly. There are thus few reliable predictors of the risk of obstetric problems.

If a classification of risk is used, the woman's care should still be individualised. However, she should also be referred to a medical practitioner or higher level of care for assessment upon classification of high-risk status.

Table 21.1

Factors to consider as risks in the antenatal history

Demographic	General
Maternal age: < 15 or > 35 Parity: nullipara, grand multipara Marital status: single Primipaternity (pregnant with new partner) Economic status: Dependent on public transport Antenatal care: First visit after 27 weeks	Nutrition: > 20% overweight, massive obesity, > 10% underweight Poor nutrition Inadequate weight gain Excessive weight gain Smoking Drug or alcohol abuse: history of and/or in this pregnancy
Obstetric	**Medical and surgical**
Infertility factors: < 2 years Previous abortion: one or more Premature or low birth weight (LBW): history of one, two or more Previous large infant: one, two or more Previous perinatal loss: one, two or more Post-term in this pregnancy Previous Caesarean section Previous congenital abnormality Incompetent cervix (cervical cerclage) Uterine abnormality Contracted pelvis Abnormal presentation: history of and/or in this pregnancy Rh negative sensitised Polyhydramnios Oligohydramnios Pre-eclampsia: history of severe, mild and/or in this pregnancy Multiple pregnancy: history of and/or in this pregnancy	Anaemia: Hb 8–10 g/dl Anaemia: Hb < 8 g/dl Sickle cell trait Sickle cell disease (SCD) Hypertension: mild Hypertension: severe Cardiac conditions Gestational diabetes Overt diabetes Thyroid disease: history of and/or in this pregnancy Sexually transmitted infections (STIs) Syphilis: history of and/or in this pregnancy HIV status Urinary tract infection (UTI): in this pregnancy Mental health problems: history of and/or present in this pregnancy History of other medical conditions Other medical conditions in this pregnancy

Obstetric triage

Specialist midwives perform obstetric triage after taking a history, doing a physical examination and ordering appropriate special investigations (where these are available). A woman exhibiting suspicious or problematic findings should be admitted for observation for 24 hours and then only referred further if necessary. In rural areas where transport is a problem, medical practitioners may be consulted using telemedicine. Cases in which specific complications have been identified are then referred for medical care at a higher level, such as regional, tertiary or central hospitals.

21.3 Hypertensive disorders in pregnancy

Hypertension is a common disorder and a leading cause of maternal death globally. Pre-existing hypertension and gestational hypertension can occur in women of childbearing age. In a low-risk pregnancy, BP will decrease in the first trimester and then gradually rise from 20 weeks until the end of the pregnancy.

Pre-eclampsia that develops into eclampsia (life-threatening) accounts for 2 per cent of all maternal deaths in developing countries. Large studies incorporating several countries showed an incidence of 0.5–6.7 per cent for pre-eclampsia and 0.1–0.7 per cent for eclampsia (Wikipedia, 2017b). In South Africa, pre-eclampsia is the single most common direct cause of maternal death (besides HIV) (DoH, 2015a). This complex condition needs special attention in South Africa to reduce maternal deaths.

Definitions

Hypertensive disorders of pregnancy include conditions such as pre-eclampsia, essential hypertension, eclampsia and HELLP syndrome (haemolytic anaemia, elevated liver enzymes, low platelet count):

▶ *Pregnancy-induced hypertension (PIH)* includes both pre-eclampsia and gestational hypertension, which occurs when women develop hypertension for the first time after 20 weeks of gestation. PIH is related to an enlarged placenta, as in multiple gestation or hydatidiform mole, or in conditions of compromised placental blood flow, such as in diabetes mellitus. Globally, 1–8 million women will develop pre-eclampsia and 250 000 will develop eclampsia, 90 per cent of whom will be in developing countries (Preeclampsia Foundation, 2013).

▶ *Chronic hypertension* is hypertension that is present before 20 weeks of gestation. The woman will have been on antihypertensive medication before pregnancy.

▶ *Gestational hypertension* refers to hypertension in pregnancy after 20 weeks (without proteinuria).

▶ *Pre-eclampsia* refers to elevated blood pressure with proteinuria. If left untreated it has an extremely serious effect on the well-being of both the woman and her fetus. Pre-eclampsia includes:
  • proteinuria with hypertension after 20 weeks of pregnancy
  • chronic hypertension with superimposed pre-eclampsia
  • chronic hypertension and renal disease (hypertension that existed before the pregnancy)
  • chronic renal disease (proteinuria with or without hypertension)
  • unclassified hypertension or proteinuria (a combination of the above).

▶ *Imminent eclampsia* refers to signs and symptoms that indicate a woman is severely pre-eclamptic. These signs and symptoms include severe and persistent headaches, visual disturbances, epigastric pain, hyper-reflexion, clonus, dizziness and fainting and vomiting.

▶ *Eclampsia* is when a woman has tonic-clonic seizures after 20 weeks. Seizures and/or convulsions within seven days after delivery are also part of the syndrome.

▶ *HELLP syndrome* occurs with the presence of haemolysis, elevated liver enzymes and low platelets, as well as hypertension and proteinuria.

Aetiology and pathology of pre-eclampsia and gestational hypertension

Factors that predispose an individual to pre-eclampsia include:

▶ *nutritional deficiencies:* for example protein and calories, calcium, iron and vitamins

▶ *genetic disposition:* daughters of mothers who had the condition are at higher risk

▶ *uterine ischemia:* when there is not enough blood flow through uterus

▶ *parity:* mainly primigravidae or primipaternity (pregnant with new partner)

▶ *age:* younger than 18 or older than 35 years; the incidence is three times higher in women younger than 15

▶ *altitude:* there is a higher incidence at 3 100 m above sea level

▶ *smoking:* there is a lower incidence among smokers

▶ *obstetrical and medical conditions associated with placental pathology:* there is a higher incidence in cases of multiple pregnancy, hydrops fetalis, diabetes mellitus, a basal metabolic index (BMI) of ≥ 35 and hydatidiform mole

‣ *previous complications:* eg abruptio placenta, intrauterine death (IUD)

‣ *spacing of pregnacies:* 10 years or more since last pregnancy.

Contributing factors

Placental factors

Focus must be placed on the placental pathology and the trophoblastic invasion of the spiral arteries in the deciduas. There is vasoconstriction, which will lead to decreased placental perfusion, which may ultimately lead to early placental hypoxia. The muscular walls and the endothelium of the spiral arteries are eroded and replaced by the trophoblast to ensure a suitable environment for the developing blastocyst. A second phase of this erosion process occurs between 16 and 20 weeks. This is when the trophoblast erodes the endothelial cells of the spiral arteries (see Chapter 7).

There is evidence that pathological processes of abnormal placentation are linked to the occurrence of PIH. This may be a genetically predetermined maternal immune response to fetal antigens derived from the father and expressed in normal placental tissue. This maternal immune response triggers the release of factors that damage the endothelial cells. When these cells are damaged, the following occurs:

‣ There is increased vascular sensitivity to the angiotensin II.

‣ The coagulation cascade is also activated.

‣ There is production of thromboxane (causing vasoconstriction, leading to increased BP).

‣ There is increased production of lipid peroxides and antioxidant production is decreased. This is known as oxidative stress.

The combined effects of these events will cause vasospasm, which will lead to the following pathological changes:

‣ *Haematological changes:* Capillary permeability is affected by hypertension and changes in the endothelial cells. Plasma proteins leak from the damaged blood vessels, causing a decrease in the plasma colloid pressure and an increase in oedema within the intracellular space. The reduced intravascular plasma volume causes hypovolaemia and haemoconcentration, which are reflected in the elevated haematocrit. In severe cases, the lungs become congested with fluid and pulmonary oedema develops, oxygenation is impaired and cyanosis occurs. With vasoconstriction and disruption of the vascular endothelium, the coagulation cascade is activated.

‣ *The coagulation system:* Increased platelet consumption produces thrombocytopaenia and may be responsible for the development of disseminated intravascular coagulation (DIC) (comprising low platelets, prolonged prothrombin time and low fibrinogen levels). As the process progresses, fibrin and the platelets are deposited, occluding the blood flow to many vital organs, particularly the kidneys, liver and the placenta.

‣ *The renal system:* In the kidneys, hypertension leads to vasospasm of the afferent arterioles. This results in a decreased renal blood flow, which in turn produces hypoxia and oedema of the endothelial cells of the glomerular capillaries. The glomerular endothelial damage allows plasma proteins, mainly in the form of albumin, to filter into the urine, producing proteinuria. Renal damage is reflected by reduced creatinine clearance and increased serum creatinine and uric acid levels. Oliguria develops as the condition worsens, signifying the severity of the condition and kidney damage.

‣ *The hepatic system:* Vasoconstriction of the hepatic vascular bed will result in hypoxia and oedema of the liver cells. In severe cases, swelling of the liver causes epigastric pain and can lead to intracapsular haemorrhages and, in very rare cases, the rupture of the liver. Altered liver function is reflected by falling albumin levels and a rise in liver enzyme levels.

‣ *The central nervous system* (CNS): Hypertension, combined with cerebrovascular endothelial dysfunction, increases the permeability of the blood–brain barrier, resulting in cerebral oedema and micro-haemorrhaging. This will be clinically characterised by the development of headaches, visual disturbances and convulsions.

‣ *The placenta:* Owing to vasospasm, there is reduced blood flow through the decidual arteries, causing hypoxia. In an attempt to overcome this hypoxia, hyperplasia and swelling of the layers of the chorionic villi (the syncytial and cytotropic layers) occur, causing more branched villi; there is swelling of the villi and thickening of the basement membrane.

Nutritional factors

There is no evidence that dietary restrictions of any sort (water, salt, etc) are of benefit to pregnant women. The following are some guidelines:

‣ High-protein dietary supplementation should be avoided.

‣ A calcium deficiency may cause increased activity in the vascular angiotensin by stimulating prostacyclin synthesis, thus triggering pre-eclampsia. Women who are at high risk of pre-eclampsia and have low dietary calcium intake should receive calcium supplementation during pregnancy.

▶ Magnesium is known to cause vasodilatation. A deficiency may therefore be associated with pre-eclampsia.

▶ Low plasma zinc levels are associated with pre-eclampsia. Zinc competes with cadmium at various biochemical binding sites. A lack of zinc therefore exposes the pregnant woman to cadmium toxicity, which can cause vasospasm and endothelial cell damage.

Immunological factors and abnormal placentation

The aetiology is still unknown and no definite cause has been identified.

A clinical picture

A change in BP is the essential diagnostic criterion for hypertensive disorders of pregnancy. A diagnosis is based on a raised diastolic BP of 90 and above after 20 weeks of gestation. The three cardinal signs of PIH are hypertension, proteinuria and oedema. A diagnosis is made if systolic BP is 140 mmHg and diastolic BP is 90 mmHg on two or more occasions, four hours apart with no protein in the urine.

Measuring blood pressure in pregnancy

According to the WHO's guidelines for the evaluation of BP, diastolic pressure may be taken at the fifth Korotkoff's sound (WHO, 2003b). Since vasoconstriction is the pathological feature in late pregnancy, the diastolic pressure is the important measurement. The diastolic pressure indicates peripheral resistance and the systolic pressure indicates cardiac output. In 15 per cent of women, the fifth sound cannot be heard (Duggan, 1998). The systolic pressure is measured at the systolic sound one.

A woman's BP must be taken while she is resting. The woman should be placed at an angle of 15–30 degrees to the side to avoid the inferior vena cava syndrome (IVCS) effect. Use the largest possible cuff. If the woman is sitting up straight, the upper arm must be at the same level as the heart. A false high reading will be obtained if the cuff does not encircle at least three-fourths of the circumference of the arm; a wider cuff should be used when the diameter of the upper arm is greater than 33 cm. Repeat the measurement in three to four hours.

Diastolic BP

A cut-off point of 90 mmHg has been determined, since perinatal mortality is significantly increased at this level. The BP drops by 15 mmHg in early pregnancy and reaches the lowest values in the middle of the second trimester. It should remain low for the first half of pregnancy. In the third trimester, the BP rises to the same levels as at the beginning of the first trimester.

A diagnosis of pre-eclampsia is made when the BP consistently measures 90 mmHg for two consecutive readings, taken four to six hours apart. At a diastolic BP of 110 mmHg, the mother can have a cerebral haemorrhage and the fetus is in severe danger. This condition needs immediate attention and intervention.

Proteinuria

Proteinuria may appear before hypertension, in which case it may be a result of infection or renal disease. Proteinuria not accompanied by a BP of 140/90 mmHg is usually associated with infection, anaemia or renal conditions.

There is a clear correlation between diastolic BP and proteinuria. Proteinuria changes the diagnosis from PIH to the more serious condition of pre-eclampsia.

Proteinuria is defined as 300 mg of protein in urine collected over 24 hours. Using a dipstick, the following criteria can be used as a guideline:

▶ 1+ = 0.3 − 0.45 gr/ℓ
▶ 2+ = 0.45 gr/ℓ
▶ 3+ = < 3 gr/ℓ
▶ 4+ = > 3 gr/ℓ

Fetal mortality is significantly increased when the diastolic BP is 140/90 mmHg with 2+ proteinuria. It is the combination of these factors that is important.

Oedema and weight gain

Placental insufficiency (intracellular) appears to be the most frequent cause of fetal and neonatal morbidity before 35 weeks of pregnancy.

Oedema is a significant symptom of PIH. The mechanism of water retention in a normal pregnancy differs from that in hypertensive disorders. Pre-eclamptic women are hypovolaemic.

Primigravidae who develop generalised oedema with a weight gain of more than 0.57 kg/week between 20 and 28 weeks are at greater risk of developing hypertension, with or without proteinuria. Primigravidae with a low weight gain of 0.34 kg/week are less likely to develop BP problems. Rapid weight gain is also significant.

The following are guidelines for the classification of oedema:

▶ *Hands:* Rings do not fit.
▶ *Feet:* There is swelling in the morning.
▶ *Face:* Peri-orbital puffiness can easily be seen.
▶ *Body:* The fetal stethoscope leaves a mark.

▶ *Dependent oedema:* This develops when the woman is standing or walking.

▶ *Pitting oedema:* Pressing on the lower leg leaves a mark, which does not disappear within 30 seconds. A dent measured in mm can be interpreted from 1+ to 4+, as follows:
- 1+ = 2 mm
- 2+ = 4 mm
- 3+ = 6 mm
- 4+ = 8 mm

A woman on bed rest must be checked for sacral oedema. In severe cases, ascites and pulmonary oedema may develop. Both are serious complications. Deep tendon reflexes can be affected by severe oedema.

Management of gestational hypertension

A woman diagnosed with gestational hypertension at a community clinic should be referred to a medical practitioner for treatment and investigations. The following should be done by the midwife:

▶ Proteinuria, oedema and weight gain should be checked.
▶ Find out about any family history of hypertension, hypertension in previous pregnancies, stillbirths and neonatal death/s.
▶ Check the woman's dietary history.
▶ Refer the woman to a district hospital.

At the district hospital, the woman should be reassessed to confirm the diagnosis and exclude pre-eclampsia. The following should be done by the advanced midwife at the district hospital:

▶ Do ultrasound to assess the gestational age (GA) of the fetus and check fetal well-being.
▶ Test for proteinuria.
▶ Control the BP. If necessary, treat with antihypertensive therapy (methyldopa).
▶ Delivery should take place from 37 weeks' gestation (hypertension and pre-eclampsia intervention trial at term, or HYPITAT).

Postpartum care

Antihypertensive treatment with methyldopa should be stopped after delivery (as it can worsen postpartum depression). The woman should be placed on other antihypertensive medication if needed. The woman's BP should be stable for 24 hours before discharge. Follow-up must be done at a postpartum clinic (district level) after three days and again at six weeks postpartum, to evaluate the need for continuation of medication.

Upon discharge, a prescription for four weeks should be provided by the medical practitioner, if needed. The woman should be without medication for two weeks by the six-week follow-up visit so that it can be established if she is hypertensive and needs chronic medication. If more than one drug was given to control the BP, withdraw one drug at a time with more regular follow-ups, preferably at a specialist high-risk clinic.

The woman should return for care if she experiences constant dizziness or headaches.

Pre-eclampsia

Pre-eclampsia is a multisystem disease. Women with pre-eclampsia do not feel unwell until the condition is severe, at which stage the disease is life-threatening. Early detection by regular antenatal monitoring and careful follow-up of those with mild pre-eclampsia is therefore essential for the early diagnosis and treatment of severe eclampsia. Mild pre-eclampsia can progress to severe pre-eclampsia and eclampsia very suddenly, with little or no warning. This is called fulminating pre-eclampsia and is very dangerous for both mother and fetus.

The diagnosis of pre-eclampsia is difficult to make. All women presenting with an increased BP after 20 weeks need to be referred for medical assessment. A rise in BP before 20 weeks may indicate a multiple pregnancy, hydatidiform mole, kidney problems and essential hypertension.

Principles of care for a woman with pre-eclampsia and eclampsia

The cure for pre-eclampsia and eclampsia is the delivery of the fetus and placenta. However, in an unstable patient a rushed delivery is risky. It is suggested that the woman deliver only after severe hypertension has been corrected and the woman is haemodynamically stable. Refer the woman to a district or higher-level hospital. The following should be done on a medical practitioner's prescription:

▶ Treat the hypertension with rapid-acting agents if the systolic BP is higher than 160 mmHg, or the diastolic BP is higher than 110 mmHg and the patient is symptomatic. Aim to reduce BP to 130–149/90–95 mmHg.
▶ If the BP drops by more than 15 mmHg, diastolic placental perfusion is impaired. Commonly used rapid antihypertensive drugs are hydralazine, nifedipine and labetalol. In addition, prescribe methyldopa 1 g stat and 500 mg 8-hourly per os.

continued

- Reduce fluid intake.
- Take blood for full blood count (FBC), including platelets, urea and electrolytes, and liver function tests as prescribed.
- Give steroids (betamethasone) to promote lung maturity in a fetus of less than 34 weeks' GA.
- Consider the need for magnesium sulphate (MgSO₄) if eclampsia seems imminent and/or there is significant hyperreflexia and clonus (more than three beats) on clinical examination. In all cases of severe pre-eclampsia and eclampsia (fitting or convulsions), MgSO₄ is given. It more than halves the risk of eclampsia and probably reduces the risk of maternal death; however, it does not improve outcomes for the baby in the short term (Duly et al, 2010).
- The mode of delivery is decided at senior level after vaginal examination to assess the possibility of induction of labour. Always consult with your referral hospital.
- Ensure that the monitoring of vital signs occurs at frequent intervals during antenatal and intrapartum periods, and following delivery for up to 72 hours. Also ensure that monitoring is continued if the patient is going to be referred and is waiting for transport.
- All health facilities must establish an eclampsia box for the management of severe pre-eclampsia or imminent/impeding eclampsia.

Eclampsia box

An eclampsia box contains:
- MgSO₄ in sufficient quantities for the loading dose
- an infusion set (standard set)
- appropriate strapping and syringes of the right size
- calcium gluconate (10 ml of a 10 per cent solution = IVI over 10 minutes) for MgSO₄ toxicity
- 200 ml normal saline
- a flow/drip controller
- Venflows or equivalent, for venapuncture
- Foley catheter 5 ml bulb, plus sterile water and syringe
- methyldopa (1 g)
- a rapid-acting antihypertensive agent: either hydralazine or nifedipine.

Management of pre-eclampsia

Pre-eclampsia should be managed according to the *Guidelines for Maternal Care in South Africa* (DoH, 2015a).

Prevention of pre-eclampsia

Evidence to confirm that pre-eclampsia can be prevented is lacking. The lower incidence of this condition in developed countries is associated with improved standards of living and nutrition, coupled with evidence-based care protocols in an effective healthcare system. Weight gain and salt intake do not appear to have any influence on the development of pre-eclampsia. However, the following aspects of antenatal care remain important:
- Recognise severe pre-eclampsia and eclampsia.
- Provide an effective response to a woman with severe pre-eclampsia or eclampsia.
- Standards of living and nutrition should be improved as far as possible.
- Use evidence-based care protocols.
- Do not use diuretics in pre-eclampsia. The woman is already hypovolaemic and these drugs may be dangerous.

Control of hypertension

Treatment of hypertension does not prevent the progression of the condition in other respects (eg renal or hepatic dysfunction) and it may not in any way halt the progression to eclampsia. Antihypertensive medication prescribed by a medical practitioner may also interfere with placental blood supply. The woman should be admitted to hospital if there are signs that she will progress to eclampsia so rapidly that normal outpatient monitoring would not be safe, or if she lives far from medical help. (Refer to the *Guidelines for Maternal Care in South Africa* [DoH, 2015a] to initiate antihypertensive treatment in time before referral or transfer to a hospital.) When checking for signs of hypertension or pre-eclampsia, do not forget to evaluate the condition of the fetus as well.

Referral to a major obstetric unit

Controlling BP, although not treating the cause of pre-eclampsia, may reduce the severity of complications of late second- and third-stage pre-eclampsia. Generally, a BP of 170/110 mmHg or above should be controlled, keeping diastolic BP in the range of 90–100 mmHg. This can be done by using antihypertensive medications – see the *Guidelines for Maternal Care in South Africa* (DoH, 2015a). The following are guidelines for referral:
- Refer the woman the same day or the next day, especially if the patient is past 34 weeks' gestation. Do an ultrasound to assess the GA of the fetus or estimated fetal weight.
- Evaluate fetal well-being by using an antenatal cardiotocography (CTG) or fetal movement chart.

▶ Do a 24-hour protein collection, except if there is persistent proteinuria of 1+ or higher on the dipstick to confirm the diagnosis of mild to moderate pre-eclampsia.

▶ Do a platelet count, serum creatinine and serum aminotranferase (ALT) and lactate dehydrogenase (LDH) to confirm proteinuria (≥ 0.3 g/24 hours or persistent ≥ 1+).

If the condition remains stable, the woman should stay in the hospital until 36 weeks, when delivery (induction of labour [IOL]) is strongly advised. Contact a specialist health facility for further management if any acute, severe hypertension or imminent signs of eclampsia or organ dysfunction develop during her stay. These symptoms now indicate a diagnosis of severe pre-eclampsia. While in the hospital, the growth of the fetus must be plotted on the antenatal card every two weeks.

Medication

The following medications are used for eclampsia:
▶ *Short-acting antihypertensive drugs:*
  - Hydralazine dilates arteries, thus reducing resistance to blood flow. Side effects in approximately 50 per cent of users include severe headaches, palpitations, restlessness and anxiety – side effects which mimic the symptoms of impending eclampsia. Hydralazine must be given by injection, usually in a saline drip.
  - Nifedipine (a calcium channel blocker) reduces BP and can be taken orally. Headaches are even more common with this medication than with hydralazine.
  - IV administration of labetalol is also an option instead of nifedipine.
▶ *Slower-acting antihypertensive drugs:*
  - Methyldopa suppresses the hypertensive activity of the sympathetic nervous system and controls elevated BP within 6 to 12 hours. Although it causes extreme sleepiness for the first 48 hours, methyldopa is effective and is the only hypertensive drug known to have little effect on the fetus after initial sedation.
  - Beta blockers such as oxprenolol and labetalol interfere with sympathetic nervous system activity and cause fewer side effects than methyldopa. Their short-term safety for the fetus has been established.

Delivering the baby

Pre-eclampsia improves once the baby is delivered, although the improvement may be delayed by a few hours or, more rarely, days. The essential decisions to be made are, first, whether induced delivery is necessary, and, if so:
▶ when and how to deliver (vaginally or Caesarean section)
▶ whether any specific medication is required.

The answers to these questions will depend on the facilities available locally. Delivery of premature infants will be hazardous in circumstances where supplies and technological assistance are limited.

Eclampsia

Eclampsia is a serious condition, most commonly defined as seizures or coma in a patient with other indications of PIH. Eclampsia was once thought to be the endpoint of progressively worsening pre-eclampsia, but this is no longer the case. Instead, it is now recognised that some patients can develop eclampsia or eclamptic symptoms directly, without first developing any symptoms other than high BP.

Eclampsia is extremely rare before 20 weeks of pregnancy. Eclampsia is more common in teenage pregnancy and those older than 35 years. Regardless of age, eclampsia is more common in primigravidae. Patients with severe pre-eclampsia are at greater risk of seizures. Of patients with severe pre-eclampsia, 25 per cent have symptoms consistent with mild pre-eclampsia prior to the seizures (Stöppler & Davis, 2015).

Signs and symptoms of eclampsia

The signs and symptoms that most commonly indicate eclampsia are:
▶ headaches
▶ hyperactive reflexes
▶ marked proteinuria
▶ generalised oedema
▶ visual disturbances
▶ right upper quadrant pain or epigastric pain.

One or more seizures may occur and they generally last 60–75 seconds. Initially, the woman's face may become distorted, with protrusion of the eyes and foaming at the mouth. Respiration ceases for the duration of the seizure. The seizure may be divided into two phases:
1. Phase 1 lasts 15–20 seconds and begins with facial twitching. The body becomes rigid, leading to generalised muscular contractions.
2. Phase 2 lasts about 60 seconds. It starts in the jaw, moves to the muscles of the face and eyelids, and then spreads throughout the body. The muscles alternate between contracting and relaxing in rapid sequence.

Signs and symptoms of severe gestational hypertensive disease

- Systolic BP > 160 mmHg
- Rapid rise in BP
- Diastolic BP 110 mmHg
- Increased liver enzyme levels or jaundice
- Platelets < 100 000 per mm³ $(100 \times 10^{9/\ell})$
- Oliguria < 400 ml in 24 hours (16 ml/hr)
- Proteinuria 3 g/ℓ or 4+
- Epigastric pain, nausea, vomiting
- Scotoma and other visual disturbances, severe headaches
- Retinal haemorrhage
- Pulmonary oedema
- Coma
- Drowsiness

A coma or a period of unconsciousness follows Phase 2. Unconsciousness lasts for a variable period and the patient may regain some consciousness (see Table 21.2 for a scale to measure consciousness). The patient may become combative and very agitated and not be able to recall the event. Hyperventilation follows the seizure stage. This compensates for the respiratory and lactic acidosis that develops during the apnoeic phase. Seizure-induced complications may include tongue biting, head trauma and broken bones.

Table 21.2

The Glasgow Coma Scale

Test	Response	Score
Eyes open in response to	Spontaneously	4
	To speech	3
	To pain	2
	Do not open	1
Best verbal response	Orientated	5
	Confused	4
	Inappropriate words	3
	Incomprehensible sounds	2
	None	1
Best motor response	Obeys commands	6
	Can localise pain	5
	Non-movement	4
	Flexion to pain	3
	Extension to pain	2
	None	1
TOTAL		3–15

Management

Guidelines for the treatment of pre-eclampsia and eclampsia are available and midwives and obstetricians should understand the management of the two conditions.

Treatment of seizures

In women with severe pre-eclampsia, $MgSO_4$ is recommended as prophylaxis for eclampsia. A total dose of 14 g is given IMI (5 g into each buttock) and IV (4 g).

Evidence-based regimen for $MgSO_4$

Magnesium sulphate remains the drug of choice for both prevention of eclampsia and treatment of women with eclampsia. Regimens for the administration of this drug have not yet been formally evaluated. There is strong evidence from systematic reviews of randomised trials to support the use of $MgSO_4$ for the prevention and treatment of eclampsia but there is insufficient reliable evidence indicating the minimum effective dose, best routes of administration (IV or IM) or the ideal duration of therapy.

Effective regimes are based on the Eclampsia Trial and the largest study, the Magpie Trial (Duly et al, 2010). These studies used the same regimens for IM and IV $MgSO_4$ (IV: 4 g loading dose over 10–15 minutes followed by an infusion of 1 g/hour over 24 hours; IM: 4 g IV and 10 g IM as loading dose followed by 5 g IM every 4 hours for 24 hours).

- *Dosage:* The total dosage is 14 g. The initial dosage is 4 g IV in 200 ml saline over 10–15 minutes and 5 g in each buttock deep IMI (add 1 ml of 2 per cent lignocaine). Follow with maintenance dosage of 5 g IMI 4-hourly after seizure for 24 hours.
- *Toxicity:* Monitor for levels of toxicity, poor urinary output (less than 30 ml per hour), respiratory depression (less than 16 breaths per minute), drowsiness, loss of consciousness and patellar reflexes. Serum levels of higher than 3.5 mmol/ℓ indicate toxicity.
- *Antidote:* 10 per cent calcium gluconate (10 ml) administered over a 10-minute period.
- *Side effects:* Flushing, nausea, vomiting, muscle weakness, dizziness and discomfort at the area of injection.

$MgSO_4$ halves the risk of eclampsia and reduces the incidence of first seizure compared with other agents. The following is the emergency protocol for treating seizures:
- Prevent injury by using cot sides.
- Turn the patient on her side; do not constrain.

▶ Perform suction to prevent aspiration (use covered metal tongue spatulas and never your fingers) and ensure an open airway.
▶ Give oxygen.
▶ Start IV infusion.
▶ Give medication (see $MgSO_4$ regimen in the box on the previous page).
▶ After the patient has settled, assess labour and insert an indwelling catheter.
▶ Listen to the fetal heart.
▶ Do observations or high care.
▶ Transfer to the appropriate level (multi-professional team).
▶ Deliver the baby. This can be through IOL, ventouse extraction delivery or Caesarean section, depending on the duration of the pregnancy and the status of the cervix.
▶ The woman should stay in the hospital until the condition-specific BP is well controlled.

Complications

Maternal complications of eclampsia may include permanent CNS damage from recurrent seizures or intracranial bleeds, DIC, renal insufficiency, acute pulmonary oedema, hepatic failure or sub-capsular haemorrhage, transient blindness, aspiration, cardiopulmonary arrest, injuries and death.

Obstetric complications may be placental abruption due to the high BP. Factors such as prematurity, placental infarcts, intrauterine growth restriction (IUGR), placental abruption and fetal hypoxia can result in neonatal death.

HELLP syndrome

This syndrome is a life-threatening condition that may be associated with pre-eclampsia. However, it is often misleading, presenting with diffuse symptoms in pregnancy.

The clinical picture

The diagnosis of HELLP syndrome is frustrating and difficult. Some patients present with generalised malaise, some with epigastric pain, some with nausea and vomiting, and others with headache, all of these with or without proteinuria, mostly in the third trimester. The aetiology is unclear. Because early diagnosis of this syndrome is critical, any pregnant woman who presents with malaise or a viral-type illness in the third trimester should be evaluated with an FBC and liver function tests. Because of the variable nature of the clinical presentation, the diagnosis of HELLP syndrome is generally delayed for an average of eight days. Many women with this syndrome are initially misdiagnosed.

The following are the three main abnormalities found in HELLP syndrome:
1. *Haemolysis:* The haematocrit may be decreased or normal and is typically the last of the three abnormalities to appear.
2. *Elevated liver enzymes:* The serum glutamic-oxaloacetic transaminase (GOT) levels may be elevated to as high as 4 000 U/ℓ, but milder elevations are typical.
3. *Low platelet count:* This is the best diagnostic criteria (130×10^9). Class I (severe) is under 50 000/mm^3, Class II (moderately severe) is under 100 000/mm^3 and Class III (mild) is above 100 000/mm^3. A positive D-dimer test in the setting of pre-eclampsia has been reported to be predictive of patients who will develop HELLP syndrome (O'Hara Padden, 1999). The D-dimer is a more sensitive indicator of subclinical coagulopathy and may be positive before coagulation studies are abnormal.

Unless DIC is present, the prothrombin time, partial thromboplastin time and fibrinogen level are normal in patients with HELLP syndrome. In a patient with a plasma fibrinogen level of less than 300 mg per dl (3 g per ℓ), DIC should be suspected, especially if other laboratory abnormalities are also present.

Protein in the urine is of no value in HELLP syndrome, but bilirubin may be present.

Management

Women with Class I HELLP syndrome are at higher risk for maternal morbidity and mortality than patients with Class II or III. Laboratory abnormalities typically worsen after delivery and peak at 24–48 hours postpartum. The peak LDH level signals the beginning of recovery and subsequent normalisation of the platelet count. The incidence of haemorrhagic complications is higher when platelet counts are less than 40 000 per mm^3.

Patients with HELLP syndrome who complain of severe right upper quadrant pain, neck pain or shoulder pain should be considered for hepatic imaging regardless of the severity of the laboratory abnormalities, to assess for sub-capsular haematoma or rupture.

Prompt recognition of HELLP syndrome and timely initiation of therapy are vital to ensure the best outcome for mother and fetus. The treatment is immediate delivery of the baby. The risk is intra- or postpartum haemorrhage (PPH) and the woman will receive platelets before or during the delivery (usually Caesarean section). The woman will be admitted to the ICU until stable.

21.4   Hormonal disturbances in pregnancy: Diabetes mellitus

Another risk factor for pregnant women is diabetes mellitus, which may result in complicated pregnancy, labour and neonatal problems.

Diabetes mellitus is a metabolic disorder of insulin deficiency, which interferes with carbohydrate, fat and protein metabolism in the body. It is characterised by inappropriately elevated blood glucose levels (hyperglycaemia and glycosuria) and results in complications of physiology and organ function. The course of the condition is variable and depends upon both hereditary and ongoing environmental factors.

In pregnancy, diabetes mellitus can be classified as known diabetes mellitus or a family history of the condition, and gestational diabetes (a transient condition).

Gestational diabetes

If diabetes mellitus is diagnosed for the first time during pregnancy, it is called gestational diabetes. Most cases of gestational diabetes are asymptomatic at first and therefore diagnosis can be difficult until later on or after the pregnancy.

Pregnancy, carbohydrate metabolism and diabetes

Pregnancy alters the carbohydrate metabolism. Pregnancy is considered a state of accelerated starvation or a diabetogenic state. The increased levels of oestrogen, progesterone and human placental lactogen (HPL) present during pregnancy produce resistance to insulin in the maternal tissues, causing the blood glucose levels to remain raised longer than in the non-gravid state. The fetus is dependent on the mother, who actively transports glucose to the fetus. Insulin does not cross the placenta; the fetus produces its own insulin and metabolises glucose.

During pregnancy, there is normally a drop in the maternal fasting glucose level, from 4 mmol/ℓ at around 10 weeks' gestation to 3.6 mmol/ℓ at term. During the third trimester, the mother's body mobilises and utilises the fat stores that were laid down in the first and second trimesters. This increases the circulation of free fatty acids and the woman becomes ketotic more easily than in the non-gravid state.

High levels of blood glucose in early pregnancy (before 20 weeks) are associated with fetal abnormalities and spontaneous abortions. In a woman with diabetes, the amount of glucose transferred is increased and the fetal insulin response is rapid, resulting in increased fetal insulin production and lower fasting blood glucose levels, which is thought to be the cause of

macrosomia (large for gestational age [LGA]). The fluctuation of blood glucose can cause sudden IUD in the third trimester.

Although oestrogen in particular causes increased insulin output, this is counteracted by HPL, which is the major insulin antagonist in pregnancy (it reduces the cellular utilisation of insulin).

At term, when the placental hormones are at their highest levels, the body has difficulty in mobilising glucose for itself and for the fetus, even when the maternal blood glucose levels are low (hypoglycaemia).

The effects of diabetes mellitus on pregnancy

Prior to the use of insulin, women with diabetes mellitus were infertile or had habitual abortions. Often women were only diagnosed with diabetes mellitus after a period of infertility, habitual abortions or previous congenital abnormalities of the fetus, a history of IUD or large babies (over 3.6 kg).

Fluctuations in blood glucose in pregnancy lead to a higher incidence of *Candida albicans*, macrosomia (a large fetus with immature lungs and liver), placental pathology such as a large placenta with polyhydramnios, sudden IUD after 36 weeks and the risk of premature birth, hyaline membrane disease (HMD), respiratory distress, jaundice and infections in the newborn. Hyperglycaemia often leads to UTI.

The woman with diabetes mellitus has a higher risk of pre-eclampsia and obstetric interventions and/or birth trauma due to the large fetus that could lead to PPH with resultant maternal death.

Pathophysiology

The control of diabetes mellitus is difficult due to increased placental hormones, oestrogen and cortisol (which are insulin antagonists) that constantly increase as the pregnancy progresses and the placental function increases. There is also a loss of glucose in the urine throughout pregnancy, due to an increased glomerular filtration rate and a lower glomerular ceiling for the re-absorption of glucose.

In early pregnancy, insulin requirements may drop. There is often increased early morning nausea and vomiting (hyperemesis gravidarum), which could lead to hypoglycaemia in a diabetic woman receiving insulin. The insulin and fasting blood glucose levels are reduced.

From 20 weeks, there is a gradual increased requirement for insulin. As the fetus grows, the mother requires more carbohydrates and breaks down her own fat stores, resulting in ketosis.

The fluctuation in blood glucose cannot be accommodated by the fetus, who is dependent on the mother for glucose. As mentioned, sudden IUD is a common complication of diabetes mellitus, even when under strict control.

Altered carbohydrate metabolism throughout pregnancy can change dramatically after labour. The insulin requirements drop drastically as soon as the placenta is delivered and the dosage must be reduced or hypoglycaemic coma will result. Conditions of physical activity destabilise blood glucose control.

Identification and diagnosis of diabetes mellitus

History

The history of diabetes mellitus includes:
- a family history of diabetes mellitus
- a history of infertility or abortions
- obesity
- unexplained stillbirths late in pregnancy
- congenital abnormalities
- previous polyhydramnios
- previous macrosomia or large babies over > 4 kg
- previous infections or history of *Candida albicans* infections
- polydipsia
- hypertension.

Physical examination

The physical examination includes glycosuria and obesity or weight loss.

Special examinations/tests

These include the following:
- A *routine urine test* should be done at each antenatal visit. If glycosuria is present on two consecutive visits, further tests are warranted.
- *Random fasting blood glucose* or a modified glucose tolerance test (GTT) can be done for cases under suspicion.
- In terms of *screening after birth*, all women should be tested if they are infertile, have aborted, have had a baby with congenital abnormality, have experienced IUD of unknown cause or have had a macrosomic baby over 4 kg. A HbA1C (glycosolated haemoglobin) gives a retrospective history of the blood glucose over a period of a month. The HbA1C remains high for weeks post-delivery, making it useful for diagnosis.

The modified GTT

For three days before the test, the patient is instructed to have no alcohol or coffee and to increase her carbohydrate intake to

300 g per day. The patient then starves from 22:00 the previous night. In the morning, a fasting blood glucose is performed and the urine is tested for glucose. Thereafter, a glucose load of 75-100 g (as suggested by the WHO) is given orally and blood is taken at one, two and three hours. (The amount of glucose ingested varies from centre to centre.)

The following are guidelines for interpreting the results:
- The normal fasting values for blood glucose should be below 6.1 mmol/ℓ (110 mg/dl). Values above 7.0 mmol/ℓ (126 mg/dl) are diagnostic of diabetes.
- At one hour, a blood glucose level below 10 mmol/ℓ (180 mg/dl) is normal.
- At two hours with 75 g intake, a blood glucose level below 7.8 mmol/ℓ (140 mg/dl) is normal, while values above 11.1 mmol/ℓ (200 mg/dl) are diagnostic of diabetes.
- At three hours, a blood glucose level of > 8.1 mmol/ℓ is abnormal.

Elevation of blood glucose levels in the third trimester is associated with macrosomia.

Care of the diabetic woman in pregnancy

Specialised care is required for a diabetic woman. The following are important:
- A team approach is most important in this condition. The team includes the internal medicine specialist, the specialist obstetrician, the patient, the midwife, the paediatrician, the dietician and the social worker.
- If diabetes mellitus is present and recognised, it is important to reduce blood glucose to a normal level before the patient becomes pregnant. Management should ideally start before conception.
- During pregnancy, maintain strict control of blood glucose in order to prevent complications. The aim of the treatment is to control the blood glucose level so that it never rises above 7 mmol/ℓ and never goes below 3.5 mmol/ℓ (prevent fluctuations).
- Carefully monitor fetal well-being in pregnancy. Perform an early ultrasound to confirm that the fetus is normal and to exclude the possibility of a multiple pregnancy. On follow-up ultrasounds, monitor the growth and development of the fetus.
- Prevent or treat complications or UTI and pre-eclampsia promptly.
- Decide upon the time and the mode of delivery in advance.
- Care for the newborn baby in a neonatal unit.
- Ensure post-delivery contraception.

Health education is extremely important. This must include both parents, so that the woman and her husband or partner can understand the importance of strict control of the condition, particularly during pregnancy, and the long-term implications.

Careful control and maintenance of blood glucose levels within acceptable levels may decrease the prevalence of many of the maternal and fetal complications associated with diabetes mellitus. Pregnant women with pre-existing diabetes mellitus should achieve tight glucose control before conception and throughout pregnancy. Control includes blood glucose monitoring, adherence to diet, moderate exercise and strict adherence to prescribed insulin. It is important that the woman wait for six to 12 months to stabilise the condition before becoming pregnant. She must also understand that she will need insulin therapy during pregnancy.

Nutrition is the single most important way to control blood glucose. Pregnant diabetics require the same nutrients and weight gain as non-diabetic pregnant women. Daily activities and the home environment should be investigated. The woman should visit the dietician in hospital. Protein intake should be 100 g, carbohydrate intake 200 g and fat intake 60–89 g per day. The woman's weight gain should not exceed 10–12 kg in total. Meals should consist of three main meals a day, with snacks at 10:00, 15:00 and 22:00. Constant intake is important, but with no refined sugars. There should be increased fibre intake to prevent constipation and weight gain.

Teach the woman to monitor her blood glucose and give herself insulin. Also teach her to monitor the signs and symptoms of hypo- and hyperglycaemia and to observe the well-being of the fetus (kick chart after 26 weeks of gestation).

Oral hypoglycaemics

Oral hypoglycaemics are not given during the first trimester of pregnancy, as a low level of this crosses the placenta. Instead, insulin therapy should be given. After 20 weeks' gestation, oral hypoglycaemics may be given. Glyburine may be unassociated with an increase in neonatal complications.

Start with glyburine 2.5 mg once or twice a day. Increase to a maximum of 20 mg per day. Metformin is not associated with an increase in perinatal complications compared to insulin, but 46 per cent of women in a clinical trial required conversion to insulin (Frier, McKay & Carty, 2017). Metformin is given at 500 mg once or twice daily. Increase to a maximum of 2 500 mg per day.

The infant's exposure to oral hypoglycaemic agents through breastmilk is minimal; mothers on these agents should therefore be encouraged to breastfeed.

Insulin therapy

Human insulin is an alternative therapy of choice during pregnancy, as the mother does not produce antibodies to this type of insulin and it does not cross the placenta. There are two types of insulin that can be used during pregnancy, namely:
1. short-acting insulin (Actrapid®), which lasts from 30 minutes to 6 hours
2. intermediate insulin (Monotard®), which lasts 2–12 hours and is given twice a day (in the morning and again in the evening).

The woman's insulin requirements are determined and prescribed by the specialist, who will change the regimen depending on the woman's and fetus's requirements.

While in hospital, the woman's blood glucose is tested one hour before a meal or snack and two hours after each meal or snack. Long-acting insulin is given twice a day and short-acting insulin is given on a sliding scale. When the woman's blood glucose is stable, she is allowed to go home. However, she needs to be warned that her higher levels of activity at home will influence her insulin requirements. The patient must monitor her own blood glucose and work according to the sliding scale to inject herself.

Unstable blood glucose may be caused by infections such as UTIs or changed activities or lifestyle and may be a reason for readmission.

Fetal compromise

From 32 weeks, ultrasound is done weekly, including the fetal biophysical profile. Fetal kick counts are carried out by the patient at home. If fetal movements are reduced, a cardiotocograph (CTG) non-stress test (NST) is carried out at 32 and 34 weeks. The medical practitioner may decide to do an amniocentesis to check the fetal lung maturity before delivery. Lecithin sphingomyelin (LS) ratio is not accurate in diabetes mellitus and the phosphatidylglycerol ratio (PGR) gives a more accurate result.

Critical periods

It is recommended that the blood glucose is checked fortnightly up to 28 weeks' gestation and weekly up to 34 weeks' gestation and then twice weekly up to delivery. Women are often readmitted for the period 34–36 weeks – which is when unexplained IUD usually occurs – for control and observation.

Delivery

The time and mode of delivery

This is decided upon by the obstetrician and the internal medicine specialist and depends upon the general condition of the woman and the fetus.

Caesarean section is avoided because of the risk of infection and poor wound healing in diabetes mellitus. The maturity of the fetal lungs is particularly important and corticosteroids are administered between 32 and 34 weeks. If the phosphatidylglycerol result is positive, labour can be induced. If complications should arise before term, the baby is delivered at about 38 weeks' gestation. If there is little or no control of the diabetes, the baby is delivered as soon as lung maturity is confirmed.

Specific protocols during labour

Labour is physically demanding. This places demands on glucose metabolism. If birth is planned, long-acting insulin is discontinued in labour and the blood glucose is controlled by:
- an IV infusion of dextrose and saline
- blood glucose laboratory tests hourly
- administration of short-acting insulin on a sliding scale.

The following protocols are observed in each stage:
- *The first stage:* An IV infusion with 5 per cent dextrose is in place during labour. Hourly blood glucose levels are taken. The goal is to try to keep the blood glucose levels between 4.4 and 5.5 mmol/ℓ, within a range of two to four hours. The intermediate insulin is discontinued the day before and short-acting insulin is given on a sliding scale in labour. Constant monitoring of the labour and fetal condition is essential. If labour is induced, it may be necessary to ripen the cervix first with prostaglandins. Labour is not allowed to last longer than eight hours.
- *The second stage:* The perineal phase must be shortened. The woman is delivered in the lithotomy position to manage any possible shoulder dystocia occurring with the large infant. An episiotomy may be necessary. Assisted delivery will be performed by the medical practitioner where necessary.
- *The third stage:* Active management of the third stage of labour (AMTSL) is the preferred method.

Neonatal care

The fetus of a woman with diabetes mellitus is at risk, as is the neonate. A paediatrician should be present at the delivery. At delivery, the baby's blood glucose is checked, which is repeated every three hours after delivery until the baby's condition is stable. The baby is at risk of hypoglycaemia and hypothermia. Hypoglycaemia occurs because of the increased insulin produced by the baby's pancreatic beta cells during intrauterine life in response to the high maternal blood glucose levels, which are now no longer received by the baby.

Early feeding is commenced and the mother may breastfeed. The baby may have an IV infusion with dextrose until the blood glucose stabilises.

The baby is admitted to high care and observed for potential complications which are more prevalent in diabetes mellitus, such as HMD, jaundice, infection, hypothermia, hypocalcaemia, hypomagnesaemia and macrosomia. Other potential problems are congenital abnormalities (an enlarged heart due to myocardial hypertrophy, enlarged liver and adrenals), immaturity, macrosomia (large, overweight baby), flabbiness, lethargy, neuromuscular excitability and difficulty in feeding.

Postnatal care of the mother

After birth there is a sharp reduction in maternal insulin requirements; requirements are re-assessed by the doctor after delivery.

A diabetic who is poorly controlled does not lactate adequately, so neonatal progress must be carefully assessed. The patient must be monitored for hypoglycaemia by checking for sweating, drowsiness, tachycardia, disorientation, slurred speech and coma. Before discharge, the patient must be stabilised on insulin therapy and diet control.

The mother must be given health education. She is prone to infections and any pyrexia must be noted. She needs to continue to visit the diabetic clinic after delivery, so provide a follow-up date. She must be given advice on baby and self-care to prevent infections.

When discussing contraception, remember that combined hormonal contraceptives may not be suitable and that an intrauterine contraceptive device (IUCD) increases the risk of infection. However, an IUCD is the best contraceptive, as it lacks metabolic properties. Sterilisation might be chosen if future pregnancies pose a grave risk for the woman or if she does not desire any further pregnancies.

21.5   Thyroid disease in pregnancy

The physiological and hormonal changes in pregnancy alter thyroid function. Thyroid function tests should be interpreted carefully in pregnancy, as an increase in plasma protein increases thyroid stimulating hormone (TSH) while the free T3 and T4 remain the same. Thyroid function in pregnancy is normal when all the thyroid tests are normal.

The thyroid may enlarge by 10–15 per cent in pregnancy (not clinically noticed), but goitres are mainly associated with iodine deficiency. An ultrasound examination will identify abnormalities. In the first 12 weeks, the baby is totally dependent on the mother for thyroxin. By the end of the first trimester, the fetus will start to produce its own thyroid hormones. The fetus remains dependent on the mother for iodine.

Graves' disease (hyperthyroidism)

The most common disease (80 per cent) of the thyroid is hyperthyroidism, which occurs in 1:500 pregnant women (Shomon, 2016). Very high levels of human chorionic gonadotrophin (hCG) associated with hyperemesis gravidarum may cause hyperthyroidism. The diagnosis is made based on history, clinical examination and blood tests. Thyroid scanning is contraindicated due to the high radioactivity.

Effects on the mother

Besides the associated hyperemesis gravidarum, the woman is at risk of developing early-onset pre-eclampsia. The woman can also develop an acute crisis called a 'thyroid storm'. The condition improves in the third trimester and worsens postnatally.

Effects on the fetus

Uncontrolled maternal hyperthyroidism has been associated with fetal tachycardia, prematurity, stillbirths, congenital malformations and IUGR.

Antibodies called thyroid stimulating immunoglobulin (TSI) cross the placenta and interact with the fetal thyroid. This can cause fetal hyperthyroidism. A test in the third trimester will indicate the condition.

If the mother is on treatment, the fetus will be normal. In cases where the mother has a history of previous radioactive treatment, the condition may be missed and the fetus will be affected. Drug therapy in pregnancy is safe and beneficial for the fetus. The mother on treatment can breastfeed, but the baby needs to be tested from time to time.

Hypothyroidism in pregnancy

This autoimmune disease is called Hashimoto's thyroiditis. Approximately 2.5 per cent of women will have a slightly elevated TSH of greater than 6, and 0.4 per cent will have a TSH level higher than 10 during pregnancy (Wikipedia, 2017c).

Effects on the mother

Untreated or inadequately treated severe hypothyroidism has been associated with maternal anaemia, myopathy (muscle pain, weakness), congestive heart failure, pre-eclampsia, PPH, placental abnormalities and LBW infants. Most women with mild hypothyroidism may have no symptoms.

Effects on the fetus

The thyroid hormone is critical for brain development in the baby. Children born with congenital hypothyroidism (no thyroid function at birth) can have severe cognitive, neurological and developmental abnormalities if the condition is not recognised and treated promptly. These developmental abnormalities can largely be prevented if the disease is recognised and treated immediately after birth. Consequently, all newborn babies need to be screened for congenital hypothyroidism so they can be treated with thyroid hormone replacement therapy as soon as possible.

Clearly, women with established hypothyroidism should have a TSI test once pregnancy is confirmed. Once hypothyroidism has been detected, the woman should be treated with levothyroxine to normalise her TSH and free T4 values.

21.6   Cardiovascular system conditions

Cardiovascular disease is one of the leading causes of maternal mortality associated with pregnancy. It is therefore important to know what the pathology is and how to manage this.

Anaemia and haemoglobinopathies in pregnancy

The cardiovascular changes in pregnancy are hyperdynamic. The woman's blood volume increases gradually, with a peak volume at 32 weeks. The red blood cells (RBCs) also increase, but not to the same degree. This has a diluting effect on the blood and a drop in Hb, known as the physiological anaemia of pregnancy. The ideal Hb in pregnancy is between 12.0 and 14.0 g/dl. An Hb lower than 11 g/dl is seen as anaemia.

Normal haematological values in pregnant women
Hb range: 12–16 g/dl
Platelets: 130 000–400 000 x 109/ℓ
Serum iron: 11.6–31.3 µmol/ℓ

Anaemia in pregnancy is mostly due to nutritional problems or diseases that cause anaemia. Fifty per cent of women are anaemic in pregnancy, which has serious consequences for the outcome of the pregnancy. The two main types of anaemia are iron deficiency and megoblastic or folic acid insufficiency. Folic acid insufficiency is based on a poor diet that lasted over an 18-week period or interference in absorption due to medication. Hyperemesis gravidarum, if longstanding, may cause anaemia.

The physiological changes in pregnancy predispose a woman to anaemia. Conditions that cause pathological processes include infections, poor nutrition, pregnancies that follow too soon (less than two years apart), antepartum haemorrhage (APH) and PPH and inherited blood disease.

Complications of anaemia in pregnancy (irrespective of cause)
An Hb of 7 g/dl is associated with a high maternal mortality and cardiac failure. Other complications include: ▶ preterm labour ▶ premature rupture of membranes (PROM) ▶ fetal distress ▶ infections ▶ APH ▶ PPH ▶ placental abruption.

Anaemia increases the risk of maternal mortality five-fold and the incidence of stillbirth increases six-fold. It is important to identify anaemia early to prevent complications.

Table 21.3 gives an overview of the different types of anaemia that can be found in pregnancy.

Diagnosis of anaemia

Anaemia is a deficiency in either quality or quantity of RBCs. There is some debate about the level of Hb below which anaemia may be diagnosed in pregnancy. However, WHO guidelines (2006a) use a level higher than 11 g/dl as an indication that there is no clinical anaemia, levels of 7–11 g/dl as an indication of mild anaemia and lower than 7 g/dl as an indication of severe anaemia. These guidelines are used in conjunction with clinical signs such as pallor, breathlessness and fatigue. An Hb level of 6 g/dl is associated with a high mortality.

Table 21.3

Anaemia in pregnancy

Classification	Iron deficiency	Folic acid (megoblastic); B12	Sickle-cell anaemia	Beta–thalassaemia (minor) (Cooley's anaemia)
Definition	Anaemia due to depletion of iron	Deficiency of folic acid	Inborn genetic defect	Autosomal recessive condition
Cause	Malabsorption Breastfeeding and children too close: < 2 years apart Infections Blood loss Depleted iron stores	Poor diet over an 18-week period Malabsorption Intake of folic acid antagonist	Inherited Common in West Africa where 1:10 carries the gene sickle-cell trait 0.3% of black people are carriers (Grosse et al, 2011) Begins in childhood and is lifelong One-third of all indigenous inhabitants of sub-Saharan Africa carry the gene	A high incidence among Mediterranean people
Pathology	A mature woman has a total body iron content of 3 500–4 500 mg in Hb: 20% in body stores (ferritin) and 5% in muscle and enzymes. Iron status is not static.	Folic acid and vitamin B are needed for the formation of haeme, the pigmented, iron-containing portion of the Hb in RBCs (erythrocytes).	Haemoglobin S causes erythrocytes to take a sickle-cell shape. Capillaries become occluded and lack of oxygen to tissue occurs.	Alpha thalassaemia (affected fetus has one gene from each parent) cannot synthesise Hb = hydrops fetalis.

continued

Classification	Iron deficiency	Folic acid (megoblastic); B12	Sickle-cell anaemia	Beta–thalassaemia (minor) (Cooley's anaemia)
Pathology (continued)	The life of an erythrocyte is 100–120 days. Non-pregnant women need an intake of 2 mg of iron per day. To replace dead skin and cells daily, 2.7 mg is needed. Non-anaemic women need 2 mg per day. Pregnant women need 425 mg over 40 weeks (4.5 mg/day). The fetus needs 300 mg and the placenta 25 mg. More is needed in the last 10 weeks. A diet of animal products gives 12 mg/day.	A deficient intake of folic acid impairs the maturation of young RBCs, which results in anaemia. The disease is also characterised by leukopaenia (a deficiency of white blood cells [WBCs], or leukocytes), thrombocytopaenia (a deficiency of platelets) and ineffective blood formation in the bone marrow.	Some people are without symptoms; others have life-long complications. During stress, hypoxia, acidosis, pyrexia, dehydration, emotional and physical stress occur.	Only one gene (carrier with mild symptoms). In beta thalassemia, the baby will be anaemic and require blood transfusions to survive. This results in problems throughout life such as paleness, degrees of jaundice, hepatosplenomegaly with retarded growth and development.
Management	The WHO recommends 120–240 mg iron and/500 µgr folic acid. Prophylaxis: routine supplementation of pregnant women with oral iron. Ferrous sulphate 300 mg/day with vit C 500 mg (Fefol). Nutrition very important. Best absorption when taken with orange juice in-between meals. The average woman cannot manage more than 600 mg/day. Ferrous gluconate 500 mg 3 x/day.	Prophylactic treatment is very important for all mothers in pregnancy. Treatment should begin three months prior to pregnancy. Reduces the risk of open neural tube defects (NTDs) by 50%.	Hb varies between 6–8 mg%. Management is symptomatic. Higher risk for abortion, stillbirth, neonatal deaths and preterm labour. 10–20% of women have an acute crisis in pregnancy due to anaemia. Cardiomegaly or cardiac failure may occur. Mortality 25%.	Iron intake contraindicated. Not responsive to routine treatment. Higher risk for infection.
Treatment	Oral iron treatment to raise Hb in four weeks	Folic acid 5 mg per os	Blood transfusions may be needed for the mother.	Repeated blood transfusion is needed to maintain life.

continued

Classification	Iron deficiency	Folic acid (megoblastic); B12	Sickle-cell anaemia	Beta-thalassaemia (minor) (Cooley's anaemia)
Treatment	IV or IM iron treatment in last trimester Blood transfusion of packed cells in last trimester		Children born with sickle-cell disease will undergo close observation by a paediatrician and will require management by a haematologist to ensure they remain healthy. These patients will take a 1 mg dose of folic acid daily for life. From birth to 5 years, penicillin should be taken daily due to the immature immune system that makes them more prone to early childhood illnesses. Bone marrow transplants have proven to be effective in children. Folic acid therapy for life.	Removal of spleen seems to be beneficial.

Prevention of anaemia

The most common cause of anaemia in pregnancy is iron or folate deficiency. This can be compounded by short birth intervals, HIV infection, hookworm, schistosomiasis or other parasitic diseases.

Iron and folate deficiencies are mainly nutritional in origin, so it is very important that midwives and other health professionals give correct, culturally sensitive nutritional advice. Midwives must encourage the healthy pregnant woman to absorb enough iron and folic acid from a balanced diet. However, to prevent anaemia, all pregnant women should receive prophylactic iron and folic acid. Blood Hb levels are monitored during pregnancy and labour. If the levels are too low, therapeutic iron is prescribed or administered in a total dose infusion or, if needed, a blood transfusion is done.

The following WHO protocol is recommended:
- Midwives and other healthcare professionals should be trained to give advice on dietary intake and to recognise anaemia so that appropriate action can be taken.
- Facilities should be available for estimating Hb concentration levels accurately.
- Iron, folate and vitamin C supplements (where appropriate) should be available for pregnant women.
- Facilities should be available for screening for malaria and other parasitic diseases.
- Malaria should be controlled in affected areas.
- Appropriate referral systems should be in place.

Assessing Hb concentration

It is clear that the successful management of anaemia in pregnancy depends on reliable techniques for the detection of anaemia, with subsequent reliable monitoring of the response to treatment.

In developing countries, Hb levels may be difficult to estimate, making clinical screening for anaemia extremely important. Although clinical signs may be considered subjective and less sensitive, they can still aid clinicians in their diagnosis. Signs include paleness of conjunctivae, skin and nail beds. Symptoms of severe anaemia might include tiredness and shortness of breath.

Two quick and simple tests are the Tallquist test and the copper sulphate method. These tests use finger-prick blood, are easy to carry out and the results are rapid, visible and suitable for clinicians working in rural areas. Major obstetric units use more sophisticated and expensive methods but the technology used may not be applicable to developing countries, as the instruments may require skilled technicians to provide frequent maintenance and to ensure correct calibration.

Management and referral of anaemia in pregnancy

All pregnant women are given routine iron and folic acid supplements in pregnancy. They need to understand how to take these and the importance of the daily dose. The role of the midwife is the early identification of risk factors for anaemia. History taking will reveal women at risk. All women need to have an Hb test at the first antenatal visit. A low Hb in the first or early second trimester needs to be rechecked by a laboratory FBC test. The Hb test is repeated in the second trimester of pregnancy.

If the pregnant woman does not respond to oral therapy, further investigations are needed for accurate diagnosis. Refer the woman for medical intervention. Table 21.4 details the referral actions that need to be taken based on Hb results.

Table 21.4

Hb in pregnancy and referral criteria

Hb (g/dl)	Level of care
11	Antenatal follow-up more regularly than according to the schedule
Less than 10 at 36 weeks' gestation or more	Transfer to hospital for antenatal care and delivery
Hb 8–9	Transfer to high-risk clinic if no improvement after one month of treatment
Hb 6–7.9	Urgent transfer to hospital if symptoms such as tachycardia, breathing problems, dizziness present
Hb lower than 6	Immediate transfer to hospital

Blood tests for iron studies, folic acid and other genetic conditions may be needed. Treatment of anaemia is specific to the type of anaemia diagnosed. The aim is to have an Hb of not less than 9 g/dl at birth. Every woman's Hb is tested on admission for labour and compared with previous results. A woman with an Hb of 7 g/dl and below may receive a blood transfusion in the hospital. Low Hb is a risk factor of placental abruption, APH and PPH and fetal distress in labour. A pregnant woman is never given whole blood in pregnancy, unless she is bleeding and hypovolaemic. Packed cells are the treatment of choice.

Physiological changes in the cardiovascular system in pregnancy

Blood volume changes:
- Plasma gradually increases by 50 per cent by end of the second trimester and reaches peak volume at 32 weeks.
- This provides an increased vascular bed for mother and baby.
- In a multiple pregnancy, there is a similar increase for each fetus.
- RBCs increase (18 per cent) but not at the same rate as plasma, predisposing women to physiological anaemia resulting from haemodilution.

A guide to laboratory values indicating anaemia in pregnancy

- Hb: 11 g/dl
- Haematocrit: < 0.371/ℓ; 32–33%
- Mean cell volume (MCV): < 70 fl (hectolitres) at most always indicates iron deficiency (microcytic anaemia), rarely thalassaemia
- Mean cell Hb concentration (MCHC): < 33 suggests iron deficiency (hypochromic anaemia)
- Serum ferritin: < 50 µg/ℓ indicates that anaemia is likely to develop, < 10 µg/ℓ indicates severe depletion.

Cardiac conditions in pregnancy

Women with known cardiac problems are usually under supervision from the beginning of pregnancy. However, it is not uncommon for cardiac problems to be identified for the first time during pregnancy, as the pregnancy places a demand on the cardiovascular system. (The changes in the cardiovascular system during pregnancy are described in Chapter 14.)

During the third stage of labour, 500 ml of blood is forced back into the cardiac system with each contraction and there are further haemodynamic shifts of the placenta during delivery. These cardiovascular changes can be accommodated by a woman with a healthy heart, but pose a serious risk to a woman with cardiac disease.

The classification of cardiac disease (the New York classification)

The classification of cardiac disease is made by a cardiologist or a team of cardiologists based on symptoms and functionality:

▶ *Grade I:* There are no symptoms of cardiac disease. Although cardiac damage is present, there is no limitation on physical activity.
▶ *Grade II:* The person is comfortable at rest (and on slight exertion). Normal (ordinary) physical activity causes tachycardia, dyspnoea and fatigue.
▶ *Grade III:* The person is comfortable at rest. Slight exertion or any activity causes tachycardia, dyspnoea and angina.
▶ *Grade IV:* The person has dyspnoea at rest and symptoms of cardiac insufficiency.

The effects of cardiac disease on pregnancy

Cardiac disease is extremely important to be aware of in pregnancy, because it raises maternal morbidity and mortality rates. Fetal and neonatal death rates are also higher in women with cardiac disease. Two-thirds of the deaths occur in the first 48 hours after delivery. Three-quarters of the deaths are from:
▶ congestive cardiac failure
▶ acute pulmonary oedema (the main cause of death in the puerperium, occurring mainly in the first 24–48 hours after delivery)
▶ bacterial endocarditis
▶ rheumatic fever prior to pregnancy, resulting in valve incompetence (mitral stenosis)
▶ peripartum cardiomyopathy (PPCM).

The effects of pregnancy depend to some extent upon the grade of cardiac disease before pregnancy.

The effects of cardiac disease on the fetus

The adverse fetal conditions associated with cardiac disease in pregnancy are due to maternal hypoxaemia, especially if cyanotic heart disease is present. This results in placental insufficiency, causing:
▶ IUD or IUGR and small-for-gestational-age (SGA) babies, asphyxia neonatorum and possibly neonatal death
▶ preterm labour and preterm babies, with all the associated complications.

In rheumatic heart disease, the clinical deterioration is slower and more predictable, whereas in other cardiac conditions the change can be dramatic (from any grade to sudden cardiac failure and death). In addition, a woman who has congenital heart disease has a 2–4 per cent chance of delivering a baby with a congenital heart defect (Medscape, 2017).

Causes and incidence

The physiological condition of pregnancy alone can burden the heart and result in cardiac problems.

Congenital cardiac defects account for 75 per cent of cardiac problems in pregnancy. Congenital anomalies include patent ductus arteriosus (PDA), ventricular septal defect (VSD), atrial septal defect (ASD), tetralogy of Fallot, pulmonary stenosis, VSD with an over-riding aorta and hypertrophy of the left ventricle, and Eisenmenger complex (pulmonary stenosis, VSD and ASD). Not many women with untreated congenital heart disease reach childbearing age.

In the high-income group, the most common cardiac diseases in pregnancy are rheumatic diseases (25 per cent) (Medscape, 2017).

Other cardiac conditions include:
▶ endocarditis (including damage to the mitral valve and/or disease of the mitral valve) and carditis
▶ myocarditis: a viral infection associated with malnutrition
▶ bacterial endocarditis
▶ cor pulmonale: hypertensive cardiac disease
▶ PPCM found in women without a cardiac problem (primigravidae and young women) from the last month in pregnancy and first six months postpartum with a 15 per cent mortality (Medscape, 2017).

Factors that aggravate cardiac conditions are:
▶ anaemia
▶ respiratory infection
▶ febrile disease
▶ excessive exercise
▶ emotional upset
▶ hypertension
▶ pre-eclampsia
▶ other infections.

Diagnosis in pregnancy: Cardiovascular assessment

In pregnancy, women with a known cardiac condition will be under the specialist care of a cardiologist.

Often, pregnancy is the first time that possible cardiac disease is suspected, noted and diagnosed. The midwife needs to be able to recognise new or previously undiagnosed cardiac symptoms. A history of previous rheumatic fever, tiredness, low BP or shortness of breath should alert the midwife.

The skilled midwife with post-basic training is educated in specialised history taking and general examination of the chest and lungs and will be able to detect and refer appropriately. The physical examination includes vital signs, BP, body mass and the mid-upper-arm circumference (MUAC). Investigations include urine testing.

Medical diagnosis

When cardiovascular problems are suspected, the woman is referred to an obstetrician and a cardiologist. Table 21.5 shows the factors on which the diagnosis will be based.

Assessment is more difficult in the second half of pregnancy; therefore it is better to try to assess the condition early in pregnancy.

Treatment and care

Women with diagnosed cardiac problems and newly identified cases in pregnancy will be under the supervision of a multidisciplinary team with a cardiologist or specialist obstetrician as supervisor.

Ideally, the cardiac patient should have pre-conception counselling. Surgery will be advised in selected cases. Some women are advised against pregnancy altogether.

The aims of treatment in a pregnant woman with a cardiac condition are to:
 ▶ prevent congestive cardiac failure
 ▶ assess the need for prophylactic treatment against subacute bacterial endocarditis
 ▶ prepare the patient for labour
 ▶ provide the correct treatment throughout pregnancy, labour and the puerperium
 ▶ return the woman to at least the cardiac grade she was in before pregnancy.

Table 21.5

Medical diagnosis of cardiovascular problems

History	Physical examination
Previous heart failure, with syncope during exertion Previous heart failure during pregnancy Age, parity, socioeconomic status, type of work and the type of cardiac lesion	Any murmurs Any extra sounds (third heart sound) Displaced apex beat (from the fourth intercostal space and to the left)
Other signs and symptoms	**Cardiac observations**
Oedema Crepitations in lung bases Cough and haemoptysis Orthopnoea (breathlessness, particularly when lying down) Progressive dyspnoea on effort (progressive difficulty in breathing) Paroxysmal nocturnal dyspnoea (nocturnal attacks of breathlessness, caused by fluid in the lungs when lying down) Fatigue Cyanosis Chest pain	Bounding pulse or thin, thready pulse Irregular pulse Tachycardia (at rest 100 bpm or more) Clubbing of fingers (chronic cardiac disease)
Specific heart abnormalities	**Special investigations**
Specific heart murmurs Irregular heart rhythms Heart enlargement Pulsation or thrill in chest Signs of congestive cardiac failure, which include cyanosis, turgid neck veins and enlarged, tender liver, due to engorgement	Electrocardiogram (ECG) Chest X-ray Echocardiography Exercise tolerance test Respiratory gases Cardiac reserve test

The woman must attend an antenatal clinic every two weeks until 28 weeks. Thereafter, she must attend every week until hospitalisation is necessary. A careful watch is kept for:

▶ hypertension (superimposed pre-eclampsia or any rise in BP)
▶ anaemia
▶ infection of any kind
▶ emotional stress, such as fear and anxiety
▶ multiple pregnancy
▶ polyhydramnios
▶ preterm labour
▶ tachycardia
▶ cardiac arrhythmias
▶ oedema.

The midwife must watch out for signs of congestive cardiac failure and/or pulmonary oedema, which can be sudden and dramatic. These signs include the following:

▶ *Congestive cardiac failure:* Increasing dyspnoea and cyanosis, oedema and tachycardia. Abdominal discomfort (due to liver engorgement as a result of blood backing up in the hepatic veins) may be present, with cold clammy skin, fatigue and a distended jugular vein.
▶ *Pulmonary oedema:* This is usually as a result of left-sided heart failure. Signs and symptoms include cyanosis, dyspnoea and orthopnoea, frothy sputum and haemoptysis, grunting and wheezing, and paroxysmal nocturnal dyspnoea.

Women with dental caries and poor mouth hygiene (which could result in bacterial endocarditis) must be referred to a dentist. All infections must be treated promptly. An antibiotic is prescribed if required. Any surgical procedure (such as dental extraction) is dangerous because of the risk of infection and bacterial endocarditis. In some cases women are on lifelong prophylaxis with penicillin. Women are hospitalised for any infection, for example a UTI.

Grade I and II cardiac pregnant women are assessed every two weeks and preterm labour is excluded by assessing the cervical score. Grade III and IV cardiac pregnant women are assessed throughout the pregnancy and certainly from 28 weeks' gestation. No strict hospitalisation is needed for those women.

Pharmacological treatment

All medication must be prescribed by a cardiologist or specialist obstetrician. This will include medication specific to the pregnancy and chronic cardiac medication.

Principles and protocols of midwifery care

The midwife must pay attention to the factors detailed in the following subsections.

Health education

It is particularly important that the woman knows and understands her condition and the health consequences, the importance of regular antenatal attendance and the signs and symptoms of congestive cardiac failure. She should report to the clinic immediately if any of the following occur:

▶ Dyspnoea (progressive)
▶ Cough
▶ Symptoms suggesting anaemia
▶ Haemoptysis
▶ Palpitations
▶ Fainting (syncope)
▶ Paroxsymal nocturnal dyspnoea
▶ Orthopnoea
▶ Any infection.

Rest

The woman is encouraged to get 10–12 hours' rest at night and two hours in the afternoon. She will require reassurance, understanding and support from the midwife. Relaxation should be encouraged and she is advised to avoid any strenuous effort or work.

Assessment of the woman's personal circumstances

The woman's home circumstances, her financial status, the help available at home, the transport facilities near her home, the nearest clinic and the woman's occupation must all be assessed.

Nutrition

A dietician will help the woman with advice on a balanced diet and weight control.

Medication

Stress the importance of taking prescribed medication and highlight the side effects so that the woman can seek help if these occur.

Exercise

The level of exercise depends on the severity (grade) and type of the disease. The woman should avoid undue exertion at 28–32 weeks because of the peak in blood volume during this period and the risk of cardiac failure. Hospitalisation is encouraged if circumstances at home will not allow for bed rest and support.

Compression stockings

These can be prescribed and must be worn to improve venous return and cardiac stability and to prevent deep vein thrombosis (DVT).

Admission

The woman will be admitted near term, as women with cardiac disease often deliver very quickly when labour starts. They also often have small fetuses. The woman should deliver in hospital under specialised medical and obstetrical observation and care. Depending on the severity of the condition, for safety, a woman with cardiac disease should be hospitalised until the condition is stabilised in case any complications occur. Complications can include:

▶ cardiac symptoms and bacterial endocarditis
▶ infections such as UTI, vaginal infections or chorioamnionitis
▶ HIV or other STIs
▶ pre-eclampsia
▶ obstetric problems such as multiple pregnancy or placental insufficiency, IUGR and placenta praevia.

Care

The patient is kept on bed rest in Fowler's position until the condition is stabilised. In a cardiac patient, the heart must always be higher than the rest of the body. Medication is given as prescribed. The woman is encouraged to get plenty of sleep and rest. Observations are those specific to cardiac failure and pulmonary oedema and infection, such as:

▶ pyrexia
▶ tachycardia
▶ tachypnoea, dyspnoea
▶ sore throat
▶ any local inflammation
▶ pain
▶ oliguria.

Risk

The woman is at risk of cardiac decompensation if she develops an infection. She is particularly at risk from commensals (normal bacterial inhabitants) of the genital tract, such as Gram-negative anaerobic streptococci. Routine septic work-ups include urine microscopy, culture and sensitivity (MC&S), vaginal and throat swabs, rapid plasma reagin (RPR), HIV status and FBC. Constipation is prevented through a balanced diet and prescribed medication. The risk of thrombosis is increased with bed rest; therefore compression stockings should be used.

The birth processes

A vaginal delivery is the safest way for a woman with a cardiac condition, as long as there is expert obstetric, medical and nursing management available and there are no obstetric complications. Obstetric complications such as cephalopelvic disproportion (CPD), IUGR, placenta previa and breech presentation may warrant a Caesarean section, if possible under epidural or spinal anaesthesia.

Specific complications of Caesarean section in women with cardiac disease include infection, post-operative thrombosis and pulmonary complications due to difficulty with coughing and breathing, as well as the after-effects of general anaesthesia, which also causes increased pulmonary complications.

First-stage care protocol

Type of delivery

Labour is allowed to start spontaneously. Induction is not advised. Analgesia and sedation are given to reduce pain and anxiety. Epidural analgesia is ideal. However, it can also be dangerous in certain cardiac conditions due to vasodilatation and the drop in BP. The epidural or spinal anaesthesia is performed by a qualified anaesthetist. Anaemia must be treated before birth and the ideal Hb is 10 g/dl or more.

Fluid balance

An IV patent line is established, but it is important that fluid is restricted in labour. A micro-dropper and buretrol are used to monitor fluid intake (with a dial-a-flow or device to control fluid intake), particularly if oxytocin is administered. A Swan-Ganz cardiac catheter may be passed so that pulmonary arterial and wedge pressures and left atrial pressures can be monitored.

Medication

Pulmonary oedema should be prevented by controlling and limiting IV fluids and giving diuretics early in labour if there is any suspicion of the condition. The medications used are furosemide, morphine and digoxin.

Antibiotic prophylaxis is given to all patients with cardiac conditions. After normal birth, AMTSL is recommended for all women with cardiac conditions.

Anticoagulants may be administered, particularly with previous valve surgery, prosthetic valves, the presence or incidence of thrombosis in pregnancy and tachyarrhythmias. Women on anticoagulants are usually admitted at 37 weeks and change to IV heparin therapy. Heparin is used in the first trimester – particularly during organ formation – because it does not cross the placenta, and at 36 weeks. Heparin is stopped at the start of labour (or two hours before Caesarean section), as it has a tendency to cause postpartum haemorrhage.

Anticoagulant therapy is started again with warfarin or heparin 12 hours after delivery, unless there is excessive bleeding.

Adequate pain relief is needed to prevent exhaustion. An epidural may be valuable if not contraindicated.

Observations

Standard observations of labour and the fetus are carried out. Additional observations include intake and output, a cardiac monitor to measure the apical pulse beat and to watch for arrhythmias in serious heart conditions, plus oximetry for oxygenation observation. Fluid management is essential. A microdropper, infusion pump or dial-a-flow is used to control fluids in labour.

Unnecessary vaginal examinations and the early artificial rupture of membranes are restricted and are only performed when indicated due to the risk of infection.

Oxygen is administered by face mask at 4–6 ℓ per minute. The emergency trolley is on hand and the woman is cared for in the second stage room (delivery room) ready for the birth, with a midwife in constant attendance. The woman is never left alone.

Position in labour

The woman is nursed in an upright position in bed or in a high Fowler's position and the heart is always higher than the rest of the body. The woman cannot lie flat for abdominal palpation or vaginal examination.

Second-stage care protocols

The second stage places an extra burden on the heart, as it is overloaded with each contraction of the uterus as well as during bearing down. Trauma, shock and haemorrhage need to be prevented. A paediatrician is usually present for the delivery.

The labour is very carefully monitored and assessed. In the second stage, adequate analgesia (if no epidural is performed), such as a pudendal nerve block, or local anaesthetic (without adrenaline) is infiltrated into the perineum, after which an episiotomy is performed if necessary.

Assisted delivery using vacuum extraction and forceps delivery is usually indicated to minimise bearing down and to shorten the second stage. The woman is never placed in a lithotomy position. A high Fowler's is maintained in the second stage. The woman's knees must always be lower than her heart, to prevent venous return that overloads the heart.

If the woman needs fluid replacement in case of haemorrhage, a haematologist should be involved if there is clotting abnormality. The Hb, haematocrit and coagulation, as well as the central venous pressure, are carefully monitored.

Third-stage care protocols

The third stage of labour carries the highest risk of cardiac failure, when the uterus contracts and 500–1 000 ℓ of blood is pushed back into the cardiovascular system after the delivery of the placenta.

Oxytocin is the drug of choice for AMTSL and no post-delivery ergometrine is given. Ergometrine has an effect on the smooth muscle of the heart, thereby returning large amountS of blood back into circulation. After delivery, the uterine contraction is maintained with an IV infusion of 20 U oxytocin in 200 ml IV fluid controlled with a paediatric dropper.

Note that a diuretic is sometimes given very slowly intravenously post-delivery on prescription.

Postpartum care

At this stage there is increased venous return to the heart, caused by the removal of vena caval compression, and due to the extra blood and vascular fluid in the general circulation from the contracted and retracted uterus.

The woman must be under strict observation for the fourth stage (six hours) and nursed in the ICU for 48 hours post-delivery because of the danger of acute pulmonary oedema, cardiac failure and death. The following principles are followed:

- The woman is on bed rest and encouraged to get as much sleep and rest as possible.
- The woman is nursed in Fowler's and semi-Fowler's position and given oxygen if necessary.
- Deep breathing and passive exercises are encouraged, to prevent pulmonary complications.
- Early ambulation after 24 hours is also encouraged once the woman's condition is stable, to prevent thrombosis.
- The intake and the output of fluids is carefully measured because of the risk of pulmonary oedema.
- Breastfeeding is encouraged, unless contraindicated in Grade IV or in cardiac failure.

Grades I and II who are well compensated after delivery may use contraception. However, grades III and IV are discouraged from using contraceptives and may be advised to consider tubal ligation. If the patient chooses a tubal ligation and has an epidural, the operation can be performed while the epidural is *in situ*, to avoid a second anaesthetic.

It may be necessary to refer the patient to a social worker. Help at home must be arranged to allow the patient to rest as much as possible. Women are only discharged when cardiovascular stability is confirmed.

Peripartum cardiomyopathy

This is a condition presenting in late pregnancy and after birth, in which women may develop life-threatening cardiac failure. Symptoms of cardiac failure may develop in the last month of pregnancy and up to five months post-delivery in women who have never had cardiac problems. This often starts with a cough and flu-like symptoms and is often overlooked. PPCM can occur in any woman, at any age during reproductive years, and in any pregnancy.

The cause is unknown, but it is thought to be auto-immune damage to the left ventricle. The redistribution of blood to the breasts after birth places a burden on the heart and breastfeeding is contraindicated in these cases.

The incidence is 1:1 000 in South Africa and is genetic in origin. A study taken in Soweto showed that mortality was 15 per cent and only 23 per cent of women fully recovered after six months of standard treatment (Sliwa et al, 2010).

Midwives need to have a high index of clinical suspicion and screen women appropriately during the antenatal period, focusing on the third trimester and early postnatal period. Women are referred for follow-up care to the cardiac clinic for observation and re-evaluation of medication.

Note: Midwives in primary healthcare (PHC) centres need to look out for PPCM in women without previous cardiac problems at six weeks postnatally.

21.7 Surgery during pregnancy

Pregnant women may need general surgery for non-pregnancy-related conditions. If the condition is life-threatening, the surgery will be carried out during pregnancy. The fetus is usually not affected by the general anaesthesia, but the use of medication and potential infections and hypovolaemia may carry a risk for the fetus.

The following principles are to be considered for surgery in pregnancy:

- The mother's life always takes preference over that of the fetus.
- Changed anatomy and physiology can mask the diagnosis. The organs are in a new relation, masking symptoms.
- Under stress the maternal homeostasis will favour her well-being at the cost of the fetus.
- The fetus is completely dependent on the mother and hypotension and hypovolaemia must be corrected fast and effectively.

- Owing to the hyperdynamic cardiovascular system and enlarged blood vessels, bleeding will be profuse and fast.
- After 20 weeks' gestation, the enlarged uterus will cause IVCS, which will complicate matters.
- The changes of the sphincters and the displacement of the stomach increase the risk of aspiration during induction of anaesthesia. The stomach takes 12 hours to empty in pregnancy, therefore induction of anaesthetics must be adapted.
- The fetal heart rate (FHR) must be determined before any operation, because its absence may modify the procedure.
- The effect of emergency medication on the fetus must be considered.
- Women might not always know that they are pregnant when presenting with problems. If X-rays are unavoidable, the abdomen is screened.

Pre- and post-operative care needs to be adapted for pregnant women. The woman will be in a gynaecological ward if she is under 14 weeks pregnant. The woman needs to be observed for contractions and the fetal heart should be observed. In late pregnancy, she may be in high care depending on the surgery risks.

Surgery during pregnancy could result from obstetric emergencies that affect the woman or the fetus. Severe APH due to placenta praevia, particularly in the case of Grade III and Grade IV, warrant Caesarean section because of cervical os occlusion by the placenta. Other obstetric emergencies that require surgery in the form of Caesarean section include:

- cord prolapse and not fully dilated
- cord presentation while not fully dilated
- obstructed labour
- CPD diagnosed during labour.

21.8 Epilepsy in pregnancy

Epilepsy is a common chronic neurological condition that can also affect some pregnant women. An epileptic seizure is a paroxysmal discharge of the cerebral neurons, resulting in a clinical event, which may or may not be apparent to the subject and/or an observer. Epilepsy can be classified according to causation:

- Symptomatic epilepsy results from a specific identified mode, such as head injury or the development of a brain tumour.

- Idiopathic epilepsy presents as a result of an anonymous reason or a medical feature:
  - Grand mal epilepsy is characterised by a loss of consciousness with widespread tremors.
  - Petit mal epilepsy is characterised by a blurring of consciousness with no widespread tremors.
  - Jacksonian epilepsy could start in one group of muscles then either spread to other groups or remain localised. It could include a loss of consciousness.
- Primary epilepsy is caused by hereditary factors, as it occurs during the first two weeks of life or in puberty.
- Secondary epilepsy is caused by infections, brain tumours or trauma etc. It could begin during childhood or after the age of 30.
- Abdominal epilepsy is characterised by repeated occurrences of abdominal pain with lack of tremors.
- Akinetic epilepsy presents with no movement and the person does not lose consciousness.
- Focal epilepsy is characterised by minor tremors of one side of the body.
- Myoclonic epilepsy is hereditary in nature and is characterised by quick bouts of muscle tremors and shock-like twitches of a limb or the whole body that often occur in the morning.
- In psychomotor epilepsy, tremors prevail soon or later after head injury and might or might not recur.
- Status epilepticus is characterised by repetitive epileptic tremors in rapid sequence with no recovery in-between.

The better the disease is controlled prior to pregnancy, the less likelihood there will be of further deterioration during pregnancy. If the patient suffers from seizures, a neurologist should be consulted.

The effect of pregnancy on epilepsy

Women with known epilepsy must consult a neurologist for a reassessment of medication for the condition while pregnant. Women with secondary generalised and partial complex seizures are most likely to have an increase in seizures during pregnancy. The effect of pregnancy on the condition varies greatly and depends on the degree of control.

Drug absorption

Drug absorption from the bowel may be reduced during pregnancy. Fluid retention in pregnancy increases the available volume for distribution of anticonvulsant drugs. Therefore, the dilution tends to lower the serum levels of the drug. The liver develops an increased capacity for hydroxylation of some anticonvulsants, such as phenytoin. Therefore, increased clearance and changes in volume of distribution may result in a fall in serum levels.

Epilepsy medication may cause lowered serum folate concentrations. Megaloblastic anaemia (folic acid deficiency) occurs occasionally. The long-term use of phenytoin and phenobarbitone induces clinical osteomalacia and rickets, although hypocalcaemia is more common because these drugs increase the hepatic metabolism of vitamin D. Those patients requiring medication should be given as low a dose as possible and serum and/or salivary levels of the drugs should be checked during pregnancy. The patient must be carefully observed for status epilepticus.

The effect on the pregnancy and fetus

The effect of the seizures on pregnancy and on the fetus can include:

- an LBW baby
- a reduced circumference of the head
- an increased stillbirth rate
- fetal hypoxia due to the trauma of the seizures, especially with prolonged seizures or during a status epilepticus period
- increased risk of preterm birth.

The effect of drugs on the newborn

There is an increased incidence of haemorrhagic disease. This is due to deficiencies in clotting factors II, VII, IX and X as well as vitamin K caused by epileptic drugs. Vitamin K given to the mother in pregnancy could prevent this.

Impaired suckling occurs with drug withdrawal. Other effects include:

- hyper-excitability
- occasional seizures
- tremulousness
- slower weight gain
- failure to thrive
- increased perinatal mortality.

Phenytoin should be avoided in pregnancy, as it will lead to the baby developing fetal phenytoin syndrome. This syndrome includes:

- craniofacial anomalies
- IUGR
- mental restriction
- digital hypoplasia.

The children of women with epilepsy have an increased risk of developing epilepsy in later life, except in cases where the epilepsy is caused by head trauma or infection.

Management and care

Pre-pregnancy management

It is advisable that a woman with epilepsy consult a medical practitioner before pregnancy. Supplements of folate (folic acid) and vitamin D may be necessary due to the effect of the medication on the absorption of vitamins. Before pregnancy, the medical practitioner can start with a slow withdrawal of anticonvulsants if the patient has had no attacks for about three years.

There is a significant risk of teratogenesis with some drugs used to control seizures, particularly during the first trimester, as epileptic drugs cross the placenta. The potential fetal abnormalities include cleft lip, cleft palate and congenital heart disease.

Care during pregnancy

Care for the pregnant woman diagnosed with epilepsy is delivered at the higher level, as the pregnancy is classified as high risk. High-risk pregnancy requires the attention of specialist members of a multidisciplinary team, including the midwife, the obstetrician and the internal medicine specialist. The internal medicine specialist is responsible for the epilepsy, as it is assessed with each visit, while the obstetrician supervises the progress of pregnancy. The midwife offers the woman and her family support throughout pregnancy, including referral for risk assessment in order to detect or exclude possible challenges that could result from the epilepsy.

The management of seizures is provided for in the same manner as for any other patient, except that fetal well-being is evaluated through the use of CTG as soon as convulsions cease. The care given during fits is very similar to that given during an eclamptic fit. However, magnesium is not used; instead, anti-epileptic drugs such as benzodiazepines are used.

The differential diagnosis of an epileptic fit includes:

▶ eclampsia
▶ hypoxia
▶ hypernatraemia
▶ hypoglycaemia
▶ tetany
▶ drug withdrawal.

Labour

The woman can give birth normally, unless there is an obstetric problem. The midwife should remain watchful for any signs of epileptic attack, as the stressful nature of labour could sensitise convulsions. Anti-epileptic treatment is continued as prescribed. The patient requires reassurance, encouragement, support and a positive outlook.

The puerperium

Anti-epileptic treatment is continued. In the absence of any contraindication, postnatal visits are scheduled in the same manner as for any other postnatal woman. However, at the six-week visit the woman is referred to the internal medicine specialist for re-evaluation of anti-epileptic medication.

The woman is allowed to breastfeed, provided that her condition is well controlled. The mother should be made aware that barbiturates can cause drowsiness in breastfed babies. The baby should be assessed throughout the hospital stay for irritability, as this could be a withdrawal symptom (Wylie & Bryce, 2008).

Contraception advice is offered before discharge from the hospital and the mother is counselled to seek medical care before the next pregnancy to avoid teratogenicity on a future fetus or baby.

21.9 Tumours in pregnancy

Tumours of the breast: Pregnancy-associated breast cancer

Pregnancy-associated breast cancer (PABC) is breast cancer which occurs during pregnancy or in the postpartum period. Approximately 6.5 per cent of women 40 years and younger develop tumours in the breast, and 0.03 per cent of women do so during pregnancy (Keyser et al, 2012).

Clinical picture

Tumours in the breast are indicated by itching, pain, nipple discharge or bleeding, lumps in the breast or under the arm.

Diagnosis

All women should have a bilateral breast examination during pregnancy and are encouraged to do self-examination on a monthly basis. Check for a family history of breast cancer, parity and previous breastfeeding. Examine the breasts on each visit and in the postnatal ward. Ultrasound can be done if a lump is detected.

Medical management

The management depends on the type of tumour, whether it is benign or malignant and whether it has already spread to other body parts. Fine needle aspiration biopsy is carried out, with further investigations if the lump is malignant.

Treatment may be by lumpectomy or mastectomy, with removal of axillary nodes. Further treatment includes radiotherapy and chemotherapy, which may be delayed until after birth.

Cancer of the cervix

Cervical cancer is found in one in 3 000–5 000 women at routine Pap smear. One in 200 women attending antenatal clinic will show abnormal cell changes of the cervix (Karam, 2017).

Clinical features

The woman will have a watery, bloodstained discharge from the cervix and frank bleeding.

Medical management

All women should have a Pap smear in pregnancy before 28 weeks or at the six-week postnatal examination. Pregnancy is not an ideal time to screen women for cancer of the cervix. The hormones of pregnancy affect the cells of the cervix after 28 weeks and abnormal cells will be found.

If the Pap smear is suspect, a repeat test is done. Thereafter, colposcopic assessment may be done by an experienced colposcopist. A punch biopsy can be done, and the following results could be found:

- Normal epithelium
- Dysplasia
- Carcinoma-in-situ
- Invasive carcinoma.

The patient must be assessed by a specialist. The treatment depends on many factors and is individualised. The patient and her partner require counselling.

If cervical intraepithelial neoplasia (CIN) is *in situ*, it is usual to wait until after pregnancy to treat it. (The degree of CIN is determined by the extent to which the neoplastic cells involve the full thickness of the cervical epithelium.) Other treatments include cryotherapy, diathermy and laser or cone biopsy.

If the cancer is invasive, radical treatment with radiotherapy is given. The woman and her family need empathy, support, information and encouragement. A postpartum follow-up is essential.

Complications

The abortion rate is 20 per cent. There is an increased incidence of preterm labour. Haemorrhage from the cervix occurs in 15 per cent of cases – sometimes immediate, sometimes delayed until the later stages of the disease (Karam, 2017).

Vulval and vaginal cancer

These forms of cancer are rare in the reproductive age group. Very occasionally, the intraepithelial type may occur.

Ovarian cancer

The occurrence is 1:1 500 (INCIP, nd). This is also uncommon in the childbearing period, but is slightly more common in older primigravidae.

There are many types of ovarian cancer and an accurate diagnosis can be difficult. The size of the tumour is unaltered in pregnancy. Displacement is evident on palpation. Torsion may occur, and during pregnancy and labour the tumour may be incarcerated in the pouch of Douglas, where it may cause an obstruction. There is a risk of preterm labour.

Once ovarian cancer is diagnosed, an oncologist will determine the options of care.

21.10 Conclusion

Certain conditions such as hypertensive disorders, anaemia, diabetes mellitus, thyroid disorders, cardiac disease, epilepsy and cancers may complicate pregnancy. Women with established conditions will generally be managed by specialists, but midwives need to be able to recognise these diseases and refer appropriately.

Obstetric haemorrhage

22.1 Introduction

Obstetric haemorrhage is a leading cause of preventable maternal death worldwide and includes early antepartum, intrapartum and postpartum bleeding (up to 42 days post-delivery). It includes all bleeding related to the placenta and the uterus.

Obstetric haemorrhage can occur from early pregnancy to 42 days after birth. The *Saving Mothers 2014* report indicated that 16.1 per cent of maternal deaths can be related to obstetric haemorrhage, with 1.8 per cent related to ectopic pregnancy and 3.5 per cent being cases of miscarriage (DoH, 2015b). Blood loss of 500 ml in the third trimester is considered serious.

Advances in obstetric care have provided physicians with the diagnostic tools to detect, anticipate and prevent severe life-threatening maternal haemorrhage in most women who have had prenatal care. In an optimal setting, women at high risk for haemorrhage are referred to tertiary care centres, where multidisciplinary teams are prepared and ready to care for and deal with known potential complications. However, even in the face of the best prenatal care, unexpected haemorrhage occurs. Unforeseen and suspected obstetric haemorrhage can be averted by the implementation of basic and comprehensive emergency obstetric signal functions. This chapter highlights factors that predispose women to severe bleeding. The chapter also explains the management of severe bleeding and the most recent treatment guidelines.

22.2 Early (first trimester) obstetric haemorrhage

Early obstetric haemorrhage is the term used for bleeding from the genital tract occurring before 26 weeks of pregnancy (or, in South Africa, before viability). This bleeding can be the result of many conditions, but the main conditions that present as bleeding from the genital tract in early pregnancy are implantation bleeding, ectopic pregnancy, threatening or spontaneous miscarriage, cervical lesions and placental abnormalities such as hydatidiform mole.

Implantation bleeding

Implantation bleeding occurs at the time that the syncytial layer of the trophoblast (the fertilised ovum) embeds into the endometrial lining of the uterus. The bleeding usually occurs a few days before the menstrual period is due and can easily be mistaken for a period, thus confusing the estimated date of delivery (EDD). Careful history taking is important to avoid this problem.

This condition usually settles down quickly, within three to four days, once the blastocyst has completely embedded and is covered by endometrial cells.

Miscarriage

Miscarriage is the interruption of pregnancy before 26 weeks' gestation, after which the fetus is said to be viable. The peak time for miscarriages is weeks 6–10 of pregnancy.

Classification of miscarriages

Miscarriage can be classified as:
- *spontaneous* first trimester and second trimester miscarriage
- *inevitable miscarriage:* vaginal bleeding and pain with cervical dilatation
- *threatening miscarriage:* vaginal bleeding with closed cervix and no pain

- *incomplete miscarriage:* only part of the products of conception are expelled
- *complete miscarriage:* complete expulsion of the products of conception
- *habitual miscarriage:* three or more consecutive spontaneous miscarriages, usually after 14 weeks' gestation
- *missed miscarriage:* the fetus dies and is retained *in utero*, together with the placenta and membranes
- *septic miscarriage:* infection of the uterus following miscarriage
- *induced miscarriage:* interruption of pregnancy on demand
- *therapeutic abortion:* for medical reason(s)
- *criminal abortion:* illegal termination of pregnancy (TOP), usually referred to as a 'backstreet' miscarriage
- *tubal abortion:* termination of a tubal pregnancy.

Spontaneous miscarriage

The incidence of spontaneous miscarriage is not truly known, because not all women who abort will see a medical practitioner or will be admitted to hospital. Spontaneous miscarriage is the most common complication of early pregnancy and in clinically diagnosed pregnancies varies between 8 and 20 per cent (Tulandi & Al-Fozan, 2017). The number of unreported miscarriages is unknown.

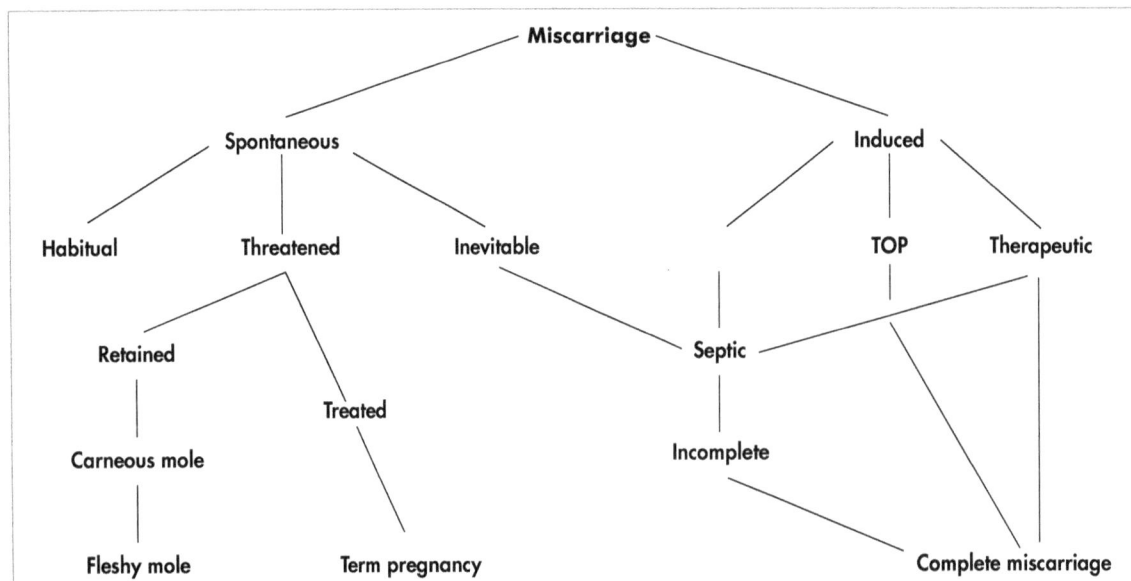

Figure 22.1 Classification and algorithms of outcomes of miscarriage

Therapeutic abortion and TOP

A therapeutic abortion is an induced abortion for medical reasons, including mental or physical danger to the mother or the fetus, with congenital defects of the fetus as the main reason.

Choice of termination of pregnancy (CTOP) is a legal abortion before 20 weeks of pregnancy, requested by the pregnant woman. In South Africa, midwives are trained to terminate unwanted pregnancies of up to 12 weeks, while medical doctors terminate unwanted pregnancies up to 20 weeks' gestation, as requested by any pregnant woman.

Habitual or recurrent miscarriage

Habitual miscarriage could be interspersed with normal deliveries, but can also associated with late or mid-trimester miscarriage occurring between 22 and 24 weeks' gestation. Warning signs for habitual miscarriage are lacking. The sudden rupture of membranes and expulsion of a fresh abortus occur after the gradual, painless dilatation of the internal cervical os.

The cause of habitual miscarriage is usually mechanical, such as uterine abnormality or cervical incompetence. However, there may be a psychological, immunological, infective or chromosomal underlying cause, all of which would require specialised investigation and care.

Causes of miscarriage

The causes of miscarriage are unknown, but are related to an abnormal uterine environment (including hormonal problems). Contributing factors include:
- abnormal development of the embryo; Rubio et al (2003) found that chromosomal abnormalities is an important cause of miscarriages in the first trimester and has a higher incidence in reoccurring miscarriage (RM).
- abnormalities of the placenta, such as hydatidiform mole
- maternal causes such as hormonal insufficiency of progesterone to support the implantation of the ovum
- maternal infections, including toxins, microorganisms that cross the placenta, high temperatures and hypoxia
- endometritis and abnormalities of the decidua
- retroflexion of the uterus, which may cause miscarriage in rare cases
- thyroid disease, which may also interfere with the ability to conceive and carry a fetus to term
- abnormalities of the uterus and cervical incompetence
- extreme emotional stress, which releases pituitary hormones, affecting uterine function; an episode of severe pain, grief, fright or distress after accidents may lead to a miscarriage

- multiple pregnancies: the more fetuses in the uterus, the higher the risk for complications, including miscarriages.

The mechanism of miscarriage

In the first six to eight weeks, the whole ovum covered by the decidua (see Chapter 7) is expelled if the cervix is dilated.

In the case of a miscarriage during the third and fourth months of pregnancy, the fetus in an intact sac and the placenta may be expelled, with minimal bleeding. Intervention is not needed. If the membranes are ruptured, the cervix is closed and the placenta is retained, bleeding may be profuse and intervention will be needed.

In miscarriage, the contractions are the same as in labour and the dilatation of the cervix is the same. Lactation can also follow.

Donnet et al (1990) found that although there is some disturbance of endocrine function in the first cycle after spontaneous miscarriage, the majority of women have a rapid return to ovulation, making the early use of contraception necessary for those wishing to avoid conception. The risk of pregnancy is very high after an evacuation.

Signs and symptoms

Signs and symptoms of miscarriage include:
- vaginal bleeding
- uterine contractions (low abdominal or back pain)
- pain and shock (in the case of an ectopic pregnancy)
- septic shock (in the case of septic miscarriage)
- hypertension before 20 weeks of pregnancy
- hydatidiform mole.

Obstetric management

The management and care will depend on the gestational age (GA) of the fetus, the gravidity and parity of the woman and the cause and extent of the vaginal bleeding.

Ultrasound is used for diagnosis in early pregnancy. The diagnosis of the condition of the ovum, placenta, implantation, bleeding and cervix will determine the path of care.

Intervention is required if there is a blighted ovum (empty sac), partial or full separation of the placenta, hydatidiform mole or an ectopic pregnancy, as well as if the products of conception are partially retained. The interventions are aimed at stopping bleeding and contraction of the uterus, pain relief and removal of the products of conception.

Miscarriage with intact or ruptured membranes

The surgical evacuation of the uterus may be needed in miscarriage before 12 weeks of pregnancy.

Management of inevitable miscarriage

A miscarriage is inevitable if the pregnancy can no longer continue. Some women with vaginal haemorrhage seek care in the primary healthcare (PHC) setting. In these settings, manual vacuum aspiration (MVA) is used in women experiencing bleeding with retained products of conception as a result of incomplete miscarriage. MVA is an emergency obstetric signal function that must be practised by registered nurses and midwives in PHC settings to avert maternal death that could result from haemorrhage. If bleeding persists despite MVA, evacuation of the uterus is executed in hospitals.

Habitual miscarriage and medical intervention

Medical intervention to prevent habitual miscarriage includes:
- referral to a specialist for diagnosis of the cause of a previous pregnancy loss
- a period of total bedrest in some cases
- hormonal treatment to maintain the pregnancy
- the insertion of a Shirodkar or McDonald stitch or cervical cerclage in the cervix, around 16 weeks of gestation or later in the pregnancy, followed by hospitalisation for 24 hours to assess the body's response to the stitch
- education on safe sexual practices to avoid unnecessary cervical stimulation; however, research evaluating the consequence of sexual intercourse on the risk of second trimester pregnancy loss among women with a Shirodkar or McDonald stitch or cervical cerclage is lacking
- instructions to shower rather than taking a bath, to exclude pressure being exerted by the growing fetus on the lower abdomen, which could exacerbate cervical opening
- admission to hospital around 36 weeks' gestation for the removal of the stitch in preparation for birth.

Specific nursing care in case of miscarriage

Nursing management will largely depend upon the duration of the pregnancy, gravidity and parity, loss of blood and the condition of the woman. The aims of management are to:
- determine the cause of the bleeding
- preserve the life of the woman
- stop the bleeding
- administer pain relief if needed
- maintain the fetal life if possible
- suppress contractions
- provide for bed rest.

The principles of care include the following:
- Assess and stabilise the woman's condition by determining her vital signs: pulse, respiration rate and BP as well as abdominal assessment for tenderness and size of the uterus.
- Assess the general appearance of the woman in terms of colour, hydration and any signs of shock.
- Determine the GA and condition of the fetus (is the fetus safe or expelled?). If under 12 weeks, an ultrasound will be done. If more than 16 weeks, the fetal heart may be determined using a Doppler.
- Stop the vaginal bleeding and prevent infections.
- Preserve all blood loss and expelled products for the medical practitioner's inspection.
- Collaborate with the medical practitioner for the appropriate diagnosis and intervention. This may include bed rest and treatment, surgical evacuation or removal of the Fallopian tube in case of an ectopic pregnancy.
- Offer emotional and psychological care, suppress lactation if necessary and be aware of the emotional condition of the woman. A miscarriage can be a devastating occurrence in a woman's life. She may experience feelings such as depression, anxiety, guilt, shame, a sense of failure and of worthlessness and, if she is married or in a partnership, she may feel she is not capable of providing her husband or partner with a child. The midwife who is aware of these problems should be able to provide support, encouragement, understanding and empathy when caring for women after miscarriage. The midwife should be a good listener, and should allow the patient to express her feelings, fears and anxieties.
- Give anti-D treatment within 72 hours of miscarriage to Rh-negative women to prevent isoimmunisation.
- Prevent complications from infection and think about infertility, depression and choriocarcinoma in case of hydatidiform mole.

A consent form in case of surgery (evacuation for ectopic pregnancy) is obtained and completed, should this be necessary. An IV infusion is started if the patient's condition is unsatisfactory. The patient is kept warm and is prepared for the operating theatre. Pain relief is given per medical prescription.

After the miscarriage and/or surgery, vulval toilet is carried out four-hourly for the first 24 hours. When the patient has sufficiently recovered, she is taught to continue her own vulval toilet or Sitz baths.

Complications

A miscarriage may lead to complications, such as:
- haemorrhage resulting in hypovolaemia
- sepsis after missed miscarriage, in the case of retained products of conception or after an illegal miscarriage

- depression after pregnancy loss
- complications of surgery, such as perforation of the uterus
- choriocarcinoma following hydatidiform mole
- maternal isoimmunisation, in the case of an Rh-negative woman
- maternal death due to severe haemorrhage.

Hydatidiform mole (gestational trophoblastic disease)

A hydatidiform mole is the abnormal development of the primitive chorion, where hydropic or cystic degeneration of the centre of the villi occurs. These distended chorionic villi form vesicles of variable size. The choriodecidual spaces are obliterated and there is no circulation of the maternal blood. The products of conception resemble a large bunch of grapes. The embryo is absorbed and no fetus or placenta can be identified.

The proliferation of the trophoblast results in large increases in the level of human chorionic gonadotrophin (hCG), large amounts of which are excreted in the urine. Stimulation of the ovaries by the high levels of hCG may result in the formation of large lutein cysts. If hCG remains in the bloodstream after the miscarriage or if the levels rise, choriocarcinoma is suspected.

The incidence of hydatidiform mole is varies greatly and is 1: 1 200 pregnancies in the USA and 1: 5 000 in Paraguay (Moore, 2016). In South Africa, Snyman (2009) reports an estimate of 1.2/1 000 pregnancies. The pregnancy rarely reaches 18 weeks. Problems develop at around three to four months. The age of the woman does not appear to be important and any pregnancy could be susceptible.

Signs and symptoms

Vaginal bleeding may be the first sign of the condition. Excessive nausea and vomiting (due to high levels of circulating hCG in the blood) and hypertension (for the same reason) may develop before 20 weeks of pregnancy.

The uterus will be large for the period of gestation and soft and bulky. No specific fetal parts can be palpated, no fetal heart is heard and fetal movements are not felt by the woman, even though these are expected in the second trimester of pregnancy.

The diagnosis is confirmed through a blood test and ultrasound.

Medical care

An evacuation of the uterus is performed as soon as possible after a diagnosis is confirmed. If the pregnancy is less than 12 weeks, dilatation and curettage is performed. If the pregnancy is more than 12 weeks, oxytocin is first used to expel the mole and then an evacuation by suction is performed.

A strict follow-up regimen is carried out because of the possible complication of choriocarcinoma. Serum hCG levels are monitored post-operatively. The hCG levels usually only return to normal after eight weeks. The tests are performed every month for a year, and then at three-monthly intervals for a year.

Complications: Choriocarcinoma

Choriocarcinoma is a malignant growth of the trophoblast that sometimes follows hydatidiform mole. It can also follow an early miscarriage. This rare condition can be fatal because of the rapid growth of the trophoblast. The growth invades the uterus and the vagina and eventually, via the bloodstream, also the liver, lungs and brain.

If the hCG levels remain high after miscarriage, choriocarcinoma is suspected. Women are therefore advised to continue with the blood tests until it is normal. Any follow-up pregnancy is postponed for two years.

Previously, the final outcome of choriocarcinoma was frequently the death of the patient and, without treatment, this took place very shortly after the choriocarcinoma was first diagnosed. However, today, with treatment, this condition is often successfully cured. A cure is defined as the complete absence of all clinical evidence of the disease for a period of five years.

Ectopic pregnancy

An ectopic pregnancy is a condition where the fertilised ovum is embedded outside the uterus, as it failed to reach the uterus before implantation took place. The pregnancy therefore develops in a Fallopian tube or, in extremely rare cases, in the abdomen (an extra-uterine pregnancy or abdominal pregnancy).

Incidence

The incidence of ectopic pregnancy varies, from 13 to 20 out of 1 000 pregnancies (Luesley & Kilby, 2016). The majority of cases are in the ampulla and isthmus of the Fallopian tube, but unusual sites of implantation include the fimbriated ends of the Fallopian tubes, the interstitial portion of the Fallopian tubes, the ovary (0.5 per cent) and the abdominal cavity (0.1 per cent) (Badr et al, 2013).

Mechanism

The ovum only implants when the zona pellucida is completely or almost completely shed. Therefore, any factor that slows the passage of the ovum along the tube to the uterus can result in an ectopic pregnancy. The implantation may occur at any point along the tube.

If the ovum dies, it is re-absorbed completely, forms a tubal mole or is aborted into the abdominal cavity.

If the ovum survives, the trophoblast enlarges and erodes into the tissues of the Fallopian tube. The endometrium thickens, the uterus enlarges, the muscles of the tubes thicken and the ovarian and uterine arteries become twisted (as in a normal pregnancy). The tube stretches as the ovum develops and enlarges. As a result, there are repeated bleeding episodes.

Eventually, the Fallopian tube can stretch no further and the tube ruptures. The ovarian artery and vein can be torn as a result of the rupture, which will cause severe internal and external bleeding. The rupture can either be subacute, which is difficult to diagnose immediately, or acute, in which case the signs are dramatic. An acute rupture will result in collapse due to internal haemorrhage and excessive pain.

Aetiology

The causes of an ectopic pregnancy include:
- congenitally narrowed Fallopian tubes
- pelvic inflammatory conditions
- chronic salpingitis
- endometriosis
- tuberculosis
- tubal surgery
- intrauterine contraceptive devices (IUCDs).

Signs and symptoms

The classical symptoms of an ectopic pregnancy are:
- amenorrhoea
- lower abdominal pain (occasional sharp, stabbing pains)
- vaginal bleeding
- nausea and vomiting.

If tubal rupture occurs, the signs are:
- sudden, excruciating abdominal pain
- fainting
- signs of shock, which include pallor, cold clammy skin, tachycardia and vomiting.

Management and care

Women generally present at a medical practitioner's rooms or at an emergency unit with signs and symptoms of abdominal pain or discomfort. Women may also come to PHC clinics with signs and symptoms that are diffuse. This may be missed or misdiagnosed, with serious consequences for the woman.

If signs of shock and pain are present, the woman will be treated as an emergency. An accurate diagnosis can be made using ultrasound.

All women with a history of amenorrhoea and pain or vaginal bleeding are referred for medical care. The following are routine medical interventions carried out by the medical practitioner:
- Assess the patient's condition.
- Take an accurate history.
- Examine the patient thoroughly for rigidity, guarding and rebound tenderness.
- Carry out special investigations, including Hb, packed cell volume (PCV), white cell count test (WCC), erythrocyte sedimentation rate (ESR) and a pregnancy test.
- Perform a full urine test.
- Perform an ultrasound scan.
- Take blood for cross-matching. Blood or replacement therapy is given if necessary.
- Consider IV therapy.

Abdominal pregnancy

An abdominal pregnancy is a rare condition that occurs if the conceptus develops in the distal end of the uterine tube and becomes attached to the fimbriated ends of the tube, or is aborted into the abdominal cavity, where it attaches itself to the ovary and/or abdominal organs. The fetus can die and calcify (a lithopaedion) or it can grow to term, usually suffering from compression deformities and growth restriction.

The diagnosis of an abdominal pregnancy is made by findings on abdominal palpation and confirmed by ultrasound. On abdominal palpation, the fetus is found to be not in the uterus. It may be in an unusual position and is felt more clearly due to the lack of abdominal wall.

After confirmation of the diagnosis by ultrasound scanning, a laparotomy is performed to deliver the baby. The pregnancy rarely reaches term. If the pregnancy reaches term, the fetus will be delivered by laparotomy. The placenta and membranes are left *in situ* to avoid haemorrhage; these are reabsorbed by the body.

Other causes of vaginal bleeding in early pregnancy

If a woman presents with vaginal bleeding in early pregnancy, it is important to identify the cause and severity of the problem and assess the risk of miscarriage. The most accurate investigation is ultrasound.

If the fetus is intact and in the uterus, other causes for the vaginal bleeding are considered:
- *Cervicitis:* Inflammation of the cervix may cause vaginal bleeding after coitus.
- *Cervical or uterine polyps:* These are small, bright-red, fleshy, pedunculated, benign growths originating in the cervical canal. They may become malignant, causing bleeding.

▶ *Cervical cancer:* The Papanicolaou (Pap) smear is performed routinely in the antenatal period.

▶ *Trauma:* The vagina is very vascular in pregnancy. Trauma of the vagina can happen during rough sexual intercourse and high vaginal tears may occur.

22.3 Antepartum haemorrhage

The definition of antepartum haemorrhage (APH) is bleeding from the genital tract after 24 weeks of gestation. The incidence is 2–5 per cent of all pregnancies beyond 24 weeks (DoH, 2014). Currently it is the third most important cause of maternal death in South Africa (DoH, 2015b). The highest risk of death occurs in the first 24 hours after birth.

Causes

The causes of APH range from cervicitis, vasa praevia and more commonly, placental abnormalities, placenta praevia or placental abruption. The two major causes of APH are:

1. *placenta praevia*, which is defined as a placenta that is partially or totally implanted in the lower segment of the uterus
2. *placental abruption*, which is accidental haemorrhage where the placenta has separated partially or completely from the uterine wall (when normally implanted in the upper segment). Low Hb, in particular, plays a role in placental abruption.

A proactive approach should be used for patients at high risk of haemorrhage, since pre-operative preparedness can improve the outcome.

Complications

The complications that can arise due to APH include:

▶ hypovolaemic shock (see Chapter 35), which can result in Sheehan's syndrome (pituitary gland necrosis due to lack of blood flow)
▶ a Couvelaire uterus in placental abruption – the myometrium is full of blood and cannot contract – which may lead to a hysterectomy
▶ the development of disseminated intravascular coagulation (DIC); clotting factors are depleted and obstetric haemorrhage will occur
▶ a greater risk of premature delivery
▶ fetal hypoxia
▶ sudden fetal death, making APH an even greater risk to the fetus than to the mother
▶ postpartum haemorrhage (PPH), which usually follows APH
▶ maternal death
▶ perinatal mortality.

Table 22.1 details the different types of APH, and their causes, symptoms, management and complications.

Table 22.1

Haemorrhage in pregnancy

Criterion	Placental abruption	Placenta praevia	Vasa praevia	Other
Incidence (Bakker & Smith, 2016)	0.5–2.0%	0.5% of pregnancies	1 in 2000 to 1 in 5000	
Pre-existing factors or causes	Often hypertensive conditions Pre-eclampsia Often anaemic Short cord (30 cm) Trauma Decompression of uterus (polyhydramnios) Multiple pregnancy Uterine abnormalities Poor nutrition and social conditions Smoking	Multiple pregnancy Previous Caesarean section Maternal age Placenta implanted in lower segment Grand multipara	Often low-lying placenta Velamentous insertion of the cord	Vaginal infection Cervical lesions Hydatidiform mole

continued

Criterion	Placental abruption	Placenta praevia	Vasa praevia	Other
Onset	More common after 28 weeks Sudden and stormy Retroplacental clot may develop over a period of time	Bleeding is thought to occur in association with the development of the lower uterine segment in the third trimester Lower risk after 28 weeks and high risk after 36 weeks: • 10% after 28–31 weeks • 30% after 31–35 weeks • 60% after 35 weeks Small warning bleeding Severe second episode	During third trimester or onset of labour Blood vessels over internal os	Any time during first or second trimester
Symptoms	Pain with or without external and concealed vaginal bleeding Shock not related to visible blood Increased pulse and drop in BP	Painless vaginal bleeding Clear, fresh blood Fetal movements normal Can coincide with the onset of labour	Fetal bradycardia associated with vaginal haemorrhage	Fresh bleeding or spotting with or without pain
Examination	Pain: uterus hard and tender Increased uterine tone Fetus large for expected dates Difficult to feel baby or hear fetal heart Anaemia not related to blood loss	No pain Tone of uterus normal Malpresentation or high presenting part Anaemia related to blood loss Fetal heart present	No maternal problems Poor prognosis for the baby Vessels may be damaged with vaginal examination (PV – *per vagina*) and amniotomy Compression from presenting part APT test (fetal haemoglobin test) to determine the origin of the blood	No uterine tenderness Stable vital signs Usually from cancer If there is pain, is miscarriage threatening?
Nature of bleeding	Dark clots if not concealed bleeding	Bright red blood from low-lying placenta	Bright red blood from the cord or vagina	Spotting, or old or fresh blood from cervix or miscarriage
Ultrasound	Fetus may be dead Retroplacental clot Normal implantation of placenta	Placenta implanted in lower segment: Grades 1–4 (see Figure 22.3 on page 325)	Ultrasound may reveal abnormalities	Normal or signs of miscarriage or hydatidiform mole

continued

Criterion	Placental abruption	Placenta praevia	Vasa praevia	Other
Intervention	IV therapy Oxygen Pain relief Strict observation Deliver if mother or baby is compromised: vaginally or by Caesarean section	*No vaginal examination* until position of placenta has been confirmed Speculum examination in theatre ready for Caesarean section If the woman is at home: transfer to hospital as emergency Depends on amount of bleeding, grade of placenta praevia and duration of pregnancy	Caesarean section if baby is in danger If baby is dead, preferred route is vaginal delivery	Treat according to cause Hydatidiform mole: surgical curettage
Complications or outcomes	Perinatal death: 30–52% (Shrivastava, Kotur & Jauhari, 2014) Hypoxic-ischemic encephalopathy (HIE) with neurological damage Couvelaire uterus (blue discolouration of uterus) due to bleeding in myometrium Sheehan's syndrome Clotting defects Atonia of uterus PPH Hypovolaemic shock Low fibrinogen and factors II, V and VII DIC and renal failure	PPH Hysterectomy if bleeding cannot be controlled Prematurity	Fetal distress Death of the newborn	Miscarriage if contractions were present Sepsis Choriocarcinoma in the case of hydatidiform mole

Placental abruption (accidental haemorrhage)

Abruption complicates about 0.5–2.0 per cent of pregnancies (Leunen et al, 2003) and is the leading cause of vaginal bleeding in the latter half of pregnancy. Known risk factors include hypertension, pre-eclampsia, advanced maternal age, multiparity, polyhydramnios, maternal or paternal tobacco use, cocaine use, trauma, premature rupture of membranes (PROM) and chorioamnionitis.

Placental abruption can happen at any point in pregnancy and during the intrapartum period. Sometimes a woman can have a small abruption that goes unnoticed and the pregnancy recovers and continues. The fetus might have had an episode of stress *in utero* and there could be evidence of old meconium.

The clinical classification of abruption placenta is as follows (Deering & Smith, 2016):

▶ Class 0: Asymptomatic
▶ Class 1: Mild (represents approximately 48 per cent of all cases)
▶ Class 2: Moderate (represents approximately 27 per cent of all cases)
▶ Class 3: Severe (represents approximately 24 per cent of all cases).

Vaginal bleeding may be present or hidden. The nature of the bleeding, when visible, is usually dark clots. This is due to the body trying to clot the blood to control the haemorrhage.

On abdominal palpation, uterine tenderness and severe abdominal pain are present. The uterus is hard and contracts to control the bleeding. Rapid contractions may be present, but are difficult to feel because of the tone of the uterus. The fetal heart rate is abnormal but difficult to pick up. (Figure 22.2 shows the cause and types of haemorrhage).

Placenta praevia

This is the implantation of the placenta in the lower segment of the uterus. It is classified as placenta praevia grades 1–4, as shown in Figure 22.3. The anterior, lateral or posterior position of the placenta can further complicate the outcomes. The reasons for and symptoms of placenta praevia are given in Table 22.1 on pages 321–323.

The bleeding is clear and painless and occurs after 28 weeks of pregnancy. Usually, there is a warning bleed before the serious bleeding starts. The lower segment starts to develop after 28 weeks of pregnancy and pulls away from the placenta.

Vasa praevia

This is the presentation of umbilical or fetal blood vessels that run in the membranes and lie in front of the cervical os. The incidence is 1:2000 to 1:5000 pregnancies (RCOG, 2011). Vasa praevia can be a complication of placenta praevia. If the blood vessels rupture, clear blood is visible and the fetus may lose blood fast. Because the fetal blood volume is around 80–100 ml/kg, the loss of relatively small amounts of blood can have major implications for the fetus, so the delivery should be without delay. There is no mechanism to control blood loss as a result of vasa praevia.

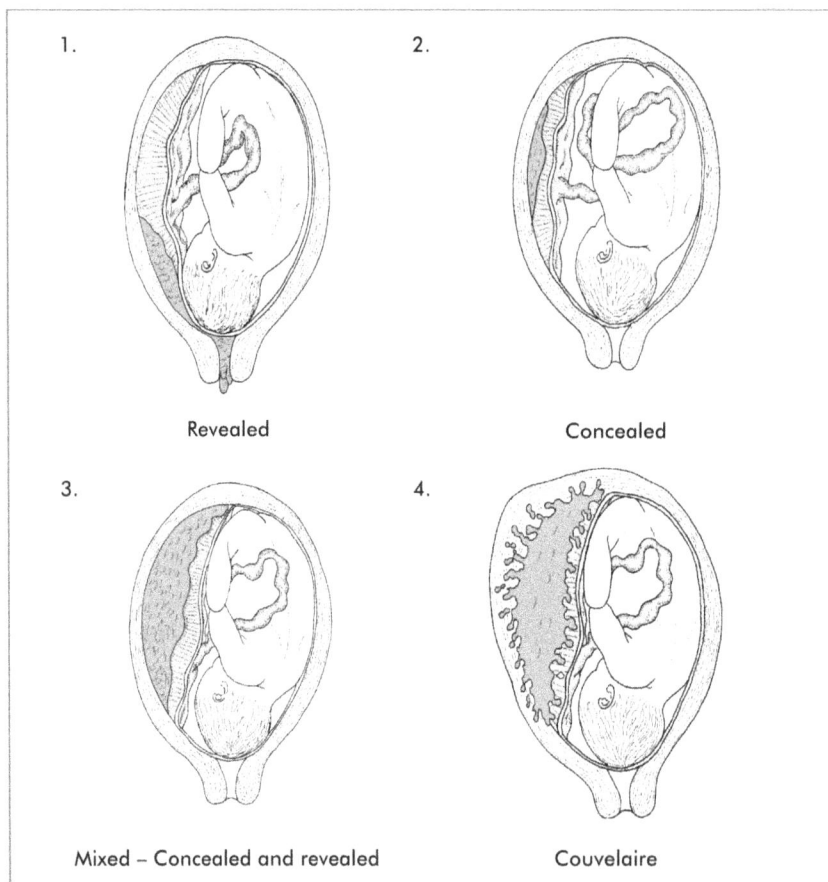

Figure 22.2 Placental abruption: 1 = marginal separation with revealed haemorrhage; 2 = central separation with concealed haemorrhage; 3 = complete separation; 4 = Couvelaire uterus

Grade 1

Low-lying placenta

Dips into the lower segment

Grade 2

Marginal placenta praevia

Reaches the edge of the internal os

Grade 3

Partial placenta praevia

The edge of the placenta covers the internal os when undilated, and up to 4 cm dilatation

Grade 4

Total placenta praevia

The placenta completely covers the internal os

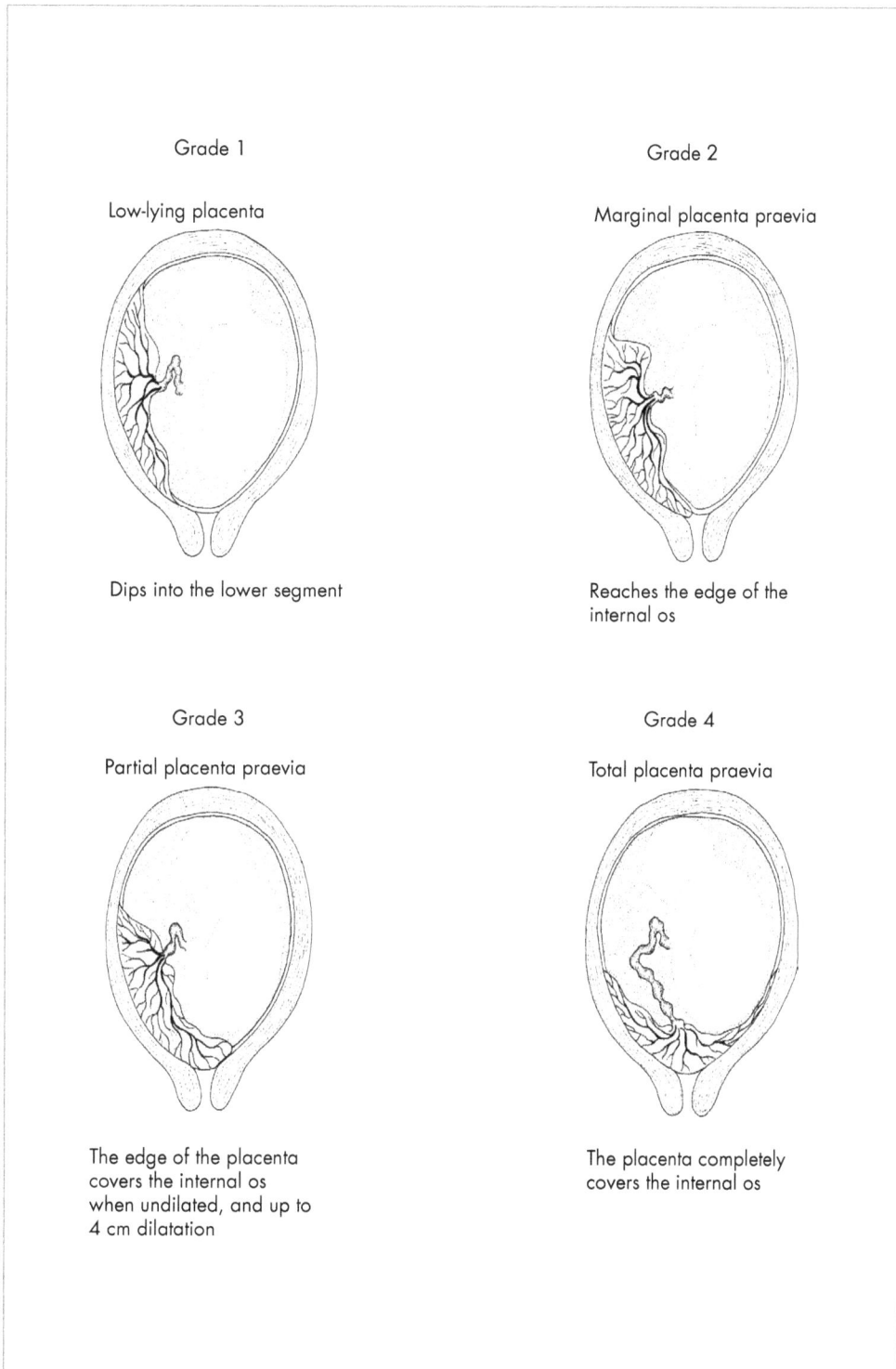

Figure 22.3 Grades of placenta praevia

The management of obstetric haemorrhage

If a pregnant woman experiences bleeding, a midwife should be called or the woman should be taken to the nearest health centre where maternity services are available. Speed is required, even if only a small amount of blood is being lost. This is true particularly in late pregnancy, since some of the haemorrhage may have been concealed (see placental abruption in Table 22.1 on pages 321–323). It is important to keep the woman calm, as anxiety may raise her BP and cause further bleeding. The woman should be kept nil per os in case she has to have an anaesthetic later.

Care for the patient with obstetric bleeding should follow an algorithm that goes through a rapid and successive sequence of medical and surgical approaches. The aim is to stem bleeding in order to decrease maternal morbidity and mortality.

Specific interventions will be required depending on the underlying cause of the haemorrhage, but several basic steps are essential in the initial and continued management of any patient with obstetric haemorrhage. The basic guidelines for the management of massive obstetric haemorrhage are to:
- organise the multidisciplinary team
- restore blood volume via a large cannula for access, using fluid and blood
- correct defective coagulation with blood products and factors
- evaluate response to treatment by haemodynamic and laboratory assessment
- treat the underlying cause of the bleeding.

Another therapeutic goal in the treatment of severe obstetric haemorrhage is avoidance of myocardial ischaemia by increasing the myocardial supply–demand ratio (see Chapter 35). A significant percentage of patients with haemorrhagic shock experience electrocardiographic signs of ischaemia and decreased contractility that correlate with the severity of the haemorrhage.

Given that most maternal morbidity and mortality is due to underestimation of blood loss, inadequate volume replacement and delay in intervention, every delivery unit should have a management protocol for the treatment of obstetric haemorrhage that initiates a sequence of conservative and operative interventions. The success of each treatment should be rapidly assessed, with the swift institution of the next intervention if it has failed. Prompt communication between anaesthesiology, obstetric gynaecology, nursing, the laboratory and the blood bank is essential for effective evaluation and management of excessive blood loss.

Prevention of and preparation for obstetric haemorrhage

All pregnant women should be informed early in their pregnancy that any amount of bleeding is abnormal, except for the 'show'. Therefore, any bleeding requires referral to a healthcare professional with midwifery skills.

Specific preventive measures include the following:
- Identify all women at risk for APH and PPH and refer for birth at a referral hospital (eg women with multiple pregnancies, polyhydramnios, grand multiparous women, history of previous Caesarean section and previous PPH that required blood transfusion).
- Iron supplementation should be routinely provided during pregnancy. Anaemia needs to be detected, treated and followed up during pregnancy.
- Facilities at all levels of care must take steps to ensure that they are prepared for the emergency care of a woman with massive obstetric haemorrhage. A standard protocol for managing obstetric haemorrhage must be known by all healthcare providers at institutions that provide care for pregnant women. In order to keep staff's obstetric skills up to date, compulsory attendance of Essential Steps in Management of Obstetric Emergencies (ESMOE) training, followed by regular performance of skills drills (Emergency Obstetric Simulation Training, or EOST) by all involved in maternal and newborn care is recommended. Being prepared entails ensuring the implementation of basic and comprehensive emergency signal functions in healthcare facilities that are responsible for maternal and newborn care. In addition, adequate supplies of IV fluids, oxytocic agents, necessary equipment and emergency blood must be available. Skilled personnel must be available on a 24-hour basis.
- An effective and functional ambulance transport infrastructure must exist in all provinces. Obstetric haemorrhage must always receive the highest priority for emergency transport.

Resuscitation

Any patient with signs of shock (tachycardia, low BP and oliguria) due to haemorrhage requires two IV infusions with large-gauge needles (at least size 16), and rapid infusion of rehydration fluid (plasmalyte B, Ringer's lactate) and/or crystalloids (Haemaccel or Voluven). Details of all fluids given – with times specified – must be documented on an input/output chart. The resuscitation is extremely important and ideally requires a staff member to take primary responsibility, while others are assessing the cause of the haemorrhage, measuring blood loss and performing measures to arrest the bleeding. The PPH box must be brought in to execute resuscitation with speed.

In Level 1 hospitals, emergency blood should be given, as this is a comprehensive signal function applicable at this level of care. Frozen dried plasma should also be available. In Level 2 and 3 hospitals, cross-matched blood should be given as well as additional blood products. If the estimated blood loss is greater than 1 500 ml, a central venous pressure (CVP) line is useful for monitoring fluid balance and blood volume.

Clinical management of placental abruption

Placental abruption is an obstetric emergency. Action depends on the clinical assessment of the woman and on if the baby is still alive. The priority is to deliver the fetus as soon as possible without putting the mother's life at risk.

Active resuscitation and prompt referral to a Level 2 or 3 hospital is mandatory after the diagnosis of placental abruption with an intrauterine death (IUD). Blood group O-negative blood and frozen dried plasma can be administered in the hospital.

Vaginal birth is the preferred route for delivery in the event of placental abruption with an IUD, unless there are obstetric indications for Caesarean section. If the fetus is alive, an emergency Caesarean section is indicated. With the addition of potent uterotonic agents and the advent of minimally invasive interventional radiological techniques, such as angiographic embolisation and arterial ligation, conservative management is now possible in an attempt to avoid hysterectomy in patients with severe APH. If these interventions are inadequate to control the bleeding, the decision to proceed to hysterectomy must be made expeditiously.

Management of bleeding associated with placenta praevia

The principles for the management of placenta praevia are the following:
▶ Admit the woman to hospital for bed rest.
▶ Assess the degree of shock and treat (replace blood loss as appropriate).
▶ Identify the cause of the bleeding. The uterus is soft and the presenting part is high because the placenta is in the way. No vaginal examination should be performed until the position of the placenta has been determined by ultrasound.
▶ Treatment will depend on the grade of placenta praevia, the GA and the amount of blood loss. The fetus is not in the same danger as in the case of placental abruption. Treatment can be conservative, to give the baby a chance to grow to maturity.

• Bed rest in or out of hospital is in order if the placenta praevia is grade 1 or 2. However, the woman should be educated that coitus is contraindicated, as it will aggravate bleeding.
• Women with placenta praevia grades 3 or 4 are hospitalised and delivered if the condition warrants intervention.
▶ Corticosteroids are administered to mature the baby's lungs to prevent hyaline membrane disease (HMD). The pregnancy seldom reaches 36 weeks in grades 3 and 4 placenta praevia.
▶ The mode of delivery is usually by Caesarean section. Women with grades 1 and 2 may deliver vaginally if the baby is in the correct cephalic position and the presenting part engaged normally.
▶ In Grade 4 or in malpresentation (breech or high head), Caesarean section is indicated.

22.4 Intrapartum haemorrhage

Any of the conditions mentioned in Section 22.3 can occur or present during labour. Placental abruption may occur with induction of labour (IOL) and overstimulation of the uterus. A sudden decompression of the uterus in polyhydramnios may cause a placental abruption. A short cord may cause a placental abruption as the fetus descends in the pelvis.

The treatment will depend on the condition of the mother and fetus, the amount of blood lost and the stage of the labour.

Measuring blood loss during and after birth

A leading cause of maternal deaths and morbidity is the failure to recognise and measure excessive blood loss during childbirth. The inaccuracy of the visual estimation of blood loss is widely acknowledged: health professionals may over- or underestimate the amount of blood lost. Large volumes (greater than 1 000 ml) tend to be underestimated and smaller volumes generally result in overestimation. The outcome is that management of the woman is flawed because it was based on an imprecise measurement of the blood lost.

Despite active management of the third stage of labour (AMTSL) to reduce uterine atony and subsequent blood loss, PPH may occur within the first 24 hours after childbirth. Overestimation of blood loss results in costly, invasive and unnecessary treatments (blood transfusions), whereas an underestimation can lead to delays in delivering lifesaving interventions.

Obstetric care has changed in an attempt to decrease blood loss, yet PPH has a rapid onset and represents danger if left untreated.

PROCEDURE Measuring blood loss intrapartum

Unreliable methods of estimating blood loss
There are various methods to estimate blood loss. However, most methods are impractical or not very reliable, including the following:
▶ The visual estimation of blood loss is most inaccurate when there is a large amount of blood; the continued use of this method in clinical practice is likely related to ease of use and tradition rather than serving any clinical value.
▶ The direct measurement of blood loss is probably the oldest reported method of determining blood loss during childbirth, because of the limited equipment necessary.
▶ Weighing the blood by collecting all contaminated linens, pads, towels or swabs and then deducting the dry weight of the items only requires an accurate scale. However, weighing does not discriminate between blood and other types of fluid, such as amniotic fluid or urine. Note that other fluids inadvertently collected would affect the final results and that the weights of pre-weighed items may vary, affecting final results. Remember that drapes must be weighed quickly to limit evaporation loss. This method can be easily taught, but is both time- and labour-intensive.
▶ Objective data, such as vital signs and haematocrit changes, are helpful in the clinical management of patients with large blood loss over time. However, objective data do not assist in the measurement of blood loss in clinical practice or research.
▶ Hb and specific gravidity are not reliable methods of determining acute blood loss in pregnant women.

Recommended method of measuring blood loss
The quantification of blood loss is an objective method to measure blood loss after childbirth. This method uses the following principles:
▶ Items (dry) used during the delivery that may become saturated with blood are weighed.
▶ Blood lost during the birth must be collected from the drape under the maternal buttocks to provide an indication of the amount.
▶ Most of the fluid collected prior to the birth from the placenta consists of amniotic liquor, urine, cleaning lotions and faeces.
▶ Blood loss is estimated by weighing the saturated drapes on a calibrated scale and by subtracting the weight from the weight of the dry item.
▶ After placental delivery, the primary fluid lost is blood. The saturated drapes and blood clots are weighed to determine the cumulative volume of blood loss.
▶ The equation used when calculating blood loss using a blood-soaked item is:
  • wet item (weight in grams) minus dry item (weight in grams) = millilitres of blood within the item
  • 1 g of blood loss equals 1 ml.

Procedure
During the intrapartum period, do the following:
▶ Suction and measure amniotic liquor if membranes rupture during birth (to deduct from the weight of the measured drapes).
▶ After delivery of the placenta, measure the amount of blood lost in the drapes.
▶ Weigh all the blood-soaked materials and clots. Calculate the weight and convert it to millilitres.
▶ Add the volume of quantified blood calculated by weight to the volume of quantified blood in the suction canister to determine the quantified blood loss.

Recording and interpretation
▶ Document all findings in the obstetric records.
▶ Communicate findings to healthcare professionals.
▶ Document all interventions.

22.5 Postpartum haemorrhage

The definition of PPH is excessive vaginal bleeding of 500 ml or more post-delivery until 42 days after giving birth. It can be classified as primary PPH if bleeding takes place within 24 hours post-delivery and secondary PPH if bleeding happens after 24 hours and up to 42 days post-delivery.

Primary PPH is divided into:
▶ atonic PPH
▶ traumatic PPH
▶ uterine rupture, usually catastrophic.

Various factors need to be considered, namely:
▶ APH and intrapartum blood loss
▶ Hb levels and haematocrit
▶ cardiovascular competency or compromise
▶ the woman's physical condition and body weight
▶ other factors such as coagulation defects
▶ contextual factors, such as staff, skills and equipment available.

It is important for a unit to develop an accurate standard to measure blood loss over a 24-hour period after birth (see the procedure box on pages 330–331). Blood loss in theatre should also be recorded. Accumulated blood loss may exceed 500 ml. A soaked pad changed every two hours postnatally indicates heavy blood loss.

Types of primary postpartum haemorrhage

There are two major types of PPH, as discussed in the following subsections.

Atonic postpartum haemorrhage

Atonic PPH occurs mainly within the first 24 hours post-delivery. It is characterised by clear blood gushing from the vagina, with a relaxed uterus. It occurs as result of:
▶ an overstretched uterus in a grand multipara woman, multiple pregnancy or polyhydramnios and/or a uterus that is tired after a prolonged or obstructed labour
▶ abnormalities of the uterus such as myomata and bicornuate uterus
▶ congenital factors such as blood coagulation defect conditions
▶ retained products of conception and placental pathology
▶ obstetric interventions such as IOL, anaesthesia and Caesarean section
▶ a low Hb
▶ a full bladder.

Traumatic postpartum haemorrhage

Traumatic PPH may be masked at the beginning of bleeding. The signs and symptoms of traumatic PPH are a well-contracted uterus, with clots coming from the vagina. Bleeding is not active. Predisposing factors include forceps delivery, vacuum/ventouse extraction, a large baby and precipitate labour. Traumatic PPH includes high vaginal tears, cervical tears, incomplete uterine rupture and inversion of the uterus.

Prevention

The following are guidelines to be following in order to prevent PPH:
▶ Good antenatal care with improved nutritional status of pregnant women and routine supplementation of iron, folic acid and vitamin C can prevent PPH.
▶ All women at risk for PPH should be delivered in the relevant clinical setting (at least Level 1 or higher).
▶ Women with previous history of PPH or retained placenta are at risk, as well as those with low Hb, a large baby, and abnormalities of the uterus and placenta.
▶ Early detection of PPH by routine monitoring after delivery and after Caesarean section, especially of high-risk patients, is essential.
▶ All women at risk for PPH should routinely have an IV line during labour. Ensure an empty bladder. Execute AMTSL for all women.
▶ Carry out routine management of the fourth stage of labour with strict observation of the uterus and blood loss. Putting the baby to the breast can be useful in mild cases.
▶ An IV infusion with 20 IU of oxytocin in 1 000 ml Ringer's lactate is continued for 24 hours post-delivery or until stable.

Diagnosis

The diagnosis of PPH is made if 500 ml of blood is lost from the genital tract post-delivery. The importance of the volume of blood loss depends on the woman's Hb level. With a low Hb, the loss may be fatal irrespective of the amount of blood lost. The cause and stage of the condition need to be determined and acted upon. Life-threatening haemorrhage occurs in more than 1:1 000 deliveries (Wikipedia, 2017d).

Clinical manifestations

The clinical picture may vary depending on the severity of the blood loss and the ability to compensate. Aggravating factors for PPH are:
▶ APH with the current pregnancy
▶ low Hb

- cardiac conditions
- pre-eclampsia.

The following progression of the condition can occur if it is not arrested (all are compensatory responses) (grade I + II):
- Vasodilatation to increase blood volume to the heart
- Restlessness and anxiety
- Tachycardia
- Increase in diastolic BP
- Decrease in urine output
- Nausea and vomiting.

The progressive state (1 500–2 000 ml; 30–40 per cent; grade III) is characterised by:
- overwhelming compensatory responses
- severe dysrhythmia and myocardial ischemia
- hypotension, a late sign of shock.

The refractory stage (more than 2 000 ml; 40 per cent; Grade IV) is characterised by:
- the failing of compensatory mechanisms
- the shutting down of the kidneys

- tissue necrosis caused by low BP
- pituitary gland necrosis (Sheehan's syndrome)
- air hunger.

Management

If PPH occurs in a PHC setting and is caused by retained placenta, the midwife should call for help to mobilise all personnel to assist during the resuscitation. The activities for treatment of PPH as a result of retained placenta are as follows:
- The midwife or the registered nurse should remove the placenta to arrest haemorrhage.
- Skill and execution of AMTSL is needed following every birth. This has been shown to reduce PPH.
- Always check the placenta and membranes for completeness and then record and report.
- A Foley catheter is inserted to keep the bladder empty. A full bladder displaces the uterus with resultant sub-involution.

High-risk cases should routinely receive an IV administration of 20 IU oxytocin for at least 24 hours after birth.

| PROCEDURE | Managing postpartum haemorrhage |

Indications
Blood loss must be measured and recorded:
- during the intrapartum and postpartum period
- during and after a Caesarean section
- for the first hour in all women who have given birth. Most blood loss related to childbirth occurs within the first hour after birth due to uterine atony.

Principles
- Risk assessment in the antenatal period does not effectively predict those women who will experience PPH.
- Normal maternal Hb levels determine how the body tolerates a given volume of blood loss.
- All postpartum women must be closely monitored to determine those who are experiencing PPH.
- Continuous slow bleeding or sudden bleeding are both regarded as an emergency. Early and aggressive intervention is needed.

The general management of a woman presenting with PPH includes:
- mobilising all available health professionals
- performing a rapid evaluation of the general condition of the woman (pulse, BP, respiration, temperature)
- managing shock and initiating treatment
- massaging the uterus to expel blood and blood clots
- following the prescribed protocol for management of the haemorrhage.

Measuring blood loss
During the postpartum period, firstly determine the amount of blood loss, using the following guide:
- *Heavy amount:* The perineal pad has a stain larger than 10 cm in length within one hour: 30–80 ml blood loss. Reassess the source of bleeding, uterine tone and degree of bladder distension.

continued

> ▶ *Moderate amount:* The perineal pad has a stain less than 10 cm in length within one hour: 25–50 ml blood loss.
> ▶ *Small amount:* The perineal pad has a stain less than 8 cm in length after one hour: 10–25 ml blood loss.
> ▶ *Scant amount:* The perineal pad has a stain less than 2 cm in length after one hour or lochia only on tissue when the woman wipes.
>
> If the woman reports heavy bleeding or clots, apply a clean perineal pad and reassess in one hour. Assess clots passed into the toilet during voiding. Manage PPH according to protocol (DoH, 2015a).
>
> **Recording and interpretation**
> ▶ Document all findings in the obstetric records.
> ▶ Communicate findings to healthcare professionals.
> ▶ Document all medications and interventions.

The management of PPH follows the progression of the condition in steps, as described in the following subsections.

Step 1: Grade I

Grade I is characterised by 15 per cent blood loss of 500–750 ml. Compensatory mechanisms are adequate and the woman may be symptom-free. A PPH box is brought in urgently. Interventions include instituting measures to contract the uterus by:
▶ rubbing up the uterus
▶ inserting a urinary catheter
▶ putting the baby to the breast.

Step 2: Grade II

Grade II is characterised by a compensatory stage blood loss of 750–1 500 ml (15–30 per cent). Compensatory responses are present and the cardiac output drops. Interventions include:
▶ rapid IV fluid with 20 IU of oxytocin
▶ continuing to rub up the uterus
▶ considering the transfer of patient from a lower to a higher level of care using the situation, background, assessment and recommendation (SBAR) clinical report form.

Note: Steps 1 and 2 are always done, irrespective of the cause of PPH.

Up to 30 per cent of blood loss (1 500 ml) can be replaced by a colloid solution (the haematocrit is reduced to 30 per cent). The replacement of fluid is now essential.

Step 3: Grades III and IV

The progressive stage is characterised by a loss of 30–40 per cent (1 500–2 000 ml). Interventions include:
▶ lifting the foot end of the bed to improve venous return
▶ giving oxygen: 6–10 ℓ

▶ IV ergometrine or syntometrine 0.2 mg to 0.4 mg, 6–12-hourly but not for longer than 48 hours, IM 0.2 mg 2–4 hourly x 5 doses (except for cardiac, pre-eclamptic and bicornuate uterus) or misoprostol 600 micrograms rectally.

Step 4

Suture vaginal or cervical tears if present.

Step 5

The refractory stage is characterised by blood loss greater than 40 per cent (2 000 ml). Refer to next level if bleeding persists (it is definitely not recommended to send off an unstable patient).

Note: An atonic PPH that does not respond to steps 1–4 needs bimanual compression of the uterus while the woman is being transferred. A midwife must accompany the patient to the hospital. Paramedics need to be trained to give the appropriate care.

If the placenta is still *in utero* and bleeding, try to remove it while resuscitating the woman. Pain medication (pethidine, 50 mg) is given during manual removal of the placenta following the unit's protocol. If the placenta has not separated, manual removal is indicated under general or spinal anaesthesia. Morphine can be used on medical prescription if anaesthesia is not possible. IV oxytocin 20 IU is administered in 1 ℓ of Ringer's lactate. Antibiotics are administered and the woman is transferred to high care until stable.

The following are guidelines in case of persistent bleeding:
▶ If bleeding continues, it should be managed by skilled staff in a Level 2 or 3 facility.
▶ Bimanual compression of the uterus can be done when the uterus is not contracting.

Step 6

Review the diagnosis. Potential conditions are intractable uterine atony, retained products, rupture of the uterus or coagulation disorders.

Step 7

Cross-match blood, order and administer.

Condom catheter

A condom is inserted into the uterus and 600 ml of saline is infused into the condom using a Foley's catheter to create pressure on the bleeding uterus. If bleeding is arrested and the woman is in a PHC setting, she is transferred to the hospital with the condom catheter *in situ*. The saline is drained by first withdrawing 50 ml and observing if any bleeding recurs. In the absence of bleeding, 50 ml is drawn hourly until all the fluid is drained out. If bleeding persists, 50 ml of saline infused into the catheter is drained and it is not removed until after six hours.

Hypovolaemic shock in obstetrics

Whenever blood or plasma is lost from the body, whether accidentally or during planned surgery, the possibility of shock should be considered (see Chapter 35). Death due to the loss of blood is caused by a lack of intravascular circulation rather than a deficit of red blood cells (RBCs).

The first priority is the replacement of fluid. Haemaccel (1 000 ml) (a volume expander) increases the cardiac output by 45 per cent and CVP by 35 per cent. It does not draw fluid from the interstitial spaces. Alternatively, voluven or crystalloid fluid (Ringer's lactate or plasmalyte B can be used).

The level at which an individual becomes compromised varies depending on age, body mass, Hb and haematocrit condition (a drop of more than 10 per cent) of the cardiovascular system and the volume of loss of plasma or blood (above 500 ml).

Pathological processes in acute hypovolaemic shock include increased blood viscosity, which results in tissue hypoxia due to decreased blood flow. Coagulation and haemostatic changes occur. Reflex cardiovascular mechanisms reduce the flow to the kidneys and a drop in BP and sympathetic vasoconstriction lead to oliguria and anuria. In obstetrics, the defibrination syndrome (Factor II, V, and VII) develops. Fluid is shifted from the interstitial space to the intravascular space. BP drops.

In obstetrics, death can occur with frightening speed. Principles to consider are:
- an accurate estimation of blood loss and replacement
- the prompt recognition of clotting disorders
- the early involvement of a haematologist to consult on Hb and haematocrit
- the involvement of an anaesthetist for resuscitation if needed
- the availability of a PPH box with an adequately sized cannula
- the close monitoring of venous pressure.

The clinical status of the woman is assessed by monitoring:
- cardiac rate (by electrocardiogram, or ECG)
- arterial pressure or BP
- CVP
- respiratory function (for risk of pulmonary oedema)
- temperature of the extremities that indicates blood perfusion and vasoconstriction
- level of consciousness
- urine and blood electrolytes.

Danger signs

The following are warning signs of progressive obstetric haemorrhagic shock:
- There is persistent, significant bleeding.
- The woman says she is light-headed, sees stars, faints or acts in a strange way.
- The woman acts anxiously, with air hunger, and wants to sit upright.
- The skin colour changes to ashen or greyish.
- The skin temperature is cool and clammy.
- Tachycardia occurs, combined with a dropping BP.

Complications

Complications of hypovolaemia include:
- acute renal failure
- pituitary necrosis
- DIC
- death.

22.6   Conclusion

Obstetric haemorrhage remains the main cause of maternal death globally. A woman's highest risk of death is in the first 24 hours after birth and is related to blood loss. Midwives and obstetricians can underestimate blood loss during birth by 100 per cent. It is thus of the utmost importance to have standards for blood loss estimation, evidence to establish the loss, and interventions to prevent or manage blood loss if this occurs.

Pre- and post-term birth

LEARNING OBJECTIVES
On completion of this chapter, you must be able to:
▶ define pre- and post-term birth
▶ demonstrate competency in identifying the risks for pre- or post-term birth
▶ demonstrate competency to provide care in pre- and post-term birth using best practice guidelines
▶ demonstrate knowledge of and skill in the use of drugs related to the suppression of uterine contractions
▶ demonstrate knowledge and skills to prevent or manage complications related to pre- and post-term birth.

KNOWLEDGE ASSUMED TO BE IN PLACE
The management of normal pregnancy and birth
The assessment of gestational age (GA) and fetal surveillance
The ability to identify risk factors in pregnancy

KEYWORDS
preterm birth • post-term birth • betamimetics • low birth weight (LBW) • corticosteroids • surfactant • tocolytics • intrauterine growth restriction (IUGR)

23.1 Introduction

Complications related to pre- and post-term birth add considerably to adverse outcomes in the infant. Preterm birth is the single most important cause of perinatal morbidity and mortality. The care of preterm infants has financial implications for healthcare planning, with health risks for the child that may continue into adulthood. One of the main objectives of antenatal care is the prevention and early detection of cases where preterm birth occurs, and evidence-based intervention in these cases. Post-term birth is less common, but also has a high incidence of complications.

These two conditions are related to the accuracy of the determination of duration of pregnancy. In many cases, more sophisticated investigations such as an ultrasound may be required to make a better determination of the duration of a pregnancy. In the absence of ultrasound investigations, the clinician relies on the history, antenatal visits and clinical findings. The symphysis fundal height (SFH) measurement of the uterus is only reliable between 20 and 36 weeks, when multiple pregnancy and polyhydramnios are excluded.

23.2 Preterm birth

Preterm birth is defined as birth that occurs after fetal viability (in South Africa, 28 weeks of gestation is still the legal period acknowledged for viability) but before 37 completed weeks of pregnancy. However, many infants survive after only 20 weeks' gestation as a result of sophisticated interventions. Viability is defined as from 500 g in developed countries (22 weeks) and from 1 000 g (28 weeks) in developing countries.

Birth can be spontaneous or induced before term if the mother's health is threatened.

The survival of a preterm infant depends on factors such as developmental stage, weight, the presence of complications such as placental abruption or infections, and the care received. In neonatal care, a differentiation is made between the care of early preterm (less than 34 weeks) and late preterm babies. Early preterm babies generally have problems, while the latter usually do well with standard or minimal extra newborn care.

The incidence of preterm birth

Accurate information on the incidence of preterm birth is not available. In 25 per cent of cases the cause of preterm birth is unknown (WHO, 2014a). The overall mortality for infants weighing 500 g and above is 55/1 000, with a difference between urban and rural areas: urban being 35/1 000 and rural being 100/1 000 (WHO, 2014a).

In South Africa, 59 per cent of births occur at community healthcare clinics (CHCs) or district level and the highest perinatal mortality is found in both these settings (DoH, 2015b). The perinatal mortality rate (PNMR) is the highest on district level for immature infants and attention should be focused on prevention and improved standards of care for preterm birth, with a particular emphasis on improved intrapartum care.

Factors contributing to preterm labour/birth

The following are conditions that may contribute to preterm birth. Contributing factors can be maternal, fetal, obstetrical and/or iatrogenic, and include:

▶ maternal causes associated with known and unknown infections that cause pyrexia, such as urinary tract and vaginal infection, appendicitis, pneumonia or amniotic fluid infection syndrome (AFIS)

▶ conditions such as pre-eclampsia, diabetes, cardiac conditions, hypertension, thyroid disease (see Chapter 21) and antepartum haemorrhage (APH)

▶ causes related to the fetoplacental unit, including over-distension of the uterus as in multiple pregnancy or polyhydramnios, as well as congenital abnormalities of the neonate

▶ obstetric causes associated with APH, such as abruptio placenta or placenta praevia

▶ previous preterm births

▶ cervical incompetence or previous cervical surgery or cone biopsy

▶ obese or underweight women; inadequate maternal nutrition

▶ tobacco smoking, use of illicit drugs

▶ psychological stress

▶ low socioeconomic status

▶ idiopathic or unknown causes.

Signs and symptoms of preterm labour

Clinical signs and symptoms of preterm birth include:

▶ the spontaneous onset of regular, rhythmic uterine contractions, as in normal labour

▶ membranes that may or may not rupture spontaneously; if ruptured, this is usually followed by the onset of painful, regular contractions

▶ a history of vague backache or low-grade abdominal discomfort, heavy pressure in the pelvis, or abdominal or

back pain; the same symptoms can be caused by urinary tract infection (UTI), hence it is important to rule this out

▶ vaginal bleeding in the third trimester

▶ premature cervix dilatation without pain or perceived contractions.

The diagnosis of preterm labour

Preterm labour is diagnosed when there is a history of regular, rhythmic uterine contractions before 37 completed weeks of pregnancy. Occasionally there is an accompanying descent of the presenting part and dilatation of the cervix.

The diagnosis can be very difficult, but is based on the above signs and symptoms as well as the documentation of prematurity. The diagnosis of preterm birth is confirmed by the observation of uterine contractions through abdominal auscultation or an electronic uterine activity assessment using a cardiotocograph (CTG) to confirm the presence of contractions.

Vaginal examinations are usually not performed, as these stimulate contractions. The performance of a vaginal examination will be indicated if a woman has strong contractions and there is no medical practitioner available or if the woman is in a primary healthcare (PHC) unit and needs to be transported to a higher level of care. Vaginal examination is avoided if the membranes are ruptured and the contractions are mild.

An ultrasound scan can determine the condition of the fetus and the amount of amniotic fluid, which will guide management.

Best practice guidelines for management of preterm labour/birth

The management and treatment of preterm birth depends on an accurate diagnosis of preterm labour and the co-morbidities that are present. In 70 per cent of cases in South Africa, the midwife will identify the condition in the PHC setting or in the maternity CHC (DoH, 2015b). Early recognition and swift intervention are the keys to successful management of this condition. It is important to establish the gestational age of the fetus and to diagnose labour. Thereafter, prompt referral to the appropriate level of care can improve outcomes. If in a remote setting, arrangements are made to transfer the patient to a healthcare facility that offers emergency obstetric care. If the birth is imminent, the situation is managed in the remote setting.

The care of a woman in preterm labour involves not only general clinical care but a great deal of support, comfort and information. It is a period of great distress and the woman may be stressed and not hear or take in what she is told. Midwives need to be present, assist and stay with the woman until she is comfortable, the diagnosis is made and the course of action is mapped. Preterm labour may be suppressed using tocolytics.

Indications for suppressing labour

Preterm labour can be suppressed if:
- the membranes are intact and the cervical os is less than 3 cm dilated
- no major congenital abnormality is present
- the fetus is alive and no fetal distress is present
- gestational age (GA) is less than 36 weeks and the risks of prematurity exceed those of infection
- there is no infection or severe maternal disease present
- there is no intrauterine growth restriction (IUGR).

Tocolytic drugs are administered to stop contractions. These are prescribed by a medical practitioner and may include the following:
- Calcium-channel blockers are increasingly used to promote tocolysis, such as nifedipine 30 mg oral stat dose, followed by 20 mg 6- to 8-hourly for seven days.
- Antiprostaglandins (eg Indomethacin®, a non-steroidal anti-inflammatory drug) have been used as tocolytics. Indomethacin® can be given orally (25 mg) or as a suppository (100 mg). *Caution:* A total daily dosage of 200 mg should not be exceeded in 24 hours. Caution is needed because the administration of Indomethacin® is known to cause premature closure of the ductus arteriosus in the more mature fetus.

Contraindications to the use of tocolytics

Some of the contraindications to the use of tocolytics to arrest preterm labour are:
- evidence of fetal maturity
- intrauterine infection (evident by raised temperature and raised pulse rate)
- intrauterine death (IUD)
- IUGR
- severe pre-eclampsia
- active APH, except in placenta praevia
- cardiac disease – an absolute contraindication
- diabetes mellitus, as this condition is aggravated and keto-acidosis results
- preterm rupture of membranes.

Side effects of the use of nifedipine and Indomethacin®

Potential side effects with the use of tocolytics include:
- tachycardia
- palpitations

- feelings of anxiety and nervousness
- hypotension
- pulmonary oedema (if tocolytics are administered with steroids)
- hypokalaemia
- anaemia
- fetal tachycardia
- neonatal hypoglycaemia and hypokalaemia.

Tocolytics should be discontinued if any of the following occur:
- Hypertension
- Tachycardia of more than 120 beats per minute (bpm)
- Chest pain
- Pulmonary oedema.

Other drugs administered are:
- prophylactic antibiotics to prevent infection in the neonate (see Chapter 49)
- pethidine 50–100 mg IMI; as a rule, the use of narcotics is avoided in preterm birth but a stat dosage of pethidine 50–100 mg IMI may be prescribed by a medical practitioner for pain relief if needed.

Failure to suppress labour

If labour is not arrested despite the use of tocolytic drugs, labour is allowed to progress and closely monitored to exclude fetal distress. The aim is to deliver the baby at the appropriate level of care for the GA, where a paediatrician and a neonatal unit are available with specially trained neonatal staff. Transport of the mother is only advised if she will not deliver on the way. It is a requirement in South Africa that all medical practitioners and advanced midwives working in maternity should be able to intubate a preterm baby. This requires training and certification.

The following are general guidelines for labour in this context:
- Labour should be monitored using a partogram.
- An IV line should be in place.
- Delayed cord clamping by 30–120 seconds seems to be associated with less need for blood transfusion and less intraventricular haemorrhage in the neonate.

Use of steroids

Steroids are indicated in the management of preterm labour if the GA is less than 34 weeks and membranes are intact. Urinalysis should be performed prior to administration of steroids.

The administration of corticosteroids to the mother to prevent hyaline membrane disease (HMD) is an evidence-based intervention that is accepted as best practice globally. Any mother at risk for preterm birth should receive corticosteroids IM in two dosages one week apart.

Corticosteroids are given IMI (eg Celestone Soluspan® 3 mg/ml, betamethasone disodium phosphate, dexamethasone phosphate 4 mg/ml) to stimulate lung maturity if the gestation is less than 34 weeks. Steroids appear to be of benefit only from 28 to 34 weeks' gestation. Corticosteroids take 24 hours to be effective in the fetus and suppression of labour is often aimed at getting the full value of the corticosteroids. The dosage is repeated in 24 hours. Dexamethasone 5 mg 6-hourly IV has been used to stimulate lung maturity for 24 hours prior to delivery if the gestational period is less than 34 weeks. It can also be given in two dosages 24 hours apart.

General principles of care

▶ Give sedation in order to allay anxiety and pain.
▶ Administer drugs as per a medical practitioner's prescription or protocol (some form of pain relief may be needed).
▶ Do not perform a digital vaginal examination (except a speculum examination) to note the state of the cervix.
▶ Ensure an accurate diagnosis and appropriate intervention based on the diagnosis.
▶ Monitor uterine contractions half-hourly or continuously until the danger has passed.
▶ Observe for presence of show or rupture of membranes.
▶ Monitor vital signs as per protocol of the institution (BP, pulse, temperature and respiration).
▶ Monitor fetal heart by CTG or intermittent auscultation half-hourly.
▶ Allow the woman to go home if labour is successfully suppressed but give health advice.

Indications to allow labour to continue

The woman is usually allowed to deliver if:
▶ the cervix is 4 cm dilated or the woman is in active labour
▶ the fetus is more than 36 weeks' gestation, which means there is a good chance of survival
▶ there is infection or severe maternal co-morbidities, such as diabetes mellitus
▶ there is IUGR, IUD or gross fetal malformation
▶ the membranes have ruptured and liquor is draining or has drained out
▶ there is placental insufficiency.

The following must be observed when a woman is in preterm labour:
▶ Membranes should be preserved and remain intact until the second stage of labour to minimise ascending infection.
▶ Adequate pain relief is essential. This should preferably be non-pharmacologic or an epidural to prevent preterm bearing down.
▶ Narcotics should be avoided by all means *and only administered on a medical practitioner's prescription.*
▶ Close fetal heart monitoring and an emergency Caesarean section should be performed in the case of fetal distress.

Mode of delivery

Preterm delivery is associated with high perinatal mortality and morbidity; therefore a team of skilled attendants should be available at delivery. The team should include midwives, an obstetrician and a paediatrician to provide care for both the mother and the baby.

Normal vaginal delivery is encouraged unless there are other complications such as multiple pregnancy or breech presentation, in which case a Caesarean section will be performed.

Resuscitation equipment should be prepared. A Resuscitaire® or a warm environment should be prepared. The staff in the special baby nursery unit should be asked to prepare for admission of a preterm infant. If the woman has delivered in a remote facility, transport equipped with resuscitation equipment and a warm environment should be ready and available to transfer the preterm infant to the appropriate level of care. It is preferable to transport the mother and baby together and not to separate them.

The following is essential and should be provided for the baby:
▶ Warmth, as the baby is prone to hypothermia
▶ Gentle handling, as the baby is preterm and hence fragile
▶ Oxygen (however, some babies will not require oxygen).

Airways should only be cleared if necessary. The baby should be transferred to a special baby unit as soon as possible.

Complications of preterm labour

Spontaneous preterm labour
Spontaneous preterm labour and premature rupture of membranes (PROM) are associated with higher perinatal mortality and morbidity; maternal problems emanate mainly from the interventions carried out to stop the contractions.

The birth process in a preterm baby may be complicated because the soft parts of the baby do not put enough pressure on the cervix and there is slow dilatation. Preterm birth can be complicated by malpresentations, breech or a prolapsed cord. It may take longer to be fully dilated and the breech may prolapse before full dilatation.

The *Guidelines for Neonatal Care* by the Department of Health (DoH) (2008) give norms and standards of neonatal care for South Africa.

There are various possible complications in babies weighing 1 000 g or less, namely:

- birth asphyxia
- respiratory distress syndrome (RDS)
- jaundice
- hypoglycaemia
- hypothermia
- feeding problems
- infections (septicaemia, pneumonia or meningitis)
- intraventricular haemorrhage
- congenital malformations.

See Chapter 42 for care of the preterm baby.

23.3   Premature membrane rupture

PROM is defined as the spontaneous rupture of membranes before the onset of labour, regardless of the period of gestation. It occurs in 3–4 per cent of all pregnancies and 33 per cent of preterm deliveries (Jazayeri, 2016).

Predisposing causes

In many cases, the causes of PROM are unknown. Some factors which can predispose a woman to PROM include:

- the weight of the fetus causing herniation of the membranes, which are then exposed to the vaginal flora; this weakens the membranes and they rupture
- malpresentations due to herniation of the membranes as a result of a badly fitting presenting part
- premature bearing down
- twins and polyhydramnios, resulting in increased intra-abdominal pressure leading to rupture of the membranes
- cervical factors such as cervical incompetence due to surgery or trauma.

Signs and symptoms

The following would indicate PROM:

- There is vaginal discharge or liquor draining from the genital tract.

- If infection is also present, the patient may present with:
  - lower uterine tenderness
  - pyrexia over 37 °C
  - maternal tachycardia
  - leukocytosis.

Diagnosis

The following procedure is followed to diagnose PROM:

- Take the patient's history.
- Do a sterile speculum examination to observe liquor in the vagina.
- *Nitrazine test:* If the fluid is alkaline, there is rupture of membranes.
- *Nile test:* The fluid is stained with Nile blue. If the cells from the fetal skin are stained orange, the fluid is liquor.
- *Ferning:* A drop of fluid is placed on a slide. Once dry, the slide is examined under a microscope. Sodium in the liquor crystallises on drying, showing a fern-like pattern.
- *Smell:* Liquor has a distinctive odour.

Management

Midwifery management

Management will depend on the period of gestation and the neonatal facilities available.

A balance must be kept between the risks of infection and the risks of prematurity. Approximately 50–70 per cent of patients with PROM commence labour within 72 hours of the rupture. The midwife does the following:

- Obtain an accurate history from the patient.
- Conduct a detailed physical examination to detect problems.
- Carefully assess the data obtained.
- Provide accurate, prompt investigation and treatment where necessary.

The midwife also establishes:

- the time of rupture of the membranes
- the amount of liquor draining: if the pads are soaking, or just damp, or not wet at all
- whether there is any urine draining
- the colour of the fluid draining
- whether there is any fluid running down the patient's legs.

Finally, place a clean, sterile pad on the vulva and keep the patient at bed rest.

Management at the primary healthcare centre

At PHC level, the following must be done by the midwife:

▶ Provide healthcare education to all pregnant women regarding the dangers of membrane rupture and the importance of reporting to the hospital should the membranes rupture early.

▶ Carefully screen all high-risk patients to detect potential problems. These patients require careful counselling, frequent monitoring and, if needed, hospitalisation for investigation.

▶ Detect problems early and refer promptly to a hospital.

▶ Establish a good midwife–patient relationship to instill confidence in the woman so that she will visit the clinic regularly.

▶ Treat all vaginal infections, sexually transmitted infections (STIs) and general infections promptly.

▶ Maintain strict asepsis for any pelvic examinations.

▶ If necessary, make arrangements to transfer the patient to hospital as soon as possible.

Management in hospital

Depending on the circumstances, management may be active or conservative. Conservative treatment may include the following:

▶ Bed rest is prescribed. Temperature is monitored four-hourly, plus the pulse and fetal heart.

▶ Take blood for a white cell count (WCC).

▶ Vaginal examinations are not done.

▶ Ultrasound can be done weekly to establish liquor volume, cord position, fetal growth and fetal breathing.

▶ Steroids may be given at 26–33 weeks in suspected preterm labour and/or PROM.

▶ Any underlying infection is treated.

▶ The patient is closely observed for the onset of contractions, and when they do occur, the frequency, duration and strength are noted.

▶ Urinalysis is performed and a midstream specimen of urine is sent to the laboratory for microculture and sensitivity.

▶ A non-stress test (NST) may also be ordered.

▶ The mode and the time of delivery will have to be planned.

The patient requires support, reassurance and encouragement.

Complications

The following maternal complications could occur:

▶ The first stage of labour can become prolonged, due to the absence of a fluid wedge.

▶ A prolapsed cord can occur due to malpresentation, hydramnios and disproportion.

▶ The uterus moulds around the fetus, because there is no liquor to separate them.

▶ Chorioamnionitis and generalised sepsis can result.

▶ In labour, the anterior lip of the cervix is nipped, causing pain, oedema and delay.

▶ There is often uterine irritability, causing spasms and constriction rings.

▶ Maternal death can occur if sepsis is severe.

The fetal complications that could occur include:

▶ prematurity, with its complications
▶ respiratory distress
▶ infection, leading to sepsis and even to death
▶ anoxia and death as a result of a prolapsed cord
▶ increased perinatal mortality.

23.4 Intrauterine fetal growth restriction

Preterm and small-for-gestational-age (SGA) infants are one of the major causes of perinatal deaths. Those who survive may have life-long problems as a result of poor development *in utero*, including cerebral palsy and neurological defects and learning disabilities. This condition should be detected early in pregnancy and appropriate interventions put in place.

Definition

IUGR refers to a fetus whose estimated weight is below the tenth percentile, *in utero* or at birth.

Classification

IUGR can be classified as one of two types:

1. *Symmetric IUGR* refers to a fetus whose body is proportionally small. In other words, there is a symmetrical reduction of the fetal body and head, because the restriction started early in the second trimester, possibly due to fetal chromosomal disorders.

2. *Asymmetrical IUGR* refers to a fetus who is undernourished and is directing most of its energy to maintaining the growth of vital organs, such as the brain and the heart, at the expense of the liver, muscle and fat. This means that the condition started late in the second and the third trimester, usually due to placental insufficiency. The body is thin, but the growth of the head is according to norms for the GA.

Indicator of intrauterine growth restriction

The most sensitive sign of both types of IUGR is a fetal abdominal circumference below the 25th percentile on ultrasound.

Diagnosis of intrauterine growth restriction

IUGR is diagnosed by following this procedure:

▶ *History:* A detailed history is done, looking for high-risk factors such as the following:
  • *Fetal:* perinatal infections and congenital abnormalities
  • *Maternal:* smoking, nutrition, physical exercise and manual labour, or maternal disease
  • *Placental:* maternal hypertension, auto-immune disease (lupus) and vascular disease or diabetes mellitus.
▶ *Ultrasound and biometry:* The measurements most commonly used are:
  • biparietal diameter (BPD)
  • head circumference
  • abdominal circumference
  • femur length.

Note: Ultrasound and biometry should be performed not later than 20 weeks, ideally at 8 and 13 weeks, as it is only accurate during this time. Do not make the error of changing the patient's due date based on third trimester ultrasound. Serial measures of the SFH at all antenatal visits are done for comparison.

Assessment of potential problems in labour

This involves assessment of fetal well-being with a combination of the NST and:

▶ a Doppler ultrasound
▶ maternal weight gain.

A meticulous record of maternal weight gain or mid-upper-arm circumference (MUAC) is essential. The normal MUAC is 23–33 cm.

The early detection and identification of IUGR during the antenatal period is an important function and competency of midwives, and essential to facilitate early referral. Referral to a higher level of care is needed for more sophisticated care.

The following factors may suggest potential problems during labour. A woman should thus be referred to a higher level of care for medical opinion in the case of:

▶ previous stillbirth
▶ previous perinatal deaths
▶ poor weight gain
▶ poor abdominal growth (SFH)

▶ reduced fetal movement
▶ a non-reassuring NST.

23.5 Post-term pregnancy and post-maturity

Pregnancy is usually considered to be post-term when it exceeds 42 weeks, or 294 days from the first day of the last normal menstrual period, when early ultrasound dating is used as an indicator of GA. An average pregnancy is 40 weeks or 280 days. The term 'post-dates' means that the patient has gone past her estimated due date for delivery, that is, she is 'post-term'.

The incidence of post-term pregnancy is approximately 3–12 per cent of all pregnancies (Caughey, 2016).

The effect of post-term pregnancy on the pregnant woman

Post-term pregnancy will have an effect on the pregnancy and the pregnant woman in terms of her psychological and physical well-being.

Psychological effects

The woman begins to worry about the health and condition of the baby. As her anxiety increases, she begins to worry about her pregnancy. She begins to lose morale and becomes depressed as the days go by and labour has not begun. Arrangements which have been made for delivery are disrupted, causing possible extra expense and inconvenience. The woman becomes depressed and tired.

Physical effects

The uterus increases in size, causing more discomfort to the woman. She does not want to move and does not sleep well at night. Often, she develops oedema of the ankles.

Later, in labour, there is often inefficient uterine action. There is also an increase in traumatic delivery and intervention. There is a greater incidence of occipitoposterior (OP) positions and malpresentation, further prolonging labour and causing greater risk to the fetus.

Effects on the fetus

A post-term pregnancy can affect the fetus in the following ways:

▶ The functional capacity of the placenta decreases after term. The placenta deteriorates from 36 weeks of pregnancy, causing IUGR due to placental insufficiency.

- The liquor decreases and the fetus enlarges, leaving very little space within the uterus for the fetus to move around. This may possibly delay the progress of labour.
- In all conditions that are associated with placental dysfunction, prolonged pregnancy is an added risk, resulting in possible fetal anoxia and IUD.
- The risks of perinatal mortality and morbidity are increased. The increased size of the fetus may result in prolonged and/or obstructed labour due to cephalopelvic disproportion (CPD).
- There is less fetal Hb after term and the oxygen saturation decreases. This results in the real danger of intrauterine hypoxia or anoxia. Fetal anoxia can lead to polycythaemia.
- There is a high incidence of meconium-stained liquor.
- Meconium aspiration may occur.
- There is a high incidence of cord compression, leading to fetal distress and to alterations in the fetal heart rate (FHR) patterns, such as tachycardia and variable decelerations.
- There is a relatively high incidence of neonatal respiratory distress at birth.
- Developmental and behavioural disturbances can occur after birth and later in life.
- The fetal mortality rate is doubled after 42 weeks and trebled after 43 weeks.
- About 20–40 per cent of babies born post-term suffer from 'post-maturity syndrome'.
- There is a possibility of meconium aspiration syndrome (MAS) either in labour or at delivery, resulting in pneumonitis, RDS and pneumonia. There is often injury to the fetus as a result of traumatic delivery, for example shoulder dystocia.

Diagnosis of post-term pregnancy

The accurate diagnosis of the duration of the pregnancy is dependent on accurate information from the mother and early measurements (history, serial SFH measures and ultrasound before 20 weeks).

This can be a problem, because many patients have poor memories regarding dates and these are often incorrect. They also have irregular menstrual cycles and lactational amenorrhoea. It is therefore important that the midwife takes an accurate and detailed history from the patient at the very first antenatal visit before 20 weeks of gestation, for a good baseline reference when the dates appear to be post-term.

The history of previous ultrasound is important. The midwife must consider when this was performed in the pregnancy and whether it was an early scan (before 20 weeks, as these are accurate to within seven days). The crown–rump length (CRL) can be measured from 6 to 14 weeks and the BPD from 9 to 28 weeks. This is then plotted on a graph; serial scans will reveal the rate of growth and the gestation estimation (see chapters 7 and 18).

If no previous ultrasound was done, the following information is important:
- BPD can be measured.
- Doppler studies can be done to determine placental function and fetal well-being. One of the purposes of an ultrasound is to look for fetal abnormalities and malpresentations. The fetus plays a role in the onset of labour and prolonged pregnancy may be due to conditions such as anencephaly or other neural tube conditions.
- Serial NSTs can be done to determine fetal well-being.
- The Bishop's score determines the status of the cervix for induction of labour (IOL).
- Amniocentesis determines lung maturity.

Management

The delivery of the fetus after 42 weeks of pregnancy depends on the condition of the fetus and the cervix. IOL will be done when there is certainty about the GA. If this is uncertain, the woman is reviewed weekly with kick charts, cervical assessment, ultrasound for amniotic fluid volume and CTG. If the fetal condition is still fine, the woman can wait another week until she goes into labour herself or an abnormality is found in those parameters.

The pregnancy can be managed conservatively, but IOL is usually done (by a medical practitioner) if the condition of the fetus allows it and the Bishop's score is favourable. There is strict monitoring of the fetal condition with CTG throughout the labour.

Manage the mother by:
- providing IV Ringer's lactate
- preventing supine hypotensive syndrome
- preparing for possible resuscitation of the infant
- offering epidural analgesia, which is the preferred analgesia in labour
- giving additional reassurance, support and encouragement during labour.

A Caesarean section is considered if:
- the patient has a history of previous large babies
- the baby is large (over 4 kg)
- the cervix is unripe
- there is insufficient placental reserve

- there is gestational proteinuric hypertension
- the NST or Doppler study indicates fetal distress or reduced placental blood flow.

Special consideration is given to the baby after birth for hypothermia and hypoglycaemia. If meconium is present in the liquor, care is taken to clear the airways. The increased incidence of fetal distress in post-term infants requires immediate intervention and management of asphyxia in the newborn. (See Chapter 42 for care of the baby.)

23.6   Conclusion

Neonatal immaturity or post-maturity are major causes of perinatal mortality and morbidity in South Africa. This is aggravated by the co-morbidities that complicate perinatal health outcomes, in particular the HIV pandemic. The *Saving Babies* report (Pattinson & Rhoda, 2014) indicated that the highest perinatal mortality occurs at district level. This warrants an improvement of the skills and competencies of nurses, midwives and medical practitioners as well as the improvement of the quality of care, specifically intrapartum care.

Standard best practice protocols for the care of immaturity and hypoxia intrapartum have been set and should be part of each professional practitioner's competencies. In addition, the norms and standards of staffing and equipment need enforcement for quality of care (as suggested by the *Saving Babies 2008–2009* report). Lastly, the organisational and administrative processes in healthcare must support care.

24

Pregnancy-related complications

LEARNING OBJECTIVES
On completion of this chapter, you must be able to:
- ▶ recognise pregnancy-related conditions that complicate pregnancy
- ▶ show competency in identifying and diagnosing pregnancy-related factors that complicate pregnancy and birth
- ▶ show competency in preventing pregnancy-related complications
- ▶ show competency in the treatment and specific care, including evidence-based protocols/regimens of medical care for obstetric conditions that complicate pregnancy and birth.

KNOWLEDGE ASSUMED TO BE IN PLACE
The knowledge and competency to assess and care for low-risk pregnant women

KEYWORDS
hyperemesis gravidarum • fetoplacental unit • disseminated intravascular coagulation (DIC) • intrauterine death (IUD) • elderly primigravidae • grand multiparity • adolescent pregnancy • multiple pregnancy • Rh haemolytic disease • ABO incompatibility • amniotic fluid abnormalities • parity • gravidity • obesity

24.1 Introduction

This chapter will focus mainly on common obstetric complications, such as Rh haemolytic disease, ABO incompatibility, hyperemesis gravidarum, disorders of the amniotic fluid and placenta, intrauterine death (IUD) and multiple pregnancy. The effects of age and parity are also mentioned because of their importance as contributing factors in maternal deaths in South Africa.

24.2 Rh haemolytic disease

This is also known as Rh isoimmunisation and Rh incompatibility. In the past, Rh haemolytic disease in the newborn was a very serious problem, and the cause of much misery and distress for many Rh negative (Rh–) women.

Prior to the use of Rh (D) immunoglobulin (human) – or anti-D, as it is more commonly known – 1:200 pregnant women were affected (Gandhi, 2016). However, the introduction of Rh prophylaxis has caused a sharp decline in the occurrence of this condition.

Today, haemolytic disease of the newborn occurs when Rh (D) immunoglobulin is not given post-delivery or post-abortion, or when protection fails due to the development of anti-D before delivery, as occasionally occurs in mismatched blood transfusions and in ineffective or inadequate prophylaxis. The disease can also be caused by other antibodies, such as ABO incompatibility (see Section 24.3), anti-C or anti-Kell antibodies or other factors in the blood.

Greatly improved obstetric management and neonatal intensive care facilities have reduced the number of deaths from Rh incompatibility by about 90 per cent.

Incidence

The incidence of Rh disease is approximately 3 per cent lower in Africans, as fewer African women are Rh negative. In women of European descent, the incidence is 13 per cent of the Rh-negative women who are sensitised with their first pregnancy (Wikipedia, 2017e).

The inheritance of the Rh factor

The Rh factor refers to the D antigen of the Rh blood group system. People either do or do not have this antigen. Rh positive (Rh+) indicates that the person has the D antigen, while Rh negative (Rh−) indicates that the person does not have the D antigen.

The Rh factor is transmitted by a genetic factor denoted as D for Rh+ and d for Rh−. Each person has a pair of these genes. People with two dominant genes (DD) are Rh+. Those with one D and one d – that is, Dd (heterozygous) – will test Rh+ because of the dominant gene. Those with two dd genes are Rh−. If both parents are Dd, they will both test Rh+, but they can produce children with the combination DD, Dd or dd.

Rh factor pathology

Rh incompatibility develops as a result of antibody formation in an Rh− person. In midwifery, we are concerned with the pregnant woman who is Rh−. If her husband or partner is also Rh−, there is no problem. However, if the husband or partner is Rh+, then problems can arise.

During her first pregnancy, and if the baby she is carrying is Rh+, small haemorrhages, known as 'fetal leaks', can occur. This will result in fetal Rh+ blood entering the circulation of the Rh− mother. These haemorrhages may also occur during procedures such as amniocentesis, during antepartum haemorrhage (APH) and during the separation of the placenta when the maternal sinuses are left open in the third stage of labour, and/or after a miscarriage or an ectopic pregnancy. The haemorrhages can vary, from small leaks to as much as 50–400 ml of red blood cells (RBCs).

Once the fetal blood enters the maternal circulation in significant amounts (see figures 24.1 and 24.2 overleaf), it stimulates an antibody response in the maternal circulation, resulting in the formation of maternal serum Rh antibodies. These Rh antibodies remain in the mother's blood and also make a template or memory of the antibody response. Very small haemorrhages may not produce an antibody response, whereas a large bleed is more likely to result in a more intense antibody response, with clinical consequences.

During a subsequent pregnancy, maternal Rh antibodies can cross the placenta. This results in the haemolysis (breaking up) of the fetal RBCs. (See figures 24.1 and 24.2.) The mother's Rh antibodies attack the baby's RBCs, which causes anaemia in the fetus and leads to erythropoietin increase, especially in the fetal liver and spleen. This may disrupt the fetal hepatic circulation, leading to portal hypertension, reduced production of albumin and – in cases of severe haemolysis – a condition known as hydrops fetalis (cardiac failure).

Hydrops fetalis

There are various degrees of severity of Rh isoimmunisation, and hydrops fetalis is the most severe form of this condition. The clinical features include:

- a large, pale infant
- subcutaneous oedema
- ascites
- pleural and pericardial effusions
- anaemia
- hepatosplenomegaly
- petechial haemorrhages
- cardiac failure.

The placenta is large, pale and oedematous. The liquor and the vernix caseosa are both golden yellow.

Prevention

Today, Rh incompatibility can be prevented. Routine blood specimens should be taken from all women attending antenatal clinics to ascertain their blood group and Rh factor at the first visit. If the woman is Rh−, the husband or partner's blood is taken for grouping and the genotype is identified.

If the woman is Rh− and has positive antibodies in titres of less than 1:32, the test is repeated at 30 and 36 weeks' gestation. If the woman is Rh−, a direct antiglobulin test (Coomb's test) is done to look for antibodies. Blood is taken at 24 weeks and then every two weeks thereafter, to determine whether the antibody titre is rising or not.

All women's Rh status must be known at birth. If not, maternal and cord blood is taken and tested. All Rh− women's blood is taken after birth, along with a cord sample to test the baby's blood type, Rh factor, bilirubin and antibodies (Coomb's test). A positive Coomb's test indicates sensitisation.

All Rh− women who have not been sensitised should receive high-titre anti-Rh globulin within 72 hours after an incident (APH, amniocentesis or birth). This must be given after each incident or pregnancy. The serum destroys fetal cells that cross the placenta into the maternal blood circulation. The failure rate is 1–2 per cent, as sensitisation occurs in pregnancy rather than at birth (Wikipedia, 2017e). Therefore, all pregnant Rh− women with a negative Coomb's should receive a 300 µg dosage of anti-D at 28 weeks, which will protect them for six months. In addition, anti-D will be repeated after birth if the baby is Rh+.

Prophylactic anti-D immunoglobulin 300 µg can be given at 28 and 34 weeks' gestation, at least in the first pregnancy, as antenatal prophylaxis.

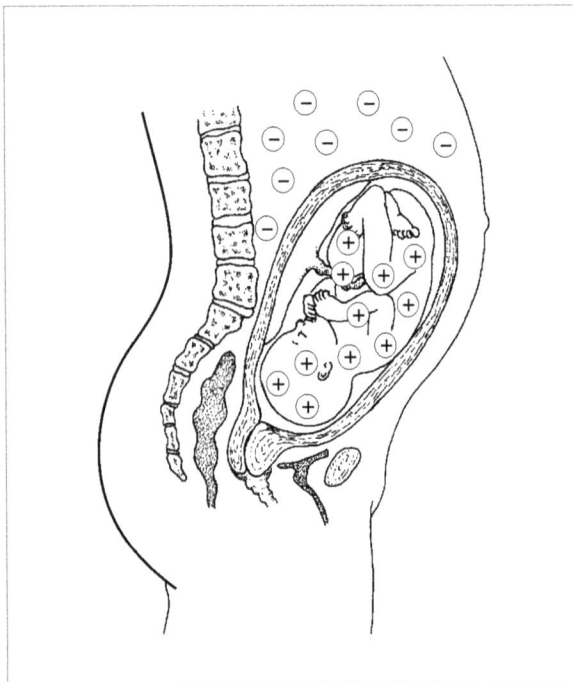

A: Mother not sensitised against baby's blood type

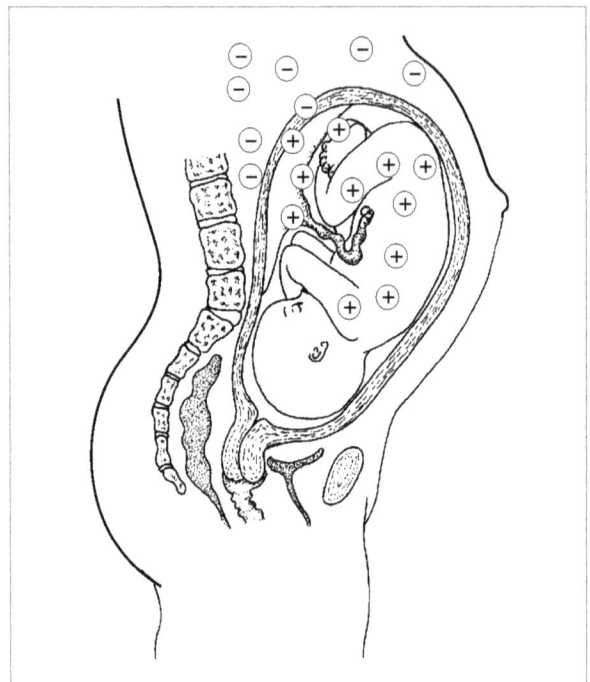

B: First exposure of mother to baby's blood after an incident

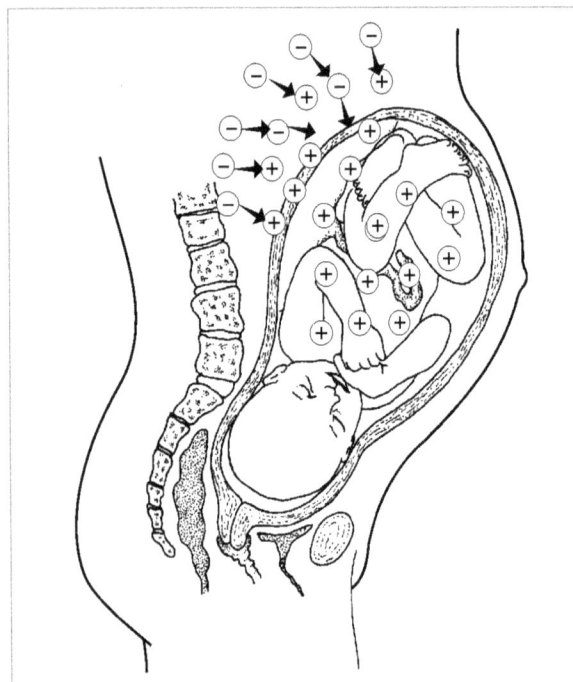

C: Maternal antibodies formed against baby's blood type

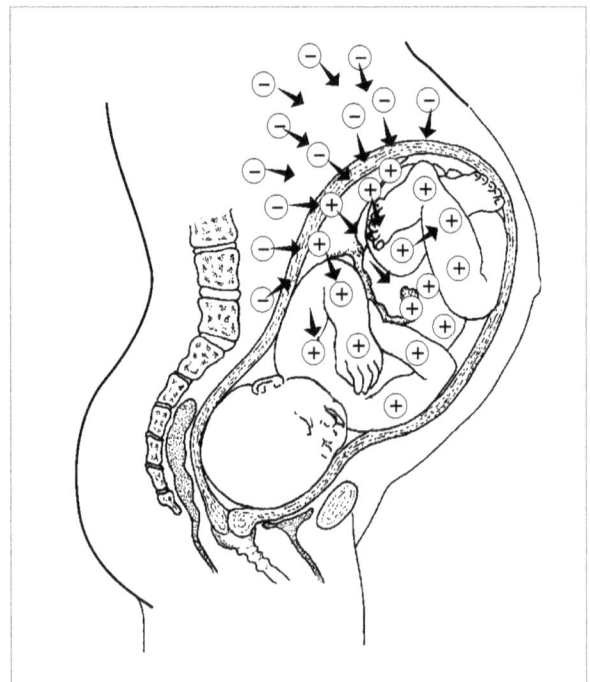

D: Maternal antibodies cross placenta and haemalyse fetal blood if any contact with fetal blood occurs (second exposure)

Figure 24.1 Schematic diagram of development of ABO/Rh incompatibility during pregnancy

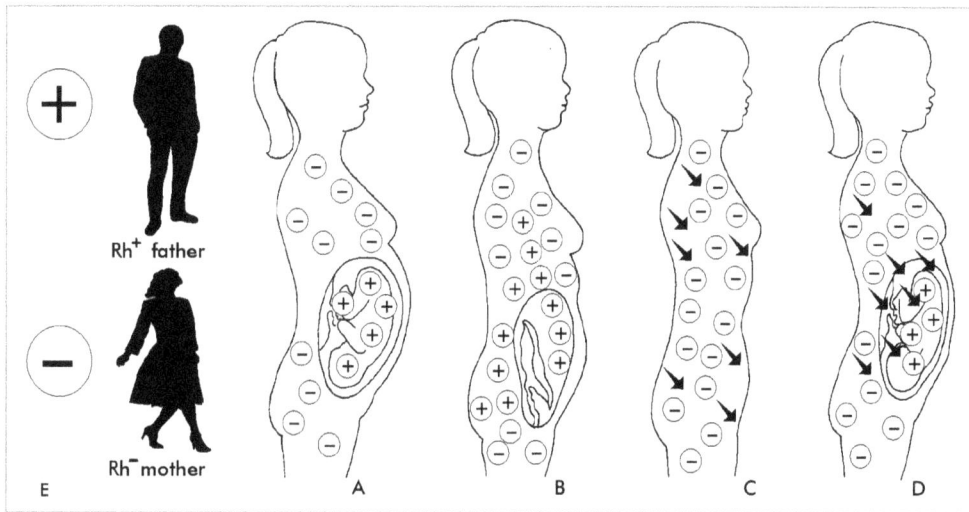

Figure 24.2 Schematic diagram of development of ABO/Rh incompatibility in a follow-up pregnancy.
A: Mother's and baby's blood is incompatible, without contact during pregnancy.
B: Positive fetal blood enters maternal circulation at birth. C: Mother develops antibodies.
D: First contact with incompatible fetal blood during any of the following pregnancies
results in release of antibodies that cross the placenta and haemolyse fetal blood.

Sensitised women

Titres indicating Rh incompatibility are of limited use in
already sensitised women, but they are useful in women who are
at risk but not yet sensitised. If the titre is 1:32, amniocentesis
is indicated to determine the bilirubin concentration in the
amniotic fluid every two weeks from 28 weeks.

If a woman is already sensitised, Doppler studies are done
from 26 to 30 weeks to determine the severity of the disease
in the fetus. If the fetus is affected, intrauterine exchange
transfusion can be done at two-week intervals or the baby can
be delivered as soon as it is safe.

Rh immunoglobulin (anti-D)

Rh immunoglobulin (anti-D) is given to women:
- who have given birth to an Rh+ infant
- after miscarriage, whether spontaneous, threatened or
  therapeutic miscarriage
- after an ectopic pregnancy
- after a chorionic villus biopsy
- after abruptio placenta and/or abdominal trauma
- after IUD
- after external cephalic version (ECV)
- after manual removal of the placenta.

continued

An IV anti-D can also be issued from the blood bank once
cross-matching has been done with a fresh specimen of the
patient's blood. Dosage:
- Less than 20 weeks' gestation: 50 µg (250 IU)
- More than 20 weeks' gestation 100 µg (500 IU).

The effects on the fetus and neonate

If Rh haemolytic disease is not prevented, it results in serious
consequences, such as:
- IUD
- hydrops fetalis
- icterus gravis neonatorum (grave jaundice of the
  newborn), which manifests within 24 hours of birth and
  can result in kernicterus and death if untreated
- haemolytic anaemia
- anaemia, caused by the breakdown of fetal RBCs (if left
  untreated). The fetal bone marrow releases immature
  RBCs. The red blood cell lysis releases bilirubin, which
  builds up in the fetus. Dangers of high bilirubin *in utero*
  include hearing loss, mental retardation and kernicterus
  for the neonate.

24.3 ABO incompatibility

The most common blood groups are the ABO groups. There are four main blood groups, namely A, B, AB and O (with 200 subgroups that can cause incompatibility):

▶ Blood group A has the antigen A on the RBCs.
▶ Blood group B has the antigen B on the RBCs.
▶ If neither of these antigens are present, the blood group is O.
▶ If both these antigens are present, the blood group is AB.

These antigens, also known as polysaccharides, are situated on the outer membranes of the RBCs. The ABO antibodies occur in different blood groups as follows:

▶ People of blood group A develop anti-B antibodies in the plasma.
▶ People of blood group B develop anti-A antibodies in the plasma.
▶ People of blood group AB develop no antibodies in the plasma.
▶ People of blood group O develop both anti-A and anti-B antibodies in the plasma.

The pathophysiology of ABO incompatibility

This type of incompatibility is common if the mother is of the O blood group and the fetus is group A, B or AB. The fetus can inherit one or more group factors from the father, which are absent in the mother. Group O mothers have anti-A and anti-B antibodies in their serum. If the fetus is group A or group B and any of the fetal RBCs leak into the maternal circulation, they are coated with an antibody in the reticuloendothelial system and destroyed by the maternal anti-A and/or anti-B haemolysins.

The chances of sensitisation are reduced, as haemolysins anti-A and anti-B antibodies do not normally cross the placenta – they are too large. However, immunoglobulins such as IgG can cross the placenta from the maternal to the fetal circulation. If IgG does cross the placenta, it attaches itself to the fetal RBCs and destroys them, causing haemolytic disease. First-born babies can thererefore be affected in this way, as can babies born in subsequent pregnancies. (See Figure 24.2 on the previous page.)

ABO factors cause the greatest number of incompatibilities: three to four times greater than Rh incompatibility. Table 24.1 details the differences between ABO and Rh incompatibility.

ABO incompatibility is now the most common cause of isoimmune haemolytic disease of the newborn, since prophylaxis with anti-D gamma globulin has reduced the incidence of Rh incompatibility.

Table 24.1

Differential diagnosis of ABO and Rh incompatibility

ABO incompatibility	Rh incompatibility
Antibodies may not be detected during pregnancy.	Antibodies are detected during pregnancy.
Mother and baby may both be Rh–.	The mother is Rh– and the baby Rh+.
Amniotic fluid and placenta are normal.	Amniotic fluid and placenta are abnormal.
Infant of first pregnancy can be sensitised and may manifest the condition.	Infant of first pregnancy is not usually sensitised.
Coomb's test is usually positive, but may be negative.	Direct Coomb's test is positive.
The disease is milder.	The disease is more severe.

Effects of ABO incompatibility on the fetus

At birth, the baby is usually healthy. Soon thereafter (on the day after delivery) the baby becomes jaundiced. The jaundice is progressive and can be unpredictably severe in some cases.

Diagnosis

This is done by evaluating the neonate who has developed jaundice during the first week of life. Antenatal antibody blood test screening for ABO incompatibility is not done, as the results do not correlate well with ABO haemolytic disease.

If an infant is suffering from ABO incompatibility, the direct Coomb's antiglobulin test is positive. Hb is normal. Free anti-A or anti-B antibodies are seen in the fetal serum. Nucleated RBCs and spherocytes and reticulocytes are seen in the blood smear. The diagnosis is thus based on the following:

▶ The infant is jaundiced within 24 to 36 hours.
▶ The mother's blood group is O.
▶ The baby's blood group is A, B or AB.
▶ The direct Coomb's test is positive.

Care

Care for infants suffering from ABO incompatibility includes:

▶ phototherapy (see Chapter 44)
▶ exchange transfusion, only if the serum bilirubin reaches danger levels:
  • 340 µmol/ℓ (20 g/dl) in a term baby
  • 260 µmol/ℓ (15 g/dl) in a preterm baby.

24.4   Hyperemesis gravidarum

Definition and incidence

Hyperemesis gravidarum is defined as severe vomiting that persists after the first trimester and becomes excessive and pathological. However, it can also occur before 14 weeks.

This condition occurs in less than 2:1 000 pregnancies. The rate of re-occurrence in a next pregnancy is 25 per cent (Wikipedia, 2016a).

Aetiology

The cause of hyperemesis gravidarum is unknown, but certain conditions are associated with it, such as:

▶ a previous unsuccessful pregnancy
▶ first pregnancy: primigravidae are more often affected than multigravidae
▶ hyperthyroidism
▶ psychogenic elements (certain personality types): women who are nervous and anxious, have emotional stress at home, are obese, have a prior or family history of hyperemesis gravidarum or suffer from an eating disorder.

Hyperemesis gravidarum is more common in conditions with increased human chorionic gonadotrophin (hCG), such as:

▶ multiple pregnancy
▶ hydatidiform mole
▶ pyelonephritis
▶ trophoblastic disorder.

Pathophysiology

Vomiting is controlled by two centres in the brain, which are sensitive to the rise in oestrogens and hCG levels.

Diagnosis

Vomiting, which becomes increasingly persistent and severe, occurs at any time of the day or night, and persists after 14 weeks' gestation. There are signs of dehydration, including:

▶ a dry, furred tongue
▶ cracked, sore lips and mouth
▶ sunken eyes
▶ a loss of 5 per cent of mass or more than 2 kg.

Blurred vision is a serious sign, indicating decreased intraocular pressure. Headaches and depression are common, followed by diplopia, nystagmus, delirium, coma and oliguria, with concentrated urine with proteinuria, ketones or bilirubin. Liver damage occurs due to a reduction in vitamin B absorption. The woman may also show tachycardia (a weak, rapid pulse) with symptoms of hypotension. There is increased urea in the blood (uraemia), with some renal damage.

The woman may show physical and emotional signs of the stress of pregnancy on the body and experience difficulty with the activities of daily living.

Treatment and care

The interventions depend on the severity of the condition:

▶ Take a full history and do a thorough physical examination to identify the cause of the vomiting.
▶ Start with dry, bland food and oral rehydration. Medical care is needed in most cases. Hospitalisation is needed in some cases and hyperemesis gravidarum is treated as an emergency.
▶ In the beginning, the woman is nil per mouth until she is stabilised. A mouth wash is given.
▶ If necessary, use anti-emetic medications and IV rehydration. An IV infusion 1 000 ml saline dextrose, 125 ml per hour, is started with an anti-emetic and sedation. Intake and output are measured.
▶ The electrolytes are checked and corrected. Vitamin B complex and vitamin C are given, with calcium gluconate, to protect the liver.
▶ There is a gradual return to oral fluids and when food is tolerated, IV therapy is discontinued.
▶ A special diet is given, which includes small, frequent, attractive meals. Fatty, spicy foods should be avoided.
▶ Thromboembolic stockings or low-molecular-weight heparin may be used as measures to prevent the formation of a blood clot.
▶ A calm atmosphere is created. Provide reassurance and arrange psychotherapy if required.
▶ Visitors are restricted. The woman is placed in a private room or side ward.

Investigations

▶ Urine is taken for microscopy, culture and sensitivity (MC&S), specific gravidity, ketones and bilirubin. Any urinary tract infection (UTI) must be treated.
▶ Blood tests may include electrolytes and liver function tests.
▶ Ultrasound should be done to exclude hydatidiform mole or multiple pregnancy.

Complications

If the condition is very serious and there is no improvement with treatment, a termination of the pregnancy may be considered in the case of:

▶ persistent, severe jaundice
▶ persistent albuminuria

▶ pyelonephritis
▶ neurological symptoms, such as delirium and coma
▶ rising temperature and tachycardia
▶ cardiac symptoms.

24.5   Amniotic fluid abnormalities

Amniotic fluid abnormalities can take the form of an excessive amount of fluid (polyhydramnios) or an insufficient amount of fluid (oligohydramnios).

Polyhydramnios

Polyhydramnios is a pathological condition, characterised by an excessive amount of amniotic fluid for the period of gestation. The liquor can increase to 2 000–3 000 ml. In very severe cases, the liquor may increase to 15 ℓ. Once the volume reaches 3 000–4 000 ml, there are abnormal clinical signs.

Amniotic fluid gradually increases in pregnancy to 1 000 ml at term. The normal amount of liquor at term is between 400 ml and 1 500 ml, and is usually about 600 ml. Approximate amounts at given gestation periods are as follows:

▶ at 10 weeks = 30 ml
▶ at 20 weeks = 300 ml
▶ at 30 weeks = 600 ml
▶ at 38 weeks = 1 000 ml
▶ at term = 600 ml.

Amniotic fluid is produced by the amniotic epithelium and its volume is related to the fetal weight in the first trimester. It is the same concentration as fetal intracellular fluid and is a filtration of maternal plasma, which also contains fetal urine.

Amniotic fluid is not static. There is a rapid turnover of amniotic fluid in the third trimester; about 500 ml is exchanged each hour. At term, the fetus swallows the same amount as the feeding requirements after birth (500 ml per day).

Incidence

The incidence of polyhydramnios is 0.2–1.6 per cent of all pregnancies (Carter, 2015). The rate may be higher in women with diabetes mellitus.

Aetiology

Polyhydramnios is caused by any condition that is involved in the overproduction of amniotic fluid or which prevents the circulation of amniotic fluid through the fetus, for example if the gastrointestinal (GI) canal is blocked (duodenal atresia and oesophageal atresia) or in neurological conditions in which the fetus may not be able to swallow. Table 24.2 lists various types of factors that can cause polyhydramnios.

Table 24.2

Causes of polyhydramnios

Maternal conditions	Diabetes mellitus: responsible for 25% of cases (Carter, 2015) Rh incompatibility: responsible for 10% of cases (Wikipedia, 2017f) Liver and kidney disease Infections: toxoplasmosis, other, rubella, cytomegalovirus, herpes simplex (TORCH); cardiac problems
Fetal conditions	Congenital abnormalities, 20% of which are neurological: anencephaly, open neural tube, spina bifida, encephalocele, meningocele, meningomyelocele GI: gastrocysis and oesophageal atresia Tumours of the neck Cystic fibrosis
Obstetric	Multiple pregnancy: 10% (uniovular twins) Large placenta Pre-eclampsia Twin-to-twin transfusion Chorioangioma of the placenta
Idiopathic	35% of cases (Carter, 2015)

Classification

Polyhydramnios may develop gradually or acutely. Table 24.3 details the two types.

Table 24.3

Classification of polyhydramnios

Acute polyhydramnios: 2%	Chronic polyhydramnios
Second trimester onset Rapid increase: > 2 000 ml Preterm labour is common Abdominal pain, dyspnoea, oedema of abdomen and lower extremities, nausea and vomiting Amniocentesis is done to relieve maternal discomfort	Develops late in pregnancy, at 32–42 weeks A gradual increase, causing discomfort if abnormalities are present, with poor perinatal outcomes

Table 24.4

A comparison of factors present in polyhydramnios and multiple pregnancy

	Polyhydramnios	**Multiple pregnancy**
History	No excessive fetal movements No twins in family Not necessarily one of a pair of twins Minor disorders not necessarily exaggerated Drugs not necessarily used for fertility Diabetes, pregnancy-induced hypertension (PIH) Congenital abnormality	Excessive fetal movements Twins in family One of a pair of twins Exaggerated minor disorder Drugs used for infertility Not necessarily any incidence of diabetes mellitus or PIH Not necessarily any congenital abnormality
Physical examination	Exaggerated pressure symptoms Oedema Acute dyspnoea Palpitations Distressed	Exaggerated pressure symptoms Oedema Dyspnoea Palpitations Uncomfortable at 24 weeks, not distressed
Abdominal inspection	Round, globular No movements seen Skin shiny, taut and over-stretched Appears as a 'tumour' tilted to one side	Large, irregular Multiple movements seen Muscles relaxed Appears as a pregnant abdomen and a fibroid
Abdominal palpation	Small fetus Difficult to feel parts Two poles felt, unstable lie Abdominal girth enlarged Malpresentation common Fluid thrill Height of fundus enlarged Small head Ballottement can be easy or difficult	Uterus large for dates Many fetal parts, multiple limbs present Three or more poles present Abdominal girth enlarged Malpresentation present No fluid thrill Height of fundus enlarged Two small heads felt Ballottement difficult
Abdominal auscultation	Difficult due to amniotic fluid volume Fetal heart difficult to hear	Two fetal hearts heard at different sites by two midwives (at least difference of 10 beats per minute
Ultrasound	One baby seen	Two babies seen
X-ray	One baby seen	Two babies seen

Clinical features and diagnosis

The clinical features will depend upon the period of gestation, the amount of amniotic fluid and the rapidity of the accumulation of the fluid.

There is often a history of exaggerated minor disorders of pregnancy such as nausea and vomiting, abdominal discomfort, abdominal distension, pain and oedema, dyspnoea and orthopnoea and oedema of the vulva and legs.

On examination, the following may be observed:
- The uterus appears large for dates.
- The uterus is globular in shape.
- The skin of the anterior abdominal wall is taut, stretched and shiny.

On auscultation, the fetal heart is muffled. The following may be found on palpation:
- The uterus is tense and tender.

- A 'fluid thrill' can be demonstrated. (The palm of one hand is placed against one side of the abdomen while the fingers of the other hand flick the uterus on the other side. Waves of movement are transmitted through the excess fluid and are felt on the palm of the hand against the abdominal wall on the opposite side.)
- The whole fetus is ballotable. Fetal parts are not easily felt.
- It is difficult to palpate the fetus, because the uterus is filled and overstretched with amniotic fluid, making it impossible to grasp or feel the parts.

When an ultrasound is done, the amniotic fluid is found to be excessive and evident throughout the uterine cavity. Large pockets of fluid, more than 8 cm in vertical diameter, indicate polyhydramnios. Fetal abnormalities may be detected.

Table 24.4 on the previous page shows a summary of the abovementioned clinical features found in polyhydramnios when compared with multiple pregnancy (discussed in Section 24.6).

Complications

The complications of polyhydramnios are associated with the cause of the condition, the gestational period and the classification. Common complications are preterm labour, abruptio placenta due to overstretching or rapid decompression when the membranes rupture, and maternal distress from discomfort and symptoms.

In labour, there is a high risk of prolapse of the cord with the rupture of membranes due to malpresentations and the poor application of the presenting part. Abnormal uterine action and prolonged labour occur due to the overstretched atonic muscles. Postpartum haemorrhage (PPH) occurs due to ineffective contractions, caused by an atonic uterus from overstretched muscles.

In the postnatal period, sub-involution and infection may occur. The woman is referred for medical care.

The fetal complications are those of the preterm neonate and those with congenital and genetic abnormalities.

Treatment and care

- The patient is admitted to hospital on bed rest or semi-bed rest in an upright position.
- Any associated condition is determined and treated.
- If the fetus is mature, labour is induced.
- If the fetus is abnormal, the choice of termination or delivery will depend on the kind of defect.
- If there is need for genetic counselling, this is arranged.

- If the fetus is normal and premature labour can be suppressed, beta-sympathomimetics may be used to reduce uterine activity.
- The woman is made as comfortable as possible and reassured and supported emotionally.
- All her personal hygiene is attended to.
- The symptoms of polyhydramnios are treated and relieved where possible.
- Draining amniotic fluid (amnioreduction) by amniocentesis (drawing 500 ml of amnion liquid per hour) is done to relieve the signs and symptoms. However, this is not without risk. Amniotic fluid is quickly replaced and the risk of infection is increased. The procedure must be repeated three to four times a week.

Oligohydramnios

Oligohydramnios is a condition in which the amount of liquor is grossly deficient. It could be reduced to less than 300 ml or even to a few millilitres of dark, thick fluid.

Aetiology

Premature rupture of membranes (PROM) is the main cause of oligohydramnios. Other conditions that are associated with oligohydramnios are renal agenesis or obstruction in the fetal urinary system. Babies with renal agenesis often present with Potter's syndrome. Other causes include:

- prolonged pregnancy and the resultant reduced placental function
- a post-mature fetus
- intrauterine growth restriction (IUGR)
- placental insufficiency in PIH.

Complications

Early oligohydramnios can result in:

- fetal damage caused by amniotic bands winding around a part of the fetus (amniotic band syndrome), as there is little liquor to keep the amnion away from the fetus
- maldevelopment or amputation of toes, fingers or limbs
- cord constriction and obstruction, causing fetal hypoxia or anoxia
- pressure deformities due to the extremely confined intrauterine space
- pulmonary hypoplasia due to compression by the uterus on the chest wall, preventing expansion of the chest wall; this will also inhibit lung growth and cause intrinsic lung defects
- the fetal skin becoming dry, leathery and wrinkled
- meconium-stained amniotic fluid.

The abovementioned fetal deformities are severe and often result in IUD or neonatal death. In severe cases, irreversible deformities can result in the child.

Late oligohydramnios will result in pressure deformities, such as:
▶ pressure or obstruction of the cord
▶ signs of fetal distress or compromise, with abnormal heart rates and rhythms and thick meconium in the sparse liquor
▶ a distorted face, flattening of the nose, micrognathia and squashing of the limbs resulting in talipes, dislocated hips or scoliosis (due to the fetus being squashed in the uterus).

Most of these deformities improve with time and the body may return to a normal shape and function.

Clinical signs and symptoms

The uterus is irritable on palpation. The uterus appears small for the gestational age (GA). Palpation is difficult, as the uterus is moulded around the fetus and the head cannot be balloted. There are reduced fetal movements and a possible malpresentation, such as breech presentation.

Investigations

Ultrasound will show reduced liquor. Amniotic fluid is decreased, with small pockets of fluid less than 5 cm in vertical diameter. Fetal abnormalities and features of IUGR may be visible. Fetal growth, PROM, placental insufficiency and IUGR must be assessed.

Treatment and care

The following treatment and care is required for the woman during pregnancy:
▶ The woman is referred for medical attention. Admission to hospital is needed to investigate causes, fetal status and a treatment plan.
▶ Tests for placental function, including oestriol values (seldom performed now) and/or cardiotocograph (CTG) tracings for placental reserve are performed.
▶ If no or only slight abnormalities are found, the pregnancy is allowed to go to term under close observation of the fetal status.
▶ If there are gross abnormalities, the pregnancy may be terminated or delivered based on the GA, fetal status and placental function.
▶ If the fetus is distressed, it is delivered by Caesarean section in a level of care where neonatal care is available.

The following treatment and care are required during labour:
▶ Constriction rings may be present and may cause problems during delivery; therefore, an obstetrician should deliver the baby.
▶ The fetal condition is carefully observed through continuous electronic monitoring.
▶ The mother needs information, extra support and reassurance during labour.
▶ If fetal abnormalities are present, a paediatrician is involved to carefully explain to the parents about the abnormality, its management and the prognosis for the baby.
▶ The patient requires firm reassurance, kindness and understanding.

24.6 Multiple pregnancy

A multiple or plural pregnancy is when there are two or more fetuses in the uterus at the same time. Twin pregnancy (two fetuses) is the most common. Triplets occur in 1:7 600 pregnancies (Wikipedia, 2017g).

Incidence

The incidence of multiple pregnancy is relatively constant, with variation between different demographic groups (Fletcher, 2015):
▶ Black: 1:50 viable pregnancies
▶ White: 1:85–100 viable pregnancies
▶ Asian: 1:150 viable pregnancies.

Multiple pregnancy is also associated with infertility treatment. The use of substances to stimulate ovulation influences and increases the incidence of multiple pregnancies in most developed countries.

Highest record number of babies in multiple pregnancies
The official record of number of children born naturally to a woman is 69. A woman in Moscow bore 16 sets of twins, seven sets of triplets and four sets of quadruplets in 27 pregnancies, of which 67 children survived (McWhirter & Russell, 1988:13).

Whether the multiple birth is natural or caused by infertility treatment, it is imperative that the midwifery and nursing personnel are completely conversant with the care of a mother with multiple pregnancy and with the management of twin delivery. This is particularly important, as this type of pregnancy has an increased risk of perinatal morbidity and mortality, related to the risk of premature birth.

The perinatal morbidity and mortality rates increase considerably with each extra fetus. There is also increased risk during delivery of the second and every subsequent baby.

Types of multiple pregnancy

Multiple pregnancy can be twins (two babies), triplets (three babies), quadruplets (four babies), quintuplets (five babies), sextuplets (six babies), septuplets (seven babies) or octuplets (eight babies).

For every extra baby in the womb, the risk for complications increases. Quadruplets and higher numbers are rarely conceived normally. The most common natural multiple pregnancy is the twin pregnancy. There are two main types of twins: uniovular and binovular twins.

Uniovular twins

Uniovular twins are also referred to as monovular, monozygotic or identical twins. In uniovular twins, only one ovum is fertilised (by one sperm). During its early development, the zygote divides into two or more similar, separate zygotes. The reason for this separation is not known, but may be environmental or genetic.

The babies who develop from these zygotes are very similar in appearance and are the same gender, with very similar or even identical fingerprints and electroencephalograph patterns.

In most instances (64 per cent), the two fetuses share one placenta and one chorion, but each has its own amnion, as shown in Figure 24.3 (Wikipedia, 2017g). Less often, they will each have their own placenta, chorion and amnion, and less often still they will share all three. The circulations of the fetuses may anastomose to a greater or lesser degree, which can be seen on the fetal surface of the placenta after delivery. This can result in the cardiovascular system of one twin developing disproportionately more than that of the other twin.

Conditions such as inherited disorders will affect each twin, but the time of appearance of the disorder may depend on environmental factors. Developmental anomalies are more common in monozygotic twins, resulting in a high abortion rate, and if the zygotes do not separate completely, conjoined twins can result.

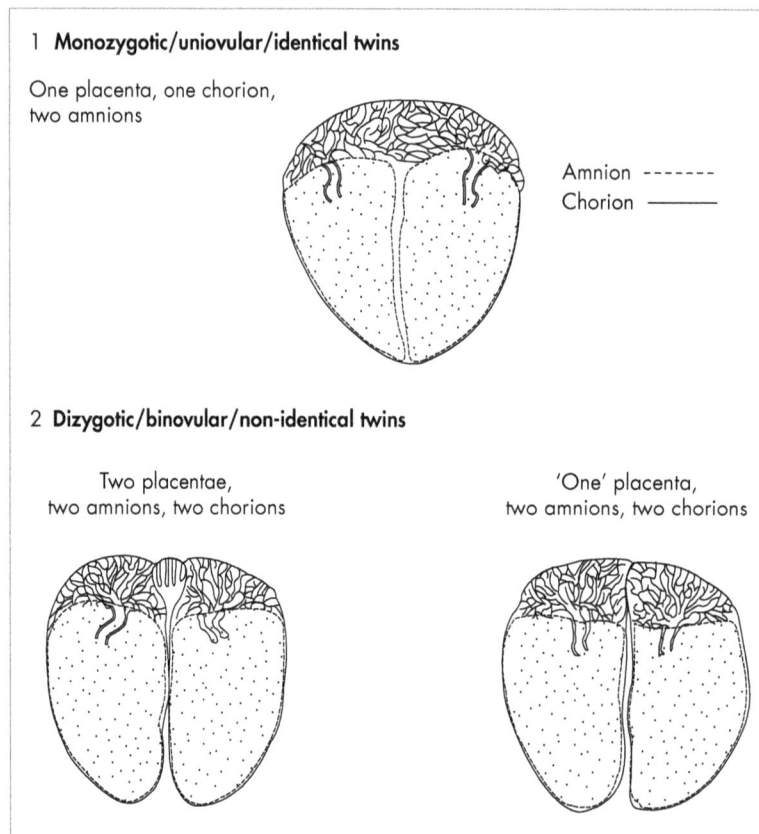

1 **Monozygotic/uniovular/identical twins**

One placenta, one chorion, two amnions

Amnion - - - - - - -
Chorion ————

2 **Dizygotic/binovular/non-identical twins**

Two placentae, two amnions, two chorions

'One' placenta, two amnions, two chorions

Figure 24.3 Multiple pregnancy – placentae of monozygotic and dizygotic twins

Uniovular twins are usually of a more similar mass, unless there is an anastomosis of the circulations, when one could be much bigger and heavier than the other. Even when the pregnancy goes to term, the weight of each twin is almost always less than that of a normal singleton baby, which is the result of IUGR in the third trimester due to placental insufficiency. This occurs in both uniovular and binovular twins, although the combined weight of uniovular twins tends to be less than that of binovular twins.

Binovular twins

Other names for binovular twins are dizygotic or non-identical twins. In this type of multiple pregnancy, two or more ova are each fertilised by a separate sperm. The babies may be the same sex or of a different sex. The incidence of binovular twins is three times greater than that of uniovular twins. Superfecundation is where two or more ova were fertilised with sperm from two different men. The gestational period will be the same as ovulation is from the same menstrual cycle.

There is a definite familial background with binovular twins, although older mothers also tend to have a greater incidence of dizygotic twins. Drugs for infertility also produce multiple ova.

Although binovular twins each have their own placenta, chorion and amnion (see Figure 24.3), the placentae may fuse and appear as one. With careful examination after delivery, two chorions and two amnions (four layers of membrane) can be demonstrated. The fetal circulations do not mix.

Conjoined (Siamese) twins

Conjoined twins arise when the separation in uniovular twins is not complete. The degree of union can vary greatly, from joining of the skin only, to sharing the thoracic cage and even the internal viscera.

The success of the separation of conjoined twins by surgery depends upon the degree of union and the involvement and sharing of internal organs, as well as the degree of expertise and the equipment available. The survival of the twins depends on the time of separation and the organs that are shared. There are documented cases of conjoined twins who were never separated and survived for more than 50 years.

Aetiology

The causes of multiple pregnancy are as follows:
- *Inherited:* There is a trend in families for twins, usually from the mother's side.
- *Demographic group:* Black women have a higher incidence of twins.
- *Maternal age:* There is an increased risk with age.
- *Parity:* There is in increased risk with increasing parity.
- *Other factors:* These include nutrition, the use of substances and infertility treatment (chlomiphene and gonadotrophins).

Infertility

Infertility is the inability to fall pregnant after one year of regular coitus. Primary infertility refers to the inability to fall pregnant at all and secondary infertility refers to a woman who has had previous pregnancies and fails to fall pregnant again.

Delayed fertility can be due to infertility or sterility. Couples may resort to advanced reproductive technology to conceive a genetic child or a child genetically related to one of the parents through donor sperm or surrogate pregnancy. When advanced technology is used to stimulate pregnancy, there is always a high risk of multiple pregnancy.

Twin-to-twin transfusion syndrome

This condition occurs in uniovular twins and is due to the anastomosis of the fetal circulations when a placenta is shared. The one twin derives most of the blood and therefore also the nourishment, while the other is deprived of blood and nourishment. There is a great disparity in mass (weight). Both twins are at great risk of fetal demise, but for different reasons.

At birth, the recipient twin may:
- be bigger and weigh more
- suffer from polycythaemia
- be plethoric
- have congestive cardiac failure
- have respiratory distress
- be prone to arterial thrombi
- have a high risk of mortality, both intrauterine and neonatal.

The donor twin may:
- be the smaller, lighter twin, who is very small for the GA
- be anaemic
- have hypoglycaemia
- have a risk of high mortality, both intrauterine and neonatal. If the amount of blood is seriously diminished, the deprived fetus will die *in utero*, but the donor twin can survive if the circulation has not been too grossly overloaded.

The effects of multiple pregnancy

The effects on the pregnancy

For every extra fetus in the womb, the risk of complications is increased. The following general risks are increased for multiple pregnancies:

▶ The minor disorders of pregnancy, such as morning sickness, heartburn or backache, are accentuated.
▶ There is an increased incidence of hyperemesis gravidarum due to the increased hCG.
▶ There are often increased pressure symptoms in the third trimester, such as:
  • varicose veins in the legs and the vulva
  • haemorrhoids
  • oedema of the lower limbs
  • difficulty in breathing
  • sleeplessness because of the inability to get comfortable with the grossly distended abdomen.
▶ There is an increased abortion rate.
▶ The incidence of pre-eclampsia and eclampsia is greatly increased in multiple pregnancy.
▶ Placental abruption and APH are increased. Placenta praevia is increased because of the large placenta, with resulting APH.
▶ Polyhydramnios is greatly increased, both acute and chronic, with the resultant complications.

▶ There is a risk for fetus papyraceous: when one twin dies *in utero* as a result of twin transfusion syndrome, or because the heart and the circulation have not developed normally, the fetus shrinks, becomes flattened, compressed, pale and paper-like and is known as a fetus papyraceous, as shown in Figure 24.4.
▶ There is an increased risk of IUGR and twins are usually smaller than singleton babies, although the combined mass is more than a singleton.
▶ Anaemia is prevalent because of the increased fetal demands for iron, and the Hb is below 10 g/dl in many instances of twin pregnancy.
▶ There is a high percentage of fetal abnormalities.

The effects on labour

There is a high incidence of Caesarean section. In some communities, this has almost become the accepted way of delivering twins, because of the complications involved. However, in developing countries, where a uterine scar can be dangerous in subsequent pregnancies, Caesarean section is only resorted to in case of:

▶ a previous Caesarean section
▶ severe pre-eclampsia
▶ undiagnosed twins or multiple fetuses
▶ malpresentation, particularly a transverse lie
▶ conjoined twins or locked twins
▶ gross pelvic deformity, cephalopelvic disproportion (CPD).

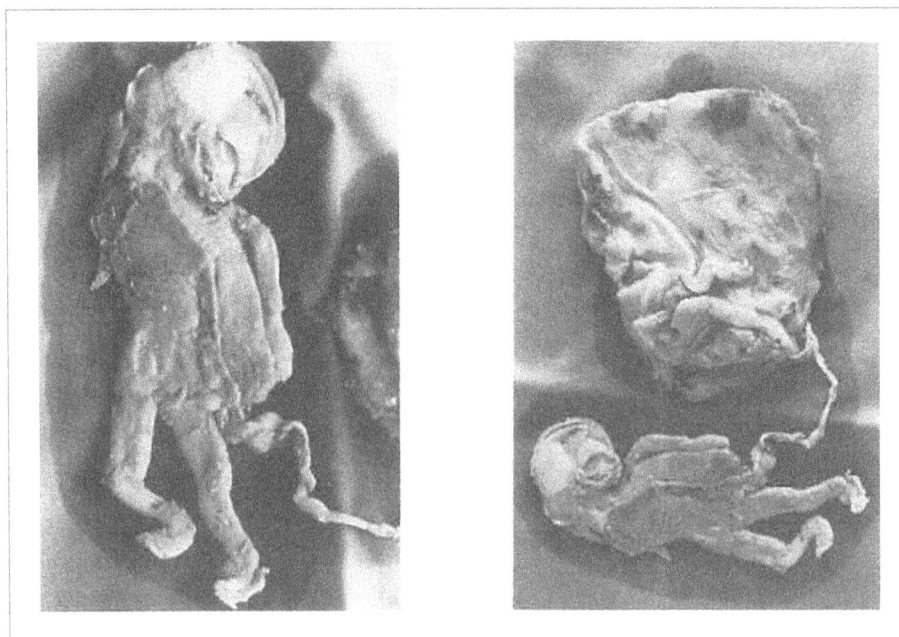

Figure 24.4 Fetus papyraceous

There are increased stillbirth and neonatal morbidity and mortality rates, especially for the second twin, due to a reduction in the placental circulation when the volume of the uterus is reduced after the birth of the first twin and due to early separation of the placenta.

Uterine inertia may occur before the birth of the second twin because of atony of the uterus due to the distended uterine muscles, particularly if the first stage was prolonged. This may cause a delay in the birth of the second twin. The cervix may start to close, causing the woman to undergo a second labour before the second twin can be delivered.

There is great variety in the lie and presentation that can arise in twins, as shown in Figure 24.5. The main combinations are two cephalic presentations (in 40 per cent of twins), followed by a cephalic and a breech presentation. Some of these abnormal lies and presentations can cause serious complications in labour.

Locked twins also present a serious problem when the first twin begins to descend down the birth canal. This could arise, for instance, when the first twin is a breech and the second is cephalic, and the head of the second twin prevents the head of the first twin from entering the pelvis.

If the second twin is not in a longitudinal lie, obstructed labour could result, as shown in Figure 24.6 on the next page. Fetal abnormalities are often present, with the accompanying difficult and prolonged labour.

Intrapartum haemorrhage from early separation of the placenta, after the birth of the first twin and before the birth of the second twin, can occur.

PPH is common, due to:
- uterine atony and inertia
- anaemia
- previous APH
- a large placental site.

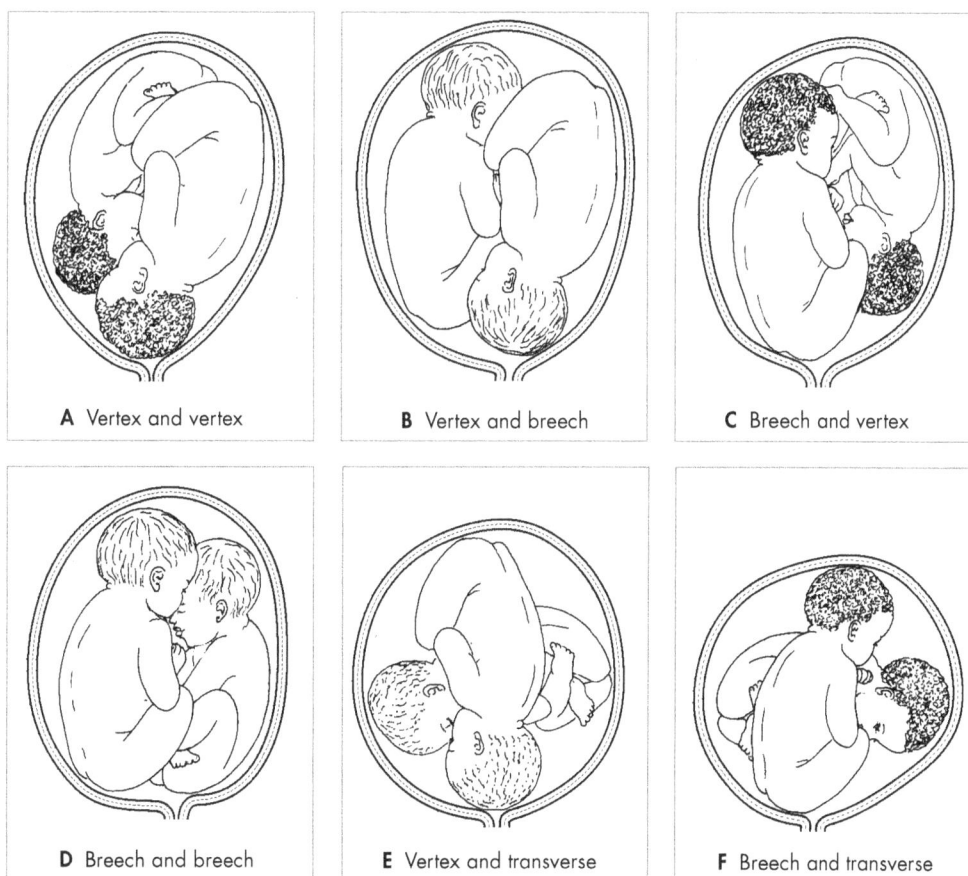

| A Vertex and vertex | B Vertex and breech | C Breech and vertex |
| D Breech and breech | E Vertex and transverse | F Breech and transverse |

Figure 24.5 Presentation of twins before delivery

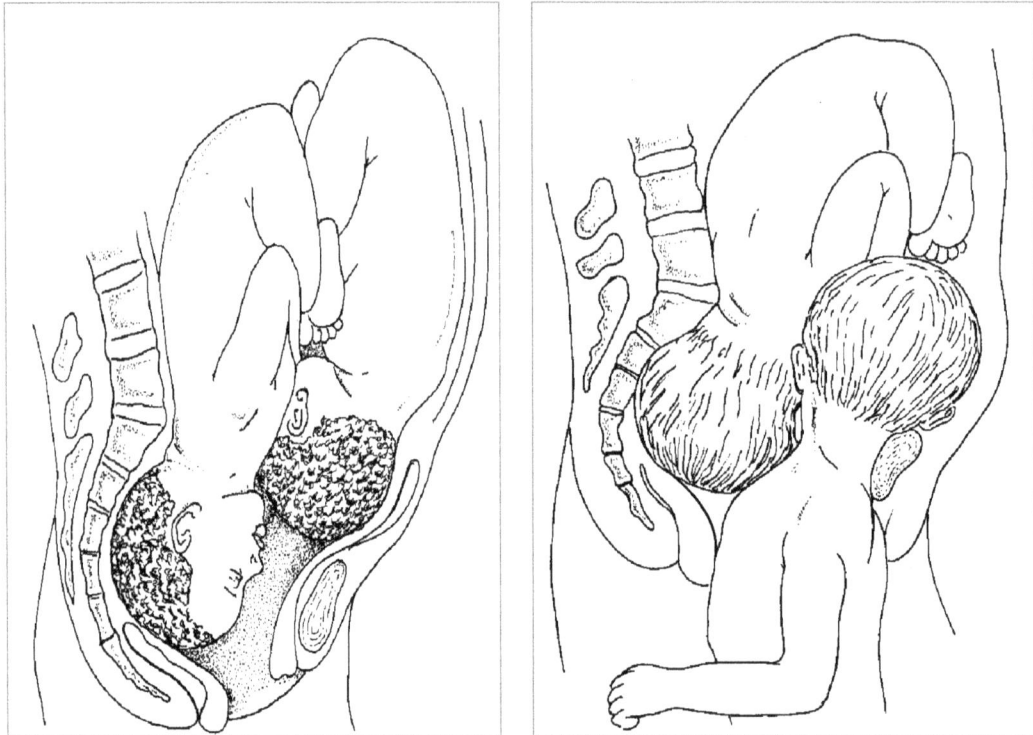

Figure 24.6 Locked twins

A uterine constriction ring may develop after the birth of the first twin, causing active retention of the second fetus.

The effects on the babies

Certain abnormal fetal conditions occur only in multiple pregnancy. The incidence of other conditions is also greatly increased, such as:

▶ a high perinatal mortality rate (PNMR) related to preterm birth
▶ twin-to-twin transfusion syndrome
▶ asphyxia neonatorum
▶ small-for-gestational-age (SGA) babies and the accompanying complications
▶ birth injuries, particularly due to manipulations which may be necessary for malpresentations
▶ fetal malformations and conjoined twins.

Diagnosis of multiple pregnancy

History

The following factors are important:

▶ Determine the woman's demographic group and her home situation.

▶ Find out if there are twins in the family.
▶ Find out if the woman has had a previous twin pregnancy.
▶ Take a very careful history of the current pregnancy so that a correct estimated date of delivery (EDD) can be arrived at.
▶ The woman may complain of increased minor disorders of pregnancy, or later in pregnancy the woman may complain of the abdomen being larger than expected and of excessive pressure symptoms.
▶ Hyperemesis gravidarum may be present.

Abdominal examination

The abdominal inspection is extremely important and may, in early pregnancy, be the only real indication of twins. Serial measures of the symphysis fundal height (SFH) are needed to determine the GA between 20 and 36 weeks.

Inspection

▶ The uterus will be broad and round (rather than oval).
▶ The uterus will look larger than expected for the EDD.
▶ More than the usual amount of fetal movements may be seen.

Palpation

▶ The SFH is measured and found to be higher than the period of gestation warrants (particularly in the first and the second trimester, before IUGR occurs). There is a correlation between the GA and the SFH.

▶ Two heads may be felt, which is diagnostic of twins. The heads could be at any place within the uterus. In 40 per cent of twins, both fetuses are cephalic presentations. (The fetal head is usually identified by 30 weeks of gestation.)

▶ If the second twin is a breech presentation, the head could be tucked up under the maternal ribs and very difficult to palpate.

▶ If only one head is palpated, it will feel small in comparison with the size of the (enlarged) uterus.

▶ An unusual number of limbs may be felt.

▶ In many twin pregnancies, polyhydramnios is present. This could make the palpation and a positive diagnosis very difficult (see Table 24.4 on page 349).

Auscultation

Two fetal hearts may be heard. However, in order to be reasonably sure there are two different heartbeats, a difference of at least 10 heartbeats with a silent area in-between should be discernible. This is not a reliable sign of twins.

Special examinations

It is recommended that all women have at least one ultrasound during pregnancy, in order to detect any possible abnormality. The optimal time is 12 weeks and 20 weeks:

▶ A positive diagnosis of multiple pregnancy would be possible at both 12 and 20 weeks.

▶ Two fetal sacs can be distinguished at eight weeks' gestation.

▶ Two heads can be seen at 15 weeks.

▶ The position of the placenta is important.

▶ The fetuses are checked for congenital abnormalities at 20 weeks' gestation.

Without ultrasound, the diagnosis of multiple pregnancy is made almost entirely on a good history and on the clinical examinations at each antenatal visit. Therefore, the importance of women attending antenatal clinics early and regularly must be stressed. The importance of this must be emphasised by health education in the communities, and the whole family should be included.

Blood testing should be done to check:

▶ levels of hCG, which may be quite high

▶ alpha-fetoprotein (AFP)

▶ levels of a protein released by the fetal liver and found in the mother's blood, which may be high when more than one fetus is present.

Obstetric and midwifery management of multiple pregnancy

Normal antenatal care applies, with additional specific medical and midwifery care. The management of multiple pregnancy is based on:

▶ pregnancy, overall health and medical history

▶ number of fetuses

▶ tolerance for specific medications, procedures or therapies

▶ expectations for the course of the pregnancy

▶ opinion or preference.

The most important factors to be addressed in multiple pregnancy are:

▶ early diagnosis of the condition

▶ screening patients at risk and referring them to the nearest hospital and an obstetrician.

Women are seen more often for the early identification of potential problems such as:

▶ the high incidence of IUGR and how to diagnose this

▶ the high incidence of preterm labour and how to prevent this (see Chapter 23)

▶ the high incidence of anaemia, pre-eclampsia, polyhydramnios, fetal abnormalities, abnormal presentations, APH and the complications that result from all these conditions. Most of the abovementioned conditions are interrelated and affect one another. (See chapters 21 to 23 for the diagnosis and management of these conditions.)

It is essential that the diagnosis of a multiple pregnancy be made early, in order to have a baseline from which to work. The baseline will assist the obstetrician in making an early diagnosis of IUGR. The obstetrician will also try to assess the degree of IUGR and the rate of degeneration of the fetus (the diagnosis and assessment of IUGR are very difficult to estimate) in order to decide the optimum delivery date.

Health education by the midwife and the social worker should stress the necessity for each pregnant woman to present herself at the antenatal clinic as early in her pregnancy as possible. In developing countries, because of the lack of expensive equipment and laboratory investigation, the diagnosis of IUGR has to be made entirely based on the clinical skills of the obstetrician and on meticulous antenatal care and recording.

Unless there are complications, women with multiple pregnancies are treated as outpatients at antenatal clinics because of the disruption of family life and the expense involved.

Prevent or treat any of the complications which can be treated. Prescribe diet supplements such as vitamins and iron, and advise the woman on diet. Advise the woman to reduce her activities at home and to avoid enemas and laxatives. She should also avoid coitus – or at least deep penetration – because both the physical irritation and the natural prostaglandins may induce preterm labour.

The woman must attend the antenatal clinic regularly. She and her husband or partner are warned of the danger of preterm labour, educated about signs of preterm labour and advised to come to the hospital immediately if these are noticed.

The obstetrician decides on the type of delivery. The woman is usually told to come to hospital at about 38 weeks, in case of early labour. If complications arise, she is admitted immediately.

Care and birth plans are developed in collaboration with the mother and the multidisciplinary team or a skilled midwife. These include:

▶ regular Hb checks
▶ observations for pre-eclampsia and UTIs
▶ checking of the abdominal girth at the level of the umbilicus (the fundal height is not reliable after 32–34 weeks)
▶ monitoring of fetal well-being through a non-stress test (NST) (simultaneously for two fetuses, with different NST machines), ultrasound and biophysical profiles.

Delivery of multiple fetuses

The decision for a vaginal birth depends on the lie, presentation (see figures 24.5 and 24.6 on page 355 and 356) and size of the fetuses, previous deliveries and the parity of the woman. If complications such as anaemia, pre-eclampsia and placenta praevia are present or the fetuses are compromised, vaginal delivery is contraindicated.

In a percentage of women, the second baby may only be diagnosed after the first one is born. If it is a known twin pregnancy, it is advisable that the woman deliver in an institution where medical assistance is available, with a theatre and a neonatal unit. In the case of triplets or more fetuses, special care is required, with a paediatrician and midwife for each baby.

The first stage

It is essential that the delivery takes place in a hospital, where all the necessary personnel and equipment are at hand should any emergency arise. Induction of labour (IOL) is usually undertaken because of evidence of better outcomes if the delivery occurs at 37–38 weeks.

The position and presenting part of the leading twin is important if a vaginal birth is considered. The uterine contractions may be hypotonic due to the overstretched uterus, yet dilatation may be good if the presenting part is a vertex and it is well applied (see Figure 24.5 on page 355).

Common complications include:

▶ delay in the delivery of the second twin
▶ transverse lie of the second twin
▶ intrapartum haemorrhage between the delivery of the first twin and the second twin (see Chapter 22)
▶ cord prolapse.

Because of these possible complications, the following should always be done:

▶ The midwife and the medical practitioner must carefully palpate the patient and make sure that the lie of both twins is longitudinal.
▶ There should be continuous fetal monitoring.
▶ Blood should be sent for cross-matching.
▶ An IV infusion is started and the type and the amount of fluids are given according to the medical practitioner's orders. (A vacolitre of IV fluid with oxytocin is erected 'piggy-back' so that it is available if and when it should be necessary.) Oxytocin is avoided, if possible, before the birth of the first twin.
▶ The operating theatre should be available at all times for a possible emergency Caesarean section.
▶ Large doses of analgesia and heavy sedation are to be avoided. Epidural analgesia is the best means of analgesia in this instance, as any necessary manipulations can then be easily carried out.
▶ Very careful observations are made frequently, using a partogram. Any abnormalities are immediately reported to the medical practitioner.
▶ Position the woman to avoid inferior vena cava syndrome (IVCS).
▶ When the membranes rupture, a vaginal examination must be done to:
  • exclude cord prolapse
  • determine the presenting part
  • determine the effacement and dilatation of the cervical os.
▶ Preparations are made for the delivery and all the necessary equipment made available for the babies, who may very well be preterm and/or SGA. This includes

resuscitation equipment, suction and oxygen, incubators and name tags, and a midwife and paediatrician per baby.

▶ The woman is prepared mentally and physically for the delivery. She is reassured and the procedure is carefully explained to her.

▶ Consent is obtained for an operation, should this be necessary. The patient is carefully put into a wedged lithotomy position and the bladder is emptied, if she has been unable to pass urine.

▶ In twin delivery, the labour is usually shorter than normal: about six hours. If the progress is slow, the cause must be identified and remedied.

The delivery

A multiple pregnancy should be delivered by an obstetrician or skilled midwife. If more than two babies are in the womb, or in the case of abnormal presentation, the birth is usually by Caesarean section. However, if no medical practitioner is available, the midwife must know exactly what to do. A paediatrician should be present at the delivery.

The procedure is as follows:
1. An episiotomy is performed for preterm or breech delivery.
2. The first baby is delivered and the time is noted.
3. The baby is identified as number one, and the name is checked with the mother.
4. The umbilical cord is immediately clamped in two places and cut between the clamps. This is very important should there be uniovular twins.
5. Once the first baby is in a satisfactory condition, the mother's abdomen is immediately palpated to determine the lie of the second twin.
6. If the lie is longitudinal, the presentation and position are determined.
7. The fetal heart is checked.
8. The woman is kept warm and the conditions of the mother and fetus are carefully observed while waiting for the contractions to recommence.
9. The contractions usually recommence soon after the first baby is born. However, if they have not recommenced after five to seven minutes, the mother's abdomen is again palpated to make sure the lie is still longitudinal. The delay in the onset of the contractions of the second twin may be up to two hours as long as the fetal heart is normal. If the presenting part is not descending, the bladder is emptied and the doctor will turn on the IV oxytocic infusion, which will cause the uterine contractions to recommence.
10. A vaginal examination is done to make sure of the presentation.

11. The membranes are ruptured carefully, to ensure the cord does not prolapse. This should also stimulate the uterus to contract.
12. The second baby is delivered and the time noted. This baby has been deprived of some oxygen while *in utero* after the birth of the first twin and, in addition, this twin has passed rapidly through the dilated cervix and down the distended birth canal, so the staff should be prepared for an asphyxiated baby. The second twin is nearly always at greater risk than the first twin and therefore receives special attention and care during and after the delivery.
13. The baby is identified as number two, the cord is cut, the airways cleared and respiration established.
14. A final abdominal palpation should be done to ensure that there are no further babies before the active management of the third stage of labour (AMTSL) is undertaken.
15. For medicolegal reasons, the end of each baby's cord must be clearly identified (ligature and clamp) to enable identification of the cord blood of each baby after delivery.

The third stage

There is a very real danger of PPH and the third stage must be actively managed. A very careful watch is kept for bleeding in the first 24 hours, as there is a very large placental site and often at least part of the placenta is in the lower segment, where there are fewer criss-cross muscle fibres to control postpartum bleeding. Any episiotomy or perineal tears are sutured.

Care of the babies

The following special care is given in line with the standard care of newborns:
▶ These babies are frequently SGA as well as preterm and therefore must be nursed in a high-care unit until their condition is satisfactory.
▶ A full examination is carried out on each baby for any birth injury and for any congenital abnormality.
▶ A full examination is also made of the placenta and the membranes, to try to determine whether the twins are uniovular or binovular.
▶ If the babies are preterm at birth, the use of artificial surfactant may be necessary to prevent or minimise hyaline membrane disease (HMD).
▶ The mother will require extra care when breastfeeding or when bottle-feeding these babies.

Emergency care in an undiagnosed or unplanned delivery

The following procedure should be followed if no doctor is available or in the case of an unexpected or unplanned twin delivery:

1. If the mother should present at the clinic in labour with the first twin almost delivered as either a vertex or a breech and with the second twin as a transverse, the first twin should be delivered.
2. Immediately after, if a spontaneous version to a longitudinal lie has not taken place, an ECV must be attempted at once, taking great care not to rupture the membranes.
3. Once the lie is longitudinal, a vaginal examination is performed to make sure of the presentation.
4. If it is a vertex (or a breech), the membranes are ruptured and the head allowed to enter the pelvis.
5. If ECV is unsuccessful and the lie is still transverse, the midwife should send for a doctor urgently, or immediately transfer the woman to a hospital.
6. If the membranes have ruptured while attempting the ECV, but the version is unsuccessful and the baby is still a transverse lie, the midwife should immediately do an internal podalic version (IPV) and deliver the baby as a breech.

Intrapartum haemorrhage

When intrapartum haemorrhage occurs, the objective is to deliver the second baby as quickly as possible. This is done both for the sake of the baby, who will suffer from a lack of oxygen, and for the mother's sake, as she could bleed to death.

The first baby has already been delivered, the placenta has started to separate, and the second baby is preventing the uterus from contracting and retracting in order to control the bleeding:

▶ If no medical practitioner is available, the midwife must make sure the lie of the second twin is longitudinal and then rupture the membranes immediately.
▶ The woman is encouraged to bear down and the baby is delivered. Fundal pressure may have to be used to help get the baby out quickly, if the bleeding is excessive.
▶ In very rare instances, the birth of the first twin is immediately followed by the birth of the placenta. This will result in extensive bleeding, as the uterus will be unable to contract, and the second baby must be delivered immediately.
▶ IM ergometrin is given immediately after the birth.
▶ AMTSL is performed.

▶ An oxytocin infusion 20 IU in 1 ℓ Ringer's solution is *in situ*. Alternatively, misopostrol 600 mcg can be administered rectally.

24.7   Intrauterine death

Definition and incidence

IUD is the death of the fetus after viability and before or during labour. This is called a stillbirth. If the fetal heart was present at the start of birth, it is called a fresh stillbirth.

Early IUD (before 20 weeks' gestation) usually leads to a spontaneous abortion. However, occasionally the dead fetus is retained. This is called a missed abortion.

The stillbirth rate is included in the PNMR, but when considered separately, it is estimated at 29/1 000 births in developing countries versus 3/1 000 live births in developed countries (WHO, 2006b).

Causes and predisposing factors

The predisposing causes of IUD can be divided into those that occur during pregnancy and those that arise during labour:
▶ During pregnancy:
  • *Maternal:* chronic conditions such as gestational diabetes, chronic nephritis, infections, TORCH, HIV and others, for example sexually transmitted infections (STIs), typhoid, malaria, cholera, Rh incompatibility (isoimmunisation) and medication
  • *Obstetric:* chorioamnionitis, accidents or trauma during pregnancy
  • *Placental pathology:* APH, placental abruption, oligohydramnios and amniotic bands, placental insufficiency.
▶ During labour:
  • *Cord factors:* short cord, cord around the neck, cord prolapse, true knots
  • *Complications:* prolonged and obstructed labour, malpresentations, anaesthetics, uterine rupture and maternal death.

Pathology

The fetus dies when the placental blood circulation to the fetus ceases and the fetal heart stops. Stasis of the blood at the placental site causes the clotting of blood and fibrinogen is activated to protect the mother from the clots. Eventually, the fibrinogen will be exhausted and disseminated intravascular coagulation (DIC) may develop within a period of weeks.

Maceration of the fetus starts within six hours after IUD. Aseptic autolysis takes place and pockets of dark-coloured fluid accumulate under the skin of the fetus. The tissue gradually disintegrates, causing the skin to peel off the tissue. The placenta and fetus may be green due to the presence of meconium. Fluid gradually accumulates in all the tissues and gas accumulates in the circulatory system. The longer the fetus remains *in utero*, the more grossly macerated it becomes. The skeleton of the fetus collapses, as there is no longer any tissue to hold it together. The fetal skull bones begin to overlap one another.

At some stage during the three weeks after IUD has occurred, in 70–90 per cent of cases labour starts spontaneously and a macerated fetus is expelled. If spontaneous labour does not occur within four weeks, there is an increased risk of maternal DIC, which can result in severe maternal bleeding.

Diagnosis

History

▶ There is a history of decreased or no fetal movement (kick chart).
▶ Sometimes, a brownish vaginal discharge is present.
▶ There are predisposing factors present, such as pre-eclampsia, infections and congenital abnormalities.
▶ The NST is non-reassuring.

Clinical findings

▶ The size of the uterus is less than that suggested by the EDD.
▶ The uterine size (the height of the fundus) has failed to increase since the previous visit (no increase in abdominal girth around the umbilicus).
▶ Depending on the period of death, the fetus may not be felt on abdominal palpation.

Confirmation of death

▶ No fetal heart can be heard with the Pinard fetoscope.
▶ In cases where IUD is suspected and the fetal heart is not audible, ultrasound is indicated (see below).
▶ The use of sonicaid and CTG to hear the fetal heart creates enormous anxiety in the woman and is not conclusive. If ultrasound is not available, X-rays will be diagnostic (see below).

Ultrasound

A diagnosis is made when the following signs are present:
▶ The fetal heart is not detected, there is no fetal breathing and there is no fetal movement.
▶ The biparietal diameter (BPD) shows no increase in growth at weekly intervals after 30 weeks.
▶ There is a 'fluffy' contour and/or a double skeleton outline.

▶ There is loss of fetal structure, with a collapsed thorax and misshapen skull.
▶ Multiple intracranial echoes appear; a double skull.
▶ There is an abnormal reduction in liquor.
▶ Gas is seen in the fetal circulatory system, commonly in the heart, the aorta, the portal veins and the umbilical veins. This may be seen as early as 12 hours after IUD. The nature and the origin of this are uncertain, but the gas is probably carbon dioxide. This is known as Robert's sign. The gas can also be seen in the heart, the liver, the cord, the abdominal cavity and the large blood vessels.
▶ There is loss of muscle tone and the fetus appears 'rolled up', with either hyperextension of the head or angulations of the fetal spine. This is known as Ball's sign: the thoracic cage collapses, the ribs concertina together, there is hyperflexion of the spine and softening of the ligaments.

X-rays

A diagnosis is made when the following signs are present:
▶ A positive Spalding's sign is seen: there is overlapping and angulation of the cranial bones. This may also be apparent after a week of IUD. Later, there is gross overlapping of the skull bones due to shrinkage of the brain.
▶ The 'halo' sign may be seen, where a halo is evident around the skull of the dead fetus. However, this may also be observed in erythroblastosis fetalis in a live fetus. The cause of this image on X-ray is the infiltration of fluid beneath the scalp.
▶ There is gas visible in the gastrointestinal system.

Treatment and care

Identify the women and fetuses at risk and intervene in time to prevent IUD. The woman needs to know early warning signs and to come to the clinic if any of these occur. Women at risk are admitted to hospital under medical supervision.

Quality antenatal care protocols, early access, standard screening, referral for medical care and vigilant monitoring of fetal well-being is needed to prevent stillbirths. In spite of the highest quality of antenatal care, fetuses sometimes die for unknown reasons in pregnancy. When a fetus dies in labour (a fresh stillbirth), this generally indicates poor-quality care.

Refer for a medical opinion immediately if IUD is suspected. The doctor can diagnose and confirm the death by ultrasound. The midwife supports the patient. Once the death of the baby is confirmed, the midwife must follow protocol and medical management. She will have to provide the patient and her husband or partner with all the psychological support they might need.

Obstetric management

There is no medical urgency for the delivery of the fetus if no risk factors, such as hypertension, are present. If the woman is near term or the cervix is favourable, IOL can be done. A Caesarean section is seldom performed for a dead fetus, unless the mother's life is in danger. A woman can be given the choice of waiting for birth to start spontaneously. If she does not go into labour within the first three weeks after the fetus has died, the medical practitioner will terminate the pregnancy because of the danger of a severe clotting defect arising.

Allowing the woman to go into labour spontaneously may have the psychological advantage of giving the mother time to mourn the loss of the baby. The disadvantage is the risk of DIC and the maceration of the fetus, making it difficult for the parents to see the fetus at birth. A fetus delivered within 24 hours of death may still look normal.

Blood is taken for platelets and fibrinogen levels. A fibrinogen level of less than 1 (100 mg/dl) is abnormal. If there is a defect, appropriate blood component therapy is given before the pregnancy is terminated.

In most instances, induce labour by first giving prostaglandins to ripen the cervix. Misopostrol is used to start labour. The midwife must monitor the patient very carefully because large doses may be necessary and there is a danger of uterine rupture.

Delay amniotomy until the patient is in well-established labour. This is done to avoid the risk of infection, as these patients often have long labours and this keeps the pressure on the cervix equal. The birth tends to be more painful. The presenting part collapses on the cervix and does not open the cervix fully. A part of the fetus may be expelled before the woman is fully dilated. Provide the woman with analgesia, such as morphine 10–20 mg IM and promethazine 25 mg IM 4-hourly if necessary. Antibiotics are given if the membranes have been ruptured for more than 6–12 hours.

General management and care during labour

All the normal principles of care in labour still apply. The significant person or partner or husband is allowed to attend the birth if they wish to do so.

After delivery, the parents are offered the chance to see the baby, with support from the staff. The baby is then removed, examined and weighed, as are the placenta and membranes. Histological examination of the fetus and the placenta may be required to establish the cause of death. The baby and the placenta will be sent to the nearest laboratory for investigation. The placenta and membranes are examined for completeness. If incomplete, a uterine evacuation will be done. The cervix and perineum are inspected for any tears.

The baby, if viable by definition, will be treated as a stillbirth. All the necessary forms will have to be filled in and signed and the baby will have to be buried. If the baby is not viable by definition, it does not have to be buried – unless the parents wish to do so – but can be incinerated. The parents must give permission and complete the legal forms.

The mother can be discharged within six hours depending on her condition. Lactation should be suppressed. The woman is told of the importance of attending a postnatal examination in six weeks' time, when she can also discuss family planning and, if necessary, be referred for genetic counselling.

The local health clinic is notified about the stillbirth, so that they can visit the mother and check up on her progress and condition.

24.8 Parity, gravidity, obesity and teenage pregnancy

Grand multiparity

Grand multiparity refers to women who have had five or more viable babies. These women are also known as 'dangerous multiparae' and form part of the high-risk group of patients. They are susceptible to a number of serious complications, which are often unsuspected. It is extremely important, therefore, that they deliver in hospital under expert obstetric and midwifery care.

Complications of grand multiparity

During the antenatal period, the following complications can occur in grand multiparae:

- *Age:* These are often older women, who are more likely to develop complications and genetic disorders, for example babies with Down's syndrome.
- *Obesity:* These patients can be obese, making assessment of the EDD difficult. Physical examinations are difficult. Obesity leads to lordosis and, together, these problems carry increased risks.
- *Social conditions:* These women are more likely to be poor, overworked, tired, anaemic and malnourished. They often neglect themselves and subsequently suffer from dental caries, infections, and so forth.
- *Medical problems:* There is a great risk of developing hypertensive disease in pregnancy, diabetes, chronic renal disease, thromboembolism and cardiac disease.
- *Abortion:* There is an increased risk of abortion due to malnutrition.

▶ *Problems with the placenta:* Placental abruption and placenta praevia occur more frequently in this group of women.

▶ *Preterm birth:* This group is at great risk of going into early or preterm labour.

▶ *Disorders:* The minor disorders of pregnancy are often exaggerated.

▶ *Multiple pregnancy:* This is more common, greatly adding to the risks.

▶ *Anaemia:* Due to poor diet and repeated hydraemias (haemodilution) of pregnancy, which is a physiological state, anaemia occurs more frequently. However, with advancing maternal age, poor spacing of pregnancies and breastfeeding for many years with no break, iron deficiency anaemia can become a problem.

▶ *CPD:* Babies tend to grow larger with each pregnancy, causing CPD.

▶ *Malpresentations:* These are common, due to a pendulous abdomen. This can lead to PROM.

▶ *Older age group:* Women in the older age group are susceptible to cancer of the cervix.

During labour, grand multiparae can suffer from the following complications:

▶ *Malpresentations:* Brow, face and transverse lie are relatively common and lead to prolonged and obstructed labour.

▶ *PROM:* This is a result of malpresentation and can lead to a prolapsed cord and to acute fetal distress, thus increasing the rate of perinatal mortality.

▶ *Precipitate labour:* This may occur, leading to traumatic PPH and possible cerebral damage to the fetus if the delivery is uncontrolled.

▶ *Shoulder dystocia:* This occurs because of large babies (on the whole, each successive baby is a little bigger than the last).

▶ *Haemorrhage:* PPH can occur due to tired and overstretched atonic uterine muscles.

▶ *Obstructive labour:* This may result from a large fetus or pendulous abdomen with a malpresentation.

▶ *Rupture of the uterus:* The uterus can rupture as a result of strong contractions and obstructed labour, leading to an increased maternal mortality rate.

▶ *Placenta:* Adherent placenta is common.

▶ *Surgical interventions:* There is an increased Caesarean section rate due to CPD as a result of the larger babies.

The following complications can arise in grand multiparity during the puerperium:

▶ *Infection:* Sepsis is common due to the high incidence of complications and the consequent interference and manipulations in labour.

▶ *Breastfeeding:* There is a reduced ability to breastfeed successfully, due to tiredness, anaemia and the complications of pregnancy.

▶ *Maternal mortality:* Complications such as shock and PPH increase the maternal mortality rate.

Care and management

Women who are grand multiparae need to be seen regularly during pregnancy to exclude complications associated with grand multiparity. The women are referred to deliver in a hospital with a medical practitioner, a theatre and a neonatologist due to high perinatal mortality and morbidity.

The patient is taught possible danger signals (without alarming her unduly) and she is encouraged to watch for these and to report promptly at the clinic should she be concerned at any time. Friendly, helpful, caring and concerned midwives will help to allay this patient's fears and to build up her confidence in the midwife's ability to care for her and the family.

Specific considerations in labour include the following:

▶ IV therapy is started once the patient is in labour. The medical practitioner may want to take blood for cross-matching in case a blood transfusion should be necessary, depending on how the labour progresses.

▶ Careful, accurate monitoring of the mother and continuous electronic monitoring of the fetus are essential.

▶ Oxytocin is seldom administered to a multigravid woman in labour, due to the risk of the uterus rupturing. However, should the need arise, great care must be taken to monitor the contractions. A low dosage of 2 IU oxytocin in 1 ℓ is used and controlled by the use of an infusion pump.

▶ Labour is monitored using the partogram. Any problem, or suspected problem, must be reported to the medical practitioner immediately.

▶ Caesarean section is performed if there is no progress in labour, or if CPD develops.

▶ The third stage of labour is actively managed, and careful observations are carried out with regard to PPH. An infusion with 20 IU oxytocin is maintained for 24 hours.

In the puerperium, specific considerations regarding care include the following:

▶ Observe for PPH.

▶ Check for anaemia before discharge.

▶ Observe for thrombosis.

▶ Help, advise and support with breastfeeding and with baby care are necessary. Plenty of sleep and rest, followed by exercises, are encouraged.

▶ Family planning is discussed. If consent is obtained, tubal ligation can be performed while the patient is still in hospital.

Elderly primigravidae

First-time pregnancy is always considered a risk, regardless of age and other contributing factors. High-risk primigravidae should be encouraged to deliver in a hospital. Primigravidae have a higher risk for long labour, may require more pain relief, experience more abnormal uterine activity and need more surgical interventions.

The elderly primigravida is a woman who is having her first child when she is over the age of 35 years. Advanced maternal age refers to women giving birth at an advanced age and it carries several risk factors. This woman is part of the high-risk pregnancy group of women.

This pregnancy is usually very important for a number of reasons. One of the main reasons is that the woman is less likely to fall pregnant subsequently, so this pregnancy is probably very important to her and to her partner.

Women have their first baby late in life for two main reasons: infertility, or delayed motherhood due to late marriage or because the woman chose to develop her career first.

Complications of the elderly primigravida

During the antenatal period, the following complications can occur:

▶ *Age:* As previously stated, there is a reduced chance of the woman having more pregnancies due to her age.

▶ *Problems with the placenta:* There is an increased risk of placental insufficiency, resulting in IUGR.

▶ *Medical problems:* These women are at risk for developing hypertensive disease in pregnancy.

▶ *Disorders:* There is an increased risk of chromosomal or genetic disorders resulting in a congenital abnormality, for example Down's syndrome (see the box on this page).

▶ *Uterine fibroids:* These are more likely to be present.

The elderly primigravida might present with the following complications during labour:

▶ *Risk:* There is an increased risk of operative deliveries and manual removal of the placenta.

▶ *CPD:* This is common, resulting in an increased incidence of Caesarean section.

▶ *Prolonged labour:* Due to joints not being able to give well during labour, there is an increased chance of a prolonged labour.

▶ *Uterine inertia:* This is more likely to occur in the elderly primigravida.

▶ *Birth injuries:* Owing to the increased risk of operative deliveries and/or manipulations, there is also an increased risk of birth injuries to the baby.

In the puerperium, the elderly primigravida might present with complications related to the following:

▶ *Breastfeeding:* There is a reduced ability to breastfeed, which is associated with increased breast and breastfeeding problems in the puerperium.

▶ *Maternal factors:* If the pregnancy was delayed due to career choices, the risk of postnatal depression may exist.

Care and management

It is important that the elderly primigravida is identified early in pregnancy and that a careful watch is kept on her progress antenatally. Prenatal screening is important. Specific attention is given to the 16 weeks Triple test, the fluorescent *in situ* hybridisation (FISH) test at 20 weeks or amniocentesis to rule out Down's syndrome or other abnormalities for women over the age of 37.

The risk of a Down's syndrome child
The risk of having a Down's syndrome child increases with maternal age. A woman 45 years of age is 100 times more likely to have an affected child than a 19-year-old. The global incidence for Down's syndrome in 1:800 births (Psychology Wiki, nd).

Ideally, ultrasound is done at 12 or 20 weeks to rule out fetal abnormalities. Any complications must be identified promptly, so they can be assessed and treated by the medical practitioner as early as possible. Amniocentesis is often carried out at 16 weeks to check for fetal abnormalities.

The elderly primigravida should not be allowed to go post-dates and needs to be referred for medical care if birth has not spontaneously commenced.

Care during labour

The elderly primigravida should always deliver in hospital. Since elderly primigravidae are not allowed to go post-term, they are often induced (if no contraindications exist) to avoid additional risks to the mother and the fetus. Labour is monitored in the usual way. Analgesia is provided according to the woman's wishes, and a birth companion should be present if she so wishes.

Care after birth

The elderly primigravida should be encouraged to breastfeed and be provided with support where necessary.

Gross obesity

Obesity is a body mass of 20 per cent in excess of normal weight for height. However, during pregnancy a pre-pregnant weight of 90 kg or more is considered to be obese. There is no evidence of increased maternal or perinatal mortality related to obesity, but there may be several difficulties with the birth and the postnatal period.

The complications of gross obesity

The risks associated with obesity relate to medical complications and complications in birth and during the postnatal period.

There is the possibility of miscalculation of the EDD in obese women due to irregular menses. There are also difficulties with accurate abdominal palpation and pelvic assessment due to adipose tissue. Other complications are:

▶ increased incidence of malpresentations and difficulty diagnosing this because of the obesity
▶ difficulty hearing the fetal heart
▶ hypertension and pre-eclampsia
▶ diabetes mellitus
▶ large babies (usually) and therefore an increased incidence of prolonged labour
▶ the increased risk for surgical interventions, complicated by the risks of general and regional anaesthesia
▶ an increased risk of thromboembolism, as obese women are relatively immobile
▶ a possible failure to lactate adequately
▶ poor wound healing, if complications of diabetes mellitus and infections are present
▶ hypoxia because of soft tissue obstruction and difficult endotracheal intubation.

Obstetric management risks

▶ The patient is referred to a dietitian for nutritional counselling. Carefully explain to the woman that she should gain no more than 0.25 kg a week.
▶ An assessment is done to make sure that the date of the last menstrual period (LMP) and therefore the EDD are accurate.

▶ An early ultrasound is performed, if possible, at 18–20 weeks to confirm the diagnosis of pregnancy and to confirm the EDD.
▶ A glucose tolerance test (GTT) is done to eliminate the possibility of diabetes mellitus.
▶ Thorough examinations are done frequently to identify complications.
▶ A repeat ultrasound is done at 32 weeks.
▶ Re-evaluate the patient's eating habits. Give advice on diet and eating habits, to reinforce the counselling of the dietitian. It may be necessary to admit the patient to hospital and place her on a diet.
▶ Encourage, support and reassure the patient.
▶ Check the woman's social history and deal with any problems with hygiene.

Management risks in labour

▶ Palpation and auscultation are difficult in labour. There is often soft tissue dystocia, with uterine inertia, leading to prolonged labour.
▶ A delayed diagnosis of obesity in pregnancy can lead to rupture of the uterus and shoulder-girdle dystocia because of large babies.
▶ An IV line should be set up.
▶ There is an increased incidence of Mendelson's gastric aspiration syndrome because of increased volume and acidity of the gastric juices and difficulty intubating if required.
▶ There is often prolonged recovery from general anaesthetic.
▶ There may be protracted post-anaesthesia analgesia, due to fat solubility of anaesthetic agents.
▶ There are technical difficulties with spinals and epidurals.
▶ The third stage of labour must be actively managed to prevent PPH.

Management risks in the puerperium

▶ Early ambulation is encouraged, to prevent complications such as thrombosis.
▶ Referral to a physiotherapist may be necessary for deep breathing exercises.
▶ Specific attention is given to breastfeeding.
▶ If surgery was performed, pay attention to wound care and be alert for thrombophlebitis, pulmonary embolus, post-operative infections, post-operative atelectasis, pneumonia, a longer recovery period and wound dehiscence.

Teenage pregnancy (early motherhood)

Definition and incidence

Early motherhood, also referred to as adolescent pregnancy, is pregnancy before 18 years of age. (The ideal period – physiologically – for reproduction is 19–35 years.)

The incidence of teenage pregnancy in South Africa is 25 per cent or 350:1 000 births, with figures varying between urban and rural populations (Wikipedia, 2016b). Increased sexual activity among adolescents is manifested in increased teenage pregnancies and an increase in STIs.

Risks of early motherhood

Pregnant adolescents are at risk due to their physical, psychological, social and economic circumstances. Pregnant teenagers face many of the same obstetric risks as other pregnant women, but with more intensive risks. Teenagers under the age of 15 have additional medical concerns, as their physical development is not mature enough to sustain a healthy pregnancy or to give birth. Risks for teenagers aged 15–18 are higher than in normal pregnancies of older mothers, with socioeconomic factors likely to play a role.

A pregnant adolescent also presents a special case of intensive nutrient needs, as the teenager may already have a poor diet. Many teenagers enter pregnancy with a deficiency of nutrients that puts themselves and their fetus at risk. Adequate nutrition is thus an indispensable component of the special care for pregnant teenagers. They need emotional support and counselling as well and close monitoring.

The risks associated with teenage pregnancy include the following:
- *Obstetric risks:* These include low birth weight (LBW), miscarriage, stillbirth, premature labour and pre-eclampsia, which can cause cardiovascular and kidney problems in later life. Caesarean section is also more common, as well as maternal death.
- *Medical risks:* Teenagers are more likely to suffer from anaemia and hypertension, as well as a deficiency of nutrients that puts themselves and their fetus at risk.

Pregnant teens are less likely to receive prenatal care, often seeking it only in the third trimester.
- *Socioeconomic and psychological risks:* A pregnant teenager's financial status and support systems are often poor. Malnutrition is a risk, as the majority of adolescents tend to come from lower-income households and have poor eating habits. If the teenager has to drop out of school, this ultimately threatens future opportunities and economic prospects.
- *Neonatal:* Teenage mothers have a tendency to prematurity, with LBW newborns.

Management of teenage pregnancy

The management of teenage pregnancy is that of any normal (or abnormal) pregnancy. However, prevention is important and family planning advice needs to be given while the girl is at the clinic or in hospital.

The focus should be on addressing the underlying reasons for adolescent pregnancy, such as poverty, gender inequality, social pressures and coercion. To address this, comprehensive sexuality education should be included for all young people, in an effort to prevent child marriage, sexual violence and pressure. This will also help to ensure access to sexual and reproductive health information for adolescents as well as give them information on services that welcome them and facilitate their choices.

As mentioned before, a pregnant adolescent may already have a poor diet, and therefore has special nutrient needs.

24.9   Conclusion

The common conditions that can complicate pregnancy were presented in this chapter. These include Rh haemolytic disease, ABO incompatibility, hyperemesis gravidarum, polyhydramnios and oligohydramnios, multiple pregnancies, grand multiparity, elderly primigravidae, obesity and teenage pregnancy. All pregnancy-related risks need to be referred for medical assessment, supervision and care.

Section Five

Birth

The physiology of the stages and processes of birth

LEARNING OBJECTIVES

On completion of this chapter, you must be able to:
- explain the physiology of the birth processes
- explain the onset of labour
- explain the physiology of all the stages of birth.

KNOWLEDGE ASSUMED TO BE IN PLACE

Physiology of pregnancy and normal reproductive physiology (see chapters 5 and 14)

KEYWORDS

spontaneous onset • show • engagement • latent phase • active phase • fundal dominance

25.1 Introduction

Labour and childbirth herald another developmental phase in the life of a woman and her family. The processes that occur are both physiological and psychological. Different women anticipate labour differently and so behave differently during labour.

The transition from pregnancy to motherhood is an enormous and unique physiological and psychological change in each woman. The physiological and anatomical changes in both the mother and fetus for the process of labour and extrauterine life will be discussed in this chapter.

25.2 The physiology of normal labour

Spontaneous onset of labour occurs between 37 completed weeks and 42 weeks, with the fetus presenting in the vertex. Ideally, normal labour will be completed within 18 hours, with both the mother and the infant in good physical and psychological condition. Various factors determine the duration of labour. Normal delivery is the natural physiological process of birth, with limited or no intervention.

The process of normal labour

Labour is a process in which the products of conception (fetus, placenta and membranes) are expelled from the birth canal.

The process is expected to occur at term, although it may occur before (preterm) or after term (post-term) (see Chapter 23).

The stages of labour

The duration of labour varies and is affected by both maternal and fetal factors such as parity, birth interval, psychological state of the mother and the type of pelvis, the type of contractions, the presentation and the position of the fetus.

Normal labour should not exceed 24 hours in a primigravida and 11 hours in a multipara. In general, primigravidae have longer first and second stages of labour than women who have already had at least one viable child and a vaginal delivery; this is because the tissue of the cervix, vagina and vulva and all other soft tissues in the pelvis, as well as the pelvic muscles, have not previously been subjected to the stretching that occurs when the fetus passes through the birth canal.

There is a typical time-related biological process in all normal labour, as shown in Figure 25.1 on the next page. This scientific observation assists with the interpretation of the process of labour and is the basis for the partogram.

Normal dilatation is predictable. It is important that midwives are able to competently assess that the phases and stages of birth are progressing normally. The use of the partogram to monitor labour assists midwives and other skilled birth attendants to identify deviations, such as prolonged and obstructed labour, early on.

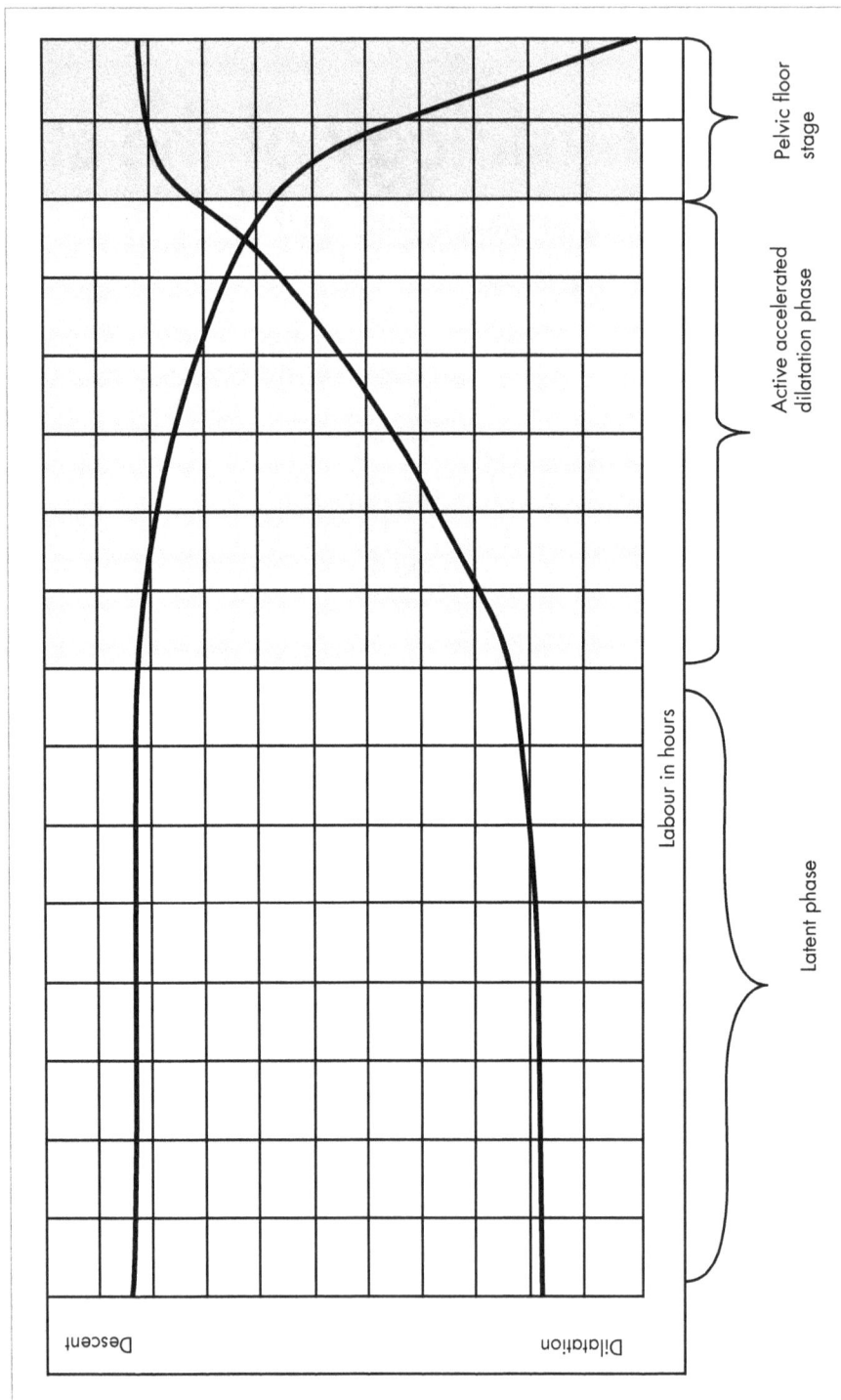

Figure 25.1 The typical parameters and functional divisions of labour illustrated on a time scale (adapted from Greenhill and Friedman, 1974)

Depending on the literature reviewed, three to four stages of labour are described. See Table 25.1 for a description of the four stages. Defining the stages of labour allows midwives and other skilled attendants to identify whether the progress of labour is normal or delayed.

Table 25.1

Stages of labour (Greenhill & Friedman, 1974)

Stages of labour	Duration
Stage 1 This is the period between the onset of labour up to full dilatation of the cervix. It is divided into two phases: *Phase I: Latent phase* – from the start of labour up to when the cervix is fully effaced and 3–4 cm dilated. *Phase II: Active phase* – from when the cervix is fully effaced to when the cervix is fully dilated.	Primigravidae: Lasts 8–18 hours Multiparae: Shorter Primigravidae: At a rate of 1 cm per hour Multiparae: At a rate of 1.5 cm per hour
Stage 2 This begins when the cervix is fully dilated and lasts until the time of the delivery (pelvic floor and perineal phases).	Primigravidae: Up to two hours Multiparae: Up to 45 minutes (30 minutes bearing-down effort)
Stage 3 This begins when the baby is delivered and lasts up to when the placenta and membranes are completely delivered, including control of vaginal bleeding.	The duration varies with the method used to manage the third stage. With active management, it is 5–15 minutes; with passive management it is up to 45–60 minutes.
Stage 4 This the period after the delivery of the placenta up to one hour post-delivery.	One hour

The four stages of labour are discussed in detail in sections 25.3 to 25.6.

The Ps of labour (also see Chapter 8)

The passage: The bony pelvis and related soft tissues should be adequate to accommodate the fetus.

The passenger: The size of the fetus in relation to the type of pelvis and degree of flexion (in a cephalic presentation) are of importance.

The powers: The uterine contractions should be rhythmic and must increase in duration and intensity.

The psyche/pain: Previous labour and childbirth experiences may affect the emotional well-being of the woman; tension can interfere with birth.

The physiological well-being of the mother and fetus: Risk factors can alter the course of labour.

continued

Professional assistance: Appropriate assistance of care by a skilled midwife or medical practitioner (referred to as skilled attendance) and a well-resourced environment that supports prompt intervention should the need arise will determine the outcome of care.

Factors that influence the onset of labour

The onset of labour is the most important phase in the management of labour, since it is on the basis of this that decisions are made that will guide the appropriate management of labour. A combination of hormonal and mechanical factors are involved. The midwife has an important role to play in providing the woman with information that will help her to recognise the signs of true labour, as explained in Table 25.2 on the next page.

Once the woman recognises the onset of labour, she must make contact with the skilled attendant.

> ### Signs of true labour
>
> Signs of true labour include regular rhythmic contractions accompanied by cervical effacement (in primigravidae) and dilatation of the cervix with or without rupture of membranes.

Table 25.2

Signs of true and false labour

Signs of true labour	Signs of false labour
The contractions are regular, rhythmic and painful and increase in intensity.	Contractions may be painful but not regular and do not increase in intensity.
While contractions increase in intensity, the intervals between contractions gradually shortens.	The interval between contractions varies.
Contractions intensify when the woman is up and about.	Pain from uterine contractions is often relieved by walking.
Show is present, as the operculum is shed.	Show is absent.
Effacement of the cervix takes place, accompanied by progressive dilatation of the cervix.	Effacement of the cervix takes place, but there is no accompanying dilatation of the cervix.

Hormonal effects

Certain hormones are involved in the onset of labour. The placenta produces progesterone and oestrogen during pregnancy. Progesterone has a relaxing effect on the uterine muscles, thereby inhibiting contractions.

As pregnancy reaches term, biochemical changes cause a decrease in the availability of progesterone to the uterine muscles and there is an increase in oestrogen, which has an effect on uterine contractions. Oestrogen increases the sensitivity of the myometrium to oxytocin and stimulates the production of prostaglandins. The synthesis of prostaglandins in the decidua, amnion and chorion, promoted by oestrogen, results in stimulation of uterine contractions because of the effect of prostaglandins on the smooth muscles.

Emotional and physical stressors stimulate the maternal hypothalamus, triggering the release of oxytocin. The mutually co-ordinated effects of oxytocin and prostaglandins on the smooth muscles initiate the rhythmic uterine contractions of true labour.

The fetal adrenal glands secrete large quantities of cortisol, which possibly cause the release of prostaglandins. Large quantities of prostaglandins are found in the amnion and are thought to originate from the membranes as well as from the decidua.

Mechanical stimulation

Uterine activity also occurs as a result of stimulation of the uterus and cervix. Smooth muscles usually contract when stretched; hence, the uterine muscles become sensitive to distension and contraction. The increased stretching of the uterine muscles by the increased intra-amniotic volume (enlarging fetus, placenta and the increased amounts of amniotic fluid) has an effect as pregnancy progresses.

The uterine muscles become more sensitive in the case of multiple pregnancy, polyhydramnios or when the presenting part is well applied to the cervix. Twins are often born two to three weeks earlier than a single fetus, which could partly be due to the increased stretch of the smooth muscle of the uterus as well as the double fetoplacental factors.

Cervical irritation and stretch

It is thought that cervical irritation and stretch of the lower segment play an important part in starting uterine contractions. When the presenting part is pressing onto the cervix and dilatation of the cervix is taking place, impulses are conducted to the neurohypophysis, causing the release of oxytocin (the Ferguson reflex).

When artificial rupture of the membranes (AROM) is performed, either to induce or accelerate labour, the presenting part is brought into direct contact with the cervix. This usually stimulates uterine activity. A well-fitting presenting part, exerting an even pressure and therefore a greater area of pressure on the cervix, appears to cause the best stimulation of uterine contractions.

False labour

Many women may experience strong, frequent, but irregular painful contractions. These are Braxton-Hicks contractions. They are real contractions which have not yet settled into the rhythmic pattern of true labour but which do cause discomfort to the woman. The contractions are not accompanied by effacement or dilatation of the cervix.

Earlier in pregnancy, all women should be told about these contractions so that they will not mistake them for true labour. Women who experience false labour should be reassured and they should be advised on when to report to hospital.

Descent of the head

Front view

Side views (from the right side)

Engaged

Increased flexion

On perineum

Front view

Note the twist in the neck

Descent of the head in the left occipitolateral (LOL) position changing to left occipitoanterior (LOA) position when the head reaches the pelvic floor.

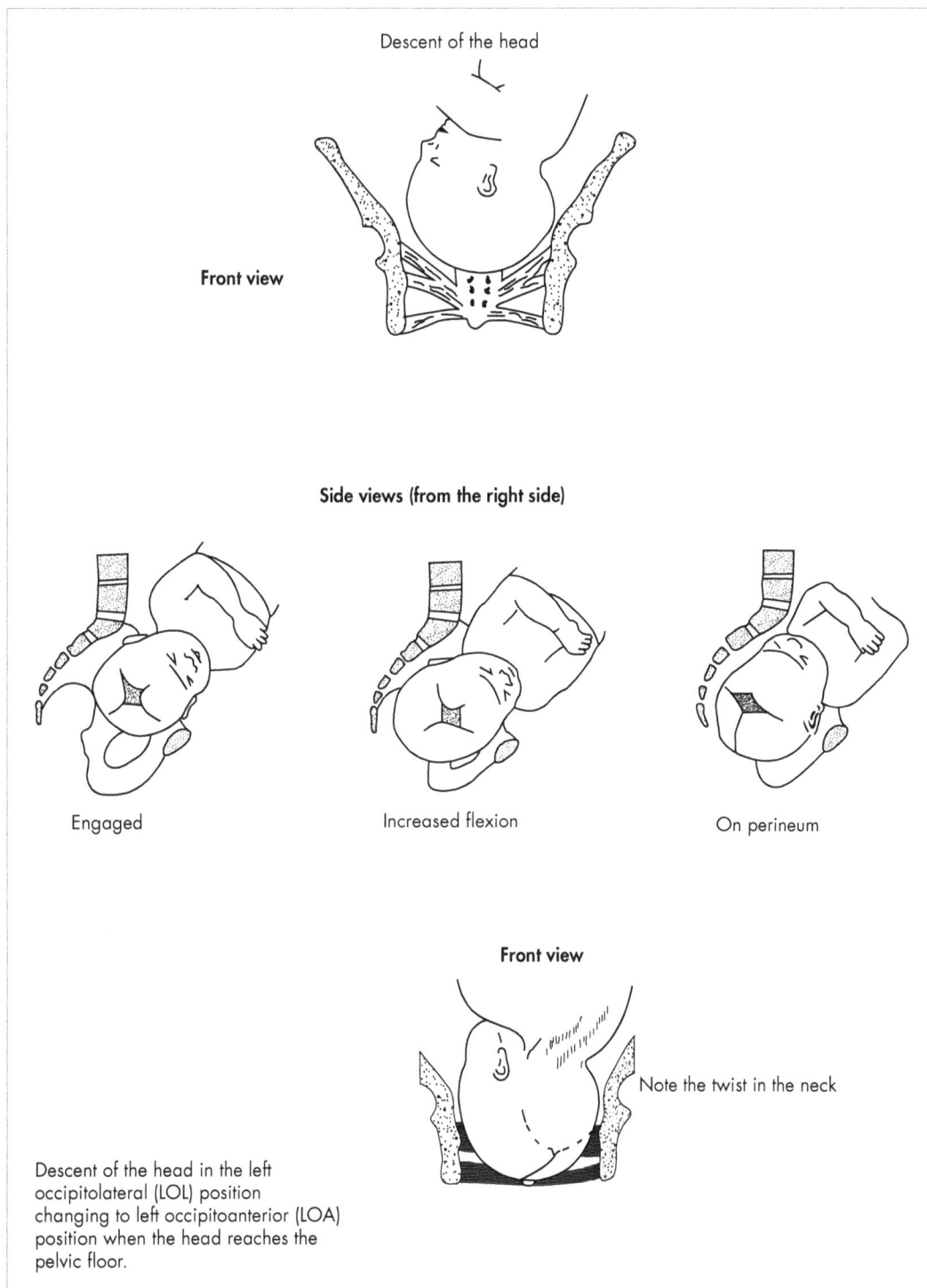

Figure 25.2 Mechanism of labour: Descent of the head with increased flexion (redrawn from Garrey et al, 1974)

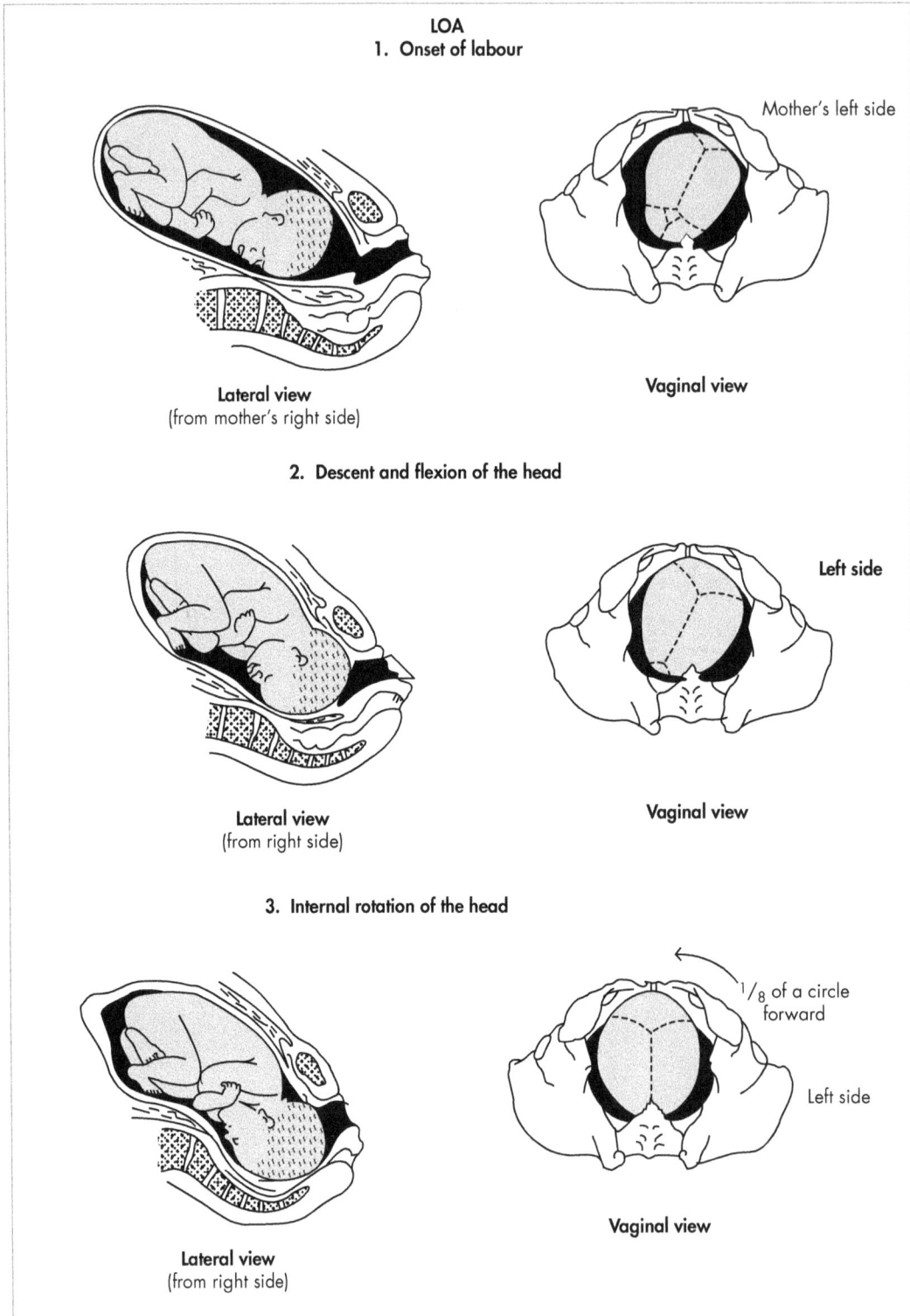

LOA
1. Onset of labour

Lateral view
(from mother's right side)

Vaginal view

Mother's left side

2. Descent and flexion of the head

Lateral view
(from right side)

Vaginal view

Left side

3. Internal rotation of the head

Lateral view
(from right side)

Vaginal view

¹/₈ of a circle forward

Left side

Figure 25.3 Mechanism of normal labour: LOA position

continued

4. Extension and crowning of the head

Lateral view
(from right side)

Left side

Vaginal view

**5. Birth of the head
(by extension)**

Lateral view
(from right side)

6. Restitution of the head

$^1/_8$ of a circle back

Left side

Vaainal view

7. External rotation of the head together with internal rotation of the shoulders

Lateral view
(from right side)

A further
$^1/_8$ of a circle
back

$^2/_8$ ($^1/_4$) of a
circle

Left side

Vaginal view

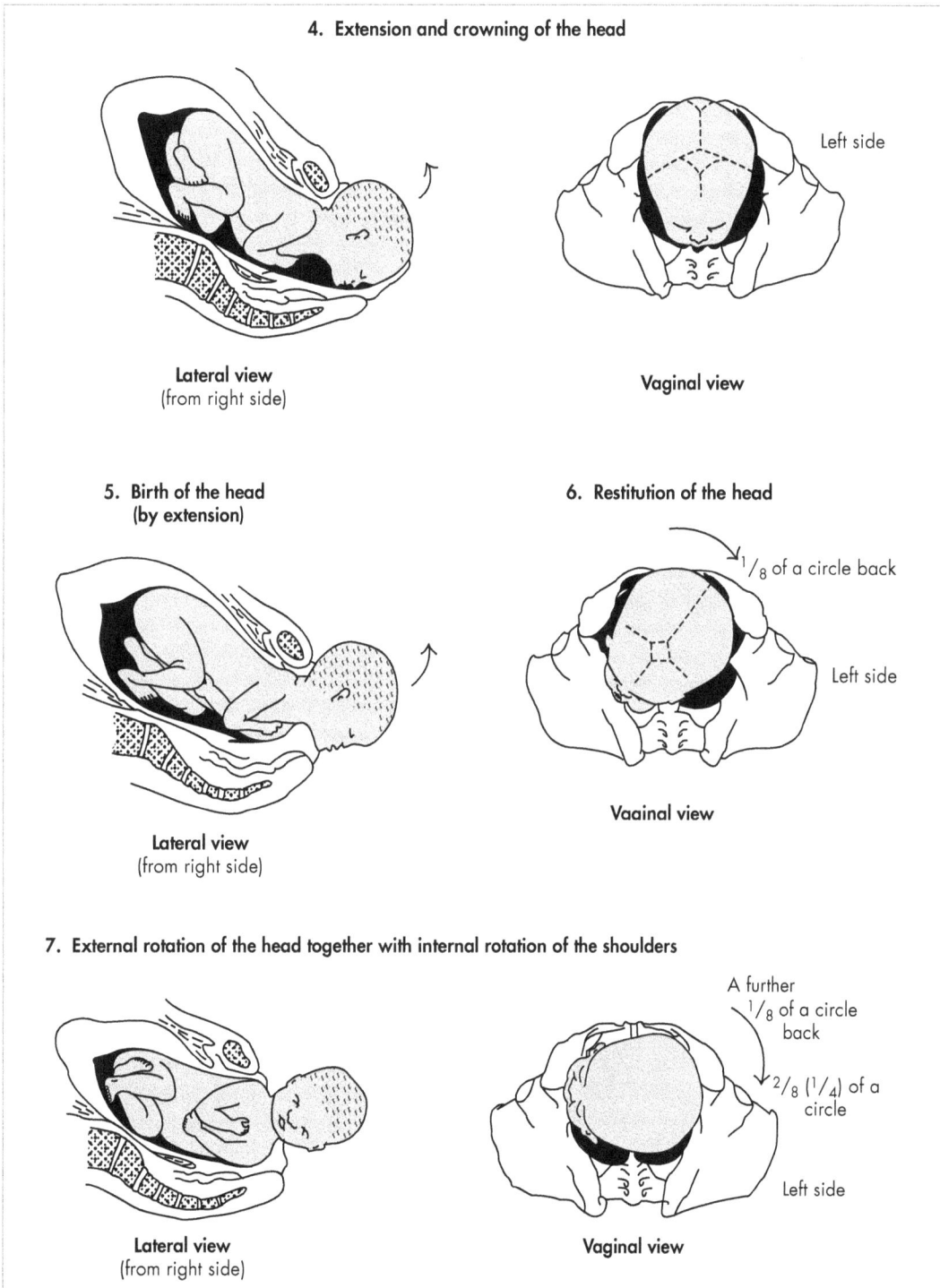

Figure 25.3 Mechanism of normal labour: LOA position

continued

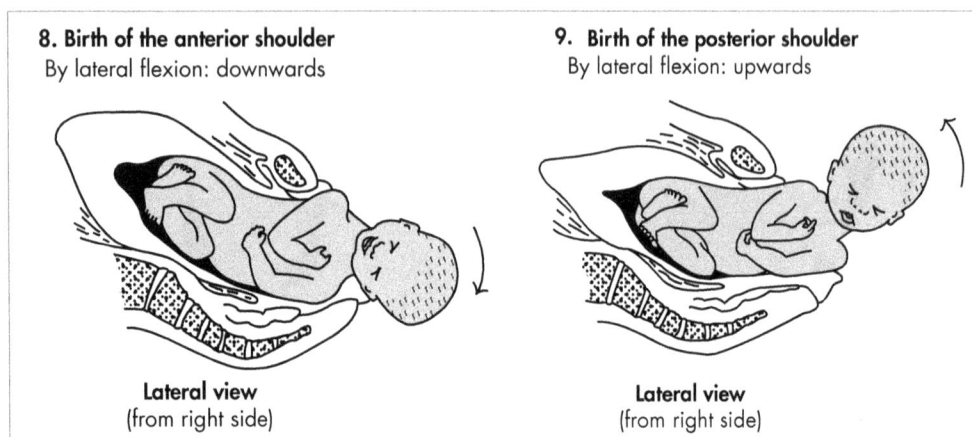

Figure 25.3 Mechanism of normal labour: LOA position

25.3 The physiology of the first stage of labour

From the seventh month of pregnancy, the uterus undergoes physiological changes in preparation for labour. Once labour has started, further changes occur in response to the action of uterine contractions. The first stage of labour starts with the onset of labour and lasts up to the time the cervix is fully dilated. The onset of labour starts when the woman experiences regular and rhythmic contractions, accompanied by dilatation of the cervix. Occasionally, some women complain of lower abdominal pain or backache. The dilatation of the cervix is expressed in centimetres (0–10 cm).

As shown in Table 25.1 on page 371, this stage is divided into two phases:

1. The *latent phase* is the period between the onset of labour to cervix dilatation of 3–4 cm. The cervix becomes fully effaced during this period. Cervical effacement (taking up of the cervix) is a process in which the cervix shortens and becomes incorporated into the lower uterine segment. Taking up of the cervix starts towards the end of pregnancy in a primigravida and is only complete by the end of the latent phase, while in multiparous women effacement and dilatation of the cervix may occur simultaneously. Therefore, progress of cervical dilatation in nulliparous women is only possible when the cervix is fully effaced. In a primigravida, the latent phase lasts 3–8 hours; this phase is shorter in multiparous women.

2. The *active phase* starts from the time the cervix is 4 cm dilated up to when the cervix is fully dilated, which is 10 cm. During this phase, the cervix dilates more rapidly: at a rate of 1 cm per hour in a primigravida and 1.5 cm in a multipara. Dilatation of the cervix is accompanied by increased descent of the presenting part. The contractions become stronger in intensity. They also increase to a duration of 40–60 seconds with a frequency of two to three contractions in 10 minutes.

Uterine actions

Fundal dominance

Each uterine contraction starts in the pacemakers, situated on either side of the uterus near the cornua, and spreads across and down the uterus. The contraction is more intense and lasts longer in the fundus, but the peak of the contraction is reached simultaneously over the whole uterus. This pattern allows the cervix to dilate and the fundus, which is contracting strongly, to expel the fetus.

Polarity

Polarity refers to the neuromuscular harmony that occurs between the two poles or segments of the uterus (the upper uterine segment and the lower uterine segment) throughout labour. The upper uterine segment contracts strongly and retracts to expel the fetus while the lower uterine segment contracts slightly and dilates to allow expulsion of the fetus to take place. If polarity is disorganised, there is no noticeable progress of labour and progress may be inhibited.

Contraction and retraction

During labour, the uterine muscles do not relax completely following contraction. They retain some form of shortening, called retraction. Hence, they do not completely return to their original length after contraction. Retraction assists in expulsion of the fetus, because the cavity of the uterus is reduced as the upper uterine segment becomes shorter and thicker.

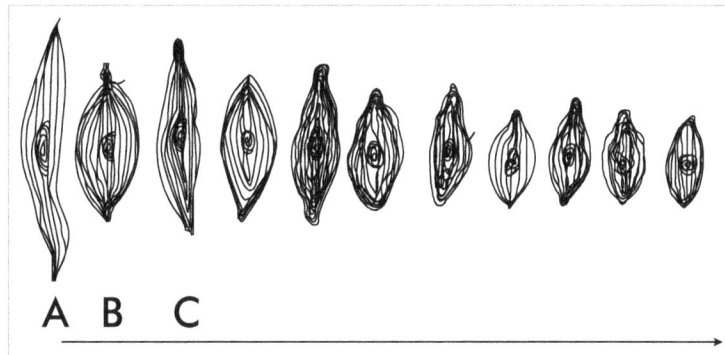

Figure 25.4 Progressive contraction and retraction of the uterine muscle fibres reducing the cavity: A = relaxed muscle fibres; B = contracted muscle fibres; C = retracted muscle fibres

Contractions are regular, rhythmic and occur over a specified period of time. Initially, they are weak. In early labour, uterine contractions may last about 30 seconds (weak or mild) and occur every 15–20 minutes. As labour progresses, contractions increase in intensity, duration and frequency. Moderate contractions last up to 35 seconds and strong contractions last 35–60 seconds. By the end of the first stage of labour, contractions may occur at intervals of two to three minutes and last 50–60 seconds. During the second stage of labour, they become strong and expulsive.

The upper and lower uterine segments and the retraction ring

By the end of pregnancy, the uterus is divided into the upper and lower uterine segments (see Figure 14.1 on page 200). The lower uterine segment has developed from the isthmus. The upper uterine segment is thick and muscular to enable it to contract and expel the fetus during labour, while the lower uterine segment is thinner to allow for distension and dilatation during labour and childbirth. The longitudinal muscle fibres are responsible for contraction and retraction, while the circular muscle fibres are responsible for distension and dilatation.

During labour, the upper uterine segment contracts and retracts, pulling on the lower uterine segment and causing it to stretch. A ridge forms between the upper and lower uterine segments, called the retraction ring. This is a physiological ring which occurs as a result of the contraction and retraction of the muscle fibres, coupled with distension and dilatation of the lower uterine segment.

The retraction ring gradually rises as the upper uterine segment contracts and retracts while the lower uterine segment contracts and dilates. Once the cervix is fully dilated and the fetus is expelled through the birth canal, the retraction ring rises no further. An exaggerated retraction ring is called

a Bandl's ring and is found when labour is obstructed. See figures 25.6 and 25.7 on the following pages.

Cervical effacement

During effacement, the muscle fibres around the internal os of the cervix are drawn upwards and merge into the lower uterine segment. The cervical canal widens at the level of the internal os. If the cervix has not been completely taken up during the last days of pregnancy, then this happens during labour. This commonly occurs in primigravidae, while in multigravidae the external os may begin to dilate before effacement. Effacement and dilatation of the cervix occur simultaneously in multiparae.

Dilatation of the cervix

Cervical dilatation is the process whereby the cervix opens (from a small aperture to an opening large enough to allow passage of the fetal head) to allow passage of the fetus during childbirth (see Figure 25.7 on page 379). Dilatation occurs as a result of uterine action and counter-pressure applied by the bag of membranes and the presenting part on the cervix. Pressure applied evenly to the cervix stimulates the uterine fundus to respond by contracting. In other words, a well-flexed head closely applied to the cervix favours efficient cervical dilatation. (Also see Figure 26A on page 396.)

Show

When the cervix dilates, the operculum – which formed the cervical plug during pregnancy – falls off and is shed. This is called 'show'. The mucous plug is mixed with blood from ruptured capillaries where the parietal decidua has detached.

The woman will give a history of a blood-stained mucoid discharge a few hours before or after labour starts. Frank bleeding may occur and is considered abnormal, while red blood may herald the second stage of labour.

Formation of the forewaters

As the lower uterine segment stretches, the chorion is detached from it and becomes loose. The intrauterine pressure causes the loosened part of the sac to bulge downwards into the internal os. The well-flexed head fits into the cervix and cuts off the fluid in front of the head from that which surrounds the body. The fluid in front of the head is known as the forewaters, while that which surrounds the rest of the body is known as the hindwaters.

The separation of the forewaters prevents the pressure that is applied to the hindwaters during contractions from being applied to the forewaters as well. This assists the membranes to remain intact during the first stage of labour, thereby providing a natural defence against ascending infection.

General fluid pressure

General fluid pressure describes the pressure that is exerted by the uterine contractions on the amniotic fluid during labour. As the fluid cannot be compressed, this pressure is equalised throughout the uterus and over the fetal body. If the membranes rupture and a significant amount of fluid is lost during uterine contractions, the placenta and umbilical cord become compressed between the uterine wall and fetus, causing diminished oxygen supply to the fetus. If membranes remain intact during labour, this may enhance oxygen supply to the fetus and also assist to prevent intrauterine infection if prolonged labour occurs.

Rupture of membranes

The best time for the membranes to rupture is at the end of the first stage of labour, when the cervix is fully dilated and delivery of the baby is imminent. This helps to minimise intrauterine and fetal infection, especially in cases of HIV and gonococcal infection.

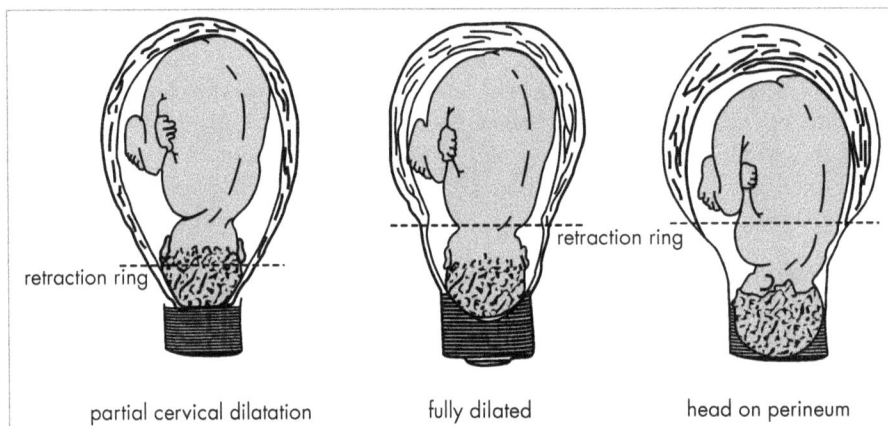

partial cervical dilatation   fully dilated   head on perineum

Figure 25.5 Normal or physiological retraction ring of the uterus

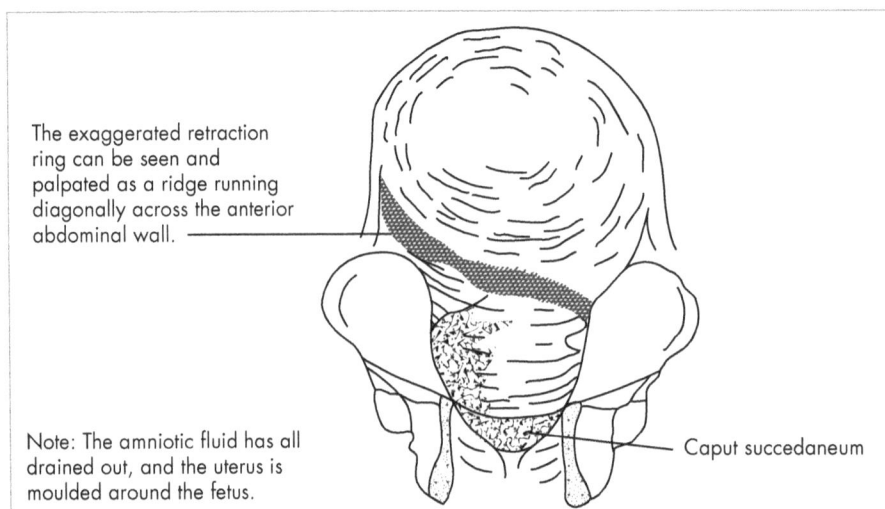

The exaggerated retraction ring can be seen and palpated as a ridge running diagonally across the anterior abdominal wall.

Caput succedaneum

Note: The amniotic fluid has all drained out, and the uterus is moulded around the fetus.

Figure 25.6 Bandl's ring

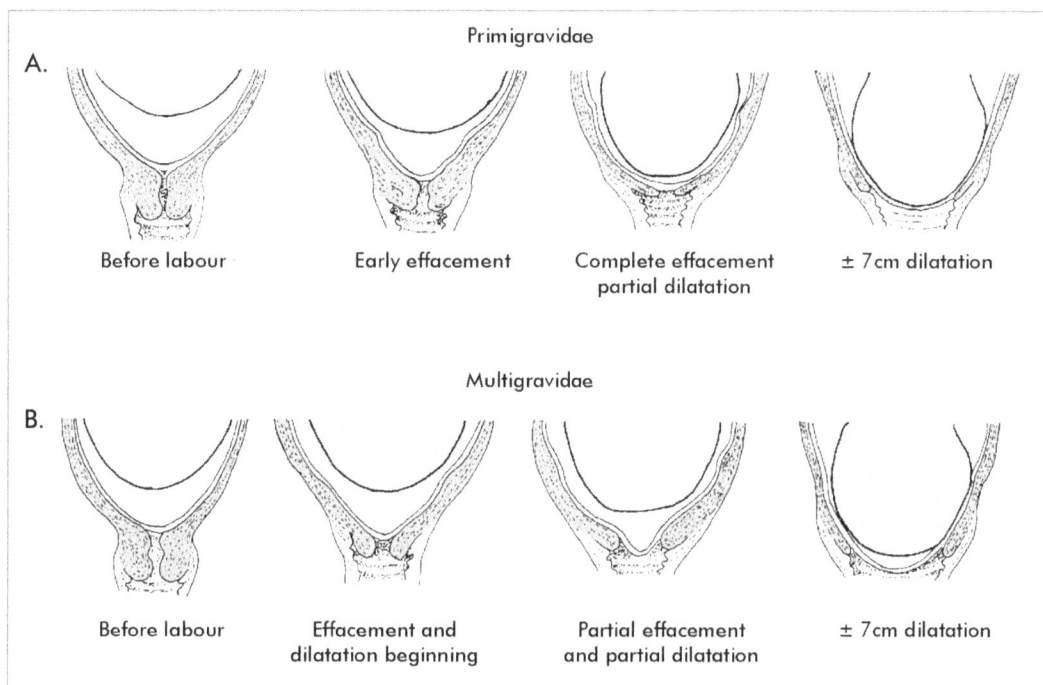

Figure 25.7 Effacement and dilatation of the cervix: A = primigravidae; B = multigravidae

During labour, the membranes may rupture early if the presenting part is poorly applied to the cervix, resulting in the forewaters not being properly cut off from the hindwaters.

In certain cases, the membranes do not rupture. Instead, they appear at the vulva in the second stage of labour as a sac covering the fetal head. Occasionally, membranes may rupture days before labour begins; there may be no reason for this. The premature rupture of membranes (PROM) predisposes the fetus to infection and may lead to fetal distress.

General physiological changes in the woman during the first stage of labour

Besides the extensive changes to the urogenital system during labour, the most important changes that occur – mainly as a result of energy expenditure – are related to the respiratory system, the gastrointestinal system (GI), the cardiovascular system, the acid–base balance, fluids and electrolytes and temperature.

Changes to the respiratory system

During pregnancy, there is the tendency to mild hyperventilation. In addition, because more CO_2 is exhaled with each breath, there is a subsequent decrease in carbon dioxide tension ($PaCO_2$). Occasionally, there might be hypoventilation. These changes result in changes in the acid–base balance.

Hyperventilation tends to increase if the woman is anxious or in pain, which may occur during the later part of the first stage of labour and may result in mild respiratory alkalosis. During labour, both the rate and the depth of respiration are increased, causing a further decrease in the $PaCO_2$ levels, particularly towards the end of the first stage of labour. This results in a mild respiratory alkalosis.

If hyperventilation is severe, the $PaCO_2$ levels can fall too low and will manifest as maternal dizziness, tingling in the fingers, numbness around the mouth and, if extreme, as a carpopedal spasm. The resulting alkalosis may interfere with the release of oxygen from the maternal blood to the fetus, resulting in fetal asphyxia. In order to increase the woman's $PaCO_2$, encourage her to pant and to take frequent deep breaths. If shallow respiration is overdone, the tidal volume will be low and too little oxygen will be taken in. This can result in fetal hypoxia.

It is important to note that the level of oxygen consumption increases as the contractions intensify, which may lead to an increase in labour pain due to myometrial hypoxia and subsequent stimulation of anaerobic metabolism, resulting in metabolic acidosis.

Gastrointestinal changes

Prior to the onset of labour, there is a certain degree of metabolic acidosis and a reduced ability to utilise glucose as the main fuel source for the fetus. The metabolic (energy-releasing) processes require glucose as an initial ingredient and, as there is considerable energy expenditure during labour, the glucose requirement is increased.

If the woman does not have a sufficient glucose intake, other methods to supply energy are utilised by the body, such as the oxidation of accumulated fats. However, fat oxidation results in metabolic acidosis. A mild metabolic acidosis may develop towards the end of the first stage and during the second stage of labour, but it is to some extent compensated for by the mild respiratory alkalosis. However, it is essential that the woman receives an adequate intake of glucose and fluids. It is also necessary to undertake urine tests for ketones (ketonuria) at set intervals during labour in order to diagnose maternal ketoacidosis as soon as it arises or occurs.

If labour is prolonged or if the contractions are very strong and frequent, and if the woman does not receive adequate hydration and sufficient glucose, ketoacidosis can develop very quickly. Although mild maternal ketosis is now thought to be of little importance, severe maternal ketoacidosis is dangerous and will be followed shortly by fetal acidosis, which can have serious consequences for the fetus. (Fetal acidosis, however, can also occur without the initial maternal acidosis.) Severe maternal ketoacidosis is recognised by the presence of pyrexia, tachycardia, dehydration and blood and urinary evidence of acidosis.

During labour, GI motility and absorption are reduced and the contents of the stomach may be retained for up to 48 hours. Factors that exacerbate delayed gastric motility include the consumption of food high in carbohydrates and fats, fear and pain as well as use of opioid drugs during labour. Nausea and vomiting may also occur in advanced labour due to maternal acidosis.

Changes in the cardiovascular system

There is increased cardiac activity during labour and this is especially marked during each uterine contraction. The cardiac output increases by about 20–30 per cent during the first stage of labour, but towards the end of the first stage and during the second stage, the increase may be even greater. Therefore, labour increases the strain already placed on the heart by pregnancy, but a woman with a healthy cardiovascular system has adequate reserves to compensate for this.

The increased cardiac output contributes to the rise in the BP and a raised pulse rate. In the first stage of labour, there is little change in BP between contractions, but there is an average rise of 10 mmHg systolic pressure and 5–10 mmHg diastolic pressure during contractions. There is a slow but progressive rise in the pulse rate during the first stage. However, the pulse should not exceed 100 beats per minute (bpm), unless ketoacidosis has developed. The pulse rate will be accentuated by prolonged labour, dehydration, haemorrhage, anxiety, unrelieved pain, infection and by certain medications such as those inhibiting labour.

The acid–base balance

As explained in the sections on the physiological changes to the respiratory and GI systems, the acid–base balance is very delicately poised during labour. Conditions such as starvation, a lack of adequate glucose and fluids, as well as prolonged, difficult and/or painful labour can result in metabolic acidosis. The pH of the blood just prior to labour is ± 7.42, as it is normally slightly raised towards the end of pregnancy. It usually decreases to ± 7.35 during labour. (The non-pregnant blood pH is ± 7.40.)

Fluids and electrolytes

There is an increased secretion of corticosteroids during labour, which leads to progressive changes in the serum electrolyte pattern. With the extra energy expenditure, there is increased heat production and subsequent fluid loss from sweating and panting. This is aggravated by reduced gut absorption and also by the tendency to vomit in advanced labour. As a result, there is a degree of haemo-concentration and a fall in the plasma levels of sodium and chloride.

Temperature

There is often a slight drop (by 0.5 °C) in the woman's body temperature a day or two before the onset of labour. During labour there is normally a gradual, slight rise in temperature, but this should not exceed 37.8 °C unless ketosis has developed. Factors that may contribute to a change in the woman's body temperature include the room or atmospheric temperature as well as prolonged, difficult and/or painful labour.

25.4 The physiology of the second stage of labour

The second stage is transitional and lasts from the moment the cervix is fully dilated up to when the fetus is completely expelled from the birth canal. Two phases of the second stage of labour are identified:

1. The *pelvic floor phase* is when the cervix is fully dilated, the head is not yet on the perineum and there is no urge to bear down. Bearing down at this stage is discouraged, as there is no evidence that it may expedite delivery. Premature bearing down may cause the uterine ligaments, vaginal and perineal muscles to become strained.

2. The expulsion phase, also called the *perineal phase*, is when the head is pressing on the sacral nerves to the rectum and there is a desire to bear down. The fetal head becomes visible at the perineum and the woman will experience a compulsive urge to bear down. The midwife may also encourage the woman to bear down and advise her on when to push and when not to push. Factors that determine the duration of the second stage of labour include the nature of the contractions, the maternal and fetal condition and the degree of descent. Descent of the presenting part is made possible by the combination of the increased intensity of the uterine contractions and intra-abdominal pressure.

The duration of the second stage of labour

As mentioned previously, the duration of the second stage of labour is 45 minutes for multiparous women and up to two hours for primigravidae. In South Africa, the primigravida is allowed 45 minutes while the multipara is allowed 30 minutes as the duration of the second stage of labour. The limitation of the duration of the second stage of labour must not be limited to time alone but must also consider the progress of labour, the condition of the mother and the condition of the fetus. In addition, the length of the second stage will depend on the size and position of the head and the presence of strong uterine contractions.

During this stage, the stronger contractions interfere with the placental circulation and the fetal head is subjected to compression (200 mmHg) as it enters and descends in the pelvis. If there is a loop of cord around the fetal neck, it can become tightened as the head descends. For these reasons, the second stage of labour is much more hazardous to the fetus than the first stage.

During pregnancy and in the first stage of labour, the pressure of the contractions is partially absorbed by the amniotic fluid, which more or less equalises the pressure over the whole uterus. The purpose of these contractions is initially to bring about the formation of the upper and lower uterine segments and subsequently to bring about the effacement of the cervical canal and the dilatation of the cervix. However, in the second stage, the purpose of the contractions is to force the fetus through the birth canal and to expel the infant from the uterus through the vaginal orifice.

The uterine contractions

The involuntary uterine contractions are the primary force that pushes the baby out. If the membranes have not ruptured previously, they usually rupture at the beginning of the second stage of labour. Much of the liquor amnii drains out, bringing the uterus into closer contact with the fetus. This causes additional stimulation of the uterine muscles, resulting in stronger contractions (Ferguson reflex). These are then further enhanced by reflex stimulation due to the stretching of the pelvic floor and the vagina as the fetal head descends. This results in the uterine contractions becoming stronger, longer and expulsive in nature. The contractions are very painful, but when the woman bears down or 'pushes' during a contraction, this significantly decreases the pain. The combined forces of the secondary powers (see below) and the uterine contractions force the fetus to descend through the birth canal. The upper uterine segment continues to contract and retract in an effort to expel the fetus from the uterus.

The secondary powers

The descending fetus exerts pressure on the rectum and pelvic floor, giving the woman the urge to bear down. The urge may be controllable for a while. However, at a point the woman will suddenly feel she cannot control it and be overwhelmed, and she will begin to bear down. The secondary powers that come into effect are the abdominal muscles and the diaphragm.

The ancillary or auxiliary muscles of the second stage

Certain voluntary skeletal muscles, the abdominal muscles and the diaphragm aid in expelling the fetus from the uterus in the second stage of labour. These are brought into play when the woman bears down or 'pushes'. She can control these muscles.

In normal circumstances, the bearing-down reflex, or the urge to bear down, is experienced by almost every woman in the second stage of labour. In fact, a woman may experience this urge even before the cervix is fully dilated. However, this should be guarded against, as premature bearing down can result in the cervix becoming nipped between the pelvis and the fetal head, with the danger of causing an oedematous lip of the cervix. While bearing down, an increase in the intrauterine pressure can also occur, causing a reduction in oxygen to the fetus. The woman should only be encouraged to bear down when no cervix is felt on vaginal examination. In addition, the woman should only be encouraged to bear down during contractions in the second stage, because bearing down between contractions – as with bearing down before full dilatation – can result in stretching of the uterine supports, which could later lead to uterine prolapse.

Towards the end of the second stage, when the head is on the perineum, the woman often experiences a feeling similar to the reflex to defecate. If the woman requests a bed pan in the second stage, it may indicate that the fetal head is well down in the pelvis and the woman is about to deliver the baby.

Changes to the pelvic floor and pelvic organs

As the fetal head descends, there is pressure on and stretching of the soft tissues and organs of the pelvis.

The bladder is drawn upwards and becomes an abdominal organ, making more space in the pelvis for the fetus and lessening the risk of damage to the bladder. However, in the second stage the urethra is frequently nipped between the bony prominences of the fetal skull and the pelvis.

The descending head stretches the vagina and may cause small lacerations of the vaginal mucosa, which may be seen as a trickle of blood from the vagina.

The posterior part of the pelvic floor is pushed downwards and is elongated and thinned out. The rectum is compressed by the descending head and faecal material may be forced out of the anus. The anus will start to pout and then to gape, revealing the anterior rectal wall.

The vaginal introitus will start to gape and the presenting part will then be seen in the vagina. At first, this may slip back out of sight between contractions. The perineal body and perineum are also pushed downward and elongated. As the head is crowning, the vaginal orifice, which is directed upwards towards the subpubic arch, is stretched to allow the head to pass out of the vagina. Tearing of the tissues around the orifice may occur, usually in the perineal area, but occasionally laterally or upward into the clitoris.

The birth of the baby

(See Figure 25.8.) The head is flexed as it passes out from under the pubic arch. As the widest presenting circumference of the fetal head distends the vaginal introitus, the head is said to be crowned by the perineum. When the head has almost crowned, the woman should stop bearing down and should pant – in small, sharp breaths – in order to allow the head and then the remainder of the infant to be born slowly and with control. This will help to prevent bad perineal lacerations.

In addition, if the head remains well-flexed during crowning, then the smallest presenting diameter, the suboccipito frontal diameter of 10 cm, will distend the vaginal orifice. This will also lessen the chance of perineal lacerations. Only when this diameter, together with the biparietal diameter (BPD), has been born, should the head be allowed to extend.

The head then extends at the neck and the perineum slips over the baby's forehead and face, and the mouth and chin emerge from the vagina. The head is then born and there is a pause before the next contraction, when restitution (the undoing of the twist in the baby's neck, as in step 7 in Figure 25.8) takes place. With this next contraction, the shoulders are forced onto the pelvic floor and the anterior shoulder rotates forward, forcing the shoulders into the anteroposterior (AP)

diameter of the pelvis and at the same time causing the head to rotate externally so that the sagittal suture lies in the transverse diameter of the pelvis, as illustrated in step 8 in Figure 25.8. (The baby now faces the mother's thigh, either the left or the right, depending upon the baby's original position in the uterus.) With the following contraction, the anterior shoulder escapes from under the pubic arch, the posterior shoulder slips out from behind the perineum and the rest of the body follows. These processes are explained in greater detail in Section 25.7, where the mechanism of labour is described.

The remainder of the amniotic fluid is also expelled with the fetus. The mother, usually exhausted, relaxes for a few minutes, her attention directed towards the baby, which gasps convulsively once or twice and then cries vigorously. With the complete birth of the infant, the second stage has ended and the third stage commences.

25.5 The physiological processes in the third stage of labour

The third stage of labour begins when the baby is delivered and lasts up to the complete expulsion of the placenta and membranes and the achievement of haemostasis. The events include separation and expulsion of the placenta and membranes as well as control of bleeding.

With active management of the third stage of labour (AMTSL), this stage lasts 5–15 minutes. With passive management (spontaneous delivery of the placenta), it lasts 45–60 minutes. Anything beyond that is considered to be a prolonged third stage of labour.

The delivery of the placenta firstly entails its separation from the uterine wall. This is followed by the descent of the placenta into the lower uterine segment and then its expulsion from the uterus and vagina.

The physiology of placental separation

During pregnancy, the endometrium becomes known as the decidua of the uterus and develops into specialised layers. The inner basal layer is separated from the spongy layer by the fibrinous layer of Nitabuch, which is also known as the postage-stamp layer. This layer prevents the chorionic villi of the trophoblast from penetrating into the basal layer of the decidua and so into the myometrium. It is also this layer that allows the uniform separation of the placenta from the decidua during the third stage of labour. Hence the name 'postage-stamp' layer: it allows the placenta to shear off from the uterine wall like a postage stamp from an envelope.

1. Anteroposterior slit

2. Oval opening

3. Circular opening

4. Crowning of the head

5. Extension of the head

6. Birth of the head

7. Restitution of the head

8. External rotation of the head

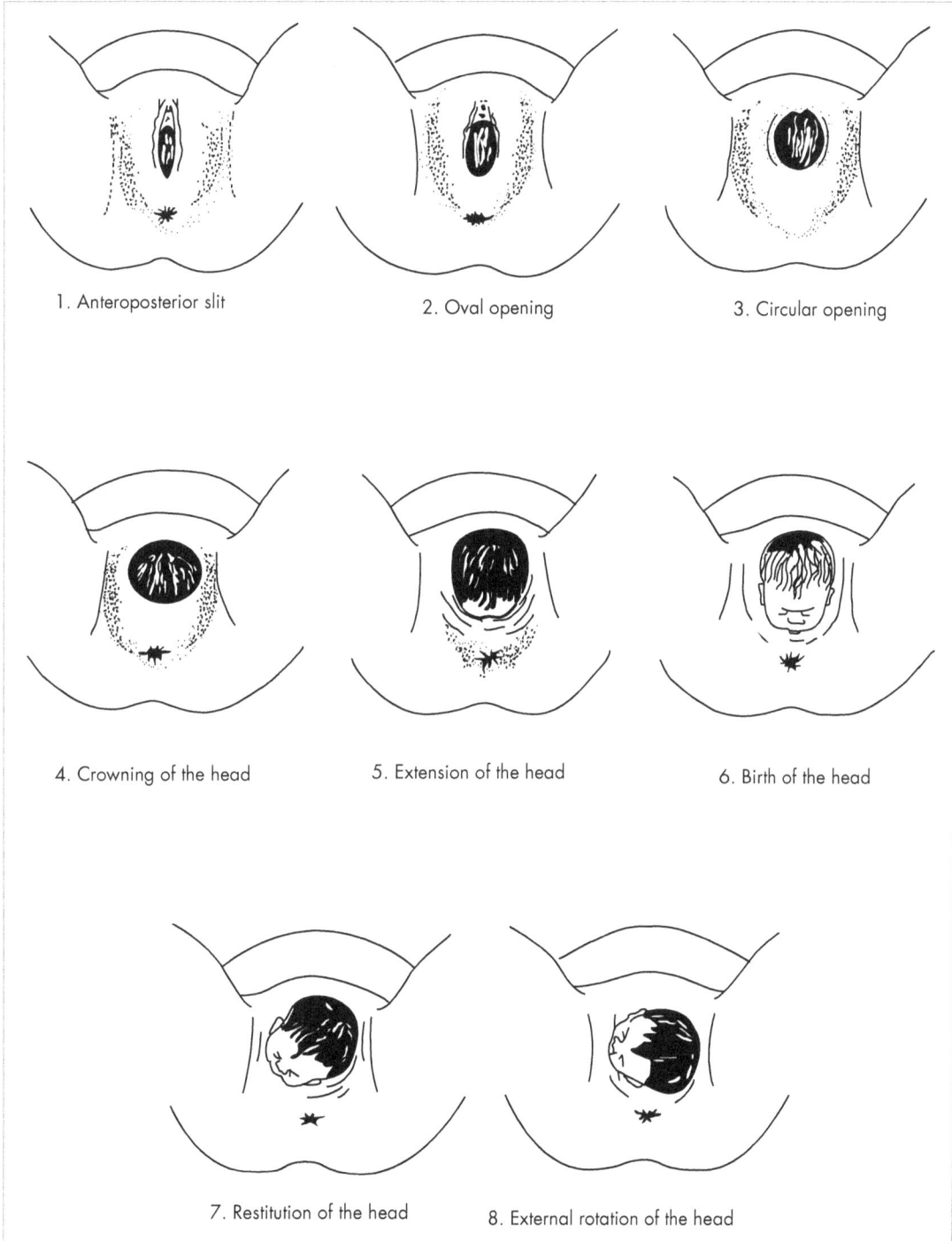

Figure 25.8 Labour: the birth of the head – dorsal position

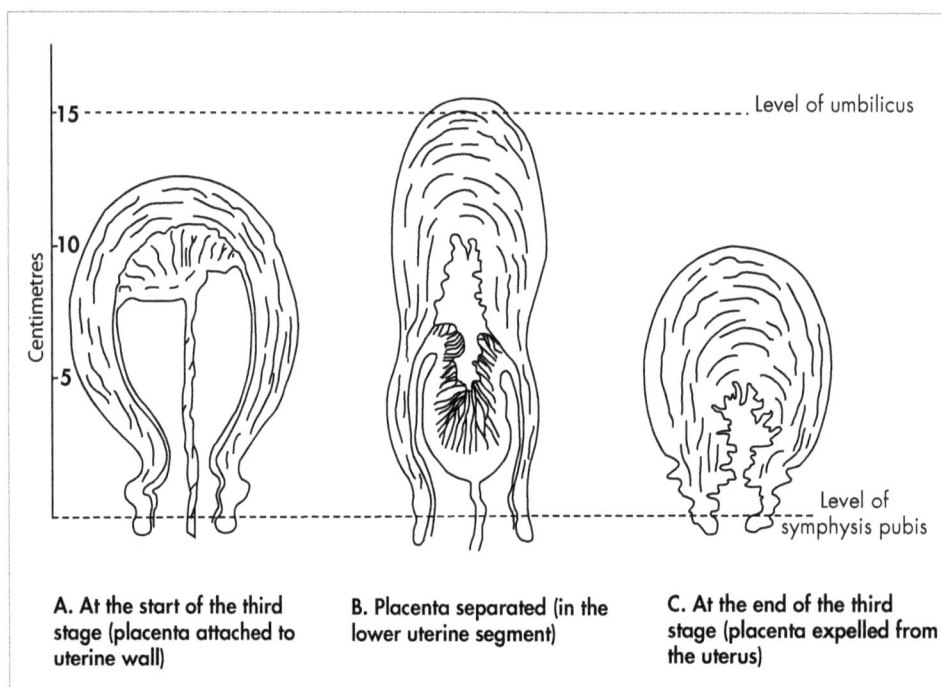

A. At the start of the third stage (placenta attached to uterine wall)

B. Placenta separated (in the lower uterine segment)

C. At the end of the third stage (placenta expelled from the uterus)

Figure 25.9 Separation of the placenta

The separation of the placenta is facilitated with the expulsion of the baby from the uterus at birth. The surface area of the inner uterine cavity is greatly decreased when the uterine muscles continue to contract and retract. The placental site starts to diminish in size by the beginning of the third stage of labour. The placenta is squeezed and blood in the intervillous spaces is forced back into the spongy layer of the decidua. This has the effect of causing a portion of the placenta, which is unable to contract with the muscle, to become detached from the uterine wall at its implantation site, where a shearing-off of the placenta from the uterine wall occurs. (The process is rather like a piece of inelastic material stuck to the surface of a stretched piece of elastic. When the elastic is allowed to contract, the piece of inelastic material becomes detached from the surface of the elastic because it is not able to contract with the elastic.)

When a portion of the placenta becomes detached from the uterine wall, blood vessels from the uterus, which carry blood to and from the maternal side of the placenta, are ruptured and there is an outflow of blood between the decidua and the maternal placental surface. This extravasation of blood causes further detachment of the placenta from the uterine wall.

The uterine muscles, if functioning efficiently, will continue to contract and retract, and will complete the detachment of

the placenta from the uterine wall. The placenta will fall into the collapsed lower segment of the uterus and the contracting and retracting uterus will then push the placenta into the vagina.

The membranes are usually detached from the uterine wall merely by the weight of the placenta descending in the birth canal, causing traction on the membranes and thereby stripping them off the decidua.

The signs and symptoms of placental separation and expulsion are the following:

▶ The uterus is tightly contracted and retracted and becomes hard and round (like a cricket ball).

▶ The uterus can be palpated abdominally through the maternal anterior abdominal wall, between the rectus abdominis muscles. It also rises in the abdomen because it is trying to push the placenta out.

▶ A fresh trickle of blood is noted vaginally.

▶ Finally, the placenta is expelled from the birth canal by maternal effort.

The placenta separates in one of two ways – according to the Schultze method or the Matthews-Duncan method – and the manner of the separation prescribes the way in which the placenta will emerge from the birth canal.

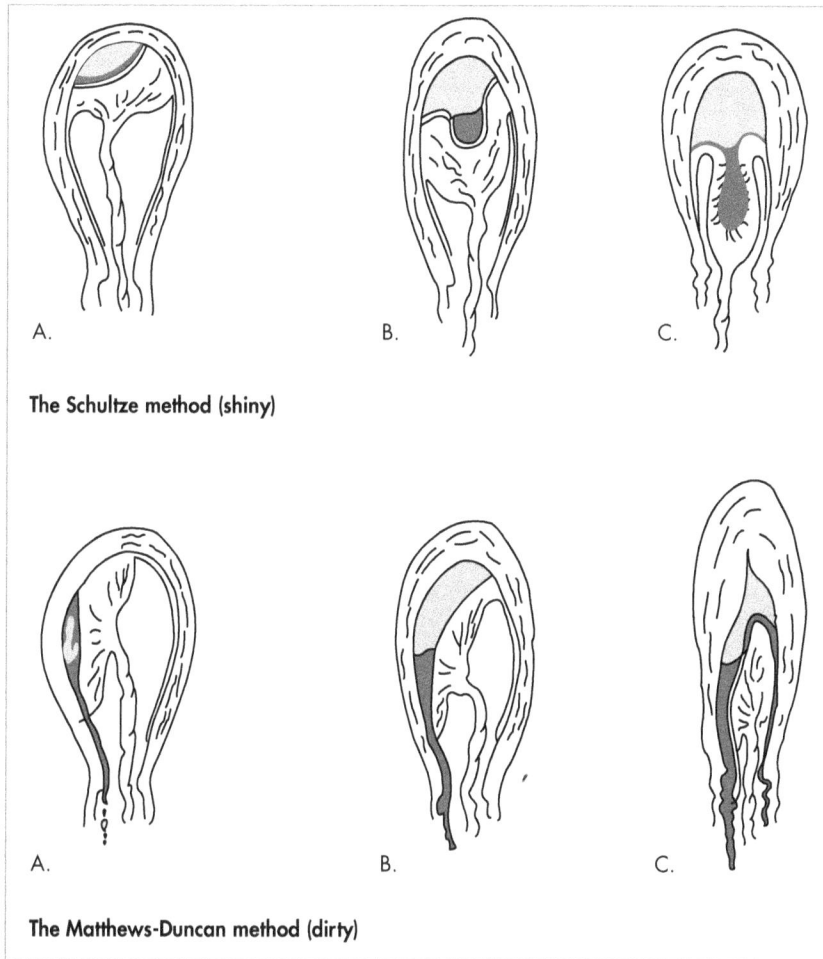

A.   B.   C.

The Schultze method (shiny)

A.   B.   C.

The Matthews-Duncan method (dirty)

Figure 25.10 Types of placental separation

The Schultze (shiny) method

This type of separation usually occurs when the placenta is implanted high up near or in the uterine fundus. Here, the centre of the placenta separates from the uterine wall first, resulting in the formation of the retroplacental clot. This clot causes an increase in weight, which will facilitate the peeling off of the membranes from the uterine wall. The retroplacental clot collects in the centre of the placenta and causes the placenta to invert as it descends in the uterus and birth canal. The shiny fetal surface emerges from the vaginal orifice first, with the blood clot contained within the membranes. Very little blood is spilt. The membranes are usually intact, except for the hole through which the baby was born.

The Matthews-Duncan (dirty) method

This type of separation may occur where the placenta is implanted in the side of the uterine body. Here, the lower edge of the placenta separates from the uterine wall first. This causes bleeding, which dislodges the membranes below the bleeding. Blood escapes from the uterus into the vagina and eventually out of the vaginal orifice. The separation continues upwards. When it is complete, the lower edge of the placenta slips through the cervical os and emerges from the vaginal orifice first, often together with a gush of blood. This is followed by the maternal surface of the placenta and torn and ragged membranes.

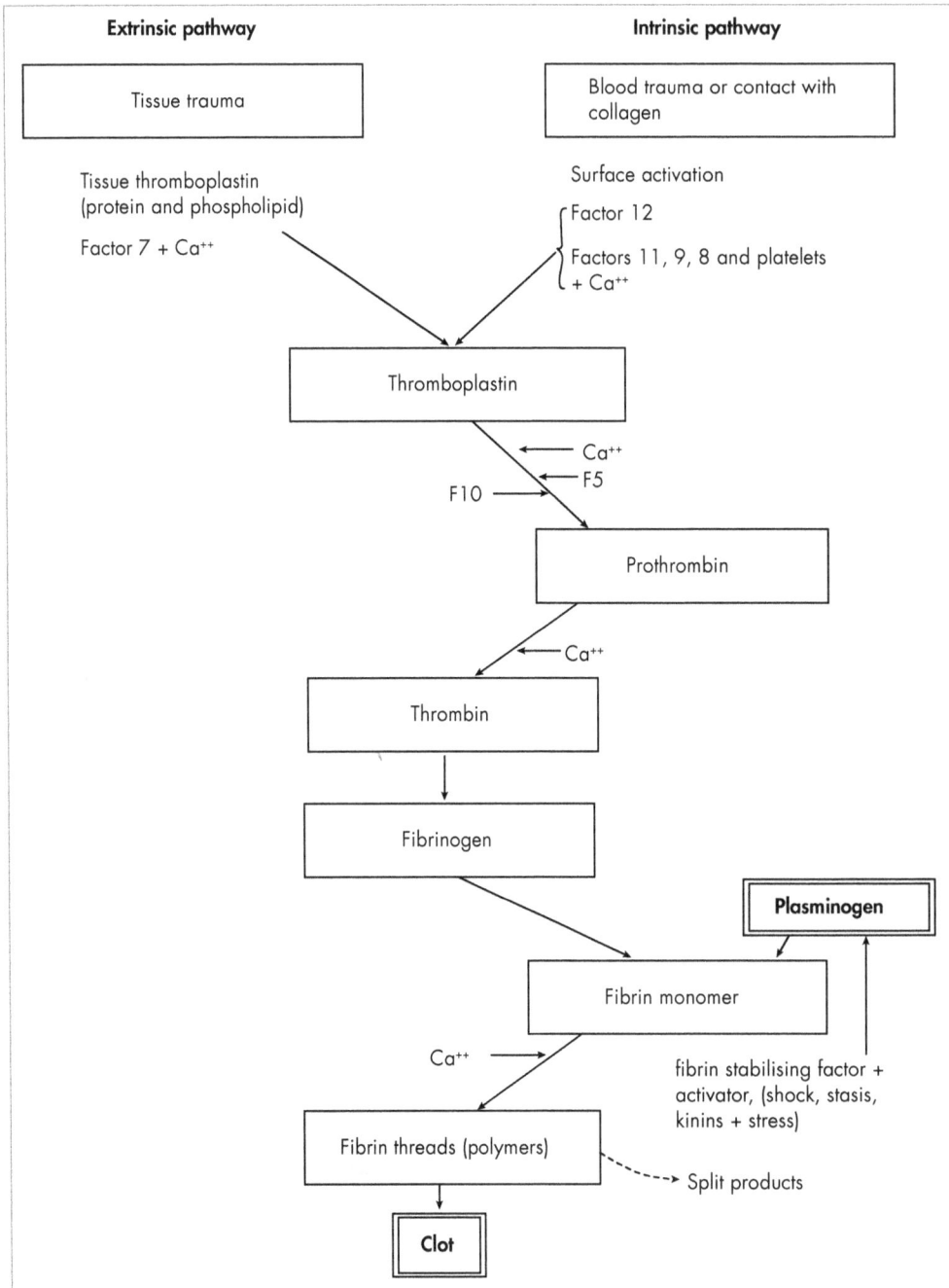

Figure 25.11 The normal coagulation process of the blood (the formation of a blood clot)

The physiological process of haemorrhage control in the third stage

The average amount of blood loss in a normal third stage of labour is 150–250 ml.

The control of haemorrhage in the third stage of labour is brought about by two main physiological processes: the normal coagulation process of the blood and the constricting effect of the uterine muscles. The coagulation process – from the release of thromboplastins through to the formation of fibrin – occurs with any wound (see Figure 25.11).

The smooth muscle fibres of the uterine musculature are arranged in figures of eight around the blood vessels as these vessels pass through the uterine wall (the so-called 'living ligature' effect). The contracting and retracting of the criss-crossing uterine muscle fibres, after the birth of the baby and the separation of the placenta, controls the bleeding from the exposed blood vessels that had previously supplied blood to the placenta, as shown in Figure 25.12. (If there is no separation of the placenta, there will be no bleeding from the placental site.)

The failure of either of these physiological processes will result in uncontrolled haemorrhage. If the uterus is able to contract but there is a failure of the coagulation process, there will be continued bleeding, which in itself will eventually prevent the uterus from contracting efficiently. Conversely, if the coagulation process is normal but the uterus is atonic, severe haemorrhage can result. In fact, the efficiency of the uterus is directly proportionate to the efficient separation of the placenta and the efficient control of haemorrhage, if the clotting mechanism is normal.

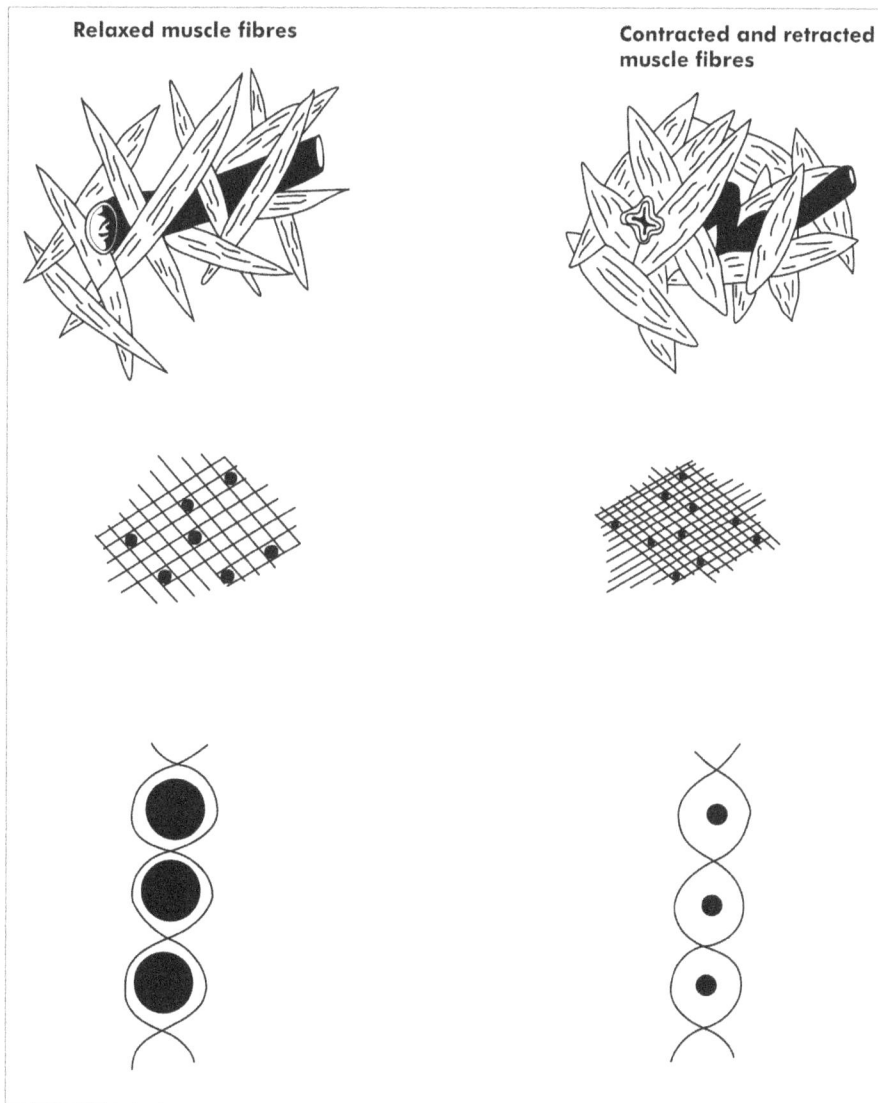

Figure 25.12 The constricting effect of the uterine muscles on the blood vessels

25.6   The fourth stage of labour

The fourth stage of labour is the period after delivery of the placenta up to one hour post-delivery. During this time, the mother's vital signs are checked and recorded and any abnormalities managed appropriately. Breastfeeding is initiated within the hour following birth. The placenta is examined for abnormalities and the baby is examined to exclude any abnormalities and congenital malformations.

25.7   The mechanism of labour

The fetus has to undergo a series of movements in order to pass through the birth canal. This is known as the mechanism of labour. Knowledge of the female pelvis, the pelvic floor, the fetal skull and the physiology of normal labour is essential to understand the mechanism of normal labour. The midwife should also have knowledge of the different terms used to describe the fetus in relation to the pelvis during pregnancy and childbirth.

Labour progresses normally in most women and the mechanism follows a set pattern of movements. In the mechanism of normal labour, the lie is longitudinal, the presentation is cephalic, the attitude is that of complete flexion and the denominator is the occiput. In certain circumstances, there is a variation in this set pattern of movements, which results in an abnormal mechanism of labour. This is attributed to an abnormal relationship of the fetus to the uterus and pelvis.

The movements of the mechanism of labour

The series of movements that constitute the mechanism of labour are a continuous process, but for convenience they are divided into different stages, depending upon the different movements that the fetus undergoes. These stages are described in the following subsections.

Engagement

Engagement occurs when the widest part of the presenting part enters the pelvic brim. In a primigravida, engagement occurs at 36 weeks of pregnancy and in a multigravida, it usually occurs after the onset of labour. In a cephalic presentation, the widest diameter is the BPD (9.5 cm). Engagement demonstrates that the pelvis is likely to be adequate for the size of that particular fetus to allow for vaginal delivery.

Descent

In each plane of the pelvis, the fetus turns in order to take advantage of the largest available space, for example the transverse diameter at the pelvic brim and the AP diameter at the outlet.

In a primigravida, the descent of the fetal head begins before the onset of labour. It usually occurs during the latter weeks of pregnancy as a result of tight abdominal muscles. In a multigravida it may not occur until the onset of labour.

Descent occurs when there is a softening of the cervix and other pelvic organs, as well as some effacement of the cervical canal. Contraction and retraction of the uterine muscles aid descent during the first stage of labour. The descent is more rapid in the second stage of labour, because when the woman bears down, the abdominal muscles and the diaphragm assist the muscle action of the uterus.

Flexion

With descent, increased flexion of the fetal head takes place throughout labour. At the beginning of labour, the fetal head is in an attitude of natural flexion. There are several theories as to how this increased flexion comes about. One theory suggests that in a normal vertex presentation, the long axis of the fetus lies parallel to the long axis of the mother and the fetus is already in an attitude of general flexion, with the occiput slightly lower than the sinciput. As the fundus of the uterus presses against the fetal buttocks in the upper uterine pole, the vertex meets the resistance of the now cone-shaped cervical canal and the head is further flexed.

In conjunction with this, the lever theory states that as the spinal column is articulated to the head nearer to the occiput than to the sinciput, any force transmitted through the spine to the head of the fetus will cause the short occipital protuberance to dip down in advance of the sinciput.

In a normal vertex presentation, the sub-occipitofrontal diameter of 10 cm lies at the pelvic brim before labour. With increased flexion of the head, the smaller sub-occipitobregmatic diameter of 9.5 cm (together with the BPD of 9.5 cm) enters the pelvic brim and the occiput becomes the leading part of the fetal head.

Internal rotation of the head

The rule is that the part to reach the pelvic floor first rotates forwards due to pressure from the contractions and muscular diaphragm, coupled with resistance from the pelvic floor muscles. The resistance from the pelvic floor causes the occiput to glide forwards. In vertex presentations, when the head is well flexed, the occiput leads and meets the pelvic floor first and rotates. The occiput rotates anteriorly one-eighth of a circle along the left side of the pelvis towards the symphysis pubis. This causes a slight twist in the neck of the fetus (see Figure 25.8 on page 383). The AP diameter of the head lies in the AP diameter of the pelvic outlet (13 cm).

The distance which the occiput rotates in a vertex presentation depends upon its position at the pelvic brim at the onset of labour:

▶ In an occipitoanterior (OA) position, the occiput will rotate forward one-eighth of a circle along the side of the pelvis (45 degrees).
▶ In an occipitolateral (OL) position, it will rotate forward two-eighths of a circle along the side of the pelvis (90 degrees).
▶ In an occipitoposterior (OP) position, it will rotate forward three-eighths of a circle along the side of the pelvis (135 degrees).

Crowning

Crowning occurs when the occiput escapes under the symphysis pubis (see step 4 of Figure 25.8 on page 383). The BPD is born (9.5 cm). The head no longer recedes between contractions. If flexion is maintained, the sub-occipitobregmatic diameter distends the vaginal orifice. Crowning of the head refers to the stage at which the largest presenting diameter of the fetal head passes through the vulval orifice.

Extension of the head

The movement of extension is the opposite to that of flexion. Following crowning, the fetal head becomes extended on the neck, releasing the sinciput, face and chin. The sinciput, face and chin sweep the perineum and the head is delivered by a movement of extension (see step 5 of Figure 25.8). In a normal vertex presentation, the sub-occipitofrontal diameter (10 cm) distends the vulva and the head is born by a movement of extension (see step 6 of Figure 25.8).

Restitution

Restitution (see step 7 of Figure 25.8) is the untwisting of the twist in the fetal neck that occurred during the internal rotation of the head. In a normal vertex delivery, the occiput moves one-eighth of a circle back along the side of the pelvis (from which it came before the internal rotation of the head) and so undoes the twist in the neck.

During delivery, it is very important that the midwife who is delivering the baby waits for restitution to take place. This will indicate the position of the fetus. It will, first of all, prevent the midwife from turning the fetal head in the wrong direction, which may result in large diameters presenting and cause trauma to fetal tissues. Secondly, it will help to prevent both shoulders from passing through the vulva simultaneously, and so decrease the risk of perineal lacerations and reduce the incidence of shoulder dystocia.

Internal rotation of the shoulders and external rotation of the head

The internal rotation of the shoulders takes place in a way similar to that of the head, except that the rotation will be on the opposite side of the pelvis. The shoulders are at right angles to the sagittal suture. The anterior shoulder reaches the pelvic floor first and rotates anteriorly to lie under the symphysis pubis. This means the long axis of the shoulder is now lying in the AP diameter of the pelvis.

As the shoulders rotate anteriorly, this movement is accompanied by an external rotation of the head (see step 8 of Figure 25.8). This is because the long axis of the head has to be at right angles to the long axis of the shoulders and therefore, when the shoulders turn one-eighth of a circle, the head also has to turn one-eighth of a circle in the same direction. The movement occurs in the same direction as restitution and the fetal occiput now lies laterally. This allows for smaller diameters of the fetus to present at the outlet.

Birth of the shoulders

With a further contraction, the anterior shoulder is delivered first. The anterior shoulder slips under the pubic arch while the posterior shoulder sweeps the perineum, reducing the size of the presenting diameters. The shoulders are born by a movement of lateral flexion.

Delivery of the rest of the body

Ideally, within the same contraction and continuing the movement of lateral flexion, the rest of the body is born by lateral flexion. This occurs because the fetal body follows the curve of Carus, which directs it over the symphysis pubis and onto the mother's abdomen. The midwife facilitates delivery of the baby over the mother's abdomen to promote bonding.

Factors affecting the fetus during labour

The birth process is not an easy or gentle experience for the mother, but it is an even more traumatic experience for the fetus. However, the physiological reserves with which the fetus normally enters labour enable it to withstand the effects of labour and birth. There are many factors that are involved in this journey from the safety of the uterus, through the birth canal and into the outside world.

The fetus also experiences major changes during labour, which may cause stress, so it is important to monitor fetal well-being. Fetal heart monitoring can be through intermittent auscultation by a fetal stethoscope (fetoscope), by a sonicaid or by continuous fetal heart monitoring using a cardiotocograph (CTG) during normal labour. The following sections detail factors which may affect fetal well-being during labour.

The uterine contractions (powers)

During normal uterine contractions, there is compression of the placenta in the upper uterine segment. This can retard the amount of oxygen to the fetus to a greater or lesser degree, especially during the peak of the contraction. Thus, even in normal labour the fetus is subjected to a certain amount of hypoxia. This can be noted when monitoring the fetal heartbeat during contractions. Hypertonic or inco-ordinate uterine action or prolonged labour may lead to fetal anoxia.

The passages

The passages refer to the birth canal that the fetus must pass through during the process of childbirth. There are various factors which help to make the path through the birth canal larger and therefore easier. These include the smooth dilatation of the cervix, the intact membranes and an average amount of liquor, an adequately sized pelvis (in relation to the size of the fetus), a pelvis that is normally shaped and inclined, the pelvic joints, the softening of the pelvic tissues and the elasticity of the perineum. If any of these factors are changed, this can lead to a more difficult labour and delivery.

The passenger

The fetus itself dictates to some degree whether the labour is comparatively easy or difficult. Factors that suggest that labour is likely to progress well include:

- a term pregnancy at the onset of labour
- a normal-sized fetus
- adequate pelvic capacity (including the soft tissues and the pelvic floor muscles)
- normal presentation (cephalic) and position at the onset of labour.

An OA position, coupled with the ability of the fetal skull to mould during passage through the birth canal (but not excessive, rapid or upward moulding), will contribute to less trauma to both the fetus and the mother. If the fetus is at term, the necessary reserves will have been built up to enable it to withstand a certain amount of hypoxia and trauma. If, however, the fetus is post-term (42 weeks' gestational age or more), it will not necessarily be at a greater advantage. In this case moulding is less likely to take place due to ossification of the skull bones. In addition, the placenta may have started to degenerate, leading to placental insufficiency and fetal hypoxia.

The changes to the fetal systems that are affected by labour are as follows:

- *Changes to the fetal cardiovascular system:* The fetal heart rate (FHR) normally stays within a range of 120–160

bpm, but in practice 110–160 is accepted as a normal range, considered as the baseline FHR. During normal contractions, there is only a slight variation in the baseline FHR, with the heart rate remaining within a normal range of plus or minus 20 bpm. An increase in the FHR at the peak of the contraction (beyond the acceptable baseline variability) indicates that there is compensation for mild hypoxia. If the baseline FHR were to increase by more than 20 bpm to over 160, or to slow down by more than 20 bpm to less than 110, this would indicate moderate to severe hypoxia and fetal distress. The rhythm of the fetal heartbeat is fairly constant, with a baseline showing a characteristic fluctuation of about 5–10 bpm over a selected time interval. This is known as the beat-to-beat variation or baseline variability. The loss of this variability may indicate either loss of cardiovascular adaptability to stress or the depression of the cardiac reflex centre in the brain.

- *Acid–base balance (fetal acidosis):* There are normally sufficient glucose reserves to compensate for the effects of fetal acidosis caused by hypoxia during uterine contractions. However, if the placenta has not been functioning efficiently for the last few weeks of pregnancy, or if the labour is preterm, there would be diminished glycogen reserves and the fetus may be unable to compensate for any reduction in the supply of glucose or oxygen which may occur in a prolonged or difficult labour. Maternal ketoacidosis could also aggravate the degree of fetal acidosis and the use of excessive amounts of analgesia may cause a reduction in the amount of oxygen transferred to the fetus.

25.8   Conclusion

Understanding the mechanism and physiology of labour can contribute to reducing complications related to childbirth. Knowledge of the normal mechanism of labour allows midwives and other skilled birth attendants to identify, at an early stage, any deviations from normal and take appropriate action. An abnormal mechanism can result in obstructed or prolonged labour due to large diameters of the presenting part. Knowledge of the physiology of labour also allows for appropriate interventions to be implemented. For instance, the contractions must be regular, rhythmic and increase in intensity as labour progresses to facilitate descent and dilatation of the cervix. In the absence of effective contractions, labour can be augmented.

Management and care during the first stage of labour

LEARNING OBJECTIVES

On completion of this chapter, you must be able to:
- explain the role of the midwife during the first stage of labour
- explain the process of admission of a woman in labour
- explain the general care and management of the woman during the first stage of labour
- explain the use of the partogram in the management of labour.

KNOWLEDGE ASSUMED TO BE IN PLACE

The physiology of labour
Guidelines and principles as set out in the *Guidelines for Maternity Care in South Africa* (DoH, 2015)

KEYWORDS

partogram • skilled attendance • intrapartum records • baseline variability (BV)

26.1 Introduction

Every woman going through labour and childbirth must receive individualised, holistic care from a skilled attendant in a safe environment.

Many women experience stress and physical pain during labour. Midwives need to be skilled in the management of discomfort in line with the woman's desires and cultural beliefs, for example what the woman thinks about, wants and has planned for natural birth. The role of the skilled birth attendant, whether it is a midwife or medical practitioner, is supportive. The attendant intervenes only when circumstances demand it.

Adequate and relevant information will allow the woman to make relevant, informed decisions. Good communication among healthcare professionals and with the woman is established by keeping accurate records and developing a rapport with the labouring woman in a present and supportive manner. The continuous presence of a skilled professional and high-quality care in labour helps to reduce stress and fear.

Psychological comfort

Women who are pregnant for the first time (primigravidae) tend to experience fear of the unknown, while multigravidae might have bad memories from previous births. This may result in fear and anxiety, which may affect the smooth progress of labour. As a preventive measure, midwifery care should focus on providing emotional support, alleviating labour pain, providing comfort and allowing the significant person (husband/partner, relative or friend) to be present during the labour process and childbirth if the environment and policy of the healthcare facility allows.

26.2 The role of the midwife during the first stage of labour

The midwife is the preferred skilled caregiver in midwifery. The midwife gives the appropriate evidence-based technical care and creates a supportive environment for birth by listening and giving appropriate responses to the woman's requests and needs. The outcomes and level of satisfaction of a natural and uncomplicated delivery will depend upon the care and support that the woman receives from the midwife. Caring communication will give her confidence in herself and labour is likely to progress well and last a shorter time. Fear, tension and anxiety – all associated with a prolonged labour – are likely if the mother is shown an uncaring or even rude attitude. 'Humane care', as expressed in the midwifery model of care, spells out the best practice in childbirth and creates choice, continuity of care and autonomy – principles that give the woman control over the events. This means that a known caregiver listens, acknowledges and is in close proximity (not more than one metre from the labouring woman) giving evidence-based care and psychological support.

26.3   Diagnosis and assessment of labour

The diagnosis of the first stage of labour is based on the signs and symptoms experienced by the mother and confirmed by findings obtained on vaginal examination. There are certain signs and symptoms that collectively may suggest the onset of labour. Some of these are presumptive, while others are confirmatory.

Diagnostic (conclusive) signs

The following are the diagnostic signs of the start of the first stage of labour:

▶ *Regular uterine contractions.* At the onset of the first stage of labour, uterine contractions of 40–45 seconds occur every 20 minutes in a regular pattern. This may coincide with the presence of discharge, or 'show', or the rupture of membranes. The contractions gradually become more frequent (every 10 minutes or less), increase in intensity and last longer (45–60 seconds). Occasionally, the woman may complain of lower back pain. These symptoms are experienced by the mother and confirmed on abdominal palpation. The direct observation of the contraction by abdominal feeling is the most accurate measure, as the cardiotocograph (CTG) is dependent on the operator and other factors (such as obesity of the mother), for effect.

▶ *Dilatation and effacement of the cervix.* Regular, rhythmic contractions are accompanied by cervical dilatation. Cervical dilatation is noted on vaginal examination and is measured in centimetres. In a primigravida, cervical effacement occurs first, while in a multipara cervical effacement occurs simultaneously with cervical dilatation.

▶ *Show.* This is a thick, mucoid, blood-stained plug of the cervix which is expelled from the cervix when it dilates. It is known as the operculum. The operculum, which formed during pregnancy, is the mucus plug that has been

protecting the fetus and the genital tract from ascending infection. Birth usually commences within 24 hours after the 'show'.

The midwife confirms the onset of labour by objectively assessing the events communicated by the woman. The midwife will examine the abdomen to assess the nature of contractions and perform a vaginal examination to assess the state of the cervix and cervical dilatation. The rupture of the membranes is not a sign of labour and can happen any time when the woman is not in labour.

Decision making in the first stage of labour

The midwife assesses the woman on admission and refers the woman if there are factors that indicate particular risks. The midwife is obliged to use a partogram to monitor labour and if any problems arise that put the mother and baby at risk, the mother is referred for medical care.

Quality control

The clinic manager or unit manager does weekly audits of the partograms and institutes an in-service programme to ensure a high quality of care in labour.

26.4   The admission of the woman in labour

All women with high-risk pregnancies should be delivered in a facility that offers emergency obstetric care or with the means to urgently transfer the woman for emergency obstetric care should the need arise. Potential high-risk pregnancies include (DoH, 2015: 66):

▶ the primigravida
▶ any woman presenting with risk factors or an abnormality who has not been seen by a medical practitioner prior to the onset of labour (unbooked cases)
▶ the grand multipara
▶ any woman with a history of obstetric complications
▶ any identified risk factor or any abnormal condition of the fetus
▶ a woman younger than 16 or older than 35 years of age.

All women attending an antenatal clinic should be screened for high-risk and risk conditions and relevant action should be taken.

First impressions

The midwife should welcome the mother and give her a brief explanation of the activities that will take place to confirm whether she is in labour or not. The woman's expectations, desires and wishes are discussed; this information will assist with the planning of further management. The way in which the professional midwife interacts and attends to the woman will put her at ease.

The midwife then proceeds to an assessment of the woman.

Immediate status determination

It is essential to ascertain immediately what the status of the pregnancy and labour is. If the woman has a maternity card or case record, this will give the needed information. The following questions need to be asked:

▶ Is this your first pregnancy?
▶ At what stage have you attended antenatal care?
▶ When is the baby due?
▶ Is the baby still moving?
▶ When did the contractions start?
▶ How far apart are they now?
▶ Is there any vaginal bleeding?
▶ Are there any problems you know about?

If the birth is not imminent, the midwife can continue to gather information.

Observation

The general status of the woman can provide information on her well-being. It is important that the midwife assesses the woman's psychological, emotional and physical condition immediately. Listen to the way she answers any questions and note her attitude. Observe her physical condition, height, gait, size of feet, size of hands and any signs of a pendulous abdomen. Emotional instability may predispose the woman to puerperal psychosis, while abnormalities of the spine and pelvis may affect the capacity of the pelvis to allow for normal delivery.

Observe for any signs that the woman is undernourished, obese or very thin, including any signs of apparent dehydration. Note if she looks fresh or tired and ask how she has been sleeping lately and in particular what sleep she has had over the past 24 hours. Niggling, painful contractions can cause the woman to have disturbed sleep just prior to labour and she may be very tired. Allow the woman time to talk or ask questions.

Review or take a history

The woman should be seated in a comfortable chair during the history-taking, depending on her condition. However, if she is experiencing severe labour pains, it may be necessary for her to lie on the admitting couch. She should lie on her side whenever possible, to avoid supine hypotensive syndrome.

The antenatal notes are reviewed, if available, with special attention to any abnormalities recorded in the woman's notes. Specific attention is given to the past medical history and the history of the present pregnancy. This is recorded on the labour notes and any problem or abnormality is highlighted. Particularly, note:

▶ the woman's age
▶ parity
▶ type of previous labour and any operative delivery
▶ the outcome of any previous pregnancy
▶ any evidence of cephalopelvic disproportion (CPD)
▶ maternal disease such as cardiac disease, diabetes mellitus, pregnancy-induced hypertension (PIH) and/or anaemia
▶ the last Hb count (after 36 weeks)
▶ HIV status.

Take a full history if the above information is not available.

Obstetric details of the present pregnancy and labour are very important and they must be carefully noted and recorded:

▶ *Reason for seeking admission.* Is she in labour? Have her membranes ruptured? Is she not feeling well?
▶ *Menstrual period.* Confirm the first day of the last menstrual period (LMP) in order to work out the estimated date of delivery (EDD).
▶ *Fetal movements.* Ask about the nature of the fetal movements. Is the amount of fetal movement the same as it has been throughout the pregnancy? Are the fetal movements reduced, normal or excessive?
▶ *Uterine contractions.* At what time did contractions commence? When did they start to get stronger and more frequent? Are they regular now? How often are they coming (frequency) and how long do they last (length)? Are they much stronger than at first (strength)? Do they cause discomfort or pain and where is the pain felt?
▶ *Membranes.* Have the membranes ruptured? What time did they rupture? Did a lot of amniotic fluid come out? Is there any amniotic fluid draining? If so, check the colour of the liquor.
▶ *Show.* Has there been a mucus and blood show? When did it start? How much bleeding was noticed?

Written informed consent

Labour has an unpredictable outcome. In certain circumstances, written informed consent should be obtained on admission in case of emergency intervention such as surgery or anaesthesia. Obtaining consent on admission depends on the policy of the institution and the patient's age and general condition.

The birth plan

All women are encouraged to have a birth plan, which is developed with the assistance of the midwife during pregnancy. The admission period provides an opportunity to review the birth plan, which might be documented in the case notes or separately. The following issues need to be addressed or reviewed, if not discussed before:

- The presence of a birth companion, if the environment and the facility protocol allows
- Ambulation
- Position for delivery
- Pain relief
- Cutting the umbilical cord
- Infant feeding after birth
- Transfer to a postnatal ward.

Baseline observations

Do a physical examination, as described in Chapter 17 (also see DoH, 2015: 46). The observations and examinations are similar to those carried out at the first antenatal visit. Temperature, pulse, respiration and BP should be checked and any deviations should be reported immediately or appropriate action taken at once. A midstream specimen of urine should be obtained for urinalysis to exclude proteinuria and ketones.

The abdominal examination is performed as during pregnancy (see Chapter 18), with special emphasis on:

- engagement
- descent of the presenting part
- uterine contractions
- the fetal heart rate (FHR)
- response to uterine contractions: Is the woman calm and relaxed and coping with the pain? Is she restless and obviously in great pain and distress?

The vaginal examination

A vaginal examination is an intimate procedure that should be conducted in an environment where the woman's privacy and dignity is respected. The *Guidelines for Maternity Care in South Africa* (DoH, 2015: 48) propose that these examinations are done four-hourly during the latent phase of labour and two-hourly during the active phase.

During labour, plotting the information obtained from a vaginal examination onto a partogram will provide information about the progress of labour. Key decisions to be taken to manage labour, such as accelerating labour or deciding on a Caesarean section if progress is not optimum, will be based on this information.

PROCEDURE Vaginal examination during birth

Definition
Digital vaginal examination is a routine examination performed to assess the risks and progress of labour. It is done at two- to four-hourly intervals. Women prefer vaginal examination to the rectal examination (Downe et al, 2013).

Prerequisites
This procedure is only performed by professional midwives and doctors. Privacy must be ensured. The woman must give verbal consent.

Indications
The procedure is done to:
- confirm the onset of labour
- identify the presentation, position and engagement of the fetus
- assess progress or delay in labour
- artificially rupture membranes or determine if they have already ruptured
- exclude prolapse after membrane rupture (especially if FHR abnormalities occur or if the presenting part is ill-fitting)
- assess cervical progress prior to administering analgesia
- confirm full dilatation.

Contraindications
Vaginal examination is *not* be carried out in case of:
- ruptured membranes in women who are not in labour (perform a speculum examination)

continued

- the presence of active herpes simplex virus (HSV) lesions in a woman with ruptured membranes, unless the woman is in labour
- unknown placental localisation, or known placenta praevia
- unexplained vaginal bleeding – there is a risk of causing a major haemorrhage if the woman has placenta praevia
- the woman not giving consent
- female genital mutilation (FGM) – only an experienced healthcare professional familiar with the care of such women may perform a vaginal examination in this case, as intrapartum vaginal examination or catheterisation is difficult or impossible.

Observation

An intrapartum vaginal examination provides valuable information about cervical dilatation and effacement, membrane status, characteristics of amniotic fluid, fetal position and situation.

Principles and preparation (pre-examination)

- The woman is informed of the need for the examination and is offered an explanation in a way that she can understand. If required, an interpreter is used to ensure valid consent to the examination.
- Any emergency situation and any circumstances that make the woman unable to consent are documented in the obstetric record.
- The woman has the right to request the presence of a female chaperone during the procedure. The chaperone's name and designation are documented in the obstetric notes.
- Remember that hand hygiene and gloves, as well as eye protection if there is a risk of splashing, are universal precautions.

Setting up the examination

- Respect cultural and religious considerations regarding being exposed during the examination. For example, Muslim women may not be examined by a male healthcare professional.
- The woman is placed in a comfortable position, with her thighs flexed and abducted. The heels of her feet are positioned together. If the woman is at ease, her muscles will be more relaxed, which will reduce maternal discomfort.
- The woman's bladder must be empty.
- The woman is not exposed and is covered with a sheet.
- An abdominal palpation is done before the vaginal examination, to confirm findings.
- After the abdominal palpation, the FHR is determined by fetoscope, Doppler or CTG.

During the examination

- The intrapartum vaginal examination is performed between contractions to minimise pain and discomfort.
- Keep verbal and non-verbal communication relevant and appropriate.
- Avoid interruptions and discussions with other staff members.
- Minimise the time of exposure.
- Pay particular attention to non-verbal cues by the woman indicating discomfort and pain. Victims of physical and sexual abuse, rape or FGM may be particularly anxious during the examination.

The procedure: External inspection

Inspect the perineum and the condition of the vulva before the actual vaginal examination:

1. Inspect the external genitalia (labia, perineum, any scars) and make a note of any warts, lesions, discharge, liquor or blood.
2. Note that perineal scars are usually secondary, due to tears or episiotomy during childbirth.

The procedure: Internal inspection and assessment

1. Using the gloved dominant hand, gently part the labia to inspect the introitus.
2. Note the presence of any discharges, ulceration, oedema or varicose veins.
3. Assess the vaginal muscle tone, dryness and heat, which could indicate dehydration or prolonged labour.
4. Cleanse the vulva and vagina with chlorhexidine 25 per cent.
5. Open the vagina by holding the labia apart with the middle and index fingers of one hand.

continued

6   Insert chlorhexidine (or any approved disinfectant agent according to protocol) into the vagina as a precautionary measure for prevention of mother-to-child transmission (PMTCT) of HIV.

7   Position the gloved hand with the wrist straight and the elbow tilted downward to gently introduce two fingers of the dominant hand into the vagina until the second and index fingers touch the cervix.

8   Palpate for an opening in the cervix and estimate the diameter to identify the amount of dilatation (see more details below and Figure 26A).

9   Identify the position of the posterior fontanelle to determine fetal descent (see more details on the next page and Figure 26B).

10 Withdraw the hand gently and assist the woman to cover herself.

11 Explain the findings.

Estimation of dilatation

1   Pass one finger through the external os, and then through the internal os if the cervix permits.

2   Determine the length and thickness of the cervix in centimetres.

3   Determine the consistency of the cervix (hard, soft).

4   Determine the position of the cervix (anterior, posterior, central).

5   Determine the extent of application of the cervix to the presenting part.

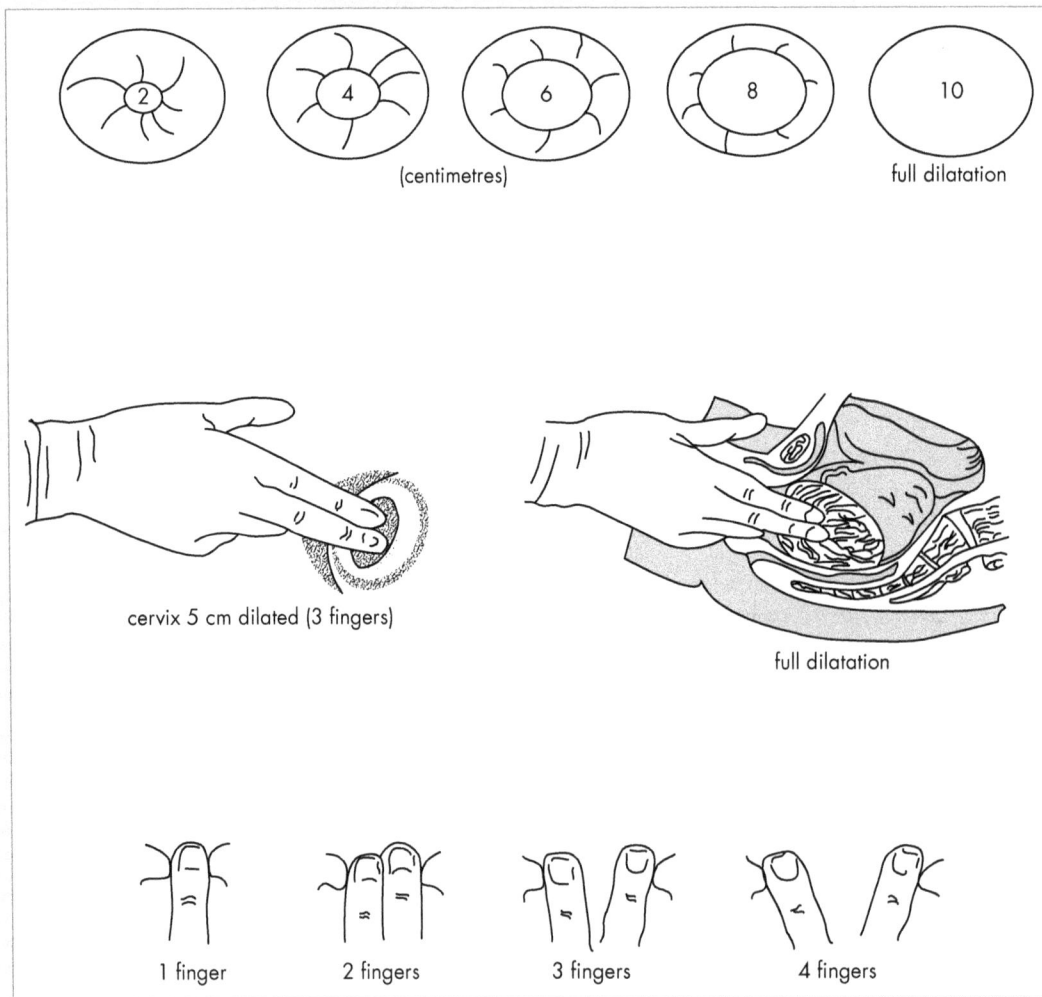

Figure 26A Cervical dilatation

continued

Palpating the cervix

1   Assess the state of the membranes (intact, bulging or smooth).
2   Note the colour or the amniotic liquid (clear or meconium-stained) and its odour (offensive or musky).
3   If premature rupture of membranes (PROM) is suspected, test the liquor during a speculum examination for a fern test:
   ▶ Do not use lubricant for the fern test; use water sparingly to lubricate the speculum (lubricant interferes with the fern pattern formation).
   ▶ Insert a sterile cotton-tipped swab or wooden spatula into the pool of fluid in the posterior vagina and then apply the fluid to a glass slide.
   ▶ A typical fern pattern confirms the presence of amniotic liquor.
4   Feel for the application of the presenting part on the cervix. If this is poor, feel for the existence of a presenting or prolapsed umbilical cord if the membranes have ruptured.
5   Palpate the presenting part and membranes.

See Figure 25.7 on page 379 for effacement and dilatation of the cervix. Also see Figure 18.6 on page 250.

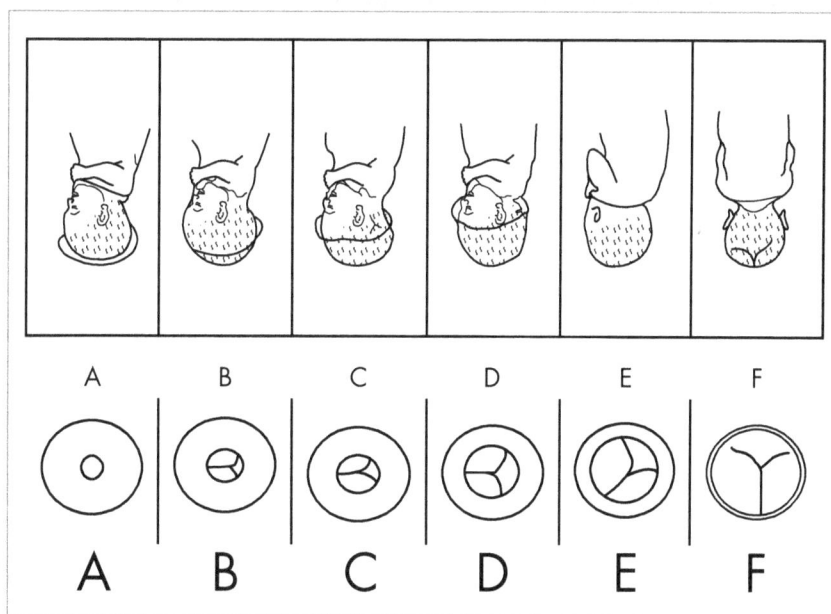

Figure 26B Descent of the presenting part showing the suture lines and posterior fontanelle determining the position in an anterior position

Determining descent

Determine fetal descent and station by identifying the position of the posterior fontanelle:

1   Draw an imaginary line between the two ischial spines.
2   Estimate the lowest part of the presenting part against this line.
3   If the lowest part of the presenting part is still above the imaginary line, it will be indicated in negative symbols (eg −2).
4   If the lowest level of the presenting part is on the level of the imaginary line, it will be indicated as a station of 0.
5   If the lowest part of the presenting part has passed the ischial spines, the station will be indicated in positive symbols (eg +2).

continued

Auscultation

Auscultate the fetal heart correctly and accurately to assess the condition of the fetus and obtain baseline data. A baseline non-stress test (NST) is done to determine the fetal status. If there are irregularities in the FHR, the medical practitioner must be informed and appropriate interventions implemented.

Referral

The midwife who cared for a woman in a satellite clinic may continue with the care of the woman if no abnormalities are found. In case of an abnormality, the midwife must immediately report the abnormality to a medical practitioner or obstetrician, or refer the woman to the nearest hospital.

If the woman is being delivered in a hospital under the supervision of the hospital medical practitioner, a GP or an obstetrician, then the medical practitioner should be informed of the admission of the woman and should receive a report on the woman's condition. See the SBAR forms for referral in *Guidelines for Maternity Care in South Africa* (DoH, 2015: 27).

26.5 Evidence-based, general principles of care during the first stage of labour

The admission of a woman in labour should only be undertaken by a qualified, experienced midwife who is able to assess whether or not the birth is proceeding normally and refer appropriately if it does not.

Environment

The physical environment should be clean, warm, safe and supportive. The Batho Pele principles dictate that all women should know their caregivers by name.

Companion in labour

The woman should have the option of having a chosen companion in labour. This may be her husband or partner, mother or other relative, or a friend. The midwife should explain everything to both the woman and her companion throughout the labour. This is currently an option in selected midwife obstetrics units (MOUs) and institutions.

Privacy

An effort should be made to maintain privacy by not examining the woman in front of other carers. If others are present, then the midwife should explain the presence of these people to the woman. Avoid too many people entering and leaving the room, as this may cause or increase the woman's stress and thus have a negative impact on quality of care.

Prevention of infection

It is essential that every precaution is taken to prevent the occurrence of infection, irrespective of the place of birth. Interventions during labour provide possible vehicles for infection and should be kept to a minimum and performed using full aseptic technique. Vaginal examinations should only be performed when absolutely necessary and with sterile equipment.

If the midwife is suffering from any infection, she must not attend a woman in labour but must make other arrangements for the woman's confinement. In HIV-positive women, vaginal examinations are avoided and done only when necessary. The membranes remain intact as long as possible in HIV-positive women.

Position and mobility

During the early first stage of labour, the woman may be ambulant if not contraindicated or if the membranes are intact. This will allow for the descent of the presenting part and also relieve the intensity of pain by diverting the woman's focus. She may even have a shower or bath. She can sit or lie in any comfortable position, except supine. The various positions that women can adopt in the different stages of labour will be discussed in Chapter 28.

Intake of food

The process of labour depletes the woman's energy resources. Oral fluids and light meals should be allowed during labour in low-risk pregnancies.

Women with high-risk pregnancies should have their oral intake restricted in case they require surgical interventions. In the case of mild dehydration, sips of fluids may be permitted.

Care of the bladder

All urine passed is measured and tested for glucose, protein and acetone. Any abnormalities are reported. All findings are documented.

Care of the bowels

Enemas are no longer routinely used in labour.

Comfort measures

Pain during labour and birth can be caused by both physical and emotional factors. Various methods can be used to relieve pain, ranging from natural methods to the use of opiates or an epidural. The presence and support of a midwife can relieve pain and increase comfort. (Pain relief methods will be discussed in more detail in Chapter 27.)

Monitoring the progress of labour

The progress of labour is monitored using the partogram (see Figure 26.1 on the next page). A partogram is a graphic record of the observations made of the progress of labour as well as the condition of the mother and fetus. The record of labour is a legal document and observations must be accurately recorded as soon as any event has occurred. An accurate record of the early stages of labour provides a basis for making objective decisions as labour progresses or fails to progress.

26.6   The partogram

The partogram, also called partograph or cervicograph, has been widely accepted as a tool to monitor the progress of labour. In under-resourced settings, the partogram is a cost-effective tool to monitor labour.

The chart is designed for recordings at 30-minute intervals, although the time may vary with institutions or local protocol. There are three main sections, namely sections for recording:
1. *fetal condition:* FHR, moulding in cephalic presentation and colour of liquor
2. *the progress of labour:* effacement and dilatation of the cervix, descent, flexion, rotation and presentation
3. *maternal condition:* vital signs, urinary output or vomitus, contractions.

Also see Figure 26A on page 396.

The advantages of using the partogram

The partogram:
▶ reduces complications from prolonged labour and obstructed labour for the mother (postpartum

haemorrhage [PPH], sepsis, uterine rupture and its sequelae) and for the newborn (anoxia, infections and death)
▶ provides information at a glance to assess the progress of labour
▶ reduces maternal mortality and morbidity caused by obstructed labour
▶ reduces the occurrence of prolonged labour, augmentation of labour and Caesarean sections
▶ helps healthcare personnel working in peripheral centres make referral decisions.

Principles for the use of the partogram

The following must be borne in mind when using the partogram:
▶ The latent phase of labour should not last more than eight hours.
▶ The active phase of labour starts when the cervix is 4 cm dilated.
▶ During the active phase of labour, the cervix should dilate at least 1 cm per hour.
▶ The duration between vaginal examinations should be at least four hours. The duration may vary with healthcare facilities, with some facilities allowing four hours during the latent phase and two hours during the active phase.

The partogram and African women's labour

Studies have shown that African women have a dilatation rate twice as long as other women, but their second stage of labour is shorter and quicker. Hence, if an African woman arrives late for admission, her time of admission is noted as zero (Farrell & Pattinson, 2005).

Key legal considerations when using the partogram

All skilled attendants are responsible for their own acts of omission and commission. Obligations include:
▶ correct and comprehensive recordings
▶ identifying abnormalities in recordings
▶ interpreting findings correctly
▶ identifying warning signs of abnormalities and preventing further development of these abnormalities
▶ acting on abnormalities in recordings
▶ the timely referral of women in case of abnormalities.

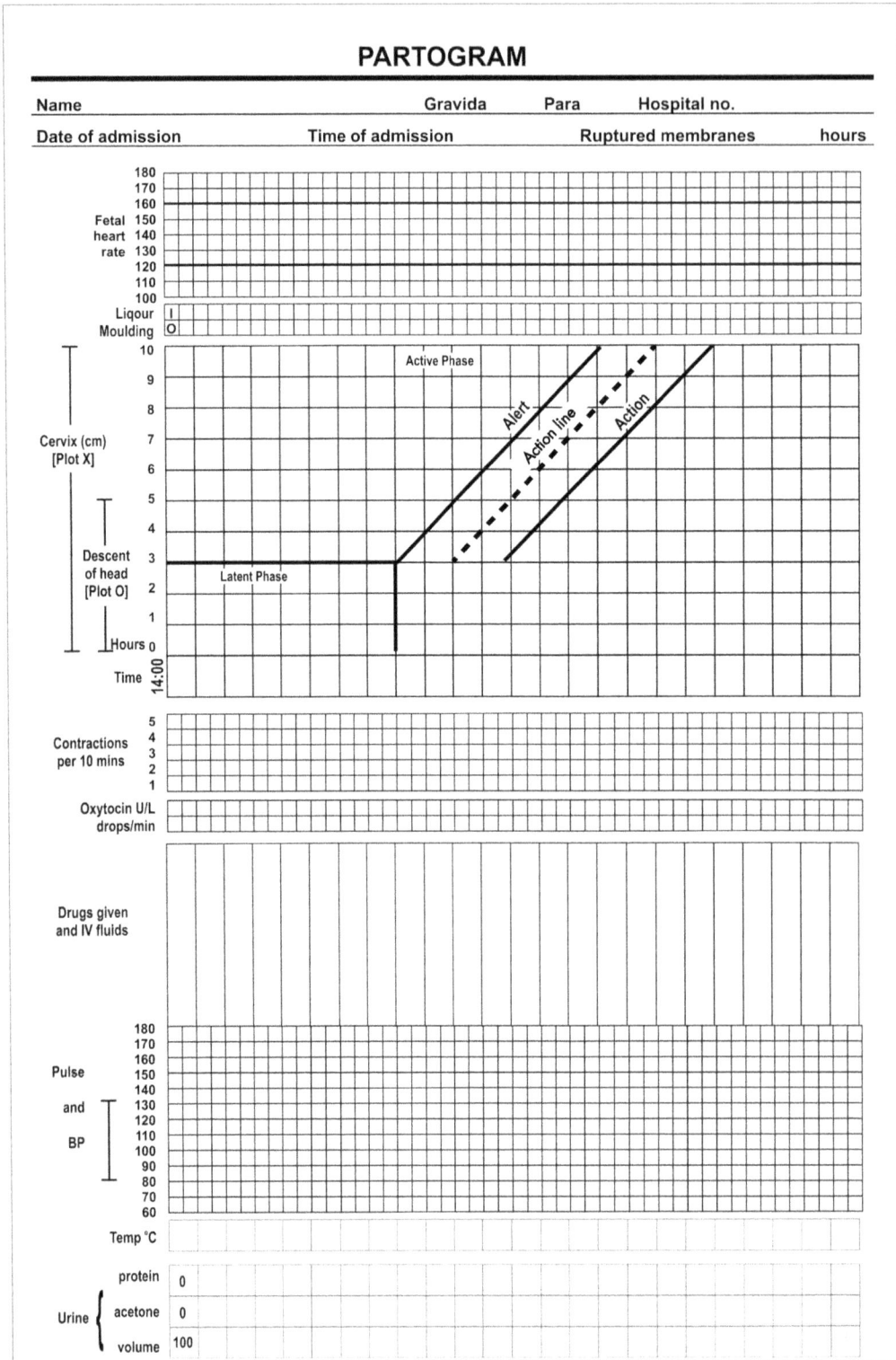

Figure 26.1 A blank partogram

PARTOGRAM

Name **Mrs Esther Kgololo**   Gravida 1   Para 0   Hospital no. **2435**

Date of admission   Time of admission   Ruptured membranes   hours

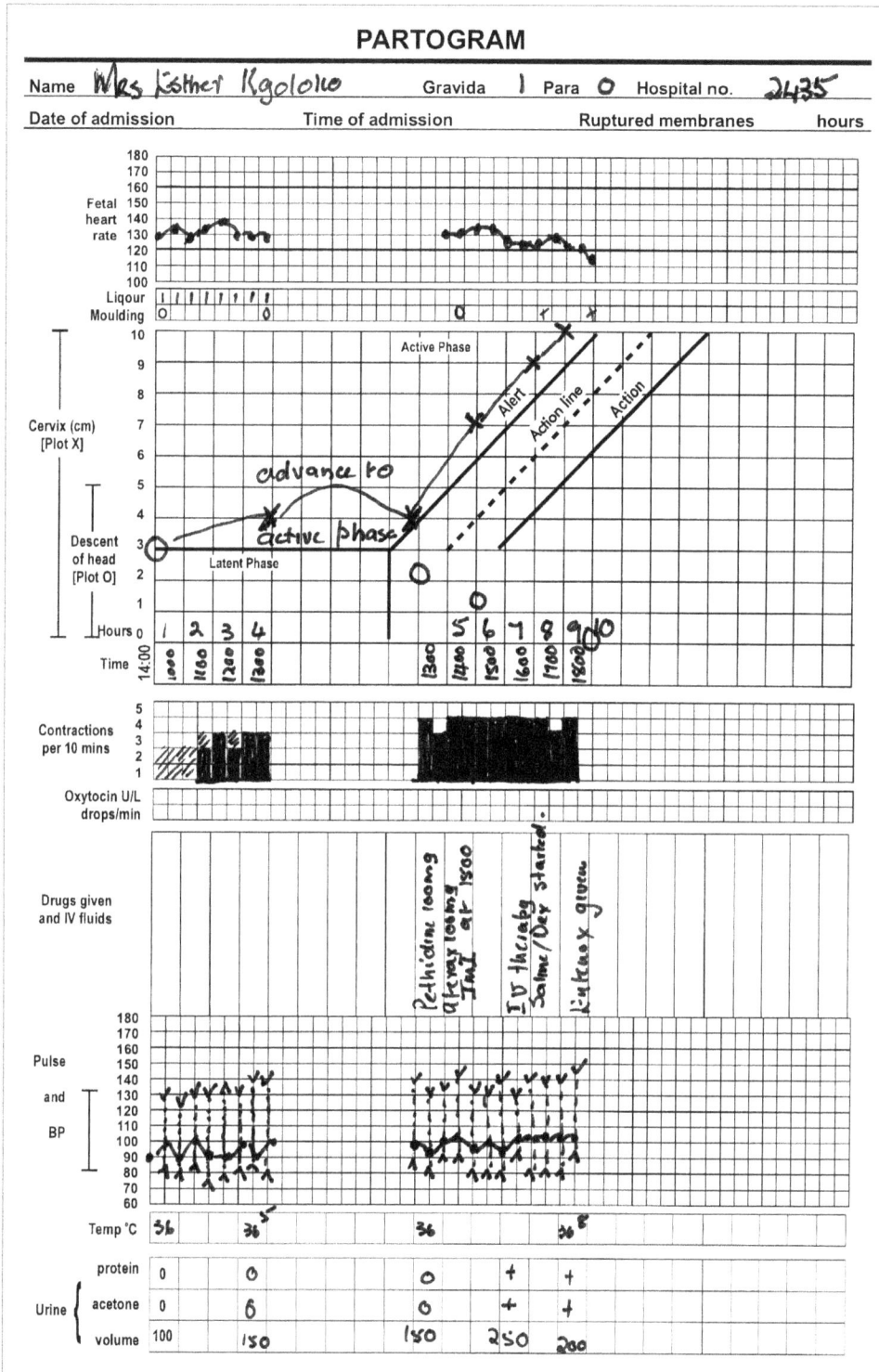

Figure 26.2 A completed partogram

Assessment of the fetal condition

After the determination of the normal baseline FHR, the FHR is checked every 30 minutes and recorded. It should be checked before, during and after a contraction over a full minute and correlated with the maternal pulse each time. In case of a multiple pregnancy, both heart rates are observed at the same time using a Doppler and a fetoscope. There should be at least 20 beats per minute (bpm) difference between babies.

Continuous fetal heart monitoring can be done using a fetal and maternal CTG. In this case, the fetal heart is monitored in response to the uterine contractions, which provides a graphic record of the response of the fetus to the uterine contractions.

The fetal section on the partogram is the part used to plot the monitoring and assessment of the fetal condition during labour. The condition of the fetus during labour is assessed using FHR, the state of the membranes and the colour of the liquor (if membranes have ruptured) and the moulding of the fetal skull bones. The baseline FHR must be recorded

including any variability (irregularities) and periodical changes (fast or slow heart rates) or deviations observed.

Assessment of fetal heart rate

Normal FHR is characterised by a rhythmic and regular baseline rate of 120–160 bpm. The CTG includes normal heart rate, variability and periodical changes, as explained in this section.

Deviations

Deviations are as follows:

▶ Fetal tachycardia is a baseline heart rate above 160 bpm. Baseline tachycardia is common in prematurity and may also reflect maternal tachycardia due to infection, high temperatures and/or ketoacidosis. These deviations should always be excluded. It can be a compensatory mechanism indicating undetected placental problems and possible hemorrhage.

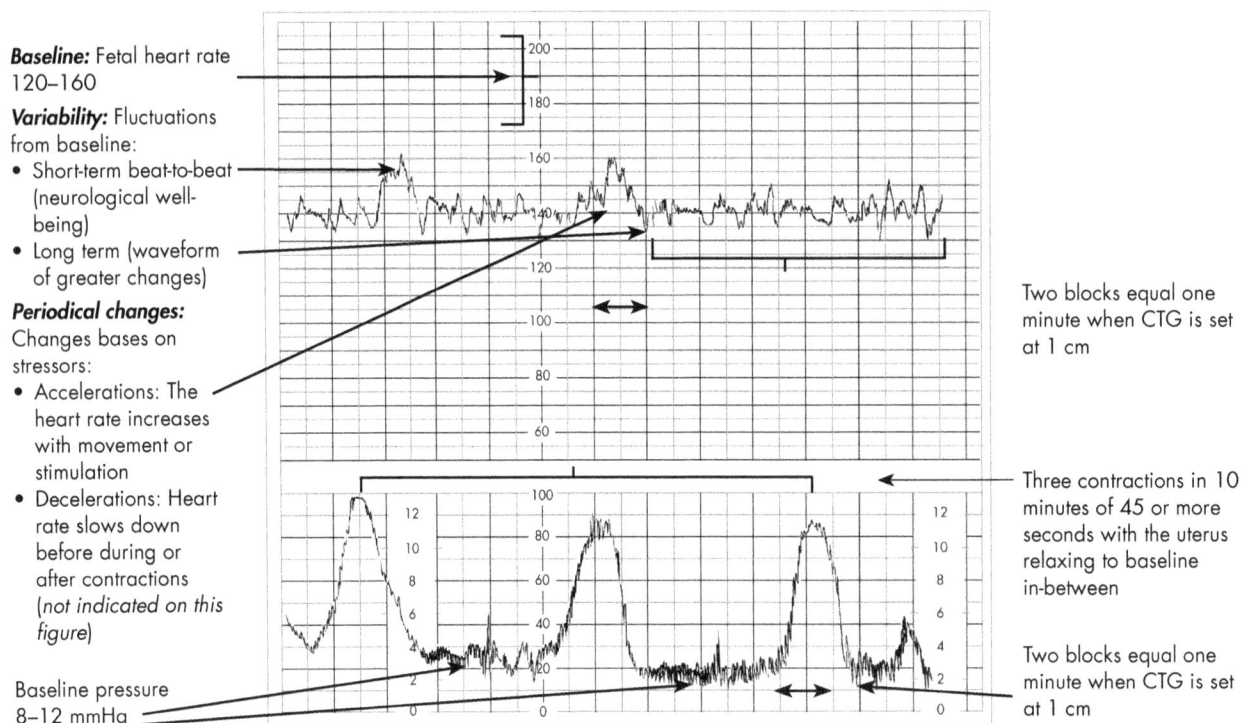

Figure 26.3 Terminology used to describe FHR patterns

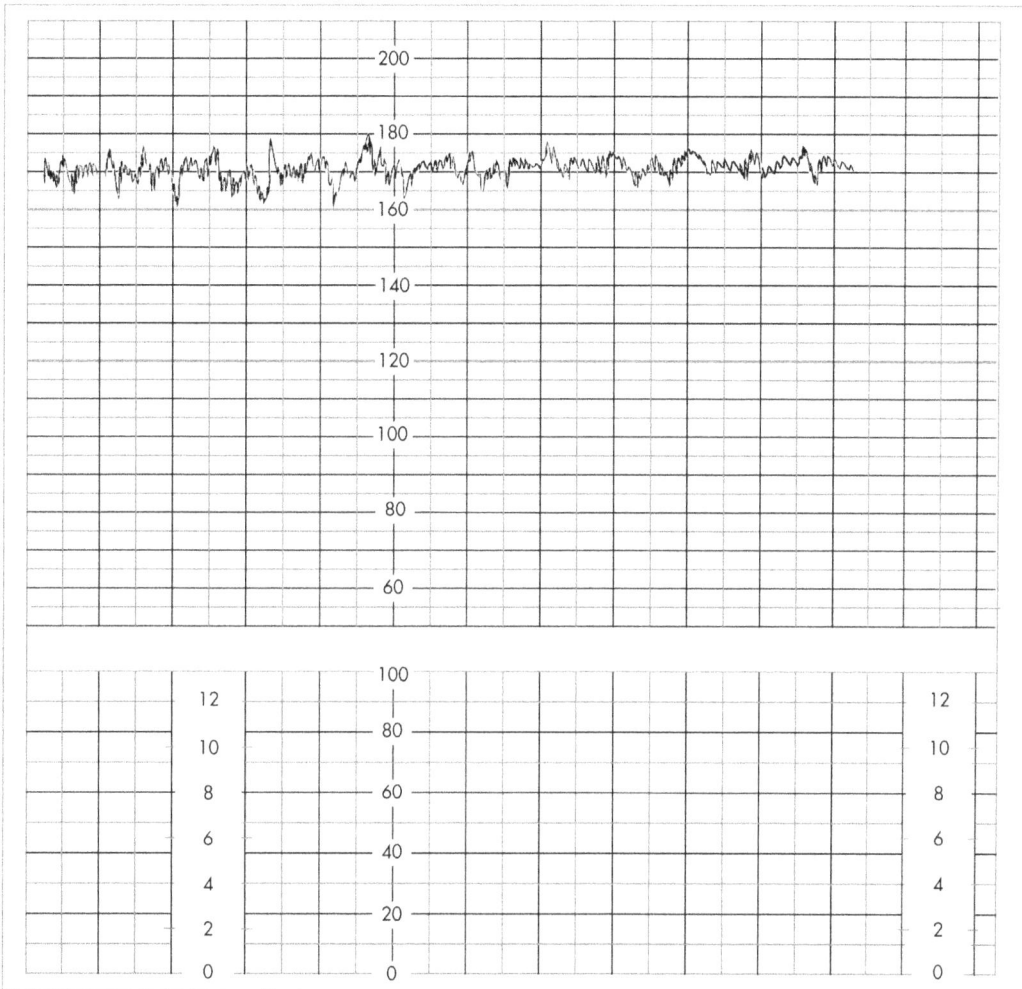

Figure 26.4 Suspicious pattern: Baseline tachycardia

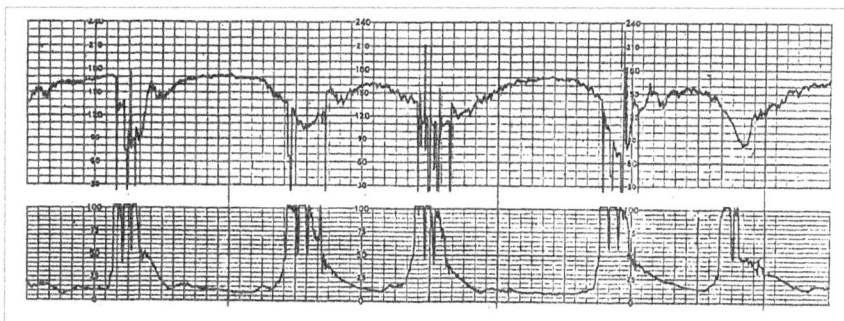

Figure 26.5 Asphyxial pattern: Complicated tachycardia

▶ Fetal bradycardia is characterised by a baseline FHR of less than 110 bpm. The maternal pulse rate is checked against the fetal heart. Fetal baseline bradycardia may be due to congenital abnormalities, drugs or fetal distress.

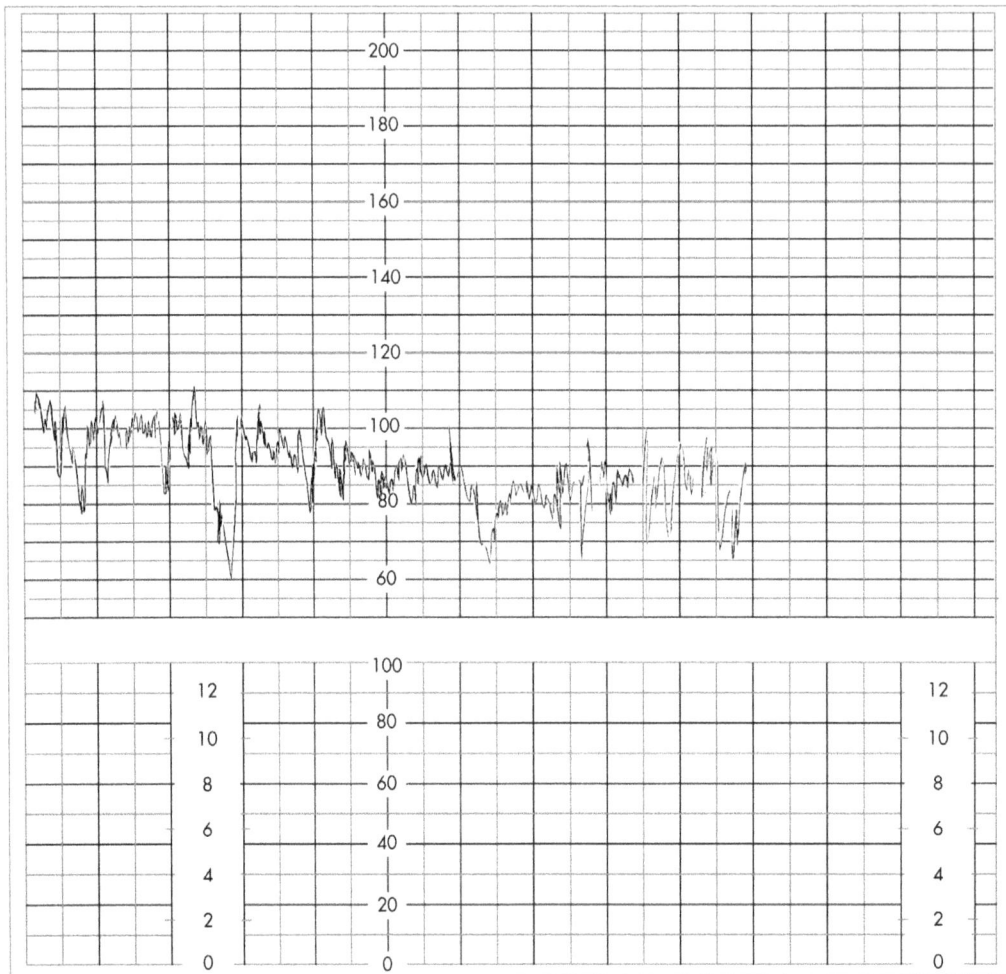

Figure 26.6 Safe pattern: Baseline bradycardia

Baseline variability

The fluctuations of the beats from the baseline are referred to as the beat-to-beat variation. This is the difference between the sympathetic and parasympathetic systems of the fetal heart and indicates the neurological well-being of the baby. Pain medication and other substances may reduce variability.

Periodical changes

▶ *Acceleration.* This is characterised by a transient increase in the FHR at the start of a contraction, with a return to the baseline by the end of the contraction or shortly after. This pattern is generally taken to indicate good reflex responsiveness of the fetal circulation to the stress of uterine contractions.

▶ *Deceleration.* There are two types of decelerations, called early and later decelerations (see the following subsection

for more on later decelerations). Early decelerations are associated with the reduction of the fetal heart pattern mirroring the contraction. The fetal heart recovers to the baseline as soon as the contraction is over. Early decelerations are related to the fetal heart slowing due to:

- pressure of the fetal head on the cervix
- poor blood supply to the baby due to placental perfusion reduction at the peak of the contraction
- the cord being around the neck.

Non-reassuring patterns

▶ *Variable decelerations (uncomplicated).* With variable decelerations, the shape and time of the deceleration varies. This pattern is thought to be due to umbilical cord compression. Persistent variable decelerations may therefore be associated with progressive fetal asphyxia.

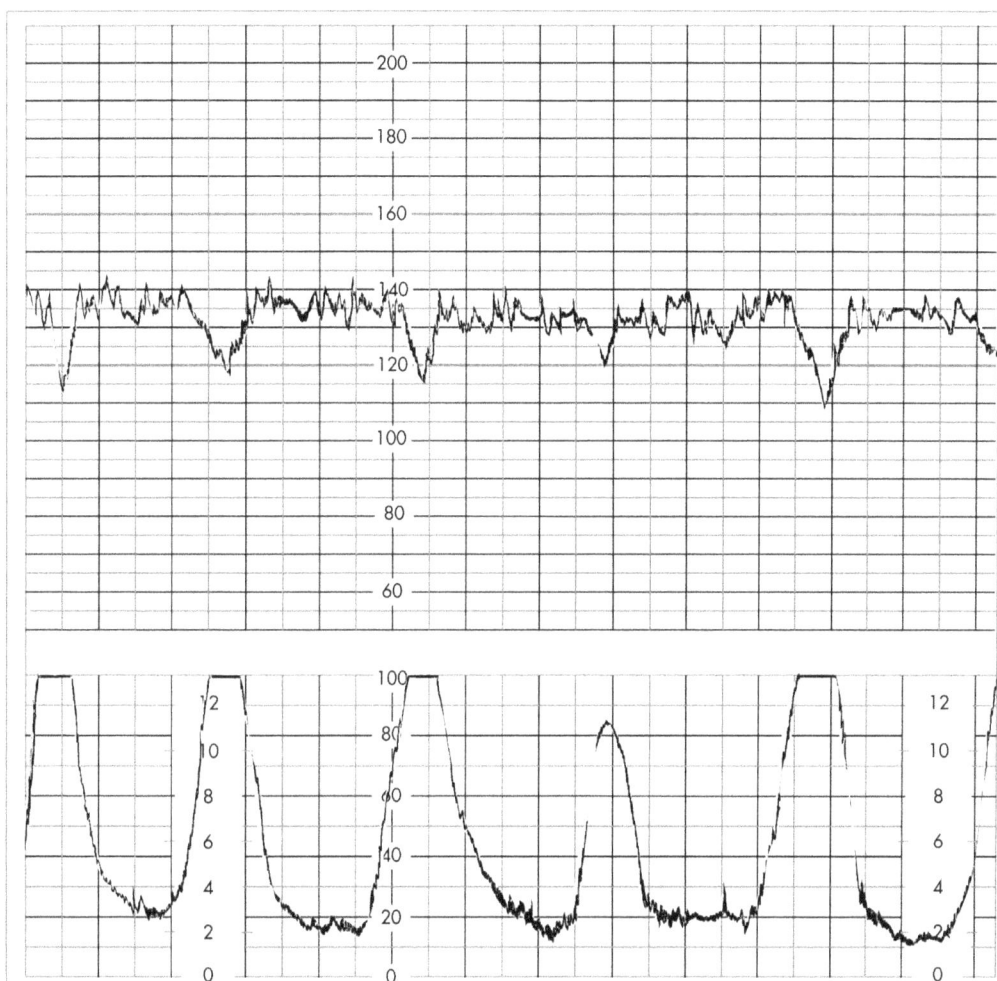

Figure 26.7 Suspicious pattern: Early deceleration

- *Late decelerations (asphyxia).* A late deceleration is any decrease in FHR after the peak of the contraction (that is, a deceleration with lag). The FHR only returns to the baseline after the contraction is ended. This type of deceleration is usually associated with asphyxial stress. In general, the greater the lag, the more serious the degree of fetal asphyxia. Late decelerations may be very shallow, with an amplitude of only 10–20 bpm, or they may be very deep.

- *Loss of beat-to-beat variation.* A loss of beat-to-beat variation is characterised by a baseline FHR variability of less than 5 bpm. This is of significance when combined with decelerations or tachycardia or bradycardia. It is due to a reduced fetal cardiac autonomic tone and may result from a variety of causes. The most important cause is the effect of asphyxia on the medullary centres. It may also be observed when the fetus is asleep or as a result of drugs such as diazepam and narcotic analgesics administered to the mother.

- *Prolonged deceleration.* Prolonged deceleration or a baseline shift may be indicated by placental abruption. The BP is checked, position changed to the left side and oxygen is administered. If the woman is induced, the induction is discontinued. If she is fully dilated, the baby is delivered. If not delivered, the woman needs an emergency Cesarean section.

Moulding

Moulding (see Figure 8.15 on page 137) is the overriding of the fetal skull bones during labour in a cephalic presentation. The level of moulding is assessed four-hourly and recorded.

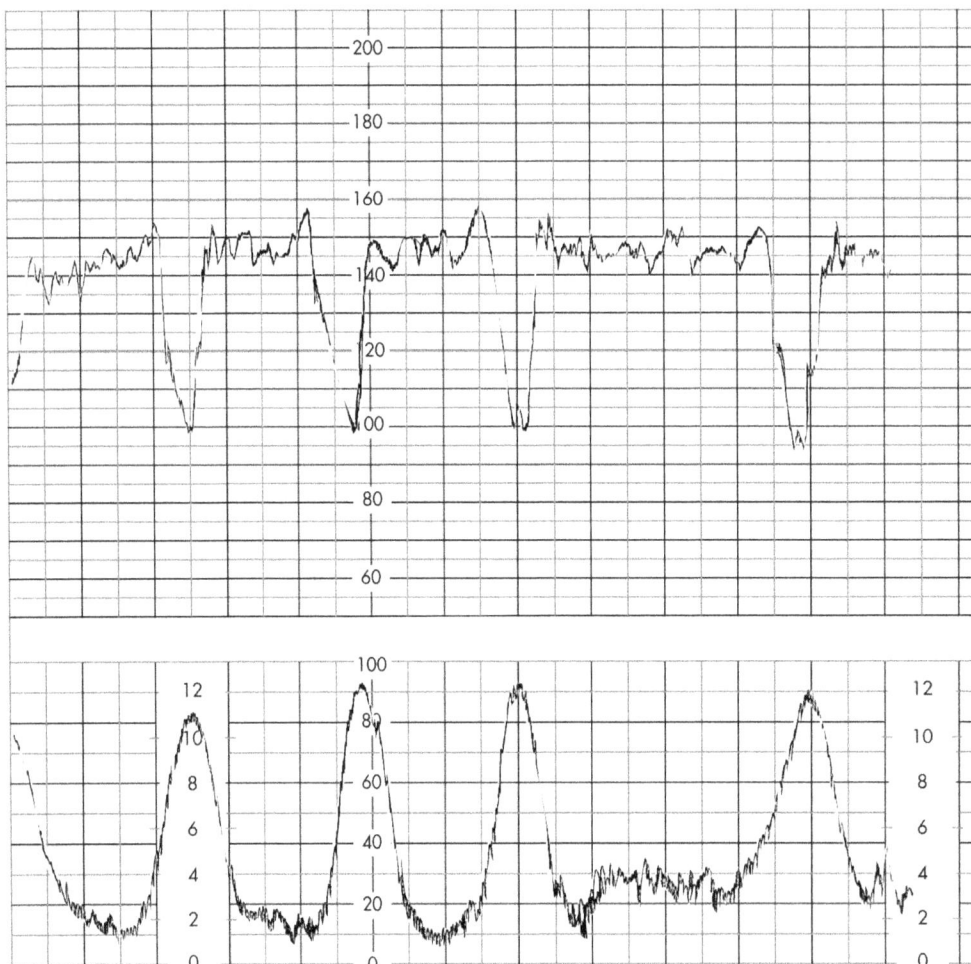

Figure 26.8 Suspicious pattern: Variable deceleration (uncomplicated)

Moulding protects the brain from compression, as long as it is not excessive or rapid or in an unfavourable direction. Increasing or excessive moulding with the head high in the pelvis is a warning sign of CPD. The bones that overlap are the occipital over the parietal, and the parietal over the parietal. The ability to mould is diminished after 40 weeks. Table 26.1 details the degrees of moulding and how to identify them.

Membranes and liquor

It is important to record if and when the membranes rupture. Early rupture of membranes exposes both the woman and the fetus to the risk of infection, so it is important to indicate the time that the membranes ruptured, particularly in HIV-positive women. The administration of antibiotics if needed is per protocol.

Table 26.1

Assessment of moulding during labour

Description	Degree of moulding
The bones are separated and sutures are felt easily.	0 (no moulding)
The bones are just touching each other.	+
The bones are overlapping, but reducible when digital pressure is applied.	+ +
The bones are overlapping and non-reducible with digital pressure.	+ + +

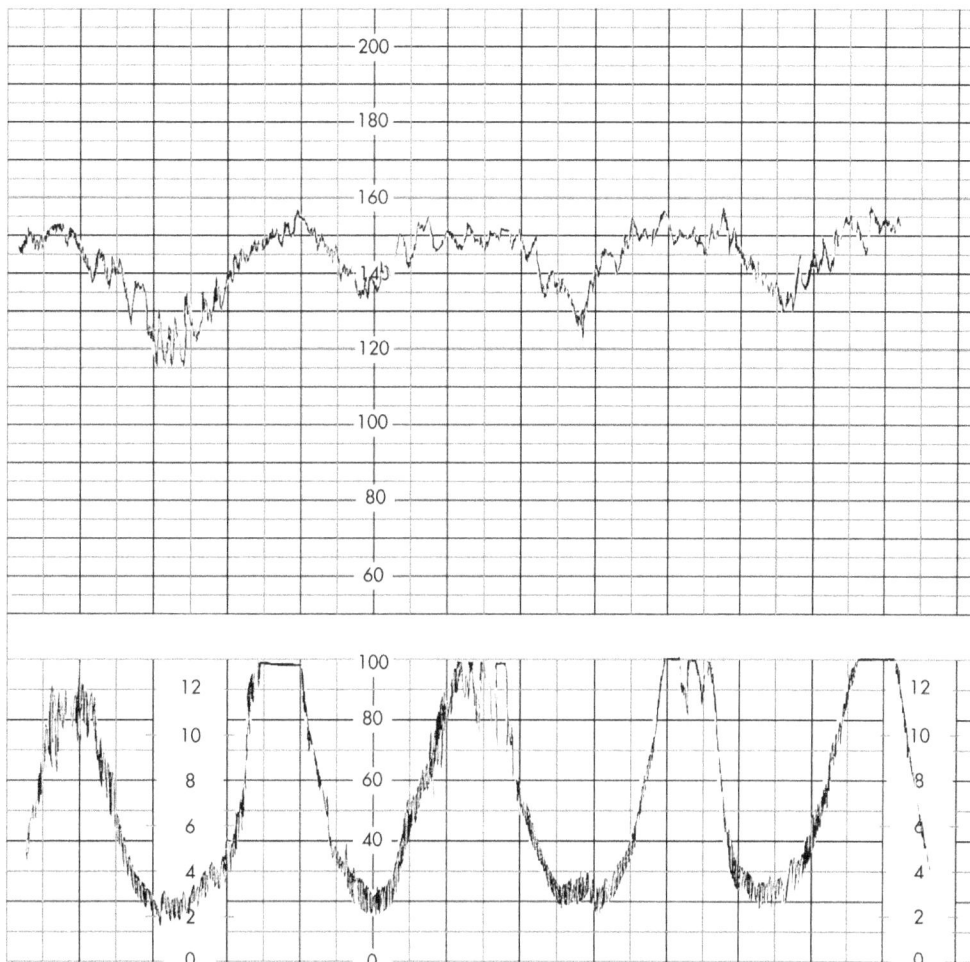

Figure 26.9 Asphyxial pattern: Subacute hypoxia leading to progressive distress

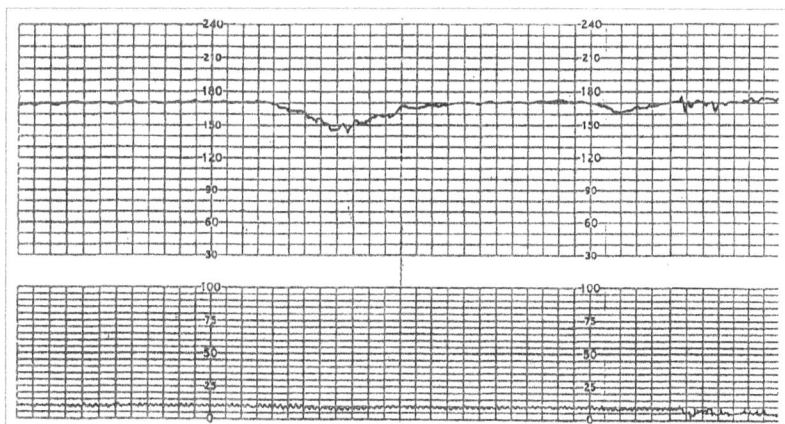

Figure 26.10 Asphyxial pattern: Loss of beat-to-beat variation

If membranes are intact, the information is recorded as an 'I' on the partogram. If membranes have ruptured, indicate the colour of the liquor with the letter that describes that colour, for example 'M' for meconium-stained liquor or 'C' for clear liquor. If meconium is present, it is interpreted as fresh or old (thin or thick) meconium.

Progress of labour

The progress of labour is determined by cervical dilatation, the level of descent of the presenting part, the fetal position and uterine contractions.

The cervicograph

The progress of labour is recorded on the middle part of the partogram. This section is referred to as the cervicograph and is defined as a graph of cervical dilatation marked against time. It is divided into the latent and active phases of labour. The latent phase lasts 0–8 hours, while the active phase starts at the eighth hour and may last up to the tenth hour, depending on parity. The descent of the presenting part is documented on the cervicograph in fifths if the presentation is cephalic. Descent can also be related to cervical dilatation when assessing the progress of labour (see Figure 26A on page 396).

Interpretation of findings

The cervicograph in the partogram is based on the principles that when recording dilatation, each block is one hour, and that birth is a time-related biological process. In the active phase, the cervix in a primigravida should dilate 1 cm each hour. The first line is called the alert line and is the pathway that the labour should take. If the woman's labour crosses the first line, the midwife is alerted and takes precaution for improved assessment. The action line is four hours later. If the woman reaches the four-hour action line, there should be interventions to deliver the baby.

In cases where the woman is not in a hospital, the two-hour line is called the transfer line, giving time to transfer the woman to the nearest centre for intervention. (The form called the SBAR, which stands for situation, background, assessment and recommendation, needs to be completed.)

Vaginal examination

Cervical dilatation is checked four-hourly (see the procedure box on pages 394–398). The cervix should dilate by 1–1.5 cm per hour in the active phase, depending on parity. The cervix dilates from 0 to 10 cm and is considered fully dilated at 10 cm. The nature of contractions and the degree of application of the presenting part to the cervix has an effect on the rate at which the cervix dilates (see Chapter 8). Particular attention must be paid to strong contractions with no or poor cervical dilatation.

Contractions

The midwife may feel the contraction before the woman is aware of it, as the contraction is felt when the uterine pressure exceeds 25 mmHg. This difference between manual palpation of the contraction and the woman feeling the contraction can be 20 seconds. If a woman feels a contraction before it is palpated by a midwife, if the contraction does not show on a CTG, or if the woman complains of pain after the contraction has subsided, abnormal uterine function is suspected.

During a normal uterine contraction, the intrauterine pressure, which is called intensity or amplitude of the contraction, increases. The contraction rises sharply and has a slow decline. The frequency of the contractions is the number of contractions in 10 minutes and is scientifically measured in Montevideo units (MVU). In clinical practice, three to four contractions of 60 seconds equals 275 MVU and are required for labour as measured by abdominal palpation or external CTG. The uterine tone needs to return to the baseline or relax completely between contractions for at least 40 seconds.

Calculating Montevideo units

This is the peak strength of contractions in mmHg, measured by an internal monitor, multiplied by their frequency per 10 minutes.

1 Measure the peak amplitude of each contraction, in mmHg = A
2 Count the number of contractions in 10 minutes = N
3 MVU = A x N

For example: contractions of 60 mmHg, with four in 10 minutes = MVU of 240.

In a retrospective report, 91 per cent of women in spontaneous active labour achieved contractile activity greater than 200 MVU and 40 per cent reached 300 MVU (UTHSCSA, nd). (See also Figure 8.17 on page 140.)

The mean force to initiate cervical change should reach 275 MVU.

The contractions are monitored abdominally and classified as mild, moderate or severe. Mild contractions last 20 seconds or less and are plotted with faint dots on the partogram. Moderate contractions last 20–35 seconds and are plotted as lightly shaded lines. Strong contractions last 35–60 seconds and are plotted as dark shaded areas on the partogram (see Figure 26.1 on page 400).

When contractions last more than 60 seconds, they are referred to as hypertonic uterine contractions. They may cause maternal and fetal distress and sometimes contribute to rupture of the uterus. If substances are used to stimulate the uterus, they need to be revised immediately.

Assessment of maternal condition

Maternal condition is assessed based on the nature of contractions, vital signs, hydration, urinary output, the woman's emotional stamina and response to labour.

Administration of drugs

Any drugs administered to the mother during labour should be recorded on the partogram, including any drugs for induction of labour or pain relief. This includes IV fluid, pain relief and other medication.

Vital signs

The woman's temperature is checked four-hourly or according to local protocol. The temperature should remain normal. Pyrexia may indicate infection, especially in the presence of PROM, ketosis or maternal dehydration. There may be a slight increase in temperature with an epidural anaesthetic.

Pulse is recorded every 30 minutes and is expected to remain normal. Tachycardia may be associated with anxiety, infection, pain, haemorrhage or a reaction to medication.

BP is checked every hour and is expected to remain normal in the absence of essential hypertension or PIH. A supine position may induce hypotension.

Urinalysis

The woman should be advised to empty her bladder every hour, as a full bladder can interfere with the progress of labour.

If she fails to pass urine and the bladder is full, a once-off catheter should be inserted.

All urine passed should be recorded and tested for glucose, proteins and ketones. Ketones may be a sign of maternal distress or starvation if the woman has been in labour for some time without having adequate nutrition. An IV infusion with saline and dextrose is commenced. A trace of protein may be a sign of infection or contamination by amniotic fluid if the membranes have ruptured. Also exclude pre-eclampsia in the presence of significant proteinuria.

Alert
A full bladder is associated with: ▶ delay in descent of the presenting part during the first stage of labour   ▶ a prolonged second stage of labour   ▶ uterine atony after delivery of the baby, causing PPH.

26.7   Conclusion

Effective communication between healthcare professionals and the woman during labour, as well as the presence of a labour companion, is associated with less anxiety, less labour pain and reduced interventions during childbirth. Labour progresses well in the presence of good uterine contractions, progressive descent of the presenting part as well as progressive dilatation of the cervix. The role of the midwife is to ensure that both maternal and fetal conditions remain stable throughout labour.

Comfort and pain management in labour

27.1 Introduction

One of the pregnant woman's greatest concerns is the pain that she will experience during labour and whether or not she will be able to cope with it. In primigravidae, expectations of pain depend on reports from others, and in women who have already given birth it is determined by previous experience.

Factors that will influence the woman's experience are the intensity of labour pain, the length of time that labour lasts, the environment in which she gives birth and the support that she receives from her companion and/or caregiver. Each woman's labour is unique. Some women need little or no pain relief, while others find that pain relief gives them better control over their labour and delivery.

Pain in childbirth is a universal expectation in all societies and cultures, but women may interpret, perceive and respond differently to the management and practices to cope with the pain. Thus, pain perceptions may be culturally defined, but within cultures there are diverse individual experiences of pain.

Weber (1996) found a strong association between culture and a woman's belief and behaviour with regards to pain in childbirth. Coping mechanisms may thus be culturally based. For example, in some cultures, birth pain is viewed as an essential experience to face and endure as part of becoming a woman; in such cultures, pain intervention is frowned upon. Midwives and healthcare professionals need to understand the meaning of pain, women's perceptions of pain and culturally bound pain behaviours in order to facilitate a satisfying birth experience and empower women of diverse cultural backgrounds.

A supportive environment, with caring professionals skilled in pain assessment and management, will give the woman a sense of control through increased options and participation in decision making in pain management. It is important to provide health information, starting from the antenatal period. An open approach in labour allows for support of the woman's choices without prejudice and judgement.

> **Recommended reading**
>
> Weber, SE. 1996. 'Cultural aspects of pain in childbearing women.' *J Obstet Gynecol Neonatal Nurs*, 25(1): 67–72. https://www.ncbi.nlm.nih.gov/pubmed/8627405 (Accessed 22 August 2017).

27.2 The psychology and physiology of pain

In most languages, the process of giving birth uses words that describe a *process of work* (labour) rather than pain. Referring to contractions in labour as 'labour pains' is discouraged. It is important that midwives adopt concepts and practices that steer away from disempowering language and support women. One of the ways to do this is by referring to birth and contractions rather than 'labour pains'.

Childbirth is more than a physiological process. Coping with birth is an emotional and complex process that can result in feelings of fulfilment and achievement.

Psychological factors of pain in labour

The components which determine an individual's reaction to pain are not fully understood. Much seems to depend upon what is known as the pain threshold. Each individual has his or her own pain threshold, which will vary according to the person's psychological and physical state at a given time. A low pain threshold means that pain is experienced when the person is subjected to relatively light and/or small amounts of stimuli, while a high pain threshold indicates that pain is only experienced with relatively stronger and/or greater amounts of stimuli. Cultural, religious and family backgrounds are also factors in setting pain thresholds.

Table 27.1

Factors that influence a woman's perception of pain during labour

Factors that would have a positive influence	Factors that would have a negative influence
Attending childbirth education classes Compiling a birth plan Reading about pregnancy Regular aerobic exercise during pregnancy	No birth preparation or birth plan to cope with pain Cultural influences and expectations Lack of information and preparation Myths ('old wives' tales')
The presence of a significant person or a doula	Being left alone A sense of isolation and helplessness
The presence of a skilled and attentive midwife	No skilled attendance
A supportive environment	An uncomfortable environment, such as wet or soiled linen on the bed, the room temperature being too hot or too cold
Receiving physical care	Physical abuse such as pinching or slapping
Self-help skills to cope better with pain, ie position change, relaxation techniques, music, etc	Poor coping skills
Privacy Confidentiality Respectful care	No privacy Feeling unsafe Feeling disrespected
The caregiver gives encouragement, for example by assuring the woman that every contraction discomfort brings her nearer to the end, etc.	No reassurance is given. Staff criticise or shout at the woman.
The caregiver displays her skills and knowledge and explains all procedures or interventions as well as the progress of labour to the patient. The caregiver communicates with and listens to the woman when decisions are made; this allows the woman to feel she is in control.	The woman feels unsafe because the caregiver does not explain interventions, or neglects to meet her needs. There is emotional neglect, eg the caregiver ignores the woman when she asks for support or information, or the caregiver criticises, shouts at or blames the woman.
The caregiver uses various non-pharmacological pain relief methods. The caregiver offers and administers analgesia on request, before the woman reaches the stage where she loses control.	The caregiver does not use non-pharmacological pain relief methods such as back massage and breathing techniques. The caregiver is ignorant of the need for pain relief and neglects to offer or administer pain relief.

Factors that may lower the pain threshold include worry, anxiety, insecurity, fear, ignorance, fatigue, intense heat or cold, poor general physical condition, malnutrition and starvation and dehydration. Continuous or severe pain experienced over an extended period, either intermittent or continuous –¹ such as in hypertonic uterine action or prolonged labour – can also lower the pain threshold.

Factors that can raise the pain threshold may be divided into emotional, psychological and physical factors – all aspects of the woman's make-up. In addition, the introduction of an outside substance such as an analgesic will raise the pain threshold.

Table 27.1 details some factors that will influence the way a woman experiences pain during labour. These factors include aspects such as the woman's preparation, the birth plan, the environment during labour and the care provided during labour.

Physiological causes of pain in labour

Pain during labour is related to contraction of the uterus, as shown in figures 27.1 and 27.2. In normal labour, the pain is intermittent. It starts as the uterus contracts, becomes more severe as the contraction reaches its peak and disappears when the uterus relaxes. Pain is usually only experienced when the intra-amniotic pressure reaches 20–25 mmHg. Pain might manifest as cramping in the abdomen, groin, lower back or thighs.

Other causes of pain might include pressure on the bladder and bowels by the baby's head, stretching of the lower segment of the uterus and vagina, and pressure on the nerve ganglia in and around the uterus. The nature of labour pain has been described as cramping, burning, sharp, excruciating, throbbing and similar to dysmenorrhea but much worse.

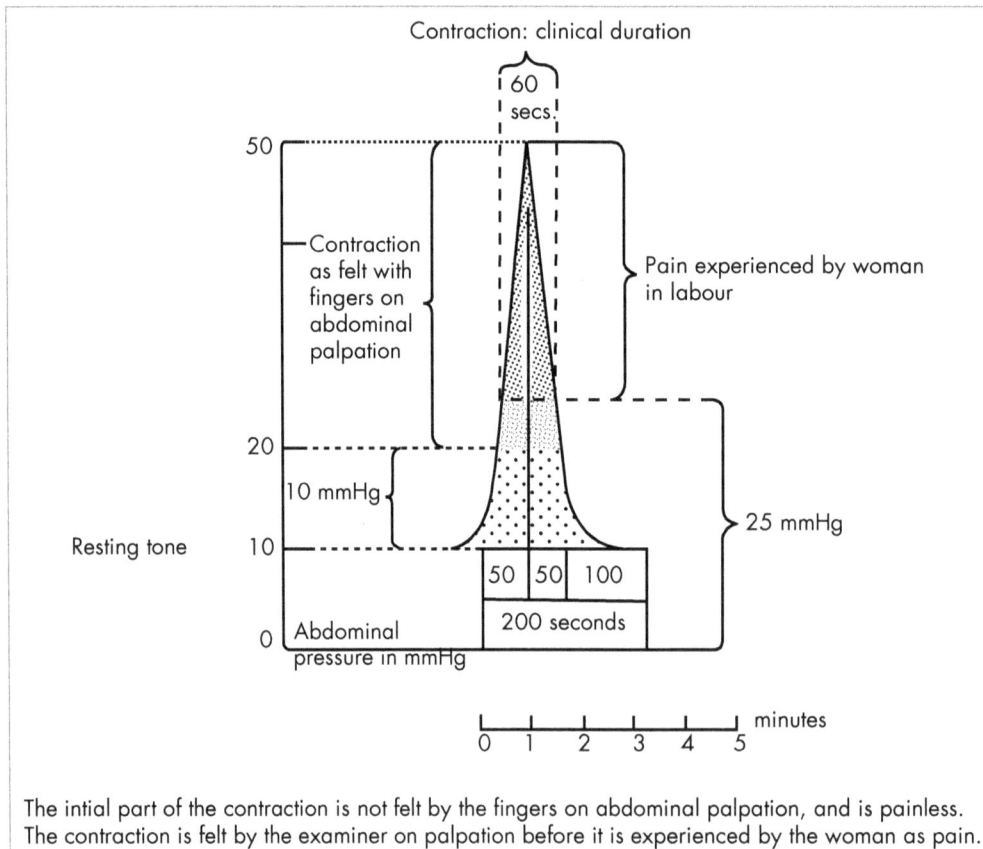

The intial part of the contraction is not felt by the fingers on abdominal palpation, and is painless. The contraction is felt by the examiner on palpation before it is experienced by the woman as pain.

Figure 27.1 Pain as experienced during a uterine contraction in established labour (redrawn from Llewellyn-Jones, 1982: 345)

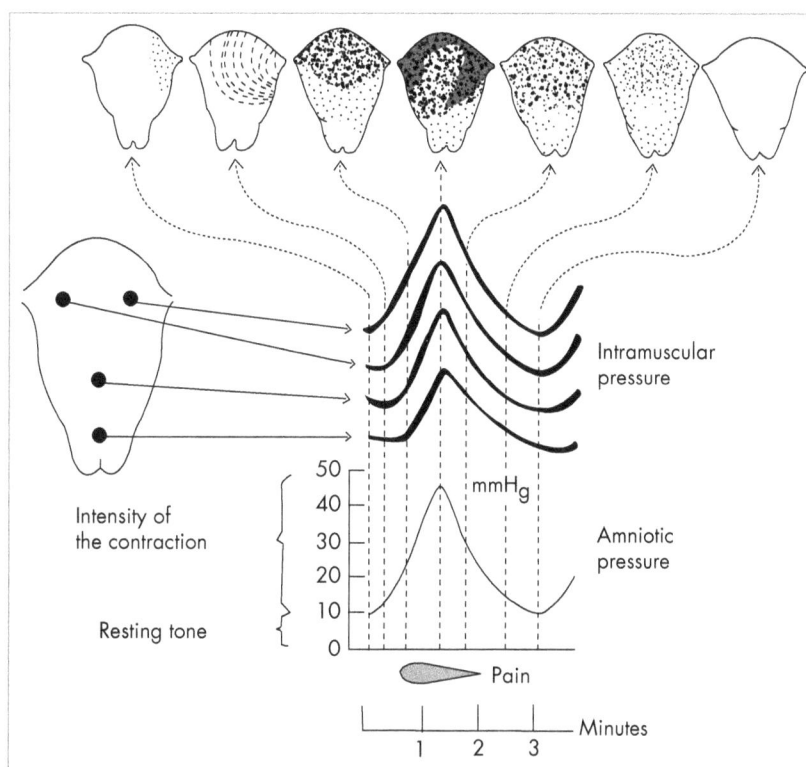

Figure 27.2 Normal labour pain

The degree of pain varies in different women, in the same woman during succeeding labours and at different stages in the same labour. In a small proportion of women, the contractions are painless.

As the uterine contractions increase in intensity, duration and frequency, the pain experienced during labour is possibly due to:

▶ the distension of the lower pole of the uterus during contractions, particularly the dilatation of the cervix

▶ the stretching of the ligaments adjacent to the uterus and other adjacent issue

▶ pressure on or stretching of the nerve ganglia around the lower part of the uterus and pressure on the bladder and the rectum

▶ contraction of the muscle while it is in a relatively ischaemic state (similar to angina pectoris). Adequate amounts of blood do not reach the uterine muscles and they become anoxic. This occurs especially when:

• the uterus has a high tone at the peak of contractions

• the contractions are too frequent

• the contractions last too long.

Pain in the lower abdomen

Pain in the lower abdomen (see Figure 27.3 on the next page) seems to be related to the activity in the upper uterine segment and is present when labour is progressing well.

Pain in the back

Pain in the back (see Figure 27.3) is related to tension in the lower uterine segment and the cervix. Backache is common in posterior positions of the vertex and is severe when there is inco-ordinate uterine action, particularly when the cervix is abnormally resistant. In general, the less backache the woman experiences, the more efficient the uterus is. However, primigravidae tend to have more back pain than multiparae.

Dystocia

Dystocia means difficult and painful labour. It can be due to faults in any of the three Ps of labour, as described in Chapter 8, namely the passenger, the passages or the powers. There may also be a combination of one or more factors at work, including the psychological make-up and outlook of the woman. Also see Table 27.1 on page 411 for factors that can contribute to dystocia.

413

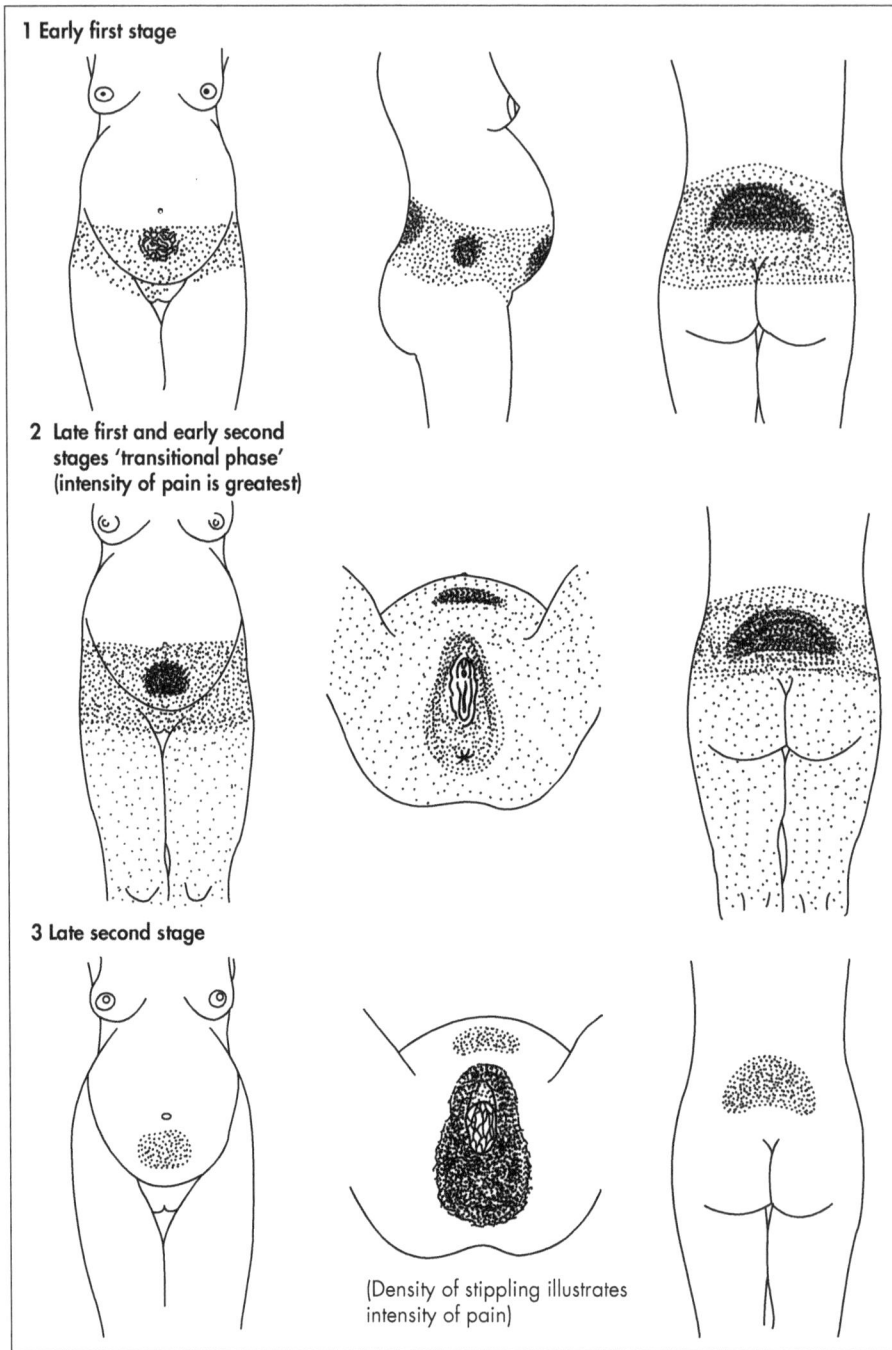

1 Early first stage

2 Late first and early second stages 'transitional phase' (intensity of pain is greatest)

3 Late second stage

(Density of stippling illustrates intensity of pain)

Figure 27.3 The distribution of pain in the various stages of labour (redrawn from Beischer & Mackay, 1981: 347)

The duration of labour

Under normal circumstances, a woman is able to successfully deal with pain for up to six hours. However, after six hours, the pain becomes progressively less bearable. Therefore, in normal circumstances, because the first labour is likely to be almost twice as long as any subsequent labours, with greater discomfort and pain, primigravidae are much more likely to require analgesics for pain relief than are multigravidae.

27.3 Theories of pain relief during labour

There are several theories on the origin, psychology and physiology of pain in general and pain in labour in particular. Understanding the cause and origin of pain will help the midwife to offer appropriate pharmacological and non-pharmacological measures of pain control.

The endorphin system theory

Endorphins (endogenous opiates) are natural opiate-like substances, similar to morphine and heroin, but not as potent. Endorphins are manufactured by our bodies in the presence of pain and act as a natural analgesic. When a person feels a certain level of pain, the brain stem and pituitary gland release endorphins. The endorphins act by travelling to the opiate receptors, where they fit like a key in a lock and block the transmission of the pain impulse. This local release of endorphins stops some of the pain messages reaching the brain, decreasing the person's sense of discomfort.

The levels of endorphins are much higher in women in labour than in women who are not in labour. Endorphins are the main reason that women in strong labour look 'sleepy' and often feel relaxed and drowsy. Endorphins can provide internal protection against the intensity of labour and giving birth. Some women even experience an amnesic affect (forgetting the pain) after birth. However, if the woman in labour feels that her or the unborn baby's life is in danger, her body releases adrenalin to trigger the 'fight-or-flight' response. This in turn causes the endorphin levels to decrease.

The gate control theory

The gate control theory was first described by Melzack and Wall (1965). According to this theory, a person can block a painful stimulus by using touch, heat or cold application on the body (Dubin & Patapoutian, 2010).

The neural fibres that transmit pain are thin in comparison with those that transmit other sensations such as touch, heat and cold. Therefore, when the larger A-beta skin nerves (which sense touch, heat, cold and pressure) are stimulated, they are capable of overriding the smaller A-delta and C-fibres that sense sharp, burning or aching pains. The larger nerve fibres carry the sensory message to the spinal cord more rapidly and get priority, shutting the 'gate' to the pain messages being carried by the smaller fibres (see Figure 27.4 on page 420). This is the reasoning behind our natural instinct to rub or massage our bodies when we hurt ourselves. It is also the reason why therapies such as massage and cold or heat packs can change or modify the pain of labour.

If the pain intensifies, however, the 'gate' is pushed open, increasing the sensation of pain. This usually happens during labour as the woman reaches the transitional phase of the first stage, just before it is time to push.

Other ways to stimulate the gate control is by changing position, walking, standing, hugging, rolling the hips and rocking the pelvis. All these activate receptors in the woman's joints to help reduce the pain.

Cognitive control theory

The fear that women experience in labour causes tension, which in turn causes the body to react in ways that increase pain. Mental and emotional preparation can assist in developing coping mechanisms to reduce anxiety, tension and pain. Coping with labour pain is an emotional and complex process and can give the woman feelings of fulfilment and achievement.

The descending inhibitory pathways can be enhanced by the following cognitive coping strategies:

▶ The woman replaces feelings of anxiety and fear of pain with knowledge of childbirth. This includes reading up on childbirth, educating herself, acting out different scenarios of births, looking at informative videos and building a trusting relationship with her care provider.
▶ The woman controls her mind and body activity through relaxation, music and self-hypnosis.
▶ The woman's reaction to pain can also be modified through techniques such as conscious release, attention focusing, guided imagery, distraction or physical activity.

27.4 Assessment of pain in labour

Pain management is discussed with the woman in the antenatal period and on admission. The midwife supports the patient's plan and provides the woman with available options.

The administration of pain relief during labour is given in accordance with the practitioner's guidelines and is guided by the need for pain relief as expressed and requested by the labouring woman. Hospitals and birthing units will have protocols to guide the care and non-pharmacological pain control measures employed by midwives or requested by women in labour. However, when pharmacological measures are needed, it can only be prescribed by a medical practitioner for each particular woman based on her condition and need at that time.

It has been documented that there are often disparities between how nurses rate pain and how the childbearing woman experiences pain. Studies indicate that midwives and health professionals underestimate women's pain experience, particularly when it is severe (Baker et al, 2001). The assessment of pain in labour can be done using a pain rating scale.

Pain rating scales used in clinical practice

There are different kinds of pain questionnaires that measure the type of pain, its intensity, its duration and precipitating or relieving factors. These can be used to identify and express levels of pain and responses, document experiences to prescribed treatments and improve pain control.

Four commonly used one-dimensional scales are the following:
1. *Visual analogue scales* are highly sensitive to changes in pain levels, which can make them difficult to use.

2. *Numerical rating scales* are easy to understand and simple to use. It is also not difficult for the midwife to explain to the woman how to use the tool, to score and to document results.
3. *Verbal rating scales* are dependent on the person's interpretation and understanding of the descriptive terms and thus lack the sensitivity and perhaps the accuracy of other rating scales.
4. The *pain faces rating scale* was initially designed for use with children, but is well accepted by patients with learning difficulties or language barriers. Six faces are shown, ranging from a happy, smiley face to a sad and crying face.

Recommended reading

Several pain assessment scales have been developed for labour. Dr M Yazbek developed and tested a scale for women in labour in the following study:

Yazbek, M. 2016. 'Development of a labour pain assessment instrument'. *Africa Journal of Nursing and Midwifery*, 18(1):4–26. https://journals.co.za/content/ajnm/18/1/EJC192144 (Accessed 22 August 2017).

PROCEDURE **Labour pain assessment**

Indications
It is necessary to assess, manage and record pain using a standard pain-screening tool during the first stage of labour.

Contraindications
Professionals unfamiliar with pain assessment or who are not yet trained and competent in the use of the tool should not continue with the procedure.

Principles
A simple, standardised tool for pain assessment should be part of the patient's documents, and should be used four times during labour. The midwife's structured observations are compared with the patient's experience of the pain, using the patient's verbal self-reported scale from 1 to 10.

Procedure
1 Baseline data are collected and recorded, for example as per the partogram.
2 Assessment is done four times during the first stage of labour:
   a) On admission
   b) On progress assessment
   c) Before and after administration of pain relief
   d) When severe pain is present, as observed or on patient request.
3 Baseline data is monitored and progress of labour in terms of duration and dilatation is recorded.
4 The midwife observes the woman as per the scale, in terms of pain intensity, pain quality, psychological behaviour, fatigue and emotional support (see Table 27.2).
5 The midwife asks the patient to give a rating from 0 to 10 of the discomfort or pain she is experiencing, with 0 being 'no pain' and 10 being 'worst pain'.
6 The midwife's observations are compared against the score given by the patient.

continued

Table 27.2

Pain assessment tool

Intensity	0 1 2 3 4 5 6 7 8 9 10	0 No pain 2 Mild pain 4 Moderate pain 6 Severe pain 8 Very severe pain 10 Worst pain possible	
	0–3	**4–7**	**8–10**
Quality	Uncomfortable Tender	Hurting Intense	Exhausting Unbearable
Psychological behaviour	Happy Relaxed	Restless Anxious	Crying Vomiting
Fatigue	Normal eating Breathing	Silent Rapid breathing	Fatigue No eating/drinking
Emotional/social support	Sufficient support Normal interaction Anticipation	Frustrated Fear of the unknown Focused	Discouraged Fear of being alone Reduced interaction

Recording and interpretation

Record all the data on the score card, including the patient's comments. Interpret the pain in terms of it being moderate or severe.

Actions

Take the needed actions according to the patient's preference, the birth plan and the midwife's clinical guidelines. Alternatively, refer for medical intervention.

Recommended reading

Baker, A, Ferguson, SA, Roach, GD & Dawson, D. 2001. 'Perceptions of labour pain by mothers and their attending midwives'. *Journal of Advanced Nursing*, 35(2): 171–179.

27.5 Methods used to relieve pain in labour

Methods to reduce or manage discomfort or pain should start in the antenatal period. These range from education to the administration of pharmacological substances. Pain management techniques include the following:

▶ *Psychoprophylaxis.* This includes emotional, psychological and physical antenatal preparation.
▶ *A supportive care environment.* The personal attention that the woman in labour receives is undoubtedly the first and most important consideration in the reduction of pain. This includes the presence of a midwife skilled in pain assessment and management as well as the presence of a significant person or doula.
▶ *Non-pharmacological methods.* A holistic approach to labour by the woman and her family is recognised as one of the best ways to reduce pain and anxiety around labour.

Non-pharmacological methods of pain management include natural methods such as back rubbing, hydrotherapy and movement.

▶ *Pharmacological methods.* It may be necessary to use medication or substances for the relief of pain in labour, particularly in first labours and for complications.

Psychoprophylaxis: Preparation for childbirth

Antenatal preparation is now offered in many forms. It is essential that neither the midwife nor the medical practitioner do or say anything to influence the woman's faith in her chosen regimen, even if they themselves are not enthusiastic about the method. However, this must be a recognised regimen, which in no way compromises the health of the mother or the fetus.

Antenatal preparation includes the midwife gaining the woman's attention and building up her faith in the method she chooses – or inspiring her to develop a usable plan. It includes classes on motherhood and fathering, and classes that prepare the woman and her partner for labour. This should include relaxation, breathing, focused concentration, distraction, bearing down, good posture and other exercises, all of which help to raise the woman's pain threshold.

However, it is also most important to avoid making a promise of painless labour to any pregnant woman – if she then does experience pain, she will immediately lose faith in the regimen. It is far better to tell the woman that the regimen is aimed at making pain in labour 'bearable'. In this way, a large proportion of women will receive a most valuable reduction in the amount of pain they experience during labour.

Different ideas and methods for the relief of pain that can be incorporated into antenatal preparation or which can be used during labour, other than the administration of drugs (analgesics and anaesthetics), are considered below.

A birth plan for coping with birth and the discomfort needs to be discussed in the antenatal period or on admission. This includes aspects such as the choice of provider, hospital, method of delivery, preferred significant person to attend and pain control preferences.

Natural childbirth or childbirth without fear

Dr Grantly Dick-Read's classic ideas (1959) remain the basis for the emotional, psychological and physical antenatal preparation taught today. His concept is that normal labour need not be painful and that the cause of the pain is the fear–tension–pain syndrome.

The La Leche League of Franklin Park

The principle of natural childbirth is that birth is a normal bodily function and should normally cause bearable discomfort in a woman in labour (who has the co-operation and encouragement of her husband or partner, or significant person). Natural childbirth is a fearless, trained, relaxed, easier, satisfying childbirth, especially if the mother is supported and given choices and allowed to give birth to her baby consciously without too much discomfort, instead of 'being delivered' and instructed while almost unconscious.

Natural childbirth is not necessarily painless childbirth nor an endurance test. It is not a failure if an anaesthetic is used or if the birth ends up being assisted. Natural childbirth is not a step backward nor a denial of the importance of the medical practitioner for medical care during pregnancy and labour, but rather reflects the belief that psychological care is also important. Natural birth is not a cult, nor does it have any religious, political or racial affiliation or bias. It is based on the principles of:

▶ a confident and loving woman, healthy in mind and body
▶ birth in a safe environment to welcome the baby in the great event of birth
▶ the birthing woman's understanding of what is happening to her and to her baby during the process
▶ knowledge of how to relax during labour when this is needed
▶ knowledge of how to work with the forces of labour when this is needed
▶ support and encouragement from those who attend the woman in labour.

Psychoprophylaxis: Lamaze

The concept of psychoprophylaxis, developed in France by Lamaze and Vellay (Michaels, 2010) has the conditioned reflex as its basis. These men believed that most women have been conditioned by their social environments to accept that labour is painful.

Psychoprophylaxis focuses on deconditioning women out of the belief that uterine contractions are painful, which is then followed by reconditioning to the idea that uterine contractions are a normal process and that the pain can be managed. Great emphasis is placed on active participation by the woman and her partner. It is based on the principles of establishing new conditioned reflexes and performing mental and physical activities with the intention of raising the pain threshold.

The specific aims during labour are to achieve the maximum amount of work with the minimum amount of effort, to conserve energy and to raise the pain threshold. To achieve these aims, the conditioned reflex is used for two basic techniques: first, selective relaxation, which is learning to relax each part of the body separately and together, and secondly, controlled conscious breathing, which acts mainly as a distraction from pain.

A supportive environment for birth

Creating a supportive environment for birth influences the outcomes and levels of satisfaction. Note that a supportive environment includes both the place of birth and the skilled birth attendant of choice.

One-on-one skilled attendance

The most important aspect in dealing with pain in labour is the personal attention that is given to the woman; every expectant mother should be guaranteed continuous personal attention throughout labour. No woman should ever be left alone at any time during labour. The presence of a birth attendant of choice requires a prolonged engagement with one-on-one caregiving, which exists in private practice but is more difficult to maintain in the public health sector.

Birthing rooms

The concept of birthing rooms has become very popular. In birthing rooms or birthing centres, the surroundings are adapted to resemble a home, with a normal bed, easy chairs and home-type furnishings. The husband or partner and any other chosen attendant may be present. Even children or siblings may be present, depending on the woman's wishes.

The woman is acquainted with the midwife and the medical practitioner who are to attend her during the birth. In the ideal situation, they have attended her throughout her pregnancy and will attend her in the puerperium.

Adjacent to the birthing room, there must be an emergency ward to cope with any complications that could arise during the birth.

After the birth, when both the mother and the baby have been examined and are in a satisfactory condition, the woman may go home. She will be attended daily at home by the midwife until both she and the baby no longer need this supervision (one to two weeks).

The Leboyer milieu

The Leboyer concept of 'birth without violence' is based on an increased awareness and understanding of the wishes and needs of the mother and child. This approach promotes a peaceful and serene atmosphere or milieu for the birth.

Leboyer (1975) (Conley, 2010) advocated delivery in a quiet, semi-darkened room on an ordinary bed, in surroundings that are familiar to the mother. In other words, what is required is the opposite of the typical hospital labour ward, where there is noise and loud talking, bright lights, strong hospital smells, stark white surroundings, high surgical beds, instruments and machines.

Water birth and hydrotherapy

Leboyer's ideas on non-violent birth have been taken further by Travkovsky (1960) (Balaskas & Yehudi, 1992: 14), who advocated water delivery as less damaging to the mother and to the baby's brain. In terms of pain relief, a warm bath or shower (40 °C) can assist with relaxing the mother.

In some birthing centres and hospitals, the woman can sit in a special bath with warm water, which seems to help relieve the pain of the contractions. However, because of the risks involved, underwater births are only undertaken in specially screened women who are attended by specially trained staff.

Non-pharmacological methods of managing the discomfort of birth

There are many other proven ways of creating comfort and reducing the effects of the birthing process perceived as painful. Some of these are discussed in the following subsections.

Hypnosis

Hypnosis may be induced by a medial practitioner trained in the technique, or the woman may practise self-hypnosis. The woman should be of reasonable intelligence. She lies down and relaxes in quiet, comfortable surroundings. A state of suggestibility is induced without the use of gimmicks or gadgets. Under hypnosis, the woman can be told that labour pains will be bearable or only slightly painful. The success rate for pain relief is claimed to be as good as that for psychoprophylaxis. This method is similar to the methods used for relaxation classes.

White sound

The use of white sound is a way of distracting the woman's mind from the pain. It is a mixture of many frequencies of sound (just as the colour white is the mixture of all the colours of the rainbow). It is likened to the sound of steam being released under pressure or of rushing water. It is self-manipulated; the woman increases the volume of the sound during contractions. Its use appears to be limited.

Acupuncture

This method of relieving pain has been used in China for over 5 000 years. Needles are placed in points along certain meridians in the body and then vibrated. Acupuncture is claimed to restore the normal balance of energy flow, which thereby relieves pain. However, in labour, there seems to be very limited pain relief and acupuncture is seldom used in China for the relief of pain in labour.

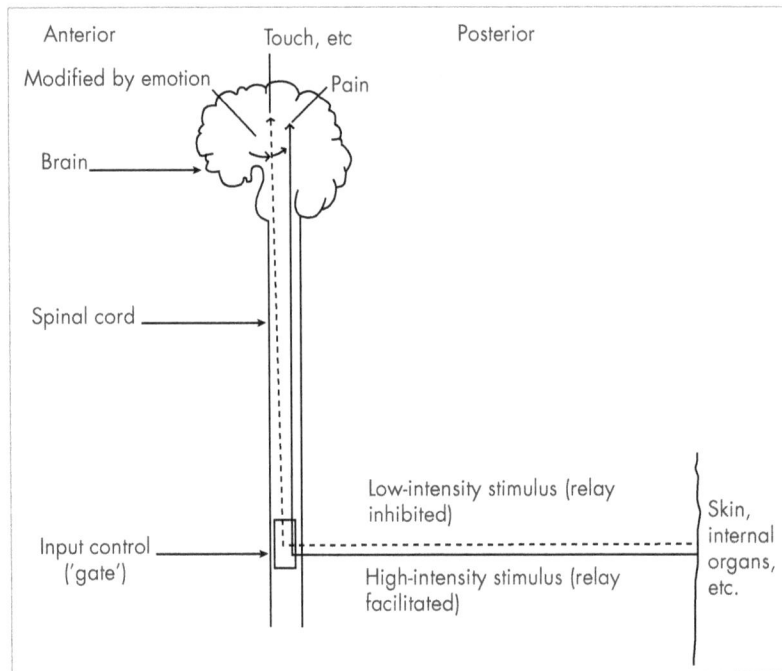

Figure 27.4 Pathways involved in the perception of pain (adapted from Trounce, 1983: 352)

Transcutaneous electrical nerve stimulation

Transcutaneous electrical nerve stimulation (TENS) is administered by an apparatus that delivers both low- and high-frequency currents. The low-frequency current is used in early labour and probably stimulates the production of endorphins (endogenous opiates). It takes about 40 minutes to become effective. It is interesting to note that TENS analgesia is partly reversible by naloxone, the narcotic antagonist, which tends to support this theory.

The high-frequency current is believed to close the gate in the spinal cord so that pain impulses carried by the slower unmyelinated nerve fibres are not transmitted onwards. This is used in advanced labour. The apparatus is self-manipulated and the pain relief is variable, most women obtaining some benefit. The apparatus is relatively inexpensive.

27.6 Pharmacological methods of pain relief

The use of analgesic and anaesthetic preparations is absolutely essential in the practice of midwifery and obstetrics. Painful labour increases the output of the catecholamines, adrenaline and noradrenalin, which have an adverse effect on uterine action and which inhibit contractions. Effective analgesia reverses this effect and therefore can shorten the duration of labour by promoting more efficient uterine action. The problem has been and still is to find the ideal preparation and the ideal method and time of administration.

Definitions of terms used in pharmacology

The following terms are used to classify medications according to the actions which the medications are capable of producing in the recipient:

▶ A *sedative* is a substance that induces a feeling of calmness and drowsiness and in this way often relieves anxiety. When given in a large dose, a sedative is capable of inducing sleep (it has a hypnotic action).

▶ A *tranquilliser* is a substance that is capable of relieving anxiety. There is not a great deal of difference between a sedative and a tranquilliser, although the tranquilliser does not necessarily cause drowsiness.

▶ A *hypnotic* is capable of inducing sleep which resembles natural sleep. A sedative given in a large dose may act as a hypnotic.

▶ A *narcotic* is a substance which, if given in sufficiently large doses, is capable of producing a deep sleep, stupor, unconsciousness or insensibility, and which at the same time may relieve pain.

- An *analgesic* is a substance that is capable of relieving pain without producing unconsciousness. An analgesic may produce total or only partial relief of pain. The relief of pain may be general or regional, depending upon the medication used and the manner of administration.
- An *anaesthetic* is an agent that is capable of producing insensibility or the complete loss of feeling. An anaesthetic may produce general anaesthesia and unconsciousness or it may only produce regional or local anaesthesia, depending upon the medication used and the method of administration. (In pharmacology, the term 'anaesthesia' implies a reversible state of depression of all the senses.)
- *Amnesia* means the loss of memory. With the administration of certain substances, the recipient, while able to feel or experience pain at the time, is unable to remember or recall the suffering later.

Indications for analgesia

Analgesia is indicated:
- when there is severe unrelieved pain, for whatever reason – it is essential that pain should be relieved before maternal and/or fetal distress becomes evident
- in prolonged labour, which is usually brought about by abnormal conditions of the powers and/or the passages and/or the passenger, for example posterior positions of the vertex in primigravidae, especially persistent occipitoposterior (POP) positions, inco-ordinate uterine action, cephalopelvic disproportion (CPD), large babies or an abnormal lie of the fetus
- if labour has to be induced or augmented, as the contractions brought about by the administration of oxytocics are generally considered to be more painful than the contractions of spontaneous labour
- in assisted deliveries such as forceps and vacuum deliveries
- for the incision and suturing of the perineum
- during manipulative procedures, such as internal versions, manual removal of the placenta, and so on
- post-Caesarean section.

The ideal medication for normal labour

The desired properties of the 'ideal analgesic' in labour include the following:
- The preparation and/or the method of administration should not be dangerous or potentially dangerous to the mother.
- The preparation and/or administration should not be dangerous or potentially dangerous to either the fetus or the newborn baby.

- Uterine activity should be enhanced and not adversely affected by the administration of the ideal medication.
- With the administration, sufficient analgesic effect should be obtained to make labour as easy as possible and to reduce the pain to the level at which it is acceptable (bearable) for each individual woman. At the same time, the woman's co-operation, particularly in the second stage, should not be diminished and she should be able to participate in the birth and feel, see and hear her baby at birth.
- It should be available to any woman in need of pain relief in labour and it should be easy to administer.
- There should be no need for medical or midwifery specialists or for specialised and expensive technology or equipment to monitor the progress of labour. (In the total abolition of pain in labour, specialist personnel and technical instrumentation are prerequisites for the care of the woman in labour and the fetus.)
- It should be relatively quickly and easily excreted by the body of the woman and the newborn baby.
- Its action should be easily reversible should it be necessary to discontinue it.
- It should be financially within the means of any woman who requires it.

The ideal medication in normal labour and its administration for the relief of pain has not yet been found, although Entonox® (combined with good antenatal preparation for labour) comes closest at the present time. The commonly accepted analgesia used in labour in South Africa is pethidine, a synthetic opioid that is morphine-like, belonging to the phenyl piperidine class. Both of these analgesics are discussed in Section 27.7.

The potentially harmful effects of unrelieved pain

The potentially harmful effects of unrelieved pain in labour, which can be reversed by the timely and effective use of analgesics, are:
- an increased cardiac output of up to 50 per cent, due to a raised BP and an increased heart rate
- maternal and fetal metabolic acidosis
- raised adrenaline and noradrenaline (catecholamines) concentrations, which can lead to abnormal uterine action and prolonged labour. This in turn leads to:
  - raised corticosteroid concentrations when a woman hyperventilates, which may cause a reduction in intervillous blood flow that may result in fetal anoxia if not corrected
  - increased oxygen consumption
  - nausea and vomiting.

Severe, unrelieved pain lowers the pain threshold, causing an increase in the intensity of the pain.

Methods of pharmacological intervention

The main types of medication used for pain relief in South Africa and the route of administration are grouped as in the subsections below.

Systemic medications

These medications may be administered by IM injection or intravenously. They include sedatives, hypnotics and tranquillisers, which may be given early in the first stage of labour, and narcotics and analgesics, which are given towards the middle of the first stage of labour.

Inhalation analgesics

This is the administration of anaesthetics by inhalation in subanaesthetic doses, given in the late first stage and during the second stage of labour, such as nitrous oxide and oxygen (Entonox®), discussed in Section 27.7.

Local analgesics

These analgesics are administered by the injection of a local anaesthetic. They include a paracervical block in the late first stage of labour, a pudendal nerve block in the second stage of labour and direct perineal infiltration with a local anaesthetic in the perineal phase of the second stage of labour.

Regional analgesia

▶ *Epidural (extradural/peridural) analgesia* is administered by injecting a local anaesthetic into the epidural space of the lumbar region of the spine. This may only be administered by a medical practitioner. Epidurals are not freely available at the primary healthcare (PHC) level or Level 1 public hospitals.
▶ *Spinal (subarachnoid, intrathecal, intradural) analgesia* is administered by the single injection of a local anaesthetic solution into the subarachnoid space. This type of anaesthetic may be used by medical practitioners for breech and forceps deliveries and for Caesarean section.

General anaesthesia (IV and inhalation anaesthesia)

The administration of general anaesthesia in the private healthcare context is almost exclusively the task of the specialist anaesthetist. All medical practitioners are required to be skilled to perform general anaesthesia in lower-level facilities and particularly so in obstetrics, should an emergency Caesarean section become necessary.

The administration of pharmacological pain relief in labour

Measures used to relieve pain in labour start with antenatal preparations to raise the psychological pain threshold and continuous personal attention to the woman in labour. However, these may not be sufficient to reduce the pain to a bearable level. Alternatively, the woman may not have had antenatal preparation, there may be complications in the pregnancy, or the situation may arise where it is necessary to obliterate all pain.

Legislation on the administration of analgesics by the midwife
The professional regulation of midwifery practice does not address pain relief. The Medicines and Related Substances Act 101 of 1965 and Regulation 24727 of 10 April 2010, Government notice R510, regulate the obtaining of pethidine or preparations or admixtures thereof by registered midwives. This replaces regulation R 777 of 10 April 1981 (Govement gazette 7636). A midwife may not prescribe but may administer pethidine and other substances when taking on a case as an independent midwife practitioner if the midwife has the required permits. If a midwife works as an employee of an institution, the rules of the institution in combination with the scope of practice apply. As a rule, a medical practitioner needs to prescribe pain relief.

Precautions relating to pharmacological substances

The midwife should take certain precautionary measures when administering pharmacological substances to the labouring woman. The midwife should always:
▶ refer to the written institutional policy
▶ refer to the verbal or written prescription issued by the medical practitioner
▶ be trained and competent in pain management
▶ respond to the woman's request for pain relief.

The midwife may advise on the use of pain relief based on the assessment of observed severe pain during labour. The woman may also give verbal or written consent to the form of pain relief advised by the midwife and as prescribed by a medical practitioner.

Note that pain relief is not to be given against the woman's wishes. However, if the woman refuses pain relief and the midwife feels that the woman is suffering unduly and unnecessarily, the midwife should refer to a medical practitioner.

Principles to consider in pharmacological pain management

If medication is prescribed by a medical practitioner, it is usually the midwife, being in constant attendance, who judges when the woman needs relief from pain. The optimal time for administering analgesia is determined by many factors, including the *careful observation, assessment and evaluation* of the woman in labour. This is done taking into account:

- whether the woman is a primigravida or a multigravida
- if the woman is experiencing normal or abnormal uterine action
- the dilatation of the cervix (the stage of labour)
- the woman's pain tolerance
- any obstetric conditions that may lead to severe pain (such as occipitoposterior positions, hypertonic or inco-ordinate uterine action, and CPD)
- co-morbidities contraindicated to the experience of severe pain as it would be deleterious to her condition (such as pre-eclampsia, eclampsia and any cardiac condition).

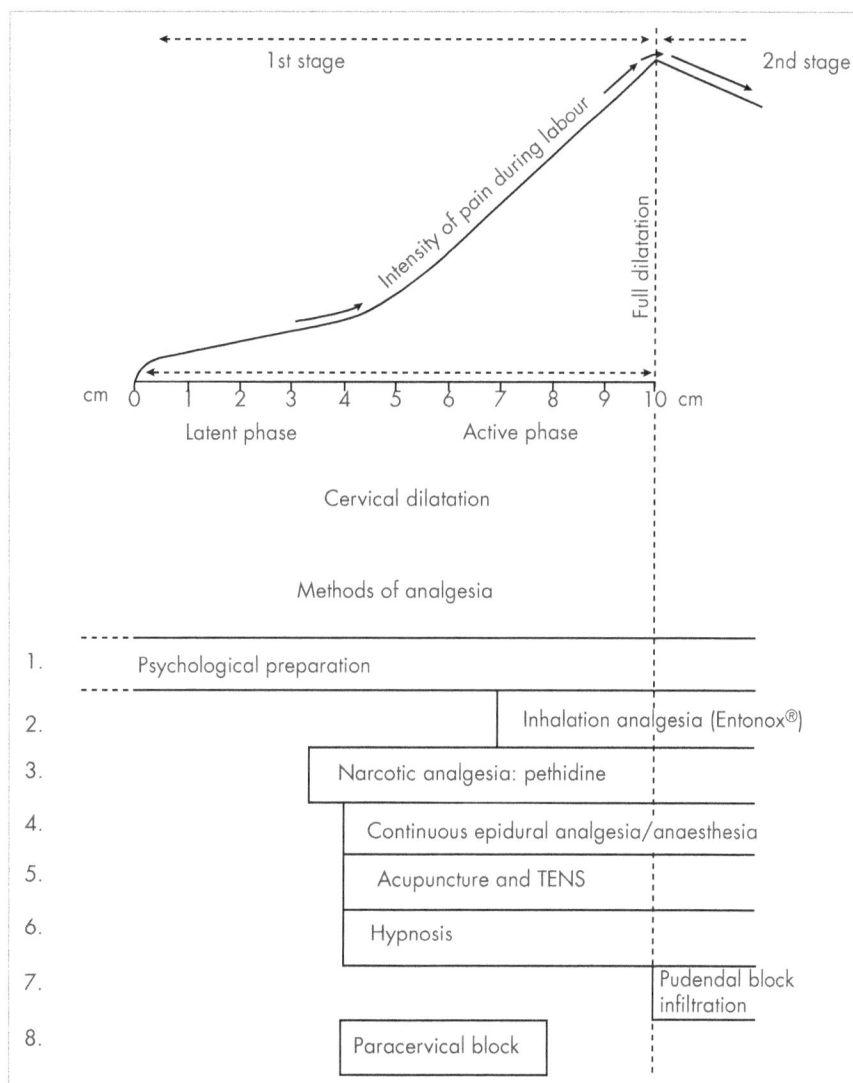

Figure 27.5 A representation of the timing of various methods of analgesia in relation to pain and cervical dilatation (redrawn from Moir, 1986: 356)

The appropriate time for the administration of each of the different types and routes of medication depends upon the type and route of the medication prescription. There is an appropriate time during labour for the administration of each type of analgesic, depending upon its effectiveness in relieving pain, the route of administration, the time it takes to become effective, the length of time it is effective, and the manner and time of its excretion from the body of the mother and of the newborn baby. These facts will be expanded upon when various medications are outlined in Section 27.7.

To obtain adequate pain relief in labour, it may be necessary to use more than one medication. The use of more than one medication should be extremely carefully assessed. While there is the possibility of a dangerous and even fatal reaction occurring from the administration of a single medication, there is even greater likelihood of a problem due to drug interactions.

27.7   The administration of specific pharmacological substances

It is important to note that not only is there a wide variety of tolerance to pain; there is also a wide variety of effects and tolerance to pharmacological preparations such as sedatives, hypnotics, tranquillisers, narcotics, analgesics and anaesthetics. Every woman has a different reaction to a given medication and some women may be extremely sensitive or even allergic to a certain preparation, while the same medication may have little effect upon other women. This must be borne in mind whenever any medication is administered to a woman in labour. The effect of the medication administered should be carefully observed and recorded in each instance. Each woman must be considered individually.

The midwife should have a sound knowledge of all pharmacological preparations that she is likely to have to administer. She should be familiar with:

- the type of medications she may administer
- the routes of administration she is allowed to use
- the specific dose of each medication according to the effect required
- the contraindications to the use of these medications
- the side effects of the medications
- the interaction with other medications.

The objective is to administer the minimum amount of any medication prescribed to obtain the maximum amount of pain relief. It is also very important that the most suitable medication is given at the correct stage of labour. Continuous personal attention, together with the power of suggestion on the part of the midwife, helps to increase the effectiveness of the medication.

To obtain the best effects from the administration of a medication, certain principles should be followed, as detailed in the following subsections.

Systemic medications

With the acknowledgement and more widespread use of antenatal psychological and physical preparation for birth, systemic medications such as sedatives, tranquillisers and hypnotics are now less frequently used in labour in general. In PHC, the use of such substances is mainly for emergencies.

Sedatives, tranquillisers and hypnotics

The sedatives, tranquillisers and hypnotics commonly prescribed and used in midwifery and obstetrics are hydroxyzine and promethazine. A sedative or hypnotic is often administered in false labour. This calms the woman and, if given in a large enough dose, will induce sleep. Invariably, when the woman wakes up, the painful but irregular contractions will have ceased, or in some instances true labour will have started.

Hydroxyzine (Aterax® – scheduled substance)

Hydroxyzine is an antihistamine that is often prescribed by the medical practitioner as a pre-anaesthetic medication. It also acts as a tranquilliser, sedative and anti-emetic. It produces minimal circulatory and respiratory depression and does not prolong anaesthesia.

This medication can be used in false labour and in early labour (the latent phase) when the cervix is slow in dilating, to calm an anxious woman. Hydroxyzine may, on medical practitioner's prescription, be administered in labour in combination with pethidine hydrochloride; this combination is effective for relieving pain and for helping to normalise uterine contractions in women with inco-ordinate uterine action.

Dosage

Hydroxyzine is given in labour as an IM injection 50–150 mg.

Side effects

It causes drowsiness and it potentiates the effects of narcotics.

Promethazine (Phenergan®)

The phenothiazine derivatives are tranquillisers and also have anti-emetic and antihistamine properties. They may be prescribed by the medical practitioner. Promethazine is sometimes given with pethidine, in which case the dosage of pethidine can be reduced. Promethazine has a longer duration of action and so would not be given with a second dose of pethidine.

Dosage

Promethazine hydrochloride (Phenergan®) is often used during labour. This may be given by IM injection in doses of 25 mg four- to six-hourly on prescription with a maximum dose of 50 mg, not exceeding 100 mg in 24 hours. It can be given alone or in combination with a reduced dosage of analgesia. When labour is established, the dosage can be reduced. It has the potential to cross the placenta and cause respiratory distress of the newborn and thus needs to be used with caution (Bettercare.co.za, nd).

When administered in combination with pethidine, the dose of pethidine is reduced by about a third, or even halved.

Where an anti-emetic action is required, promethazine or metoclopramide (Maxolon) are used.

Side effects

In some women, these medications have a sedative effect, while in others, euphoria, nervousness, insomnia and tremors may manifest. Other side effects may be tinnitus, dizziness, inco-ordination, blurred vision, dryness of the mouth and throat, cough, urinary frequency or dysuria, palpitations, hypotension, headaches, tightness of the chest, tingling, heaviness and weakness of the hands, epigastric distress with nausea and vomiting, constipation or diarrhoea.

The phenothiazines do not inhibit uterine contractions. They also do not depress respiration in the doses used in labour and are relatively safe medications. However, although they do not depress respiration in the newborn, they may depress reflex responses, such as the sucking reflex.

Narcotic analgesics

Pethidine hydrochloride (scheduled substance)

Pethidine (an opiate) is a synthetic analgesic agent traditionally used during labour. The analgesic effect it provides is relatively ineffective and the perceived benefit comes from the sedation and euphoria. Although it exhibits some of the pharmacological effects of morphine, it is chemically quite dissimilar.

The analgesic effect of pethidine is experienced 20–30 minutes after an IM injection and lasts approximately four hours. An IV injection takes effect about two to three minutes after administration. It causes respiratory depression in both the mother and baby, and should best be avoided four hours before delivery. Naloxone must be available should it become necessary.

Women may complain of drowsiness and loss of self-control while under the influence of pethidine. This may be resented by the mother if it interferes with the performance perception, control, controlled breathing and selective relaxation.

Indications

Severe pain in labour is the main indication for the administration of pethidine hydrochloride. However, a careful evaluation of the progress of labour must be made and the rate of dilatation of the cervix must be assessed. Pethidine does not inhibit the action of well-established labour; in fact, when pethidine is given at the right time, it often results in a more rapid dilatation of the cervix and the acceleration of labour, even in inco-ordinate uterine action. This is probably due to the reduction of fear and pain rather than directly relaxing the cervix.

Precautions

Pethidine administered too early in labour may prolong labour. Pethidine should not be given in the late active phase of labour because of the possibility of respiratory depression of the baby. If the analgesic is administered too close to the second stage of labour, the analgesic effect of the pethidine will not have reached its maximum and will therefore not be of value in pain relief. The mother may also be too drowsy to bear down effectively.

Contraindications

Pethidine should not be administered to any woman who is on monoamine oxidase inhibitors (MAOIs), as serious reactions such as coma, profound hypotension and severe respiratory depression may result, with the possible death of the woman and/or newborn. Care must be taken when giving pethidine following the previous administration of any sedatives, hypnotics, tranquillisers or other narcotics and analgesics.

Dosage

An IM injection of 50–100 mg is given, which may be repeated on medical practitioner's prescription only.

Pethidine may be combined with hydroxyzine (Aterax®); this combination is effective for relieving pain and for normalising labour when there is inco-ordinate uterine action. When these medications are combined, the dose of pethidine can be reduced by half. This is only done with a medical practitioner's prescription.

An IV injection of 25 mg of pethidine may be given by the medical practitioner, or *in an emergency, by the midwife on prescription of a medical practitioner*. It should be given slowly over 5–10 minutes and it should be diluted before injected. This could be used in obstetrical emergencies such as retained placenta requiring manual removal where no operating theatre facilities are available or in acute inversion of the uterus. The IV injection of opiates is considered risky.

Side effects

Patient-controlled-analgesia (PCA) used after birth with morphine provides slightly better analgesia, but the side effects are similar to those of pethidine. The side effects include the following:

▶ *Respiratory system.* Pethidine depresses respiration. The peak respiratory depression is observed within one hour after IM injection. It starts to decrease after two hours, but may last up to four hours. Naloxone, nalorphine and related opiate antagonists can reverse the respiratory depression and are specific antagonists for morphine and pethidine. Naloxone 0.4 mg to 0.8 mg can be given intramuscularly or may be given intravenously to the mother as a single dose or titrated. IV naloxone takes effect almost immediately after administration. Possibly the greatest danger in the use of pethidine during labour is that it freely crosses the placental barrier and may therefore cause respiratory depression in the newborn baby, preventing the establishment and/or the effective maintenance of respiration at birth.

Naloxone to prevent neonatal respiratory distress

Established respiratory depression in the newborn due to pethidine administered to the mother within the last two hours or more can be treated with naloxone. Usually, the blood level of pethidine in the newborn baby is approximately 70 per cent of the maternal blood level at delivery.

It is essential that neonatal naloxone (0.01 mg/kg body weight) is only given intramuscularly once perfusion is established. If naloxone is administered intravenously to the woman shortly before delivery, it will help prevent narcotic-induced respiratory depression in the newborn, but the preferred method is to administer neonatal naloxone directly to the infant at birth (see page 717).

The effects of an IM injection of neonatal naloxone to a newborn baby is delayed if there is respiratory depression and thus the only really satisfactory method of administration in these circumstances is by the umbilical vein.

▶ *The cardiovascular system.* If the woman remains in bed after an IM injection of pethidine, hypotension may occur when she sits or stands (orthostatic hypotension). Hypotension may also occur when single IV injections are administered; hence the need to give the injection very slowly with a contraction or over three minutes. Pethidine, administered together with or soon after a phenothiazine

derivative or other hypnotics or narcotics, may also result in hypotension.

▶ *The gastrointestinal (GI) system.* Nausea and vomiting is a common occurrence. Hydroxyzine or certain phenothiazine derivatives with anti-emetic properties may be used in the prevention or treatment of nausea and vomiting.

▶ *The liver.* In severe liver disease, the breakdown of pethidine may be impaired, causing the action of the pethidine to be intensified and prolonged. In the newborn baby, the liver is unable to break down pethidine effectively and it may remain in the body of the newborn for as long as three days. Because pethidine depresses reflex activity, reflexes such as sucking may be delayed for two to three days after birth.

Morphine and papavertum (scheduled substances)

The administration of morphine is not recommended during pregnancy or labour unless the potential benefits outweigh the potential risks to the developing fetus *in utero*.

Neonatal respiratory depression is possible when morphine is used in labour. Equipment for neonatal resuscitation should be available if morphine must be used in labour.

These opiates may be used in labour as analgesics after Caesarean section. In case of an intrauterine death (IUD) or in manual removal of the placenta after birth, morphine is a useful drug to reduce pain.

Inhalation analgesia

Inhalation analgesia is used in advanced labour (towards the end of the first stage and in the second stage). Nitrous oxide and oxygen (Entonox®) are administered using a single cylinder of premixed gases with the Entonox® apparatus.

Nitrous oxide and oxygen: The Entonox® apparatus

Nitrous oxide is a weak anaesthetic but it has a relatively strong analgesic action. Stored in cylinders under pressure, nitrous oxide becomes a liquid, but when it is mixed with oxygen at room temperature, it becomes a stable gaseous mixture.

Although the mixture of nitrous oxide and oxygen is a good option, it is not widely used in South Africa. The mixture is inhaled through a mouthpiece or a mask and brings swift relief when inhaled as soon as a contraction is felt. The mask should be taken off the face between contractions. Entonox® is a rapid-acting substance and is only effective while being breathed.

The analgesic effect of nitrous oxide is produced very rapidly, as analgesia is experienced approximately 20 seconds after inhalation commences and reaches its maximum after about 45 seconds. The depth and rate of respiration will influence the amount of nitrous oxide taken up through the lungs; this will therefore affect the rate of onset of analgesia.

The 50 per cent nitrous oxide mixed with 50 per cent oxygen which is administered by the Entonox® apparatus provides analgesia that is found to be satisfactory for most women in labour. It is entirely free from harmful effects and can be safely used for up to 12 hours; there are no real contraindications to or side effects from the use of Entonox®. In fact, the administration of nitrous oxide and oxygen by means of the Entonox® apparatus has multiple benefits.

The midwife needs a prescription from the medical practitioner for the administration of Entonox®.

The benefits of using Entonox®

As the Entonox® apparatus is self-administered, the woman is actively participating in her own pain relief. This in itself helps to distract from the pain of labour. The woman cannot be given an overdose, or anaesthetic dose, of nitrous oxide – if the build-up of nitrous oxide becomes too great, she will not be capable of holding the mask over her mouth and nose. For this reason, the midwife should never hold the mask on the woman's face.

Uterine contractions are not inhibited, but the relief from pain and the relaxing effect of the nitrous oxide help to facilitate normal uterine action. This in turn helps to reduce the duration of labour.

Entonox® is almost odourless and seldom causes nausea.

Nitrous oxide is excreted from the mother's body almost as quickly as it is taken in and therefore there is very little likelihood of a build-up to a dangerous level with the correct use of the Entonox® apparatus. However, in spite of the relative safety of Entonox®, the midwife must always observe the correct methods of use.

Indications

Entonox® can be given if the labour is progressing normally and the cervix is 8 cm or more dilated in the primigravida and 6 cm dilated or more in the multigravida, but there is a definite need to relieve pain. In normal labour, without CPD, most women who are not coping with the pain towards the end of the first stage of labour should find that Entonox® gives sufficient relief if their emotional, psychological and physical needs have already been met. It is also very useful for relieving pain in the second stage of labour and for helping the woman to keep control in the perineal phase, when the head is crowning.

Entonox® is also a means of providing additional oxygen to the fetus during labour. More than double the amount of oxygen that is present in the air is taken in when the Entonox® machine is used.

Another advantage is that it is very useful in instances where the woman is unable to prevent herself from bearing down when the cervix is not fully dilated. This may occur in posterior positions of the vertex, particularly in the primigravida. An oedematous lip of cervix can result from this premature bearing down.

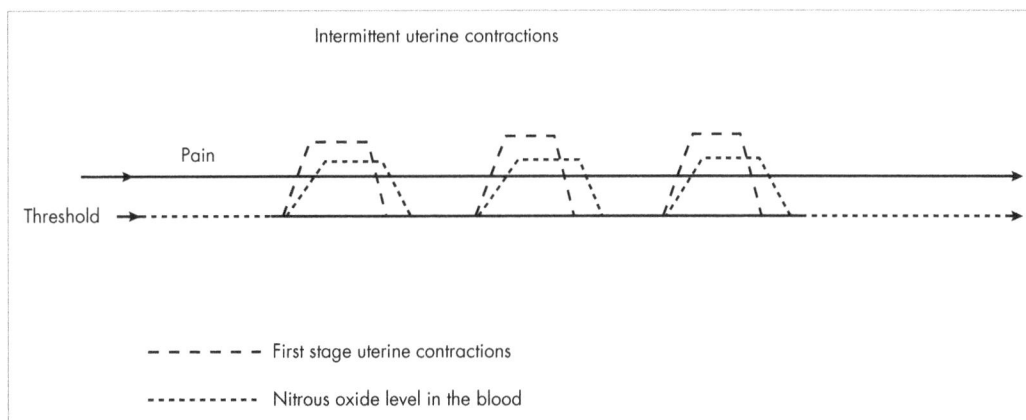

Figure 27.6 The nitrous oxide in the blood when Entonox® is correctly used in labour (50:50 mixture of nitrous oxide and oxygen) (redrawn from Moir, 1986: 359)

Contraindications

There are virtually no contraindications or side effects if the apparatus is correctly used. However, the following must be noted:

▶ The woman's consent and co-operation must be obtained before Entonox® can be used.
▶ Occasionally, a woman experiences feelings of suffocation when using the mask for the first time. However, this can be avoided if, during antenatal preparation, visits are arranged to the maternity unit and the woman is shown how to use the Entonox® by face mask or mouth piece.
▶ The woman may feel dizzy. In this case she should be confined to bed.

Local anaesthesia and nerve blocks

The term 'local anaesthetic' is applied to substances which, when injected into the body, bring about analgesia although the sensations of touch and temperature may not be affected. If most or all sensation is occluded, then it is anaesthesia. Local anaesthetics block the conduction of impulses along the nerves. (See Chapter 33 for spinal anaesthesia.)

Midwives and local anaesthetics
The local anaesthetic that is generally used for local infiltration of the perineum is lignocaine 1 per cent. The concentration should never exceed 1 per cent and the maximum amount is 20 ml.

The use of adrenalin together with a local anaesthetic is to be avoided in obstetrics. It is capable of causing severe cardiovascular effects if inadvertently given intravenously and it suppresses uterine contractions in epidural anaesthesia.

Local anaesthetic is particularly dangerous if the solution enters a blood vessel, and may result in:

▶ a toxic reaction
▶ suppressed vital centres of the brain stem, resulting in anxiety, shivering and hypotension
▶ inadequate respiration and reduced cardiac output
▶ cerebral excitation – fine muscular twitching, especially of the facial muscles, generalised convulsions
▶ loss of consciousness, with the associated obstruction of the airway and inhalation of vomitus
▶ hypoxia or anoxia of the mother and/or the fetus
▶ death.

To prevent this danger, the syringe plunger should be withdrawn before the solution is injected, to check for blood.

If a dental syringe is used, then the solution should be injected while withdrawing the needle.

Local anaesthetics are transferred fairly freely via the placenta to the fetus. Local or regional analgesia (excluding epidural analgesia) is obtained by the following means:

▶ *Pudendal nerve block.* This may only be performed by a medical practitioner. It is an aseptic procedure. It is seldom used in South Africa today, but may be done for forceps delivery, together with infiltration of the perineum.
▶ *Local infiltration of the perineum.* Direct perineal infiltration with a local anaesthetic can be used in the latter part of the second stage of labour to perform an episiotomy, or in the third stage for suturing the perineum. A midwife is allowed to perform this procedure according to Regulation 2488.
▶ *General anaesthesia.* In modern obstetrics, general anaesthesia is now used only for Caesarean section, and even this use has receded with the more frequent use of spinal anaesthesia. Maternal deaths can occur due to the complications which arise with general anaesthesia, such as Mendelson's syndrome. Most of these maternal deaths occur as a result of general anaesthesia used for emergency Caesarean section. (See Chapter 33.)

Epidural and spinal analgesia is discussed in Chapter 33, which deals with obstetric interventions.

Spinal anaesthesia is mainly used for Caesarean section. Its uses in obstetrics are:

▶ for severe, unrelieved pain in labour
▶ to exclude pain during certain procedures, such as forceps delivery and vacuum extraction.

27.8   Conclusion

Midwives practice within the legal framework for pain management – for the safety of women and for self-protection against malpractice. This requires that midwives stay abreast of the latest developments through continuous professional development (CPD) to maintain competence.

Clinical skills require that midwives be competent to assess discomfort and pain and able to comfort women. They must be able to find effective measures to support women through pain management and take them safely through the birth experience.

The midwife must always consider the rights and wishes of the labouring woman, her family and cultural customs. It is also necessary to maintain a good relationship with the medical practitioner.

Management and care of the second and third stages of labour

LEARNING OBJECTIVES
On completion of this chapter, you must be able to:
▶ explain the second and third stages of normal labour
▶ describe the positions that are utilised during the second stage of labour
▶ give details of the care during the second and third stages of normal birth
▶ clarify the role of the midwife in normal labour
▶ describe the role of the midwife in conducting a birth.

KNOWLEDGE ASSUMED TO BE IN PLACE
The anatomical and physiological changes in pregnancy in preparation for birth
The physiology of the stages of labour
Psychosocial preparation for birth
The first stage of labour

KEY WORDS
normal birth • pelvic floor stage • perineal stage • Apgar score

28.1   Introduction

The second stage of labour is usually the most painful and distressing period of the whole labour and the woman needs the full attention and co-operation of the midwife during this time. The midwife needs to know how to manage this situation. Subsequently, in the third stage, it is important to manage the delivery of the placenta as well as control any haemorrhage. In this chapter the duration, challenges and management of both these stages of labour are described.

28.2   The duration, dynamics and challenges of the second stage

In a primigravida or nullipara, the average duration of the normal second stage of labour is 40 minutes; it should not exceed one hour. In a multigravida/primipara or multipara it is 15–30 minutes; it should not exceed half an hour. These times apply when the woman is actively bearing down, and include the phase of descent and the perineal phase.

The duration of the second stage may depend on:
▶ the strength and co-ordination of the uterine contractions (the powers)

▶ the mother's ability to bear down, which will be affected by her general condition and the length of the first stage (her psychological and physical fortitude)
▶ the resistance of the soft tissues of the pelvis, which will be affected by whether the labour is a first or subsequent delivery (the passages)
▶ the size and shape of the mother's pelvis (the passages)
▶ the lie, presentation, position, attitude and size of the fetus (the passenger)
▶ whether it is a first labour or whether the woman has previously given birth to a viable infant
▶ the size and position of the head.

Strong contractions, the effort exerted during bearing down, the weariness caused by anxiety, as well as the length of the first stage and the pain endured, can all lead to maternal exhaustion and distress if the second stage is prolonged. Maternal distress also leads to fetal distress. A prolonged second stage may also be an indication of some abnormal obstetric condition, such as cephalopelvic disproportion (CPD), deep transverse arrest or some other abnormal condition causing delay of the birth of the infant.

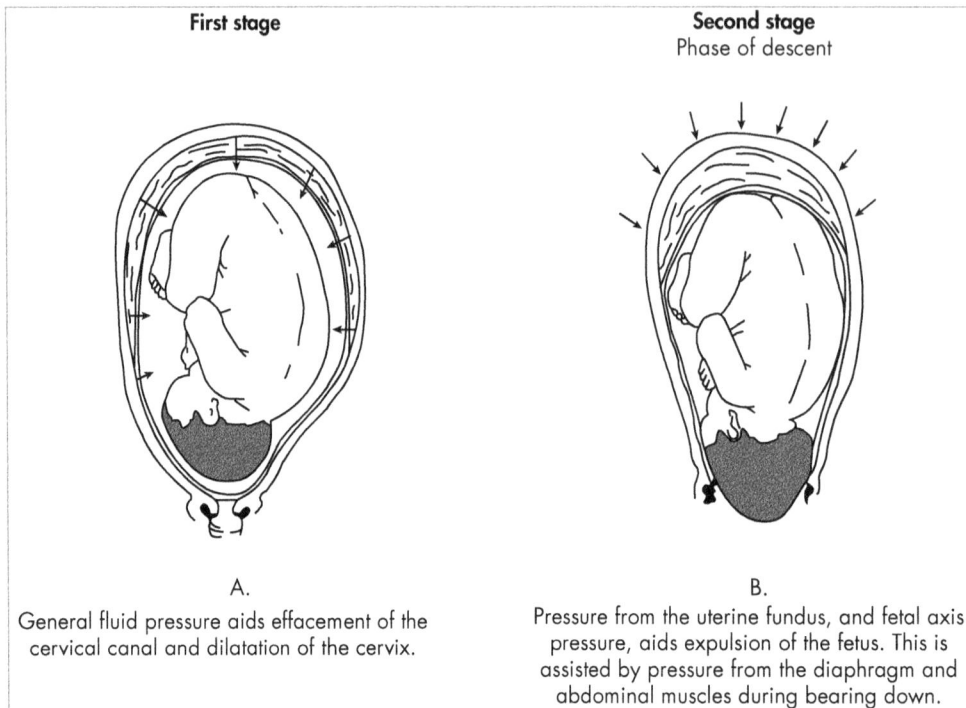

First stage

A.
General fluid pressure aids effacement of the
cervical canal and dilatation of the cervix.

Second stage
Phase of descent

B.
Pressure from the uterine fundus, and fetal axis
pressure, aids expulsion of the fetus. This is
assisted by pressure from the diaphragm and
abdominal muscles during bearing down.

Figure 28.1 Pressure on the fetus during labour

The duration of the second stage of labour is not so important if the mother is not actively bearing down, for instance with epidural analgesia.

The effect of the fetus on the second stage of labour

During the second stage of labour, the fetal head descends in the pelvis and reaches the pelvic floor. The fetal head makes certain passive movements, known as the mechanism of labour (discussed in Chapter 25), which allow the fetus to pass down the pelvic canal and through the pelvis and the vagina for birth.

The uterine fundus acts as a piston during contractions. As the normal placental site is near the fundus, the placental circulation can be interfered with, particularly if the membranes have ruptured. This increases fetal risk during the second stage of labour.

The surrounding voluntary skeletal muscles and diaphragm are brought into play when the woman bears down. This increases the pressure of the uterine fundus onto the fetal buttocks, which are normally in the upper pole of the uterus. The expulsion of the fetus is brought about by means of so-called fetal axis pressure, where, although there is greater flexion of the fetal head, the fetal spine straightens out and the fetus is elongated as it is forced through the pelvis. This

elongation of the fetal body results in the fundus remaining above the umbilicus, although the head may have descended well into the pelvis, as shown in Figure 28.1. Flexion and rotation allow the smallest diameters of the fetal head to pass through the pelvis.

The uterine muscles alone are capable of expelling the fetus from the uterus even if the muscles from the waist downwards have been weakened and the woman is unable to bear down. This is of particular significance when the woman has been given an epidural analgesia and she is unable to utilise her abdominal muscles properly because they are affected by the local anaesthetic and the bearing down reflex is diminished. This is also of importance in conditions where the woman has some form of permanent paraplegia (paralysis of the lower part of the trunk and limbs) due to poliomyelitis or accidental trauma to the spinal cord. The uterus will expel the fetus unaided, making the use of forceps unnecessary. It will just take longer.

Towards the end of the second stage, when the head is on the perineum, the woman often experiences a feeling which is similar to the reflex to defecate; this may indicate that the fetal head is well down in the pelvis and the woman is about to deliver the baby.

28.3 The diagnosis of the second stage of labour

The diagnosis of the second stage of labour (the phase of descent, followed by the perineal phase) is based on:

- symptoms experienced by the woman
- findings on general examination
- findings on abdominal examination and palpation
- findings on examination of the vulva and anal regions
- findings on vaginal examination.

It is only on vaginal examination that the diagnostic or conclusive sign of the start of the second stage of labour can be made. This is full dilatation of the cervix.

There are psychological and physical signs and symptoms that are suggestive of the commencement of the second stage of labour. As the woman should not be allowed to bear down before the cervix is fully dilated, these signs should be taken collectively in order to help in the diagnosis of the commencement of the second stage and as an indication of when the vaginal examination should be undertaken in order to substantiate these findings.

Physical signs of the start of the second stage of labour

Changes in the uterine contractions

At this stage, the uterine contractions become very strong and of long duration and are expulsive in character. These contractions are very painful unless the woman bears down during the contractions. The urge to bear down becomes compulsive and the woman cannot control herself.

Spontaneous rupture of the membranes

If the membranes are intact at the end of the first stage, they very often rupture spontaneously when the woman starts to bear down. This is, however, a very unreliable indication of the commencement of the second stage unless taken together with the other signs.

The fetus

The fetal heart rate (FHR) patterns often change with the expulsive type of contractions. If recorded during contractions, the fetal heart may be found to fade altogether and may take longer to return to normal after contractions. The FHR drops to 80 but recovers immediately after a contraction. It is extremely important that the fetal heart is monitored diligently after each bearing-down effort during the second stage because of the high risk to the fetus.

If the fetal heart rate pattern is causing concern (dropping below 80 and recovering slowly) and at the same time the progress of the fetus becomes delayed, a skilled midwife or a medical practitioner must be notified. Forceps or the ventouse may then be used to hasten delivery.

A trickle of blood

There may be no bleeding at all. However, a trickle of blood may be noticed at the vaginal orifice. This could be due to a slight laceration of the cervix in the transitional stage, when the fetal head is forced through the external cervical os, and/or slight lacerations of the vaginal mucosa as the head descends in the pelvis.

The tension between the coccyx and the anal margin as the head descends in the pelvis (the phase of descent) is directed backwards at first (following the curve of Carus) and compresses the rectum and the region between the coccyx and the posterior margin of the anus; faeces may be expelled from the anus.

If the midwife gently presses this area with the palmar aspect of her middle finger (postanal palpation), she may notice a tenseness or hardness, which is the hard fetal skull pressing on the soft pelvic tissue. If the hard fetal head is felt, it is a fairly reliable indication that the head is at or below the level of the ischial spines and that the cervix is probably fully dilated. It is important to notice the position of the fontanelles and the sagittal suture.

Pouting and gaping of the anus

Shortly after the tenseness is noticed in the anal region, the anus will start to pout as it is pushed outwards. As the head descends even further, the anus will gape and the shiny anterior rectal wall may be seen through the distended anal aperture. This is also a fairly reliable sign of the second stage.

Gaping of the vulva

When the head reaches the perineum (the perineal phase), it is directed forwards and upwards (following the curve of Carus) and the vulva starts to gape. This usually means that the presenting part is below the ischial spines and the cervix is fully dilated.

The appearance of the presenting part

The presenting part appearing at the vaginal orifice, as shown in Figure 25.8 on page 383, is an almost positive sign that the cervix is fully dilated. If the presenting part is the fetal head, it is almost conclusive.

If there is excessive caput and moulding, however, this may just be visible in the vagina, although the actual bony skull of the fetus may still be above the ischial spines and the cervix not yet fully dilated. This is unlikely, but it can occur.

Bulging of the perineum

The hard fetal head compressing the perineum when the woman bears down during contractions can cause bulging of the perineum. If this is seen and can be felt by pressing on the perineal area, it is almost always an indication that delivery is imminent. Tearing of the tissues around the orifice may occur, usually in the perineal area, but occasionally laterally or upward into the clitoris.

At this stage, it may occasionally be necessary to perform an episiotomy to prevent a third-degree tear of the perineum or to aid in the hurried expulsion of the fetus if there is fetal distress. However, an episiotomy should only be performed at the optimum time and only when absolutely necessary, after infiltration with a local anaesthetic.

PROCEDURE Performing an episiotomy

Definition

An episiotomy is a surgical incision into the perineum in order to enlarge the introitus. It is the most common of all operations. However, routine episiotomy is discouraged, because clinical trials do not support the claims that it reduces perineal trauma or prevents genital prolapse in later life. An episiotomy shortens the second stage of labour in a primigravida.

Various types of episiotomies may be performed, but the mediolateral type (see Figure 28A) is recommended by the Department of Health (DoH) (2015). The perineal muscles are incised just before delivery.

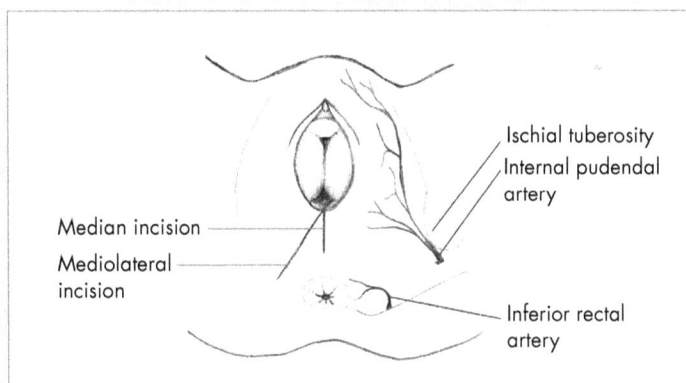

Figure 28A Different types of episiotomy

Indications

A Caesarean section should be considered in cases where excessive perineal trauma is expected. However, performing a Caesarean section is not always possible. An episiotomy is indicated:
- to shorten the second stage of labour, due to a tight or rigid perineum preventing delivery, especially in the case of fetal distress and maternal exhaustion
- in complicated vaginal delivery (breech, shoulder dystocia, forceps, vacuum extraction)
- in cases of scarring due to female genital mutilation (FGM) or poorly healed third- or fourth-degree tears
- in preterm delivery, to decrease pressure on the fetal skull
- when the mother suffers from hypertension, diabetes or cardiac conditions, to minimise maternal effort
- where a significant risk of perineal tearing exists because of a tight perineum or where a large baby is expected
- in abnormal presentations and positions.

Contraindications

An episiotomy should not be performed:
- routinely, as it has not been shown to reduce perineal trauma or bladder prolapse
- if the mother is HIV positive, as it can increase the possibility of mother-to-child-transmission (MTCT) of the virus
- if the midwife in attendance lacks the necessary knowledge and skills to repair the episiotomy safely.

Principles
- Hand washing and gloving is necessary to prevent cross-contamination and to minimise the risk of contact with bodily fluid and blood.

continued

▶ Strict antiseptic measures are mandatory.
▶ Local anaesthesia is mandatory. Lignocaine 1 per cent solution (maximum 20 ml) must be used to infiltrate the perineum before cutting the episiotomy. Early anaesthesia is needed to provide sufficient time for effect because if anaesthesia is administered:
  • too late, it fails to prevent lacerations and protect the pelvic floor.
  • too early, it leads to needless blood loss.
▶ The correct time is when the perineum is bulging, when a 3–4 cm diameter of fetal scalp can be seen and when the presenting part will be delivered in the next three to four contractions.
▶ A mediolateral episiotomy should be performed (DOH, 2015: 49), as per the procedure described below.
▶ Absorbable sutures are recommended (Polyglactin 1/0 or 2/0).
▶ A vaginal tampon placed high in the vagina to control placental bleeding must be attached with an artery forceps as a reminder to remove it after suturing.
▶ Before repair, the anal sphincter must be inspected for patency.
▶ Emotional support and encouragement is necessary during the repair.
▶ Postpartum pain relief is necessary.
▶ Prophylactic antibiotics are necessary in HIV-infected mothers.
▶ Wound healing is complicated when there is scar tissue.

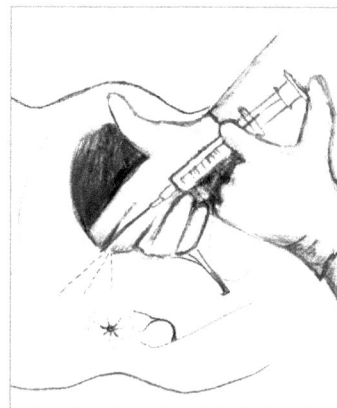

Figure 28B Infiltration of the perineum

Procedure

1 Position the woman in the dorsal position.
2 Draw up local anaesthetic solution or prepare a dental syringe.
3 Apply antiseptic solution to the perineal area. If necessary, wash the lower abdomen and perineal area with soap and water.
4 Check whether the patient is allergic to any drugs, especially local anaesthetic drugs.
5 Draw up the local anaesthetic in order to infiltrate tissue and block sensory nerves.
6 Insert the index and middle fingers of the non-dominant hand into the patient's vagina, holding the labia apart and effectively opening the vagina. Insert chlorhexidine into the vagina, using a sterile ring forceps and a gauze swab.
7 Insert the needle into the area where the episiotomy is to be done and do not withdraw it from the point of entry.
8 The needle is brought back to the subcutaneous tissue and then the direction changed (see Figure 28B).
9 Infiltrate with low concentration local (20 ml of 1 per cent Lignocaine).
10 After completion of the infiltration, wait two minutes and test for effective action.
11 With index and middle fingers between the perineum and the presenting part, an incision is made at the height of a contraction when the perineum is stretched. The cut is started in the midline in the fourchette, bearing laterally at about 45 degrees. Use a large, sharp pair of curved scissors. Note the position of the hands in Figure 28C.
12 Care should be taken not to injure the baby.

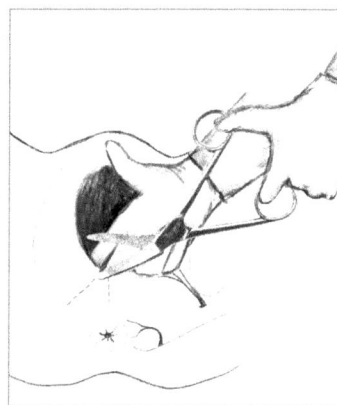

Figure 28C Cutting of the episiotomy

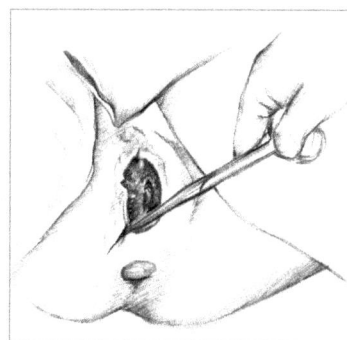

Figure 28D Visual of the episiotomy

Recording and interpretation

▶ Document the dose, the amount of anaesthesia used and the type of episiotomy that was cut in the obstetric record.
▶ Document the amount of blood loss.

Psychological or behavioural signs

Many women exhibit a change of behaviour at the start of the second stage of labour and the experienced midwife will recognise these signs.

The reason for these changes in behaviour is that the contractions have become very painful and are of an expulsive character. The woman finds that the pain is relieved to a great extent when she follows her urge to bear down. She is then no longer able to voluntarily control her actions, and with every good intention of breathing during contractions, she finds herself bearing down. She may at this stage make soft grunting noises in an effort not to bear down.

If the woman has been told not to bear down until the second stage, but the second stage has not yet been identified by the midwife, then the midwife will notice that the woman is surreptitiously bearing down because she is unable to control this urge. The woman very often becomes upset and irritated; she is no longer able to relax and breathe as before, but finds that she is pushing involuntarily. She starts to sweat and during contractions she gets a slightly 'wild' look in her eyes. She may complain of nausea and she may start vomiting. Once the midwife tells the woman that it is all right for her to bear down, she becomes 'open' and co-operative again and pushes with purpose.

Very occasionally, the woman may not have an urge to bear down at full dilatation. If this occurs, the midwife need not be concerned, because the uterus will expel the fetus eventually, without any bearing-down efforts from the mother. The only time the midwife should be concerned is if there are abnormal FHR patterns. If this occurs, a skilled midwife or a medical practitioner must be called; the mother's co-operation will be needed to deliver the baby as soon as possible with the assistance of bearing-down efforts, despite her having no urge to bear down. The skilled midwife or the medical practitioner may decide to apply forceps or the ventouse.

During the transitional stage, the woman may become flushed and/or sweat, or shivering may be noticed. The woman may perspire with the effort of bearing down, especially in high atmospheric temperatures. On the other hand, she may shiver between contractions if the atmospheric temperature is low. The woman may become flushed if she is dehydrated; this may be a sign of maternal distress.

Some women vomit at the onset of the second stage. This is probably due to the very painful contractions experienced at this time or the stretching of the ligaments.

28.4 Management of the second stage of labour

The woman and the accompanying person should be informed about the second stage of labour and what to expect.

Ensure that the bladder is empty before the woman starts bearing down, as a full bladder will affect the descent of the presenting part and also cause uterine inertia, predisposing the woman to postpartum haemorrhage (PPH). The necessary equipment is prepared when the woman is in advanced labour but before the cervix is fully dilated. Monitor the maternal pulse every ten minutes. Any signs of maternal distress should be noted and relevant action taken. Auscultation of the FHR is performed after every contraction if the fetal heart is not being monitored electronically. The woman's comfort is considered throughout the process. Aseptic technique should be observed during delivery.

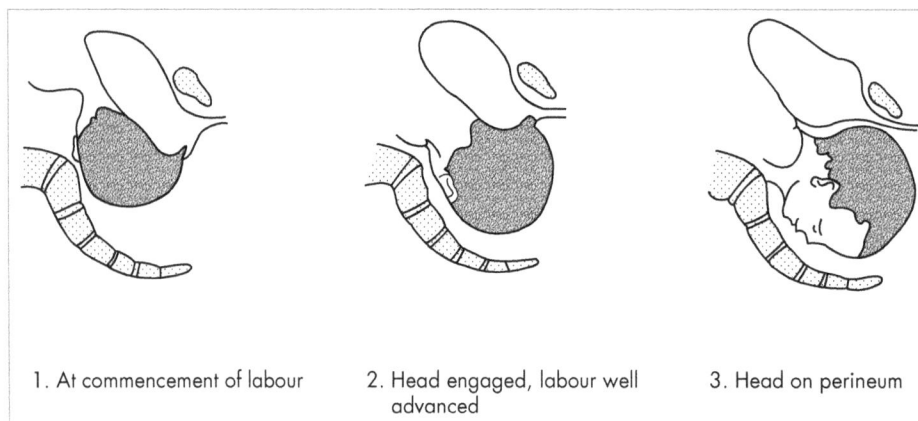

1. At commencement of labour   2. Head engaged, labour well advanced   3. Head on perineum

Figure 28.2 The bladder in labour

Positions that can be used during the second stage

The woman should be encouraged to choose the position that is most pleasing and comfortable to her during labour. The midwife should also consider the circumstances under which the delivery is performed, including the relevant skill of the midwife. Figure 28.3 and the following subsections detail some of the positions which the woman can be assisted to adopt during delivery of the baby.

The upright and squatting positions

The history of midwifery shows that various cultures have adopted a wide variety of positions for delivery. However, the upright and squatting positions seem to have been most frequently used, therefore reducing the length of labour and possibly decreasing difficulties or abnormalities. Up until recently, these positions have not been used in modern obstetrics, but lately there has been a change of attitude and more attention has been given to the position of the woman in labour. The upright and squatting positions are now more frequently adopted in normal deliveries.

It has been determined that expulsive efforts are more efficient in the squatting position and that the second stage is thereby shortened. It has also been shown that in the upright position, the pelvic inlet is widened and is more accessible to the descending fetal head. In addition, the force of gravity is used. All these advantages facilitate the descent and engagement of the head. The diameters of the pelvic outlet are also said to be increased in the squatting position, which would inevitably lead to an easier and shorter perineal phase.

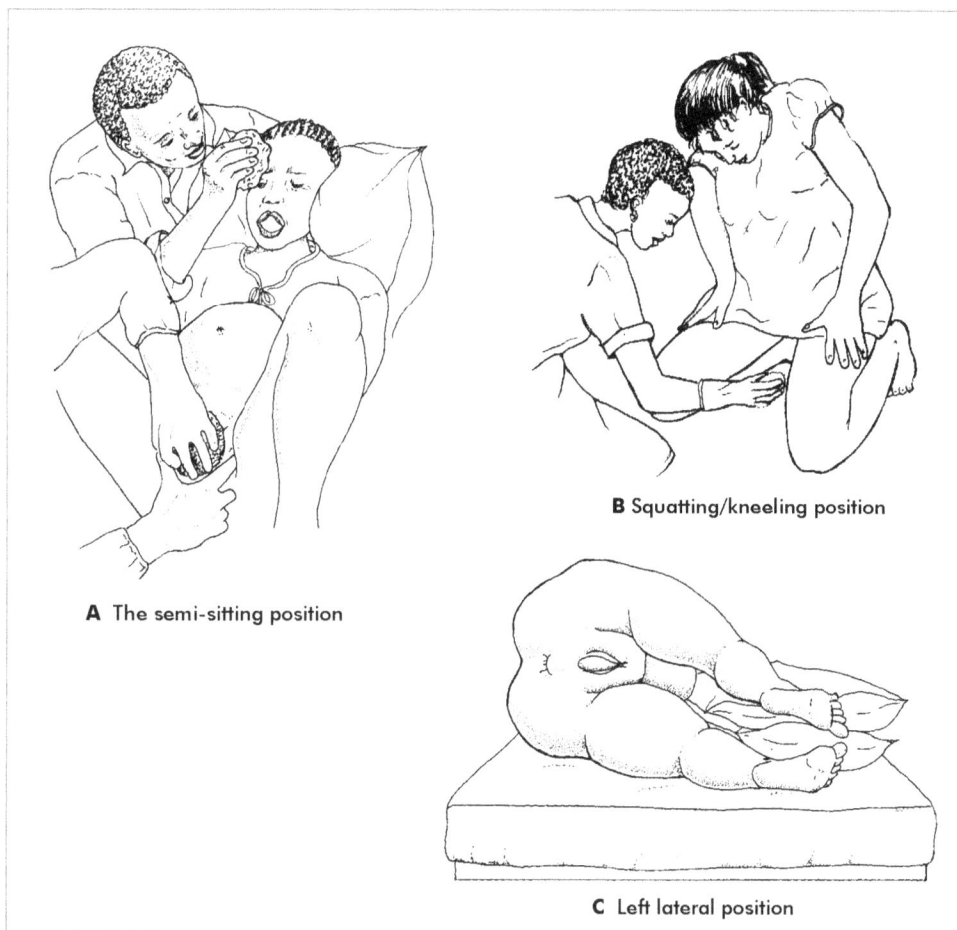

A The semi-sitting position

B Squatting/kneeling position

C Left lateral position

Figure 28.3 Maternal positions during the second stage of labour

The main drawback to these positions is that the woman is upright and mobile and that it is less convenient for monitoring the mother and the fetal heart. In addition, it is difficult for the attendant to observe the vulval area. Midwives will therefore have to learn to adjust to the various 'new' positions of the second stage of labour, with regard to the actual delivery of the baby. In Africa, women naturally deliver in the squatting position. One advantage is the improved oxygenation of the fetus, with a low incidence of inferior vena cava occlusion (which would interfere with placental blood flow).

The dorsal position

The dorsal position is sometimes known as the 'beetle on its back' position. Women have been encouraged to adopt this position since it was made popular by Queen Victoria of England. Having the woman in the dorsal position is very convenient for the midwife or the medical practitioner, because the vulval area is in full view, the fetal heart is easily accessible, contractions and the tone of the uterus are easily palpated and good eye contact is possible with the woman in labour.

However, there are very serious drawbacks to the dorsal position. The disadvantages of the dorsal position include:

▶ supine hypotension, which may lead to fetal hypoxia and subsequent fetal distress
▶ inefficient uterine action, resulting in a prolonged second stage of labour
▶ the woman's ability to bear down and the effectiveness of her efforts are diminished, as the force of gravity is not used.

It has been suggested that shoulder dystocia (impacted shoulders) is more likely to occur in the dorsal and lithotomy positions than in other positions.

The semi-squatting position

This position, also called the semi-sitting, modified Fowler's or modified dorsal position, is the ideal position for bearing down for a woman who is confined to bed. It has all the advantages of the dorsal position, with less of the dangers. The woman's bearing-down abilities are enhanced and are made more effective, as they are directed downwards towards the pelvis and the force of gravity is used. The woman is propped up by pillows, a backrest or an adjustable headpiece to the delivery bed. Her legs are abducted and bent at the hips and knees, and she grasps her shins or thighs while bearing down.

The lithotomy position

There is absolutely no need to use the lithotomy position in a normal labour. The lithotomy position is embarrassing and demoralising for the woman and is not without danger. If the staff are not careful when putting the woman into the lithotomy position and when taking her legs out of the stirrups, or if she is left in the position for a long period, it can be the cause of serious hip, leg and nerve injuries and/or circulatory problems. The lithotomy position also has all the disadvantages of the dorsal position. Women with cardiac disease should avoid this position.

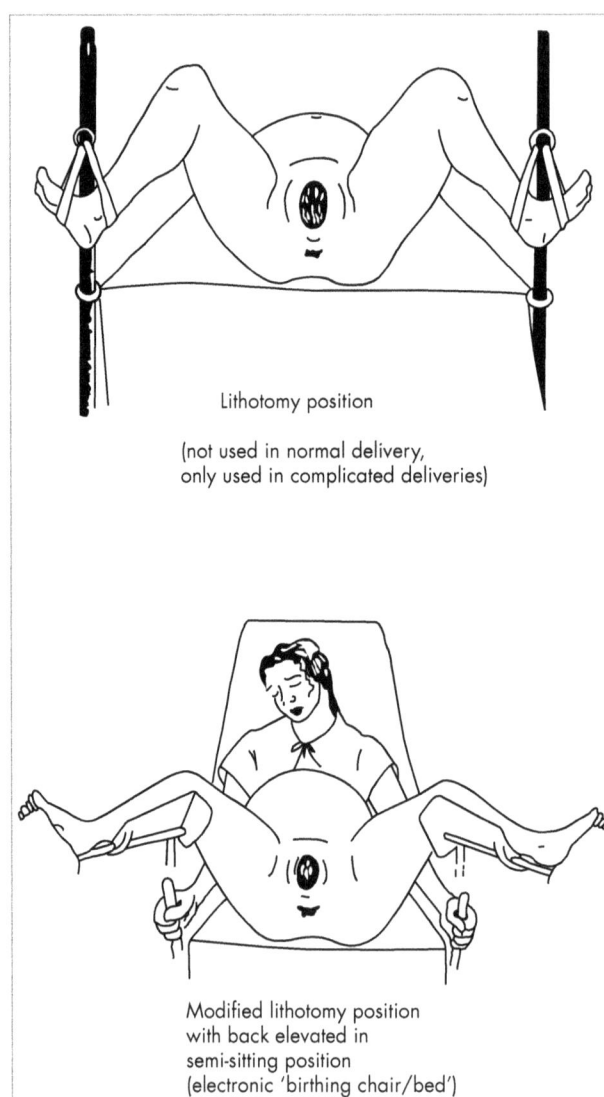

Lithotomy position

(not used in normal delivery, only used in complicated deliveries)

Modified lithotomy position with back elevated in semi-sitting position (electronic 'birthing chair/bed')

Figure 28.4 Lithotomy positions for delivery

Note: Both legs must be elevated and lowered simultaneously before and after delivery. There is a limit to the time that a woman should be in this position.

The lithotomy position does offer all the advantages of the dorsal position. In addition, there is also more space to manoeuvre the fetus, particularly during delivery of the shoulders if shoulder dystocia has occurred. It is therefore ideal for managing complications of the second stage of labour because of the easy access to the vulval area. The lithotomy position is almost exclusively used by obstetricians and skilled midwives when intervention is necessary. In addition, the lithotomy position is used for the suturing of the perineum.

It is only possible to use the lithotomy position if the necessary equipment is available, such as a delivery table or bed with facilities for the insertion of lithotomy poles. The most modern beds also have bars on either side for the woman to grasp onto during contractions and which help her to bear down; otherwise, the woman in the lithotomy position is not able to bear down very effectively.

The (left) lateral position

The (left) lateral position (see Figure 28.3 on page 435), although a good position in the first stage of labour if the woman has to remain in bed and an excellent position for the actual delivery, is not the best position for bearing down. However, if the woman is unable to bear down, for instance after epidural analgesia, then lying in a propped-up lateral position, leaving the uterus to do all the work, may be better than putting the woman into the lithotomy position too early. There is less chance of fetal distress in this position and the uterine contractions are more effective.

Maternal observations during the second stage of labour

The second stage of labour is much shorter than the first stage, but because of possible complications, it is even more imperative that frequent, accurate observations are carried out and that the progress of labour is continually assessed and evaluated. The maternal pulse should be monitored every 15 minutes and the fetal heart during every resting stage when the woman is not bearing down in-between contractions. An electronic device is useful at this stage if available.

Descent of the presenting part

Increased descent of the presenting part should occur with every uterine contraction. In a normal cephalic presentation, there should be no receding of the fetal head. Receding of the fetal head in-between contractions may indicate shoulder dystocia. Observing the fontanelles and sutures is useful to confirm the position of the presenting part.

Care of the bladder

The bladder should be empty prior to instructing the woman to bear down. If the bladder is full, the woman should be asked to empty her bladder. If the woman is not able to pass urine, the bladder should be emptied using a once-off catheter and adhering to strict aseptic technique. In the case of an indwelling catheter *in situ* (epidural), it is removed in the second stage of labour and put back after the delivery.

Maternal well-being

During the second stage of labour, the mother's general psychological and physical condition should be monitored continually. This is particularly relevant if she is a primigravida – she may be anxious and frightened because she can feel the baby descending, which is a new experience for her and she may be afraid of the possible trauma and pain.

In addition, the following observations must be made:
▶ Note her colour – whether she is flushed or pale.
▶ Note her skin temperature – whether she is sweating and how much, or whether her skin is hot to the touch.
▶ Inspect her urine for the colour and concentration and for the amount passed. Record this on the input and output chart. Test the urine for ketones.

Asepsis

Delivery of the baby is strictly an aseptic procedure. All instruments and drapes must be clean and preferably sterilised before use.

It is absolutely essential that strict asepsis and antisepsis are observed during the second stage of labour. The midwife should take every precaution to ensure that the woman is not exposed to infection or cross-infection during or after labour. It is also very important that the midwife protects herself and any other women in labour from the possible danger of cross-infection. Handwashing, using gloves and eye protection are standard preventative strategies in labour.

Monitoring the fetal heart

A prolonged second stage of labour can predispose the fetus to hypoxia. The fetal heart should therefore be checked in-between contractions immediately after the contraction, compared with the baseline FHR and any decelerations noted. Any abnormal FHR pattern should be noted. If any late deceleration is present and the heart rate takes more than 30 seconds to return to the baseline rate, the fetus needs to be delivered immediately.

Birth

The birth of the baby follows a series of passive movements through the birth canal known as the mechanism of labour (see Chapter 25).

The woman should be allowed to bear down until crowning of the head occurs; then she should be advised to pant the head out to allow for restitution. The head is born by extension in an occipitoanterior (OA) position. Once the head is delivered, the skilled attendant should check for the cord around the neck. If there is no cord around the neck, delivery should be allowed to progress. If the cord is loosely around the neck, it should be slipped over the baby's body and if it is too tight, the cord should be clamped and cut before the baby is delivered. This requires swift action, as the baby can be asphyxiated.

Restitution and internal rotation of the shoulders should occur before the delivery of the anterior shoulder. Downward traction is applied on the lateral side of the head to deliver the anterior shoulder and lateral flexion of the body to deliver the posterior shoulder. The rest of the body is delivered onto the mother's abdomen to promote bonding (see Chapter 25).

Routine suctioning of the baby is discouraged, unless the secretions are unusually thick. If secretions are few, a gauze swab is used to wipe the baby's mouth. The cord is clamped and cut (see Figure 28.5). Timing of clamping of the cord varies with local protocols. Active management of the third stage of labour (AMTSL) involves administering a uterotonic drug with delivery of the anterior shoulder of the baby or within 30–60 seconds after birth. Delaying clamping the cord for 2–3 minutes seems not to increase the risk of PPH and can improve the iron status of the infant where access to good nutrition is poor. Delaying clamping does increase the risk of jaundice, requiring phototherapy.

The newborn is identified prior to the cutting of the cord if possible or before the baby is taken from the mother, to prevent medicolegal risks. The eyes of the newborn are wiped to prevent ophthalmia neonatarum and an eye ointment is instilled according to local protocol. The Apgar score is assessed at one and five minutes. The baby is dried, wrapped in warm towels and placed on the mother's abdomen or under a radiant heater. The infant is given Konakion® (vitamin K1) according to the local protocol to prevent haemorrhagic disease of the newborn. The care and management of the newborn are discussed in greater detail in Chapter 29.

28.5   Management during the third stage of labour

The third stage of labour begins after the completed birth of the baby and ends at the completed delivery of the placenta and the attached membranes. It involves the separation and expulsion of the placenta and membranes as a result of the interplay between mechanical and haemostatic factors. The length of the third stage itself is usually 5–15 minutes, but the absolute time limit for delivery of the placenta, without evidence of significant bleeding, remains unclear.

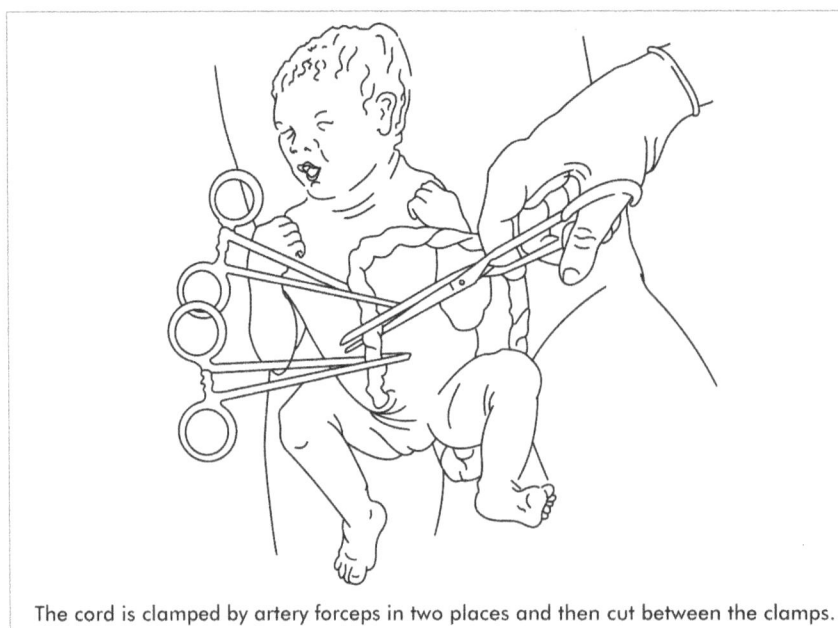

The cord is clamped by artery forceps in two places and then cut between the clamps.

Figure 28.5 Clamping and cutting of the umbilical cord at delivery

Delivery of the placenta

The *Guidelines for Maternity Care in South Africa* (DoH, 2015: 58) consider the placenta to be retained if it is not delivered from the uterus within 30 minutes of delivery of the baby. The management is greatly influenced by the clinical assessment of whether significant bleeding is occurring.

Two approaches in the management of the third stage of labour are described: the expectant or physiologic management and AMTSL (see the procedure box on the next page):

1. Expectant or physiologic management involves waiting for signs of placental separation (see Table 28.1) and allowing for spontaneous delivery of the placenta. In this natural approach, the attendants are passive and wait for the physiological process to continue unhindered. Oxytocics are not used, and the placenta is delivered by gravity and maternal effort. Note that the bladder must be empty. Intervention is only undertaken if haemorrhage or some other complication occurs. If the woman is not bleeding, this period can be prolonged to a few hours. This method is controversial, as it is known to increase the length of the third stage, the amount of blood loss and the risk of PPH.
2. A retained placenta may cause PPH, shock and death. For this reason, the DoH, the South African Nursing Council (SANC), the International Confederation of Midwives (ICM) and the International Federation of Gynaecology

and Obstetrics (FIGO) recommend active management of the third stage to reduce the incidence of PPH, the quantity of blood loss and the use of blood transfusions. AMTSL is described in the procedure box on the next page.

Stimulating uterine contractions

Rubbing up the fundus of the uterus is only done after the placenta has been delivered. The hand is gently but firmly pressed against the fundus and then rotated in tiny circular movements. This causes the uterine muscles in the fundus to contract and so helps the uterus to expel any blood or clots that may have filled the uterine cavity.

The procedure is undertaken if the fundus has risen in the abdominal cavity after the third stage of labour. However, the fundus must not be repeatedly rubbed up, as this would prevent the blood from clotting at the ends of the constricted maternal uterine blood vessels and would therefore increase the danger of PPH.

Checking the fundus means placing the hand on the fundus in a similar position in order to establish whether the fundus is well contracted and to determine its position in the abdominal cavity. However, it does not involve pressing or rotating the hand. Guarding the fundus means holding the hand over the fundus in order to prevent the uterus from filling up with blood, but does not include rotating the hand.

Table 28.1

Normal uterine consistency and the height of the fundus in the third stage

The uterus	At start of third stage (placenta attached)	Placenta in lower segment or in vagina (separated)	At end of third stage (placenta expelled)
Uterine consistency	Feels wide but firm, like a beach ball (not soft and flabby)	Feels round, smaller and hard, like a cricket ball (ballotable)	Has no specific form, but is firm and immobile (not soft and flabby)
Fundal height	About 2.5 cm below the umbilicus	At or just above the level of the umbilicus	4–5 cm below the umbilicus

PROCEDURE Active management of the delivery of the placenta

Principles
Management of the third stage of labour should be based on scientific evidence and a clear understanding of the normal physiological processes at work. The following principles must be noted:
▶ The first and second stages must be uncomplicated, as this will impact on the management of the third stage.
▶ The management of the third stage of labour is dependent on the mother's general health and well-being.
▶ The mother's preference for management of the third stage of labour must be documented during the antenatal period.
▶ Written, informed and signed consent should be obtained if the mother chooses to have expectant management of the third stage of labour.
▶ The midwife has to clarify the circumstances in which the mother's decision may be overruled.
▶ Expectant management of the third stage of labour is associated with PPH.
▶ The DoH (2015) provides guidelines for the management of the third stage of labour in South Africa.
▶ Active management includes the administration of uterotonics, controlled cord traction and uterine massage after the placenta is released.
▶ Excessive traction may result in snapping of the umbilical cord.
▶ Controlled cord traction shortens the length of the third stage of labour, but has no effect on severe haemorrhage.
▶ Squeezing, pushing on the uterus or application of fundal pressure must not be done, as it may result in uterine inversion and excessive bleeding.

Indications for placental delivery
The placenta is released when the following signs occur:
▶ The umbilical cord *lengthens* as the placenta separates and is pushed into the lower segment by progressive uterine retraction.
▶ The uterus takes on a *more globular and firmer shape* as the placenta descends into the lower segment and the body of the uterus continues to retract.
▶ The descent of the placenta into the lower segment and finally into the vagina displaces the uterus upward and the *uterus rises* in the abdomen.
▶ A *gush of blood occurs*, indicating partial or complete separation of the placenta.
▶ The *vulva* may *bulge* as the placenta descends.

Contraindications
Attempts to deliver the placenta should be aborted if:
▶ it does not deliver despite administering an infusion with oxytocin 20 IU in 1 ℓ Ringer's lactate at 120–240 ml/hour for an hour; the mother should then be prepared for manual removal of the placenta.
▶ there is active maternal bleeding without release.

Procedure
Preparation and monitoring
After delivery of the baby:
▶ The bladder should have been assessed and emptied prior to the second stage of labour; a full bladder delays uterine contraction, causing PPH.
▶ Clamp the umbilical cord close to the perineum.
▶ Wait for signs of placental release.
▶ Monitor the maternal condition every five minutes.
▶ Assess if the uterus is well contracted.
▶ Assess the mood and behaviour of the mother (eg distressed, anxious).
▶ Observe the time when the third stage of labour began.
▶ Record findings, treatment and procedures in the labour record and partogram.

continued

- Provide supportive care.
- Do not leave the mother alone.
- Ensure that 10 IU oxytocin IM was administered. (Oxytocin is administered with the crowning of the fetal head, at the birth of the anterior shoulder or after the birth of the baby, when *the presence of an undiagnosed twin baby was excluded*; or following the delivery of the placenta and membranes.)
- Await uterine contraction for two to three minutes.

Delivery of the placenta

On signs of placental release, await strong uterine contraction and deliver the placenta by controlled cord traction:

1 Grasp the clamped cord and the end of the forceps firmly with one hand.
2 Place the side of the non-dominant hand above the symphysis pubis, with the palm facing towards the mother's umbilicus. This applies counter-pressure in an upward direction to prevent inversion of the uterus during controlled cord traction.
3 Apply light, controlled and steady traction in a downwards and backwards direction (see Figure 28E), following the curve of the birth canal.
4 If the placenta does not descend during 30–40 seconds of controlled cord traction, release both cord and counter-traction and wait for the uterus to contract again.
5 After separation of the placenta from the uterine wall, it may be expelled by maternal bearing-down efforts. To facilitate this, place the mother in an upright position and flex her thighs over the lower abdomen.
6 Receive the placenta in cupped hands to prevent tearing of the membranes.
7 If the membranes do not slip out spontaneously, hold the placenta in two hands and gently twist the membranes into a rope. Gently move them up and down to assist separation without tearing them.
8 Fold the placenta with the maternal surface inwards.
9 Turn the placenta until the membranes have been delivered slowly, carefully and completely.

In case of delayed placental release

If there are no signs of placental release after 30 minutes of oxytocin administration, do the following in the absence of maternal bleeding:

1 Provided vital signs are stable, wait a further 30 minutes for spontaneous delivery of the placenta.
2 Inspect the bladder for fullness and allow the woman to void. If she is unable to do so, empty the bladder by means of a urinary catheter to assist in the delivery of the placenta and aid in the assessment and control of the uterus.

A. Exterior view (dorsal position)

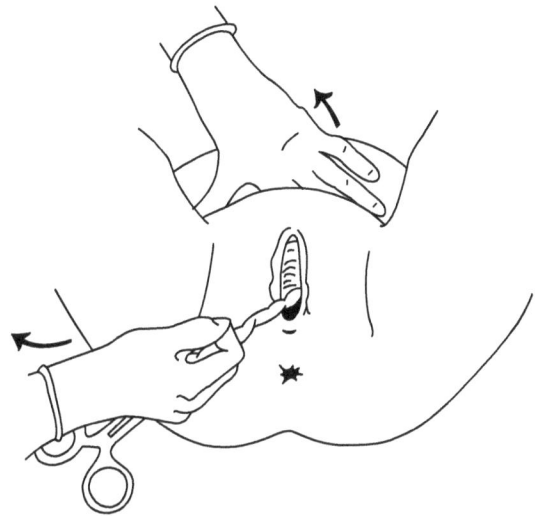

NB: Note counterbalanced traction

B. Interior lateral vlew

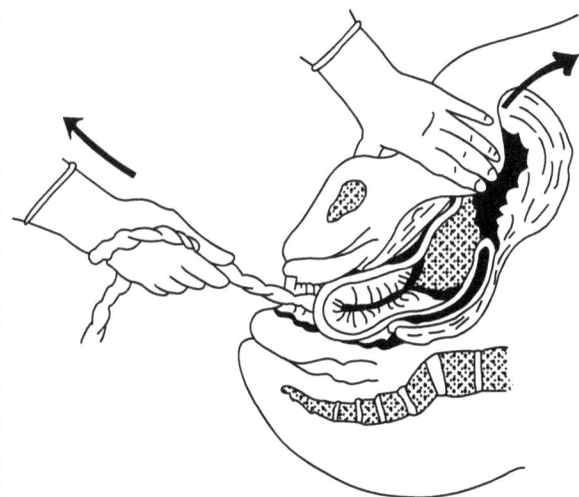

Figure 28E Controlled cord traction

continued

3   Encourage breastfeeding.

4   Repeat controlled cord traction.

If placental release does not occur, consider intra-umbilical infiltration with an oxytocic drug or substance to shorten the third stage of labour, reduce postpartum blood loss and reduce the need for manual removal of the placenta:

1   Insert a size 10 nasogastric tube into the umbilical vein; advance to the placental insertion site of the cord.

2   When resistance is met at the placental insertion site of the cord, retract the nasogastric tube by 3–4 cm to ensure the tip is not in a placental branch.

3   Inject the uterotonic solution and clamp the cord with the tube in place.

4   Saline alone or a combination of prostaglandin or misoprostol (800 mcg to oxytocin 50 IU, each in 30 ml of normal saline) may also be used.

If there are no signs of placental release after 30 minutes of oxytocin
administration, do the following in the presence of maternal bleeding:

1   Call for extra help.

2   Massage the uterus until it is hard.

3   Administer 20 IU oxytocin at 60 drops/minute via IV line.

4   Empty the bladder. Catheterise if necessary.

5   Check and record BP and pulse every 15 minutes.

6   Treat shock if present (keep the mother warm and administer fluids rapidly).

If there are no signs of placental release in another 30 minutes (one hour after delivery), prepare the woman for manual removal of the placenta in an operating room.

After delivery of the placenta

Note that membranes may tear off as the placenta delivers. Do the following after delivery:

1   Examine the placenta and membranes immediately. Check that the placenta and membranes are complete. If a portion of the maternal surface is missing or there are torn membranes with vessels, suspect retained placental fragments.

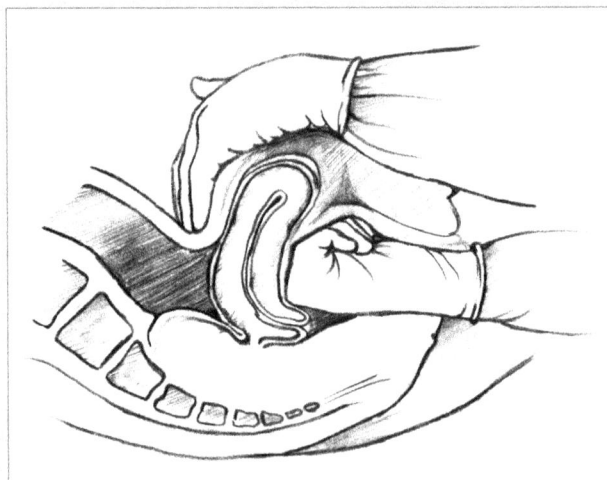

Figure 28F Uterine massage

2   If incomplete, remove placental fragments manually:

    a)   Gently examine the upper vagina and cervix with a gloved hand.

    b)   Use a sponge forceps to remove any pieces of membrane that are present.

    c)   Feel inside the uterus for placental fragments and remove by hand, ovum forceps or wide curette.

3   Massage the fundus abdominally to stimulate a contraction and express clots.

4   Repeat uterine massage every 15 minutes for the first two hours.

5   Ensure that the uterus does not become relaxed after uterine massage is stopped.

6   If bleeding continues, obtain medical help and put the baby to the breast to facilitate contraction.

7   Administer appropriate IM/IV antibiotics.

Disposal of the placenta

▶ Cultural traditions are accommodated in most hospitals.

▶ Consult the policy of the hospital regarding disposal.

▶ The clients should sign a receipt if they choose to take the placenta home with them.

continued

▶ There is currently no legislation regarding placenta encapsulation or placentophagy.

▶ There are no systematic research studies examining the risk of ingesting the placenta.

Recording and interpretation

Assess, document and report on the following:

▶ Document the time of expulsion of the placenta and membranes on the progress and obstetric reports.

▶ Document the findings on full examination of the placenta.

▶ Assess the uterus and massage it to keep it firmly contracted to prevent blood loss.

▶ Chart the presence of large clots being expelled with regards to size and amount.

▶ Weigh perineal pads, blood clots, drapes and sponges to estimate blood loss more accurately. (typically 1 g = 1 ml of blood)

28.6 Conclusion

This chapter described the management and care of women during the second and third stages of labour. Emphasis has been placed on episiotomy as well as delivery of the placenta and correct examination procedures.

29

Care of the newborn and management of the fourth stage of labour

LEARNING OBJECTIVES

On completion of this chapter, you must be able to:
- explain the physiology of the fourth stage of labour
- demonstrate knowledge and skill in the management of the fourth stage of labour
- explain all the observations to be carried out during the fourth stage and give a rationale for each observation
- show competency in using standard procedures in the examination of the placenta.

KNOWLEDGE ASSUMED TO BE IN PLACE

The physiology of the third stage of labour
Maternal–child bonding

KEYWORDS

bonding • infant feeding • placenta • ophthalmia neonatorum • infant mortality

29.1   Introduction

In the previous two chapters, the management of the first three stages of birth were described. This chapter focuses on the fourth stage of labour, which is defined as the period one hour after birth. Breastfeeding is initiated in this hour and various examinations are performed to check the well-being of the mother and the newborn baby. A careful record should be kept of all the observations and any abnormalities should be reported. This stage of labour is also very important in terms of mother–child bonding. The importance of the examination of the placenta is also described.

29.2   Basic principles of the management of the newborn

During pregnancy and labour, the mother and the fetus are monitored closely to detect the first signs of any abnormal conditions. Should any abnormality be noted, the woman is immediately referred to a medical practitioner and the woman and the fetus are treated accordingly. The cardiovascular changes at birth are explained in Chapter 40 (also see colour illustrations C12 and C13 on pages 79–80).

Care during and immediately after delivery

Careful management during delivery is extremely important in order to ensure a healthy live infant.

Preparation for delivery of the baby should be done towards the end of the first stage of labour when the second stage of labour is approaching. By this time the midwife can anticipate the possible condition of the baby at birth and make the necessary preparations. If labour is progressing well and the condition of both the mother and the fetus is satisfactory, the baby will not need any resuscitation. If the fetus has suffered intrapartum hypoxia, the baby is likely to be asphyxiated at birth and will require active resuscitation (see Chapter 46).

The environment should be warm to prevent hypothermia and the atmosphere in the labour room at the birth of the baby should be quiet and calm.

If the mother wishes to deliver the baby herself, the midwife should help her to reach down and grasp the baby around the thorax, under the arms, and lift the infant onto her abdomen. The midwife should continue to give the necessary encouragement, guidance and instruction at this time. If the mother does not wish to deliver her own baby, the midwife holds the baby around the thorax with one hand as he or she is being delivered and supports the head at the same time. The baby is very slippery at birth. The midwife must therefore use the other hand to grasp the baby firmly but gently by the ankles, keeping the forefinger between the ankles to protect them.

The time of birth should be noted. The baby is safely put on the mother's abdomen and covered.

29.3 Standard midwifery care of the newborn baby

Use universal precautions at all times. In order to give the best possible care to the infant at birth, the regimen described in the following subsections should be adhered to immediately after delivery.

Clamping and cutting the cord

The optimum time for clamping and cutting the umbilical cord remains debatable. In the normal newborn baby, the umbilical arteries go into spasm at delivery, which prevents blood from passing from the placenta to the baby. Whether it is good or bad to delay clamping of the cord until the baby has taken a few breaths in order to encourage transfusion of blood via the umbilical vein into the fetal circulation has not yet been resolved. It has been shown, however, that at three months after delivery there is no difference in the Hb content between babies with early clamping and those with late clamping of the cord. On the other hand, there is a greater incidence of neonatal jaundice where clamping has been delayed. This is of particular significance in preterm babies and in babies with Rh incompatibility.

If the baby is asphyxiated, immediate clamping and cutting of the umbilical cord is necessary, as these infants will require resuscitation.

The cord is clamped with artery forceps from the delivery pack, 5–6 cm from the baby's abdomen. The cord is clamped by a second pair of forceps about 2–3 cm above the first clamp on the placental side (see Figure 29.1). The cord is cut between these forceps with scissors from the delivery pack and protected by a gauze swab to prevent blood from spurting over the baby and also to protect the wriggling baby from the blades of the scissors. If the mother is Rh negative with antibodies, or has any other haematological condition that requires this, cord blood is taken from the placental side of the cord.

The cord is inspected to ensure that three vessels are present. (Two vessels only would indicate a congenital abnormality.) The cord is observed for haemorrhage.

Maintaining body heat

The baby should be dried as soon as possible after birth and wrapped in a warmed towel. Measures should be taken to maintain the baby's body temperature. The baby is placed over the mother's abdomen to maintain skin-to-skin contact, as this provides better warmth and promotes early bonding. The delivery room and the Resuscitaire or cot should be warmed and unnecessary exposure of the infant avoided.

If the mother needs special attention after birth, such as suturing of the perineum, the baby may be placed by the mother's side, kept warm and watched carefully or placed in a Resuscitaire. The baby should not be left alone in cold and draughty places. Cover the baby's head but make sure that the nose and mouth are open.

The Apgar score

The Apgar score, developed in 1952 by Dr Virginia Apgar, provides an accepted and convenient scoring method for reporting on the clinical status of the newborn infant at one minute after birth and the response to resuscitation if needed. It is a clinical guide used to evaluate the newborn's physical condition.

The Apgar score quantifies clinical signs of neonatal depression such as cyanosis or pallor, bradycardia, depressed reflex response to stimulation, hypotonia and apnoea or gasping respirations.

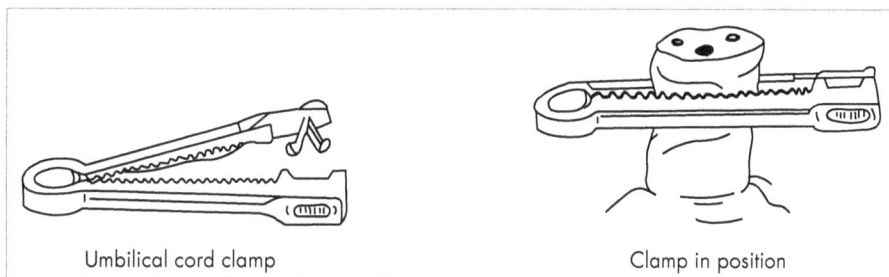

Umbilical cord clamp   Clamp in position

Figure 29.1 An umbilical cord clamp

The Apgar score alone *cannot* be considered to be evidence of or a consequence of asphyxia, does not predict individual neonatal mortality or neurologic outcome, and should not be used for that purpose.

The first examination of the newborn is done directly after birth to detect any life-threatening emergencies or abnormalities that require urgent attention. The Apgar score assessment is a clinical guide used to evaluate the newborn's physical condition. The first Apgar score indicates the need for resuscitation or not. The Apgar score is usually repeated after five minutes and gives an indication of how well the baby is adapting to extrauterine life. A re-assessment after 10 minutes may be necessary under conditions such as prolonged resuscitation. The score total is out of 10 points and consists of five clinical signs, each scoring 0, 1 or 2. The clinical signs that are evaluated are:

1. heart rate
2. respiratory effort
3. muscle tone
4. response to stimulation
5. colour.

The first examination of the newborn is done directly after birth to detect any life-threatening emergencies or abnormalities that require urgent attention. The examination is usually repeated after five minutes, and may be repeated thereafter (see the procedure box below).

PROCEDURE Assessing an Apgar score

Principles
- The score is reported at one minute and five minutes after birth for all infants. For infants with a score less than 7, the test is repeated at five-minute intervals thereafter until 20 minutes have passed.
- The first Apgar score, done directly after birth, indicates whether there is a need for immediate resuscitation, especially with a newborn heart rate of less than 100 bpm.
- The score taken after five minutes gives an indication of how well the baby is adapting to extrauterine life.
- A re-assessment after 10 minutes may be necessary under conditions such as prolonged resuscitation.
- An Apgar score assigned during resuscitation is not equivalent to a score assigned to a spontaneously breathing infant.

Procedure
Place the baby on a covered surface with adequate lighting. Evaluate the baby exactly 60 seconds after delivery, as follows:

1. Calculate the heart rate by auscultation with a stethoscope or palpation at the junction of the umbilical cord and skin. Award a score of 0, 1 or 2 depending on the rate (see Table 29.1 on the next page). During the first 10–15 minutes the heart rate increases to 160–180 bpm.
2. Determine the respiratory rate and award a score of 0, 1 or 2 (see Table 29.1). Good crying indicates good respiration. During the first 10–15 minutes, irregular respiratory efforts may be as fast as 60–80 per minute. Rhonchi, grunting, retraction and nasal flaring may be present for a brief period.
3. Determine the muscle tone by assessing the degree of flexion and resistance to straightening of the extremities. A normal term infant has flexed elbows and hips, with the knees positioned upwards to the abdomen. Award a score of 0, 1 or 2 (see Table 29.1).
4. Assess the reflex irritability by drying the baby, rubbing the soles of the feet or by suctioning the nose and award a score of 0, 1 or 2 (see Table 29.1).
5. Inspect the skin colour for cyanosis and pallor and award a score of 0, 1 or 2 (see Table 29.1).
6. Calculate the final score after one minute and again after five minutes.

Interpretation: At one minute
- A score of 8–10 indicates a newborn in a good condition who requires only nasopharyngeal suction and warmth.
- A score of 4–6 indicates mild to moderate respiratory depression. Administer oxygen by means of face ventilation.
- A score of 0–3 indicates severe respiratory depression. Cardiopulmonary resuscitation (CPR) and endotracheal intubation are necessary.
- A one-minute Apgar score of 0–3 does not predict any individual infant's outcome.

continued

Interpretation: At five minutes

The five-minute Apgar score – and particularly a change in the score between one minute and five minutes – is a useful index of the response to resuscitation. If the Apgar score is less than 7 at five minutes, the assessment should be repeated every five minutes for up to 20 minutes.

- A score of 7–10 is reassuring.
- A score of 4–6 is moderately abnormal.
- A score of 0–3 is low in the term infant and late-preterm infant and may be one of the first indications of encephalopathy.
- A score of 0–3 correlates with neonatal mortality in large populations and an increased risk of cerebral palsy.

Interpretation: At 10, 15 and 20 minutes

- The risk of poor neurological outcomes increases when the Apgar score is 3 or less at 10 minutes, 15 minutes and 20 minutes.
- Very few infants with an Apgar score of 0 at 10 minutes have been reported to survive with a normal neurological outcome. At this point discontinuation of resuscitative efforts may be appropriate.

Recording

- Document the Apgar scores and interventions (if any) on the newborn's records.
- Write an incident report in the case of low Apgar scores at birth.
- Document the presence of a medical practitioner assisting with resuscitation efforts.
- Document in full the actions taken during the resuscitation effort.

Limitations of the Apgar score

- The incidence of low Apgar scores is inversely related to birth weight and a low score cannot predict morbidity or mortality for any individual infant.
- An Apgar score alone cannot be used to diagnose asphyxia.
- The Apgar score is an expression of the infant's physiological condition at one point in time, which can be influenced by maternal sedation or anaesthesia, congenital abnormalities, gestational age (GA), trauma and lack of inter-observer reliability.
- Assessment of muscle tone, colour and reflex irritability can be subjective and partially dependent on the physiological maturity of the infant.
- The healthy preterm infant with no evidence of asphyxia may receive a low score only because of immaturity.

Table 29.1

Apgar scoring (Wikipedia, 2017a)

Sign	Score		
	0	**1**	**2**
Heart rate	Absent	Under 100 bpm	Over 100 bpm
Respiratory effort	Absent	Slow and irregular	Breathing actively or crying loudly
Muscle tone	Absent	Some flexion of the extremities	Arms and legs in flexion Active movement at times
Response to stimulation	Absent	Grimacing	Coughing, sneezing or crying
Colour	Pallor or central cyanosis	Body pink, but extremities are cyanosed	Body and extremities are pink

Initiation of respiration

The normal newborn baby should give its first cry within 60 seconds following delivery. In this case no suctioning is required. If there are any secretions, sterile gauze should be used to clear the mouth.

Suctioning

No suctioning should be carried out on a baby who cries immediately after birth or a baby with no observed secretions. However, if mucus, amniotic fluid or meconium is present in the upper respiratory passages at birth, this can be inhaled into the bronchi and could result in atelectasis or pneumonia in the neonate. In these circumstances it is therefore imperative that the air passages be cleared before the baby tries to breathe. The baby should only be suctioned if:

▶ the baby fails to initiate respiration at birth within 60 seconds

▶ there is meconium in the amniotic fluid or on the baby's skin

▶ excessive secretions are noted at delivery.

When suctioning of the newborn is indicated, it should be carried out with a soft catheter, using a low negative pressure not exceeding −10 cm H_2O, and should be gentle and brief to avoid reflex apnoea and bradycardia. Gentle, brief aspiration first of the mouth and then of the nose should be sufficient to remove any mucus or fluid. The suction catheter should not be pushed to the back of the baby's throat, as it may cause damage to the mucous membranes.

Evaluating the need for resuscitation

If the infant does not breathe well soon after birth, the midwife should provide stimulation by flicking the baby's feet with her or his fingers or by gently rubbing the baby with a warmed towel. If this does not result in adequate respiration, then 100 per cent oxygen should be administered through a face mask and the feet flicked again. In most instances a few gasps of oxygen are all that is required to establish and maintain respiration.

If, however, the baby still does not breathe adequately, then all midwives need to be competent to act in accordance with protocol to resuscitate the newborn (see Chapter 46). If the mother received pethidine shortly before delivery, then the baby may be given an IM injection of naloxone hydrochloride (neonatal Narcan®) 0.01 mg/kg (see Chapter 41).

Risk factors for neonatal resuscitation

Certain factors during labour are associated with the need for neonatal resuscitation, namely:

▶ assisted delivery, such as forceps or vacuum extraction

▶ abnormal presentations, such as breech presentations

▶ premature labour

▶ prolonged rupture of membranes (PROM)

▶ a delayed second stage of labour

▶ antepartum haemorrhage (APH), such as placenta praevia or placental abruption

▶ an abnormal fetal heart rate (FHR)

▶ cord prolapse

▶ uterine tetany due to induction of labour (IOL).

Identifying the baby

Two identification bands should have been prepared for the baby before delivery. These must bear the mother's name, the baby's sex, the birth date and time and the type of delivery. These details must be verified verbally with the mother before the birth and again when the bands are attached to the baby immediately after birth. One identification band is placed on the baby's wrist and another on the baby's ankle.

In some centres, the baby is identified before the umbilical cord is cut in order to avoid any chance of mixing up or interchange of babies. This can easily happen if the baby is not identified immediately at birth and is a serious legal safety matter. It is therefore very important to impress upon everyone concerned the necessity for immediate and correct identification of the baby. It is important that the mother notices a feature to identify her baby. A hand- or footprint of the baby is made and placed in the mother and baby's file.

Observing general condition, weighing and measuring

The baby is gently removed from the mother's abdomen, while explaining why this is necessary. The baby is laid on a safe, horizontal surface nearby, on either the left or right side. The baby's general condition is noted, in particular whether the breathing is satisfactory. (In some centres this is done while the mother is still holding the baby.) The baby is weighed and measured, as described in Section 29.4.

Care of the eyes

The eyes should be cleaned and an eye ointment applied. Eye care is provided according to local protocol. The baby's eyes are wiped with sterile cottonwool swabs and sterile water and an eye ointment is applied after the delivery of the baby to prevent the risk of ophthalmia neonatorum (gonococcal infection), which might lead to blindness. The common eye ointments used include chloramphenicol, erythromycin or tetracycline. These eye ointments are also active against chlamydia infection.

Care of the cord

A sterile, disposable plastic umbilical clamp is attached to the cord about 2.5 cm above the umbilicus and the forceps are removed. Ensure that the clasps in the clamp are tightly closed, to prevent any chance of haemorrhage from the cord. (The loss of 30 ml of blood from a newborn baby is comparable to the loss of 600 ml of blood from an adult.) The end stump of the cord is cut just above the clamp, on the placental side (see Figure 29.1 on page 445). The cord is inspected to ensure that three vessels are present. (Two vessels only would indicate a congenital abnormality.)

If this umbilical clamp is not available, the cord can be tied using sterile linen, string, silk or tape ligature, provided it is not too fine. The ligature must be capable of occluding the blood vessels but must not damage the cord at the site of the ligature. The cord is observed for haemorrhage.

29.4 Measurement and immediate examination of the newborn

Weighing the baby

The baby should be weighed without any clothes but without causing undue heat loss. The weight is documented. The recording forms a baseline for future assessment.

Observations

Several observations are carried out with the least possible exposure. Measure the baby's crown–heel length and the baby's head circumference, encompassing the occipitofrontal diameter. While these measurements are being taken, the midwife should observe the baby quickly but carefully for the following:

▶ *Respiratory distress.* Note breathing patterns and colour for signs of respiratory distress.
▶ *Hypothermia.* Temperature per axilla should be 36.5–37 °C.
▶ *Abnormal neurological features.* Features such as jitteriness, twitching, convulsions, excessive lethargy should be noted.

▶ *Blood sugar.* Blood sugar is observed and feeding established.
▶ *Anatomical abnormalities.* Abnormalities such as cleft lip and cleft palate, meningocele, exomphalos, deformities of hands and feet, and so forth, are noted.
▶ *Trauma.* Observe for any signs of birth trauma.

Chapter 41 provides complete information for a full examination of the neonate.

If the midwife is not satisfied with the baby's condition, a medical practitioner should be notified immediately.

The warmly wrapped baby is then returned to the mother or parents if the condition of both the mother and baby is entirely satisfactory. Following delivery, the baby's eyes are usually open and the baby is very alert. The parents are congratulated on the birth of their infant. Infant feeding is started within the first hour following childbirth and the mother's choice of infant feeding should be respected.

During the first 24 hours after birth, the baby is observed frequently (every half to one hour). The baby's colour, respiration and temperature should be noted. Check whether there is any mucus in the baby's mouth or nose, and check the cord for bleeding. If there are any complications, the baby should be kept under constant observation in high care and the airways aspirated whenever necessary.

Documentation

All the information regarding the baby's condition at and immediately after birth should be fully and accurately recorded as per local protocol. Report any abnormalities.

If at any time during this period the midwife is not satisfied with the condition of the newborn infant, a medical practitioner should immediately be notified.

29.5 Examination of the placenta and membranes

Examination of the placenta may yield information on the impact of maternal disorders on the fetus or the cause of stillbirth, preterm delivery, fetal growth restriction or neuro-developmental impairment. Retained products of conception are one of the main causes of postpartum haemorrhage (PPH) and infection.

PROCEDURE	Examination of the placenta and membranes

Principles

▶ Inspection of the placenta should be performed as soon as possible after birth to identify completeness and exclude abnormalities.

▶ Adequate lighting is necessary because of the intricate structure of the placental tissue.

▶ A flat surface with protection to absorb blood spillage and the wearing of a plastic apron and gloves are necessary as universal precautions against contamination.

▶ An incomplete placenta or membranes will result in uterine atony and subsequent excessive bleeding and/or infection.

▶ Health education is essential if there are concerns about the completeness of the placenta. The mother must be advised to seek professional advice from a midwife or doctor if bleeding or infections occur.

▶ If the placenta is thought to be incomplete at a home birth, the woman needs to be transferred to a hospital for evacuation of retained products of conception.

Special care and treatment of the tissue should be communicated to minimise the risk of infection in case of a lotus birth (where the placenta remains attached to the baby until the cord naturally detaches).

Indication

Examination of the placenta and membranes is done:

▶ because it is a requirement of the South African Nursing Council (SANC) under Regulation R2488

▶ in case of legal issues regarding the presence of acute versus chronic perinatal stresses and insults in case of cerebral palsy claims

▶ to determine the specific aetiologies of adverse pregnancy outcomes (fetal or neonatal demise)

▶ when there is a gestational or a neonatal pathology

▶ to identify zygosity and pathology (eg twin-to-twin transfusion)

▶ to exclude the possibility of retained products.

Contraindications

Examination of the placenta and membranes should not be carried out:

▶ in the presence of highly infectious conditions (eg Ebola), where the safety of the examiner cannot be guaranteed

▶ if no protective clothing (aprons) and gloves are available.

Pre-procedure

1   Before examining the placenta, ensure maternal comfort. Monitor blood loss and check the uterus for contraction to minimise bleeding.

2   Explain the procedure to the parents and enquire if they want to observe the assessment.

3   Make sure the placenta and membranes are examined as soon as possible before discharge or transfer to the postnatal ward.

Procedure

1   Lay the placenta with the fetal side uppermost.

2   Note the size, shape, smell and colour (See colour illustrations C6 to C11 on pages 74–78)

3   All blood vessels should stop before reaching the end of the placenta. A blood vessel radiating beyond the edge could indicate a placenta succenturiata; the extra lobe could have remained in the uterus.

4   Weigh the placenta and interpret it in terms of the baby's weight.

5   Record the colour.

Evaluation: The fetal surface

1   Identify the amnion and chorion.

2   Check the blood vessels and chorionic villi.

continued

Evaluation: The maternal surface

1 Identify, document and report missing cotyledons, infarcts, succenturiata lobes, fatty deposits or blood clots and calcifications:
   ▶ Recent infarctions are bright red and old infarctions form grey patches.
   ▶ Infarctions are only abnormal if they take up more than 50 per cent of the placenta.
   ▶ Calcification (sandy white patches) indicates degeneration of a full-term placenta.
   ▶ Any dark red areas or blood clots attached to the maternal surface are abnormal and indicate abruption placenta.
2 Retain the clots to make an accurate assessment of blood loss.

Evaluation: The membranes (for completeness)

1 Place the placenta on a flat surface, with the maternal surface facing up.
2 Insert one hand into the hole in the membranes through which the baby has been delivered.
3 While the hand is inside the membrane, stretch it out to visually gauge the completeness thereof.
4 Observe the membranes and inspect for completeness, extra vessels, lobes or holes in the surface. There should be a single hole.
5 Be cautious when holding the placenta by its cord because of the increased chance of blood splatter.
6 Peel the amnion away from the chorion to confirm the presence of both. The amnion is closest to the fetus and is thin, smooth, transparent and difficult to tear. The chorion is the inner membrane against the wall of the uterus and is thick, opaque and tears easily. Both the amnion and the chorion should be present and complete as products left behind may predispose the woman to PPH.

Evaluation: The umbilical cord

1 Evaluate the colour of the cord.
2 Measure the umbilical cord in centimetres. A cord length of less than 40 cm is considered short and may result in premature separation of the placenta or cord rupture or may have impeded descent of the fetus. A very long cord may have become coiled around the fetus, form true knots or prolapse when the membranes rupture.
3 Identify the presence of true and false knots (see Figure 7.27 on page 116). A true knot forms when the fetus passes through a loop before or during birth. A true knot may cause fetal hypoxia and death if the knot tightens. False knots are formed by an accumulation of Wharton jelly and are clinically insignificant.
4 Document the type of implantation. The cord is commonly inserted in the centre of the fetal surface of the placenta. A *lateral insertion* indicates a cord that is implanted away from the centre, yet not at the edge. A *battledore insertion* indicates a cord inserted at the very edge of the placenta (and resembles a tennis racket). A *velamentous insertion* indicates a cord implanted into the membranes of the fetal sac.
5 Identify and count the number of blood vessels (the absence of one of the arteries can be associated with renal agenesis).

Recording and interpretation

The following are guidelines for interpretation:
▶ Cloudy (pale and grey) membranes or a placenta that smells offensive suggests chorioamnionitis.
▶ Clots of blood that adhere to the maternal surface suggest abruption placenta.
▶ A placenta that is abnormally large is suggestive of:
  • congenital syphilis (if heavy and oedematous)
  • Rh haemolytic disease (if heavy and pale)
  • maternal diabetes (if heavier than expected for the weight of the infant, but with a normal appearance)
  • fetal intrauterine growth restriction (IUGR) (if lighter than would be expected for the weight of the infant).
▶ Congenital abnormalities may be present if only one umbilical artery is identified.

Do the following to wrap up the procedure:
1 Communicate abnormalities to the medical practitioner. Take action to correct or investigate.
2 Record all findings (normal and abnormal) in the obstetric documents. A photograph of the observed abnormalities can be placed in the obstetric record for future reference.

continued

3   The placenta may be stored in a separate fridge for inspection by the medical practitioner. Alternatively, dispose of the placenta into a disintegrator or incinerator or according to hospital policy (also see guidelines below).
4   Clean away equipment.
5   Wash hands.
6   Discuss the findings with the parents.

Disposal of the placenta

▶ In a healthcare facility, the institutional policies prescribe the method of universal disposal.
▶ After a home confinement, the placenta needs to be transported in a sealed container, labelled with the mother's identifying data, to a waste disposal facility.
▶ If the woman wishes to take her placenta home to bury or encapsulate it, a tissue release form for placentas should be completed and one copy filed within the woman's maternal health record.
▶ Health education and instructions for safe disposal are essential when a placenta is handed to the mother for cultural, religious or other reasons.

29.6   Transitional care in the fourth stage

Following delivery of the placenta and membranes, the midwife should palpate the abdomen to ensure that the uterus is well contracted and note any signs of uterine atony. The woman is usually tired and thirsty. A cup of tea or other drink is offered.

Women who plan to breastfeed should start within one hour of birth. The woman should be supported in her choice of infant feeding.

Observations should be carried out for both the mother (bleeding per vagina, BP, pulse, temperature and respirations) and the baby (colour, respiration, heart rate and temperature). All observations should be recorded and essential records completed. Physiologically, the temperature should be normal, the pulse less than 90 bpm and the BP lower than the values at birth. Any abnormalities are reported.

The perineum and cervix are examined for tears or lacerations. Any lacerations, tears or episiotomy should be repaired immediately to reduce the incidence of infection.

Achieving adequate homeostasis allows the midwife to prevent primary PPH. The amount of blood loss is estimated to exclude PPH. This should not exceed 500 ml or enough to cause a change in maternal condition. The woman is encouraged to pass urine, as a full bladder may contribute to uterine atony and subsequent PPH. The perineal pad is checked for blood loss before transferring the mother to the postpartum ward.

Immediately after delivery, the baby is usually wide awake with open eyes and a strong urge to suckle, while the mother and the father may be full of awe and wonder, often with strong protective maternal and paternal feelings. This is therefore a good time for the family – including older siblings, if desired – to share in the process of getting acquainted with the new addition to the family.

When transferring the mother and the baby to the postpartum ward in hospital, both the mother and the baby should be kept warm to minimise hypothermia. Ideally the mother should be holding the baby, either sitting in a wheelchair or lying down in bed or trolley, to encourage bonding.

On arrival in the postpartum ward, a comprehensive report should be given to the receiving midwife, which includes history relating to the antenatal period, labour, birth and the immediate puerperium. The woman should be examined to exclude any excessive bleeding per vagina and assess for uterine contraction.

29.7   Conclusion

Observations in the fourth stage of labour should be done according to protocol. Any abnormalities should be acted upon immediately, as delay may result in maternal or neonatal morbidity and mortality. Fetal distress is likely to occur if the woman was delivered in the supine position, especially if the second stage was prolonged. This chapter detailed the standard care of the newborn, including the Apgar score and other observations. The examination of the placenta and membranes for abnormalities was also discussed.

Malposition, malpresentation and dysfunctional labour

LEARNING OBJECTIVES

On completion of this chapter, you must be able to:

▶ identify and describe the causes of dysfunctional labour
▶ identify and describe ways to prevent dysfunctional labour
▶ identify and describe specific interventions for dysfunctional situations
▶ develop the basic competencies to assist women during labour.

KNOWLEDGE ASSUMED TO BE IN PLACE

Knowledge, competency and skill in the basic management of normal birth
The Ps of birth

KEYWORDS

dystocia • distress • dysfunction • disproportion • obstruction • prolapse

30.1 Introduction

The most commonly encountered complications directly due to obstetrical causes are presented in this chapter. A midwife should be able to anticipate and identify these conditions and refer them for medical attention.

In some cases there may be no time to refer, which will mean that the midwife needs to intervene, particularly in life-threatening conditions. Diagnosis, treatment and care are competencies and skills required for the practice of midwifery that involve the ability to use learned information in a practical way. Midwives need experience to master these skills. This chapter gives an introduction to the principles of diagnosis with guidelines for intervention. It is essential that midwives understand the terminology and definitions.

30.2 Malpresentations and malpositions

Malpresentations are deviations of the breech or fetal head, usually referring to deflexions of parts of the fetal body and/or asynclitism caused by a variety of maternal, fetal and obstetric causes. Abnormalities or malpositions of the lie of the fetus are the transverse and oblique lie. Normally the long axis of

the fetus is parallel with the long axis of the mother. (The long axes refer to the spines of the mother and fetus.)

Deviations of the presentations refer to deflexion of a part of the fetus. Normally the fetus is in an attitude of full flexion (fetal position), where all the parts are flexed. If any part of the fetus is extended, this causes complications, as the fetus must be able to rotate, flex and extend to negotiate the pelvis. These movements can be observed using abdominal palpation during pregnancy, as can the lie, position, engagement and station of the presenting part. The abdominal examination is followed by a vaginal examination to determine which part is presenting, if the presenting part is in flexion or extension, and the station of the presenting part.

In most cases of abnormal presentation or malposition, the medical practitioner is called and/or the woman is referred to a higher level of care. These births are complicated, with a high incidence of interventions as well as maternal and perinatal morbidity and mortality. Women with malpresentation and malposition need to deliver at an appropriate level of care with a medical practitioner and access to a theatre, an anaesthetist, a paediatrician and appropriately trained midwives.

The midwife's main task is early identification and referral to the appropriate level of care. Abnormalities can be identified at 36 weeks, on admission at the start of labour or during labour using a partogram. Table 30.1 gives the landmarks that will indicate abnormal presentations on vaginal examination.

Table 30.1

Landmarks of the presenting part, indicating the positions (see also Figure 30.1)

Position	Part felt on vaginal examination
Cephalic	Fontanelles and suture lines
Shoulder	Shoulder, scapula or arm
Breech	Genitalia, knee or foot
Brow	Orbital ridges and anterior fontanelle
Face	Mouth, nose and eyes
Asynclitism	Ear, felt anteriorly or posteriorly

Rules for fetal positions in labour

If the fetal head is flexed, it needs to extend for birth in the second stage. If it is extended, it needs to flex for birth to allow the best diameters to pass through the birth canal.

The best diameter is a flexed occipitoanterior (OA) in synclitism (an average-term fetus): biparietal diameter (BPD) = 9.5 cm and suboccipitobregmatic diameter = 9.5 cm.

The same diameters are found in the total extended face presentation, where the submentobregmatic diameter is 9.5 cm and the BPD is 9.5 cm. In the OA position, the head extends when delivered and in the face presentation the head flexes. All other deviations theoretically make birth more difficult (not considering other factors such as the relationship with the pelvis). These include asynclitism and partial extension (deflexion) or exaggerated extension or flexion, which allows for less favourable diameters.

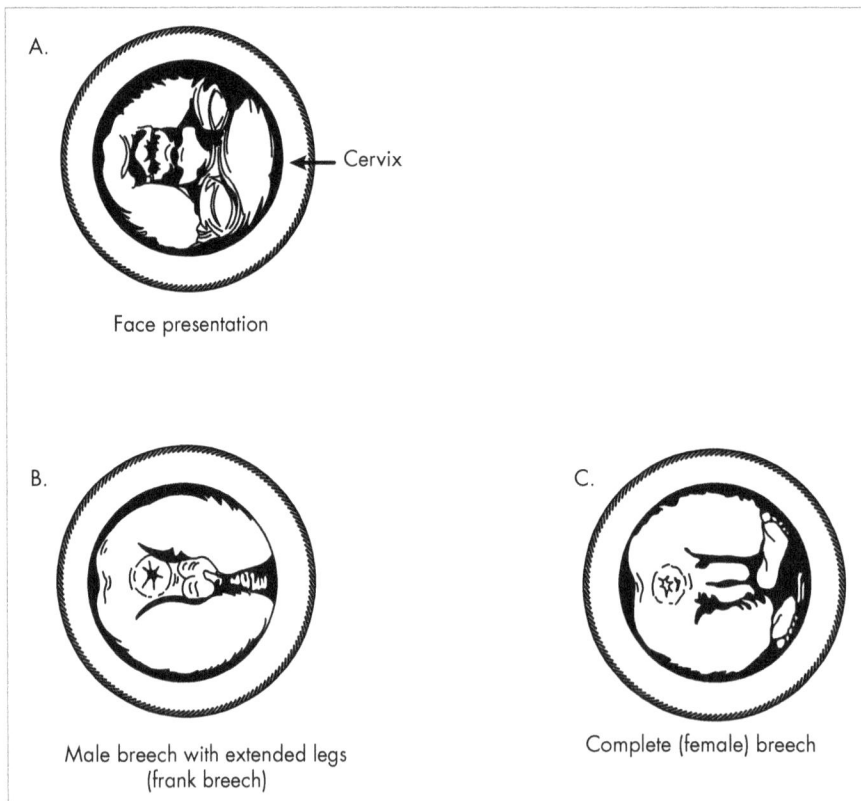

A.

— Cervix

Face presentation

B.

Male breech with extended legs
(frank breech)

C.

Complete (female) breech

Figure 30.1 Malpresentations

An abnormal lie (a transverse and oblique lie) in a fetus identified at 36 weeks cannot deliver vaginally unless corrected, and there is a high risk of cord prolapse. External version or an internal podalic version (IPV) can be performed in labour by a medical practitioner. Table 30.2 shows a comparison of normal versus abnormal findings in palpation and vaginal examination. This comparison can be used to decide whether or not a normal birth is possible. If you suspect complications, refer early.

Table 30.2

Comparison of normal versus abnormal findings in palpation and vaginal examination during labour

	Normal criteria	**Deviations**
Abdominal palpation		
Symphysis fundal height (SFH)	Correlates with the dates and grows and develops normally as plotted on a graph (only useful between 20 and 35 weeks)	Unsure or no correlation
Amniotic fluid	Adequate (allowing the fetus to be felt and moved, is ballottable) with ease on abdominal palpation	Too little or too much
Fetal movement	Present and normal (at least 10 movements a day)	Not felt by practitioner or mother
Fetal heart	Regular and heard through the posterior thorax wall of the fetus. In a cephalic presentation, the fetal heart is heard under the umbilical line	Fetal heart noticed all over abdomen, or above umbilical line
Fetal head	From 30 weeks the fetal head can be felt on abdominal palpation Only two poles felt	Difficult to feel the fetal head Three poles identified
Presenting part	From 37 weeks the presenting part may be engaged in the pelvis in a primigravida and the fetus is in position in a multigravida (sometimes only at birth)	Not engaged at birth in primigravida Unstable lie in multigravida
Vaginal examination		
Station	Presenting part at the spines or 1 cm above and fixed (not ballotting)	Presenting part above the spines
Application	Fair or good application on cervix	Cervix poorly applied, long and posterior
Bishop score	Bishop score > 5	Bishop score < 5
Synclitism	Synclitism (sagittal suture in middle)	Asynclitism (ear felt)
Landmarks	Posterior fontanelle can be felt (well flexed)	Anterior fontanelle felt (deflexed)
Pelvimetry	Diagonal conjugate 12.5 cm Ischial spines not prominent Ligaments allow two fingers Subpubic arch allows two fingers Intertuberous diameter 10 cm	Any diameter narrowed

continued

	Normal criteria	**Deviations**
Labour		
Membranes	Membranes intact with forewaters	Rupture before labour starts or bulging in vagina
Contractions	Normal contractions Normal uterine tone	Abnormal pattern (coupled, hypo- or hypertonic) Lower or higher tone
Cervical changes	Correlate with contractions Normal rate (cm/hr)	No or slow cervical changes with contractions Less than 1 cm
Position of the cervix	Cervix anterior, effacing and dilating	Cervix long and posterior or hanging like a sleeve (curtaining) or paperthin
Partogram	Follows normal guidelines	Exceeds normal criteria

Causes of malpresentations and malpositions

The causes of malpresentations or malpositions are overlapping and are in most cases related to the Ps of labour, namely the powers, the passages and the passenger.

Maternal causes

Maternal causes include:
- a pendulous abdomen resulting from lax abdominal wall muscles
- polyhydramnios, which may cause the fetus to take an abnormal position
- a contracted pelvis, which may result if the sacrocotyloid dimension or anteroposterior (AP) diameter of the pelvic brim are decreased
- spinal deformities, which may result in the fetal head being directed forwards, for example in exaggerated lordosis or in spondylolisthesis
- posterior implantation of placenta praevia
- uterine abnormalities
- neoplasm of the lower segment
- iatrogenic from an external version
- idiopathic causes that are unexplained.

Fetal causes

These are also known as primary causes and include:
- abnormalities of the fetus, such as anencephaly, tumours of the neck or other tumours
- a large head (hydrocephaly)
- coils of umbilical cord around the neck.

Brow and face presentations: Diagnosis and outcomes

This section will consider face and brow presentations, which are common malpresentations. These conditions are managed by a medical practitioner and are briefly compared in Table 30.3.

Diagnosis of brow and face presentations is difficult on abdominal and vaginal examination. Any abdominal palpation that is unclear, or a fetal heart that is heard where it is not expected, needs to be questioned and confirmed with ultrasound or X-ray if the vaginal examination is inconclusive. A high presenting part with an undilated cervix and unclear information should be a warning sign. Because the presenting part is not well applied, contractions are often poor and dilatation slow.

Brow presentation

A brow presentation is very difficult to diagnose, because the head is high and the cervix not dilated. It is thus difficult to feel the presenting part. Labour can be prolonged over days. Note that dilatation can never be the only criteria of labour. A brow presentation cannot be delivered vaginally unless the head is totally deflexed to a face presentation.

Table 30.3

Differences between brow and face presentation (see figures 30.1 to 30.6)

	Brow	Face
Incidence	1:1 400 (Marino, 2016)	1:750 (Marino, 2016)
Lie	Longitudinal	Longitudinal
Presenting part	Cephalic	Cephalic
Denominator	Sinciput	Mentum
Presenting diameters	Mentovertical diameter of 13.5 cm Biparietal 9.5 cm	Submentobregmatic 9.5 cm Biparietal 9.5 cm
Flexion or extension	Deflexed head	Total extension of head
Landmarks	Orbital ridges and root of the nose felt	Mouth, nose and eyes (no sutures or fontanelles)
Clinical diagnosis	Difficult to diagnose	Clear landmarks distinguish it from breech
Diagnosis	X-rays and ultrasound	Clinical, X-ray or ultrasound
Membranes	A bag of amniotic fluid may hang in the vagina	Intact or ruptured
Fetal heart	Heard through anterior chest pushed out	Heard through anterior chest pushed out
Vaginal examination	High head Poor application No fontanelles felt	High presenting part Application good
Mechanism	Not possible to deliver Need to flex to OA or extend to a face presentation	Mentoanterior can deliver because favourable diameters present (see Figure 30.5 on page 459) Need to extend to deliver Mentoposterior cannot deliver vaginally (see Figure 30.6 on page 460)
Effect on birth	Prolonged or obstructed labour Maternal distress	Prolonged labour Difficult second stage
Effect on fetus	Asphyxia Distress	Facial oedema and bruising Breathing difficulties
Outcomes	Caesarean section Vaginal birth if head flexed or extends to face presentation in an average infant	Mentoanterior can deliver because the diameters are favourable (see Figure 30.5) Mentoposterior can turn to mentoanterior during descent if well extended. If it stays mentoposterior there is no mechanism (see Figure 30.6)

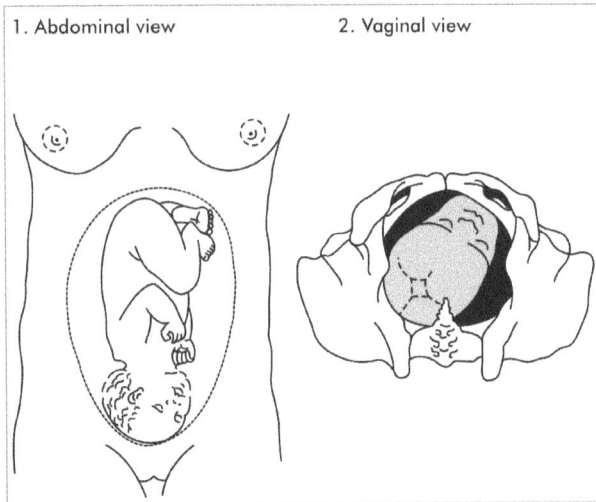

Figure 30.2 Brow presentation

Face presentation

Face presentation is more common than brow presentation. The mentum is the denominator and vaginal birth is possible, as the diameters that present are the same as the flexed cephalic anterior even though the head is in total extension. The BPD is 9.5 cm and the submentobregmatic is 9.5 cm. However, the second stage of labour is more difficult. If the baby is in a mentoposterior position, it cannot be delivered vaginally because the head cannot flex sufficiently to be born (see Figure 30.6 on page 460).

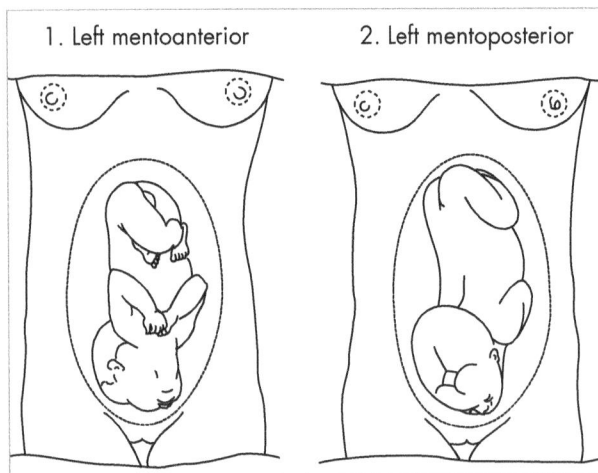

Figure 30.3 Face presentation

Complications of malpresentations

Maternal complications

Complications for the woman in labour can include:

▶ prolonged labour and maternal distress
▶ presentation and prolapse of the umbilical cord
▶ obstructed labour and all the complications that occur with obstruction
▶ uterine rupture and trauma to other pelvic organs, such as the bladder
▶ maternal death – only secondary to obstructed labour and sepsis/uterine rupture
▶ puerperal infections.

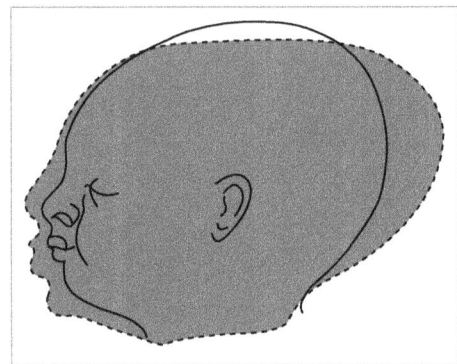

Figure 30.4 Moulding of a face presentation

Fetal complications

Note: All the complications that affect the fetus in prolonged and obstructed labour also apply here. Fetal complications arising from malpresentations include:

▶ fetal distress
▶ intrauterine death (IUD)
▶ asphyxia neonatorum
▶ birth injuries
▶ neonatal infections
▶ neonatal death.

30.3   The occipitoposterior position

The occipitoposterior (OP) position is the most common malposition that a midwife will manage. Early recognition and referral can improve the outcomes for mother and fetus. The OP position is associated with prolonged, painful labour, assisted deliveries and an exhausted mother and fetus.

Incidence

The incidence is 15–20 per cent (Holcroft Argani & Satin, 2017).

1.

Right side   Left side

Mentum to the left and anterior

2.

Descent and **extension**, making
the mentum the leading part

3a.

$^1/_8$

3b.

Lateral view

Internal rotation of the head
The mentum rotates forward $^1/_8$ of a circle and the face is born (crowning)

Birth of the head

4a.

4b.

Lateral view

The head is born by a movement of **flexion**

5.

Restitution (of mentum)

6.

External rotation of the head (mentum)
together with internal rotation of the shoulders

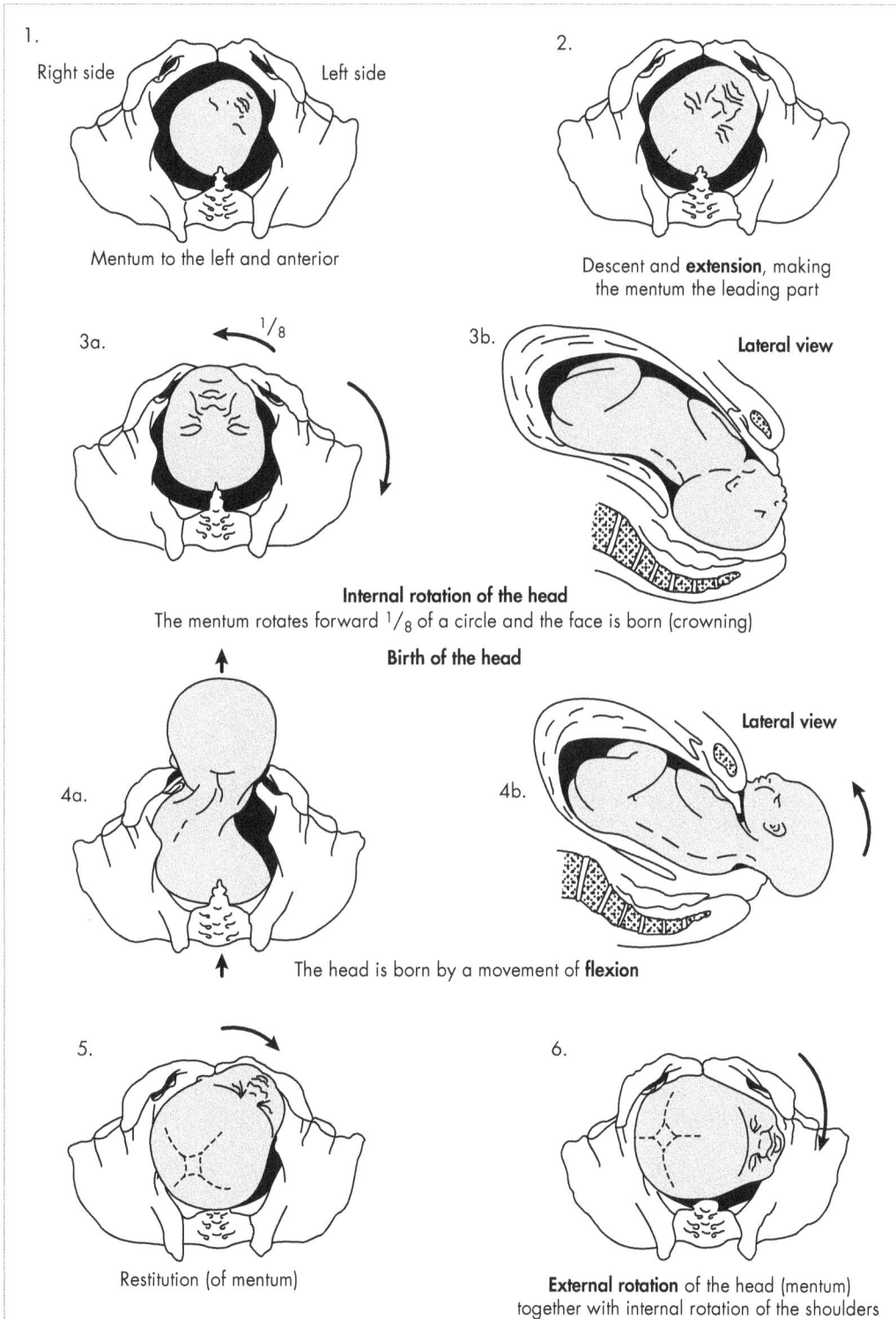

Figure 30.5 Mechanism of a mentoanterior (face presentation)

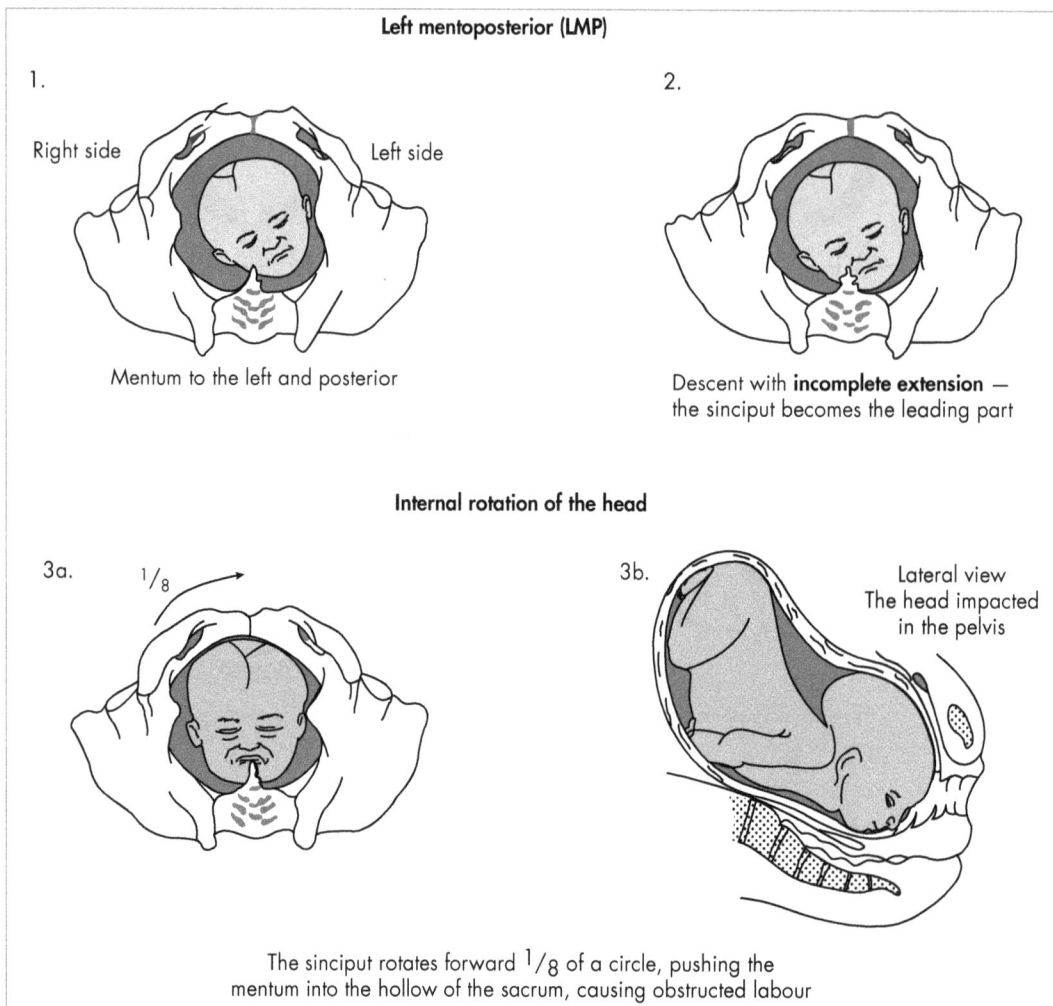

Figure 30.6 Complication of a mentoposterior (face presentation)

Definition

In an OP position of a cephalic presentation, the occiput (the denominator) lies in the posterior quadrant of the pelvis. That is, the occiput lies adjacent to either the right sacroiliac joint (a right occipitoposterior, or ROP) or, in a few instances, the left sacroiliac joint (a left occipitoposterior, or LOP). (The LOP is unusual because the descending colon lies in the left posterior portion of the pelvis.) A posterior position of the cephalic is known as a malposition, because of the problems that can arise in posterior positions (see Figure 30.7).

Causes of posterior positions of the cephalic presentation

Posterior positions of the cephalic appear to be influenced by the conditions described in the following subsections.

The shape of the pelvic brim (inlet)

The position in which the occiput enters the pelvis appears to be determined to a large extent by the shape of the pelvic brim, which allows the BPD (the widest transverse diameter) of the fetal skull to be most easily accommodated (in the largest diameter of the pelvis). For this reason, if the pelvis is an average-sized gynaecoid pelvis and the fetal head is well flexed, the head commonly lies with the sagittal suture in either the transverse diameter with the occiput lying laterally, or in one of the oblique diameters with the occiput lying anteriorly. However, where the transverse diameter of the pelvic brim is narrowed and/or where the sacrocotyloid space is narrowed, the head is more easily accommodated with the occiput lying posteriorly.

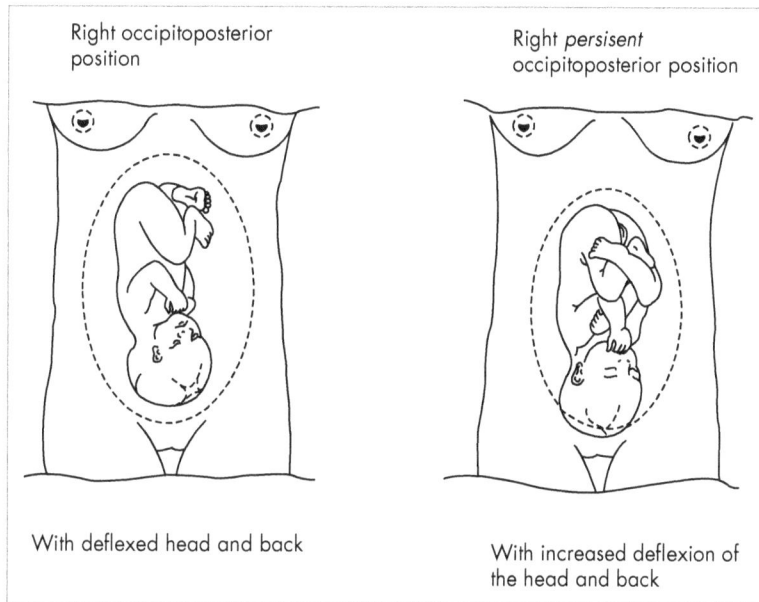

Figure 30.7 OP positions (abdominal view)

The android pelvis has a heart-shaped brim with the wider space posteriorly and a narrowed sacrocotyloid space. This allows the broader part (occiput) to be posterior. The anthropoid pelvis has a reduced transverse diameter and a wider AP diameter of the brim. Therefore both these types of pelvises can predispose to OP positions. Other types of contracted pelvis, and some spinal deformities, could also be implicated.

The shape and size of the fetal head

The shape and size of the fetal head will also affect the position of the occiput in a cephalic presentation. Conditions which could contribute to OP positions include:

▶ increased multiparity, as babies tend to get larger with each pregnancy

▶ prolonged pregnancy (fetal post-maturity), as the fetal skull is large

▶ diabetes mellitus in the mother, as the baby is larger than average.

Maternal causes

In the primigravida with tight abdominal muscles, the fetal attitude is one of less flexion of the back, namely the 'military attitude'. This could lead to the cephalic presenting posteriorly.

Obstetric causes

In placenta praevia, the fetal head takes a different position. If the umbilical cord is around the neck, the head may remain high.

Possible outcomes

There are two possible outcomes of the OP position:

1. A long rotation forward, as shown in figures 30.8 and 30.10 on page 462 and 465, ending in a spontaneous normal delivery. In 90 per cent of all posterior positions of the cephalic, the head rotates and the occiput becomes the leading part. This usually happens in the second stage of labour.

2. A persistent occipitoposterior (POP) delivery (face-to-pubis; short rotation), as shown in Figure 30.9 on page 463. This delivery occurs because the head remains in the posterior position and meets the pelvic floor first. The baby delivers face to pubis. This occurs in about 10 per cent of all posterior positions.

Complications

More complications arise in posterior positions than in anterior positions, usually due to larger diameters that rest on the posterior sacrum, causing a poor fit on the cervix. The presenting diameters are the occiput frontal (11.5 cm) and the biparietal (9.5 cm). This is not a round circle and causes poor application and dilatation. The descent of the head is slow, with pressure on the sacrum, back ache and prolonged labour. This in turn causes an increase in dysfunctional labour for the mother and the fetus.

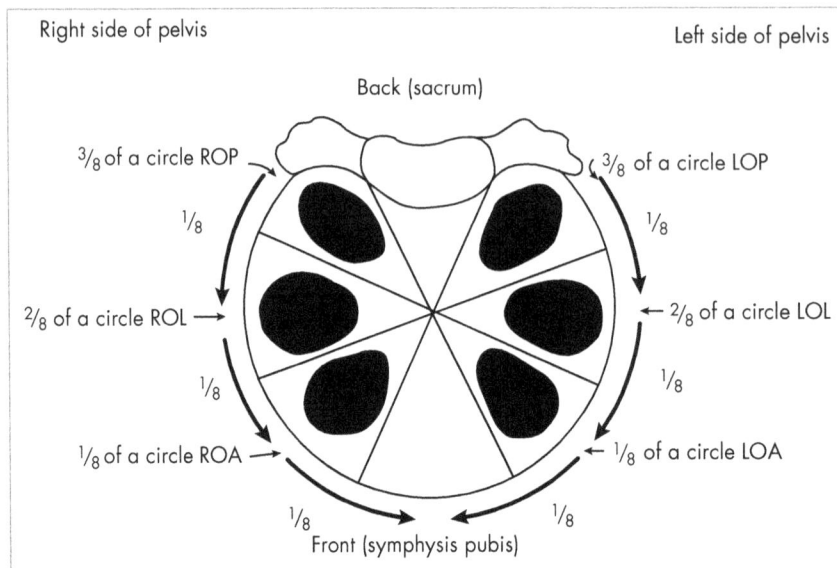

Figure 30.8 Long forward rotation of the fetal head during labour in posterior positions of the occiput

If posterior positions are not identified in labour and correctly managed, the following complications can develop:

▶ *Prolonged labour and maternal distress.* Owing to the long rotation forward of the head, the length of the first stage of labour is increased. With the larger diameters of the fetal skull passing through the pelvic cavity, both first and second stages are prolonged.

▶ *Maternal infection.* A long labour lowers the mother's resistance to infection. Frequent vaginal examinations and catheterisation may be necessary, as well as other operative measures. These, together with the early rupture of the membranes, predispose the mother to intrauterine infection, urinary tract infection (UTI) and general infection (puerperal infection).

▶ *Fetal and neonatal infection.* The early rupture of the membranes, the frequent vaginal examinations and other operative procedures may introduce infection into the uterus and so to the fetus. This infection may only manifest in the neonatal period.

▶ *Haemorrhage.* The incidence of both atonic and traumatic postpartum haemorrhage (PPH) is increased. Lacerations and damage to soft tissue are more prevalent because of the larger engaging diameters and the necessity for intervention and episiotomies. Tears of the vagina and perineum, bruising and haematomas may occur.

▶ *Cord prolapse.* The presenting part is uneven (not round) because the head is deflexed. The deflexed head has difficulty entering the pelvic brim and so remains high.

Both these conditions predispose to early rupture of the membranes and to the danger of umbilical cord prolapse.

▶ *Deep transverse arrest.* The head flexes sufficiently to allow the occiput to become the leading part and to start the long rotation forward. However, in about 15 per cent of these cases, the occiput becomes stuck at the ischial spines, with the sagittal suture in the transverse diameter of the pelvis, causing a deep transverse arrest. This condition is often associated with the android type of pelvis, which has prominent ischial spines, a long narrow pelvic cavity and a reduced outlet. A deep transverse arrest cannot be delivered vaginally. Refer to a medical practitioner immediately. Forceps are not used, as the sagittal suture should be in the AP position. If the cervix is fully dilated and the fetus is of average size, a medical practitioner may attempt to flex the head and rotate it. If this is unsuccessful, the baby is delivered by Caesarean section.

▶ *Obstructed labour.* If the fetus is large or moderate cephalopelvic disproportion (CPD) exists, obstructed labour can develop (see Chapter 31). Obstructed labour is a result of poor quality of care and should be prevented at all costs. Early diagnosis and prompt referral is essential. In the case of obstructed labour, start an IV infusion, place the woman in the left lateral position, start oxygen and call the medical practitioner immediately. Delivery will be by Caesarean section. Potential outcomes of obstructed labour are:

• *Bandl's ring.* In primigravidae, Bandl's ring or the pathological retraction ring is formed.

• *Uterine rupture.* In the multigravida the uterus may rupture.

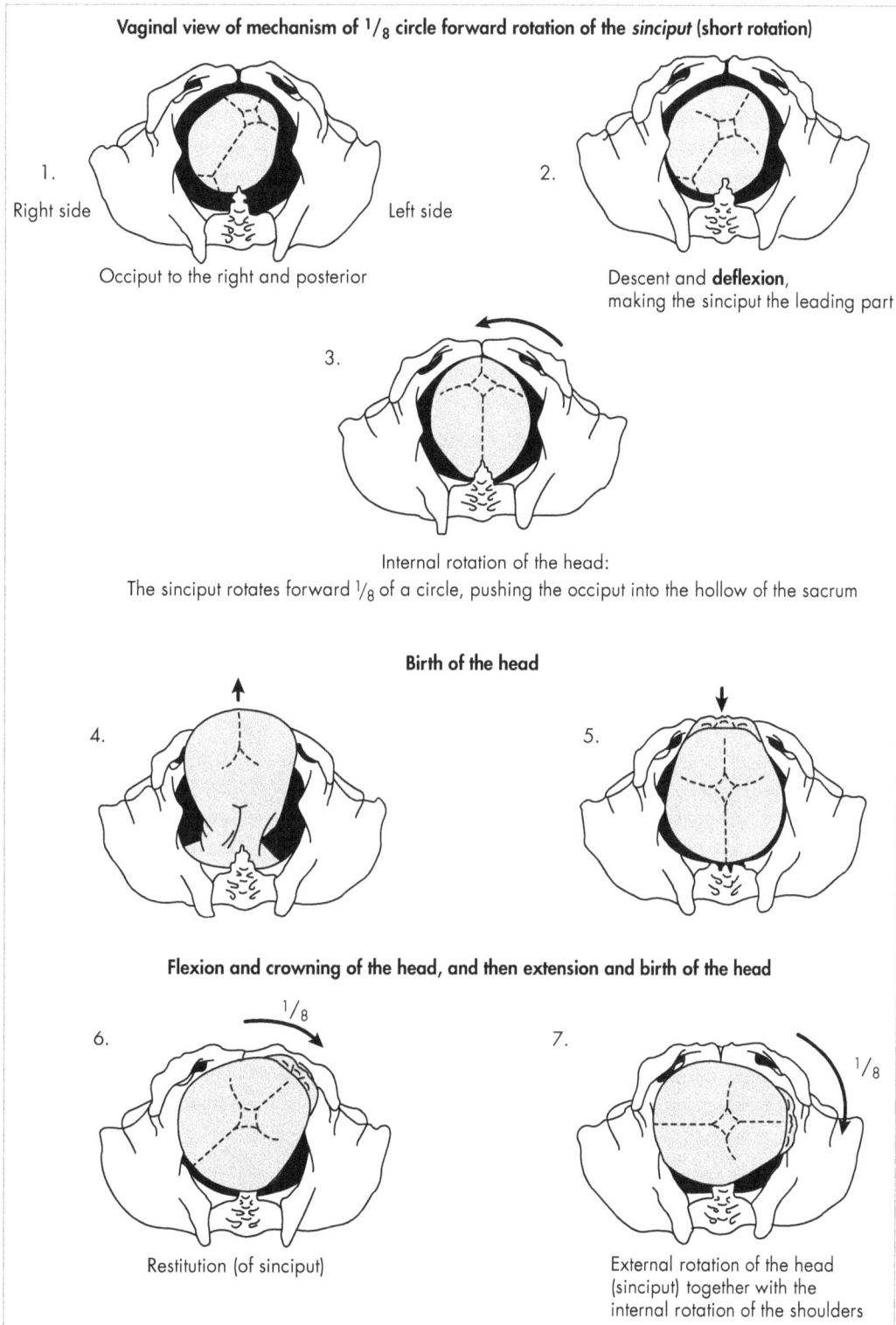

Figure 30.9 Mechanism of POP positions – right POP, short rotation

The mechanism

This section contains a typical explanation of an ROP. The reverse would apply for an LOP. Short and long rotation of the head can occur. These are explained together.

Abdominal palpation

The following are found in ROP on abdominal palpation:

▶ *Lie.* The lie is longitudinal, (vertical) parallel to the long axis of the mother, which is the maternal spinal column. The fetal back is in the right maternal flank and the small parts are anterior left or felt over the abdomen.

▶ *Fetal heart.* The fetal heartbeat is heard in the right maternal flank or over the umbilicus.

▶ *Attitude.* The attitude is flexion, which means that all the parts of the fetus are flexed and the chin is on the chest. (In OP there is a degree of deflexion.)

▶ *Position.* The occiput of the fetus points to the right sacroiliac joint and the sinciput to the left iliopectineal eminence.

▶ *Presentation.* The presentation is cephalic. The left parietal bone is right anterior in the mother.

▶ *The relationship of the denominator to the bony pelvis.* Theoretically, the occiput is in the right posterior part of the maternal pelvis and the anterior fontanelle (bregma) is anterior left near the symphysis pubis.

▶ *Presenting diameters.* The occipital frontal (11.5 cm) and the BPD (9.5 cm) are the presenting diameters. This is not a round circle and the larger diameters complicate birth.

Mechanism

The mechanism of the OP position is complicated, as shown in Figure 30.10. One of two pathways (long or short rotation) can be followed, as explained in the following steps:

1. *Descent.* This takes place with increased flexion, when the occiput reaches the pelvic floor. There is increased flexion of the head (the chin is on the chest).

2. *Internal rotation.* The pelvic floor facilitates internal rotation. One of two pathways can be followed:
   ▶ *Short rotation.* The occiput rotates through 45 degrees to the posterior to face the pubis or POP in 10 per cent of cases. The occiput is in the hollow of the sacrum. The face is under the symphysis pubis and the sagittal suture line is in the AP position. The head may still be at the ischial spines but is in the right position for birth.
   ▶ *Long rotation.* In 90 per cent of cases, mostly in multigravidae with large pelvises, the fetus may take a long rotation. This occurs mainly in the second

stage and the rotation can be seen when the head is crowning. The occiput turns 135 degrees from the OP to the occiput-transverse (OT) to the OA to the AP position, ready for delivery. The occiput thus turns from the posterior position to the anterior position and birth is normal. The anterior fontanelle is now posterior in the hollow of the sacrum and the posterior fontanelle anterior under the symphysis pubis with the sagittal suture line in the AP position.

3. *Descent and internal rotation of the shoulders:*
   ▶ *Short rotation.* The shoulder follows the head. The anterior shoulder enters the pelvis in the oblique and meets the pelvic floor. It rotates and follows the head. The shoulders should be in the AP position for delivery.
   ▶ *Long rotation.* This follows the normal mechanism.

4. The position of the fontanelles and suture lines:
   ▶ *Short rotation.* After the short rotation, the anterior fontanelle is anterior under the symphysis pubis and the face is under the symphysis pubis with the smaller diameter of the sinciput, and the posterior fontanelle is posterior in the hollow of the sacrum with the broader diameter of the occiput. The sagittal suture line is in the AP position for delivery.
   ▶ *Long rotation.* In the long rotation, the anterior fontanelle is posterior in the hollow of the sacrum and the posterior fontanelle is anterior. The sagittal suture line is in the AP position for labour.

5. *Crowning:*
   ▶ *Short rotation.* Crowning occurs when the larger diameter sweeps the pelvic floor and the perineum bulges with the head in flexion. The back is against the sacrum and birth is difficult, painful and slow. There is a high risk for perineal trauma.
   ▶ *Long rotation.* Crowning is normal and the birth is normal.

6. *Extension:*
   ▶ *Short rotation.* The head is born with extension, with the face under the pubis.
   ▶ *Long rotation.* The head is born with extension, with the face posterior.

7. *Restitution.* The head turns back on the shoulders to align with the previous position in both positions.

8. *Internal rotation of the shoulders and external rotation of the head.* These processes occur simultaneously. The shoulder reaches the pelvic floor and turns into the AP position with the back to the right.

Vaginal view of mechanism of $^3/_8$ circle rotation forward of occiput (long rotation)

1.

Right side   Left side

Occiput to the right and posterior

2.

Descent and increased **flexion**

3. $^1/_8$

4. $^1/_8$

5. $^1/_8$

Internal rotation of the head:
The occiput rotates $^3/_8$ of a circle forward until occiput is in an anterior position
(Simultaneously the shoulders rotate $^2/_8$ of a circle)

Birth of the head

6.

Extension after crowning of the head

7. $^1/_8$

Restitution (of sinciput)

8. $^1/_8$

External rotation of the head (occiput)
(Together with internal rotation of the shoulders)

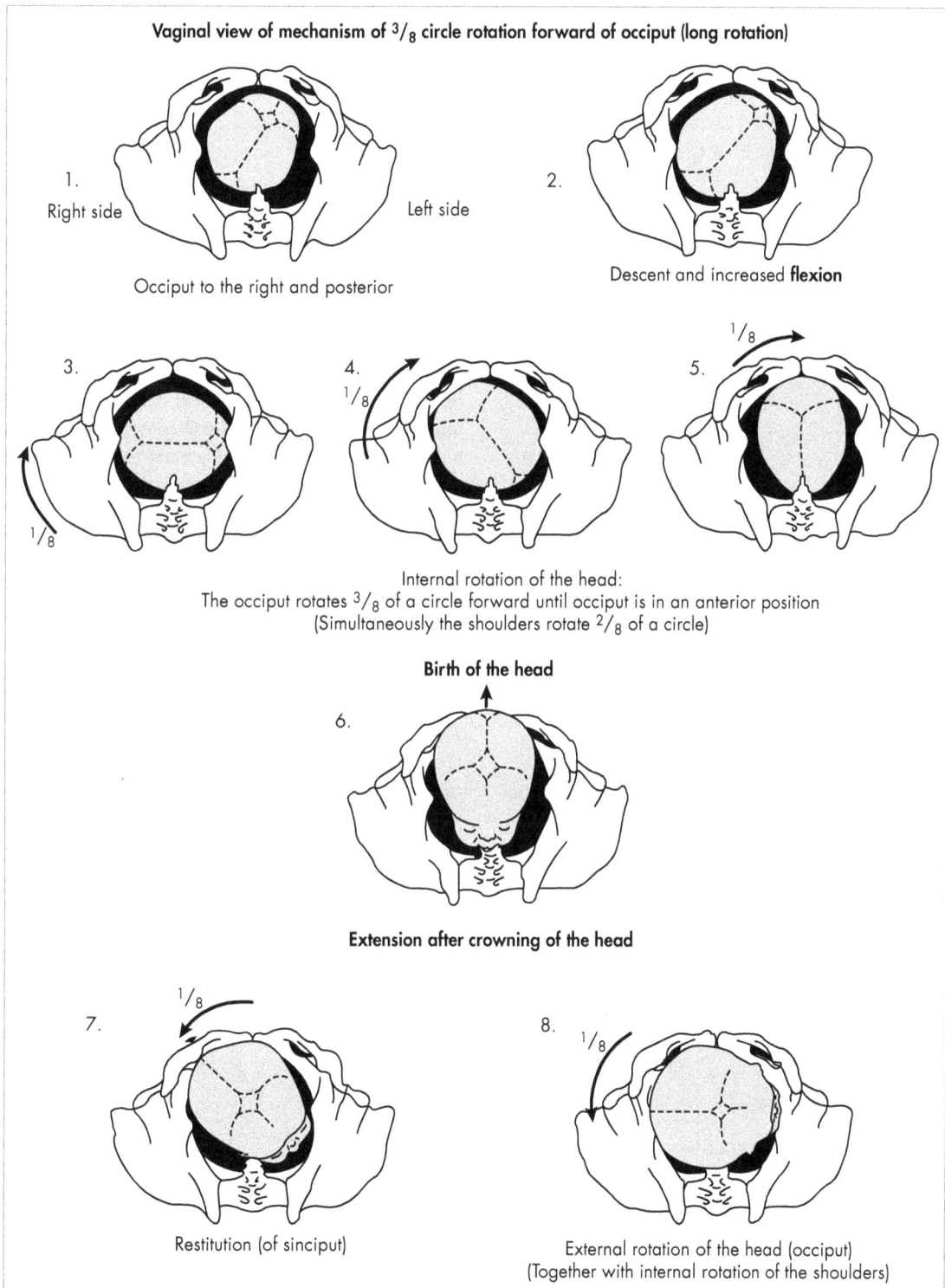

Figure 30.10 Mechanism of OP positions: ROP, long rotation

465

9. *External rotation aligns the head with the body:*
   ▶ *Short rotation.* The posterior fontanelle is now right and the anterior fontanelle left, with the sagittal suture line in the transverse position.
   ▶ *Long rotation.* The posterior fontanelle rotates right and the anterior fontanelle is left with the sagittal suture line in the oblique.
10. *Birth of the shoulders.* The anterior shoulder is born under the symphysis pubis and the posterior shoulder follows.
11. *Birth of the body.* The body is then delivered in lateral flexion over the maternal abdomen.

Self-assessment activity

Use a doll and a model of a pelvis to understand the mechanism of an OP labour.

Diagnosis

The identification of an OP position can already be made in the antenatal period at 36 weeks, when the presenting part engages in a primigravida and sure signs of OP are observable on abdominal palpation.

On admission for labour, an abdominal palpation can reveal the position of the fetus (see Figure 30.11):
▶ The shape is ovoid.
▶ There is a saucer-like indent over the umbilicus (make sure the bladder is empty).
▶ The fetal back is towards the mother's back.
▶ Small parts are felt on both sides of the abdominal midline.
▶ The fetal heart can be heard on the umbilicus.
▶ The fetal head may be difficult to palpate because the sinciput is under the symphysis and the broader occiput is in the sacrum.

The diagnosis of OP position may be difficult. Ultrasound is therefore needed.

The effects in labour

Owing to the poor application of the presenting part on the cervix, the following must be noted:
▶ The cervix may be long and posterior (not ripe).
▶ The contractions are poor and may be irregular.
▶ Membranes may rupture before the onset of labour.
▶ The presenting part may be above the spines and poorly applied on the cervix.

Management

Once an OP presentation is diagnosed, the midwife should be aware of the situation. In most cases, labour will take a bit longer but no complications will arise. In some cases, there is a risk of assisted delivery or Caesarean section. In some cases, the woman will need to be transferred for appropriate medical care. Remember to always refer early.

The partogram is used to observe the progress of labour. Application of the presenting part is usually poor and unequal. An anterior rim or a lateral rim refers to a partial dilatation where the cervix under the broader occiput dilates and the part near the sinciput remains undilated.

The position of the woman is crucial in the rotation of the presenting part. In the exaggerated lateral position (see Figure 28.3 on page 435) the woman lies on the side where the fetal back is, with the lower leg straightened and the upper leg flexed, almost lying on her stomach. This opens the pelvis and pushes the presenting part down, facilitating rotation. Alternatively, the cowboy position (over a chair with open legs, as shown in Figure 30.12) can help to promote descent, flexion and rotation.

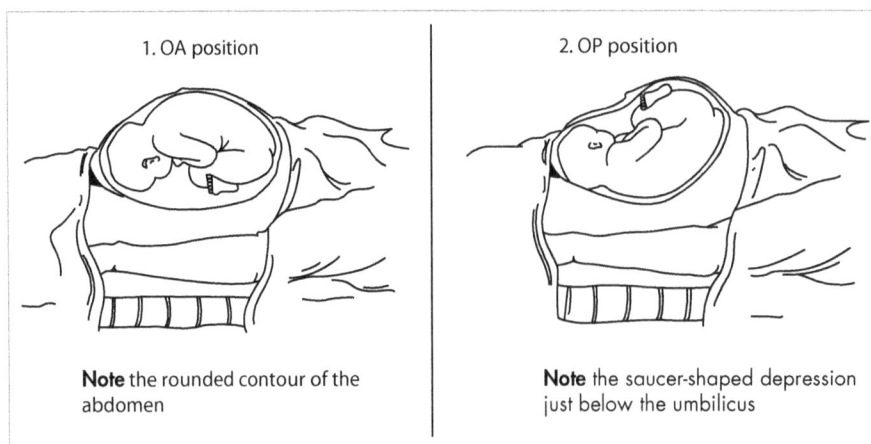

Figure 30.11 The shape of the abdomen contour on inspection

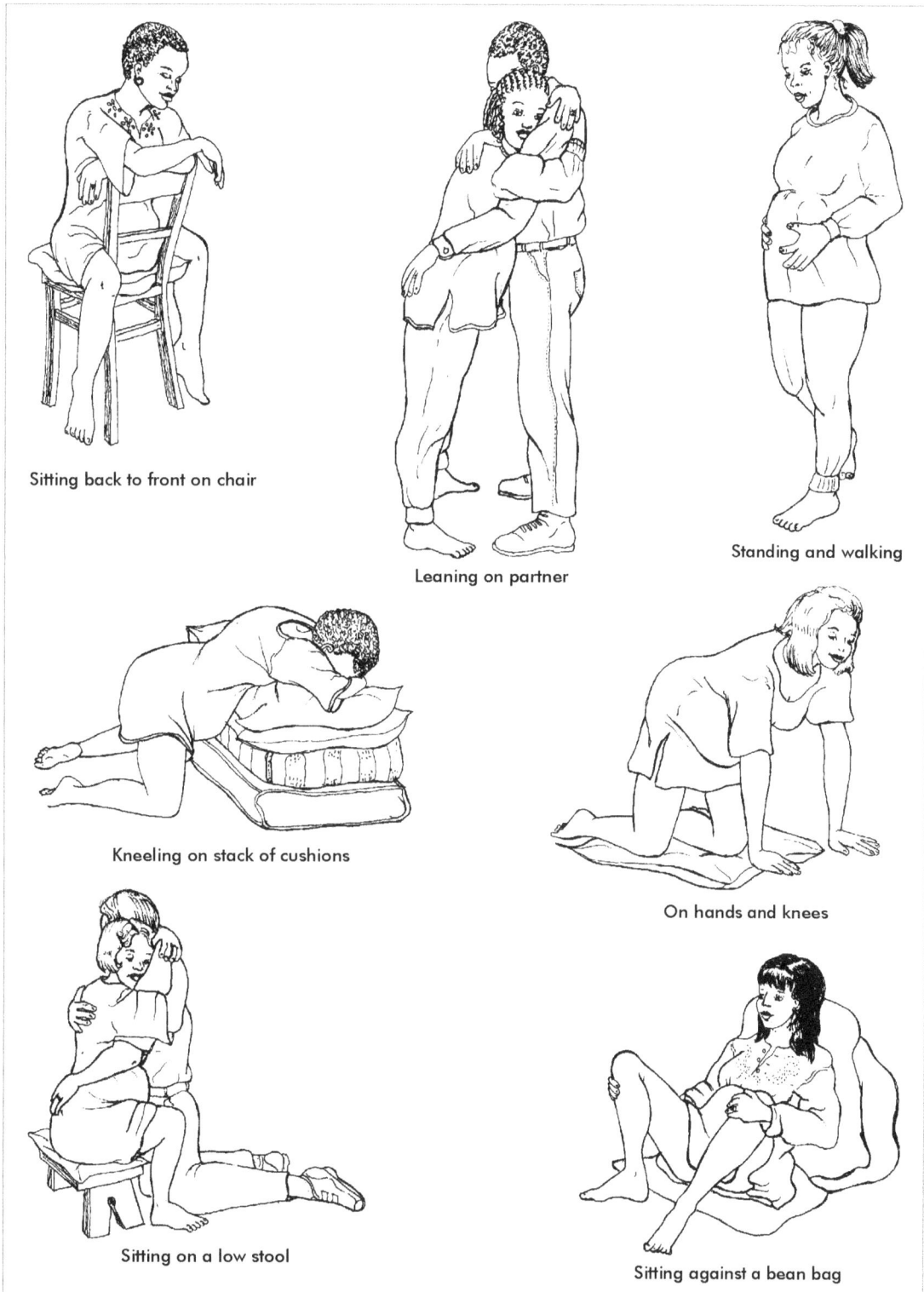

Sitting back to front on chair

Leaning on partner

Standing and walking

Kneeling on stack of cushions

On hands and knees

Sitting on a low stool

Sitting against a bean bag

Figure 30.12 Effective maternal positions during the first stage of labour

467

Medical intervention may include augmentation of labour with oxytocin. Good pain management is needed. Women with OP positions have constant pain in the back, where the fetal head is resting on the sacrum. An epidural is the pain management of choice, if available, for long and painful labour (which causes maternal exhaustion).

Dehydration is common. Once ketones are present in the urine it is difficult to reverse, so this should be prevented by starting a prophylactic IV infusion using 5 per cent dextrose in saline at 125 ml/hr.

Prolonged labour and maternal exhaustion affect the fetus. Observations of the fetus include continuous monitoring of fetal heart rate (FHR) patterns, caput and moulding and descent of the fetal presenting part. If the fetus shows signs of distress in the first stage, the second stage will be even more traumatic.

Once the membranes are ruptured, check for meconium and cord prolapse. In an OP position the membranes are kept intact as long as possible to facilitate even pressure on the cervix.

The second stage is usually not complicated, but can result in an assisted delivery and/or a Caesarean section. A large episiotomy or pelvic floor trauma is common. Neonatal asphyxia or a low Apgar score are common because of the long second stage.

30.4   Breech presentation

The breech presentation is a malpresentation that can deliver vaginally. Breech presentation can present unexpectedly and the midwife should be able to deliver the baby if medical help is not available.

Definition

In a breech presentation, the presenting part in the pelvic brim is the breech (see Figure 30.1 on page 454).

Incidence

At 32 weeks, 7–15 per cent of fetuses are in a breech presentation, which means that the incidence of breech birth is higher in preterm birth. At the start of term labour, only 3–4 per cent of fetuses are still in the breech position (Fischer, 2016).

Classification of breech presentation

The classification of a breech presentation refers to the level of deflexion of the fetal body, as shown in Figure 30.13:

▶ *A complete breech* is fully flexed and is an uncomplicated breech. A midwife can deliver an uncomplicated breech.

▶ *A frank breech* has extended legs, where the legs are extended (deflexed) at the knees. The legs are like splints and prevent the body from flexing in labour. The person delivering the fetus attempts to flex the legs at the knees during labour.

▶ In a *footling breech*, the deflexion is at the hip joint and at the knee of one of the legs, while the other is fully flexed.

▶ In a *kneeling breech*, both legs are flexed at the hip joints.

▶ When the *arms or head are extended*, a skilled practitioner is needed for a safe delivery. The extended arms and head are often complications of a podalic version and a breech extraction (see Figure 30.17 on page 476).

(Note: The more deflexion there is, the more complicated the delivery will be.)

Causes of breech presentation

Prematurity is the main cause. Other causes include:

▶ a short cord
▶ a cord around the neck
▶ placenta praevia
▶ maternal pelvis shape and size
▶ a tight uterus (in a primigravida) that does not allow the fetus to turn after 35 weeks
▶ oligo- or polyhydramnios
▶ fetal abnormalities: anencephaly and hydrocephaly and others
▶ multiple pregnancy
▶ uterine tumour and abnormalities (bicornuate uterus).

Possible outcomes

The outcome in a breech presentation can depend upon one or more of the following factors:

▶ The attitude of the fetus (type of breech presentation)
▶ Whether the legs are flexed or extended
▶ Whether the arms are flexed or extended
▶ Whether the head is flexed, deflexed or extended
▶ The size and shape of the pelvis
▶ The size of the fetus, and particularly the size or diameters of the after-coming head.

Flexed legs usually deliver spontaneously. Extended legs will usually require expert handling in order to be delivered. Once the body is delivered, however, the greatest problem may arise in the delivery of the head. As the larger diameters of the bony vault will come out last, the head may not be able to negotiate the pelvis and there is less time to allow the moulding process to occur. This may be due either to the large size of the head or to a deflexed or partly extended head with large diameters trying to pass through the pelvis.

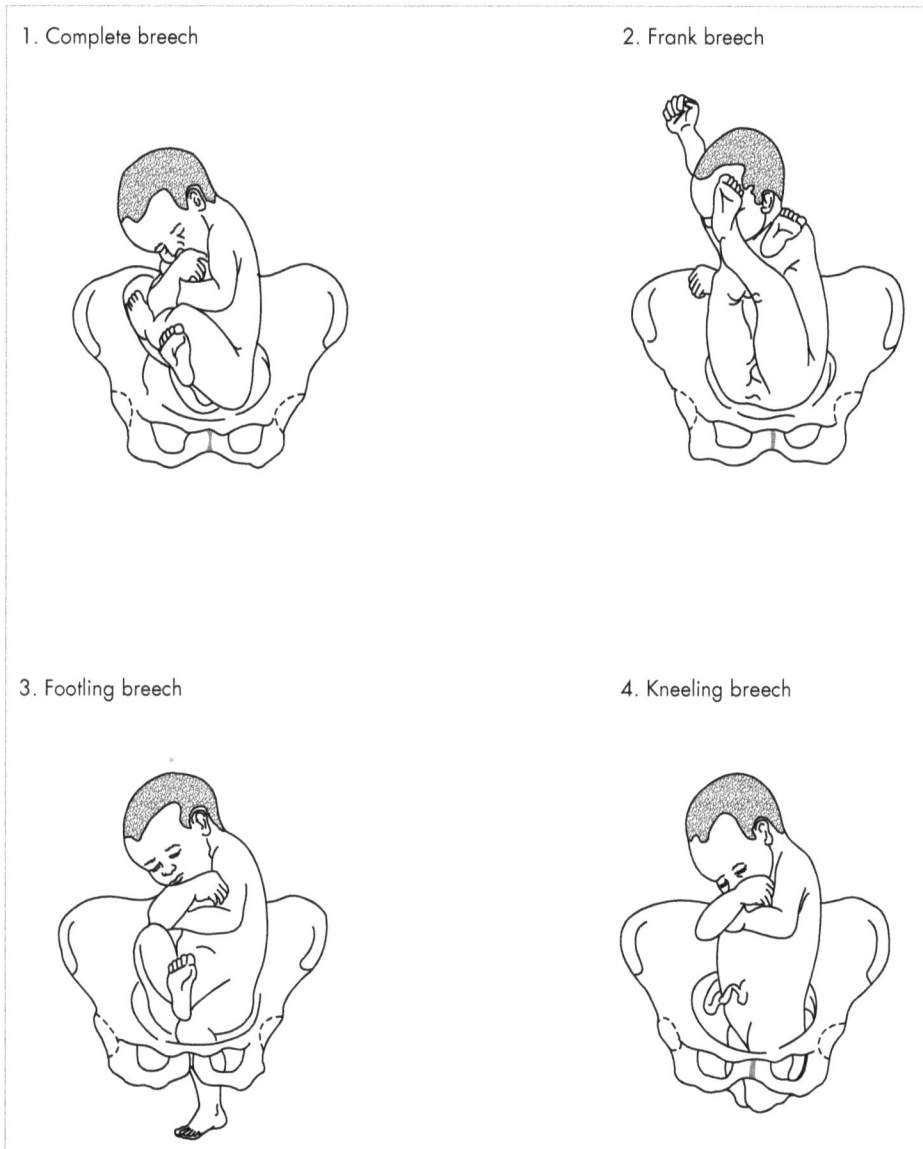

1. Complete breech

2. Frank breech

3. Footling breech

4. Kneeling breech

Figure 30.13 Types of breech presentation

In addition, if an arm or arms is/are extended, this can further decrease the area of the pelvic cavity available for the head.

In some instances, for example in a frank breech or a footling presentation, the body or the leg may slip through a partially dilated cervix, which could prevent larger diameters such as those of the head from being delivered. This will result in an obstructed labour. In a breech delivery, the head has to be delivered within seven minutes of the body if the fetus is not to become anoxic.

In preterm babies, which are more likely to be breech presentations than term babies, the head is larger in relation to the body than in the term baby. This will increase the danger of obstruction and anoxia if the body should slip through a partially dilated cervix.

In some instances, just before or even during labour, before the membranes rupture, a breech presentation may turn spontaneously and present as a cephalic presentation, surprising everyone.

Assessment for vaginal birth

The Zatuchni-Andros index, shown in Table 30.4, is used to screen women for suitability for vaginal birth.

Table 30.4

The Zatuchni-Andros score index (Schwartz, 1975)

Parameter	Score 0	Score 1	Score 2
Parity	0	1	2 >
Gestational age (GA) in weeks	39+	38	< 37
Previous vaginal birth	0	1	2
Estimated fetal weight	> 4	3.5–4	< 3.5
Cervical: 2 cm	2	3	4 >
Station of presenting part	−3	−2	−1
Score 0–4	Caesarean section		
> 5	Allow breech delivery		

The mechanism of an uncomplicated breech delivery

An uncomplicated breech refers to a fetus in full flexion. This section will examine the mechanism of an uncomplicated breech delivery in a right sacroanterior (RSA) position. The opposite principles will apply to a left sacroanterior (LSA) position. The standard mechanism is followed, as shown in Figure 30.14.

Abdominal findings

The following will be found on abdominal palpation in an RSA position:

▶ *Lie.* The lie is longitudinal podalic. The back is felt on the right side anteriorly and the small parts are on the left posteriorly. The shape of the abdomen is more ovoid and looks full in the fundus (where the head is). Two poles are identified (if the breech is not engaged). The head can be distinguished because it is hard and round and ballotted when moved (without the body moving). The fundus may be fuller and higher than expected for the birth.

▶ *Fetal heart.* The fetal heart is heard right above the umbilical line through the posterior thorax wall of the fetus.

▶ *Attitude.* The attitude is full flexion.

▶ *Position.* The sacrum is turned to the right iliopectineal line of the maternal pelvis.

▶ *Presentation.* The presentation is a breech and will be the anterior (right) buttock.

▶ *The relationship of the denominator to the bony pelvis.* The sacrum lies adjacent to the right iliopectineal eminence, thus making it an RSA position. The bitrochanteric diameter will lie in the right oblique diameter of the pelvis. The natal cleft will therefore be in the left oblique diameter of the pelvis.

▶ *Presenting diameters.* The presenting diameters of the breech is the bitrochanteric diameter (between the femur joints), which is 10 cm in the term fetus.

Mechanism

The mechanism of an uncomplicated breech, as shown in Figure 30.14, is as follows:

1. *Descent.* In a breech presentation, the anterior buttock will reach the pelvic floor first, with the anterior hip near the symphysis pubis and the posterior hip posterior in the sacrum in an oblique position. The anterior buttock becomes the leading part.

2. *Internal rotation.* The breech will rotate forward by 45 degrees for the anterior hip to lie under the symphysis pubis, pushing the posterior buttock into the hollow of the sacrum. The largest diameter of the breech is the bitrochanteric diameter of 10 cm (between the hip joints).

3. *Position.* The bitrochanteric diameter will now lie in the AP diameter of the pelvic outlet, with the anterior hip under the symphysis pubis and the posterior hip in the hollow of the maternal sacrum. The fetal sacrum is in the right sacrolateral (RSL) position with the flexed legs on the left side. The genitals of a male fetus can guide the midwife or medical practitioner during vaginal examination on the position of the fetus. In the female infant, the genital parts may be confused with a face presentation.

4. *Second stage.* When fully dilated, the mother can bear down. The breech is easier to deliver than the head and, particularly in a preterm birth, can pass through a poorly dilated cervix. However, the after-coming head may then become stuck. The mother should therefore not bear down before full dilatation.

5. *Birth of the buttocks.* The anterior buttock escapes easily under the pubic arch (in the AP position). The buttock crowns, stretching the perineum. The breech is delivered in lateral flexion. The sacrum is directed towards the mother's right thigh. The rule of care is: 'Hands off'. The body is allowed to be delivered spontaneously and may be supported by the midwife. The legs are free and are allowed to deliver by themselves.

Onset of labour

1. Right side   Left side

Vaginal view

2.

Lateral view

Descent and internal rotation of the buttocks

3. 1/8

x

Vaginal view

4.

Lateral view

Birth of buttocks by lateral flexion

5.   6.   7.

Breech is 'crowned'   Posterior buttock is born   Both buttocks and legs are born

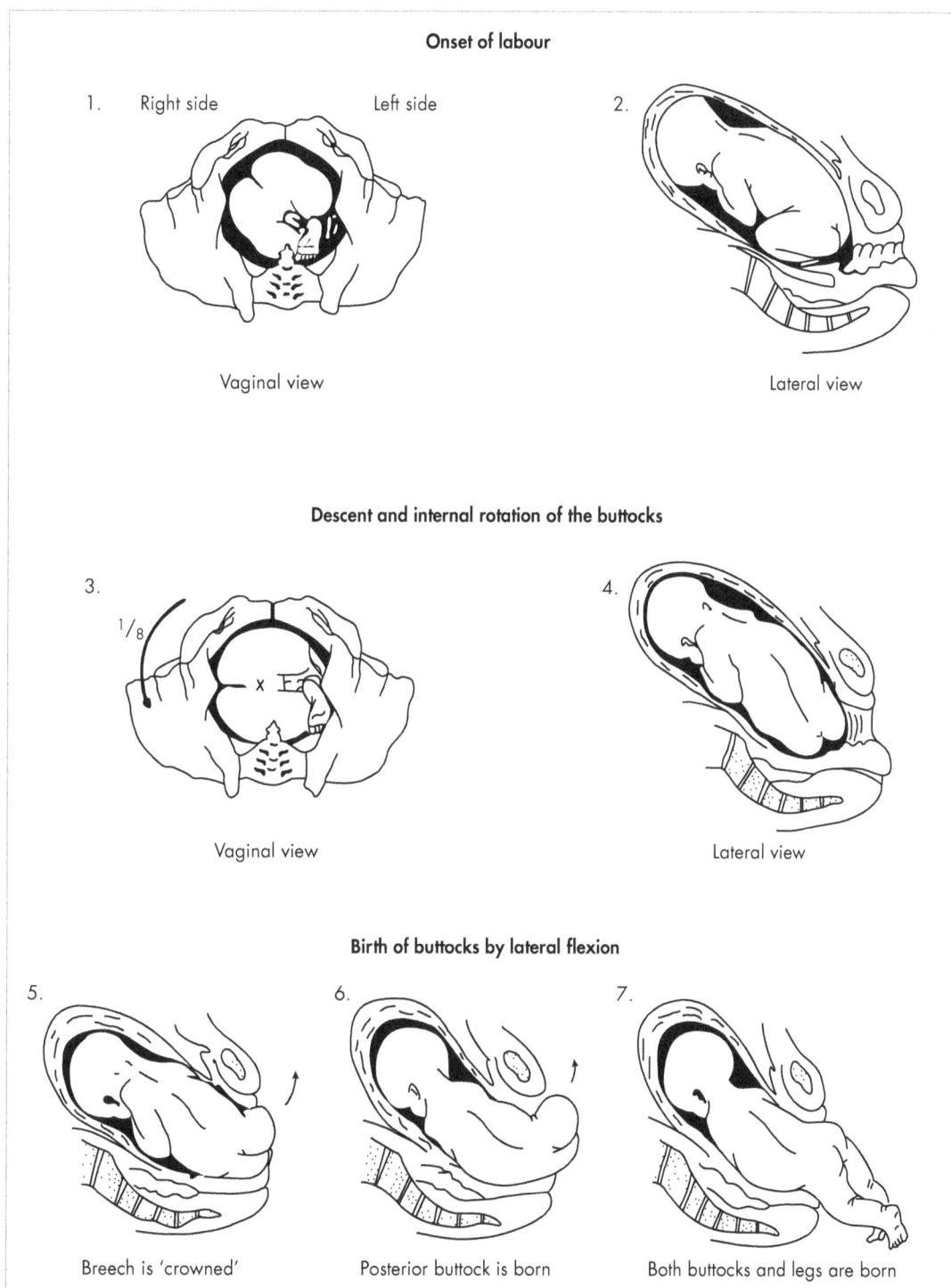

Figure 30.14 Mechanism of an uncomplicated breech

continued

Birth of the shoulders by lateral flexion

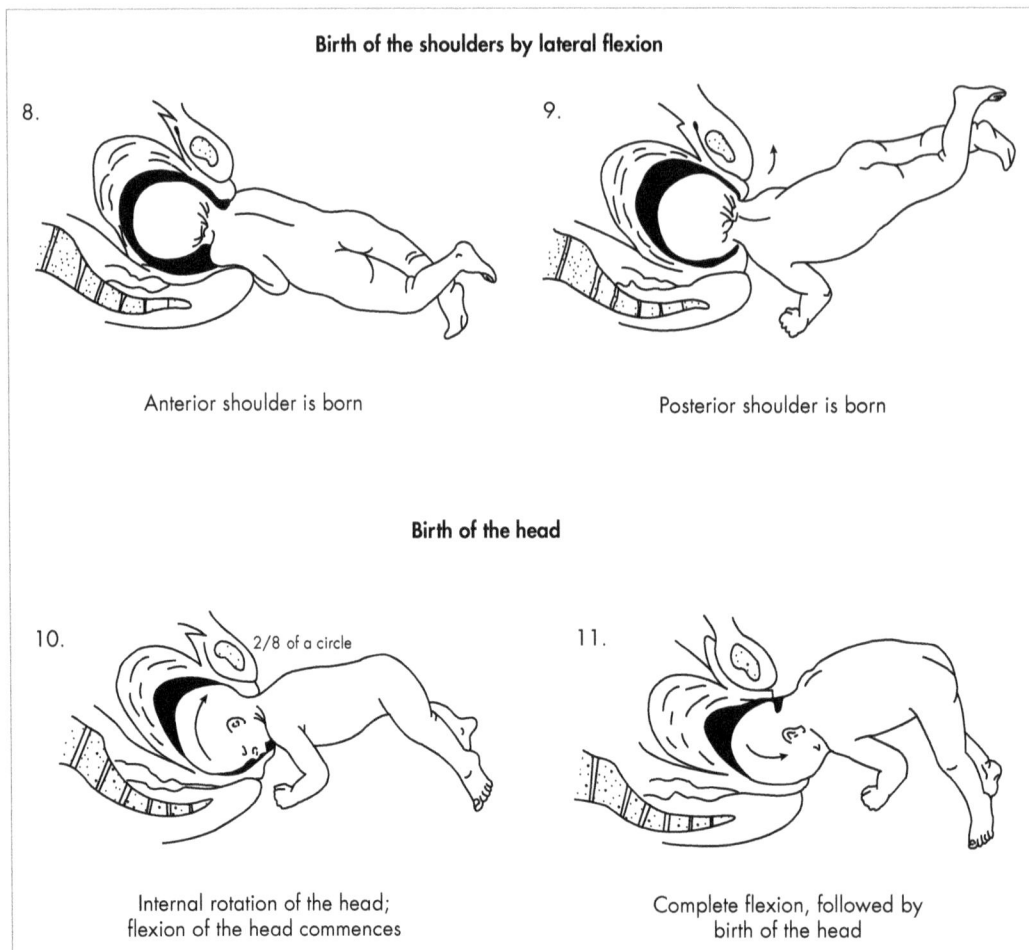

8.

Anterior shoulder is born

9.

Posterior shoulder is born

Birth of the head

10. 2/8 of a circle

Internal rotation of the head;
flexion of the head commences

11.

Complete flexion, followed by
birth of the head

Figure 30.14 Mechanism of an uncomplicated breech

6. *Loop of cord.* When the fetal abdomen is revealed at the umbilicus, a loop of umbilical cord is pulled down gently with the fingers to allow for the after-coming head. ·

7. *Restitution.* Restitution takes place in order to undo the twist in the body of the fetus. The anterior buttock rotates back 45 degrees to align with the head. The fetal shoulder and head enters the pelvis as the body is born.

8. *Internal rotation of the shoulders.* The shoulders (the biacromial diameter) also enter the pelvis in the oblique diameter. The anterior shoulder meets the pelvic floor first, rotates forward 45 degrees and comes to lie under the lower border of the symphysis pubis with the posterior shoulder in the hollow of the sacrum. (The biacromial diameter of the shoulders lies in the AP position of the pelvis.)

9. *Birth of the shoulders.* The anterior shoulder escapes under the pubic arch and then, with a movement of lateral

flexion, the posterior shoulder sweeps past the perineum and the shoulders are born. The rule is still: *'Hands off'*.

10. *Descent of the head.* The head enters the pelvis in flexion, with the sagittal suture in the transverse or oblique diameter of the pelvis. The occiput is in the right of the pelvis. The posterior fontanelle is right anterior, the anterior fontanelle is left posterior and the sagittal suture line is left oblique.

11. *Internal rotation of the head and external rotation of the body.* As the occiput reaches the pelvic floor, it rotates anteriorly forward 90 degrees to lie under the symphysis pubis. The suboccipital area of the head is under the symphysis pubis (anterior) and the face is in the sacrum (posterior). The sagittal suture line in the pelvis is in the AP position. The external rotation of the body and the internal rotation of the head are simultaneous processes. The external rotation of the body takes place with the back always turning

anteriorly to lie under the symphysis pubis. The body is now completely delivered and enough cord should be available.

12. *Birth of the head.* The body is delivered and the after-coming head must be delivered within 7–10 minutes. Start counting from the time the head is engaged in the pelvis, as the cord will be compressed from this time. The body is allowed to hang until the posterior hairline is visible. This will improve flexion of the head and allow it to descend. The pulsation of the cord can be monitored.

Methods of delivering the head

There are two methods used to deliver the head: the Burns Marshall manoeuvre and the Maurice Smellie-Veit manoeuvre.

The Burns Marshall manoeuvre

The following are steps to follow to deliver the head using the Burns Marshall manoeuvre:

1. The baby's body is allowed to hang downward, with the head inside the pelvis, for one to two minutes. (The person delivering must keep the hands near the baby's pelvis in case the head is delivered).
2. When the posterior hairline appears under the pubic arch, the baby's feet are firmly grasped in the right hand. The midwife exerts firm pressure downward and then outward and finally uses upward traction to keep the spine straight (in order to prevent damage to the spine and cord). The body is drawn upward over the maternal pubis in an arc of 180 degrees, using the fetal occiput as a pivot. While this is being done, the left hand is used to guard the perineum and to prevent the head from emerging too quickly. The baby's body is held vertically while the vault of the head remains in the vagina.
3. The mouth and the nose are then free from the perineum, the airways are gently cleaned, suctioned and cleared, and the baby can now breathe.
4. The time is noted in order to ascertain how long the delivery has taken from the delivery of the umbilicus.
5. The mother is instructed to continue breathing deeply and the vault of the baby's head is delivered very slowly and carefully over about two to three minutes. The mother pants the head out rather than bearing down. A medical practitioner may apply low forceps at this stage to control delivery of the head.

The Maurice Smellie-Veit manoeuvre

The after-coming head can be delivered slowly by the Maurice Smellie-Veit manoeuvre, as shown in Figure 30.15:

1. Lay the body on the forearm.

2. Put the index finger and middle finger on the ridges below the eye. The other hand is placed on the occiput.
3. The head is controlled and is delivered in a 180 degree circle until the mouth is open.
4. The airways are suctioned and the head slowly delivered as the mother pants the baby out

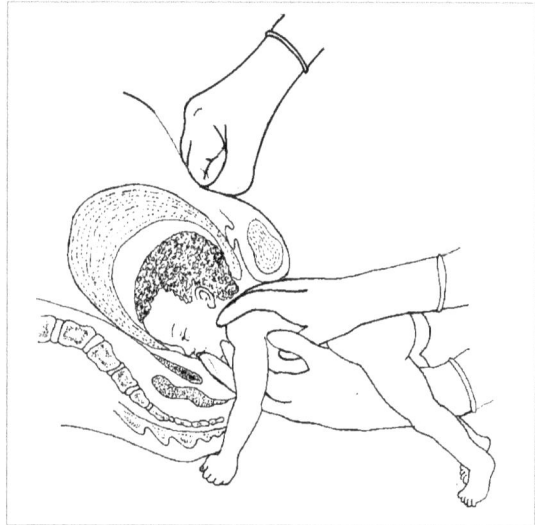

Figure 30.15 The Maurice Smellie-Veit manoeuvre

Treatment and care of a breech presentation

Determine whether the woman can have a vaginal birth using the Zatuchni-Andros score (see Table 30.4 on page 470). Early diagnosis and referral are vital. External version may be performed by a medical practitioner after 37 weeks or in early labour, where ultrasound, a theatre, an anaesthetist and a paediatrician must be available.

When in labour, the membranes are kept intact as long as possible because the cord can prolapse and this keeps even pressure on the cervix (note that the breech does not create good, even pressure on the cervix). If the membranes rupture, a vaginal examination is performed to make sure that the cord has not prolapsed. Avoid premature bearing down before full dilatation.

Analgesia is important. If epidural anaesthesia is available, this is of great value. An anaesthetist and paediatrician are alerted and on standby. An IV infusion may be needed, as labour is slow.

The following principles describe management during the second stage of labour:

▶ Make sure the cervix is fully dilated.
▶ Keep the bladder empty.
▶ Check the fetal heart regularly.

- Do an episiotomy when the breech distends the perineum.
- The hands-off approach is preferred unless there are complications.
- A loop of cord is pulled down when the body is delivered at abdominal level to make sure the cord is long enough.
- The cord is felt for pulsation. If it drops to 100 bpm, time is running out.
- The head must be delivered in 7–10 minutes.
- The head is delivered slowly and in a controlled way.
- A medical practitioner should do the delivery and a paediatrician needs to be present.
- In case of a footling breech or a breech presentation with a neonate of less than 1.5 kg, a Caesarean section should be done.

The potential complications of a breech presentation

There is increased perinatal mortality in both term and preterm babies. In term babies, the mortality rate in breech presentations is three times higher than in cephalic presentations. In the preterm breech presentation, the mortality rate is much higher.

Maternal complications

The midwife needs to be alert to the following during a breech presentation:

- Due to the high and irregular presenting part, the membranes tend to rupture early in labour and much of the liquor drains away. Because of this, there is a greater possibility that the umbilical cord will slip between the legs, resulting in a cord presentation or prolapse. The buttocks, especially in the complete breech, do not usually engage before labour and therefore the presenting part remains high. This is less likely to occur in the frank breech. Prolonged labour and possibly obstructed labour may also occur.
- There may be a prolonged first stage in the complete breech and in the footling or kneeling breech presentation. The frank breech presents a more compact and regular area, which facilitates the dilatation of the cervix. However, although the smaller circumference in the frank breech can pass through a certain cervical diameter, the larger after-coming head may become caught up in the not quite fully dilated cervix, which can obstruct further progress. This condition can also apply in the footling and kneeling breech.
- The second stage can be prolonged due to the complications that can arise with the abnormalities of attitudes (or types) of breech (for example, extended legs,

as shown in figures 30.13 on page 469 and 30.16 on the next page). Obstruction can also occur with the after-coming head if the engaging diameters are too large to pass through the pelvis at the inlet, at the mid-cavity or at the outlet.

- Extension of the arms can be a complication (see Figure 30.17 on page 476).
- The mother may become distressed with the prolonged labour, but there may also be emotional distress because she knows that the delivery is complicated. In addition, any manipulations that may be necessary will cause further distress.
- The woman is inclined to want to bear down early before the cervix is fully dilated, particularly if there is a foot or a knee in the vagina.
- There is a high risk of complications and the perineum can be severely lacerated if there is difficulty with the after-coming head. A large episiotomy is therefore a necessity. Caesarean section is often performed in preference to vaginal delivery in breech presentation. Destructive operations may be necessary if the fetus has died during delivery, usually when the after-coming head has become caught up in the pelvis.
- There is an increased incidence of both traumatic and atonic PPH. There is also a possibility of intrapartum haemorrhage due to a short cord causing premature placental separation. In addition, a loop of cord has to be pulled down when the buttocks are born so that there is no tension on the umbilicus while the head is delivering, which also contributes to the risk of intrapartum haemorrhage.

Fetal complications

The following complications can arise:

- Fetal hypoxia and compromise (distress) could occur. Asphyxia neonatorum, caused by difficulties with, damage to and delay in delivering the fetal head, including the rapid and upward moulding of the after-coming head, can result in hypoxia and asphyxia. In addition, preterm babies have a high incidence of cerebral injury (tentorial tears).
- There may be undiagnosed fetal abnormality present. A breech presentation could very well reflect some underlying fetal abnormality such as hydrocephaly or anencephaly. For this reason, any woman with a breech presentation that is diagnosed during pregnancy should have thorough investigations to detect any fetal abnormality and to find out the attitude of the fetus.
- Birth injuries
- Fractures of the spine, the legs, the arms and the clavicle due to mismanagement or difficulties during delivery

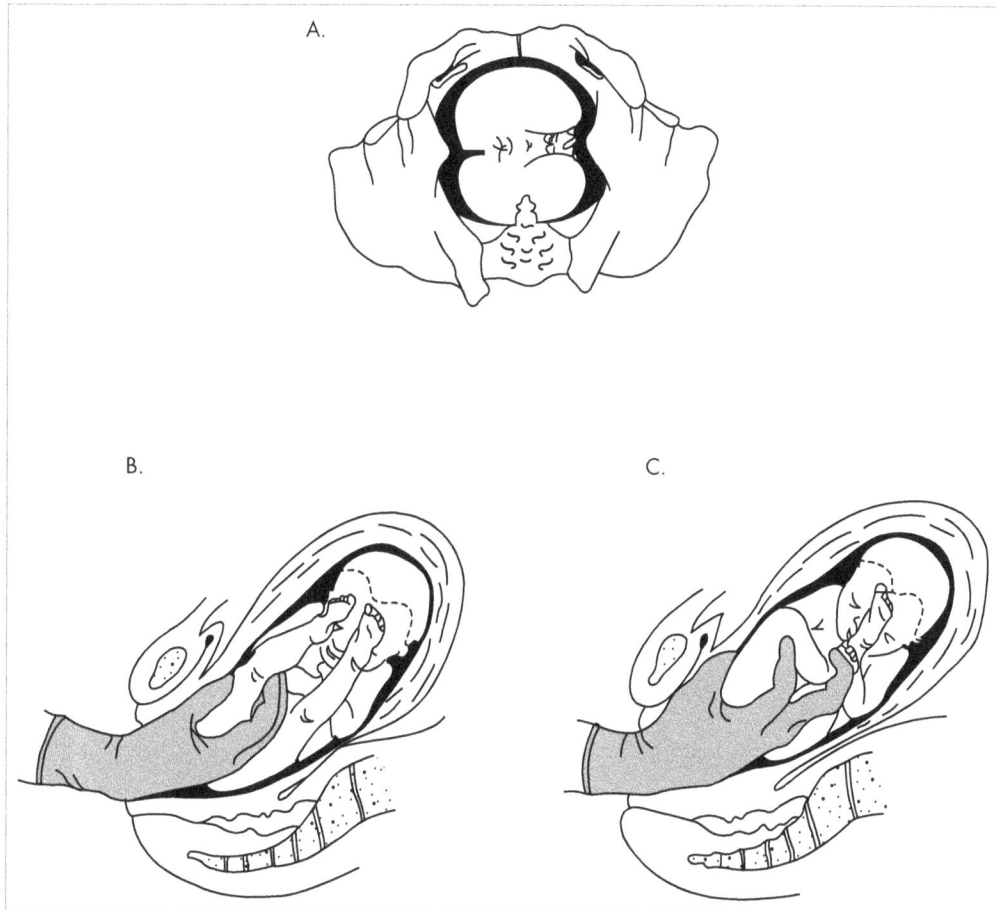

Figure 30.16 Delivery of extended legs

- Damage to the spinal cord, resulting in paralysis below the spinal injury, or the brachial plexus, resulting in the Erb-Duchenne or Klumpke types of paralysis of the arm
- Damage to, or rupture of, abdominal viscera (the liver, spleen or adrenal glands) by incorrect handling of the baby during delivery. This is even more likely in the case of a preterm baby.
- Bruising of the buttocks and the external genitalia
- Cerebral haemorrhage when the after-coming head in a breech presentation is subjected to both rapid and upward moulding (compression and decompression), which may result in intracranial haemorrhage. There is rapid and excessive compression as the head passes through the pelvis, and then there is rapid decompression if the head is allowed to be delivered quickly. Preterm babies have soft skull bones and the contents of the skull are easily damaged.

- Neonatal infection from the early rupture of membranes and from the high rate of intervention.

30.5   Cephalopelvic disproportion

The condition in which the engaging diameters of the fetal head (cephal) are too large to pass through the pelvic canal is called CPD. This means that there is disproportion between the fetal head (the passenger) and the mother's pelvis (the passages), which will affect the course and possibly the eventual outcome of the labour.

Incidence

Mild or severe CPD may be found in 1: 250 pregnancies (APA, 2015).

Extended and nuchal arm

1.

Arm extended above the head

2.

Arm in nuchal position

Løvset's manoeuvre for extended arms
(Nuchal position)

3.

180°

Keeping the back uppermost,
rotate the baby 180°

4.

Using the hand facing the baby's back and
the fingers to splint the humerus, bring the
anterior arm down across the face and chest

5.

180°

Keeping the back uppermost,
rotate the baby 180°

6.

The fingers splint the humerus
to bring the baby's other arm down,
across the face and chest

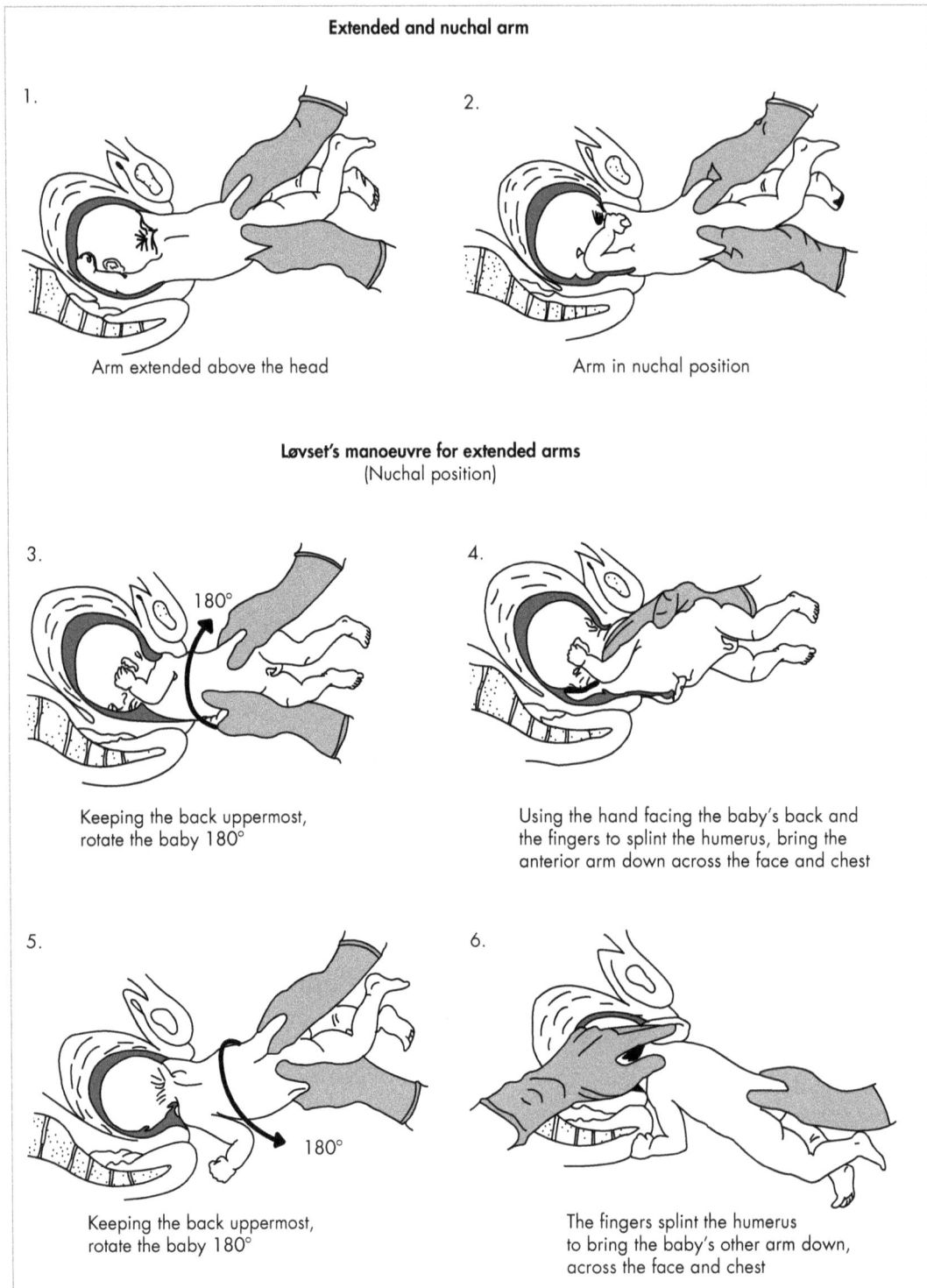

Figure 30.17 Delivery of extended arms (by a skilled midwife or medical practitioner)

Types of disproportion

There are two types of disproportion: relative and absolute.

Relative disproportion

Relative disproportion means that the attitude of the fetal head is not favourable, causing the largest diameters to present at the pelvic inlet. This leads to complications, for example OP brow or face presentations.

Absolute disproportion

Absolute disproportion means that the fetal head itself (in a normal position and attitude) is too large to negotiate the pelvis with ease, or that the pelvis is too small – or both – for example OA position.

Maternal disproportion and its effects

The causes of disproportion can be maternal or fetal. Deviations in the pelvis shape and size are common causes of CPD. One type of disproportion is a contracted pelvis, in which one or more of the average gynaecoid pelvic measurements is diminished by 1 cm or more.

The amount (degree) of disproportion will depend to a large extent upon the type (shape) and size of the pelvis. However, the degree of disproportion can only be assessed after 36 weeks' gestation, when the size of the fetal head has almost reached its maximum. The degree of disproportion may be:
- mild or minor: where a pelvic diameter is 1 cm less than normal
- moderate: where a pelvic diameter is 1–2 cm less than normal
- severe or major: where a pelvic diameter is over 2 cm less than normal.

The disproportion may occur at the inlet (brim), mid-cavity or outlet, or at two or more of these planes. The ischial spines between the mid-cavity and the outlet may cause problems if they are prominent.

Although in most instances the head is the largest part of the fetus and is usually the presenting part, other parts can be so enlarged so as to be bigger than the head and these can cause varying degrees of disproportion. For the sake of convenience, this type of disproportion is also included here. The disproportion may occur on any level of the pelvis: the inlet, mid-pelvis or outlet.

Pelvic inlet contracture

Any of the following factors may cause pelvic inlet contracture or predispose a woman to this condition:
- *Small stature.* CPD is more common in women who are less than 152 cm in height.

- *Type of pelvis (genetic).* Certain types of pelvises, such as android, anthropoid, platypelloid, justominor etc, are more prone to CPD.
- *Abnormalities of the pelvis and pelvic deformity.* This may be due to congenital abnormality (deformities or dwarfism), poor development from malnourishment (rickets), injury (fractures), disease (poliomyelitis), etc. If the woman has any noticeable type of skeletal deformity or a limp, then a deformity of the pelvis should be suspected.
- *Spinal.* CPD can be caused by spinal deformities and injuries (scoliosis, kyphosis, spondylolisthesis, etc).

The effects on the fetus include:
- non-engagement of the head
- an increase in deflexion of the head and malpositions
- an increase in malpresentations
- exaggerated synclitism and asynclitism (see Figure 8.14 on page 136)
- excessive caput succedaneum and other injuries to the skull and scalp
- an increased incidence of umbilical cord prolapse
- an increase in asphyxia neonatorum
- an increase in birth injuries, both intracranial and others
- an increase in the incidence of perinatal death.

The effects on labour include:
- prolonged labour, with slow dilatation of the cervix and descent of the presenting part
- disordered uterine action, particularly secondary inco-ordinate uterine action
- premature rupture of the membranes (PROM)
- increased malpresentations
- spontaneous symphysiotomy
- obstructed labour
- an increase in operative procedures such as forceps delivery, vacuum extraction, symphysiotomy, Caesarean section and destructive operations
- an increase in PPH
- an increase in maternal injuries, trauma to the perineum, the vagina and the uterus
- an increase in maternal infection
- vesicovaginal fistula.

Mid-cavity contracture

The android type of pelvis – with a long, narrow, less curved pelvic canal – is a contracted pelvis. This type of pelvis also predisposes to OP positions. The highest incidence of android pelvises is found among women of European descent. Black women who have suffered nutritional deficiencies in childhood may have justominor or platypelloid pelvises.

The effects on the fetus include:
▶ most of the effects of inlet contracture
▶ moulding
▶ caput formation.

The effects on labour include:
▶ most of the effects of inlet contracture
▶ the prevention or delay of the anterior rotation of the head in OP positions, resulting in POP positions and deep transverse arrest
▶ prolonged labour, which may become obstructed
▶ poor application of the cervix on the fetal head.

Pelvic outlet contracture

The conditions that may cause or lead a woman to be predisposed to pelvic outlet contracture include:
▶ a pelvis in which the distance between the ischial spines is diminished
▶ a pelvis in which the distance between the ischial tuberosities is diminished
▶ a pelvis in which the angle of the subpubic arch is diminished
▶ an immobile coccyx.

The effects on the fetus are:
▶ excessive and abnormal moulding of the fetal skull
▶ excessive caput succedaneum and other injuries to the skull and scalp
▶ an increase in asphyxia neonatorum
▶ an increase in birth injuries, both intracranial and others
▶ an increase in the incidence of perinatal death.

The effects on labour include:
▶ the prevention or delay of the anterior rotation of the head in OP positions, resulting in POP position or deep transverse arrest
▶ a prolonged second stage of labour
▶ an increase in the use of forceps. This may result in bad perineal tears such as third-degree tears, especially if the subpubic arch is narrowed, as the head is then directed backwards into the perineum. To prevent bad tears, large episiotomies are performed.

The soft tissue conditions of the pelvis are as follows:
▶ Anterior obliquity of the uterus (pendulous abdomen)
▶ Placenta praevia
▶ Tumours of the pelvic tissue (hard and soft)
▶ Abnormal uteri, congenital causes or fibroids.

Fetal disproportion

There are several fetal causes which predispose a woman towards CPD, namely abnormalities of growth, congenital abnormalities, abnormal presentations and the inability of the fetal head to mould. The effects of fetal disproportion on labour are varied, depending upon the cause/s, but they are generally much the same as the effects of maternal disproportion.

Abnormalities of growth

A fetal weight of 4.5 kg or more can cause CPD. It can be the result of:
▶ diet and eating habits in the mother
▶ familial tendencies (genetic factors)
▶ multiparity (babies tend to get bigger with each pregnancy)
▶ maternal obesity
▶ maternal diabetes mellitus (macrosomy)
▶ prolonged pregnancy (post-maturity).

Congenital abnormalities

Parts of the baby may be enlarged as a result of:
▶ hydrocephaly
▶ tumours, such as encephalocele
▶ achondroplasia
▶ conjoined twins
▶ ascites, exomphalos, atresia of ureters causing retained urine
▶ maternal diabetes mellitus causing an enlarged shoulder girdle
▶ hydrops fetalis.

Abnormal presentations

In this case the size of the fetal head is within normal limits, but the presenting diameters are large due to:
▶ presentation
▶ attitude (deflexion or extension)
▶ lie (transverse or oblique).

Inability of the fetal head to mould

In the following conditions, little or no moulding is able to take place, causing disproportion:
▶ Face presentation
▶ Post-maturity
▶ Hydrocephaly
▶ Craniostenosis.

Diagnosis, treatment and care

The main objective in the diagnosis of disproportion is to be able to correctly assess the size of the fetal head in relation to the size of the pelvis through which it will have to pass.

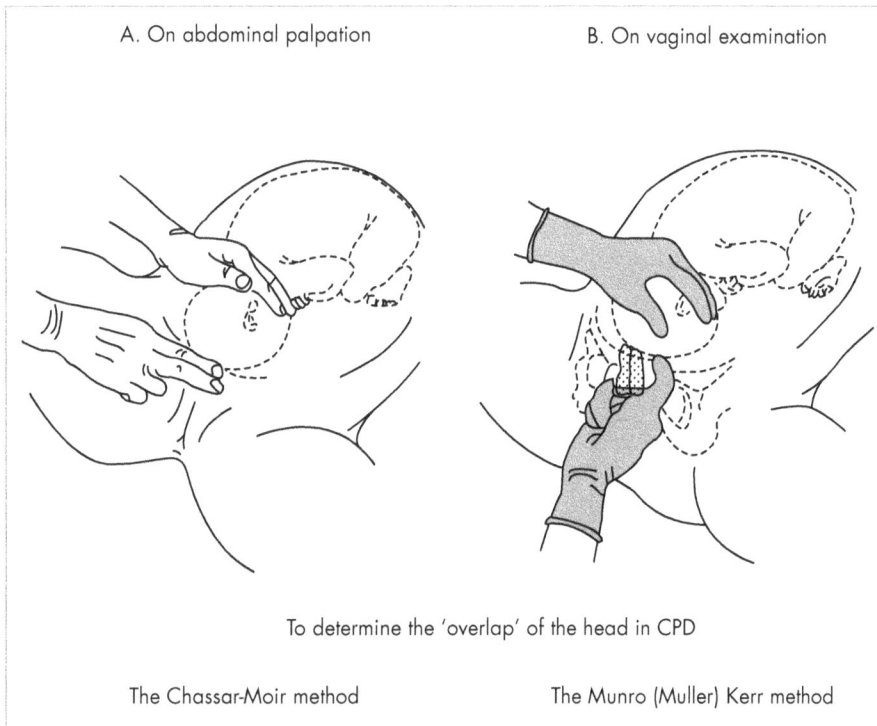

A. On abdominal palpation

B. On vaginal examination

To determine the 'overlap' of the head in CPD

The Chassar-Moir method

The Munro (Muller) Kerr method

Figure 30.18 Methods used to determine the overlap of the head for CPD

High-risk factors

High-risk factors for CPD include:
- a woman with a contracted pelvis but a normal-sized baby
- a woman with a normal-sized pelvis but an excessively large baby
- a woman with both a contracted pelvis and a large baby
- labour where the head may not be able to negotiate the pelvic brim
- labour where the head may negotiate the brim but will have difficulties in the mid-cavity
- labour where the head may negotiate the brim and the mid-cavity, but encounter difficulties at the outlet.

Borderline conditions

It is the borderline conditions that give the most trouble – those where the head may or may not negotiate the brim, the mid-cavity and/or the outlet. Severe CPD is usually diagnosed more readily.

Minor degrees of CPD may be overcome by maternal and fetal conditions. Maternal conditions include:
- efficient uterine action
- the 'give' of the pelvic joints
- the expandability of the soft tissue of the pelvis.

Fetal conditions that may help to overcome minor CPD include:
- a favourable attitude
- a favourable presentation
- a favourable position
- increased flexion of the fetal head during labour in a cephalic or breech presentation
- the ability of the fetal skull to mould. (Note, however, that excessive, upward or rapid moulding can result in intracranial injury and a reduction of 0.5 cm or more in the BPD is considered dangerous to the fetus.)

Clinical assessment

The diagnosis of CPD is usually made by the medical practitioner during labour. Unknown factors, such as prolonged pregnancy, OP positions, malpresentations, disordered uterine action and others may become evident and/or relevant during labour.

There are women who do not attend an antenatal clinic and are not examined by a medical practitioner during pregnancy. The midwife will need to manage these women in labour and know when to refer. All of those women should have a trial of labour.

The methods for diagnosing CPD that the midwife can use are detailed in the subsections that follow.

The history

The best indicator of birth is said to be the baby. If the mother has previously given birth to a baby of a particular size, under normal circumstances she should be able to do so again. However, there may be other factors, such as malposition or malpresentation that were not present before. During history taking, note:

▶ the estimated date of delivery (EDD)
▶ the stature (size) and posture of the woman
▶ if the woman is an elderly primigravida or a grand multipara
▶ if the woman has a contracted pelvis
▶ any history of:
  • skeletal injuries or disorders
  • poliomyelitis or rickets
  • diabetes mellitus
  • previous prolonged labours
  • previous operative procedures
  • large babies
  • birth trauma
  • any of the other predisposing causes of CPD.

Abdominal palpation

Palpation is done to assess:

▶ the feto-pelvic fit
▶ the lie, attitude, presentation and position of the fetus; the bladder must be empty
▶ the size and weight of the fetus
▶ the fifths of the fetal head above the pelvic brim
▶ whether the head is engaged, and if not, whether the head can engage

▶ the amount of 'overlap' (the degree of CPD) if the head cannot engage (see Figure 30.18).

Methods

It is the medical practitioner's responsibility to gauge the amount of disproportion and to decide on the course of action. However, in situations where a medical practitioner is not available and the patient may need to be transferred from a clinic to a hospital, the midwife must be able to diagnose disproportion and recognise the degree.

The following two methods are only valid if performed after 36 weeks, because the fetal head will not have grown sufficiently to provide evidence of CPD prior to this time:

1. *A trial of labour.* In all cases where mild to moderate CPD is suspected, a trial of labour in hospital can be suggested. The medical practitioner and the woman will make a collaborative decision. A trial of labour requires a normal birth within limited time with good progress (recorded on a partogram). Medical assistance is available.
2. *Elective Caesarean section.* The medical practitioner will usually do an elective Caesarean section on women with moderate to severe CPD, or if there is some other abnormal condition as well as CPD.

30.6 Conclusion

The midwife's scope of practice is normal birth. However, it is important that the midwife is able to identify abnormal labour and refer a woman for medical care in time. When a midwife works in collaboration with a medical practitioner, she needs knowledge in order to give effective assistance.

Disorders of uterine function

LEARNING OBJECTIVES
On completion of this chapter, you must be able to:
▶ identify and describe causative factors of dysfunctional uterine contractions
▶ identify and describe preventive measures and interventions of dysfunctional uterine contractions
▶ develop the basic competencies to assist women with dysfunctional uterine function.

KNOWLEDGE ASSUMED TO BE IN PLACE
Knowledge, competency and skill of the basic management of normal birth
The Ps of birth (see Chapter 8)

KEYWORDS
dysfunction • hypotonic • hypertonic • colicky • dystocia

31.1 Introduction

In this chapter, disorders of uterine function will be explained as well as how this results in dysfunctional labour. The prevention, early identification and management of these conditions are discussed. The identification of abnormal uterine function is a basic skill for the midwife. The differential diagnosis to determine the cause is more difficult. Midwives need to be able to identify abnormal uterine function and take appropriate action.

31.2 Normal uterine function

Normal uterine functions (see Figure 31.1) can be felt on palpation of the abdomen. The midwife may feel the contraction before the woman is aware of it, as the woman only feels a contraction when the uterine pressure exceeds 25 mmHg. The difference between being able to manually palpate the contraction and the woman feeling the contraction can be 20 seconds.

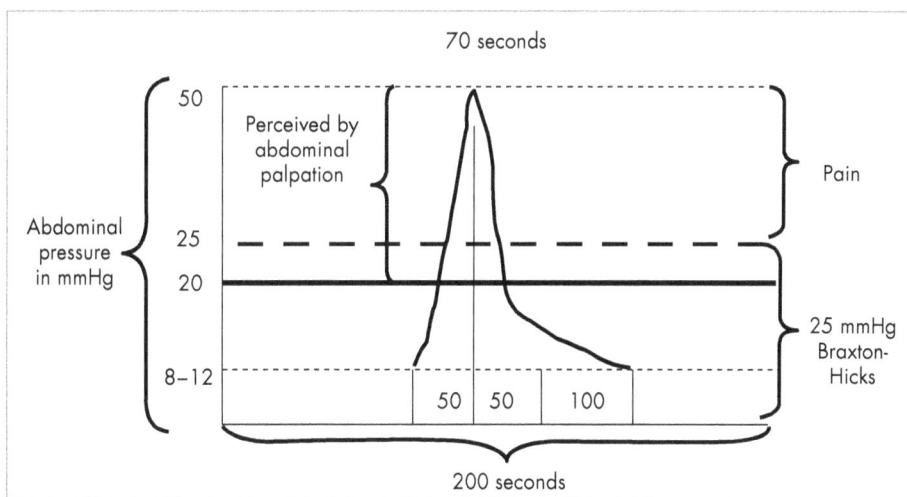

Figure 31.1 Normal uterine contractions

During a normal uterine contraction, the intrauterine pressure, which is called the intensity or amplitude of the contraction, increases. The contraction rises sharply and has a slow decline. The frequency of the contraction is the number of contractions in 10 minutes. Contractions are scientifically measured in Montevideo units (MVU). The formula is: intensity (mmHg) x frequency (per 10 minutes) = uterine activity (see the box on page 408). The mean force should reach 275 MVU.

In clinical practice, three to four contractions of 60 seconds are required for labour. These are measured by abdominal palpation or external cardiotocograph (CTG). The uterine tone needs to go back to the baseline or relax completely between contractions for at least 40 seconds.

If the woman feels a contraction before it is palpated by the midwife, if the contraction does not show on a CTG or if the woman complains of pain after the contraction has subsided, abnormal uterine function is suspected.

31.3   Uterine dysfunction

Disorders of uterine function occur when the uterine contractile pattern deviates from what is considered normal. Abnormal uterine function can manifest as hypotonic uterine function, where contractions are irregular or insufficient, or hypertonic uterine function, where contractions are very strong. The latter may lead to uterine tetany or even uterine rupture.

Incidence

The incidence is 25 per cent (Sarsam, 2014).

Classification

Ineffective uterine action can be classified as:
- hypotonic uterine actions
- inco-ordinate uterine actions:
  - colicky uterus
  - a hyperactive lower uterine segment
- constriction (contraction) ring
- cervical dystocia.

Over-efficient uterine action can be classified as:
- precipitate labour: in the absence of obstruction
- excessive contraction and retraction: in the presence of obstruction.

Causes

Eighty-five per cent of abnormal uterine function is found in primigravidae (Sarsam, 2014). Other causes include:
- mechanical causes such as:
  - minor disproportion (occipitoposterior [OP] positions)
  - cephalopelvic disproportion (CPD)
  - a large infant (those that weigh more than 3 400 g are three times more at risk)
  - a high head (lack of fundal dominance)
  - an overstretched uterus (grand multiparae, polyhydramnios and multiple pregnancy)
  - myomata
  - previous surgery to the uterus
- prolonged pregnancy
- psychological factors (fear increases catecholamine production, eg adrenaline and noradrenaline, resulting in inhibited labour)
- congenital abnormalities of the uterus (bicornuate uterus).

Table 31.1

Abnormal patterns of labour

First stage of labour	Nullipara	Multipara
Abnormal duration	> 24.7 hours	> 18.8 hours
Protracted dilation	< 1.2 cm/hour	< 1.5 cm/hour
Arrest of dilation	> 2 hours	> 2 hours
Second stage of labour		
Arrest of descent (with epidural)	> 3 hours	> 2 hours
Arrest of descent (no epidural)	> 2 hours	> 1 hour

Note: Oxytocin has a half-life of 3–5 minutes and reaches a steady state in approximately 40 minutes.

The partogram (a graphic presentation of labour) is used to detect abnormalities or dysfunctional labour, including:

▶ a prolonged latent phase
▶ a protracted active phase (slowed)
▶ a slowed descent
▶ prolonged deceleration
▶ secondary arrest
▶ arrest of descent (obstructed labour).

The uterus, fetus and pelvis work together in labour. Defects of one may affect the others. If the pelvis is abnormal, the fetal head may remain high, which may prevent the presenting part applying well to the cervix. The poor application of the presenting part delays the ripening of the cervix and the Ferguson reflex.

The uterine contractions may be insufficient and irregular, or the uterus may contract violently to try to overcome the obstruction if present.

Hypotonic uterine function

In hypotonic uterine function (see Figure 31.2), there is poor or no dilatation of the cervix. The weak (slow), short and infrequent uterine contractions cause slow dilation of the cervix, or none.

Aetiology

Various factors may be associated with this condition, such as:
▶ primigravidae
▶ psychological causes such as nervousness, emotional anxiety and fear
▶ anaemia and asthenia

▶ hormonal factors – insufficient prostaglandins or oxytocin with induced labour
▶ the inappropriate use of analgesics
▶ overdistension of the uterus
▶ developmental anomalies of the uterus, such as hypoplasia
▶ myomas of the uterus interfering mechanically with contractions
▶ malpresentations, malpositions and CPD; the presenting part does not fit in the lower uterine segment, leading to absence of reflex uterine contractions
▶ a full bladder and/or rectum.

Types

▶ Primary inco-ordinate uterine function, resulting in weak uterine contractions from the start
▶ Secondary inco-ordinate uterine function: This follows a period of good uterine contractions; an obstruction is encountered which cannot be overcome, causing the uterus to become exhausted

Clinical features

▶ Labour is prolonged.
▶ Uterine contractions are infrequent, weak and short.
▶ Cervical dilatation is slow.
▶ The membranes are usually intact.
▶ The fetus and mother are usually not affected, apart from maternal anxiety due to prolonged labour.
▶ There is greater susceptibility for retained placenta and postpartum haemorrhage (PPH) due to persistent inertia.
▶ Tocography shows infrequent waves of contractions with low amplitude.

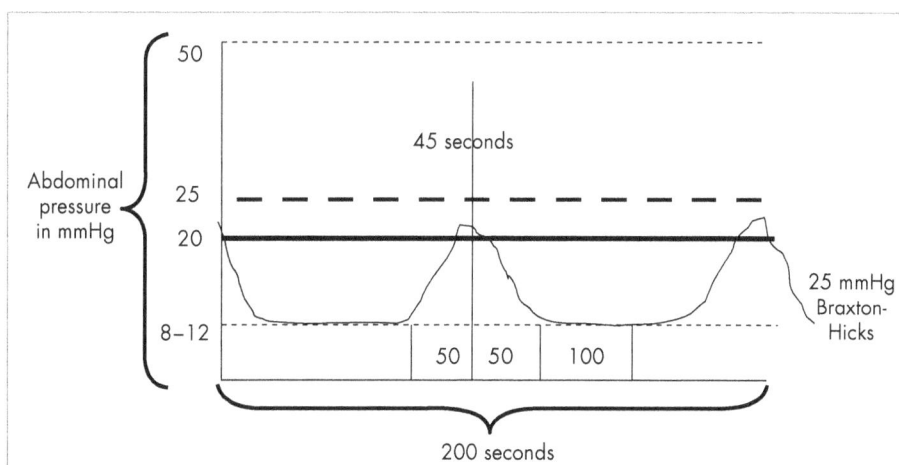

Figure 31.2 Hypotonic contractions

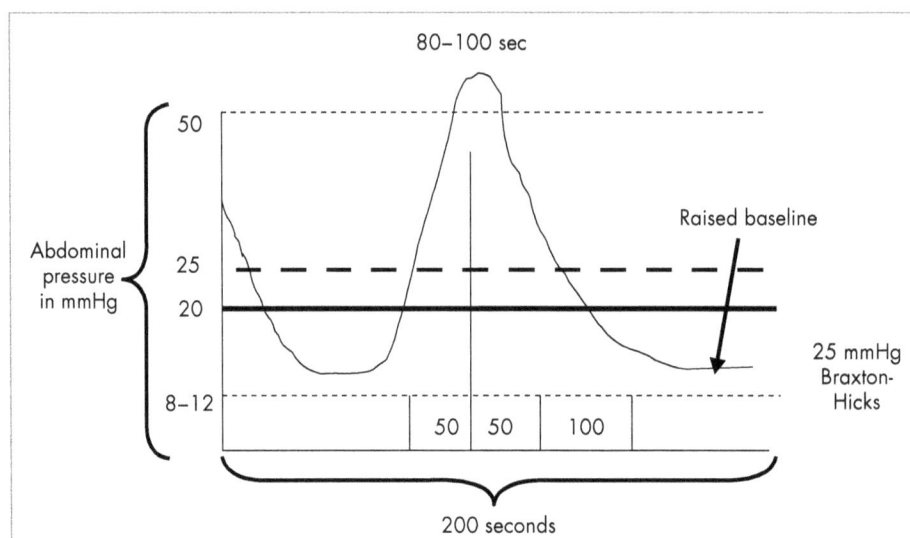

Figure 31.3 Tonic contractions (refer to Section 31.5)

Management

Antenatal preparation for labour, including antenatal classes on relaxation techniques and psychoprophylaxis, is aimed at preventing this condition. Other management aspects include the following:

1. Perform an examination to detect disproportion, malpresentation or malposition; manage according to the case:
   ▶ Ensure proper management of the first stage (see the discussion on normal labour in Chapter 25).
   ▶ If the membranes are ruptured, prophylactic antibiotics are prescribed in prolonged labour.
2. Amniotomy:
   ▶ Amniotomy can be performed if the following three prerequisites are present: Vaginal delivery is possible, the dilatation of the cervix is more than 3 cm and the presenting part is fitted well in the lower uterine segment.
   ▶ Increase the efficiency of poor uterine contractions by augmentation or acceleration of labour.
   ▶ Artificial rupture of membranes (AROM) augments the uterine contractions by the release of prostaglandins.
   ▶ When the presenting part is brought closer to the lower uterine segment, uterine contractions are stimulated.
3. Oxytocin can be used to accelerate labour.
4. Use the partogram and CTG to monitor the condition of the woman and fetus. Abnormalities in the duration of labour can be detected by using the partogram (see Table 31.1 on page 482).

5. An IV line should be *in situ* in case of abnormal uterine function to prevent maternal exhaustion.
   Assisted delivery:
   ▶ Vaginal delivery should be carried out by forceps, vacuum or breech extraction according to the presenting part and its level, provided that the cervix is fully dilated and vaginal delivery is amenable.
   ▶ Caesarean section is indicated when there is failure of the previous methods, contraindications to oxytocin infusion including disproportion, or there is fetal distress before full cervical dilatation.

Hypertonic uterine inertia (unco-ordinated uterine action)

There are two types of hypertonic uterine inertia:
1. *Colicky uterus.* Different parts of the uterus contract independently.
2. *Hyperactive lower uterine segment.* Polarity is lost, resulting in reversed polarity (a hypertonic lower uterine segment and loss of fundal dominance).

Clinical features

The condition is more common in primigravidae and is characterised by:
▶ a prolonged first stage of labour (latent and active phase)
▶ irregular and more painful uterine contractions; the pain is felt before and throughout the contraction, with low abdominal pain and backache often in an OP position

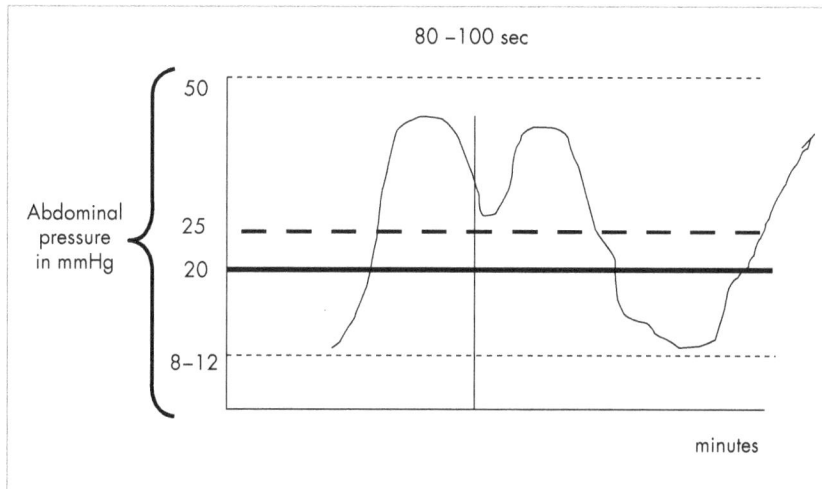

Figure 31.4 Apolarity (coupled contraction)

- a raised resting intrauterine pressure of above 8–12 mmHg (normal value is 5–10 mmHg)
- slow or no cervical dilatation
- premature rupture of membranes (PROM)
- fetal and maternal distress
- CPD or malpresentation
- decreased urine output with ketones in the urine.

Management

- Antenatal preparations for labour should have been put in place.
- Use the partogram to monitor the condition of the woman and fetus; this allows for the early detection of abnormalities.
- Notify the medical practitioner as soon as possible.
- When abnormal uterine function is suspected, place an IV line *in situ* to prevent maternal exhaustion.
- Offer analgesia, particularly epidural analgesia. Usually, labour continues well once the analgesia has taken effect. If an epidural is not possible, the woman may be sedated and given an analgesic such as hydroxyzine and/or pethidine. The woman will require support, encouragement and understanding throughout labour.
- Caesarean section is indicated in the event of:
  - failure of the previous methods
  - disproportion
  - fetal distress before full cervical dilatation.

Constriction (contraction) ring

This occurs when a group of circular muscle fibres go into spasm, usually due to irritation caused by abdominal or vaginal manipulation. It can occur at any part of the uterus, but it usually happens at the junction of the upper and lower uterine segments. It can occur at any of the stages of labour.

In this condition there is poor progress or arrest of progress in the first or second stage of labour, with constant pain. The liquor has usually drained and the uterus is moulded around the fetus. The spasm of the muscle around the fetus may prevent it from descending or the fetus may be totally or partially above the spastic fibers.

During the third stage of labour, an hourglass contraction prevents delivery of the placenta, usually at the junction of the upper and the lower segment, trapping the placenta in the uterine cavity (see Table 31.2 on the next page).

Aetiology

The aetiology of this condition is unknown, but predisposing factors include:

- manipulation, such as a version (active retention of the fetus) after correction of a malpresentation or malposition
- clumsy intrauterine manipulation under light anaesthesia
- improper use of oxytocin, for instance:
  - use of oxytocin in hypertonic inertia
  - an IM injection of oxytocin.

Table 31.2

Differential diagnosis: Constriction ring and Bandl's ring

Constriction ring	Bandl's ring
Localised ring of spastic myometrium	Formed by excessive retraction of upper segment
May occur in any part of the uterus	Always occurs at junction of upper and lower segments
Not seen abdominally	Seen abdominally
Muscle at the ring is thicker than above or below it	Myometrium is much thicker above ring than below it
Uterus never ruptures	If uncorrected, uterus may rupture
Uterus above the ring is relaxed and not tender	Uterus above ring is hard
Round ligaments are not tense	Round ligaments tense and stand out
May occur at any stage of labour	Usually occurs late in second stage
Position of ring does not change	Ring gradually rises in the abdomen
Presenting part is not driven downwards	Presenting part jammed into the pelvis
Patient's general condition is good	Patient's general condition is poor
Uterus is irritable	Uterus is contracting
Abnormal polarity	Normal polarity
Uterine action is inefficient	Uterine action is efficient or over-efficient
Results in obstructed labour	Caused by an obstruction

Diagnosis

The condition is more common in primigravidae and is frequently preceded by colicky uterus. Other signs and symptoms include:

▶ a raised resting tone; the uterus does not relax well between contractions
▶ constant pain between contractions.

An exact diagnosis is achieved only by feeling the ring with a hand introduced into the uterine cavity.

Management

In the case of colicky and hyperactive uteruses, the aim of the intervention is to effect relaxation of the constriction ring. The medical practitioner or obstetrician must be informed and the necessary interventions employed.

The management can be classified according to the stage of labour:

▶ *The first and second stage.* A Caesarean section is performed by a medical practitioner.
▶ *The third stage.* The patient is taken to the operating theatre and given a general anaesthetic to relax the uterine constriction ring. There could be severe haemorrhage if the placenta has separated.

Complications

▶ A prolonged first stage can result if the ring occurs at the level of the internal os.

▶ A prolonged second stage can result if the ring is around the fetal neck.
▶ If the ring occurs in the third stage (hourglass contraction), there is retained placenta and PPH.

Excessive uterine contraction and retraction

There are two types of retraction rings:

1. *Physiological retraction ring.* This is the separation between the upper and lower uterine segment present during normal labour, which cannot usually be felt abdominally.
2. *Pathological retraction ring (Bandl's ring).* During obstructed labour, the retraction ring rises up due to marked retraction and thickening of the upper uterine segment. To accommodate the fetus, the relatively passive lower segment is markedly stretched and thinned. The Bandl's ring is seen and palpated abdominally as a transverse channel that may rise to or above the umbilicus. (This line may be confused with a full bladder.) As the fundus rises, the round ligaments become tense and stand out. The clinical feature is that of obstructed labour with imminent rupture of the uterus. Obstructed labour should be properly treated to prevent rupture of the thinned lower uterine segment. Also see Table 31.2.

Clinical features

▶ Hypertonic contractions of the uterus may occur in obstructed labour in the multigravida.

▶ The uterine contractions increase in intensity and frequency until the maximum retraction is reached and the uterine contraction starts to seemingly disappear.

▶ The presenting part remains high, with or without moulding, and the application of the presenting part on the cervix is poor, hanging like a curtain. This is called *curtaining of the cervix*.

▶ The uterine contractile pattern is normal with resting in-between.

▶ The fetal heart is usually normal. The clinical features of obstructed labour will be present, with maternal and fetal distress.

▶ A pathological retraction ring is a complication in primigravidae and the risk of uterine rupture is increased in multigravidae (see Figure 25.6 on page 378).

Management

▶ Observe the uterine function, application of the presenting part on the cervix, dilatation rate, descent of the presenting part, caput and moulding and progress of labour, excluding malpresentations, malposition and disproportion.

▶ Observe the experience of pain of the labouring woman as well as the physical well-being of the fetus and mother. If ketones are detected in the urine, an IV infusion is indicated. It is difficult to reverse ketones and it is an indication that labour is becoming pathological. Good pain relief is required. *The use of uterine stimulants is contraindicated.*

▶ In the first stage, pethidine may be of benefit.

▶ In the second stage, deep general anaesthesia is given to relax the constriction ring:
  • If the ring is relaxed, the fetus is delivered immediately by forceps.
  • If the ring does not relax, an emergency Caesarean section is carried out, with lower segment vertical incision to divide the ring.

▶ If a woman is in the primary healthcare (PHC) setting, she should be transferred when labour crosses the alert line on the partogram. *Obstructed labour develops due to poor quality of care.*

▶ In the third stage, deep general anaesthesia and amyl nitrite inhalation are given, followed by manual removal of the placenta.

Precipitate labour

Precipitate labour is labour that lasts less than three hours.

Aetiology

Precipitate labour is more common in multiparae when there are strong uterine contractions, a small baby, a roomy pelvis,

minimal resistance of soft tissue and the misuse of oxytocics and other agents, which may cause hypertonic contractions. In the South African context, where women use traditional substances that also stimulate the uterus, adding other uterine stimulants may have a severe effect. In addition, African women's labour patterns vary from those of Western women.

In precipitate labour the uterus contracts with increased frequency, with too short resting periods in-between. This can cause both the mother and the fetus to become distressed. The risk of placental abruption is increased and hypertonic contractions may cause precipitate labour.

Complications

Maternal complications include:
▶ lacerations of the cervix, vagina and perineum
▶ shock
▶ placental abruption
▶ inversion of the uterus
▶ PPH
▶ sepsis due to lacerations and/or an inappropriate environment.

Fetal complications include:
▶ subaponeurotic haemorrhage due to sudden compression and decompression of the head
▶ fetal asphyxia due to reduced placental perfusion as a result of strong, frequent uterine contractions and/or lack of immediate resuscitation
▶ tearing of the umbilical cord.

Management

Before delivery, management is as follows:
▶ Consider the differences in women's patterns of birth and on admission take a history to determine if a woman has taken any natural or traditional remedies that may affect the uterus. This must be known before the uterus is stimulated.

▶ Women who had previous precipitate labours should be hospitalised before the estimated date of delivery (EDD), as they are more prone to repeated precipitate labour.

During delivery, management is as follows:
▶ All uterine stimulations are only administered on written prescription of a medical practitioner. Always start with the lowest dosage for safety and remember that some substances cannot be stopped once absorbed.

▶ Discontinue oxytocin therapy. If misoprostol or prostaglandin gel or tablets are used, further administration is discontinued. It is preferable to prevent the condition by good midwifery care during the administration of oxytocin and other oxytocics.

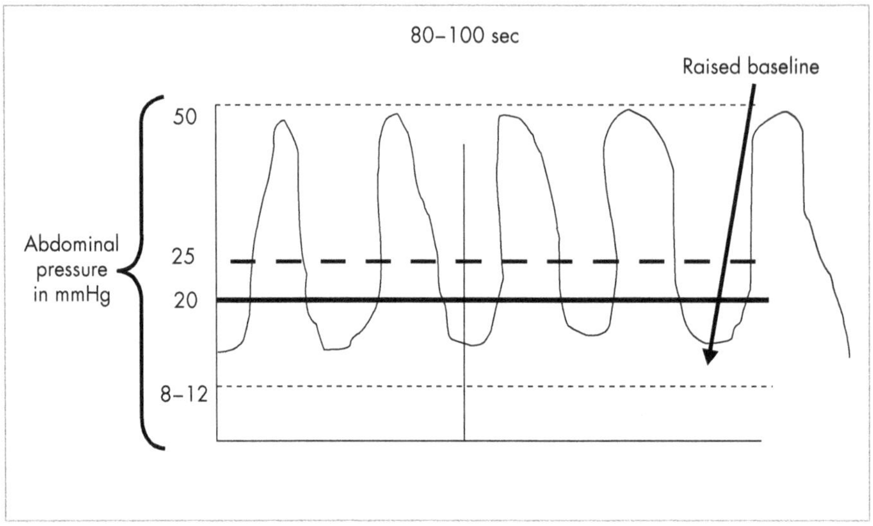

Figure 31.5 Hypertonic contractions (no relaxation)

However, occasionally, a woman may be highly sensitive to the medication and have an exaggerated response (see Figure 31.5). In such instances, discontinue the treatment immediately and call the medical practitioner. The woman is given oxygen and pain relief.

▶ Inhalation anaesthesia, such as nitrous oxide and oxygen, is given to slow the course of labour.
▶ Tocolytic agents such as salbutamol may be effective.
▶ Episiotomy may be performed to avoid perineal lacerations and subaponeurotic haemorrhage.

After delivery, examine the mother and fetus for injuries.

31.4 Cervical dystocia

Cervical dystocia refers to a rigid cervix which, despite good uterine contractions, is unable to dilate within a reasonable time.

Types of cervical dystocia

Cervical dystocia can be primary or secondary.

Primary (functional) dystocia is caused by:
▶ tenseness in a primigravida
▶ failure of the effaced external os to dilate in spite of the absence of any organic lesion; a rigid cervix which is hard and posterior.

Organic (secondary) cervical dystocia is due to:
▶ surgery or repairs to tears of the cervix, which have resulted in permanent scarring of the cervix with the inability to dilate; these include pre-malignancy or malignancy with the resultant cone biopsy, trauma during a previous labour or a Shirodkar cervical suture for an incompetent cervix (McDonald suture)
▶ oedema of the cervix, which can be caused by an anterior or posterior lip of the cervix becoming nipped between the hard fetal head and the pelvic girdle; this could occur if the patient begins to bear down before the cervix is fully dilated, particularly in OP positions
▶ organic lesions such as cervical myoma or carcinoma.

Clinical features

Inco-ordinate uterine function or strong normal contractions may be present, causing difficult and prolonged labour, tension and pain.

If cervical dystocia has not been diagnosed before labour, the labour could become temporarily obstructed by the rigid cervix. If the patient is neglected (perhaps if she is labouring at home and has not presented at a clinic or hospital until the labour has been in progress for a considerable length of time), the whole cervix may eventually slough off. This is called an annular detachment of the cervix and is a very serious condition that could require hysterectomy.

Management

Functional dystocia is managed as follows:
▶ The treatment is early diagnosis and transfer.
▶ Antenatal preparation for labour, with information and relaxation exercises, should help to prevent this condition

from occurring. However, sometimes the woman cannot restrain herself from bearing down.

▶ If the woman has a Shirodkar suture inserted, the suture must be removed at the start of labour.

▶ Manual dilatation of the resistant cervix is performed by the medical practitioner or midwife if the cervix is fully effaced and well applied to the head. Exclude disproportion.

▶ Pethidine may be effective.

▶ Caesarean section is performed if:
- medical treatment fails
- fetal distress develops.

Organic dystocia is managed as follows:

▶ All women diagnosed with a malpresentation at the onset of labour should be referred to a higher level of care in anticipation of potential problems and risk of interventions, regardless of the findings of the partogram.

▶ If the patient already has an oedematous anterior lip and the cervix is almost fully dilated with the head well down in the pelvis, the midwife will see the thick, swollen, reddish-purple tissue preceding the head. The midwife must give the woman Entonox® and try to prevent her from bearing down while she attempts to gently slip the oedematous cervix over the top of the fetal head, under the pubic arch.

▶ Caesarean section is the management of choice.

▶ If this is not possible and the labour is obstructed, the medical practitioner may cut the cervix (cervicotomy), but this could result in an incompetent cervix; the woman will then require elective Caesarean sections for subsequent pregnancies.

Complications

▶ In annular detachment of the cervix, the bleeding from the cervix is surprisingly minimal because of fibrosis and avascular pressure necrosis leading to thrombosis of the vessels before detachment.

▶ A ruptured uterus may result.

▶ PPH may occur, particularly if the cervical laceration extends upwards, tearing the main uterine vessels.

31.5 Prolonged labour

The progress of labour should be documented according to local protocol so that a skilled midwife will be able to identify at an early stage any signs of poor progress (see Table 31.1 on page 482) and take relevant action.

Poor progress of labour can progress to prolonged labour if appropriate interventions are not implemented. This can occur in both the first and second stages of labour.

Causes

Causes of prolonged labour can be described as the four Ps, often referred to as the rule of four Ps. The deviations from normal can involve the uterine contractions (the powers), the fetus (the passenger), the birth canal, bony pelvis and/or the soft tissue structures (the passage) or the pregnant woman (the patient).

The powers (uterine contractions)

The uterine contractions may be inadequate, lasting 40 seconds or less or coming at a frequency of less than three in 10 minutes, or they may be ineffective. In some cases labour does not progress despite adequate contractions and no signs indicating disproportion. Apolarity or colicky uterine contractions may be present.

The passenger (the fetus)

The fetus may be adopting an abnormal position, presentation or lie. The fetus may also be too big or have congenital malformations, such as hydrocephalus or Siamese twins.

The passage (the birth canal and soft tissues)

A contracted pelvis is the biggest cause of prolonged labour. Placenta praevia, myomata and other congenital uterine abnormalities may be present. There may be atresia of the vulva (acquired or congenital), vaginal atresia, cysts or septa, cervical stenosis, other pelvic tumours, conditions or abnormalities.

Maternal causes (the patient)

Maternal causes may be physiological or psychological:

▶ A full bladder or rectum may interfere with adequate uterine contractions as well as impede descent of the presenting part.

▶ Insufficient analgesia or dehydration may also contribute to prolonged labour.

▶ An uncomfortable maternal position may impact on labour; the position the woman adopts in labour should be comfortable and should allow her to feel in control of the situation without affecting the condition of the fetus.

▶ Previous traumatic labour and childbirth may also contribute to prolonged labour (fear and anxiety inhibit uterine functions).

Labour should not exceed 24 hours in a primigravida and less than that in a multigravida. Most women do deliver within the normal time period. However, the partogram was designed as a scientific tool to guide the duration of labour and enable the midwife to take action early should labour not progress within the specified time. This is important, because prolonged labour negatively affects the birth and outcomes for mother and fetus.

Figure 31.6 gives a graphic display of various types of prolonged labour.

Treatment and care

Identify the cause (any of the four Ps) early and correct the abnormality if possible. If the patient is at a peripheral health facility or in the community, refer. If the patient is in a healthcare facility where emergency obstetric care is available, the management will depend on the cause. The medical obstetrician should be informed and will guide further management.

Prolonged latent phase

Figure 31.6 illustrates a prolonged latent phase. Malpresentations such as a face presentation should be considered. There is great variation in the duration of the latent phase of labour. An abdominal palpation will exclude malpresentation. A malpresentation and poor application of the presenting part on the cervix, a high presenting part, breech, cord around the neck and pelvic shape may cause the presenting part to fit poorly on the cervix. The result is a poor Ferguson reflex and poor contractions, causing slow progress.

The treatment and care depends on the cause. The woman is encouraged to move around in the first stage to allow the head to 'come down'. Observation is made of the station of the presenting part, the condition of the cervix, the contractions and the changes of the cervix. Amniotomy is delayed or avoided. Keeping the membranes intact may assist with the rotation of the presenting part and dilatation of the cervix through even pressure exercised by the membranes in cases of malpresentation. Pain relief may be useful if the mother is becoming tired. Uterine stimulation is only prescribed by the medical practitioner if malpresentation and CPD are excluded.

Prolonged active phase

In the active phase of labour, cervical dilatation should occur at a rate of 1 cm per hour in a nullipara and 1.5 cm in a multipara. Dilatation of less than 1 cm per hour is considered as delayed progress.

If the powers (uterine contractions) are inadequate, labour can be augmented (if not contraindicated). Prior to administering oxytocin, CPD, malpresentation and fetal distress must be excluded. The woman should be advised to empty her bladder to allow for descent and to promote effective uterine contractions. Labour should be monitored and adequate pain relief administered (see Figure 31.6).

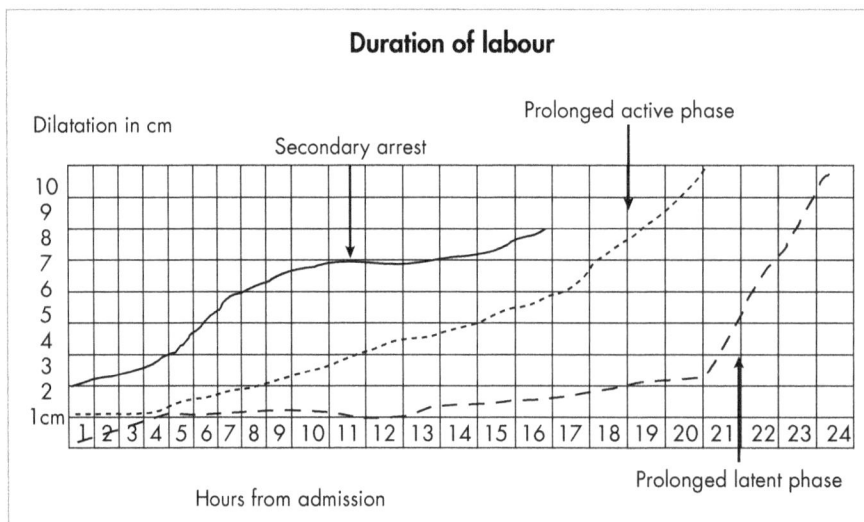

Figure 31.6 Three patterns of abnormal labour

If the alert line on the partogram is crossed, the woman should be re-assessed. The gravidity, presentation, level of the presenting part, pattern of contractions, application of the presenting part and cervical dilatation are assessed, versus the well-being of the mother and fetus. The two-hour action line indicates the need for medical attention or referral to a higher level of care.

Crossing the four-hour action line may indicate the need for delivering the baby. Ignoring these guidelines may lead to obstructed labour. The midwife should use the action line to direct further care to oxytocin, vacuum delivery or Caesarean section.

Prolonged second stage

The second stage of labour is considered to be delayed when maternal bearing-down effort is effective but delivery has not occurred within 45 minutes in a primigravida and 30 minutes in a multipara.

Causes of a prolonged second stage of labour are many and varied (see the box on this page). The cause should be identified and rectified. If the uterine contractions are poor, administer oxytocin as an IV infusion. If there is poor maternal effort in spite of good uterine contractions and no CPD, deliver by vacuum extraction. If CPD is diagnosed, deliver by Caesarean section.

The second stage of labour is a critical period for mother and fetus. A change in the position of the mother may facilitate birth. The woman may be allowed to squat or be upright to improve the process. Using fundal pressure is discouraged, as it may cause placental abruption and bruise the uterus, or cause a constriction ring.

It is possible but not desirable to transfer a woman in the second stage to a higher level of care. It is thus important to identify cases of a large infant, malpresentation or an abnormal pelvis and anticipate potential problems for early referral to a higher level where specialist care is available.

The midwife is responsible for timing the labour, for doing routine observations of mother and fetus and for their care. The medical practitioner depends on the midwife to alert him or her if there are any abnormalities. When a labour has exceeded the average time, the midwife informs the medical practitioner. However, if the labour is progressing, albeit slowly, the medical practitioner may decide not to intervene unless some abnormality arises.

Prevention of prolonged labour

Prevention requires good antenatal care, careful screening and the referral of all those at risk or with a poor obstetric history. Any abnormal condition should be recognised early and referred so that early treatment can be provided by specialists. Hospital delivery is arranged for women who have any abnormality, particularly one which could contribute to prolonged labour and would require specialised care.

Good antenatal education is given in order to eliminate fear and tension and to build up the woman's confidence in herself. Labour is only induced when absolutely necessary and then only when the cervix is or has been ripened.

Any woman admitted in false labour is given special care to increase her confidence and remove fear and tension. The signs and symptoms of true labour are carefully and kindly explained and the woman and her partner are advised to return home and await the onset of true labour.

Causes of a prolonged second stage of labour

The following are some of the causes of a prolonged second stage of labour:

▶ Ineffective maternal effort usually results from fear of the unknown, exhaustion or lack of sensation, especially if an epidural block is in use for pain relief in labour.

▶ Secondary hypotonic uterine contractions may occur, which can be relieved by the use of oxytocin.

▶ A large fetus or malposition may result in large diameters presenting or a malpresentation. A large fetus or malpresentation may require a Caesarean section.

▶ A reduced pelvic outlet, mostly in an android pelvis, is likely to cause obstruction at the outlet because of the prominent ischial spines and the narrow subpubic arch. The baby may be delivered by forceps or Caesarean section.

Midwifery management

Together with the standard midwifery care of a woman in labour, the following special care is given:

▶ *In the first stage.* Normal care and management and the observations necessary for all labour must be conscientiously carried out (see Chapter 26). Use the partogram to determine normal cervical dilatation in the first stage of labour as well as aspects such as the application of the presenting part on the cervix and the position of the fontanelles and suture lines to determine the position as well as the station of the fetal head.

▶ *In the second stage.* In primigravidae, the normal duration of this stage is one hour and should not exceed two hours. In multigravidae, the normal duration is 15–30 minutes and should not exceed one hour. If problems are anticipated, medical assistance is requested or the woman is referred.

▶ *In the third stage.* The midwife must choose the type of management carefully, according to the situation.

Risk factors for the third stage include a prolonged first and/ or second stage of labour. Complications can be unsuspected. The active management of the third stage (AMTSL) is best practice in midwifery (see Chapter 28). The normal duration of the third stage of labour is 5–10 minutes. With active management, an oxytocic is administered to the woman with the delivery of the anterior shoulder in a singleton birth and the placenta is removed by controlled cord traction.

In the passive management of the third stage, one hour may be allowed for the delivery of the placenta. If there is no bleeding, the placenta may stay in longer. A manual delivery of the placenta may be indicated if the placenta is not delivered. An IV infusion is commenced and medical assistance requested.

In all stages of labour, make sure that the woman is able to pass urine. If she is not able to, she should be catheterised.

Quality midwifery care is essential during prolonged labour, where there is a special need for vigilance, extra observations and continual reassessment of the situation. Pay attention to the fetal condition, the progress of labour and the maternal condition to ensure the early recognition of any abnormality. The midwife must be caring and instil confidence in the woman.

Lack of proper attention or relaxation of observations could lead to complications. This could be construed as negligence on the part of the midwife, because the midwife is responsible for letting the medical practitioner know as soon as possible if some abnormality has arisen.

Any maternal distress or fetal distress (compromise) is immediately reported to the medical practitioner and then treated by the midwife, pending the arrival of the medical practitioner.

If the membranes have been ruptured for 12 hours or more and there is a danger of infection, the woman may be started on antibiotics. Preparations are made for either a Caesarean section if the first stage of labour is prolonged or for an instrument delivery or Caesarean section in the second stage of labour.

Preparations must be made for resuscitation of the newborn infant and for possible complications in the third stage of labour. After a prolonged labour, the baby is observed in high care until his or her condition is satisfactory or stable.

Obstetric management

The obstetric management depends upon the cause of the prolonged labour, the duration of labour and at which stage labour is prolonged.

In order to prevent labour from becoming prolonged, active management of labour is advocated, which ensures that no woman will labour for longer than 12 hours in the active phase. Before the start of labour, the woman is given the assurance that, should the labour last as long as 12 hours, a Caesarean section will be performed in order to deliver the baby. In addition, any primigravida with hypotonic uterine function will have labour augmented by an IV infusion of oxytocin. The woman is also allocated a specific midwife to stay with her throughout the 12 hours of labour.

The first stage of labour

If the prolonged labour is due to hypotonic uterine function in the primigravida, the medical practitioner may order oxytocin by IV infusion (augmentation of labour) if CPD and pelvic abnormalities have been excluded. The mother and fetus must be well. This will strengthen uterine contractions, enhance the polarity of the uterus and so the effectiveness of the uterine contractions.

Effective pain relief is a requirement, particularly when oxytocin is administered. An epidural is the method of choice.

If the membranes have not already ruptured, the fetal condition is satisfactory, there is little or no CPD and the woman's HIV status is negative, the medical practitioner may rupture the membranes if labour is established and there is no malpresentation.

If there is little or no progress in labour, if there is obstructed labour and/or if the maternal or fetal conditions are not satisfactory, the medical practitioner will usually do a Caesarean section.

The first and/or second stage of labour

With minor CPD, if the cervix is fully dilated but the head is above the spines and the fetal condition is satisfactory, a symphysiotomy and/or a vacuum extraction may be performed. If the cervix is fully dilated, the head is at the spines and the fetal condition is satisfactory, a forceps (instrument) delivery is probable.

If there is fetal distress, if the head is high and there is more than minor CPD, or if the maternal condition is unsatisfactory or if there is placenta praevia, the medical practitioner will usually perform a Caesarean section.

If the woman has certain abnormal general conditions that contraindicate bearing down, such as cardiac conditions, respiratory conditions or severe pre-eclampsia or eclampsia, the medical practitioner will usually perform a low forceps delivery once the head is well down in the pelvis. However, if there is maternal and/or fetal distress or CPD, the baby will be delivered by Caesarean section.

In the third stage of labour

If the first two stages of labour were prolonged and the woman is very tired or if she has been heavily sedated or been given epidural analgesia, the woman may be receiving IV oxytocin in labour. However, oxytocin 10 units may be administered with the birth of the anterior shoulder to prevent PPH. The placenta will be delivered by controlled cord traction.

A continuous infusion of 20 IU oxytocin is maintained for 24 hours to keep the uterus contracted to prevent PPH. A tired uterus in prolonged labour may refuse to contract after birth.

Complications of prolonged labour

Maternal complications include:
▶ intrauterine infection, as membranes tend to rupture early due to poor application of the presenting part to the cervix and repeated vaginal examinations performed to assess progress of labour and interventions
▶ maternal distress and exhaustion due to strong uterine contractions and lack of progress
▶ an increased risk of vaginal lacerations due to prolonged pressure of the fetal head (in cephalic presentations) on the pelvic floor and vaginal walls
▶ PPH, mostly as a result of uterine atony due to prolonged labour
▶ pain and shock due to a higher risk of interventions that may result in psychological trauma, which can affect future pregnancies
▶ placental abruption
▶ pelvic floor trauma.

Fetal complications include:
▶ birth asphyxia from prolonged labour, leading to cerebral damage or cerebral palsy
▶ subaponeurotic haemorrhage due to assisted delivery
▶ intrauterine infection, manifesting as meningitis, septicaemia and/or pneumonitis
▶ admission to a neonatal unit and prolonged hospitalisation
▶ poor maternal–child bonding
▶ breastfeeding difficulties
▶ fetal death or stillbirth
▶ early neonatal death.

31.6 Obstructed labour

There is no clear definition of obstructed labour; 'dystocia' is a synonymous concept. Obstructed labour occurs when there is failure of the presenting part to descend or advance in spite of good uterine contractions and when the fetus cannot be delivered through the birth canal in spite of good contractions. Obstructed labour indicates poor quality of care in pregnancy.

Incidence

The WHO considers obstructed labour to be the most disabling condition of all. The estimated incidence for Africa is 4:100 births (Fantu, Segni & Alemseged, 2010). Obstructed labour is associated with poor quality of care and an inadequate use of the partogram, no diagnosis of abnormal labour and insufficient diagnosis and recognition, intervention and referral.

Causes of obstructed labour

Causes of obstructed labour can be attributed either to the fetus (the passenger) or the birth canal (the passage). Some of the causes of obstructed labour include:
▶ CPD: the fetus may be too large compared to the maternal pelvis, or the maternal pelvis may be grossly contracted, or a previous fracture to the pelvis may cause pelvic contraction
▶ an abnormal pelvis
▶ abnormalities in the fetus, eg hydrocephalus
▶ malposition resulting in deep transverse arrest, as in OP positions
▶ pelvic tumours, eg cervical fibroids or ovarian tumours, which may prevent engagement of the head
▶ malpresentations that make vaginal delivery impossible, eg brow presentation.

Signs and symptoms of obstructed labour

Obstructed labour should be suspected initially if there is no descent of the presenting part in the pelvis in the presence of good uterine contractions, accompanied by slow dilatation of the cervix. The poor application of the presenting part to the cervix contributes to early rupture of membranes and the cervix hangs like an empty sleeve (curtaining of the cervix).

If there is no intervention, the contractions become hypertonic and more frequent in an attempt to overcome the obstruction. In a primigravida, the contractions may cease, only to restart later with more vigour. The woman becomes distressed, anxious and looks ill due to pain. Dehydration may set in, the body temperature will rise and a rapid pulse will be palpable. Occasionally, the woman may vomit and there will be oliguria (diminished urinary output). In the final phase, the woman may become catatonic, with no response to her external environment. The contractions seem to disappear due to the state of pathological retraction of the uterus, meaning that the uterus has reached its maximum contractile ability with the upper segment bundled and the lower segment stretched to the maximum.

On abdominal examination, the uterus will be moulded around the fetus due to ruptured membranes (the liquor amnii is drained). The presenting part remains high and the uterus is hard. The difference between the upper and lower segment may be palpated abdominally as a ridge. If the obstruction is severe, a Bandl's retraction ring is noted, mainly in primigravidae (a sign that the upper uterine segment is bundled and the lower uterine segment has been overstretched due to retraction of the upper uterine segment), and uterine rupture may occur in multigravidae.

The fetal heart rate (FHR) may be normal. Often the oxygen supply to the fetus is diminished and the fetus may become distressed or die. Severe caput and moulding may be present. In a cephalic presentation, there is excessive moulding and the presence of a large caput succedaneum, which may be mistaken for a head. In some cases where the head is above the brim, no caput may be present.

At this stage, the woman is overly exhausted and may die as a result of exhaustion, haemorrhage and shock from abruptio placenta or uterine rupture. Gas may be noticed in the colon on the sides of the uterus, indicating paralysis of the gastrointestinal (GI) system. The urine is scanty and 3+ ketones are present. The woman is severely dehydrated.

Treatment and care

Prevention is better than cure. Accurate history taking, combined with the strict screening of high-risk women, should be carefully undertaken in every antenatal clinic or by the midwife in private practice:
▶ If a woman has any of the predisposing causes of obstructed labour, she should immediately be referred to the nearest hospital.
▶ All primigravidae should deliver in hospital and the labour should be treated as a trial of labour.
▶ All patients undergoing a trial of labour should undergo careful observations and attention in hospital.
▶ All women with a poor obstetric history, a previous large infant, previous assisted delivery or malpresentation should be referred for medical attention.
▶ The use of the partogram is invaluable for diagnosing prolonged labour and early obstructed labour. This enables the midwife to implement early intervention before the later signs of obstruction become evident and grave. The station and descent of the presenting part are crucial and can be assessed by abdominal and vaginal examination.

Midwifery management

Obstructed labour is an obstetric emergency. The management will depend upon whether the patient is in a clinic or a hospital. If in a clinic, the woman must be hospitalised or referred as soon as possible. If the woman is in a hospital, a medical practitioner must be notified immediately. The following guidelines apply:
▶ An IV infusion is started immediately.
▶ An indwelling Foley's catheter is inserted and the urine is tested.
▶ The woman is reassured.
▶ The woman is kept on her side and the baby is monitored continuously.
▶ The woman is given oxygen per mask.
▶ The woman is prepared for immediate Caesarean section.

This patient will require specialised care and attention during the third stage of labour and during the puerperium. There is a danger of both atonic and traumatic PPH. If the baby is alive and is successfully resuscitated, the baby should be admitted to high care or intensive care.

Obstetric management

Once/if the patient is in hospital, the following steps may be taken:
▶ The woman is rehydrated by IV fluids.
▶ Maternal acidosis is corrected by giving an IV electrolyte solution.
▶ Operative procedures depend on the cause of the obstruction, the length of labour and the condition of both the fetus and the mother.
▶ Emergency Caesarean section is performed if the baby is alive, for insurmountable CPD, all abnormal lies and pelvic tumours, and for conjoined twins. Under certain conditions, Caesarean section may also be performed if the baby is dead, especially when there are late signs of obstruction. The Caesarean section should be done by the most experienced person available.
▶ Every precaution is taken to prevent PPH in the third stage of labour and the patient is watched carefully for signs of bleeding in the post-delivery period.
▶ The medical practitioner may prescribe broad-spectrum antibiotics.
▶ The baby will require expert resuscitation and expert care in the puerperium.
▶ A symphysiotomy may be performed if the obstruction is within the pelvic cavity. This may occur with the after-coming head of a breech, or in selected cases with obstruction in OP positions when there is only borderline disproportion.

- If the baby is dead and there is no likelihood of rupturing the uterus, instead of performing a Caesarean section, a destructive operation may be performed (see Chapter 33). However, this is unlikely unless the woman lives in a very remote area (to preserve the integrity of the uterus). A destructive operation is performed in the operating theatre under general anaesthesia after adequate maternal resuscitation.

If the baby has died, the mother and her husband or partner will require a careful explanation and understanding; the midwife should supply all the support they may require or she should refer them to a specialist psychologist. The mother will require specialised care during and after the puerperium, with follow-ups if any complications were present. The woman may be very upset about not delivering normally and may require psychological support.

The woman and her husband are referred to the family planning clinic and they are warned of all the dangers of her becoming pregnant again before the damaged tissues are healed. The absolute necessity for her to attend an antenatal clinic early with any subsequent pregnancy and to deliver in hospital is also carefully explained to her and her husband or partner. She must be told of the reason for the Caesarean section so that she can relate this during future pregnancies.

Complications

In a case of obstructed labour, complications may include:
- dehydration related to inadequate fluid intake as a result of pain
- infection related to prolonged rupture of membranes and repeated vaginal examinations
- maternal exhaustion due to hypertonic uterine contractions

- Bandl's ring in the primigravida
- rupture of the uterus in the multigravida
- hysterectomy
- if there is no intervention and obstruction persists, vesicovaginal fistula related to prolonged pressure on the bladder, leading to injury and necrosis of related pelvic tissues
- maternal death due to uterine rupture
- in the fetus, intrauterine death (IUD) due to intrauterine hypoxia or trauma sustained during a difficult instrumental delivery.

31.7 General treatment and care in abnormal uterine function

The administration of uterine stimulants should be used with great caution on written prescription of a medical practitioner, who will consider all the risks and will prescribe only in a woman with a vertex presentation and with a presenting part well fitted on the cervix. The physical condition of the mother and the fetus should be normal. Induction of labour (IOL) should be performed only in settings where a medical practitioner and emergency theatre are available.

All high-risk patients should have an IV infusion during labour.

Pain relief is essential in abnormal uterine function. The use of doulas in labour is also helpful (see Chapter 27).

31.8 Conclusion

In this chapter, disorders of uterine function were described as well as their management. Correct identification and management of these conditions will reduce maternal and perinatal mortality and morbidity.

32

Obstetric emergencies

32.1 Introduction

Childbirth is considered to be a normal physiological process unless complications occur. However, complications can occur in 20 per cent of cases and may affect the mother, the fetus or both (Wikipedia, 2017b). Most conditions can occur at any stage of pregnancy and birth. Placental abruption and placenta praevia can occur in pregnancy. However, shoulder dystocia only occurs at birth, while a bleeding retained placenta happens after birth, in which case the midwife has a limited time to save the baby and the mother.

Women who are at risk should be encouraged to deliver in healthcare facilities that offer emergency obstetric care. These include women younger than 16 and older than 35, primigravidae, grand multiparae and women presenting with certain medical conditions such as diabetes mellitus and cardiac diseases. It also applies to any identified abnormal condition in the fetus, such as multiple pregnancy, malpresentations, polyhydramnios or a large infant (with a symphysis fundal height [SFH] of more than 40 cm). Care of the HIV-positive woman is discussed in Chapter 50.

Obstetric emergencies are events that require the knowledge and skill of a competent team to save the life of the fetus/newborn and the woman. Clinical competencies need to be supported by administrative standards, staff ratios, an adequate skill mix, enough and appropriate equipment, logistic support and a reliable transport system. Skills drills should be done by all responsible for maternal and child healthcare. Each midwife is responsible for developing the required skills to deal effectively with an emergency. Prevention, early diagnosis and intervention are essential.

32.2 Uterine rupture

Rupture of the uterus is an obstetric emergency that has a poor outcome for the fetus. This complication can be prevented or its occurrence minimised with effective antenatal and high-quality intrapartum care. It is a global concern, as its prevalence in developing countries remains high.

Causes

Certain circumstances can precipitate uterine rupture, including the following:

▶ *A weak uterine scar.* This is more common in classical Caesarean section but can occur in women with previous lower-segment Caesarean section, hysterotomy or any other uterine surgery. The complication can be exacerbated by impaired healing, over-distension of the uterus due to multiple pregnancies or polyhydramnios, obstructed labour or trauma following manipulation of the fetus.

▶ *High parity.* Women with high parity are likely to experience obstructed labour, resulting in uterine rupture.

▶ *Incorrect use of oxytocin.* Excessive use of oxytocic drugs can cause hypertonic uterine contractions, resulting in uterine rupture.

▶ *A severe cervical laceration.* This may be sustained as a result of premature bearing down or even a forceps delivery (applied before the cervix is fully dilated). The cervical tear may extend upwards into the lower uterine segment.

Classification

Uterine ruptures can be classified as follows:

▶ *Silent rupture:* This is the rupture of the uterus during the antenatal period. It may occur in the last four weeks of pregnancy and usually involves a previous classical Caesarean scar. The rupture can be spontaneous or traumatic.

▶ *Complete rupture:* This is the most common type of uterine rupture. The laceration is in direct contact with the peritoneal cavity and all the layers of the uterus are involved. This usually involves a previous classical Caesarean section scar (see Figure 32.1).

▶ *Incomplete rupture:* The rupture is incomplete if the laceration is separated from the peritoneal cavity by the peritoneum, which remains intact. An incomplete uterine rupture involves the endometrium and the myometrium only. This can occur in a spontaneous rupture of the uterus or when the cervical tears extend upwards into the lower segment.

▶ *Dehiscence:* This occurs as the transverse lower-segment Caesarean section scar separates, leaving a window in the lower segment. However, the rupture can spread sideways, involving the uterine blood vessels and resulting in extensive haemorrhage.

Rupture before the onset of labour

Signs and symptoms

▶ Vaginal bleeding is present.
▶ The rupture is sudden.
▶ The woman feels a sharp pain between contractions at the site of the previous scar (caused by irritation of the peritoneum due to bleeding from the uterine scar).
▶ The woman feels unusual abdominal tenderness.
▶ There is recession of the fetal head (moving back up into the birth canal).

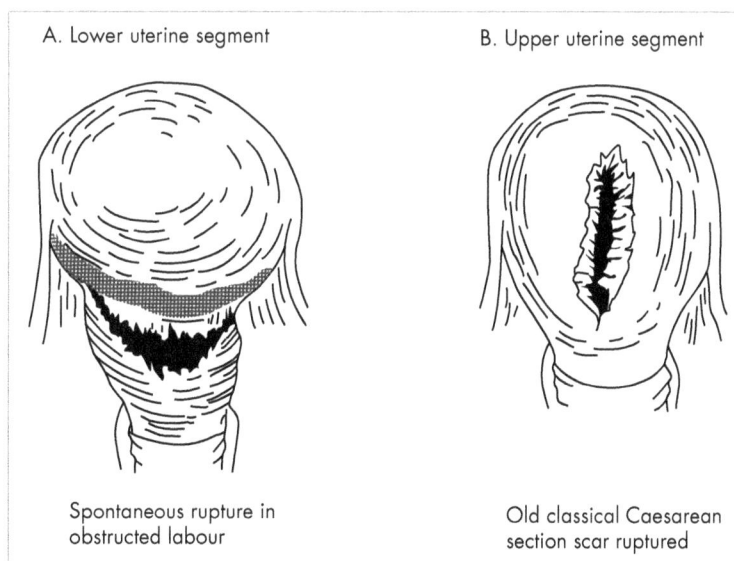

A. Lower uterine segment

Spontaneous rupture in obstructed labour

B. Upper uterine segment

Old classical Caesarean section scar ruptured

Figure 32.1 Rupture of the uterus

- Fetal parts are easily palpable all over the abdomen, as these are no longer contained in the uterus.
- The fetal heartbeat is abnormal, with variable decelerations or bradycardia; the fetus experiences severe intrauterine hypoxia resulting in intrauterine death (IUD).
- Uterine atony occurs (loss of uterine muscle tone).
- Maternal tachycardia and hypotension occur.
- Blood loss causes abdominal tenderness and shock.

Treatment and care

The woman is prepared for an urgent laparotomy. Her general condition is assessed and vital signs checked. Blood will be collected for a full blood count (FBC) and cross-matched for possible blood transfusion. Prophylactic antibiotics may be administered as per protocol.

The uterine scar will be repaired or a hysterectomy performed, depending on the nature of the uterine rupture. If the scar is repaired, the woman is advised to delay pregnancy for at least a year. Her subsequent pregnancies should be closely monitored and she should be advised to deliver by Caesarean section.

Intrapartum rupture of the uterus

Intrapartum rupture of the uterus is usually sudden. The rupture occurs at the peak of a contraction, followed by cessation of contractions and rapid shock setting in. The characteristic features include the following:

- There is a sudden onset of severe lower abdominal pain, which is persistent and becomes worse during contractions.
- There may be suprapubic tenderness.
- The woman may vomit.
- Fetal tachycardia or fetal heart decelerations may be noted, followed by cessation of the fetal heart once the uterus ruptures.
- Blood in the urine on a catheter specimen may indicate a pending rupture.
- There might be fresh blood noted per vagina, which can be mistaken for a heavy show.

A rise in maternal pulse rate may indicate danger.

If the woman is under epidural, the early warning signs may be missed. The diagnosis is usually made on the clinical picture.

Rupture as a result of obstructed labour

Vigilant management of labour through the use of the partogram may assist in the appropriate management of labour and earlier recognition of obstructed labour. The midwife must identify obstructed labour and inform the medical practitioner, who will then implement the relevant interventions to minimise complications.

Incomplete uterine rupture

This type of rupture usually occurs at the end of the second stage of labour and may be a rupture of a previous Caesarean section scar. As mentioned, the endometrium and myometrium are ruptured, but the perimetrium is not affected. Continuous vaginal bleeding is present. The baby may be delivered vaginally and will not necessarily suffer any intrauterine hypoxia.

Signs and symptoms

The warning signs of a ruptured uterus are often the same as the signs for obstructed labour. The woman complains of severe and constant abdominal pain with or without vaginal bleeding. The onset of maternal shock may be slow, depending on the extent of rupture and the amount of blood loss. Early warning signs are an increased pulse rate, a drop in BP and – if she has a Foley catheter *in situ* – haematuria. If the rupture is extensive, with severe blood loss, the woman may rapidly progress into severe shock (see Chapter 35). Diagnosis is confirmed in theatre following an exploratory laparotomy.

Fetal distress is severe and if no relief is obtained, fetal death may follow. In extensive and complete uterine rupture, fetal parts can be palpable through the abdominal wall.

Interventions for a complete or incomplete rupture

The management is the same as for complete uterine rupture. Resuscitation is critical and a blood transfusion may be necessary. Resuscitation is performed based on the degree of shock. An emergency Caesarean section is performed in an effort to save the fetus and repair the uterus.

After the birth of the baby and delivery of the placenta, the extent of the damage to the uterus is assessed and the uterus is repaired if possible. If the tear is extensive, a hysterectomy is performed. If blood loss is severe, the woman is likely to be in shock. A blood transfusion is administered depending on the amount of blood loss.

Prevention

The careful screening of pregnant women during the antenatal period can prevent subsequent uterine rupture. Preventive health education in the antenatal period should be targeted at women, their families and the community at large. Midwives should refer all women who had previous Caesarean sections to healthcare facilities to be attended to by skilled attendants during pregnancy, labour and childbirth. These women should be educated on the factors that contribute to a ruptured uterus and the possible consequences. They should be advised to deliver in health facilities where emergency obstetric care is available and to present themselves at the health facility as soon as labour starts. Women who live further away from health facilities should always have emergency transport available when the need arises.

All women with previous Caesarean sections who request a vaginal birth after Caesarean section (VBAC) must be admitted in the labour ward at the nearest hospital that has facilities to perform an emergency Caesarean section.

Other preventative measures include:
- assessing the fetal size to exclude cephalopelvic disproportion (CPD) and malposition
- using a partogram in all labours to monitor labour so that prolonged labour is identified early
- the early recognition of obstructed labour and immediate reporting and timely intervention by the medical practitioner
- avoiding the improper use of oxytocin and other uterine stimulants.

Midwifery care

A ruptured uterus is an obstetric emergency. All available resources should therefore be mobilised immediately, including the medical practitioner or obstetrician.

Together with the standard nursing care of a woman in labour, the following specific nursing care is given:
- Urgently call for help, as more assistance is required.
- The senior person (team leader) gives instructions to each person, who must report back on the execution of that action to the team leader.
- One person is responsible for time keeping and recording of all actions.
- The actions to be taken are the following:
  - An IV infusion is *in situ.*
  - An indwelling urinary Foley catheter is inserted.
  - Oxygen is administered to help the woman and the fetus.
- Obtain informed consent for an operation. This should include consent for a hysterectomy, should one be necessary.
- Monitor vital signs quarter-hourly.
- Keep the patient nil per mouth.
- Prepare the patient for the operating theatre.

The midwife must never leave the patient alone. The midwife must explain the problem and provide support and encouragement to the woman and her partner.

If rupture of the uterus has taken place at a clinic or is suspected, the patient is stabilised and then transported to a hospital as soon as possible. The hospital is notified by telephone and the expected time of arrival is given. The midwife accompanies the woman.

Complications

Complications of uterine rupture are normally severe and include:
- hypovolaemic shock
- increased fetal hypoxia or infant asphyxia
- maternal and/or fetal death.

32.3   Fetal distress

The term 'fetal distress' is widely used but poorly defined. Fetal distress is a non-specific term used to describe a non-reassuring fetal heart rate (FHR), with or without fetal acidosis. If it is not corrected, it will lead to intrauterine fetal asphyxia, which may result in decompensation of the physiological response (primarily redistribution of blood to preserve oxygenation to vital organs) and cause permanent central nervous system (CNS) damage and other damage or death (Velayudhareddy & Kirankumar, 2010). The term 'fetal distress' is commonly used interchangeably with 'birth asphyxia', which refers to acidosis resulting from progressive hypoxia in utero.

The fetal reaction to the onset of asphyxia produces characteristic FHR patterns (loss of variability, late decelerations, variable decelerations, tachycardia or prolonged bradycardia) due to the redistributed blood flow to vital organs. This enables the fetus to compensate for the distress related to poor oxygenation, unless the insult is profound or prolonged.

The monitoring of FHR can detect hypoxic episodes well before the development of asphyxia. However, fetal distress cannot be defined by electronic fetal monitoring alone, as an abnormal fetal heart tracing must be accompanied by documented evidence of fetal hypoxia, such as abnormal umbilical cord gases.

Epidemiology

Fetal distress may result in intrauterine asphyxia. Intrapartum asphyxia and birth trauma were responsible for about one in five of all deaths recorded in the Perinatal Problem Identification Programme (PPIP) database noted in 2003 (MRC Research Unit et al, 2003). More than three-quarters of the neonatal deaths due to hypoxia could be attributed to managing the pregnant woman in labour (MRC Research Unit et al, 2003). The *Saving Babies 2012–2013* report indicated that 'almost half of the deaths due to intrapartum asphyxia were thought to be probably preventable; the common problems being with fetal monitoring, use of the partogram and the second stage of labour management' (Pattinson & Rhoda, 2014: 26).

Precursors

Potential precursors to fetal distress or non-reassuring fetal status include:
- maternal anaemia
- oligohydramnios
- pre-eclampsia and cigarette smoking, both of which cause placental insufficiency
- maternal diabetes mellitus
- post-term pregnancies (42 weeks or more)
- intrauterine growth restriction (IUGR)
- preterm labour
- meconium-stained amniotic fluid
- antepartum haemorrhage (APH)
- pregnancy-induced hypertension (PIH)
- low-lying placenta
- a compressed umbilical cord
- cord prolapse
- uterine rupture.

Indications

Fetal distress can be suspected in the case of:
- non-reassuring or abnormal FHR (less than 100 bpm or over 180 bpm)
- a loss of beat-to-beat variability, late decelerations, variable decelerations, tachycardia or prolonged bradycardia (see figures 26.5, 26.7, 26.9 and 26.10 in Chapter 26)
- thick, meconium-stained liquor.

Principles

While guidelines for interpreting an FHR tracing were not included in the *Guidelines for Maternity Care in South Africa* (DoH, 2015), it is generally accepted that a full description of an FHR tracing should include:
- a qualitative and quantitative description of the baseline rate
- baseline FHR variability
- the presence of accelerations
- periodic or episodic decelerations
- changes or trends of FHR patterns over time.

| PROCEDURE | Managing fetal distress |

Determine the cause. If a maternal cause is identified (eg maternal fever), initiate appropriate treatment.

Examination

A vaginal examination is performed to identify an explanatory sign for the distress:
- In the case of intermittent or constant pain accompanied by bleeding, exclude the possibility of placental abruption.
- In the case of signs of infection (fever, offensive vaginal discharge or liquor), administer antibiotics.
- Exclude the possibility of cord compression or prolapse and manage accordingly.

Delivery

If the FHR abnormalities persist and additional signs of distress occur, expedite delivery:
- If the cervix is fully dilated and the fetal head is no more than one-fifth above the symphysis pubis, deliver by vacuum extraction.
- If the cervix is not fully dilated or the fetal head is more than one-fifth above the symphysis pubis, deliver by Caesarean section.

Intrauterine resuscitation

Apply specific measures with the aim of increasing oxygen delivery to the placenta and umbilical blood flow in order to reverse hypoxia and acidosis. Intrauterine resuscitation may be used:
- as part of the obstetric management of labour, while preparing for Caesarean delivery for fetal distress
- at the time of establishment of regional analgesia during labour in the compromised fetus
- during inter-hospital transfers.

Intrauterine resuscitation involves the following:
- Change the mother's position to left lateral.
- Ensure the mother is well hydrated by means of an IV infusion.

continued

▶ Administer maternal oxygen per facemask at 6 ℓ.
▶ Inhibit uterine contractions with subcutaneous or IV terbutaline 250 μg.

Recording and interpretation
▶ All findings are recorded in the maternal obstetric record and on the partogram.
▶ An incident report is written in all cases of birth asphyxia or low Apgar scores.

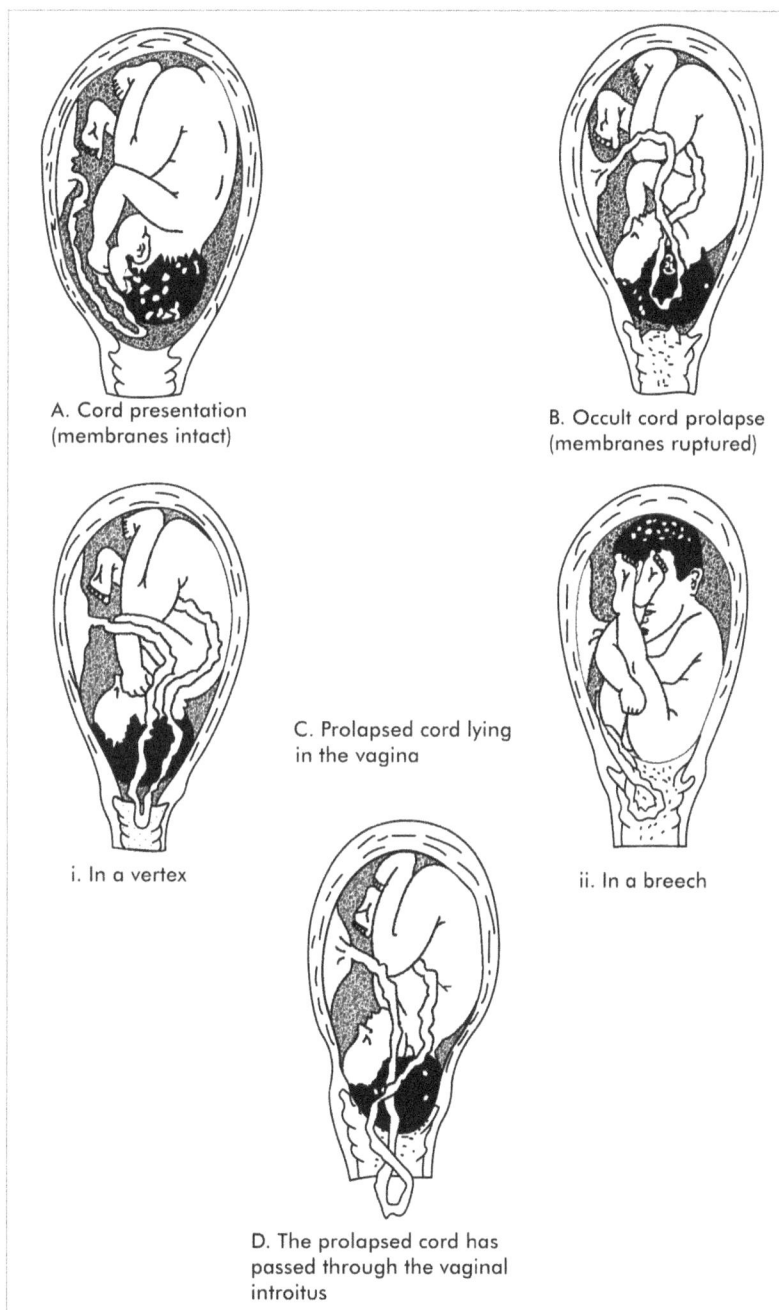

A. Cord presentation
(membranes intact)

B. Occult cord prolapse
(membranes ruptured)

C. Prolapsed cord lying
in the vagina

i. In a vertex

ii. In a breech

D. The prolapsed cord has
passed through the vaginal
introitus

Figure 32.2 Cord presentation and prolapse of the umbilical cord

32.4   Cord prolapse

Umbilical cord prolapse is an obstetric emergency where the umbilical cord passes through the cervix into the vagina at the same time as or in advance of the fetal presenting part. Although not a common obstetric emergency, it is one in which the initial response can make a difference in the neonatal outcome.

With a cord prolapse, the cord becomes trapped between the fetal presenting part and the maternal bony pelvis. The prolapsed cord may be visible at the lower edge of the vagina; however, this is quite rare. In most cases, the umbilical cord lies beside or just ahead of the fetal skull (occult cord prolapse) and may be neither visible nor palpable.

The umbilical cord transports oxygen and nutrients to the fetus and removes waste products. It is made up of three blood vessels (two arteries and one vein, as shown in Figure 32.3). The compression of the blood vessels in the umbilical cord may result in abnormal findings on FHR and fetal hypoxia. These changes may present as a severe, sudden deceleration, often with prolonged bradycardia, or recurrent moderate-to-severe variable decelerations.

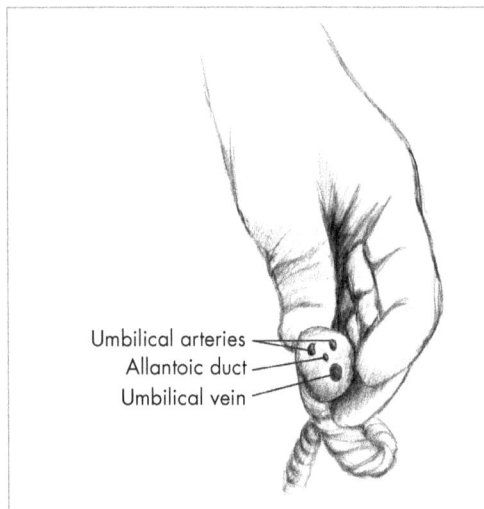

Umbilical arteries
Allantoic duct
Umbilical vein

Figure 32.3 Anatomy of the umbilical cord

Malpresentations increase the risk of cord prolapse during rupturing of membranes. Historically, cord prolapse has been associated with poor neonatal outcomes, but improved outcomes can be attributed to the increased availability of Caesarean delivery and improved neonatal resuscitation efforts.

Incidence

Umbilical cord prolapse occurs in less than 1 per cent of all births (Wikipedia, 2017c).

Risk factors

The main precipitating event is rupture of membranes (ROM), whether spontaneous, premature, during labour or performed artificially by a healthcare professional. Other factors include:
▶ artificial rupture of membranes (AROM) (especially if the fetal head or presenting part is not engaged)
▶ placement of a fetal scalp electrode or an intrauterine pressure catheter
▶ amnioinfusion
▶ attempted rotation of the fetal head from occipitoposterior (OP) to occipitoanterior (OA)
▶ external cephalic version (ECV), internal version or breech extraction
▶ fetal malpresentations (breech, shoulder, transverse, extended fetal head)
▶ fetal anomalies
▶ fetal growth restriction or small for gestational age (SGA) and prematurity
▶ uterine distension due to polyhydramnios, multiple gestation (this may result in an increased risk of malpresentations) and grand multiparity
▶ umbilical cord abnormalities such as a longer cord than usual (> 80 cm) and low implantation of the placenta.

Prevention

Preventing cord prolapse is the preferred medical approach, but there is no evidence that knowledge of risk factors can reduce the occurrence of cord prolapse. The midwife should be knowledgeable of the risks when undertaking obstetric interventions.

Preventative measures include:
▶ avoidance of an amniotomy until the fetal head is well engaged, or performing a slower, more controlled release of fluid
▶ applying mild fundal pressure during placement of a fetal scalp electrode or intrauterine pressure catheter if the vertex is not well applied to the cervix
▶ advising the mother to remain in bed after AROM until a prolapse and FHR abnormalities can be excluded.

Diagnosis

The diagnosis of a prolapsed cord is made on vaginal examination. A palpable, soft, pulsating mass can be felt within or seen visibly extruding from the vagina, necessitating an urgent Caesarean delivery. With prolapse, fetal bradycardia (< 120 bpm) and variable decelerations of the fetal heart rate will be observed. (See Figure 26.8 on page 406.)

Principles

Cord prolapse results in fetal hypoxia, and if not rapidly managed, can lead to long-term disability or death.

Prompt delivery, usually by Caesarean section within 30 minutes, has been shown to improve neonatal outcomes. If the health professional is of the opinion that a vaginal delivery can be performed more rapidly than a Caesarean delivery, vaginal delivery should be facilitated.

From the time of diagnosis until surgery can be performed, all efforts should be made to reduce pressure on the fetal presenting part. On discovery of the loop of cord, the midwife's gloved fingers are left in the vagina and the presenting part is pushed upward to relieve cord compression, as shown in Figure 32.4 and described in the procedure box below. Note that palpation of the cord causes vasospasm, potentially leading to a worse outcome.

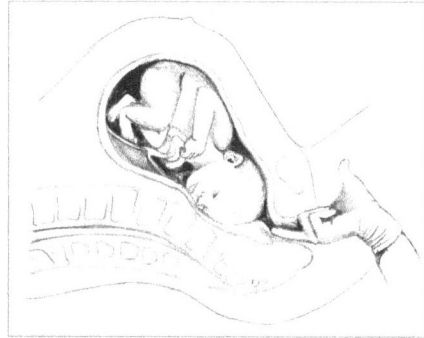

Figure 32.4 Reducing pressure on the cord

PROCEDURE	Management of a prolapsed umbilical cord

Confirm gestational age (GA) and FHR with a fetoscope or Doppler, as delivering a pre-viable or demised fetus via Caesarean provides no benefit.

If the fetus is alive (the fetal heart is heard) and viable (estimated weight ≥ 1 kg), perform a vaginal examination to diagnose the stage of labour:

▶ If the *cervix is fully dilated* and the fetal head has engaged in the pelvis, immediately deliver the baby by vacuum extraction or forceps if necessary.

▶ If the cervix is *not fully dilated*, make arrangements or let the assistant call for an urgent Caesarean section and/or an emergency transfer to hospital.

Call for help and inform the mother of the emergency.

Ask an assistant to administer 4–6 ℓ per minute via facemask and insert an IV line.

If the woman is in the first stage of labour, do the following:
1. Put on sterile gloves.
2. Insert the dominant hand into the vagina.
3. Place the other hand on the abdomen in the suprapubic region to keep the presenting part out of the pelvis.
4. Once the presenting part is firmly held above the pelvic brim, remove the dominant hand from the vagina.
5. Administer salbutamol 0.5 mg IV slowly over two minutes to reduce contractions.
6. Perform an immediate Caesarean section.

If the woman is in the second stage of labour, do the following:
1. Expedite delivery with an episiotomy and vacuum extraction or forceps.
2. Prepare for resuscitation of the newborn.

If there is a time delay in performing the surgery, do the following:
1. Place two fingers or an entire hand into the vagina to elevate the presenting part off the cord.
2. Place mother in the knee-chest or steep Trendelenburg position.
3. Consider bladder filling. In this procedure, called Vago's method, the assistant inserts an indwelling urinary catheter (at least a size 18 Foley catheter), fills the bladder with 400–500 ml of saline and then clamps. The enlarging bladder provides upward pressure on the fetus, thus alleviating the compression on the cord. This may inhibit uterine contractions, which would further relieve pressure on the cord.
4. The assistant monitors FHR to see if the cord compression is adequately relieved (the baseline will rise above 110 bpm).

continued

5   The midwife maintains the position (hand in the vagina, reducing the pressure on the umbilical cord) until the fetus is born via Caesarean section.

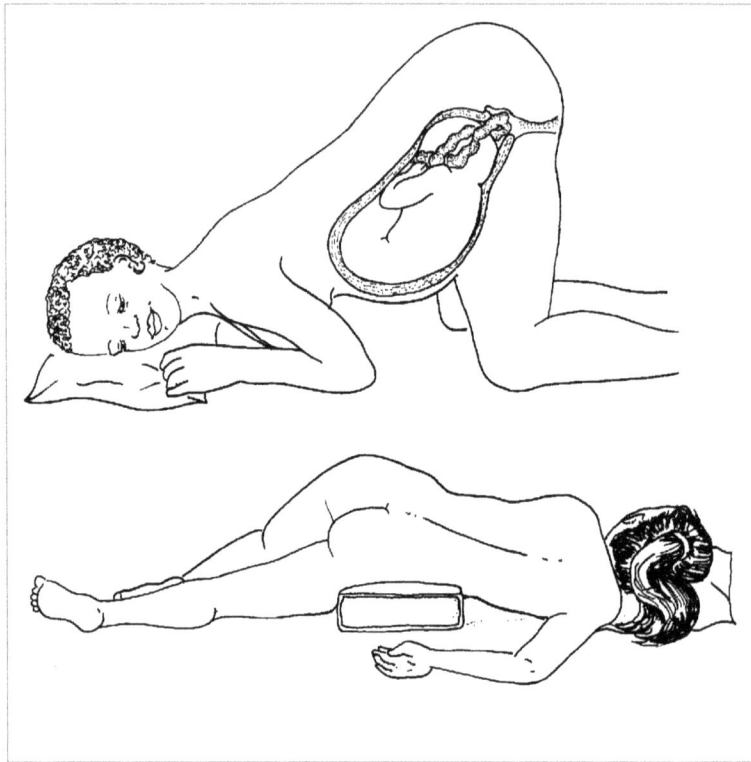

Figure 32A Knee-chest position and exaggerated Sims' position to relieve pressure on the umbilical cord

Tocolysis appears to be a useful adjunct, especially if FHR decelerations persist after the primary procedures have been performed. Administer salbutanol 250 mcg (half of a 500 mcg ampoule diluted in 20 ml saline) IV as a single dose, or salbutamol 250 mcg (half of a 500 mcg ampoule diluted in 20 ml saline) IV slowly as a single dose.

If cord prolapse is present through the introitus:
1   Replace the cord gently into the vaginal vault using wet gauze if there is a prolonged interval before delivery to prevent vasospasm and potentially worse outcomes.
2   A moist tampon or 4 x 4 gauze can then be inserted gently into the vagina below the cord to help hold it in place.
3   If cord compression is relieved, place the woman in the left lateral (Sims) position, with a pillow under the hips.

During transfer, in the delivery unit or operating room, do the following:
▶ Verify FHR and obtain a tracing.
▶ A Caesarean section is not indicated if the fetus is deceased.

Also see Figure 32.2 on page 501.

Recording and interpretation
▶ Document and date all activities.
▶ Store the cardiotocograph (CTG) tracings in a safe place.
▶ Write an incident report.
▶ Document all resuscitation efforts.

32.5   Shoulder dystocia

Shoulder dystocia is an obstetric emergency where, after the delivery of the head, the anterior shoulder of the infant fails to pass below the pubic symphysis. If the infant is not delivered, fetal demise can occur due to compression of the umbilical cord within the birth canal. Special manoeuvres are necessary in order to deliver the shoulders.

Incidence

The incidence of shoulder dystocia is between 0.5 and 1 per cent (Lerner, 2017).

Risk factors

Although there are well-recognised risk factors for shoulder dystocia, such as pre-gestational and gestational diabetes, fetal macrosomia (a birth weight of over 4.5 kg) and maternal obesity, it is often difficult to predict.

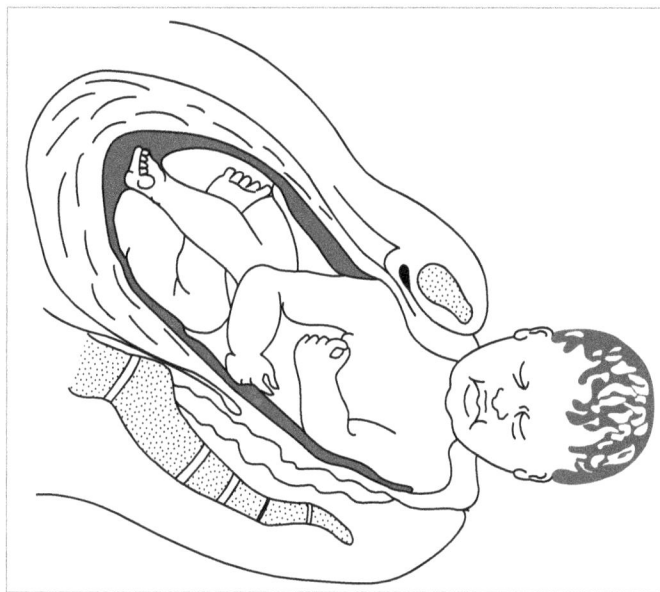

Figure 32.5 The mechanism of shoulder dystocia

Fetal macrosomia is a major risk factor for shoulder dystocia. It is not possible to accurately predict shoulder dystocia by estimating fetal size and ultrasound is not reliable in predicting macrosomia. Macrosomia is as difficult to predict in the diabetic mother as it is in the non-diabetic mother. A checklist is completed, patient data are entered and graphical and numerical estimates of personalised risk are produced.

Maternal risk factors include:
- being over the age of 35 years
- being short in stature
- a small or abnormal pelvis
- post-term pregnancy (more than 42 weeks' gestation)
- multiparity
- a previous macrosomic infant
- previous shoulder dystocia – seen more commonly with increased maternal age, obesity and multiparity

- a history of large siblings
- excessive maternal weight gain
- a fetus of the male gender.

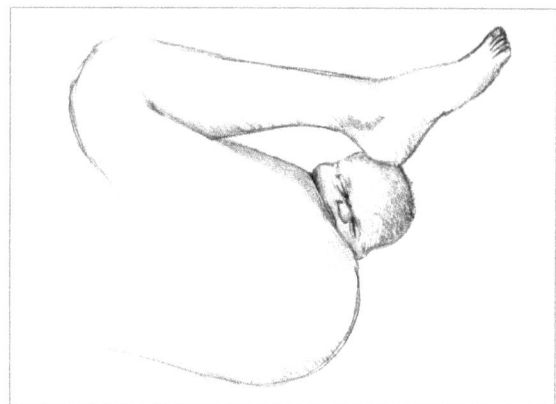

Figure 32.6 The turtle sign

Intrapartum risk factors or warning signs include:
- a prolonged or arrested first or active stage of labour
- prolonged descent of the fetal head or failure thereof
- the need for oxytocics to stimulate contractions
- the turtle sign (see Figure 32.6) and fetal head bobbing in the second stage
- a protracted second stage of labour; the need for assisted delivery
- the absence of shoulder rotation or descent.

PROCEDURE Management of shoulder dystocia

Principles

Shoulder dystocia cannot be predicted with any degree of accuracy from either clinical characteristics or labour abnormalities. Expect shoulder dystocia at all deliveries, especially if a large baby is anticipated. Note the following points:

- Several professionals are needed to help minimise maternal and fetal trauma.
- Prepare for newborn resuscitation when shoulder dystocia occurs.
- Interventions in case of shoulder dystocia should progress from least to most invasive, thereby reducing harm to the mother in the event that the infant delivers with one of the earlier manoeuvres.
- Shoulder dystocia injuries (brachial plexus or cerebral palsy, fetal demise) is an important area of medicolegal concern.

Diagnosis

- The 'turtle' sign occurs: the fetal head appears and retracts.
- There is definite recoil of the head back against the perineum and when the fetal head is delivered it remains tightly applied to the vulva.
- The chin retracts and depresses the perineum and it is often necessary to push the perineum back to deliver the face.
- Traction on the head fails to deliver the shoulder, which is caught behind the symphysis pubis.
- Due to friction with the vulva, the head is incapable of movement and therefore restitution rarely takes place.
- Traction on the head and pressure from above fail to deliver the baby.
- The baby's face is erythematous and puffy, indicative of facial flushing.

Procedure

In shoulder dystocia, the time to deliver the baby is limited because of the possibility of brain damage and death. Do the following:

1. Call for help and mobilise all available staff (midwives, medical practitioners, paediatrician).
2. Explain to the woman what is happening and ask for her full co-operation.
3. Perform a wide episiotomy to reduce soft tissue obstruction, to allow space for manipulation and to ensure a speedy delivery once the shoulder is dislodged.
4. Place the woman in an exaggerated flexed position (on her back). Hyperflex the mother's legs tightly onto her abdomen (see Figure 32B). This widens the pelvis and flattens the lumbar spine.
5. Move the mother to the side of the bed, with her buttocks hanging slightly over the edge, her legs supported by the assistants.
6. The assistants assist the woman on either side by pushing and holding her flexed thighs and knees so that her knees almost touch her shoulders. This will allow more space to apply downward pressure on the fetus.
7. If this manoeuvre does not succeed, an assistant applies suprapubic pressure (Rubin I).
8. Wearing sterile gloves, apply firm, continuous traction on the fetal head simultaneously with suprapubic pressure to assist delivery of the shoulder. *Do not apply fundal pressure*, as this will result in a further impacted shoulder and may cause uterine rupture.

If the shoulder is still not delivered, perform *anterior shoulder dis-impaction*:

1. Insert a hand into the vagina, along the baby's back behind the posterior shoulder of the fetus.

continued

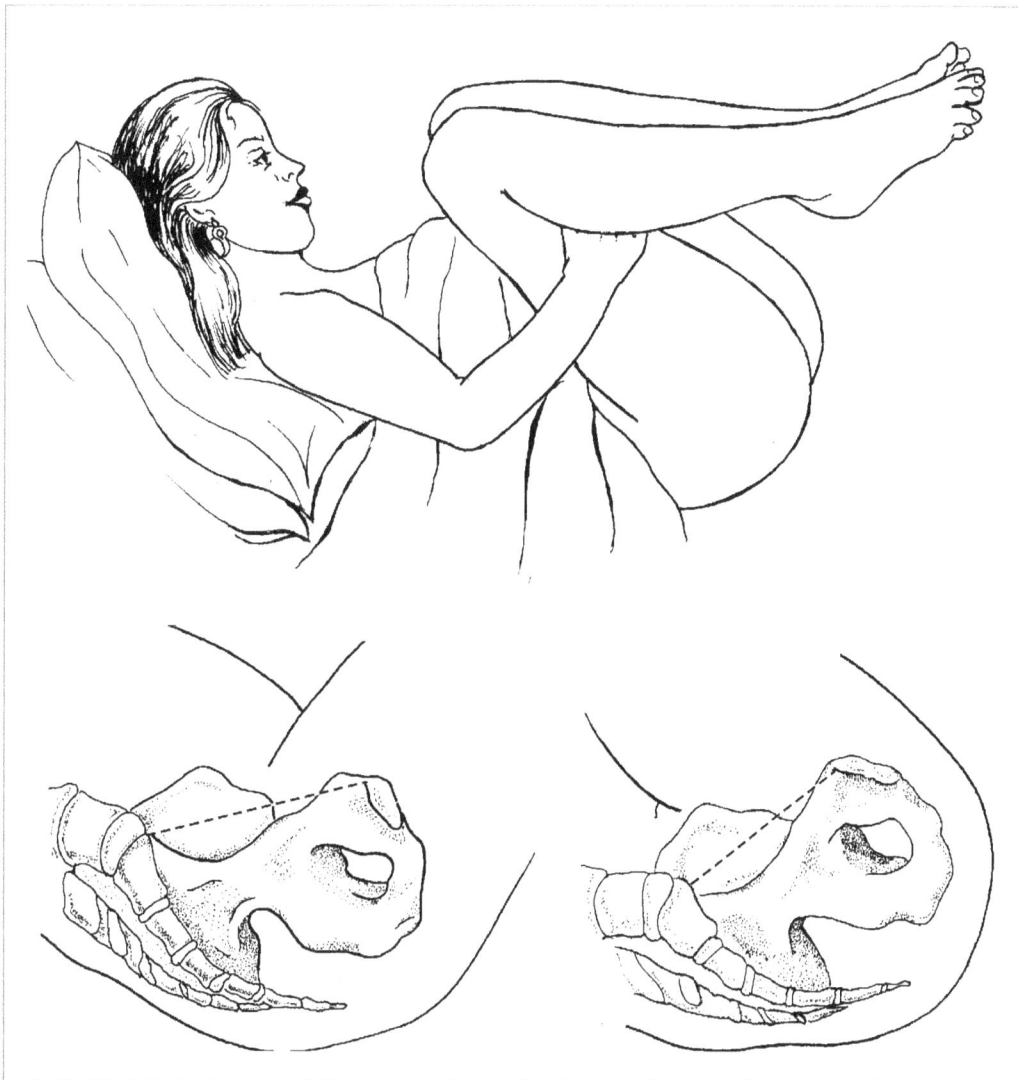

Figure 32B Technique to relieve shoulder dystocia (McRobert's manoeuvre)

2 Apply pressure to the shoulder that is anterior to the direction of the baby's sternum to rotate the shoulder and decrease the diameters of the shoulder.
3 Rotate the shoulder 180 degrees in a corkscrew manner so that the impacted anterior shoulder is released.
4 If needed, apply pressure to the posterior shoulder in the direction of the sternum.

If the shoulder is still not delivered, perform the *Rubin II manoeuvre* (manual delivery of posterior arm):
1 Place a hand behind the posterior shoulder of the fetus and locate the arm.
2 Sweep this arm across the fetal chest and deliver it.
3 With the posterior arm and shoulder now delivered, it is relatively easy to rotate the baby, dislodge the anterior shoulder and allow delivery of the remainder of the baby.

continued

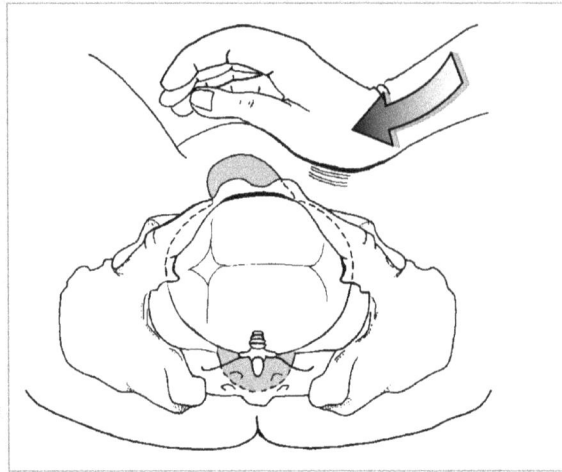

Figure 32C Correct application of suprapubic pressure

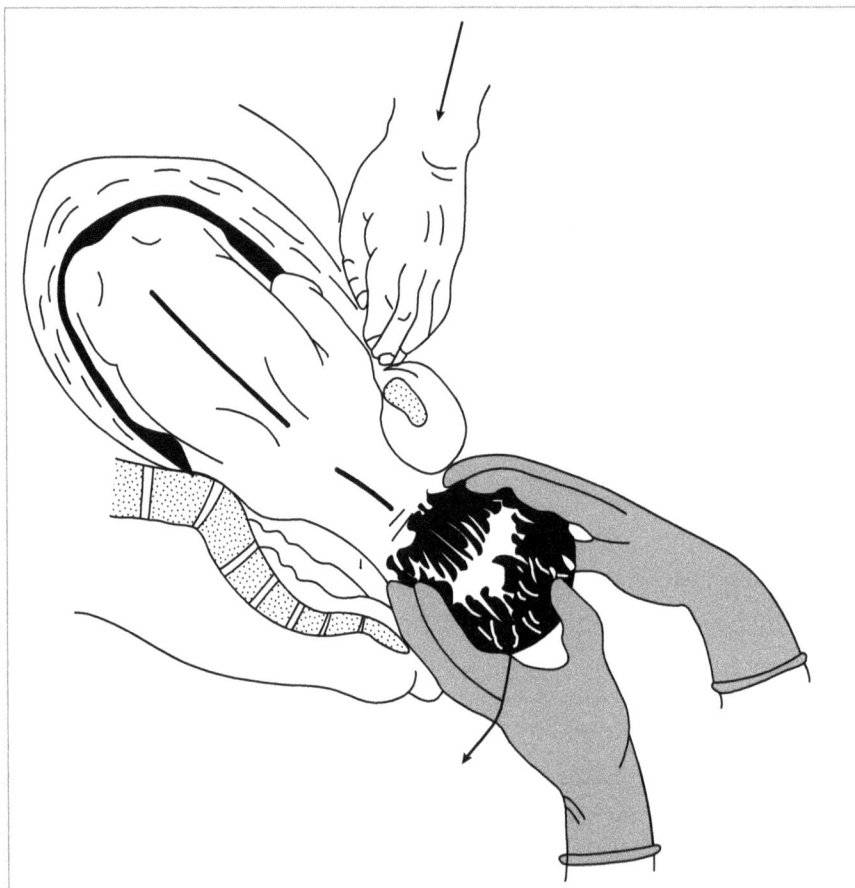

Figure 32D The management of shoulder dystocia: Backward traction of the head, together with pressure on the abdomen above the symphysis pubis, pushing the anterior shoulder downwards

continued

A.

B.

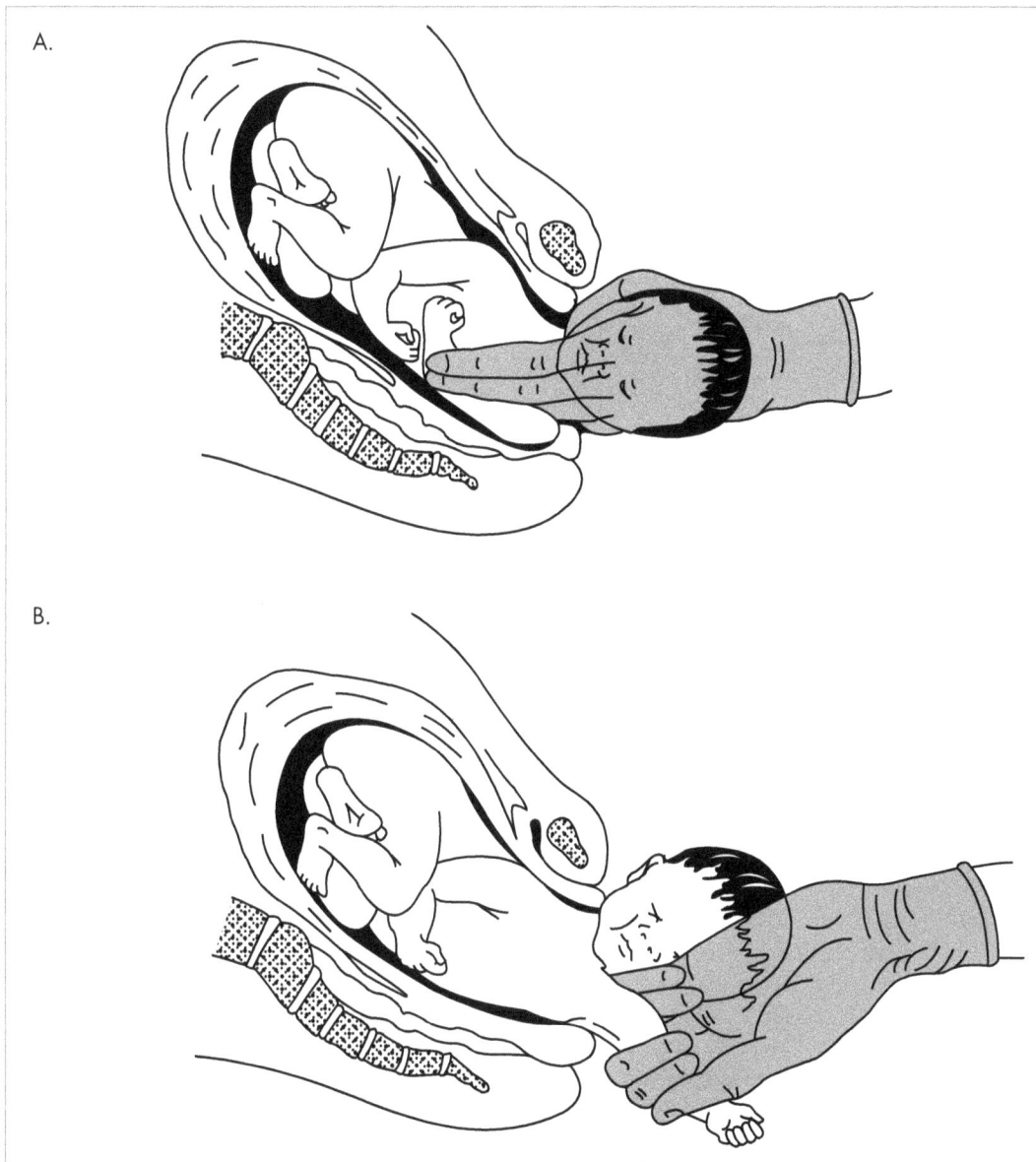

Figure 32E Extraction of the posterior shoulder in shoulder dystocia

If the shoulder is still not delivered, perform *Woods' screw manoeuvre*:

▶ The posterior shoulder is rotated progressively in a corkscrew fashion. This will release the opposite impacted anterior shoulder.

▶ In the classic description of this manoeuvre, the midwife applies pressure to the anterior surface of the posterior shoulder.

▶ The baby moves through 180 degrees through the face-to-pubis position. The posterior shoulder is brought forward and becomes anterior.

continued

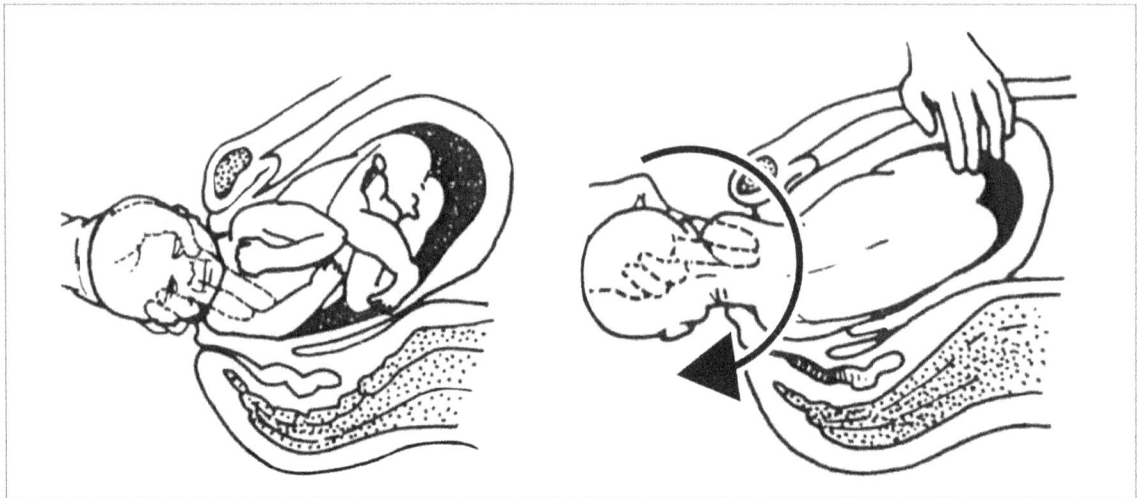

Figure 32F Woods' screw manoeuvre

Extreme measures

▶ *Gaskin manoeuvre:* This involves moving the mother onto her hands and knees (the all fours position) with the back arched, which widens the pelvic outlet to allow rotational movement of the sacroiliac joints. This results in a 1–2 cm increase in the anteroposterior (AP) diameter of the pelvic outlet, which dis-impacts the shoulder and allows it to slide over the sacral promontory.

▶ *Intentional clavicular fracture:* The purpose is to decrease the width of the shoulders and free the shoulder that is anterior.

▶ *Zavanelli's manoeuvre:* This involves pushing the fetal head back in (internal cephalic replacement) under tocolysis, followed by Caesarean section. Alternatively, internal cephalic replacement and/or a maternal symphysiotomy is done. The latter makes the opening of the birth canal larger by breaking the connective tissue between the two pubic bones, facilitating the passage of the shoulders.

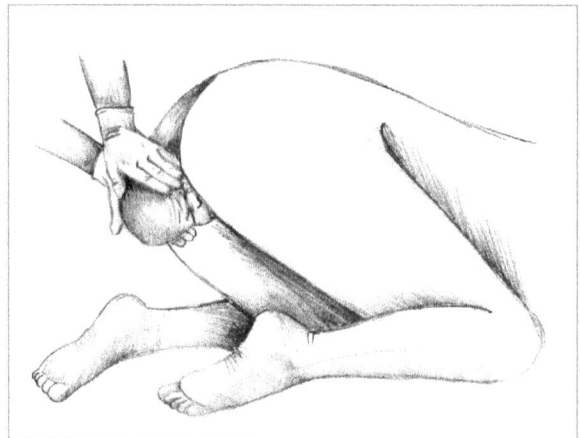

Figure 32G The Gaskin maneouvre

▶ *O'Shaughnessy abdominal rescue:* A hysterotomy facilitates vaginal delivery of the impacted shoulder.

Salvage manoeuvres

1   The posterior axillary sling traction is the procedure where a loop of a suction catheter is pushed under the armpit of the posterior arm of the fetus.
2   The edges of that catheter are used as traction to pull down the shoulder.
3   As soon as the shoulder is lowered, a hand is inserted into the vagina to deliver that particular shoulder.

Care after delivery

1   Prepare to resuscitate a severely asphyxiated baby. If the baby has suffered hypoxia, the baby's body will be limp and white, while the head will be congested and livid.

continued

2   If birth took place in the hospital, call the paediatrician.
3   If the baby is not breathing, initiate basic emergency resuscitation through the use of bag and mask. This will be followed by comprehensive resuscitation of an unresponsive newborn by the paediatrician.
4   A full examination must be carried out for injuries. The mother must be examined for lacerations and trauma of the genital tract and observed for postpartum haemorrhage (PPH).
5   The baby is nursed in the high-care ward.
6   As soon as the mother's condition is stable, she should be allowed to see and hold her baby.

Recording and interpretation
▶ Document and date all activities; also state the type of manoeuvre used to facilitate birth.
▶ Store CTG tracings in a safe place.
▶ Write an incident report.
▶ Document all resuscitation efforts.

Complications

Maternal complications include:
▶ an increased incidence of PPH
▶ uterine rupture
▶ perineal lacerations and extensions of an episiotomy
▶ the risk of postpartum infection
▶ temporary postpartum bladder atony because of the pressure directed upwards towards the bladder by the anterior shoulder
▶ occasional separation of the maternal symphyseal joint
▶ damage to the lateral femoral cutaneous nerve as a result of over-aggressive hyperflexion of the maternal legs.

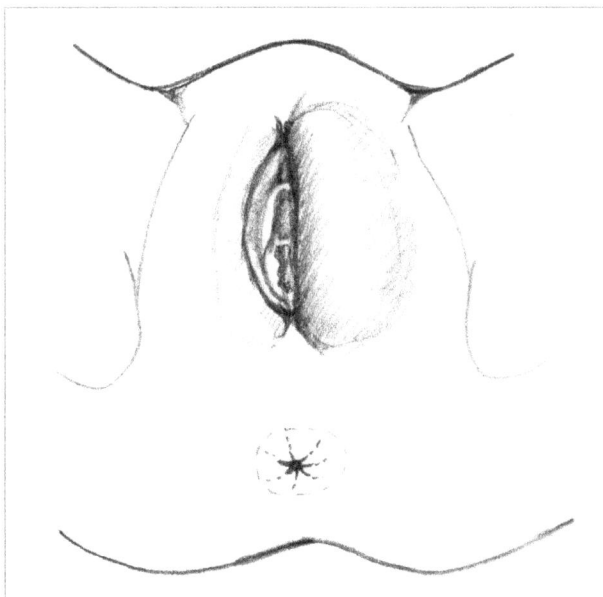

Figure 32.7 Perineal trauma and haematoma

Fetal complications include the following:
▶ Despite appropriate obstetric management, fetal injury (such as brachial plexus injury) or even fetal death may occur.
▶ Fetal asphyxia may occur, as the umbilical cord is compressed tightly between the baby's body and the birth canal; this significantly decreases or totally cuts off blood flow.
▶ If the pressure on the cord is not rapidly relieved, fetal hypoxia occurs, resulting in cerebral palsy.
▶ Damage to the upper brachial plexus nerves may occur, resulting in Klumpke paralysis and Erb's Palsy.

32.6   Acute inversion of the uterus

Uterine inversion occurs when the uterine fundus collapses into the endometrial cavity. It is a rare complication of vaginal delivery, but when it occurs, it is a life-threatening obstetric emergency. If not promptly recognised and treated, uterine inversion can lead to severe haemorrhage, shock and maternal death, depending on the degree of inversion.

Incidence

The incidence of acute uterine inversion ranges from 1:1 500 to 1:2 000 (Wikipedia, 2016).

Classification of inversion

The following different types of inversion occur:
▶ *Partial inversion:* The inverted fundus appears at the cervix.
▶ *First-degree inversion:* The fundus inverts as far as the body of the uterus.
▶ *Second-degree inversion:* The fundus reaches the vagina.
▶ *Third-degree inversion:* The fundus is turned completely inside out.

Predisposing factors

Factors which may predispose a woman to uterine inversion include:

▶ abnormalities of the uterine contents
▶ a short umbilical cord
▶ neoplasm of the uterus
▶ fundal implantation of the placenta
▶ an adherent placenta, such as placenta accreta
▶ weakness of the uterine wall at the placental site
▶ congenital anomalies of the uterus, such as bicornuate uterus
▶ a disturbance in the contractile mechanism of the uterus
▶ relaxation of the myometrium
▶ general anaesthesia, which has the potential for relaxing the uterus as well as the cervix
▶ an overstretched uterus (polyhydramnios and multiple pregnancy).

Causes

The usual cause of inversion of the uterus is mismanagement of the third stage of labour. It is brought about by the following:

▶ Undue traction on the umbilical cord in a patient with an atonic uterus – that is, instead of using *controlled* cord traction, only cord traction is undertaken – may result in inversion.
▶ Excessive fundal pressure on the uterus to expel the placenta could cause uterine inversion. (Using the fundus of the uterus as a piston should never be done.)
▶ The use of Credé's manoeuvre (squeezing or kneading the uterus) to deliver the placenta can easily cause uterine inversion. This technique is not used anymore.
▶ Hasty manual separation and extraction of an adherent placenta can cause acute inversion.
▶ Uterine inversion could occur when abdominal pressure is increased suddenly in the third stage of labour during coughing, sneezing or vomiting.
▶ Uterine inversion sometimes occurs spontaneously for unknown reasons.
▶ Failure to actively deliver the placenta could lead to uterine inversion.

The clinical picture and diagnosis

The following clinical picture unfolds as acute inversion of the uterus occurs with traction on the cord:

▶ The cord is advanced and the woman experiences increased abdominal pain.
▶ The placenta is still attached or partially attached to the inside of the uterus. It looks like a greyish-blue mass that protrudes from the vagina. This is usually accompanied by profuse vaginal bleeding, particularly if the placenta is partially or completely separated.
▶ The uterus cannot be palpated in the abdomen. (In a partial inversion of the uterus, a cup-shaped depression is palpated in the upper portion of the uterus.)
▶ The woman feels excruciating pain, combined with an 'explosive' sensation of fullness in the vagina. (The pain is caused by the stretching of the Fallopian tubes and the broad ligament, which leads to tension on the ovaries and stretching of the peritoneal nerves.)
▶ Profound shock results, manifested by sweating, pallor, tachycardia (and later bradycardia) and hypotension.
▶ Vaginal bleeding occurs, which may be watery.

If untreated, the following course of events will result:

1. With inversion of the uterus, contraction of the lower uterine segment occurs, producing a cervical constriction ring.
2. This leads to oedema of the lower inverted portion of the uterus below the constriction ring.
3. This in turn results in a reduction of the blood supply to the inverted portion of the uterus.

Complications

Uterine inversion is an extremely dangerous condition and in serious cases the patient may die from shock due to severe pain and the damage to tissues and/or from haemorrhage. Further complications include:

▶ excruciating pain
▶ profuse haemorrhage
▶ profound shock
▶ oedema of the uterus, which can lead to reduced blood supply with gangrene, necrosis and sloughing of the portion of the uterus that is constricted by the cervix
▶ air embolism
▶ infection and sepsis
▶ anuria
▶ urinary retention.

Partial inversion

Partial inversion of the uterus may not be acute and may be diagnosed immediately or over a period of hours.

In this condition, the woman complains of pain and continues to bleed vaginally, losing blood constantly. Shock is associated with the pain and hypovolaemia develops gradually. Any woman who complains of constant pain with vaginal bleeding (often watery blood) should receive attention.

Prevention

It is essential to actively manage the third stage of labour. In addition, prevention includes the following:

▶ Avoid the use of fundal pressure in the second and third stages of labour.
▶ Deliver the placenta with controlled cord traction and counteraction above the symphysis pubis and not using fundal pressure.
▶ *Never* use Credé's manoeuvre to deliver the placenta.
▶ Identify risk factors.

Interventions

Immediate interventions

Upon diagnosis, do the following immediately:

▶ Urgently send for medical assistance and an anaesthetist.
▶ Raise the foot end of the bed and try to maintain the inverted mass within the vagina (rather than allowing it to hang right out of the vagina).
▶ Withhold uterotonic agents (misoprostol and oxytocin).
▶ Avoid separating the placenta, if still attached, to decrease bleeding.
▶ Administer 40 per cent oxygen by face mask.
▶ Monitor the pulse rate and BP every five minutes and record.
▶ Start a large-bore needle IV infusion using an electrolyte solution.
▶ Catheterise the patient to empty the bladder.

If no medical practitioner is readily available, it is important to treat the profound shock first and then attempt to replace the uterus. These can be done simultaneously if an assistant is available.

Medical interventions

The ideal medical intervention is to immediately replace the uterus into its normal position. If this is not possible, other emergency treatment must be undertaken:

▶ Provide adequate analgesia. For example, Entonox® can be used or, if this is not available, pethidine or morphine could be given. A general anaesthesia, after written consent has been obtained, is the second choice of management.
▶ Elevate the foot end of the bed and place the patient in the reverse Trendelenberg position.
▶ Replace the uterus under general anaesthesia by first replacing the part of the uterus that inverted last. In other words, the portion of the uterus adjacent to the cervix (the lower segment) is replaced first, and then the upper segment, with the fundus being replaced last.

32.7 Amniotic fluid embolism

Amniotic fluid embolism is a syndrome in which there is a sudden development of acute respiratory distress, shock and collapse, caused by an infusion of a large amount of amniotic fluid into the maternal circulation. The onset is very sudden and occurs during labour or soon after delivery. The amniotic fluid enters the maternal circulation through a laceration (which may be very small) in the uterus, usually the lower segment.

Although this is a rare condition, it is very dangerous, because a large percentage (25 per cent) of women who experience amniotic fluid embolism die within an hour from respiratory distress and shock (Knight et al, 2012). Women who do survive often develop disseminated intravascular coagulation (DIC).

Incidence

The incidence of amniotic fluid embolism is 9–12:100 000 births (Knight et al, 2012). The condition is often undiagnosed.

Causes

Any condition in which the uterine muscle is cut or may tear easily, or where strong contractions bring about tearing of the uterine muscle, is a likely cause of amniotic fluid embolism. Most cases occur in women aged over 30 years. Fifty per cent of cases have antenatal complications. Specific causes are discussed below.

Relaxed and overstretched uterus

This condition could be caused by:

▶ a multiple pregnancy
▶ polyhydramnios
▶ a maternal age of over 30 years
▶ macrosomia
▶ meconium in the liquor
▶ strong uterine contractions, prolonged labour
▶ operative interventions
▶ a Caesarean section.

Manipulation and assisted delivery

Complications may follow where there is an increased incidence of manipulation and assisted delivery, such as:

▶ manual rotation of the head
▶ forceps delivery
▶ vacuum extraction
▶ uterine rupture
▶ internal podalic version (IPV)
▶ external version
▶ manual removal of the placenta

- intrauterine catheters and electrodes
- overstimulation of the uterine muscle by the use of oxytocin and prostaglandins, as in induction of labour (IOL) or augmentation of labour.

Signs and symptoms

The clinical features of amniotic fluid embolism include:

- sudden, profound, unexpected shock during or immediately after labour
- chills, shivering and pallor
- sudden extreme respiratory distress, with severe dyspnoea, cyanosis and restlessness
- a sudden, acute drop in BP
- a weak, rapid pulse
- vomiting
- the rapid onset of pulmonary oedema and acute respiratory embarrassment but with no cardiac disease
- generalised bleeding from DIC.

Amniotic fluid embolism is usually diagnosed on post-mortem examination, when components of the liquor are identified in the maternal lungs and circulation. Histology of the lungs will reveal:

- oedema
- alveolar haemorrhages
- emboli consisting of fetal squamous cells, fat, mucin, bile and lanugo
- dilated pulmonary vessels at the area of embolisation.

Differential diagnosis

Other conditions that could be confused with amniotic fluid embolism are:

- pulmonary embolism from a deep vein thrombosis (DVT)
- air or blood embolism
- fat embolism
- Mendelson's syndrome
- eclampsia

- anaphylaxis, which can be caused by hypersensitivity to medication, or mismanagement of the administration of medication
- a cerebrovascular accident
- congestive cardiac failure
- acute inversion of the uterus
- a ruptured uterus
- haemorrhagic shock.

Interventions

Send for a medical practitioner immediately and treat the patient as for shock. The medical practitioner will administer medications, such as aminophylline, to relax the pulmonary airways and vessels. If the patient survives, the medical practitioner will treat her for DIC with the administration of blood, fibrinogen and, in some specific cases, heparin.

32.8   Conclusion

Midwives are the primary caregivers of women in pregnancy, labour and childbirth, and the postnatal period. They are also responsible for the immediate care of the newborn. Emergency support may not always be available, so the midwife needs to be able to identify women at risk for emergencies in the antenatal period and early in labour and understand the principles of emergency treatment. An adult emergency trolley must always be updated and ready. All staff attending women across all stages of pregnancy – including newborn care – should attend the Essential Steps in Management of Obstetric Emergencies (ESMOE) programme annually. In addition, all staff should frequently attend and do skills drills.

This chapter reviewed emergencies that may occur in pregnancy and in labour. Other conditions that may require emergency interventions, such as eclampsia, shock, haemorrhage, infections and anaphylaxis, are reviewed in other chapters.

33

Major obstetric interventions

LEARNING OBJECTIVES

On completion of this chapter, you must be able to:
▶ identify major obstetric procedures and interventions associated with birth
▶ identify obstetric procedures and interventions that are common in all settings
▶ identify standards for obstetric procedures and interventions performed at specific levels of care
▶ develop competence in the role of the midwife in delivering a high standard of care during obstetric procedures.

KNOWLEDGE ASSUMED TO BE IN PLACE

Basic knowledge, skill and competency in the care of a normal birth

KEYWORDS

Caesarean section • general and regional anaesthetic • symphysiotomy • haemolytic anaemia, elevated liver enzymes, low platelet count (HELLP) syndrome

33.1 Introduction

This chapter details the interventions that are considered important in obstetrics and which are usually carried out in a hospital. Obstetric interventions do not fall within the scope of practice of the midwife. The midwife's scope of practice focuses on the normal. Most interventions are performed by a medical practitioner, preferably an obstetrician. Alternatively, they are prescribed by an obstetrician and the care is instituted and given under his or her direct or indirect supervision.

The role of the midwife is to:
▶ know the clinical and legal boundaries and scope of practice in South Africa
▶ have up-to-date knowledge of the clinical principles of obstetric interventions (indications, contraindications and complications)
▶ be aware of the norms and standards for procedures in the health facility's clinical manual
▶ attend regular in-service training or skills drills
▶ be experienced in the various interventions
▶ be competent in life-saving practices
▶ be aware of and use the protocols of the healthcare system and of the particular setting wherein midwifery

is practised – see the current and latest *Guidelines for Maternity Care in South Africa* (DoH, 2015)
▶ be a co-developer of norms and standards of clinical care, equipment and staff for quality and effective procedures
▶ be a manager and supervisor
▶ take responsibility for evaluation of the outcomes of care.

33.2 Caesarean section

A Caesarean, or C-section, is defined as a surgical procedure performed for the purpose of extracting a viable fetus through an incision in the abdominal wall and the uterus. The operation can be performed either under general anaesthesia or under epidural anaesthesia.

In most instances, the purpose of the procedure is to deliver a live baby. The removal of a fetus and the products of conception through the abdominal wall before viability (26–28 weeks) is called a hysterotomy.

Incidence

The WHO recommends an acceptable level of 10 to 15 per cent Caesarean sections in healthcare systems (WHO, 2015). In South Africa, the private sector has a 45 per cent Caesarean section rate and the public sector increased its Caesarean section rate from an average of 16.1 per cent in 2009 to 22.7 per cent in 2015 in district hospitals, with a variation of 41 per cent in metro areas to 8.9 per cent in rural areas (Massyn et al, 2015).

General reasons why Caesarean sections are carried out include (Massyn et al, 2015):

- arrested labour: 30 per cent
- repeat Caesarean section: 20 per cent
- breech: 10 per cent
- fetal distress: 10 per cent.

HIV is no longer a reason for doing a Caesarean section, because most women are on antiretroviral therapy (ART) and their minimal viral load makes normal vaginal delivery quite safe. Little is gained by doing a Caesarean section. However, if the viral load is high (treatment failure or untreated), a case can be made for an elective Caesarean section.

Caesarean section and mortality

Although Caesarean section is a relatively safe procedure in well-resourced settings, it remains a risk for maternal mortality in less-resourced settings, particularly at district level in South Africa. Caesarean section at this level contributes to maternal mortality in South Africa. Deaths due to Caesarean section are mainly due to anaesthetics or bleeding. Risks in low-resource settings include the *lack* of:

- experience and skill in surgical methods
- skills to suture the uterus to control haemorrhage
- blood replacement therapy to replace blood loss
- antibiotics to control infection

- experience in anaesthetics and anaesthesiology
- skilled post-operative nursing care and advocacy
- standard equipment, theatre and care.

It is important that the means and skills to perform a Caesarean section are in place when needed.

Activity: Bleeding and Caesarean section

Study the guidelines for bleeding and Caesarean section on pages 55 and 64 in the *Guidelines for Maternity Care in South Africa* (DoH, 2015).

Classification

Caesarean section is classified as follows:

- *Upper segment Caesarean:* This is an incision into the upper muscular segment. It is also known as classical Caesarean section.
- *Lower segment Caesarean:* This is an incision into the lower segment (that develops after 28 weeks of pregnancy), which is less vascular and has fewer muscle fibres. Lower-segment Caesarean section has improved outcomes for follow-up Caesarean sections.
- *Elective Caesarean:* This refers to a Caesarean section decided on before labour starts.
- *Emergency Caesarean:* This is demanded by a risk factor or a life-threatening situation that develops during labour.

Indications

Table 33.1 shows the various maternal, fetal and obstetric aspects that indicate a Caesarean section.

Table 33.1

Indications for Caesarean section

Maternal	Fetal	Obstetric
Congenital abnormality of the uterus	Fetal abnormalities	Poor obstetric history
Soft tissue scarring	Genetic disease	Cephalopelvic disproportion (CPD)
Cone biopsy	Fetal compromise	Obstructed labour
Tumours	Fetal distress	Contracted pelvis
Previous uterine surgery	Intrauterine growth restriction (IUGR)	Malpresentation or breech presentation
Hysterotomy	Multiple pregnancy	Uterine dysfunction
Myomectomy	Erythroblastosis fetalis	Cervical dystocia
Carcinoma		Antepartum haemorrhage (APH)
Previous cervical cerclage		Failed induction
Eclampsia		Elderly primigravida
Active herpes infection		Cord prolapse
Failed assisted delivery		

Advantages

Caesarean section is the safest method of delivery for many of the complications of pregnancy and/or possible complications of labour. The complications of an elective Caesarean section are 50 per cent lower than those of an emergency Caesarean section.

In addition, surgical sterilisation can be combined with Caesarean section.

Disadvantages

Overall, the rate of complications in Caesarean section is six times higher than for vaginal delivery. The risk for anaesthetic complications in obstetrics is doubled (Massyn et al, 2015).

The following aspects lead to higher costs and a longer stay in hospital, as well as a protracted recovery period:
- Analgesia and anaesthesia become necessities.
- There is post-operative pain and discomfort from the surgical incision and the general anaesthetic. However, these can now be controlled with the availability of epidural anaesthesia.
- There is an abdominal wound with scarring and risk of infections.
- It is more difficult to care for the baby after birth due to pain and discomfort.

In addition, Caesarean section reduces the woman's future childbearing options.

Contraindications

Caesarean section is major surgery and should only be performed by competent and skilled surgeons in a well-resourced environment that adheres to the norms and standards of staff and equipment for an acceptable obstetric indication.

It should be avoided, if possible, in cases of:
- cardiac disease
- diabetes mellitus
- intrauterine death (IUD)
- a fetus with immature lungs
- a preterm fetus.

Principles of treatment and care

If a Caesarean section is to be performed, the following is required:
- A competent team of healthcare professionals
- A safe environment
- Emergency blood
- A paediatrician
- Extra staff to care for the baby (or babies) and the woman after the procedure.

Pre-operative preparation

In principle, all women must give signed consent for the possibility of an emergency Caesarean section on admission. Include the woman's partner in any pre-operative preparation. Note the following points:
- In case of an elective procedure, the pre-operative procedures and preparations are explained.
- The forms for consent of the operation and administration of the anaesthetic are completed and signed.
- Allergies are recorded and highlighted.
- The fetal heart is monitored four-hourly until the woman is in theatre.
- The anaesthetist will discuss the type of anaesthesia and do a general examination. Any questions the patient may have should be discussed with the medical practitioner at this time.
- Blood tests are done when necessary, for example HIV, blood grouping and Hb.
- Urinalysis is carried out prior to surgery.
- The woman is not given anything to eat or drink for six hours prior to the operation.
- A premedication to prevent Mendelsohn's aspiration syndrome is prescribed. Some medical practitioners use metoclopramide to empty the stomach.
- Patients undergoing spinal analgesia will require IV therapy for preloading.

Intra-operative care

In many institutions, the Caesarean section theatre is part of the labour ward and the midwives are responsible for that theatre. If not, the labour ward staff is responsible for receiving the neonate and for the fourth stage of labour. If the hospital policy allows the father to go to theatre, the labour ward staff will also take responsibility for him, to show him what to do, tell him what is happening, keep an eye on him and let him hold the baby.

There needs to be accurate record keeping of the mother during the Caesarean section procedure. This includes the accurate recording of blood loss, which is important for the assessment of the woman's well-being after birth. This blood loss is added to the bleeding before the procedure and after birth and gives an accurate picture of the total blood loss over 24 hours.

If the mother and baby are well, efforts are made to maintain mother–baby skin-to-skin contact.

Post-operative care

Post-operative care includes the following:

▶ *Level of consciousness.* The patient's level of consciousness is assessed after general anaesthesia and again once the patient is fully conscious. The woman is only transferred to the ward once she is stable and conscious.

▶ *Position.* The woman is placed in Fowler's position to improve uterine drainage and reduce tension on the abdomen, reducing pain. After spinal anaesthetic, Fowler's position is required unless there was a spinal tap.

▶ *Vital signs.* The woman's vital signs (temperature, pulse, respiration and BP) are checked half-hourly for 6 hours or until stable.

▶ *Blood loss.* The intrapartum blood loss is taken into account and added to the blood loss in the first 24 hours postpartum. Changing the sanitary pad every 20 minutes indicates too much blood loss after birth. The report on the examination of the placenta and membranes is checked for completeness. The pre-operative Hb is important. Unless there is postpartum haemorrhage (PPH), the Hb is checked when the haemodynamics have stabilised, usually the fourth day postpartum.

▶ *Lochia.* The lochia is observed for colour, odour, consistency and amount. Any profuse or abnormal lochia is reported to the medical practitioner immediately. Vulval toilette is done every four hours for 24 hours. The woman is educated about personal hygiene.

▶ *Oxytocin.* Oxytocin is administered 20 IU in 1 000 ml 8-hourly for at least 24 hours.

▶ *Wound care.* The abdominal wound is checked frequently for bleeding in the first 24 hours and then daily. Report on the condition of the wound, including any haemorrhage or infection. If Portovac drainage is used to drain the wound, it is emptied 4-hourly and the drain is removed on the medical practitioner's prescription. The wound is kept as dry as possible. Some medical practitioners advocate a light abdominal dressing after 24 hours, allowing air to circulate around the wound.

▶ *Sutures or clips.* The sutures or clips are removed on the medical practitioner's prescription, usually on day five or six.

▶ *IV fluids.* These are administered as prescribed. The rate and the infusion site are checked regularly.

▶ *Diet.* The woman is allowed to eat or drink after an uncomplicated Caesarean section with general anaesthesia as soon as she is hungry and thirsty. A regular diet is started when bowel sounds are heard and flatus is passed. Water and fruit juices are encouraged to prevent constipation. In spinal anaesthesia, a normal diet is allowed.

▶ *Urine.* All fluid intake and urine output are measured and charted while the Foley catheter is in place. The amount and colour of the urine are checked and charted. The urinary catheter is usually removed after 24 hours. The patient must be encouraged to void urine every one to two hours after the removal of the catheter. The bladder is checked for distension after voiding.

▶ *Bowels.* The midwife must enquire daily whether there has been a bowel action. An aperient of natural grain only or suppositories can be given on the third or fourth post-operative day if there has been no bowel action.

▶ *Ambulation.* Early ambulation encourages the passage of flatus and a diet high in fibre, fruit and vegetables will help to avoid constipation. The woman is encouraged to be ambulant within 24 hours to prevent thromboembolism. The legs and the groin are examined daily for signs of tenderness and infection. When a patient has undergone spinal anaesthesia, the midwife must observe for the return of all sensation to the lower limbs. The woman is not allowed out of bed until all sensation has returned and then a member of the staff must accompany the woman on her first walk, until they are confident that she will not fall or faint.

▶ *Pain and analgesia.* The midwife must check on the pain that the woman experiences in terms of type, location and whether the analgesia is having the desired effect. If the patient complains of leg pains, the doctor must be notified, as this could be caused by thrombosis. Analgesia is given on the medical practitioner's prescription following principles of pain assessment and care. If the analgesia does not work well, the medical practitioner is informed and an alternative analgesic prescribed.

▶ *Physiotherapy.* Active and passive leg exercises are encouraged, as well as deep breathing and coughing.

▶ *Baby-friendly principles.* The baby is put to the breast as soon as possible after the operation. Each feed must be supervised until the woman is able to manage on her own. The baby is demand-fed and the midwife must examine the breasts for fullness and engorgement.

▶ *Infant care.* Initially, the baby is nursed by the staff in the ward or nursery until the patient is up and about and able to care for the baby herself. The baby will usually be rooming-in with the mother, but careful observations must be undertaken for any possible complications.

▶ *Rest and sleep.* Care must be taken to ensure that the patient gets good sleep at night. In addition, the woman should be able to rest and sleep undisturbed for a few hours during the day.

- *Education.* During her stay in hospital, the woman is taught how to care for herself and for her new baby. The postpartum period allows for education. The woman is advised to get as much sleep and rest as possible, and she and/or her partner should arrange for help at home for the first two weeks post-operatively if possible.
- *General care.* The woman is instructed not to lift any heavy objects until the postnatal check-up. She should also not drive a car for up to six weeks post-operatively. She should avoid climbing too many stairs at first.
- *Education.* The midwife makes sure that the woman knows the reason for the Caesarean section, particularly if it was an emergency. She must be told of the importance of delivering in hospital for any subsequent babies.

Guidelines or protocol for post-operative medical prescription in the public sector

Warning: Before administering any medication, always check the medical practitioner's prescription, hospital policy and/or the package insert.

Prescribe analgesia: Opiate, eg papaveretum (Omnopon®) 20 mg intramuscularly with prochlorperazine 12.5 mg intramuscularly 4–6-hourly when necessary for 24 hours

Indomethacin 100 mg suppository 12-hourly, or ibuprofen 400 mg orally 3 times daily (not in patients with asthma, peptic ulcer or kidney dysfunction) for 2 or 3 days when necessary.

Paracetamol 1 g orally 4 times daily when necessary.

Prescribe IV fluids: Ringer's lactate 1 ℓ with 20 units oxytocin over 8 hours, then Maintelyte® or 5% Dextrose-saline 1 ℓ over 8 hours.

Prescribe additional (therapeutic) doses of antibiotics for 24 hours to 5 days in women who have risk factors for infection, (eg all HIV-infected women; prolonged labour or prolonged ruptured membranes; Caesarean section in second stage labour; chorioamnionitis; > 5 vaginal examinations during labour; when the fetal head needed to be pushed up vaginally).

Prophylaxis for thromboembolism for women at risk (sodium heparin 5 000 units subcutaneously 12-hourly or enoxaparin 40 mg SC daily while in hospital). Risk factors to consider are advanced maternal age, obesity, HIV infection, pre-eclampsia, immobility and co-existing illnesses.
Source: DoH, 2015: 56

Complications

Since Caesarean section is major surgery, it has potential complications, particularly if it was an emergency Caesarean section.

Maternal complications

- Haemorrhage in the post-operative period, due to:
  - haematomas in the broad ligament
  - bleeding from the placental site in uterine atony
  - bleeding from the abdominal or uterine wounds
  - bleeding caused by infection due to a breakdown of sutures or to infection of the placental site
  - hysterectomy
- Anaesthetic complications
- Pulmonary collapse caused by:
  - amniotic fluid embolism
  - aspiration pneumonia
  - thromboembolism
- Infection (puerperal sepsis) of the uterus, the urinary tract, the wound, the lungs, the abdominal wall, generalised septicaemia
- Hypovolaemia
- Bladder and ureter injuries; retention of urine
- Wound dehiscence
- Gastrointestinal (GI) flatulence and vomiting
- Gut distension, causing paralytic ileus
- Incisional hernia, umbilical hernia, abdominal hernia
- Lack of mother–infant bonding
- Increased future risk of repeated Caesarean section or uterine rupture.

Fetal complications

- *Respiratory:* The infant may develop the transient wet lung syndrome as a result of amniotic fluid not being squeezed out of the chest – as occurs in a vaginal delivery – or respiratory distress syndrome (RDS) due to immaturity of the lungs.
- *Birth injuries* may occur from the use of the scalpel, obstetric forceps or other instruments, or fractures may occur due to extraction from the womb.
- *Prematurity* may result due to incorrect dates (if the Caesarean section is mistakenly performed before term).
- *Neonatal asphyxia* can be caused by a delay in the birth during general anaesthetic.

33.3 Vaginal birth after Caesarean section

Vaginal birth after Caesarean section (VBAC) is a natural vaginal birth after a previous Caesarean section. This is also called a trial of scar.

Indications

Women who had a Caesarean section for reasons such as placenta praevia, pre-eclampsia and other reasons that may not recur are allowed to have a VBAC.

Contraindications

A woman is not a candidate for VBAC if she:
▶ has a poor obstetric history
▶ has a history of perinatal death
▶ has a multiple pregnancy
▶ experienced previous PPH
▶ underwent previous assisted delivery and obstructed labour
▶ suffers from CPD
▶ is carrying a large infant
▶ has had more than one previous Caesarean section
▶ has medical problems
▶ had a previous classical Caesarean section.

Prerequisites

VBAC should only be performed under the following circumstances:
▶ This is a high-risk procedure and should only be allowed under the supervision of an obstetrician.
▶ It should be done in an institution and at a level of care with a theatre available and an anaesthetist on standby.
▶ Ultrasound should be done to assess the scar.
▶ Epidural is contraindicated.
▶ Induction of labour (IOL) is contraindicated; particularly, do not administer prostaglandins.

Principles of treatment and care

In the treatment and care of VBAC, the following principles must be adhered to:
▶ The woman must make her own decision, but she must be advised on the risks of uterine rupture.
▶ The delivery takes place in a safe setting, where a Caesarean section is possible.
▶ An obstetrician is in attendance, in collaboration with a trained and competent midwife.
▶ An anaesthetist and blood are on standby.
▶ The woman must go into labour naturally and progress must be normal.
▶ Pain relief is as natural as possible (no epidural).
▶ The woman is under continuous observation. Signs of impending uterine rupture include:
  • any vaginal bleeding
  • continuous pain between contractions

  • tachycardia
  • marked changes in blood pressure
  • blood in a midstream urine specimen.

The partogram is used to assess the progress of labour. If progress is delayed, intervention is needed. Protocol requires an immediate response if complications occur.

Complications

The main complication is the risk of rupture of the uterus, with resultant fetal or maternal death.

33.4 Anaesthesia in pregnancy and labour

There is a risk for anaesthetic complications in pregnancy and labour due to the anatomical and biochemical changes in the pregnant woman (see chapters 20 and 26).

General anaesthesia and childbirth

The motto of surgery in obstetrics is to avoid general anaesthesia as far as possible. If general anaesthesia is needed, it should be administered by a competent anaesthetist. The risk is associated with the failure to intubate.

Physiological factors to consider in general anaesthesia for labouring women include the following:
▶ *Inferior vena cava syndrome (IVCS).* A wedge or a pillow is placed under the mother's left side to lift the uterus off the inferior vena cava. The BP and pulse are monitored before the administration of the anaesthetic. The wedge or pillow is removed as soon as the baby is born or the anaesthetist can tilt the table.
▶ *The changed haematocrit, Hb and coagulation profile.* The blood loss in Caesarean section is more than in a normal birth: estimated at 1 000 ml during the procedure. The real Hb needs to be known.
▶ *GI changes.* The enlarged uterus is pushed against the diaphragm and stomach and the risk of aspiration is increased. When this occurs, it is usually a fatal condition called Mendelson's syndrome, also referred to as aspiration syndrome. Cricoid pressure is used to prevent aspiration during intubation from 12 weeks of pregnancy.
▶ *Hormonal changes.* The effects of progesterone cause relaxation of the cardiac sphincter of the stomach and the acidic contents of the stomach are easily aspirated. Premedication antacid is given.

▶ *Changes in electrolyte balance and intra- and extravascular volume.* These changes alter drug pharmacokinetics and not all pharmaceutical agents can be used. An experienced and skilled anaesthetist must be in attendance.

▶ *Normal cardiac function.* ECG changes are present because of the changed position of the heart in pregnancy and cardiac function is observed.

The anaesthetist needs to consider two patients: the mother and the baby (or babies). Anaesthetic procedures are adapted and the use of anaesthetic agents are altered to accommodate the unborn baby. The baby needs to be delivered very rapidly. As a rule, the surgical drapes are placed and the surgeon is ready before anaesthesia is induced.

The following factors must be considered:

▶ *Premedication.* The normal premedication is not administered to a woman during childbirth, as it can cross the placenta and affect the fetus. Routine premedication may include an anti-emetic to facilitate gastric emptying and prevent nausea and an antacid to neutralise stomach contents.

▶ *Risks.* Pregnancy-associated anaesthetic risks are aggravated by emergencies in which the mother and fetus are already compromised, for example hypovolaemia; disseminated intravascular coagulation (DIC); eclampsia; haemolytic anaemia, elevated liver enzymes, low platelet count (HELLP) syndrome; cardiac problems and obesity.

Regional anaesthesia and childbirth

Regional anaesthesia has become the more popular and safer option of anaesthesia in childbirth. In the private sector, regional anaesthesia is more readily available than in the public sector, where regional anaesthesia may only be available in Level 3 institutions. Spinal anaesthesia is the norm for Caesarean sections, even in emergencies, in all levels of care in the public and private sectors.

Epidural analgesia is the only intervention that can give total relief of the pain of uterine contractions. Epidural analgesia has become an extremely popular form of pain relief in labour and therefore it is important that midwives are fully conversant with it. However, it is a time-consuming procedure, requiring labour-intensive care in a busy labour ward, and if there is insufficient care and preparation by the nursing and medical staff in the delivery unit, a dangerous situation could arise.

Epidural and spinal anaesthesia carry risks and should only be administered by a skilled anaesthetist or obstetrician. Midwives in the labour ward must have a thorough understanding of anaesthetic technique, the dangers and complications that could arise and how to correct them, and how to monitor the patient effectively. Midwives must be competent in resuscitation techniques should the need arise. They should also be fully conversant with any 'topping up' ordered by the medical practitioner and with continuous epidural infusions and the legal implications and guidelines for such.

Table 33.2

Comparison of epidural and spinal anaesthesia in obstetrics

Aspect	Epidural	Spinal
Definition	This is a form of regional analgesia in which local anaesthetic is injected into the epidural space of the spinal column. The level at which the local anaesthetic is usually injected is between Ll and L4. Continuous analgesia can be obtained by introducing a polythene cannula into the epidural space to infuse a specific volume of the medication into the epidural space.	Spinal anaesthesia is the insertion of a once-off dosage of local anaesthesia into the dural space between L2 and L4.
Top-up	Given in a single initial injection (bolus dose) of a specific amount of local anaesthetic Top-ups can be given: local anaesthetic is injected at regular intervals via an epidural cannula into the epidural space	No top-ups given

continued

Aspect	Epidural	Spinal
Top-up (continued)	Given via a continuous epidural infusion of a local anaesthetic via an epidural cannula, regulated by an infusion pump, the rate of which is determined by the medical practitioner	
Indications	Maternal request Obstetric: • occipitoposterior (OP) positions or malpresentations • IOL • pre-eclampsia and hypertension • assisted deliveries • pain relief for obstetric interventions • IUD	The main indication is Caesarean section. It can be used for any emergency obstetric situation where a patient is not compromised, for example manual removal of the placenta.
Contra-indications	The woman refuses A uterine scar Cardiac or mitral stenosis Unsafe facilities or inexperienced staff Local sepsis or septicaemia A woman with a clotting disorder A woman on anticoagulation therapy Spinal deformities or kyphoscoliosis Fetal distress Drug allergies Severe anaemia	The woman refuses Neurological disease Sepsis A woman with clotting defects A woman on anticoagulation therapy Hypovolaemia Unsafe circumstances Inexperienced staff
Prerequisites	The procedure is done in an acute setting with emergency support or a theatre (not primary healthcare [PHC]). The emergency trolley and all equipment are prepared. Consent must be signed. Contraindications need to be considered. A patent IV line must be in place. A competent anaesthetist must do the procedure. A competent midwife supports the medical practitioner and provides care for the woman. Adequate staffing levels with designated competent practitioners must be available. There is a standard protocol in place. Accurate records are kept.	Consent is signed. The spinal is done in theatre before the procedure, with all practitioners in attendance. Contraindications are identified. Patent IV line is in place. Preloading of fluid is done as for epidural. The procedure is performed by a competent anaesthetist. Standard protocol is followed.
Precautions	Specific observations and precautions as well as sterile procedure are required. *Hypotension.* One of the effects of epidural is a drop in BP due to the vasodilatation of the blood vessels distal to the level of anaesthesia (the sympathetic nerve fibres in the area are blocked): • BP is observed throughout the procedure every five minutes until stable (1 hour) and with each top-up.	A sterile procedure must be followed. The spinal anaesthetic carries major risks, as the spinal needle perforates the dura and the drug is administered in the dural space. A 21–22 gauge pencil-point spinal needle is used to avoid headaches. The effects are the same as for epidural in terms of hypotension and respiratory suppression.

continued

Aspect	Epidural	Spinal
Precautions (continued)	• The woman is preloaded with 500 ml Haemaccel or 500–1 000 ml saline dextrose or Ringer's lactate before the procedure to counteract this effect. If the BP drops too much, place the woman on her side, give more fluid and give ephedrine IV as prescribed. *Motor weakness.* Motor weakness will develop in the muscles distal to the block, but the severity will depend upon the type, strength and volume of local anaesthetic used. A walking epidural allows the woman to move around, blocking only sensory perceptions. A motor block will also affect the bladder and the woman will not be able to feel the need to pass urine. A 12–14 gauge Foley catheter is inserted, with 5–10 ml of fluid in the balloon to keep the bladder empty. The woman is positioned on her side or in a Fowler's position, after which the balloon is inflated with a further 10 ml. Because sensation is blocked, the woman has no urge to push, so regular vaginal examinations are done to determine the progress of labour. *Fetal bradycardia.* Give oxygen and change maternal positions or increase BP if hypotensive. A continuous epidural carries extra risks over and above the single dose and consent is needed.	The position of the woman is important. The wedge is used to prevent hypotension with IVCS effects (see Figure 33.5 on page 530) Total motor paralysis is induced and the woman cannot move her legs. Care is taken to position the legs correctly so as not to cause pressure or injury. The woman is catheterised using a Foley 12–14 gauge catheter and the balloon inflated with 5–10 ml until after the birth.
Drugs used	Bupivacaine has the following side effects: excitation, nervousness, tingling around the mouth, tinnitus, tremor, dizziness, blurred vision or seizures, followed by depression, drowsiness, loss of consciousness, respiratory depression and apnoea. Fentanyl® is a powerful opiate. Sufentanil® is another opiate, five to ten times more potent than Fentanyl®. Ephedrine (hypotension)	Bupivacaine Opioids such as Fentanyl® Ephedrine (hypotension) Adrenaline Anti-emetics Sedatives
Method	Consent is required Position: left lateral or sitting Curve the spine (see Figure 33.3 on page 527). Identify region and infiltrate skin with lignocaine. Identify lumbar space L1–L4. Use a Tuohy blunt-tip epidural kit needle, 16 gauge. There is reduced resistance as the needle passes through the ligamentum flavum (see Figure 33.1 on page 525). No fluid or blood should be withdrawn. The catheter can be placed according to the specific marks on the catheter (4–6 cm to remain in the space). The patient may feel a prick in the leg.	Consent is required Position: left lateral or sitting Curve the spine (see Figure 33.3 on page 527). Identify region and infiltrate skin with lignocaine. Identify lumbar space L1–L4. Use Tuohy spinal needle, 12–14 gauge. There is reduced resistance as the needle passes through the ligamentum flavum (see Figure 33.1 on page 525). Move the needle until the dura is perforated and dural fluid appears. Give the total dosage.

continued

Aspect	Epidural	Spinal
Method (continued)	The needle is removed and the catheter secured. A test dosage is given (cold feeling in back). The woman is placed in semi-Fowler's position. Monitor BP and fetal heart every 5 minutes. Full dosage is given if no adverse reaction occurs. Reaction, level of effectiveness and level of anaesthesia is checked (see Figure 33.4 on page 529).	The needle is removed and the injection point is sealed with a plaster. The woman is placed on her back with a wedge under the left side. The BP is monitored. Wait 10–15 minutes to make sure the woman is stable and the desired level of anaesthesia is reached for the surgery. When the medical practitioner works on the omentum, the woman may vomit, so anti-emetics are given. Give the baby to the mother after birth. A sedative is given while suturing the abdomen.
Specific care	Fluid preload and administration are monitored. Best position is maintained. In the first half hour the woman may be changed from side to side to allow the drug to spread evenly. Check BP every 5 minutes for one hour or till stable. Check effectiveness and level of anaesthesia and respiration. Foley catheter insertion depends on the level and dosage of anaesthesia. Observe 2-hourly emptying of bladder if walking epidural. Check fetal heart. Check uterine contractions, which may subside, particularly if adrenaline was used. Start oxytocin. Observe dilatation 2-hourly. Keep accurate records. Observe and treat side effects such as itching.	Fluid preload and administration are monitored. Best position is maintained and the legs are given care during surgery. Check BP throughout the operation. Check effectiveness and level of anaesthesia and respiration before the surgery. Ensure that oximeter and ECG leads are in place. Foley catheter is inserted. Keep accurate records. Anaesthetist is in constant attendance.
Advantages	The woman is pain-free within 2–4 minutes. The first stage of labour may be shortened. The woman is more alert and co-operative. The fetus benefits from shorter birth and less exhaustion. The mother is more rested and ready to bond with and feed the baby. Manual delivery of the placenta, if needed, is not traumatic. There is no urge to bear down, which is beneficial in malpresentation and breech. Manipulations and assisted deliveries are less traumatic.	It is a safe and quick procedure, with immediate results. The woman is alert and pain-free, and can see her baby immediately after birth.

continued

Aspect	Epidural	Spinal
Disadvantages	Weak uterine contractions may result, which may necessitate an oxytocin infusion. The woman may be uncomfortable and feel out of control if she cannot feel her body. The woman cannot bear down effectively. Assisted delivery is required. Dissatisfaction will result if only partial effectiveness is experienced. Labour is intensive and more than one person is needed to assist the mother. The woman cannot get up for at least 12 hours or without assistance. Complications are very unpleasant. There is a risk of bladder infection due to catheterisation.	Requires highly skilled practitioners. A total motor block is present. The woman cannot feel or move her body distal to the anaesthetic level and will need reassurance and assistance. The woman may experience nausea due to the touching of the omentum.
Complications	Hypotension or shivering Spinal tap High block with respiratory distress or arrest Infection Bloody tap Incomplete block Death (1:100 000) (Moka, 2011) Post-epidural headaches Iatrogenic: using wrong medication Haematoma Neurological damage Fever not related to infection Fetus born with a raised temperature	Headache due to spinal tap High block with paralysis of the diaphragm Infection Segmentation (sensation retained in some areas) Hypotension Itching Death

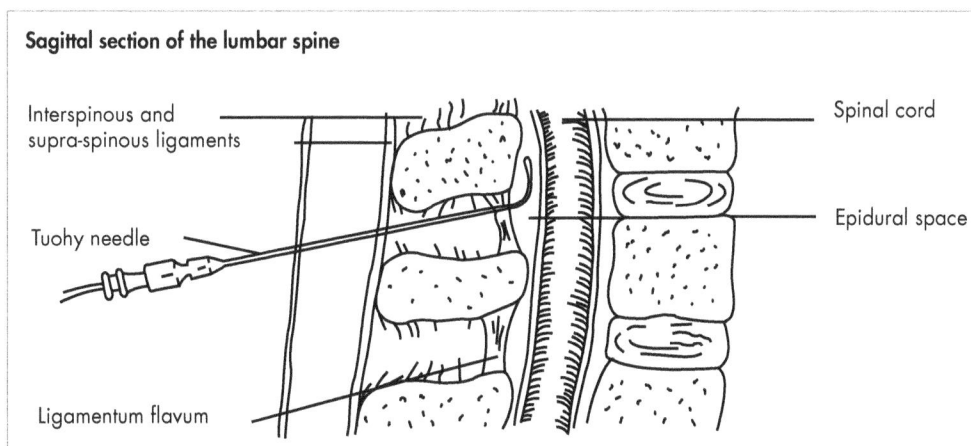

Sagittal section of the lumbar spine

Interspinous and supra-spinous ligaments

Tuohy needle

Ligamentum flavum

Spinal cord

Epidural space

Figure 33.1 Insertion of needle in the epidural space (L1–L4): Sagittal section

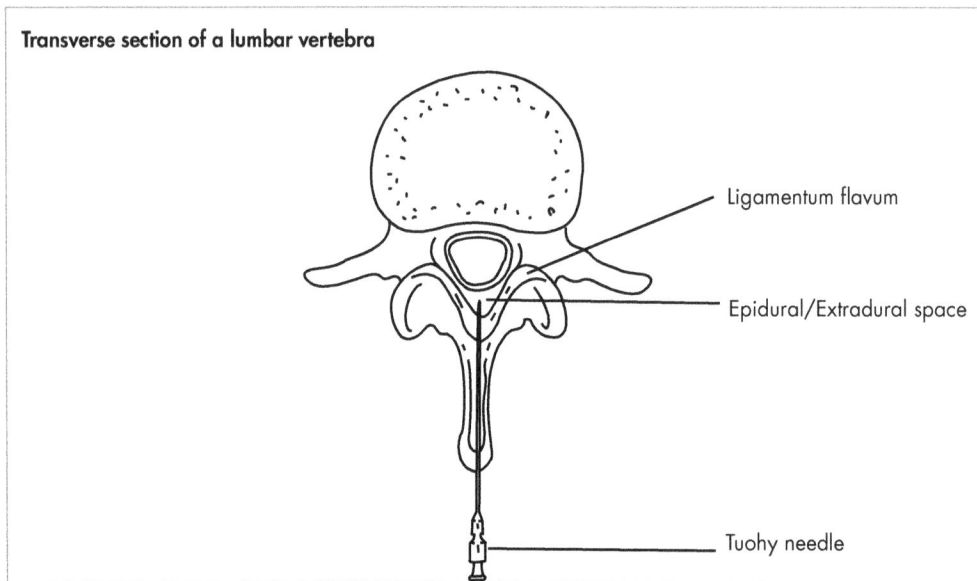

Figure 33.2 Insertion of needle in the epidural space: Transverse section

The management of the complications of epidural and spinal anaesthesia

As noted in Table 33.2, epidural and spinal anaesthesia are high-risk interventions requiring advanced skills, and several complications can occur. The patient is generally given an explanation of epidural anaesthesia during the antenatal period. If a woman has an epidural she needs to give written consent for the procedure and the possible side effects should be carefully explained to her and her partner. It is the medical practitioner's responsibility to obtain consent.

Epidural anaesthesia is only performed in a facility where medical practitioners and theatre facilities are available. It is preferable to have a room or area set aside in the labour ward for the specific purpose of epidural analgesia.

Equipment required

▶ BP monitor
▶ Stethoscope
▶ Administration sets and solutions
▶ A bucket for the discarded material near the bed
▶ An anaesthetic stool for the medical practitioner
▶ Resuscitation equipment and the emergency trolley
▶ Suction apparatus
▶ An overhead light
▶ An anaesthetic trolley containing all the medication (drugs) which are likely to be required in an emergency
▶ A correctly prepared epidural trolley; care must be taken to ensure that there is no contamination of the epidural

needles and cannula with cleaning solutions (see the box on page 528).

The midwife's duties during regional anaesthesia

The midwife needs to be competent to manage all specific care and risks associated with the procedure of giving regional anaesthesia, as discussed below.

Prevention of hypotension

Hypotension is a serious side effect of epidural and spinal anaesthesia. The effect of the drug is vasodilatation of all the blood vessels distal to the level of anaesthesia, resulting in a sudden drop in BP. This may affect placental perfusion and the fetus.

A patent IV line is mandatory for the procedure and 500–1 000 ml of Ringer's lactate, Plasmalyte B solution or Haemaccel is given. This will take about 15–20 minutes and increases the circulating blood volume, which helps to prevent hypotension. Due to the rapid administration, the fluid needs to be at body temperature or the woman will experience shivering.

Baseline BP is taken and recorded and the medical practitioner is informed before the procedure starts. There is continuous observation of the BP after the administration of the main drug dosage. Adequate explanation of all procedures must be given to the woman and her partner all the time.

A. Lying on the left side, chin on chest, knees on abdomen.

B. Sitting up on the edge of the bed

i. Side view

ii. Back view

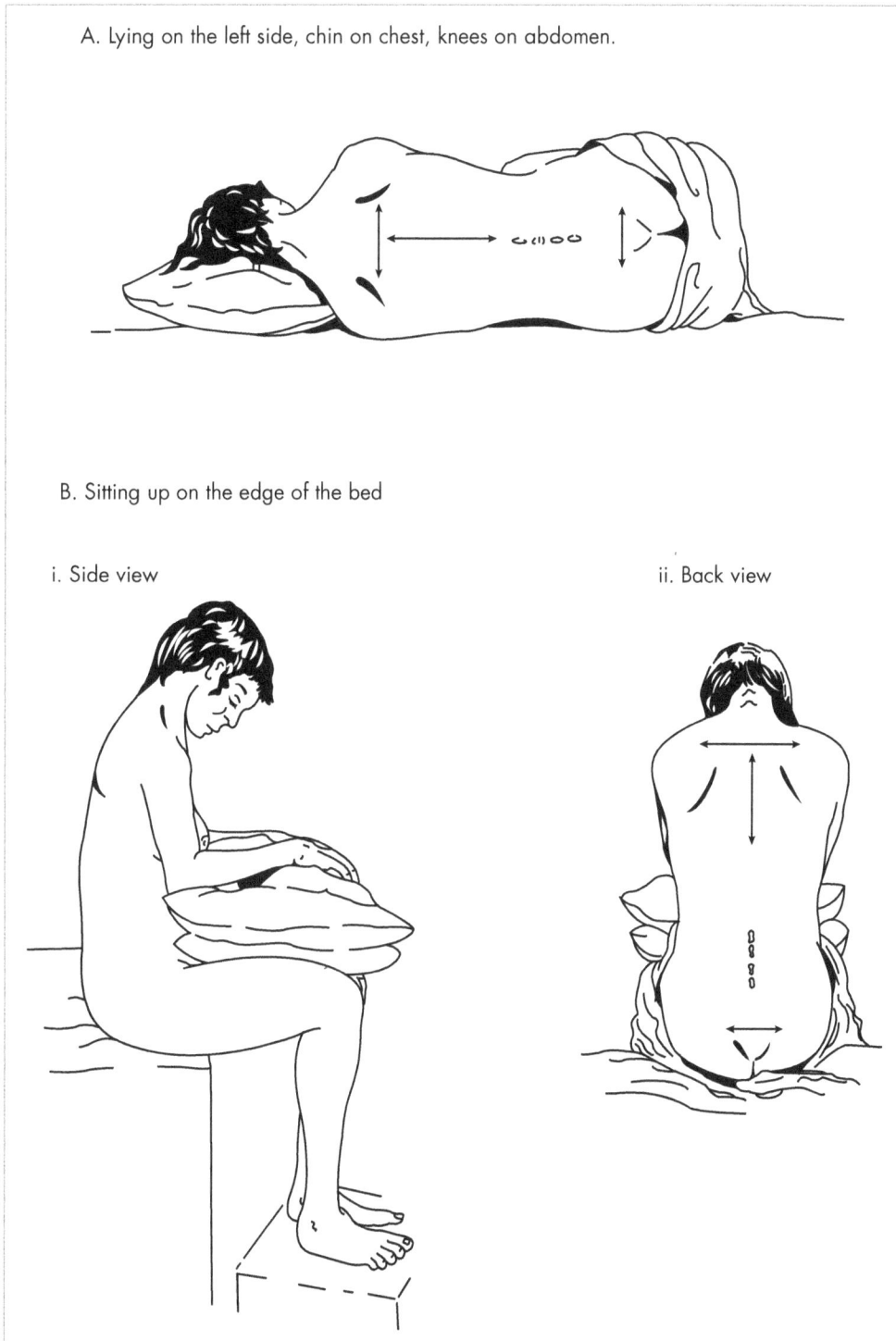

Figure 33.3 Positioning the patient for epidural or spinal anaesthesia

Once the epidural space has been located and the test dose administered, the BP is taken and recorded every minute for five minutes, and then every five minutes for 20 minutes. The medical practitioner is informed of every reading taken.

Material and instruments required for epidural or spinal anaesthesia

Note: This is a sterile procedure and full aseptic precautions must also be taken prior to starting the procedure.

The material required includes:
▶ a mask for the medical practitioner
▶ sterile gown and drapes
▶ bowls, gallipots and receivers
▶ swabs and a swab holder
▶ cleaning solution
▶ a dental syringe and needle
▶ cartridges of local anaesthetic (lignocaine 2 per cent)
▶ an epidural pack, consisting of:
  • an 18- or 16-gauge Tuohy needle (with stilette)
  • an epidural catheter
  • a disposable (Millipore) bacterial filter (pore size 0.2 microns)
  • a calibrated epidural cannula
  • a selection of injection needles of various sizes
  • a 21–22 gauge pencil-point spinal needle.

Other clean materials required include:
▶ a plastic spray
▶ a plaster
▶ local anaesthetic for injection into the epidural space
▶ a transparent plastic dressing (if available)
▶ a size 14 Foley catheter with urine bag and catheter pack
▶ drugs.

Position

The woman must be positioned correctly for the procedure and the midwife must help the woman to maintain that position during the procedure (see Figure 33.3). The woman may be placed on her side with her knees drawn up and her chin resting on her chest, with the flat plane of her back vertical and at right angles to the horizontal plane of the bed. Alternatively, she may sit upright on the edge of the bed, leaning very slightly forward, with her arms resting on pillows on her lap.

The woman may be nursed on alternate sides or sitting upright. She must not be allowed to lie flat on her back. If the woman is nursed on her side, two to three pillows can be placed under her head. One pillow must be placed between her legs to prevent pressure areas from developing and one behind her back for support. She must be turned regularly. Ensure that her legs are supported when being moved, as she cannot control them.

Bladder care

The woman must be catheterised and intake and output recorded.

Observations and support

While the procedure is in progress, the midwife becomes the means of communication between the patient and the medical practitioner. She must notify the medical practitioner of any change in the patient's condition. She must also notify the medical practitioner when a contraction begins, as they will then pause and wait for the contraction to pass. This is important, as the epidural space is narrowed during a contraction and thus difficult to locate. The midwife observes abnormalities and reports to the medical practitioner. The patient under epidural analgesia must never be left alone at any time. The medical practitioner will check the effectiveness of the procedure.

Pain relief

An effective block is indicated by immediate relief from pain, warm skin distal to the block and a sudden drop in BP, which may be accompanied by shivering, nausea and dizziness.

Complications and interventions during regional anaesthesia

The complications discussed in the following subsections (and in Table 33.2) must be anticipated and the team should have a protocol for managing them.

Total spinal block

A total spinal block may arise with frightening speed. It can occur when the injected local anaesthesia depresses the spinal cord and brainstem.

Signs and symptoms
▶ Sudden hypotension
▶ Bradycardia
▶ Difficulty breathing.

Cardiac arrest, unconsciousness and death may follow.

Interventions

The rate of the IV infusion is increased for cardiovascular support.

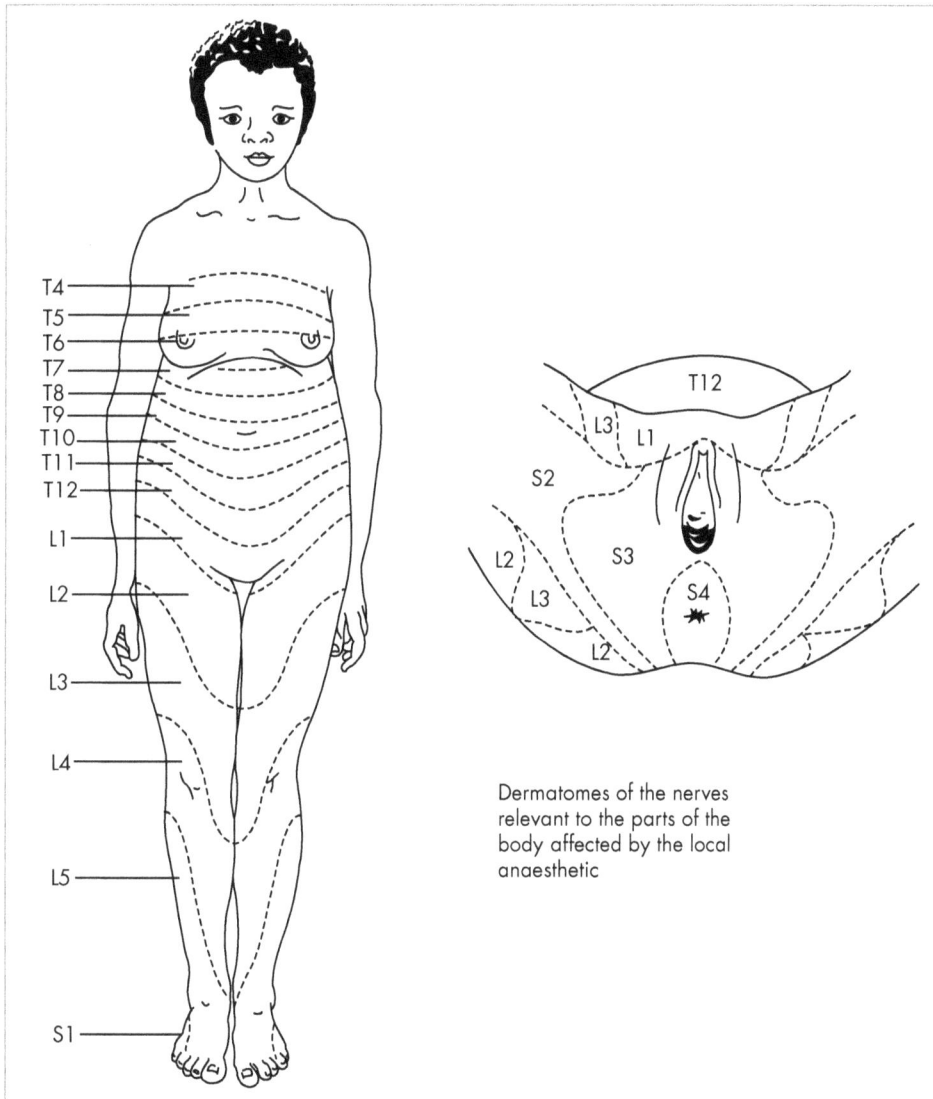

Figure 33.4 Epidural anaesthesia in the dermatone levels

Give 100 per cent oxygen immediately. The medical practitioner may give adrenalin 1 ml of 1:10 000. In some instances, intubation and ventilation will be necessary until the effects of the total block wear off. Top-ups may cause this condition, so midwives must be aware of possible complications.

Epidural IV injection in the epidural space

Epidural IV injection occurs when the needle punctures a blood vessel in the epidural space. The clinical features will arise while the medical practitioner is injecting the local anaesthetic through the cannula. A test dose should always be given before the full bolus of medication is inserted into the epidural space.

Causes

Epidural IV injection may be caused by:
- failure to perform the aspiration test
- giving an inadequate test dose
- misinterpretation of the test dose
- late IV cannula migration into one of the epidural veins.

Signs and symptoms

The effects are dose-dependent. The reaction could be mild, moderate or severe, as indicted in Table 33.3.

Table 33.3

Degrees of toxicity in epidural IV injection

Mild	Moderate	Severe
Palpitations	Nausea	Coma
Vertigo	Vomiting	Severe
Tinnitus	Hypotension	hypotension
Apprehension	Muscle twitching	Bradycardia
Confusion	Convulsions	Respiratory
Headache	Unconsciousness	depression
Metallic taste in		Cardiac arrest
the mouth		

Massive intravascular doses can result in sudden circulatory collapse within one minute. Extradural doses cause reactions within 5–30 minutes, depending upon the site of injection.

Interventions

If a reaction occurs, management is according to the emergency protocols. Give 40% oxygen by mask. The patient is turned onto her side, as this encourages optimal venous return. A vasoconstrictor is given by the medical practitioner at 45-second intervals until the systolic BP is 110 mmHg. It may be necessary to intubate and ventilate the woman.

High block

A high-level block may result in difficulty breathing, along with numbness of the hands and shoulders.

Intervention

- Place the woman in a high Fowler's position to allow the drug to flow lower.
- Discontinue the epidural infusion.
- Give oxygen by mask.
- Do not leave the woman alone.
- Increase the IV fluids.
- Ventilation may be required.

Post-dural puncture headache

The puncture may occur accidentally during epidural anaesthesia. The headache typically occurs hours to days after puncture. Post-dural puncture headache (PDPH) is caused when the dura mater is punctured and there is leakage of cerebrospinal fluid (CSF).

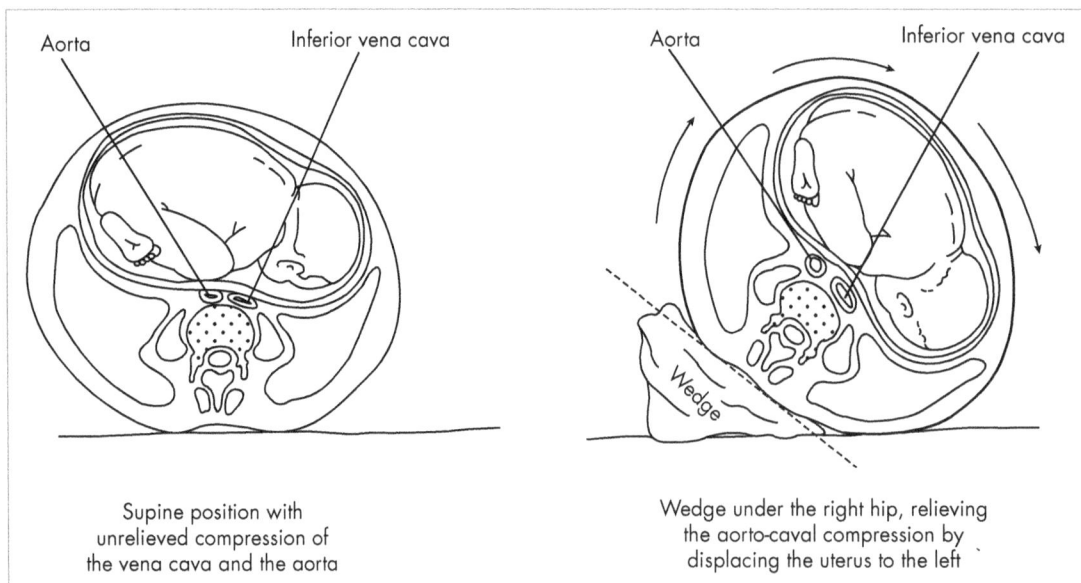

Figure 33.5 Aorta caval compression

Interventions

Some women only need analgesia and bed rest. If the headache persists, however, an epidural blood patch may be required, in which 10 ml of the woman's blood is injected into the epidural space near the site of the original puncture, by the original practitioner who did the procedure. This will seal the meningeal leak. It can be done in the ward. This is a sterile procedure that gives immediate relief.

A bloody tap

A bloody tap occurs if one of the epidural veins is punctured. Blood will track up the cannula and the epidural will have to be redone, using a higher intervertebral space.

Intervention

The procedure is abandoned. A higher level of vertebra may be attempted.

Shivering

The exact cause of shivering after epidural puncture is not known, but it may be the lowering of the core temperature. The shivering occurs within 10 minutes of the administration of the local anaesthetic.

Intervention

Fentanyl® added to the infusion as per protocol or on prescription may prevent shivering.

Haematoma formation

A haematoma may form either in the epidural or in the subdural space. These are more likely to occur if the woman is receiving anticoagulant therapy or in patients with HELLP syndrome. Symptoms depend on the site of the haematoma.

Intervention

The medical practitioner must take note of any pain that the patient complains of and, before continuing with the procedure, should closely question the patient as to the nature and extent of the pain. The medical practitioner may then decide not to continue with the epidural, to move the needle to a higher space or to give more local anaesthetic.

Routine care of the obstetric woman after regional anaesthetics

Routine observations are continued after the woman has stabilised.

Observations

Observations continue, including monitoring of the temperature and continuous pain relief. The legs and feet are warm after the administration of the first main dosage of epidural because of vasodilation. If there is a unilateral block there will be a difference in temperature between the legs and the feet.

Progress of labour

The progress of labour is observed. Vaginal examinations are performed as required. In many instances, where the patient has been in established labour prior to the epidural, there is rapid dilatation of the cervix once there is no longer any pain. It is very important, therefore, to observe the woman for signs of the second stage of labour. The woman will not be aware of the progress and in some cases the contractions cease, particularly if adrenaline-containing drugs were used. Oxytocin administration may then be required, as per medical prescription, to let the birth progress.

The midwife must check the progress of labour in the usual way and report any problems to the medical practitioner.

Maintenance of anaesthesia

Anaesthesia is maintained using either the top-up procedure or a continuous epidural infusion. The midwife is only involved in continuing observations and reporting to the medical practitioner if there are problems. A skilled midwife may be asked to top up the epidural according to the medical practitioner's prescription.

Possible problems or complications include the following:
- Inadequate analgesia can occur because the patient is lying only on one side; this should not occur with good nursing care.
- A misplaced cannula can cause a high-segment block (only TIO–T8), or too low a block (only blocking L2–L3), which would require a higher volume of the medication.
- An overdosed patient is a potential problem. With continuous epidural analgesia, the patient must be monitored continually for the level of numbness and for the degree of muscle paralysis. The level of anaesthesia should be checked hourly and recorded (see Figure 33.4 on page 529). This can be achieved very simply by supplying the patient with a small block of ice and asking her to run the ice slowly down her chest and onto her abdomen. The level at which loss of sensation is experienced is then recorded. If the patient complains of numbness above the level of T6 (the xyphisternum), the medical practitioner must be informed immediately and emergency interventions instituted.

The second stage of labour

Most patients are delivered in the lithotomy position, as they have very little control over their lower limbs. The patient's head and shoulders are propped up against pillows. As the hyperflexed lithotomy position causes postural stress, a lateral tilt must be used to elevate one hip to prevent fetal hypoxia due to venacaval compression. *Both legs must be elevated and lowered simultaneously, in order to avoid strain on the patient's lower back and hips.*

The aim of the epidural is to allow for spontaneous delivery and as long as no complications arise, this can be achieved. While the patient has no sensation to bear down and if the fetal condition is satisfactory, the presenting part should be allowed to descend onto the perineum. Thereafter, the patient is prepared for delivery and encouraged to bear down. In most instances, the baby can be delivered by uterine action alone, particularly in the multiparous woman, without any additional bearing-down efforts. This will reduce the incidence of instrumental deliveries normally associated with epidural analgesia.

If the woman is catheterised, this must be removed in the second stage before delivery to prevent bruising and trauma to the urethra during the delivery. If the patient requires an assisted delivery, the urethra could be severely damaged.

Women tend to vomit if syntometrine is administered after an epidural; it is therefore better to use oxytocin after delivery.

The third stage of labour

Take care when positioning the patient's limbs until all sensation has returned. Reassure the patient that all sensation will soon return and check for this at regular intervals.

The epidural catheter is removed on the medical practitioner's prescription. It is not usually left in for longer than 72 hours, as a fibrin pocket can develop at the tip of the catheter.

When removing the epidural cannula, the midwife must make sure that the patient is lying on her side, slightly curled up. The cannula is removed in a slow, steady movement and in an outward direction. If the cannula appears to be stuck, ask the patient to curl up a bit more. If the cannula still cannot be removed, stop immediately and notify the medical practitioner. Never use excessive traction on the cannula.

After removal, the tip of the cannula is inspected to make sure that it is complete and the insertion point is sealed with a sterile gauze and Opsite dressing or plaster.

Postpartum care

The patient is kept on strict bed rest (12 hours) until all sensation has returned to the lower limbs. She must be instructed not to get out of bed until she is able to do so. When she is allowed up for the first time, she must be accompanied by a staff member, who must make sure that she is capable of walking and is not feeling dizzy.

An indwelling catheter is left in place until all sensation has returned. The midwife must make sure that the patient is able to void urine adequately.

It is extremely important that all observations and procedures are accurately recorded in the patient's case notes.

The walking epidural

Technology in medicine has developed to the point where skilful administration of the epidural allows the woman to be pain-free and mobile during labour. These women are also able to have a normal second stage of labour. This level of skill comes with experience and is usually held by a fully qualified anaesthetist.

33.5   Symphysiotomy

A symphysiotomy is a surgical incision into the fibrocartilage of the symphysis pubis in order to permanently enlarge the pelvic girdle. The operation is performed in order to allow the fetal head to pass into the pelvis (engage), so that a vaginal delivery may be achieved. It is performed when there is:

▶ no facility for Caesarean section
▶ mild to moderate CPD
▶ an urgent need to deliver the fetus.

A spontaneous symphysiotomy can occur during a difficult vaginal delivery, in which case some of the lesser complications may also apply.

Incidence

Symphysiotomies were performed as a routine surgical procedure for obstructed labour, but became less frequent in the late 20th century. It is rarely, if ever, performed in Western countries, where Caesarean section is preferred. However, in the developing world the procedure has a place. It is usually performed by medical practitioners.

In communities where CPD is a common complication of childbirth, the procedure is relatively safe, provided that the patient is chosen well and careful attention is paid to the problems which can arise. The operator must be conversant with the indications and the contraindications for symphysiotomy, and must be skilled in the technique.

Indications

The following are indications for a symphysiotomy:
▶ It overcomes borderline CPD.
▶ It is preferable to the trauma caused by forceps delivery when used for certain clinical problems.
▶ It can be performed at the end of a careful trial of labour.
▶ It is very useful in neglected cases of obstructed labour, where a Caesarean section would be dangerous for the patient.
▶ In developing countries, where patients do not always return after a previous Caesarean section for proper antenatal care and subsequent hospital delivery, it is preferable for a symphysiotomy to be performed to correct CPD. This leaves the woman with a permanent cure for the CPD, rather than allowing the woman to run the risk of a scarred uterus from a Caesarean section and a future labour with CPD without proper care.
▶ It is useful for women whose beliefs and cultures penalise them for not delivering vaginally.
▶ It is preferable to a Caesarean section if more than four children are planned.
▶ It may permit immediate vaginal delivery in obstructed labour, while also sparing the integrity of the uterus.
▶ It can save the mother and the fetus considerable trauma, as dis-impacting a deeply impacted head at Caesarean section is difficult and dangerous.
▶ It is preferable to a difficult forceps delivery or to obstructed labour with possible uterine rupture and the resultant high fetal mortality rate.
▶ It is useful when delivering the after-coming head of a breech presentation where CPD could be a problem. In these cases there may be difficulty in delivering the head and symphysiotomy may prove to be life-saving.
▶ It could be the procedure of choice where CPD is further complicated by coagulopathy or by anaesthetic risks or allergies.

Contraindications

Symphysiotomy should not be performed:
▶ in gross CPD, with more than 80 per cent of the fetal head above the brim of the pelvis

▶ in abnormalities of the maternal spine and lower limbs
▶ in very obese women
▶ if the baby is estimated to have a mass of more than 4 kg or less than 2.5 kg
▶ if there has been a previous Caesarean section
▶ if a symphysiotomy has been previously performed
▶ if the baby is dead
▶ if the uterine action is not effective (hypotonic uterine action)
▶ if the cervical dilatation is less than 8 cm
▶ in a pelvis where the diagonal conjugate is less than 8 cm
▶ in malpresentations
▶ if the operator is unskilled or there is inadequate assistance
▶ if there is no good indication for symphysiotomy
▶ if consent has not been given.

Advantages

Symphysiotomy comes with the following advantages:
▶ It is a relatively simple procedure with few risks.
▶ The procedure takes only five minutes to perform and delivery can then be achieved very quickly, which is useful when there is fetal distress.
▶ It can be performed almost anywhere and with limited facilities.
▶ Only local analgesia is required.
▶ Vaginal delivery is achieved.
▶ There is only a small risk of infection.
▶ The operation results in a permanent enlargement of the pelvic girdle; healing takes place by the laying down of fibrous tissue.
▶ There is an increase in the transverse diameters at each plane of the pelvis, particularly at the outlet, because the lower points of the pubic bones at the symphysis become more widely separated than the upper ends.
▶ There is a minimal increase in the anteroposterior (AP) diameters.
▶ There is great improvement in the capacity of both android and anthropoid pelvises.
▶ Any following deliveries will be easier, because fibrous tissue tends to stretch more easily than does cartilage.

PROCEDURE Symphysiotomy

Prerequisites and preparation

▶ *Competence.* Symphysiotomy must only be performed by a skilled obstetrician, who must make the decision when to perform the operation. In an emergency and as a last resort, especially in order to extract the after-coming head in a breech, a skilled midwife may perform a symphysiotomy. There must be adequate assistance available, because two assistants are needed to hold the legs in the lithotomy position.

▶ *Indications.* There must be proper indications for performing this operation.

▶ *Informed consent.* The woman must be given a full explanation of the operation. The patient must be co-operative and written consent must be obtained.

▶ *Support.* It is the midwife's duty to give moral support and encouragement to the woman throughout the procedure, as the woman will be very distressed and fearful during this time. The woman is told that she has a tube in her bladder to drain the urine, and that this will ensure that she does not have to sit up or get out of bed to pass urine. The catheter is removed after four days, when she will be able to use a bedpan.

▶ *Contraindications.* The contraindications must be considered.

▶ *X-rays.* The operation is only undertaken when the CPD is borderline (mild to moderate). This must be checked by clinical and radiological estimates.

▶ *Labour.* There must be effective uterine contractions. Dilatation must be 8 cm and the head must be 80 per cent engaged.

▶ *Asepsis.* The procedure is performed using an aseptic technique.

▶ *Anaesthesia.* Adequate analgesia must be ensured. Local anaesthesia is used.

▶ *Neonatal care.* Resuscitation facilities must be available for a possibly asphyxiated infant.

Procedure

1 *Informed consent.* A careful explanation, using terminology that the woman can understand, is given to the patient regarding the incision between the two pubic bones. She should be given reassurance that the wound will soon heal and that she will only suffer minor problems for a while.

2 *Position.* Two midwives support the woman's legs against their chests. The legs must not be abducted more than 80 degrees and it is preferable to have the legs at an angle of 45 degrees.

3 *Cleaning.* The area to be operated on is swabbed and draped, using an aseptic technique.

4 *Anaesthesia.* Local anaesthetic is injected into the soft tissue over the symphysis pubis on either side, and the tissues of the perineum are then also anaesthetised for an episiotomy.

5 *Bladder care.* An indwelling Foley catheter is introduced into the bladder and kept in position until four days after the operation.

6 *Technique* (see Figure 33A):

　a) Two fingers of the left hand are inserted into the vagina. The urethra and the catheter are displaced laterally. The fingers are kept in position under the symphysis pubis to protect the urethra and the bladder, and to determine the depth of the incision.

　b) The incision is made from the upper third of the symphysis pubis downwards and then from the upper third of the symphysis pubis upwards, to complete the incision. A bistoury solid-Waded knife is used. The blade is inserted through a half-inch incision in the skin over the centre of the joint, anteriorly. All the fibres of the cartilage are completely incised from above down. The scalpel is held vertically, like a pencil, the cutting edge pointing downward.

　c) The joint is then entered at the junction of the upper and middle third and the lower two-thirds of the joint are incised.

　d) The scalpel is removed, rotated 180 degrees and re-inserted to complete the incision of the upper one-third of the joint. The separation must be less than 2.5 cm and the operator must adhere strictly to the midline to avoid osteitis pubis and subsequent difficulty in walking.

7 *Control of bleeding.* Haemorrhage is controlled by direct pressure.

8 *Leg control.* Once the incision is made, the midwives bring the legs together carefully in adduction.

continued

9 *Delivery.* A large episiotomy is performed when fully dilated so that the head is delivered as far posteriorly as possible, in order to keep the pressure of the head away from the bladder and the urethral walls.

10 *Suturing.* Once delivery is complete, the genital tract is explored for signs of trauma. The symphysiotomy skin incision is sutured.

11 *Records.* The midwife records the time of the symphysiotomy and the time of delivery.

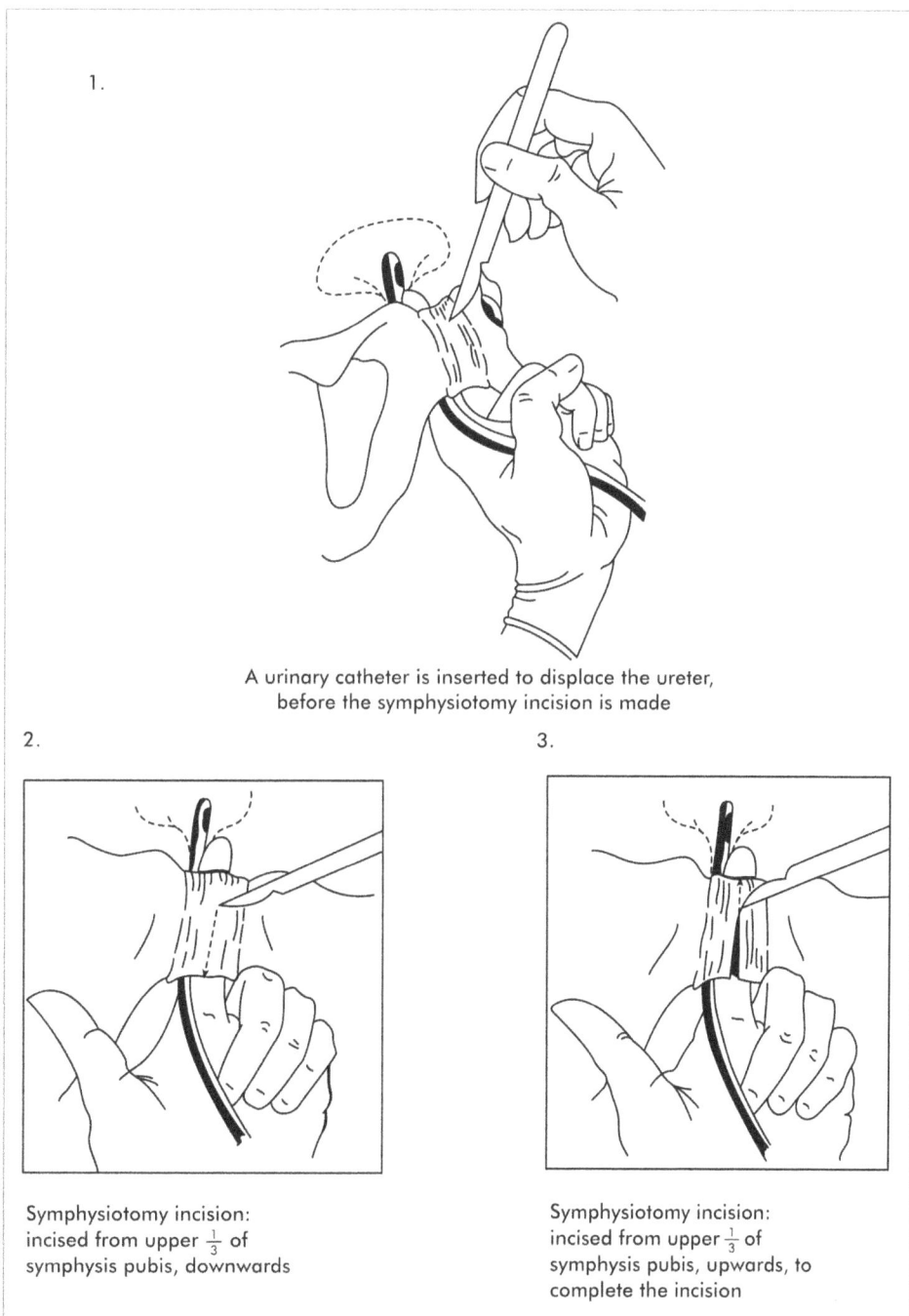

1.

A urinary catheter is inserted to displace the ureter, before the symphysiotomy incision is made

2.

Symphysiotomy incision: incised from upper $\frac{1}{3}$ of symphysis pubis, downwards

3.

Symphysiotomy incision: incised from upper $\frac{1}{3}$ of symphysis pubis, upwards, to complete the incision

Figure 33A Symphysiotomy

continued

Post-operative treatment and care

▶ *Complications.* If any complications arose during the procedure, the woman should be told exactly what to expect. She should be encouraged to comply with the nursing procedures so that optimum healing can take place.

▶ *Post-delivery care.*
  • The patient is nursed on her sides for 48 hours and turned 2-hourly by two nurses, while her legs are tied together. She must be given help in turning, especially at first.
  • The midwife must ensure that the woman is comfortable and not anxious.
  • Deep breathing exercises and leg exercises are demonstrated and encouraged. If available, a physiotherapist is called in to help the woman with the exercises.
  • The woman must be given a bed bath daily and oral and other hygiene must be provided.
  • Vulval toilette is performed 4-hourly, with the patient lying on her side, until she is able to do this for herself.

▶ *Diet.* A high-protein, high-roughage diet with plenty of fluids is given to the patient. She is given assistance with feeding, as she will find it awkward to eat lying on her side.

▶ *Fluids.* Strict records are kept of fluid intake and output.

▶ *Medication.* Some obstetricians prescribe an antibiotic cover for five days.

▶ *Breastfeeding.* The mother is encouraged to breastfeed her baby on demand, and all feeds are closely supervised. She must be reassured that the staff will take care of her baby while she is at bed rest.

▶ *Analgesia.* This is given for pain, usually in the form of IM injections for 48 hours, and thereafter oral tablets 4- to 6-hourly. The midwife must make sure that the analgesic is effective. The patient is instructed to report any excessive pain experienced and the medical practitioner is immediately informed.

▶ *Mobility.* On the fifth day, the patient is allowed to sit up, at first only on the edge of the bed for a short while. Gradually, she progresses to standing alongside the bed and finally to walking around the bed. Eventually she walks to the toilet with help from the staff and with the aid of rubber-tipped walking sticks or a walker. This is usually achieved by the sixth to seventh post-operative day.

▶ *Discharge.* The woman is allowed home on about the tenth post-operative day, provided she is confident and walking normally.

The woman is given the following advice on discharge:
▶ She must not lift or carry any heavy objects for at least three months and she should have help at home.
▶ She must not walk long distances.
▶ She must avoid any undue muscular effort where possible.
▶ She should abstain from sexual intercourse for about six weeks.
▶ She should have a full range of movement by the end of three months.
▶ She must report any abnormalities, such as difficulty in walking or excessive pain, to the nearest clinic or hospital.

Complications

Any delay in delivery after a symphysiotomy could be due to one or more of the following:
▶ Inefficient uterine action
▶ Insufficient separation of the joint
▶ An inadequate episiotomy
▶ Greater CPD than anticipated
▶ Unanticipated fetal abnormality.

Complications specific to the procedure are usually only found where the patient has not been correctly selected for symphysiotomy, the operation has been poorly performed and the aftercare and follow-up have not been adequate. Complications include:
▶ instability of the pubic joint, which may occur if the separation is excessive, causing pain and discomfort
▶ tears in the anterior vaginal wall
▶ traumatic haemorrhage at the site of the incision, resulting in the formation of haematomas, pubic pain (at the time and later) and backache (acute and/or chronic)
▶ injury to the bladder and/or the urethra, due to the incision extending through these tissues, later resulting in either a vesicovaginal fistula and/or a urethrovaginal fistula

- injury to the sacroiliac joint, causing problems with movement later
- stress incontinence (occasionally)
- osteitis of the pubic bones
- non-union of the joint, resulting in excessive pain and difficulties in walking.

Pain and difficulty in walking will often be experienced in the first few days after delivery and the difficulty in walking will be greater if a haematoma occurs.

33.6 Conclusion

Interventions in childbirth can be very traumatic and yet life-saving. The abuse of interventions in itself is a subject of debate and a global movement against unnecessary interventions exists. It is therefore important to make the right diagnosis and choose the appropriate intervention.

34

General obstetric interventions

LEARNING OBJECTIVES

On completion of this chapter, you must be able to:
▶ identify general obstetric procedures and interventions in obstetrics
▶ identify the competencies midwives need in obstetric procedures and interventions.
▶ identify the roles and responsibilities of midwives in obstetric interventions in relation to the scope of practice of midwives (SANC) (See Annexure B)

KNOWLEDGE ASSUMED TO BE IN PLACE

Basic knowledge, skill and competency in the care of a normal birth
Scope of midwifery practice SANC Regulation 786, dated 15 October 2013 (Nursing Act 33 of 2005)
The management of risks and abnormalities

KEYWORDS

uterotonics • prostaglandins • induction of labour (IOL) • termination of pregnancy (TOP) • assisted delivery

34.1   Introduction

This chapter considers further interventions that are important in obstetrics. As mentioned in Chapter 33, the midwife's scope of practice focuses on the normal and most interventions are directly performed by a medical practitioner or prescribed and supervised by an obstetrician. In some settings, task shifting may be necessary, for example where there are not enough medical practitioners available. In such cases, skilled midwives may perform certain obstetric interventions, such as an external version and assisted delivery, both of which are discussed in this chapter.

The high incidence of Caesarean deliveries, the medicolegal climate and the lack of trained professionals contribute to an unclear future for all types of instrumental delivery. However, the experienced (advanced) midwife or doctors working in a community health clinic (CHC) may be required to deliver the baby by instruments when a Caesarean section is not feasible.

The principles of the role of the midwife listed in Section 33.1 on page 515 apply to the interventions described in this chapter as well. The midwifery manager and supervisor must take responsibility for evaluation of the outcomes of care.

34.2   Induction of labour

Induction of labour (IOL) is the deliberate initiation of uterine contractions prior to their spontaneous onset. When labour is initiated after the end of the sixth calendar month (26 weeks) of pregnancy, it is known as IOL; when initiated before this time, it is known as therapeutic abortion or termination of pregnancy (TOP).

Incidence

The incidence of IOL is 9.6 per cent of all deliveries (WHO, 2011). No accurate statistics for southern Africa are available, but the induction rate is lower.

Classification

IOL can be classified according to its *purpose*. An elective induction is a planned induction, which may be performed with or without medical indication.

IOL can also be classified according *to method*:
▶ A *medical induction* refers to the administration of substances to stimulate the uterus.
▶ A *surgical induction* uses the artificial rupture of membranes (AROM) and the stretching of the cervix to release prostaglandins to start labour in a woman.

Medical and surgical inductions of labour are often used in combination.

> ### Differentiating induction of labour from augmentation of labour
>
> IOL involves initiating labour because the woman is not yet in labour. The cervix may need ripening after assessment (using the Bishop score) and oxytocin administered to initiate the onset of contractions.
>
> In augmentation of labour, the onset of labour is spontaneous but the contractions are not effective and need strengthening to facilitate progress of labour. This is done by the administration of a uterine stimulant.

Prerequisites for induction

IOL is only performed on prescription of a medical practitioner in a woman with an obstetric indication, in a setting where there is a theatre as well as a neonatal care unit available. The woman should be under supervision during the induction.

Depending on the medical and obstetric indication for the induction, the following are important prerequisites, with exceptions depending on the condition of the woman and/or the fetus (for example IOL for preterm women as well as those where the presenting part is not engaged):

‣ *The gestational period.* IOL is performed when a pregnancy is at term.
‣ *The presenting part.* The presenting part must be engaged.
‣ *The presentation.* A cephalic presentation is a prerequisite.
‣ *Fetal well-being.* A reactive non-stress test (NST) is required, as induction cannot be done on a compromised fetus.
‣ *The size of the fetus.* IOL cannot be performed in the case of macrosomia or intrauterine growth restriction (IUGR).
‣ *Maternal history.* IOL cannot be performed in the case of previous perinatal loss or obstructed labour.
‣ *The pelvis.* The pelvis should be adequate.
‣ *The placenta.* The position of the placenta must be known.
‣ *The cervix.* The Bishop score must be favourable (see Table 34.1).
‣ *Consent.* The mother must give consent to both the time and method of the procedure.
‣ *Skilled attendants.* The staff must be competent.

The Bishop score

The Bishop score is a scoring system used to determine whether IOL without cervical ripening (or priming) will be effective (ie AROM and oxytocin). The score can be used to assess the odds of spontaneous preterm delivery and labour.

The criteria for determining the score are as follows (see Table 34.1 below):

‣ *Dilatation* is a measure of the diameter of the stretched cervix. It is the most important indicator of readiness for labour. A long posterior and closed cervix is unfavourable.
‣ *Effacement* is the level to which the cervix is pulled up as part of the lower segment. Effacement is measured in centimetres. An uneffaced cervix is 2 cm long.
‣ The *station* of the denominator of the presenting part reaches the level of the ischial spines, station 0, as determined on vaginal examination. The station above the spines or below the spines is reflected in centimetres. A low head will influence cervical changes.
‣ *Consistency* refers to how tough and resistant to stretching the cervix is. A poor consistency feels like the tip of the nose, while a good consistency is as soft as the lips. If the cervix is tight (called cervical dystocia), birth may be difficult and progress delayed or induction may fail.
‣ The *position* of the cervix changes in pregnancy, particularly when the lower segment forms and the presenting part moves down. A posterior cervix indicates that the needed changes have not yet taken place. In late pregnancy, the cervix moves anteriorly.

Table 34.1

Calculating the Bishop score

	SCORE			
FACTOR	**0**	**1**	**2**	**3**
Dilatation	Nil	1–2	3–4	5+
Effacement	0–30%	40–50%	60–70%	80%+
Station	–3	–2	–1	+1
Consistency	Firm	Medium	Soft	
Position	Posterior	Mid	Anterior	

Each component is given a score of 0–2 or 0–3, as indicated in Table 34.1. The highest possible score is 13. For example:

‣ A presenting part at the spines, with a soft, anterior cervix with 50 per cent effacement and 3–4 cm dilatation gives a Bishop score of 10. This indicates what is referred to as a 'ripe cervix' and readiness for birth or a high likelihood of successful IOL. When the fetal head is well fitted (applied) on the cervix, prostaglandins are released which can cause cervical changes and the Ferguson reflex kicks in.

▶ A high presenting part with a firm, posterior cervix with poor effacement and no dilatation will give a Bishop score of 1–2.

The following are guidelines for interpreting the scores:
▶ A score of 10 or more indicates that labour will probably start spontaneously.
▶ A score of 8 is considered to be a reliable prediction of a successful induction.
▶ A score of 5 or less suggests that labour is unlikely to start without induction. A low Bishop score also often indicates that induction is unlikely to be successful, but this does not indicate that induction is not needed. Women with a low Bishop score can be induced using a catheter or prostaglandin.
▶ A poor Bishop score at term with a high head needs further consideration, for example to determine the presence of a large infant or a malpresentation. Poor application of the presenting part is suspicious.

Indications

IOL without any valid indication presents unnecessary risks to both mother and baby.

Maternal conditions

Conditions of the mother that warrant the delivery of the baby include:
▶ hypertensive disorders
▶ malignancies (if the mother needs to start chemotherapy or radiation)
▶ pruritus.

Fetal conditions

Factors that put the well-being of the fetus at risk include:
▶ macrosomia, in maternal diabetes
▶ Rh incompatibility with sensitivity
▶ IUGR
▶ antepartum haemorrhage (APH) that is not life-threatening
▶ premature rupture of the membranes (PROM)
▶ congenital abnormalities.

Obstetric reasons

Obstetric reasons for IOL include:
▶ intrauterine death (IUD) – the pregnancy is terminated
▶ post-maturity – the pregnancy is not allowed to continue to prevent complications
▶ persistent, acute renal disease
▶ APH.

Social reasons (elective induction)

Elective IOL is a very controversial subject. IOL may be requested for social reasons or for the medical practitioner's convenience. Other reasons may include the following:
▶ The woman lives some distance from the hospital.
▶ The family may be moving from the district shortly and they wish deliver to avoid not reaching the hospital on time or to avoid delivering in a new, unknown place.
▶ The woman may be experiencing discomfort.

Contraindications

There are absolute and relative contraindications for IOL.

Absolute contraindications include:
▶ the woman refusing to consent to IOL
▶ two previous Caesarean sections for cephalopelvic disproportion (CPD) or obstructed labour
▶ surgery of the uterus, eg myomectomy
▶ fetal distress (compromise) (poor kick chart or Doppler)
▶ malpresentation or malposition, eg transverse lie or brow or face presentation
▶ placenta praevia or vasa praevia
▶ cancer of the cervix
▶ active herpes infection
▶ prematurity (if no maternal indication)
▶ cord presentation or prolapsed cord, if the fetus is alive.

Relative contraindications include:
▶ previous Caesarean section for reasons other than CPD or obstructed labour
▶ a grand multipara (risk of uterine rupture)
▶ an overextended uterus due to polyhydramnios or multiple pregnancy
▶ placental dysfunction or insufficiency
▶ a frank breech, where the legs splint the body
▶ a large infant: 40 cm on the symphysis fundal height (SFH) measurement by 36 weeks (high risk of shoulder dystocia).

Complications

The complications of IOL are associated with the method of induction, the indications and risks. It is impossible to know how a woman's body and uterus will respond to the stimulation provided by the substances used in medical IOL. Known complications include:
▶ precipitate delivery with severe pelvic floor and perineal damage

- hypertonic contractions with cerebral injury in the newborn, asphyxia neonatorum and an increased perinatal mortality rate (PNMR)
- fetal distress with intrapartum death
- placental abruption with intrapartum death
- rupture of the uterus
- in the case of malpresentation or a large fetus, obstructed labour with maternal distress
- postpartum haemorrhage (PPH) due to an exhausted uterus
- allergy or hypersensitivity to oxytocin and prostaglandins, such as in asthmatic women
- maternal emotional or psychological disturbances such as post-traumatic shock.

If surgical induction is used and AROM is performed, there is an increased incidence of:
- infection of both mother and fetus
- cord prolapse, if the presenting part is not engaged and not well fitting on the cervix, with fetal distress and death
- intrauterine infections due to rupture of membranes and multiple vaginal examinations for more than 12 hours.

AROM may not initiate labour and is usually used in combination with medical induction.

Choosing a method of induction

The choice of the method of induction is made by the medical practitioner in collaboration with the woman. The following factors will guide the choice of method, the route of administration and the dosage used:

- *Gravidity and parity.* The dosage must be changed for a multigravida. In a grand multigravida, a lower dosage of uterine stimulants is used due to the risk of uterine rupture.
- *Risk of infection.* The rupture of membranes is avoided in cases of lowered immunity and vaginal and other infections.
- *Drug sensitivity.* Asthma is a relative contraindication for the use of prostaglandins.
- *Cardiac, lung and kidney problems.* Women with these conditions are prone to water toxicity associated with the administration of oxytocin.
- *Bishop score and ripeness of the cervix.* These will guide the method of induction.

Cervical ripening

IOL is less likely to succeed if the cervix is not ready (scoring 5 or less on the Bishop cervical scoring system). Before the start of either surgical or medical induction, it may be necessary to make the cervix more favourable; this is referred to as cervical ripening. The medical practitioner will prescribe medication for this purpose (see Table 34.2 and the section on medical induction on the next page).

Various hormones are involved in a complex series of interactions to stimulate the chemical reactions critical for cervical ripening. An increase in the enzyme cyclo-oxygenase-2 leads to a local increase of prostaglandin E2 (PGE_2) in the cervix. The increase in local PGE_2 leads to a series of important changes causing cervical ripening.

Prostaglandins are an important substance involved in cervical ripening. They are present in the body (the cervix) and also in semen, which means that cervical ripening can be promoted during sexual intercourse. For this reason sexual intercourse is discouraged in preterm birth and encouraged after 36 weeks. Women often have contractions after sexual intercourse. Other methods to stimulate prostaglandin release include the points discussed in the following subsections.

Stretching the cervix

The stretching of the cervix releases local prostaglandins, causing contractions. Membrane stripping, called 'stretch and sweep', is an old method used to stimulate labour. This is useful in a multigravida with an open cervix of 2–4 cm. The fingers are placed in the cervix and the membranes are separated from the lower segment through moving the fingers around the cervix between the cervix and the membranes. This will release prostaglandins and may lead to the start of birth.

Hydroscopic dilators

If the cervix is closed, it can be stretched by lamicel (seaweed). This is a tampon that is placed in the cervix. It swells as it absorbs fluid and pushes the cervix open over a period of 24 hours, releasing prostaglandins. This is useful in cases of IUD where the cervix is closed. However, it is associated with peripartum infections.

Balloon catheter

An F16–18 Foley catheter filled with saline (30–50 ml) is placed in the uterus through the cervix, if open, and the balloon is inflated. The catheter is placed extra-amniotically (between the membrane and the uterus) and is pulled down in the lower segment. It places pressure on the lower segment and releases local prostaglandins. There is no increased risk of chorioamnionitis and it is as effective as prostaglandin gel. The balloon catheter method is more useful in primigravidae and is used with IUD.

Medical induction: Antiprogesterone

Medical induction is the use of substances to start or augment labour. These include the following:

▶ *Mifepristone* (formerly known as RU 486) is a very effective antiprogesterone and antiglucocorticoid that works by binding to progesterone and glucocorticoid receptors. It is used mainly for abortions and inductions in the case of IUD.

▶ A *low-dosage oxytocin infusion* is useful with women whose fetuses are at risk of intolerance in labour, because the infusion can be closed if needed. A low dosage of oxytocin is administered in an IV infusion 1–4 mU/min (2 U at 30 drops per minutes, see Table 34.2). It compares favourably with the effectiveness of misoprostol. Nipple stimulation is a known method of releasing oxytocin in the body: the woman rubs her nipple until it contracts.

▶ Two forms of *prostaglandin E2* (dinoprostone; PGE2) are available commercially. The first is Prepidil®, which is formulated as a gel and is placed inside the cervix but not above the internal os. The application (3 g gel/0.5 mg dinoprostone) can be repeated in 6 hours, not to exceed 3 doses in 24 hours. The second is Cervidil®, which contains 10 mg of dinoprostone embedded in a mesh and is placed in the posterior fornix of the vagina. This allows for controlled release of dinoprostone over 12 hours, after which it is removed.

▶ *Prostaglandin E1 analog (misoprostol)* is a synthetic prostaglandin which is marketed as an antiulcer agent under the trade name Cytotec®. The oral dose is 50 µg orally with water, or a tablet (20-25 mcg) which can be crushed and placed on the cervix. This can induce cervical ripening and labour. It can be repeated every four hours as long as contractions are absent or not painful. The administration routes are buccal, sublingual, oral, vaginal or rectal, but vaginal administration seems to be best. It should not be given in combination with oxytocin.

Misoprostol for cervical ripening and induction of labour

The WHO advises that low-dosage oral misoprostol (50 µg) is safer than vaginal misoprostol. Although vaginal misoprostol 4-hourly 25 µg is more effective than other methods of IOL, it causes hyperstimulation of the uterus (Abdel-Aleem, 2006).

Table 34.2

Preparations for medical induction

Prostaglandins	Dosage and administration	Contraindications	Dangers and side effects
Dinoprostone PGE2 tablets Prandin® E2 gel	A powerful agent Vaginal insertion Maximum dosage: 2 mg x 4-hourly, which is 1 tab hourly x 10 A safer dosage: 4 tabs of 0.5 mg every 4 hours The preferred method of usage is the gel which is 1 mg/3 g Maximum dosage is 3 mg administered as 1 mg every 6 hours	See general contraindications for IOL A history of asthma Avoid vaginal administration when membranes are ruptured Avoid with previous Caesarean section Not used for grand multiparae	Gastrointestinal (GI): nausea, vomiting, diarrhoea Tonic uterus: fetal distress, placental abruption and pain Rupture of the uterus Hypertension Anaphylaxis
Dinoprostone Prostagladin F2 Alpha® injection, only administered by a medical practitioner	Very powerful agent Used for IUD IOL or when pregnancy is terminated for an abnormal fetus (intra-amniotic)	Fetal: When baby is alive Maternal: • Epilepsy • Cardiac, lung, kidney or liver problems • Immune-compromised • Hypertension • Glaucoma	Continuous administration for more than two days is not recommended GI: nausea, vomiting Tonic contraction of the uterus Hypotension Pulmonary oedema Tachycardia Fever Headache

continued

Prostaglandins	Dosage and administration	Contraindications	Dangers and side effects
Misoprostol Prostaglandin E1 Cytotec®	Synthetic prostaglandin E1 200 µg diluted in 200 ml and then given in 50 µg 2-hourly dosage orally or 25 µg vaginally every 4–6 hours (maximum 6 dosages) Safe to use in IUD or with PPH Useful if Bishop score is poor Misoprostol versus PE2: fewer failures to induce labour, fewer epidurals, fewer Caesarean sections and more hyperstimulation of uterus	See the general contraindications for IOL Risk of uterine rupture: 12% in previous Caesarean section (Toppenberg & Block, 2002)	Hyperstimulation syndrome Uterine rupture Fetal distress and meconium in liquor Amniotic fluid embolism Diarrhoea if taken orally plus GI effects Vaginal application may influence immune responses
Oxytocin	Synthetic oxytocin IV administration only Primigravidae: 5–10 units in 1 000 ml saline/dextrose/Ringer's Multigravidae: 2–5 units in 1 000 ml Grand multiparae: 2 units in 1 000 ml Initial dosage 5 drops/min Increase every 30 minutes with 5 drops till uterus contracts Two contractions in 10 minutes Maximum 30 drops per minute Do not exceed 1 500 ml in 10 hours	Fetal distress Hydramnios Partial placenta praevia Prematurity Borderline CPD Overdistention of the uterus Grand multiparity Placental abruption Amniotic embolism	Hyperstimulation of the uterus Maternal: • Hypertensive episode • Rupture of the uterus Fetal: • Bradycardia • Permanent damage to central nervous system (CNS) or brain • Death

Table 34.3

Guidelines for oxytocin infusion in 1 000 ml solution

Rate: drops per minute	2 units/ℓ mU/min	10 units/ℓ
1	0.13	0–66
15	2	10
30	4	20
60	8	40

Surgical induction (amniotomy)

Amniotomy is the not safest and most reliable form of IOL. It is potentially hazardous (risk of cord prolapse, infection, abruption) and irreversible. It is done with an understanding of the precautions.

In order to perform amniotomy, the cervical os must be dilated enough to introduce a finger into the cervix to rupture the membranes and the vertex must be presenting, engaged and well applied to the cervix.

Often, surgical induction is combined with a medical induction. Otherwise, if labour is not established within four hours of the membranes being ruptured, a medical induction is started.

Precautions

Amniotomy is contraindicated in cases of:
▶ a high presenting part (due to the risk of cord prolapse)
▶ HIV-positive status (membranes are kept intact as long as possible)
▶ malpresentations: the amniotic fluid is a wedge that equalises the pressure on the cervix; if the membranes rupture, the pressure on the cervix is unequal and the presenting part may deflex
▶ polyhydramnios: great care needs to be taken, as the risk of cord prolapse as well as placental abruption with the sudden decompression of the uterus is very high
▶ placenta praevia or vasa praevia
▶ active herpes genitalis, which can infect the fetus when it passes through the birth canal.

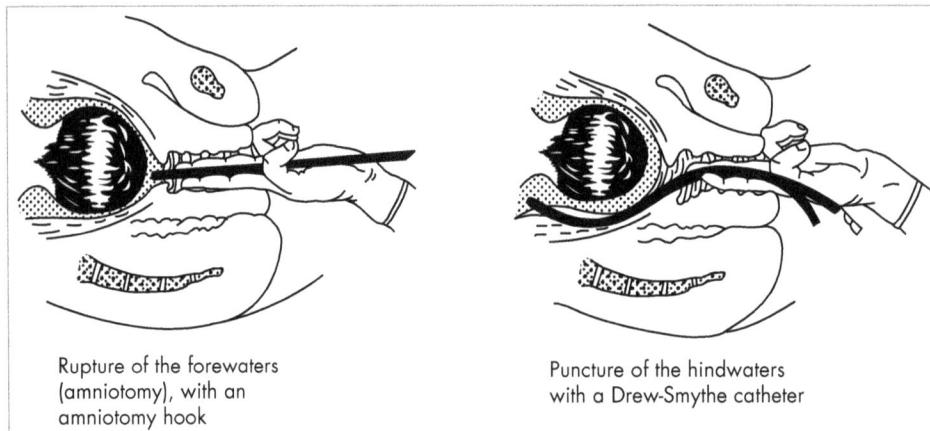

Rupture of the forewaters (amniotomy), with an amniotomy hook

Puncture of the hindwaters with a Drew-Smythe catheter

Figure 34.1 Amniotomy

Artificial rupture of membranes

It is safer to start and establish labour before an amniotomy is performed, bearing in mind the contraindications of amniotomy.

The following guidelines are observed:
▶ The patient's rectum and bladder should be empty.
▶ The patient is placed in the dorsal or the semi-Fowler's lithotomy position.
▶ A baseline fetal heart rate (FHR) is taken and recorded. It should be within normal limits (NST).
▶ An aseptic technique is maintained. Sterile instruments are used.
▶ If the presenting part is well fitted and a sac of forewaters is formed, the forewaters can be ruptured if the cervix allows a finger to be admitted.
▶ If the presenting part is not well fitted and the cervix is 4 cm dilated, a high rupture can be performed, leaving the forewaters intact. This is done by an obstetrician and is seldom performed now. Great care must be taken to avoid cord prolapse.
▶ The fetal heart is checked before and after the rupture.
▶ The volume, colour, consistency and smell of the amniotic fluid are recorded. Any meconium staining and abnormalities are reported.
▶ If all observations are normal and contractions have started, the woman should be encouraged to walk around to help the presenting part engage in the pelvis and to help stimulate contractions.

▶ Should labour not have started after an hour, the medical practitioner will review the situation and, if contractions have not started, usually order a medical induction.
▶ If the woman has not delivered within 12–18 hours, the medical practitioner may order an antibiotic that crosses the placental barrier with ease.
▶ If the patient has not delivered within 18 hours, the medical practitioner may decide to do a Caesarean section.
▶ Appropriate pain relief is administered according to prescription.

Principles of care in induction

The patient is admitted to hospital. Pain relief is essential, because induced uterine contractions have a higher peak and are more painful than normal contractions. Immediately before the IOL is started, the condition of mother and fetus must again be carefully assessed.

Midwife's liability
The midwife, on accepting the prescription to induce labour, makes sure that there are no contraindications to the procedure and refers it back to the medical practitioner if abnormalities are noted. Once she accepts the prescription, she is liable for her own actions.

PROCEDURE | Examinations in induction of labour

Preparation

1 The patient's history is reviewed: the estimated date of delivery (EDD), last menstrual period (LMP), gestational age (GA) and other risk factors.
2 The patient's emotional state and her expectations of the procedure are assessed.
3 A physical examination is carried out and the results recorded. In this way, the midwife can assess the contraindications and make baseline observations.
4 Urine tests for protein, glucose and ketones are carried out.
5 Temperature, pulse, respiration, BP and colour are checked.
6 Other tests results are considered, such as maternal blood tests and recent Hb (within seven days).
7 Ultrasound scans, NST, amniocentesis (for maternal well-being and/or fetal well-being and maturity) are done.
8 Any allergies or hypersensitivity to medication (asthma) are noted.
9 The patient signs consent for the procedure after the procedure has been explained.

The obstetric examination

An obstetric examination includes the following:

1 The reason for the IOL and the woman's preference for pain management are recorded. This assessment is similar to that which is carried out on admission of labour.
2 Abdominal palpation is done to determine the size and position of the fetus.
3 The engagement of the presenting part is determined.
4 Fetal well-being is assessed through a cardiotocograph (CTG) NST.
5 The procedure and expectations are discussed with the birth companion.

The vaginal examination

A vaginal examination is performed and a clinical pelvic assessment may be done if indicated:

1 A Bishop score is done.
2 The state of the membranes (if ruptured), the state of the liquor (clear or meconium stained) and the presence of any vaginal discharge is noted.
3 The station of the presenting part, moulding, cord presentation or prolapse and vasa praevia are noted.
4 The application of the cervix to the presenting part is noted.

Special examinations

Further tests may be requested, such as ultrasound scan; X-ray; laboratory tests of urine, blood or liquor; and NST.

Recording

It is extremely important that all the results of the examinations are carefully recorded, so that any change will be obvious once the induction has been started.

The role and function of the midwife

The following are important for a midwife involved in IOL:

▶ The midwife must have the necessary *scientific knowledge* and a thorough knowledge of the medications used for IOL: the drug, the storage of the drug, the preparation of the drug, the routes of administration, dosages, indications and contraindications, side effects and antidotes.
▶ The midwife follows the *protocols* for IOL in a well-resourced centre with adequate medical backup, theatre and neonatal support.
▶ The midwife makes sure that the drugs and emergency equipment are in place for emergencies.
▶ The midwife follows strict protocols on the prescription of drugs. Drugs are only administered on *written prescription* from a medical practitioner.
▶ The midwife is careful to identify contraindications and side effects of drugs administered.
▶ The midwife makes sure that there are no contraindications before the therapy is started.

▶ The drug is always checked with a second person before administration.

▶ Thermo-unstable substances are kept in the fridge (oxytocin and Prostin Alpha F$_2$).

▶ The treatment is always started with the lowest dosage, using the correct route of administration. Prostin E$_2$ and misoprostol cannot be counteracted once absorbed. Oxytocin can be discontinued if given intravenously and the effect stopped.

▶ The appropriate dosage is given for the parity.

▶ Care is taken when using prostaglandins (misoprostol with oxytocin for drug interaction).

▶ Careful observations are done, particularly of the uterine action. Aim for a uterine pattern close to normal labour: two contractions in 10 minutes with a normal resting tone in-between.

▶ Continuous electronic observation of the fetal heart is done.

▶ Maximum dosages are never exceeded.

▶ The woman is given sufficient pain relief. The contractions of artificial inductions are more painful than normal birth.

▶ The midwife keeps clear and accurate notes of the events.

▶ The midwife monitors the progress of labour and prevents complications such as obstructed labour, uterine rupture and fetal distress.

34.3   External and internal versions

A version involves changing the presentation or lie of the fetus in a non-labouring woman or in an emergency during labour.

In the developing world where Caesarean sections are not readily available and women do not always attend antenatal care, undiagnosed twins may present unexpectedly. Medical practitioners and skilled midwives should be able to perform versions.

External cephalic version (ECV) is also a common intervention to avoid Caesarean section. The South African Nursing Council (SANC) Regulations for Midwifery Practice (Directive 4, paragraph 2 (k)(iii) and (iv) says the following about versions (SANC, 1990): 'An external version . . . for a transverse lie should be taught in the case of a patient in early labour, and in the transverse lie of the second twin after the first has been delivered. Version in these cases is attempted only where a medical practitioner is not available.'

Incidence

The incidence of breech presentation at 28 weeks is 25 per cent, while the incidence at the onset of birth is 3 per cent. The incidence of transverse lie in twin pregnancy is estimated at 1 in 300 pregnancies (Bowes, 2010).

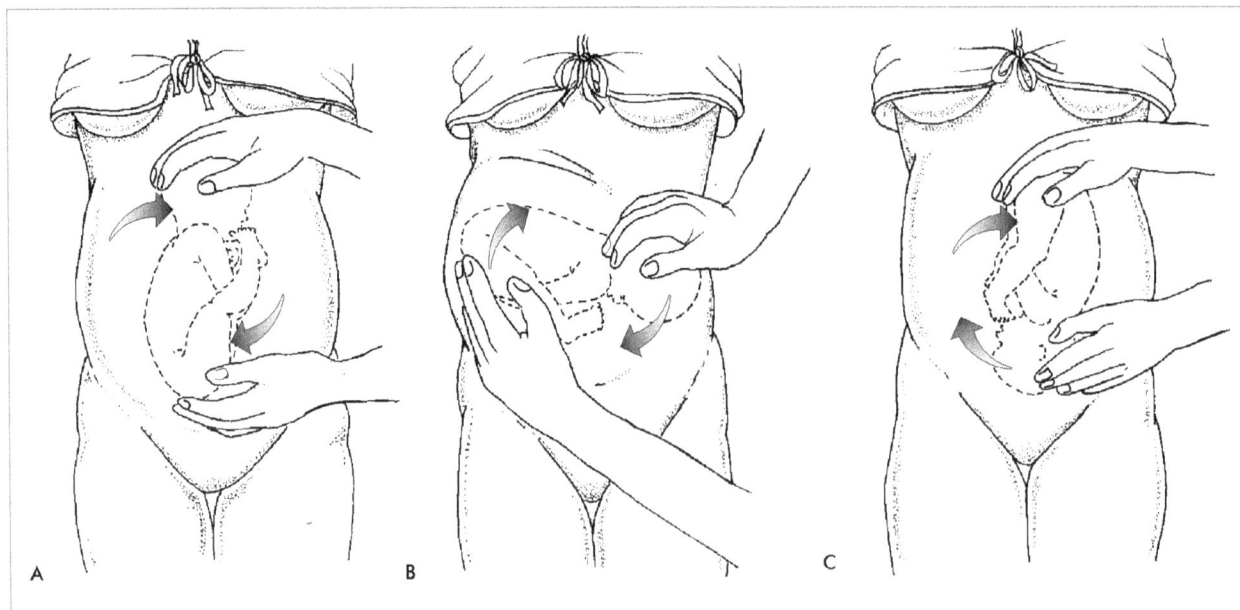

Figure 34.2 External cephalic version

Classification

A version can be spontaneous or by manipulation. Manipulation can be external or internal:

▶ An *ECV* entails changing the fetal position from a breech or transverse to a vertex, to bring the head into the brim of the pelvis. It is done using abdominal palpation (see Figure 34.2).

▶ An *internal podalic version (IPV)* entails changing the fetal position from a transverse or oblique lie to bring the buttocks over the pelvic brim (also for the second twin). It is done by placing the hand through the vagina into the uterus and using the other hand on the abdomen (see Figure 34.3).

Protocols for external cephalic version

ECV before term is of no value, because the fetus may turn back. There is evidence that fetal mortality in preterm birth is increased with ECV. In more than 50 per cent of cases, ECV can be achieved after 37 weeks with assistance of tocolysis. Leaving the woman as long as possible may lead to spontaneous version.

With ECV, the incidence of non-cephalic birth is reduced by 33 per cent and the incidence of Caesarean section by 50 per cent (Wikipedia, 2017d). There is a small risk of placental abruption and a very low risk of fetal loss. These risks must be weighed against the risks of cord prolapse, breech presentation, trauma in breech and precipitate labour.

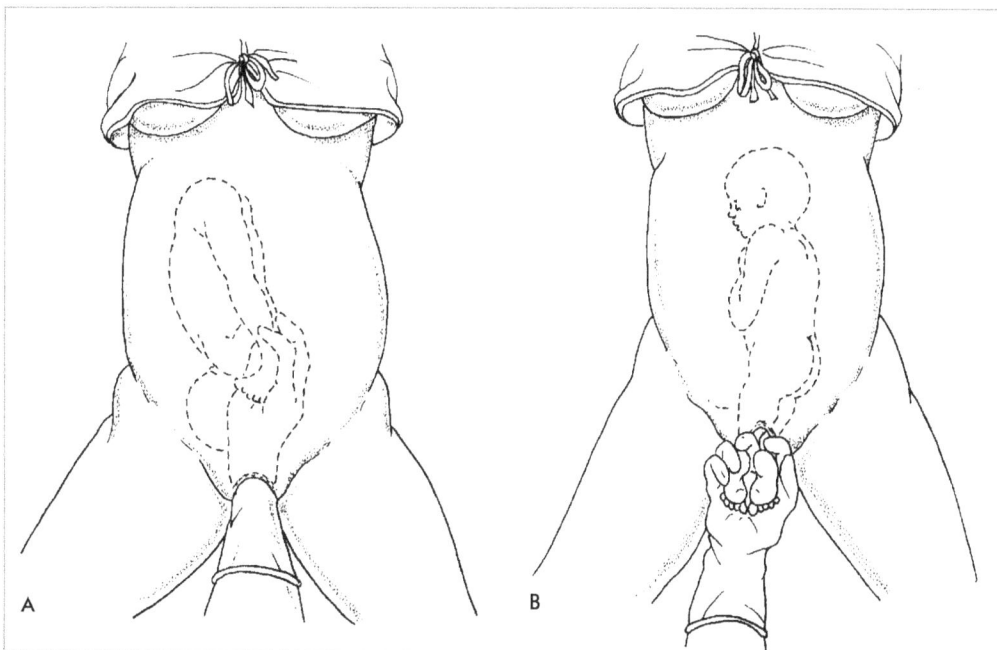

Figure 34.3 Internal podalic version

PROCEDURE   External cephalic version

Principles
The ECV is done in an appropriate level of care (with ultrasound, NST and theatre available) by skilled healthcare professionals (an obstetrician or skilled midwife). In the case of a transverse position of a second twin, if a medical practitioner is not present, a midwife may do an external version if the membranes are intact.

Prerequisites
- 37 weeks or early labour
- Ultrasound indicating normal position of the placenta
- Reactive NST
- Breech position not due to placenta praevia, a cord around the neck or CPD (sonar)
- Adequate amniotic fluid
- No uterine abnormality (eg bicornuate uterus).

Contraindications
- Prematurity
- APH
- Hypertension
- Cord around the neck
- Previous Caesarean section
- Ruptured membranes
- Vaginal birth contraindicated
- Abnormal uterus or fibroids.

Procedure
1 The woman is tilted to 45° with two pillows under her left side and two under her head.
2 The uterus is relaxed with 10 μg salbutamol slowly IV
3 The pulse rate is observed (not to exceed 120 bpm).
4 Powder is used on the stomach.
5 The patient is talked through the procedure.
6 The fetal heart is listened to every two minutes during the procedure.
7 The breech is manipulated rather than the head. The breech is lifted out of the pelvis abdominally.
8 The breech is kept in position with one hand and the fetus is allowed to readjust.
9 If this is not successful, a forward somersault is done, in which pressure is placed on the fetal head (always maintaining flexion).
10 The NST is repeated. The FHR becomes reactive after 30 minutes.
11 In an Rh-negative woman, anti-D is given to prevent transplacental bleeding and the possibility of Rh isoimmunisation.
12 The woman is discharged only when there are no contractions and the FHR is normal.
13 If complications arise, a Caesarean section is performed, as the woman is 37 weeks pregnant.

Potential complications
- Placental abruption
- Fetal distress
- Cord prolapse
- Rupture of membranes
- Uterine rupture.

Recording and interpretation
Record actions and outcomes carefully and accurately.

An IPV (see Figure 34.3 on page 547) is usually performed during birth in the case of a multiple pregnancy, where the second twin is transverse or in an undiagnosed twin with a transverse lie. IPV is done for the delivery of a retained second twin, after vaginal delivery of the first twin. A medical practitioner should perform the delivery.

There is a higher PNMR where IPV is performed. The mortality rate is associated with GA, birth weight and whether it is a singleton pregnancy or twins. The mortality rate is increased in singleton pregnancies. Currently, Caesarean section is performed for most cases of transverse lie, even for stillbirths. In settings where Caesarean section is not an option, an IPV may be needed.

A failed IPV could be followed by abruption, which can only be managed at subsequent Caesarean delivery. Fetal complications are associated with cord prolapse and the fast delivery in the breech presentation.

34.4 Assisted vaginal delivery

Births that are complicated by malpresentations and prolonged labour may require assisted vaginal delivery. The forceps and vacuum are the best-known interventions for assisted vaginal births. The use of the forceps has become less popular and requires a high level of skill.

An assisted vaginal delivery should only be performed if there is an appropriate indication. A series of criteria all need to be fulfilled before an assisted vaginal delivery can be attempted. Consider the following principles:

▶ The selection of the appropriate instrument depends on the clinical situation and the operator's preference and experience.
▶ A number of clinical conditions (potentially detrimental to the fetus) exist in which an assisted vaginal delivery should not be attempted.
▶ The risk of maternal injury is much higher with forceps compared to vacuum-assist devices (severe perineal injury, such as third- or fourth-degree perineal laceration and PPH).
▶ There is no consensus regarding minimum and maximum estimated fetal weights that preclude assisted vaginal delivery.
▶ Assisted vaginal delivery for a fetus with suspected macrosomia should be performed with caution, given the possible increased risk of fetal injury and shoulder dystocia.

▶ Paediatricians should be notified whenever an assisted vaginal delivery has been attempted because of significant fetal morbidity (scalp injuries and bleeding).

Forceps delivery
Definition

In cases of malpresentations and prolonged labour, the use of forceps may be required to assist with a vaginal delivery.

Incidence

The incidence of forceps delivery varies greatly, depending upon the community, medical practice and preference. Incidence may range from 5–15 per cent or even higher in some hospitals.

Types of forceps

There are more than 600 varieties of forceps. Forceps are designed to follow the curve of Caris and have a pelvic curvature (fitting the pelvis) and a cephalic curvature (fitting the fetal head). Forceps are made from high-quality stainless steel and are light and polished. Poorly manufactured forceps should not be used, as they can damage the mother and child.

Forceps have two blades, a shank, a lock and a handle, as shown in Figure 34.4. The forceps are made in pairs, with a left and a right blade, and have corresponding numbers inside each blade. It is essential to use blades made as original pairs. Before use, the forceps should be checked to make sure they are a fitting pair.

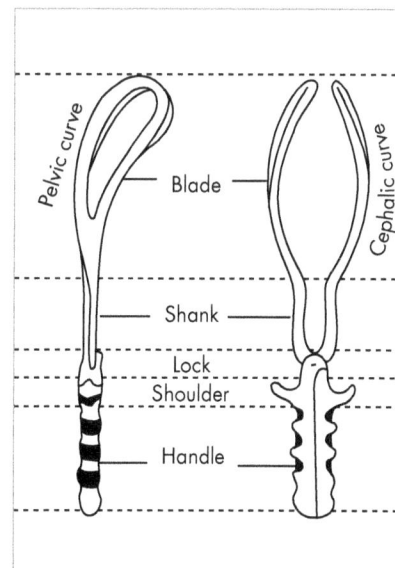

Figure 34.4 Obstetric forceps

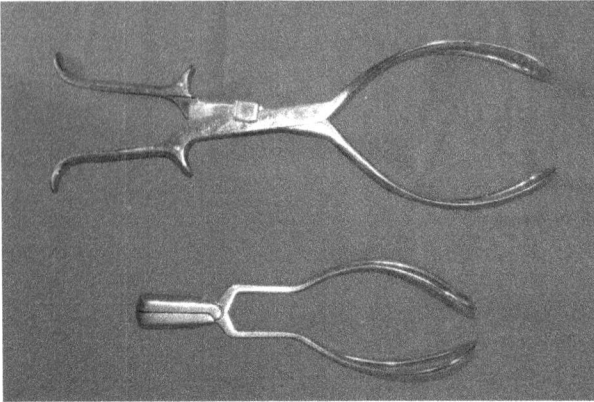

Figure 34.5 Forceps used in South Africa

The following are types of forceps commonly used in South Africa:

▶ *Low forceps or outlet forceps (Wrigley's forceps):* Low forceps may be applied when the biparietal diameter (BPD) has passed beyond the ischial spines and the vertex is visible at the vulva, without the labia being separated. The sagittal suture must be in the anteroposterior (AP) diameter, and the station +3 cm. These forceps are often used for minor degrees of pelvic outlet contraction. Wrigley's forceps are also often used to deliver the after-coming head of a breech presentation. Wrigley's forceps with a very short shank are designed to be used for delivery of a fetus with Caesarean section.

▶ *Mid-cavity forceps* are used when the fetal head is level with the ischial spines (at station 0 cm). In these instances, the BPD has passed through the pelvic brim (the head is engaged), but the presenting part has not advanced beyond the ischial spines. Examples of mid-cavity forceps are Anderson's forceps, Simpson's forceps and Neville-Barnes forceps, all of which lock just like a Wrigley's forceps. There is a wing-nut apparatus that comes with the Neville-Barnes but it is not used often.

Indications

The three classical indications for forceps delivery are:
1. maternal distress
2. delay in the second stage
3. fetal distress.

The following are *maternal indications* that assistance is required in the second stage of labour:
▶ Cardiac conditions
▶ Pulmonary disease, for example TB
▶ Pre-eclampsia and eclampsia
▶ Chronic nephritis
▶ Diabetes mellitus
▶ Chronic hypertension
▶ Poliomyelitis, with slight pelvic distortion and paralysis of the abdominal muscles
▶ Recent operations after which the patient must not bear down, such as recent eye, brain or abdominal operations
▶ Where there is poor maternal effort caused by:
  • maternal exhaustion and distress, whether mental and/or physical
  • secondary uterine exhaustion but with only mild CPD
  • after an accidental dural tap during epidural analgesia, where it is preferable not to allow the patient to bear down.

The following are *obstetric indications* that assistance is required in the second stage of labour:
▶ A delay in the second stage of more than 45 minutes in total and 30 minutes on the pelvic floor
▶ Slight outlet disproportion
▶ A rigid pelvic floor and/or perineum
▶ Failure of the presenting part to descend
▶ Failure of the head to rotate internally
▶ Fetal distress
▶ Occipitoposterior (OP) positions (including persistent OP positions and deep oblique arrest)
▶ Deep transverse arrest
▶ Face presentations
▶ A prolapsed umbilical cord in the second stage of labour
▶ The after-coming head in the breech presentation.

Contraindications

▶ Lack of skill and competence of practitioners: The risk of injury to the mother and baby requires that only skilled practitioners should attempt the use of obstetric forceps. In many institutions the use of forceps has become suppressed in favour of the obstetric vacuum and Caesarean section delivery.
▶ Any indication of prolonged labour due to a large infant, CPD or a high presenting part will be contraindications for the use of forceps.

PROCEDURE	Forceps delivery

Prerequisites

▶ The operator must have advanced skills to prevent abuse and complications during assisted delivery.

▶ There should be a good light source.

▶ The procedure is performed using an aseptic technique at all times.

▶ An assistant is necessary for the procedure.

▶ The presenting part must be engaged.

▶ The sagittal suture line must be in the AP position (for all but Kielland's).

▶ The cervix must be fully dilated.

▶ Established labour with good contractions should be present.

▶ The presentation must be cephalic.

▶ The membranes must be ruptured.

▶ The bladder must be empty.

▶ The lithotomy position is preferred.

▶ Anaesthesia, pudendal block or epidural is needed.

Preparatory examinations

A full abdominal palpation must be done prior to the forceps being applied, in order to ascertain that:

▶ the presentation is cephalic

▶ the head is flexed and the sagittal suture line is in the AP position

▶ the head is engaged in the pelvis (two-fifths above the pelvic brim, or less)

▶ the position of the baby is known

▶ there are good uterine contractions.

A vaginal examination must also be done prior to forceps delivery to confirm the findings made on abdominal palpation and to determine:

▶ the size and shape of the pelvis

▶ that the vertex is presenting

▶ the amount of caput and moulding

▶ that the cervical os is fully dilated

▶ that the membranes have ruptured

▶ the position of the fetus, by means of locating the fontanelles and sutures (the sagittal suture must be in the AP diameter of the pelvis, or the exact position of the fetus must be known)

Check that the fetal heart is normal.

Procedure

1 A full explanation is given to the woman (and to her partner, if he or she is available) and written consent is obtained. The woman should have been taught something about forceps delivery at antenatal preparation for labour. It is the midwife's duty to give support and encouragement to the woman throughout the procedure, as she may be distressed.

2 The bladder is emptied prior to the application of the forceps. If an indwelling catheter is in place, this must be removed prior to delivery to prevent damage to the urethra from the catheter bulb at delivery.

3 The patient is carefully placed in the lithotomy position for better visibility and manipulation. However, as this position is uncomfortable and undignified, the time the woman has to spend in this position should be as short as possible. (Both legs should be raised simultaneously to avoid sacroiliac joint injury and the legs should be removed from the lithotomy poles in the same manner.)

4 The medical practitioner, after lubricating the blades of the forceps, selects the left-handed blade first and inserts it into the vagina to fit snugly around the fetal head. The right-handed blade is then inserted and locked over the left one (see figures 34A and 34B on the following pages).

continued

5   At times, considerable traction is needed in order to deliver the infant; this can be dangerous in inexperienced hands. The average pull is about 18 kg for a primigravida and 12 kg for a multipara.

6   Forceps can be used to rotate the fetal head. Forceps with a sliding lock and without a pelvic curve, such as Kielland's forceps, will permit this manoeuvre.

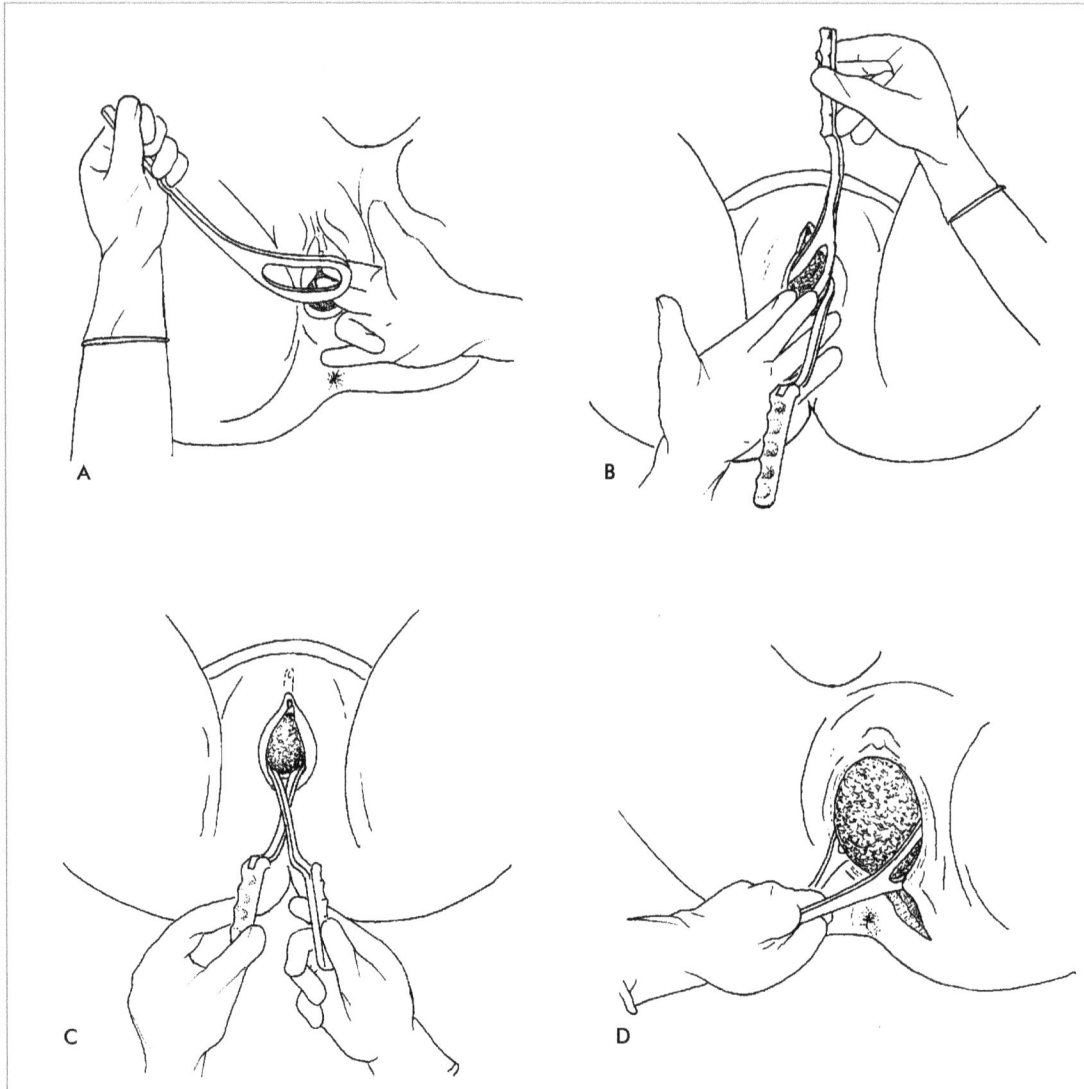

Figure 34A Forceps delivery: A = Insertion of the left blade; B = Insertion of the right blade; C = Locking of the blades; D = Gentle traction is applied to deliver the head. Episiotomy is cut when the perineum is bulging

Care after delivery

1   The baby may need to be resuscitated after a forceps delivery. All the necessary equipment must therefore be in good working order.

2   The baby may have injuries to the scalp and the face, which may require attention.

3   The baby may require high-care nursing after delivery for possible intracranial injuries.

continued

Maternal complications

▶ Damage to maternal soft tissues, such as uterine rupture, lacerations of the cervix, vagina, perineum and/or the rectum
▶ Post-traumatic stress
▶ Long-term health effects such as uterine fistulas and prolapse
▶ Infection of the birth canal
▶ Traumatic PPH due to lacerations
▶ Haematomas
▶ Injury to the bladder and the rectum
▶ Bladder atony, causing retention of urine, urinary tract infection (UTI), oedema and pain
▶ Fracture of the coccyx
▶ Injuries to nerve endings
▶ Failure of the forceps delivery.

Fetal complications

Poor application and incorrect use of the forceps can cause:
▶ intracranial damage, such as tearing of the falx cerebri and tentorium cerebellum
▶ depressed fractures of the skull, causing brain compression
▶ failed forceps delivery with risk of asphyxia neonatorum and general respiratory depression
▶ lacerations due to the use of excessive force and compression, such as cuts of the scalp, eyes, nose, lips and ears
▶ cephalohaematomas and subaponeurotic bleeding
▶ facial palsy
▶ brachial nerve injury
▶ Erb-Duchenne palsy
▶ compression of the umbilical cord
▶ fetal death.

Recording and interpretation

The midwife must record:
▶ the time of application of forceps
▶ the time of delivery
▶ all the circumstances and actions during the event, including the outcomes for mother and baby.

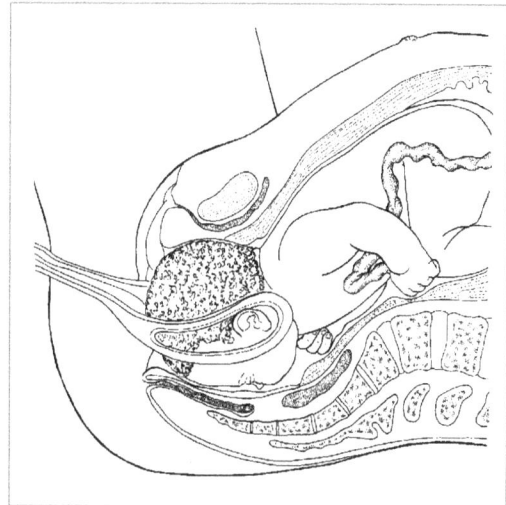

Figure 34B The relationship between the pelvis and the forceps

Trial of forceps

A trial of forceps is carried out in the operating theatre, which is set up for immediate Caesarean section in case the forceps delivery fails. A trial of forceps is attempted when a woman is fully dilated and the baby is in a favourable position and there is no fetal distress but it is not certain that the pelvis is adequate for the birth.

Vacuum or ventouse extraction

The vacuum extractor is an obstetric instrument that has progressively replaced obstetric forceps over the last years because of its relative ease of use, lower maternal morbidity and claimed safety.

The goals of a vacuum extraction are to:
▶ safeguard the well-being of the fetus
▶ assist the mother in her efforts to deliver her term, vertex baby vaginally
▶ apply traction to the fetus during uterine contractions to expedite delivery.

In order to achieve the above, a vacuum (inside the vacuum extractor cup) is applied and attached to the skin of the baby's head. The vacuum cup must be placed on the fetal scalp correctly. A vacuum of up to 0.8 kg/cm^2 is applied. This sucks part of the scalp into the cup and creates an artificial caput succedaneum (known as a chignon). The fetus is extracted by means of suction.

The function of the ventouse

The vacuum extractor is used for the following:

▶ *Flexion of the fetal head.* By the correct placing of the cup over the anterior parietal bone as far back towards the posterior fontanelle as possible, flexion of the fetal head is improved to assist the correct diameters for delivery.

▶ *Achieving traction on and rotation of the fetal head.* Rotation is also brought about by flexing the head, causing forward rotation of the fetal part on the pelvic floor. Extraction of the fetus from the birth canal is facilitated by pulling the fetus by the scalp.

Indications for vacuum extractions

Maternal indications include when there is delay in the second stage of labour due to:

▶ maternal exhaustion, with poor maternal effort after a prolonged first and/or second stage of labour
▶ failure of descent and rotation of the fetal head (OP position)
▶ deflexion of the head
▶ abnormal maternal conditions such as cardiac disease, respiratory disease, gestational proteinuric hypertension, eclampsia and asthma.

Fetal indications include:

▶ an abnormal position of the fetus, to flex and rotate the head in occipitolateral or OP position
▶ mild fetal distress during the second stage of labour, which means that the fetus needs to be delivered quickly
▶ the delivery of the second twin, when fetal distress occurs in a clinic situation.

A vacuum extractor is also sometimes used when there is a delay in the first stage due to primary uterine inertia (primary hypotonic uterine inertia). The condition for which the extractor is used is relative CPD due to deflexion of the fetal head, causing large cephalic diameters to present at the brim. The vacuum extractor is used together with a symphysiotomy in order to bring about flexion and rotation of the head.

Advantages of vacuum extraction

▶ The vacuum can be applied before full dilatation; when the head is descending the cervix will open.
▶ It takes up less space in the pelvis, as it is attached to the fetal head.
▶ It is very useful in order to flex the head.
▶ Rotation of the head will automatically take place at the optimum level in the pelvis.
▶ A vacuum extraction is relatively easy to perform.

▶ There is less discomfort to the mother than there would be in a forceps delivery.
▶ The vacuum is safer than the forceps, because it will come off if the fetus is stuck.

Disadvantages of vacuum extraction

Vacuum extraction cannot be used:

▶ on malpresentations such as a face or breech presentation
▶ in preterm birth
▶ for a macerated fetus
▶ in severe fetal distress, as it takes at least 10–15 minutes versus the 2–3 minutes of a forceps delivery.

Clinical conditions for safe vacuum extraction

All conditions should be assessed and documented:

▶ The fetus must be at term, with an estimated and documented fetal weight (more than 2 500 g and less than 4 200 g).
▶ The mother must be fully informed, co-operative and consenting.
▶ The presentation must be vertex.
▶ The fetal head must be at the zero (0) station or no more than 1/5 palpable above the symphysis pubis.
▶ The position of the presenting part must be certain.
▶ The cervix must be fully dilated.
▶ The membranes must be ruptured.
▶ The bladder must be empty.
▶ Strong uterine contractions (lasting longer than 40 seconds) must be present.

Contraindications

▶ Operator inexperience
▶ Inability to achieve a correct application
▶ Uncertainty concerning fetal position and station
▶ Suspicion of fetopelvic disproportion, evidenced by excessive moulding and heavy caput
▶ Fetal malpositioning (breech, face, brow)
▶ Known or suspected fetal coagulation defects that could predispose the fetus to intraventricular haemorrhage
▶ An underlying fetal condition such as a documented bone demineralising disease that could predispose the fetus to skull fracture
▶ Prematurity (less than 36 weeks' gestation), because of the risk of fetal intraventricular haemorrhage
▶ Known or suspected fetal macrosomia (more than 4.5 kg in a non-diabetic mother).

Types of vacuum cups

The new models for obstetric vacuum extractors have soft silicone cups and are hand-held suction pumps. The cups which fit onto the head of the fetus come in various sizes: 30 mm, 40 mm, 50 mm and 60 mm. An instrument powered by electricity is also available. New hand-operated models use silicone cups.

The following principles apply to the use of vacuum cups:
▶ Disposable vacuum cups are preferred, because of the ease of use and reliability.

▶ Soft bell-shaped cups are associated with fewer scalp injuries and no increased risk of maternal perineal injury.
▶ Soft bell-shaped cups are used for straightforward occipitoanterior (OA) deliveries.
▶ Soft or flexible vacuum cups have a higher incidence of failure than either rigid vacuum cups (plastic or metal) or forceps.

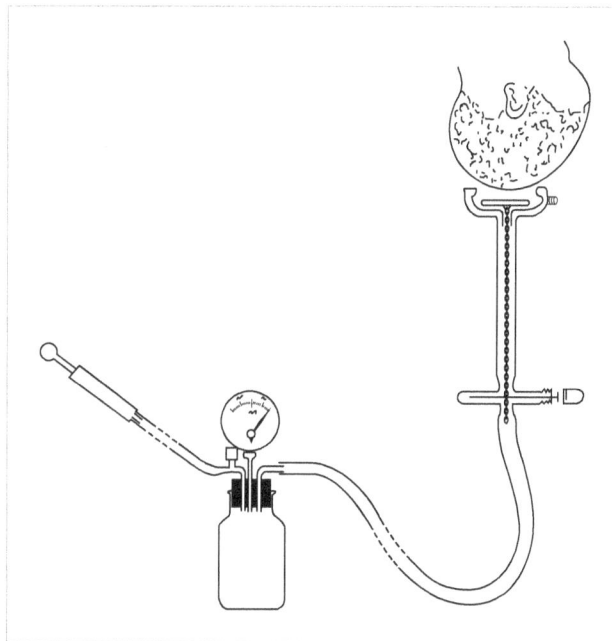

Figure 34.6 A vacuum instrument

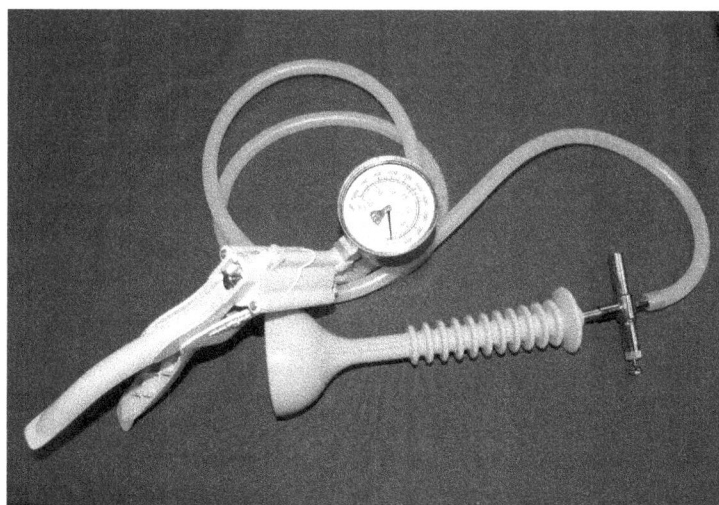

Figure 34.7 A modern vacuum instrument with plastic silicone cups

▶ A successful vacuum-assisted vaginal delivery is dependent on several factors, including patient selection and a number of technical considerations.

▶ Several features are found in all designs, including:
  • a mushroom-shaped vacuum cup of varying composition and depth

• a fixed internal vacuum grid or guard
• a combined vacuum pump or handle or a vacuum port to permit a vacuum hose attachment
• a handle, wire or chain for traction.

PROCEDURE | **Assisted delivery: Vacuum extraction**

Application and technique

Step 1: Preparation
Check all connections and test the vacuum suction on a gloved hand.

Step 2: Insertion
1 Lubricate the cup with sterile lubricant.
2 Wipe the baby's scalp clean with dry gauze and identify the posterior fontanelle.
3 Hold the cup with the fingers.
4 Separate the labia with the fingers of the other hand.
5 Remember the position of the posterior fontanelle, and press the cup downward and inward into the vagina until the cup touches the scalp. Note that if a soft cup is used, it may be partially collapsed by the midwife's hand and introduced through the labia. If a rigid cup is used, it must be turned sideways, slipped into the vagina and then positioned against the fetal head.

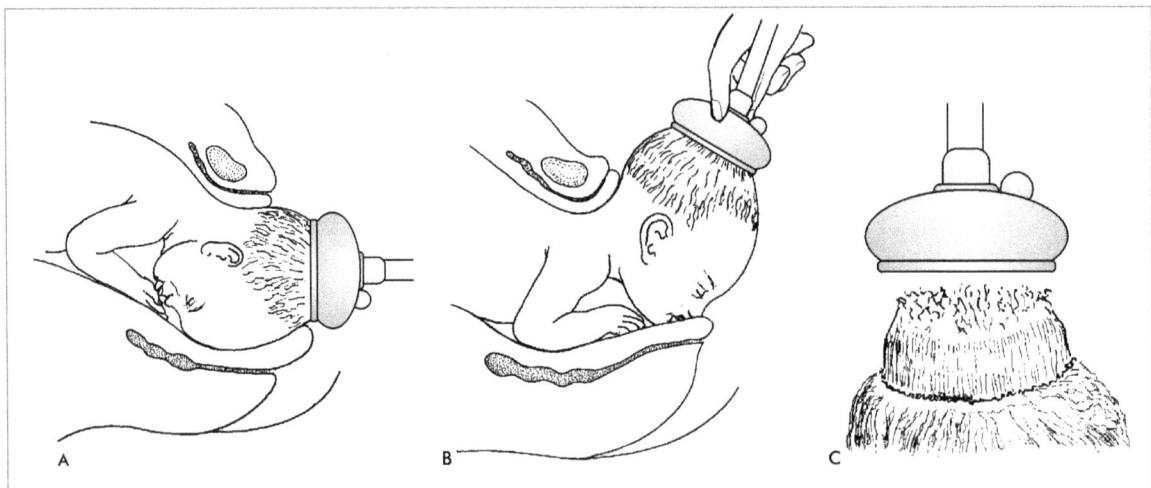

Figure 34C The application of the vacuum (metal cup)

6 Apply the largest cup that will fit, with the centre of the cup over the flexion point, 1 cm anterior to the posterior fontanelle. This placement will promote flexion and descent.
7 An episiotomy may be needed for proper placement. However, to avoid unnecessary blood loss, delay performing an episiotomy until the head stretches the perineum or until the perineum interferes with the axis of traction.
8 Pass a finger gently around the edge of the cup to be sure no maternal tissue has been caught under the cup.

continued

Step 3: Check the application

When the extraction cup is properly positioned, the fetal head will flex but neither twist obliquely nor extend as force is applied. The appropriate vector of traction is directed through the cranial pivot point as follows:

▶ Anatomically, the pivot point is an imaginary spot over the sagittal suture of the fetal skull, located approximately 6 cm posterior to the centre of the anterior fontanelle or 1–2 cm anterior to the posterior fontanelle.

▶ When properly placed with its centre over the pivot point, the edge of a standard 60 mm cup lies approximately 3 cm, or two finger-widths, behind the centre of the anterior fontanelle in the midline over the sagittal suture.

▶ In a vacuum extraction, the anterior fontanelle becomes the principal reference point for checking the instrument application.

▶ The further the cup centre is displaced from the mid-sagittal position on the fetal head over the cranial pivot or flexion point, the greater the failure rate of the fetal head extraction.

Step 4: Traction

Once the appropriate placement has been determined, aim for a negative pressure of at least –0.6 Bar to –0.8 Bar/80 Kilopascal/600 mmHg (the red zone on the disposable cups). Apply traction only during contractions.

▶ With each contraction, apply traction in a line perpendicular to the plane of the cup rim.

▶ Place the non-dominant hand within the vagina, with the thumb on the extractor cup and one or more fingers on the fetal scalp next to the cup during traction to assess potential slippage of the cup.

▶ After maximum negative pressure, start traction in the line of the pelvic axis and perpendicular to the cup. The first pull helps to find the proper direction for pulling.

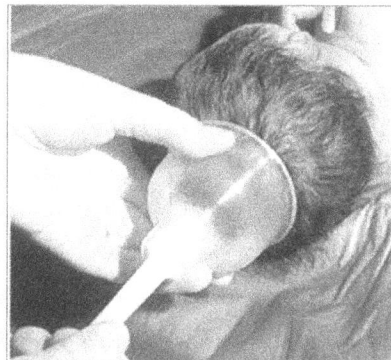

Figure 34D Placement of the soft cup as far posteriorly as possible – the centre of the cup should be over the sagittal suture

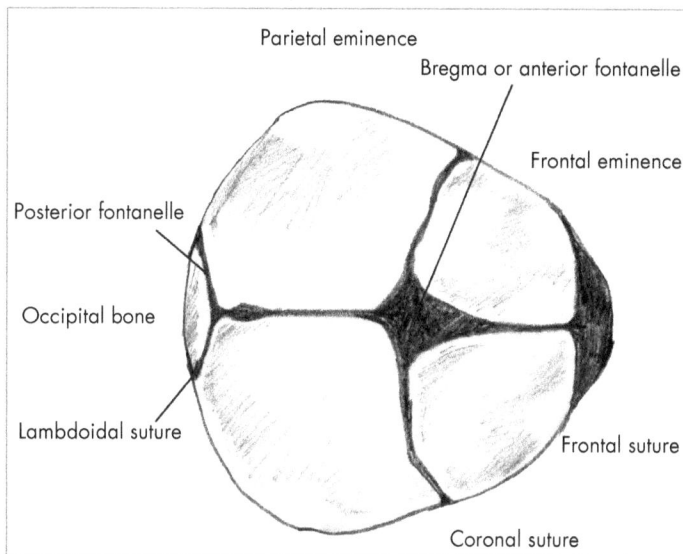

Figure 34E Imaginary spot over the sagittal suture of the fetal skull

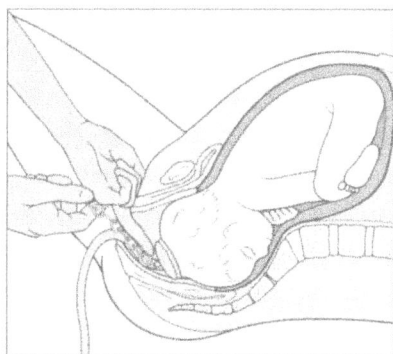

Figure 34F Placement of the non-dominant hand in the vagina

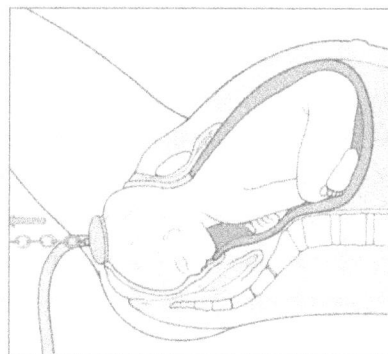

Figure 34G Traction

continued

▶ Recruit maternal bearing-down efforts to minimise failure and fetal scalp injury.

▶ As each contraction wanes, the tension on the extractor handle is relaxed.

▶ If the fetal head is tilted to one side or not flexed well, traction should be directed in a line that will try to correct the tilt or deflexion of the head. The direction of pull on the traction handle changes as the fetal head transverses the pelvic curve.

▶ Rotation of the fetal head will occur with traction.

▶ In the relaxation phase between contractions, the vacuum can either be maintained or reduced to less than 200 mmHg.

▶ Between contractions, check the FHR and application of the cup.

▶ With progress, and in the absence of fetal distress, continue the 'guiding' pulls for a maximum of 30 minutes. Repeat until the head begins to crown.

Step 5: Descent and delivery of the fetal head

▶ Bring the fetal head down with a contraction.

▶ Descent should begin with the initial traction effort, assuming proper co-ordination with the maternal bearing-down efforts and the uterine contractions:
  - Encourage long and steady pushing.
  - At the same time, pull on the handle, firmly and straight.
  - Do not twist and turn the cup, as this will cause the cup to pop off, leading to scalp injuries (bruising, bleeding, swelling).
  - The baby's head will rotate at the same speed and direction as in a normal delivery.

▶ With each contraction, the head should progress over the perineum.

▶ Do not allow the pressure to remain at maximum levels (600 mmHg) for more than 10 minutes in total. Excessive pressure can cause fetal haemorrhage into the skull or serious scalp damage.

▶ When the head begins to crown, during another contraction, with the pressure at 600 mm Hg, pull upwards.

▶ After the head has delivered, release the pressure and continue with the delivery.

Uncertain progress

▶ If the midwife is uncertain that descent has occurred, a maximum of two additional tractions may be attempted.

▶ Slow progress usually represents no progress at all.

▶ The number of tractions with the vacuum extractor should be limited to no more than two to three with soft cups and one to two with either metal or rigid plastic cups.

▶ The overall duration of the procedure should be reduced to 20 minutes.

▶ Actions between contractions:
  - Reduce the pressure to 100 mm Hg.
  - Do not pull.
  - Encourage the mother to breathe deeply and relax.
  - Have the assistant take the FHR and the mother's BP between contractions.

Aborting the vacuum procedure

▶ The decision to continue with assisted vaginal delivery must be re-evaluated continuously during each step of the delivery. The maximum time to safely complete a vacuum extraction and the acceptable number of detachments is unknown.

▶ Multiple attempts at vaginal delivery using different instruments are not supported, because of concerns about a higher rate of maternal and neonatal injury.

▶ A vacuum has failed if:
  - there is no noticeable fetal head descent during traction
  - the head has not been delivered after three pulls with functioning equipment
  - the cup has detached twice.

Reasons for failure include:
  - poor patient selection (CPD)

continued

▶ errors in application or technique (incorrect cup size, accidental inclusion of maternal soft tissues within the cup and/or incorrect placement of the vacuum cup, resulting in worsening asynclitism or extension of the fetal head)
▶ failure to apply traction with maternal pushing efforts
▶ traction along the incorrect plane.

Maternal complications

There is substantial evidence that instrumental deliveries increase maternal morbidity, including perineal pain at delivery, pain in the immediate postpartum period, perineal lacerations, haematomas, blood loss and anaemia, urinary retention and long-term problems with urinary and faecal incontinence.

The maternal complications associated with vacuum extraction are comparable to those associated with spontaneous deliveries. Complications do not vary with the type of vacuum extractor used. They include:

▶ lacerations of the vagina, cervix, uterus, labia and/or the urethra
▶ third-degree tears of the perineum, in addition to or as an extension of the episiotomy
▶ haemorrhage
▶ damage to the bladder
▶ infection of the birth canal
▶ psychological trauma.

Neonatal complications

Paediatricians should be notified whenever an assisted vaginal delivery has been attempted and whether it was successful, as serious morbidity can present several hours after birth. For this reason, such neonates should be closely observed. Vacuum extraction has not been found to result in significant intellectual or neurological disability.

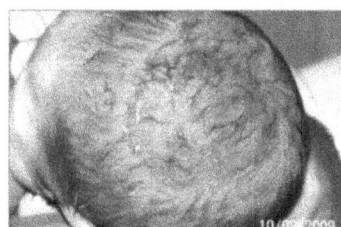

Figure 34H Scalp abrasions

Neonatal complications may include:

▶ caput formation
▶ abrasions, necrosis
▶ hyperbilirubinaemia
▶ bleeding
▶ asphyxia
▶ cerebral irritation
▶ periventricular bleeding
▶ infection
▶ subgaleal haemorrhage (boggy scalp, swelling crossing the suture lines and an expanding head circumference; symptoms include signs of hypovolaemia, pallor, tachycardia and a falling haematocrit)
▶ cephalohaematoma
▶ intracranial haemorrhage
▶ retinal haemorrhages
▶ transient neonatal lateral rectus paralysis.

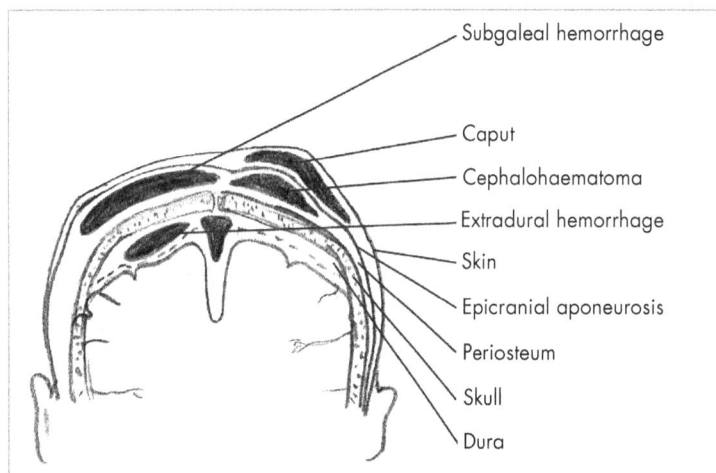

Figure 34I Fetal injuries

Recording and interpretation

Enter all the necessary information in the maternity register, including:

▶ the indication for vacuum
▶ the initial findings
▶ the number of times the vacuum was applied and the number of pulls

continued

- the cup size and type
- the infant's condition at birth.

Include drawings if necessary.

Discharge
Discharge from the clinic or hospital is possible after six hours post-delivery, provided that:
- there are no surgical, medical or obstetric problems that require attention
- the mother verbalises that she is feeling well
- there is no sign of anaemia
- the vital data is normal
- there is no uterine tenderness or excessive pain
- there is no evidence of active vaginal bleeding
- there is no incontinence or urinary retention
- infant feeding has been explained and demonstrated
- contraception has been discussed and provided
- information has been given regarding the mother's nearest clinic for immunisation and reassessment.

Cleaning the equipment
After finishing a delivery using the vacuum extractor, clean it immediately:
- Wipe the entire pump, tubes and dial with a clean, soft, damp cloth.
- If fluids went into the pump during a delivery, clean the fluids out. Do not allow fluids or water to dry inside the pump, as this may stop the pump from working.
- Wash the cup with soap and water.
- Rinse the cup very well and dry it completely.
- If you are using a reusable cup, soak the cup and tubing in antiseptic solution for 20 minutes before use.
- Handle with care. Avoid dropping.
- Store in a clean, dry and covered area.

34.5   Conclusion

Midwives should be competent in the procedures they can perform. The midwife's role and function is to create a safe environment and provide support within the medical team during interventions. In addition, the midwife should act as an advocate for the interests of the woman and the fetus.

35

Obstetric shock

LEARNING OBJECTIVES

On completion of this chapter, you must be able to:

▶ differentiate between the types of shock that will be encountered in midwifery practice
▶ identify high-risk patients for the different types of shock
▶ assess for signs and symptoms of shock
▶ determine the type of shock a patient presents with
▶ initiate a systematic approach to managing a patient with shock.

KNOWLEDGE ASSUMED TO BE IN PLACE

Normal anatomy and physiology of the cardiovascular system and respiratory system
Heart failure and pulmonary oedema
Haemodynamic monitoring

KEYWORDS

shock syndrome • haemorrhagic shock • cardiogenic shock • sepsis • anaphylaxis • atopy • colloids/crystalloids

35.1   Introduction

Shock is a severe, life-threatening emergency, since it affects all organs. Shock leads to a decrease in cardiac output, followed by compromised tissue perfusion. The cells are deprived of sufficient oxygen and nutrients, causing cellular hypoxia. If shock is not recognised and managed, cellular death may occur.

The obstetric patient in shock requires immediate attention because of the possible widespread effect on one or more body systems. Prompt interventions based on the patient's vital or haemodynamic data are essential. When faced with an emergency involving shock, it is important that the midwife assess the patient quickly and thoroughly, following the ABC approach, while at the same time being alert for subtle changes that may indicate a potential deterioration in the patient's condition. The midwife needs to have a high index of suspicion for the condition to manage and refer as soon as the condition is recognised. Ideally, a shocked woman will be managed by a medical practitioner, but the midwife needs to understand the pathology and be able to manage the woman until a medical practitioner arrives or during transfer to an appropriate facility.

This chapter focuses on the different types of shock that may be encountered in midwifery practice. These include haemorrhagic, cardiogenic, septic and anaphylactic shock.

The type of shock needs to be identified so that the specific treatment required for the effective reversal of the condition can be given. This chapter focuses on general management principles, including the use of a collaborative team approach using the ABCs to guide assessment, planning and the implementation of a systematic management approach. This chapter does not focus on the management of the obstetric patient, but rather on basic principles that should be followed when shock occurs in midwifery practice.

35.2   Shock: The clinical picture

The clinical picture of shock may include all of the following, regardless of the cause:

▶ Low BP
▶ Rapid, weak (thready) pulse
▶ Pallor
▶ Cold, clammy skin
▶ Cyanosis of the fingers
▶ Air hunger
▶ Dimness of vision
▶ Restlessness
▶ Oliguria or anuria.

Shock may be catastrophic, for example that caused by amniotic fluid embolus. The box below details the different types of shock that may be encountered in midwifery practice.

Classification of shock in obstetrics

Haemorrhagic shock is due to excessive blood loss, which may be caused by:
▶ early bleeding in pregnancy (abortion and ectopic)
▶ antepartum haemorrhage (APH) (placenta praevia and placental abruption)
▶ postpartum haemorrhage (PPH) (atonic and traumatic).

Neurogenic shock is caused by painful conditions, which may be due to:
▶ a disturbed ectopic pregnancy
▶ a concealed accidental haemorrhage
▶ forceps or breech extraction before full cervical dilatation
▶ a rough internal version
▶ Credé's manoeuvre
▶ a ruptured uterus
▶ acute inversion of the uterus
▶ a rapid evacuation of the uterine contents, as in precipitate labour and rupture of membranes in polyhydramnios. This is accompanied by rapid accumulation of blood in the splanchnic area due to sudden relief of pressure (splanchnic shock).

Cardiogenic shock is ineffective contraction of the cardiac muscle, which is due to:
▶ myocardial infarction
▶ heart failure
▶ cardiac arrest.

Endotoxic shock is generalised vascular disturbance due to the release of toxins.

Anaphylactic shock is caused by sensitivity to drugs.

Other causes of shock include:
▶ embolism: amniotic fluid, air or thrombus
▶ anaesthetic complications, eg Mendelson's syndrome
▶ postpartum pre-eclampsia-induced shock.

Shock may be caused by more than one factor, such as:
▶ incomplete abortion, which leads to haemorrhagic and endotoxic shock
▶ a disturbed ectopic pregnancy and ruptured uterus, which leads to haemorrhagic and neurogenic shock.

35.3   Shock syndrome

Shock syndrome is a condition in which the stroke volume of the heart (the amount of blood pumped per beat) is affected, which causes a decrease in the cardiac output (the amount of blood pumped per minute). This in turn leads to cardiovascular system failure, which leads to total organ failure.

Cardiac output needs to be maintained. Cardiac output is the amount of blood ejected from the left ventricle in one minute (4–8 ℓ/min). It is equal to the heart rate multiplied by the stroke volume (the amount of blood ejected with each heartbeat).

Stroke volume is the amount of blood ejected from the left ventricle with each heartbeat (approximately 70 ml). Stroke volume depends on three major factors: preload (the volume received), contractility (the ability of the muscle to contract) and afterload (the ability of the left ventricle to create enough pressure to eject the blood). These are briefly explained in Figure 35.1.

Preload is the amount of stretch or volume in the ventricle at the end of diastole, just before ventricular contraction takes place. To eject blood, the ventricle must be preloaded with blood to ensure an adequate stroke volume. Preload is determined by the:
▶ volume of the vascular space
▶ amount of venous return
▶ amount of blood in the ventricle at the end of diastole.

The type of shock that directly affects the preload in midwifery practice is haemorrhagic shock, which occurs due to an acute loss of blood in the vascular space, decreased venous return and decreased blood in the ventricle at the end of diastole, leading to a decrease in stroke volume and cardiac output.

Contractility refers to the inherent ability of the cardiac muscle to contract and eject blood into the pulmonary or systemic vasculature. In midwifery practice, cardiogenic shock develops mainly due to stress placed on the heart as a result of myocardial valve dysfunction. If a person suffers from structural and/or functional abnormalities of the valves, the heart muscle changes shape over time; at some point the patient will become symptomatic and heart failure is diagnosed. Decreased contractility leads to a decrease in stroke volume, which in turn decreases the cardiac output.

Afterload refers to the pressure that the left ventricle must generate to overcome the higher pressure in the aorta to get the blood out of the heart. The afterload can be increased or decreased. Septic shock directly affects the afterload due to vasodilation, thereby decreasing the afterload. This results in decreased venous return, stroke volume and cardiac output, which in turn produce persistent hypotension.

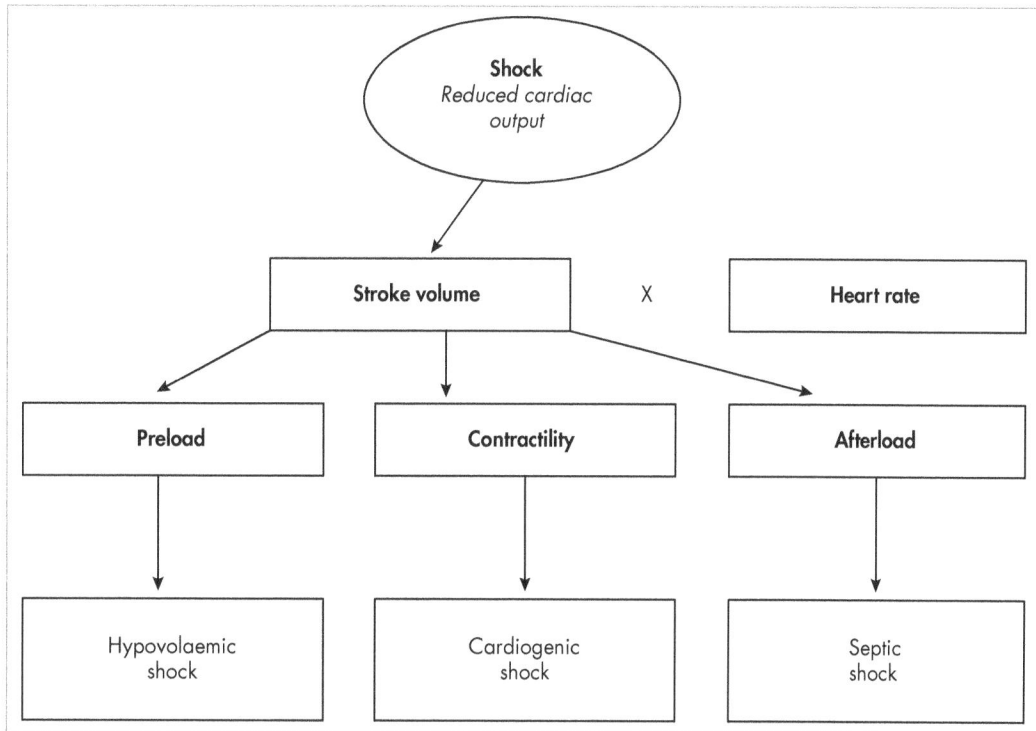

Figure 35.1 Schematic representation of shock

Compensatory mechanisms

During the initial stage of shock syndrome, the cardiac output is decreased and tissue perfusion threatened. Almost immediately, the compensatory mechanism is initiated as the body's homeostatic mechanism attempts to maintain cardiac output, BP and tissue perfusion. The compensatory mechanism is important in protecting the vital organs (brain and heart) and results in a cascade of compensatory events that affect all organ systems. Initially, the body compensates by decreasing the circulation to less vital organs such as the kidneys, gastrointestinal (GI) system and skin (resulting in paleness) in order to preserve the circulation to vital organs such as the heart and brain. This mechanism works as follows:

▶ The shunting of blood flow to vital organs is triggered by a decrease in the cardiac output, which is sensed by the baroreceptors within the aortic arch and atrium.
▶ Neural reflexes then cause a sympathetic outflow to the heart and other organs, which respond by increasing the heart rate and vasoconstriction to the non-vital organs.
▶ A hormonal response occurs and activation of the renin system leads to further vasoconstriction and the retention of water and sodium (aldosterone and antidiuretic hormone, or ADH).

▶ The anterior pituitary and adrenal medulla are stimulated to increase glucose and release epinephrine (adrenaline) and norepinephrine (noradrenaline), which further enhance the compensatory mechanism.

As a result of the activation of the compensatory mechanism, the obstetric patient will present with tachycardia, tachypnoea, cold clammy skin and an increase in diastolic BP. Table 35.1 on the next page summarises the haemodynamic changes seen in response to the effects of adrenaline and noradrenaline on the different receptors.

In the progressive stage at cellular level, a decrease in perfusion causes the cells to switch from aerobic to anaerobic metabolism as a source of energy. Anaerobic metabolism produces large amounts of lactic acid as an end product, causing metabolic acidosis. A vicious cycle of low cardiac output, sympathetic compensation, myocardial ischaemia and even lower cardiac output develops. While compensatory mechanisms initially stabilise the patient, these begin to fail if progression occurs and the oxygen demands of the already compromised heart and the compensatory mechanism become exhausted. If the cardiac output continues to decrease, damage to the cells and different body systems are inevitable.

Table 35.1

Summary of the hormonal compensatory mechanism's effect on the haemodynamic status of the patient

Receptor	Effect	Rationale	Haemodynamic changes
Skin ↑	Vasoconstriction	↑ systemic vascular resistance in order to shunt blood to vital organs	↑ diastolic blood pressure Cold clammy skin ↑ capillary refill (> 2 seconds)
Cardiac system ß₁	↑ heart rate	↑ heart rate to compensate for ↑ stroke volume in attempt to ↑ cardiac output	Tachycardia
Respiratory system ß₂	↑ respiratory rate	↑ oxygen supply Compensatory mechanism for metabolic acidosis	Tachypnoea

The patient will present with multi-organ failure:

▶ *Cerebral hypoperfusion* leads to a decreased level of consciousness, which can present as anxiety, irritability and confusion. The patient can even deteriorate to a comatose state.

▶ *Myocardial hypoperfusion* leads to decreased contractility and arrhythmias, which decrease the cardiac output.

▶ *Respiratory hypoperfusion* leads to hypoxia, because there is an increase in pulmonary capillary membrane permeability, which in turn decreases the surface area for gaseous exchange. Air hunger develops.

▶ *Renal hypoperfusion* develops due to vasoconstriction to this non-vital organ, leading to renal ischaemia and ultimately progressing to acute tubular necrosis and renal shut-down.

▶ *Gastrointestinal hypoperfusion* develops due to decreased blood flow to this non-vital organ, leading to ischaemia and presenting with decreased bowel sounds, impaired absorption and a paralytic ileus.

▶ *Metabolic dysfunction* due to hypoperfusion on a cellular level leads to an anaerobic metabolism and the formation of lactate (lactic acid).

▶ *Haematologic dysfunction* affects the clotting cascade and therefore increases the risk for bleeding and disseminated intravascular coagulopathy (DIC).

If the decrease in cardiac output is not identified and managed promptly, cellular damage will be irreversible, as the cell membrane loses its integrity. This will lead to irreversible cell damage, multi-organ dysfunction and death.

Initial management

The first rule in effective patient management is the five Ps rule, namely 'Pre-Planning Prevents Poor Performance'.

It is essential that the correct equipment and ward stock are readily available to use once shock has been diagnosed, to provide the best chance for a successful outcome.

Early recognition of shock is essential. It is vital to use the ABC approach to assess the patient's airway (patent or compromised), breathing (increase in work of breathing, nasal flaring, use of accessory muscles, crepitations) and circulation (vital signs) and to recognise subtle changes. The ABC approach should be adopted based on the identified type of shock seen in the obstetric patient.

Table 35.2 provides the general principles that should be implemented in all types of shock. The differences and specific considerations for each type of shock are delineated in table format following the discussion on each type.

35.4   Haemorrhagic shock (preload)

Haemorrhagic shock is the most common type of shock encountered in midwifery. It is regarded as a life-threatening emergency and a leading cause of death in obstetric patients. The highest risk of maternal death is related to haemorrhage within 24 hours post-delivery.

Haemorrhage can be managed effectively by recognising the condition, assessing it appropriately and performing initial management. The ABC approach is a systematic approach that ensures priorities are addressed (see tables 35.1 and 35.2).

Table 35.2

A structured approach to shock (HABCDEF)

Key principles	Interventions	Clinical notes
History	Obtain a history from the woman, relatives or friends and/or ambulance staff. Use the SAMPLE history format.	Maintain a high index of suspicion **S:** Signs and symptoms **A:** Allergies **M:** Medications **P:** Past medical history **L:** Last food or drink **E:** Events The history provides valuable information to guide the diagnosis of the type of shock.
Hazards	All team members should wear gloves, aprons or protective gowns and protective eyewear.	Reduce the risk of occupational exposure to blood-borne diseases such as hepatitis and HIV.
Help	Call for help immediately if shock is suspected.	A team approach should be followed. Call experienced staff (including obstetrician and anaesthetist). Designate a midwife to record the vital signs (every 15 minutes), urine output (hourly) and fluid and drugs administrated (continuously). Place the operating theatre on standby (if appropriate).
Airway	Assess the airway, using the 3Ps strategy: ensure the airway is *patent*, *protected* and, if not, *provide* it. *Airway patent* and *protected*: Provide supplemental oxygen via partial re-breathing mask with a reservoir bag. *Airway not protected*: If noisy breathing occurs, the woman is not able to protect her airway; perform the *chin lift manoeuvre* to open the airway. Airway not *patent* or *protected*: Initiate *bag-valve-mask ventilation*.	If the woman can speak, it can be assumed that the airway is patent. Noisy breathing indicates that the woman cannot protect her airway. The tongue falling back in an unconscious woman may obstruct the airway; she is unable to protect it. For patients who are unable to protect the airway, consider providing protection by inserting a definitive airway (eg endotracheal intubation).
Breathing	*Look*: Observe the respiratory rate, depth and difficulty. *Listen*: Briefly auscultate breath sounds bilaterally. Initiate pulse oximetry, if available.	
Circulation	Promptly insert IV line. Consider the gauge of the IV cannula, type of administration set and type and rate of fluid administration. Monitor vital signs.	Monitor and interpret vital signs vigilantly and frequently (every 15 minutes until patient is stabilised). Monitor urinary output using an indwelling urinary catheter (normal = 0.5 to 1 ml/kg/hour); minimum 30 ml/hr.

continued

Key principles	Interventions	Clinical notes
Disability	Monitor level of consciousness continuously, using the AVPU scale.	**A:** Alert **V:** Responding verbally **P:** Responding to pain **U:** Completely unresponsive
Drugs	Dopamine is the drug of choice in shock.	See Table 35.5 on page 568.
Environmental control	Keep the woman warm.	
Fetus	After the woman has been stabilised, assess the fetus with continuous cardiotocography (CTG) in the case of a viable fetus.	

History (patients at risk)

PPH is the leading cause of maternal death. Women who are anaemic, pre-eclamptic or have cardiac problems are specifically at risk. Factors that indicate a risk for haemorrhagic shock include:

▶ a history of uterine atony or an overstretched uterus in the case of polyhydramnios, multiple pregnancy or grand multiparae
▶ PPH in a previous pregnancy
▶ previous retained placenta, placenta accreta
▶ prolonged or obstructed labour or failure to progress during the second stage of labour
▶ trauma and lacerations associated with instrumental delivery, large-for-gestational-age (LGA) newborn and surgical interventions such as Caesarean section and general anaesthesia
▶ hypertensive disorders and haemolytic anaemia, elevated liver enzymes, low platelet count (HELLP) syndrome
▶ induction of labour (IOL) and augmentation of labour.

Pathophysiology

Haemorrhagic shock is usually precipitated by an event that results in an acute loss of blood from the intravascular space, causing a decrease in venous return to the heart, which in turn decreases the preload, stroke volume and cardiac output.

The placental site with the placental bed and open arteries in the uterus are not contracted, which can lead to a sudden massive loss of blood volume. A decrease in cardiac output decreases tissue perfusion, leading to a decrease in oxygen supply at a cellular level. The body's metabolic demands cannot be met and the compensatory mechanism is initiated, as discussed in Section 35.3.

Clinical signs and symptoms

The clinical manifestations of haemorrhagic shock vary depending on the amount of blood loss and the body's ability to compensate for that loss. There are four classes of haemorrhage, based on the amount of blood lost, as shown in Table 35.3. Each class has associated clinical manifestations.

The midwife should recognise that in individual patients the distinction between the different classes may not be as straightforward as delineated in Table 35.3, which gives general guidelines for healthy women. The management should rather be guided by the patient's response to the initial therapy. Consideration must be given to women with cardiac problems, anaemia and pre-eclampsia.

Principles of diagnosis, management, intervention and care

The Advanced Trauma Life Support (ATLS®) guidelines, published by the American College of Surgeons (ACS, 2017), address the initial management of haemorrhagic shock. A systematic, collaborative team approach is essential to optimise patient outcomes. This approach and its principles are also applicable in midwifery practice.

The ATLS® guidelines emphasise that diagnosis and management of shock need to occur simultaneously. Once the assessment has been done, immediately initiate appropriate management.

The first step is to stop the haemorrhage, assess blood loss and effectively replace the fluid. Replacement therapy should be started as soon as possible. The response to fluid should be monitored continuously and subsequent therapy should be based on the findings. Both crystalloids (Ringer's lactate) and colloids should be considered.

Table 35.3

Classification of haemorrhagic shock (Martel, 2002)

	Class I: Initial stage	Class II: Compensatory stage	Class III: Progressive stage	Class IV: Refractory stage
Blood loss (ml)	750	750–1 500	1 500–2 000	> 2 000
Blood loss (%)	15%	30%	40%	> 40%
Heart rate	< 100	< 100	> 120	> 140 Only carotid is felt
Capillary refill	Normal (< 2 seconds)	May be delayed (> 2 seconds)	Usually delayed (> 2 seconds)	Always delayed (> 2 seconds)
Skin	Normal	Pale, cool	Cold and clammy	Cold, pale
Respiration	Normal	Mild increase	Moderate tachypnoea	Marked tachypnoea
Urinary output (ml/hr)	> 30	20–30	5–20	Anuria
Mental status	Normal or agitated	Agitated	Confused	Loss of consciousness
BP	Normal or increased pulse pressure	Decreased pulse pressure and increase in diastolic BP	Markedly reduced	Precipitous fall Irreversible shock

The ATLS® guidelines recommend that pre-warmed Ringer's lactate be administered intravenously immediately to increase the hydrostatic pressure. An initial dose of 1–2 ℓ Ringer's lactate should be given, aiming to replace 3 ml for every 1 ml blood loss. As Ringer's lactate will increase the intravascular volume and therefore the hydrostatic pressure, it will promote the stabilisation of the vascular volume by replacing fluid losses in the interstitial and intracellular spaces.

The principles of assessment and management of haemorrhagic shock include ensuring an adequate airway, oxygenation and ventilation. Thereafter, the focus is on fluid resuscitation, which is regarded as the cornerstone of acute resuscitation. Once haemorrhage has been controlled, administration of warm IV fluids is important. All IV fluids should be pre-warmed to 39 °C before use. An increase in the intravascular volume will predictably increase the woman's cardiac output and BP, which will reverse haemorrhagic shock and restore perfusion to the vital organs. A summary of the key principles to be followed during the assessment and management of haemorrhagic shock are shown in Table 35.4 on thne next page. Only the specific difference and/or special considerations related to haemorrhage are highlighted in Table 35.4. The principles used during the ABC approach remain the same as in Table 35.2.

The midwife should monitor the woman's response to the fluid bolus, including her level of consciousness, respiratory rate, heart rate, BP, peripheral perfusion and urinary output.

Blood and blood products can be used during haemorrhagic shock. Blood products are used to restore circulating volume, replace coagulation factors and improve the oxygen-carrying capacity (Hb). Replacement of red blood cells is recommended to maintain a haematocrit of more than 30 per cent. Type-specific blood is preferred, but if this is unavailable, O-negative may be used. There are, however, disadvantages in the use of blood, as it must be cross-matched, which requires a specimen from the patient and time for processing by the blood bank. Massive transfusion can produce dilutional coagulopathy, hypocalcaemia and hypomagnesaemia. Blood-borne viral pathogens may be transferred, causing hepatitis and HIV infection.

Inotropic support can be considered once the fluid status has been optimised. Dopamine, a dose-dependent inotropic drug, is the drug of choice and may be used as a sympathomimetic agent to stimulate the adrenergic receptors and thereby increase the cardiac output and blood pressure in patients with haemorrhagic shock and hypoperfusion (see Table 35.5 on the next page).

Table 35.4

Specific considerations in the structured approach to managing haemorrhagic shock

Key principles	Interventions	Clinical notes
Circulation	Give priority to identifying and stopping the source of bleeding. Turn the woman on her left side or elevate her right hip to prevent supine hypotension. Promptly place two large-bore (14 or 16 gauge) IV cannulas and simultaneously draw blood (cross-match, urea and creatine, electrolytes, coagulation screen and full blood count [FBC]). Use a 10-drops-per-minute administration set. Administer 1–2 ℓ of warm crystalloid solution (ie Ringer's lactate) as a volume expander. This is followed by a colloid solution (ie Voluven). Give 3 ml for every 1 ml blood lost. Transfuse blood if appropriate once available.	Monitor and interpret vital signs carefully and frequently (every 15 minutes until patient is stabilised). Monitor urinary output using an indwelling urinary catheter (normal = 0.5 to 1 ml/kg/hour).
Environmental control	Keep the woman warm (warm fluid replacement and blanket) (39 °C).	

Table 35.5

Summary of the dose-dependent actions of dopamine

Dose	Effect
2–5 µg/kg per minute	Stimulates dopaminergic receptors which cause renal, mesenteric, cerebral coronary bed vasodilation, thus increasing blood flow to these tissues.
5–10 µg/kg per minute	Stimulates β_1 receptors, which increase myocardial contractility and heart rate, improving cardiac output.
>10 µg/kg per minute	Stimulates α receptors, which results in an increase in the systemic vascular resistance, which may counteract the actions of the dopaminergic and β_1 receptors.
Mixing dopamine Dilution: 6 x body weight (kg) equals milligrams to add to sufficient diluent to create a total volume of 100 ml. (1 ml/hour delivers 1.0 µg/kg per minute)	

An episode of haemorrhage can have long-term consequences for a woman. Sheehan's syndrome can be caused by an episode of hypovolaemia, when BP drops and there is poor blood flow to the pituitary gland, causing lasting hormonal disturbances. The first sign is the failure to lactate after birth, with an inability to ovulate later. The prevention of hypovolaemia – without risking overloading the patient – is essential. The accurate observation of the clinical picture, blood loss and effective replacement needs to be according to protocols and midwives need to know how to manage blood loss.

35.5   Cardiogenic shock (contractility)

Cardiac shock, also referred to as 'pump failure', is a condition of decreased cardiac output that severely impairs tissue perfusion, resulting in diminished oxygen delivery to the tissues. It leads to severe left-sided heart failure.

History (patients at risk)

A thorough history will help to predict patients at risk for development of cardiogenic shock. The obstetric patient suffering from any myocardial valve dysfunction, eg aortic, mitral or tricuspid valve stenosis or incompetence, has a high risk of developing cardiogenic shock. Patients who give a medical history of rheumatic fever or congenital cardiac conditions and cardiac dysrhythmias must also be regarded as high-risk patients.

Clinical signs and symptoms

The patient presents with anxiety, tachypnoea, cyanosis and respiratory distress. Regardless of the underlying cause, left ventricular dysfunction triggers compensatory mechanisms that attempt to increase the cardiac output and, in turn, the tissue perfusion and oxygen supply to vital organs.

The midwife should monitor patients at risk closely for any of the following signs and symptoms:
▶ *Haemodynamic findings:*
 • Systolic pressure less than 90 mmHg
 • Central venous pressure more than 12 mmHg
 • Tachycardia
▶ *Clinical findings:*
 • Decreased level of consciousness (disorientation, restlessness)
 • Distended neck veins
 • Dysrhythmias
 • Cold and clammy skin
 • Decreased urine output (less than 0.5 to 1 ml/kg/hour)
▶ *Pulmonary findings:*
 • Tachypnoea (more that 15 breaths per minute)
 • Dyspnoea
 • Abnormal breath sounds (crackles and possible wheezing)
 • Arterial blood gas indicating low PO_2
 • Use of accessory muscles to breathe.

Principles of diagnosis, management, intervention and care

Acute pulmonary oedema is probably the most important cardiac cause of death in pregnancy, hence the importance of maintaining a high index of suspicion and managing appropriately where it presents.

The major objective in treatment of this type of shock is to assist the contractility of the heart and to alleviate the causative agent.

Patients who have pulmonary congestion should not be positioned in a supine position with the legs elevated. The supine position will increase the pulmonary resistance, worsening the pulmonary oedema. The patient should therefore be placed in a semi-Fowler's position during labour.

In high-risk patients, respiratory tract infections should be managed promptly.

If anaemia is present, transfusion of packed cells should be given instead of whole blood, as the packed cells will increase the red blood cell concentration without increasing the total circulating blood volume.

IV infusions should be kept to the minimum (0.5 ml/kg/hour) to prevent an increase in the circulating volume. An increased circulating volume may lead to an increased myocardial workload and increased haemodynamic and pulmonary complications. (A microdropper and buretrol or an infusion pump is used to control the volume of fluid administered.)

The ability of the patient with heart disease to survive pregnancy, labour and the puerperium depends on:
▶ the capacity of the heart to pump (contract)
▶ the extent of the total demand to work placed on the heart during pregnancy.

Also see Chapter 21. The specific difference and/or special considerations related to cardiogenic shock are highlighted in Table 35.6 on the next page. The principles used during the ABC approach remain the same those in Table 35.2.

35.6 Septic shock (afterload)

Sepsis is a complex syndrome that occurs as a result of the systemic manifestation of infection. The human response to infection ranges along a severity continuum, from systemic inflammatory response syndrome (SIRS) to multi-organ dysfunction syndrome (MODS). Figure 35.2 on page 571 gives an overview of the sepsis syndrome.

Classification of shock

The components in Figure 35.2 can be described as follows:
▶ *SIRS:* Normally, the inflammatory response is an essential, firmly regulated and controlled protective mechanism of local response to invasion by microorganisms or to local tissue damage. In SIRS, the inflammatory response is systemic; it occurs in all body systems. The systemic result is an overwhelming and unregulated inflammation process, with widespread leakiness of the blood vessels causing the fluid to shift into the interstitial space. This leads to a maldistribution of the circulating volume (relative hypovolaemia). Furthermore, there is an imbalance in the oxygen supply and demand on tissue level and uncontrolled coagulation.

▶ *Sepsis:* Sepsis is the systemic response to infection. Sepsis is diagnosed when two or more of the following systemic responses manifest:
- Temperature: > 38° C
- Heart rate: > 90 beats per minute
- Pyrexia: > 15 breaths per minute
- White blood cell count: > 12 000 or < 4 000.

▶ *Severe sepsis:* Severe sepsis is defined as sepsis that is complicated by organ dysfunction. Severe sepsis is associated with organ dysfunction, sepsis-induced hypotension and hypoperfusion abnormalities such as lactic acidosis oliguria and acute alteration of the level of consciousness.

▶ *MODS:* This is a consequence of the inability of the body to maintain end-organ perfusion and oxygenation, resulting in cellular ischaemia and organ failure. When two or more organs become dysfunctional to the point where maintaining homeostasis requires active intervention, MODS is diagnosed.

Table 35.6

Specific considerations in the structured approach to managing cardiogenic shock

Key principles	Interventions	Clinical notes
History	When taking past medical history, specifically ask whether the patient has any underlying: • rheumatic fever • congenital cardiac conditions • cardiac dysrhythmias • cough or flu-like symptoms in late pregnancy (peripartum cardiomyopathy, or PPCM)	These patients must be regarded as high risk and monitored accordingly.
Breathing	*Look:* Observe the respiratory rate, depth and difficulty. *Listen:* Briefly auscultate breath sounds bilaterally. Initiate pulse oximetry, if available.	
Circulation	During the first stage of labour, place the woman in the semi-Fowler's position, preferably on the left side. During the second stage of labour, the woman must be positioned in an upright position. Never raise the legs above the level of the heart. Insert one 18- or 20-gauge IV cannula. Use a 60 drops-per-minute administration set. Use a 200 ml vaculitre of Ringer's lactate or normal saline at a rate of 50 ml/hour.	When sitting upright, the pulmonary pressures decrease due to gravitation pressure, decreasing the severity of the pulmonary congestion leading to pulmonary oedema. Note: The patient should be fluid-restricted, as increased circulatory volume will increase the risk of pulmonary congestion and hypoxaemia.
Drugs	Administer oxytocin (the drug of choice if needed in labour). *Do not give ergometrine during the second and third stage of labour.* Consider furosemide, digoxin and/or aminophylline post-delivery.	Ergometrine works on the smooth muscles of the heart, increasing the flow of blood into the pulmonary circulation, leading to pulmonary oedema. Furosemide is used to decrease the circulating volume. Digoxin increases the ventricular contractility, increasing the stroke volume and decreasing the pulmonary congestion. Aminophylline decreases pulmonary pressures due to pulmonary vasodilation.

Temperature > 38°C or < 36°C

Heart rate > 90 beats per minute

Tachypnoea with respiratory rate > 20 breaths per minute

White blood cell count > 12 000 or < 4 000

↓

Sepsis

SIRS resulting from bacteria, viral, parasitic, or fungal infection

↓

Severe sepsis

Sepsis that involves at least one organ dysfunction, hypoperfusion, or hypotension

↓

MODS

Two or more organ dysfunctions to the point that maintaining homeostasis requires active interventions

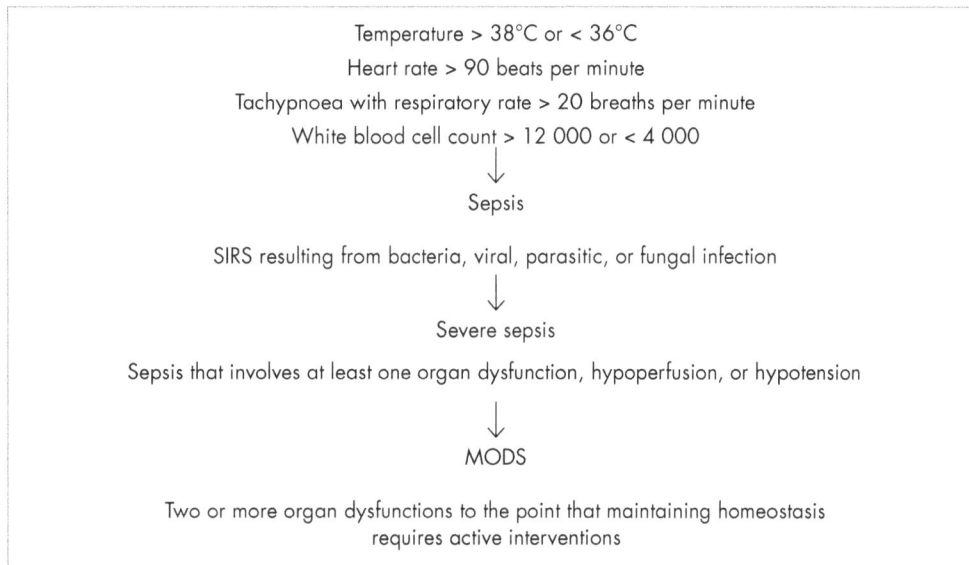

Figure 35.2 Overview of the sepsis syndrome

History (patients at risk)

The leading causes of sepsis in midwifery practice include:

- urinary tract infection (UTI), pyelonephritis and renal calculi
- chorioamnionitis and prolonged rupture of membranes
- endometritis
- necrotising fasciitis
- surgical interventions (Caesarean section, amniocentesis and episiotomy)
- septic pelvic thrombophlebitis
- anaemia
- perinatal infections
- HIV and other sexually transmitted infections (STIs)
- retained products of conception
- milk fever (mastitis)
- iatrogenic factors, such as septic abortion.

Pathophysiology

In childbirth, the risk for septic shock is increased because of the direct access of organisms to the system through the placental site via the vagina.

Sepsis begins with the entry of organisms into the bloodstream through the skin, respiratory tract, GI tract, breasts and placental site. Organisms entering the body may include bacteria, yeast, viruses and/or parasites.

The pathophysiology of sepsis is complex. It involves the activation of the inflammatory response to infection, along with activation of coagulation and impairment of fibrinolysis. An increase in inflammation and coagulation occur as a result of mediator responses, which function as part of the immune system reaction to infection.

Cytokines are released from white bloods cells (WBCs) and other cells in response to the infection in order to protect the cells from the effects of sepsis and to begin the healing process. The cytokines and WBCs trigger vasodilatation, leading to hypotension, increased capillary permeability, neutrophil activation, fever, decreased myocardial contractility and adhesion of platelets to the endothelium.

The compensatory mechanism includes the baroreceptors situated in the aortic arch and carotid arteries, which respond to the decrease in the cardiac output. The baroreceptors activate the sympathetic nervous system, which in turn stimulates the release of potent vasoconstrictors, adrenaline and noradrenaline to maintain blood flow to vital organs (the heart and the brain). Simultaneously, blood is shunted from non-vital organs such as the lungs, kidneys, GI tract and skin. Decreased blood flow to the kidneys activates the rennin system. This process eventually affects the circulatory volume, cardiac output and tissue perfusion. This leads to MODS and, ultimately, death.

Clinical signs and symptoms

The midwife should closely monitor patients at risk for any of the following signs and symptoms:

▶ *Haemodynamic findings:*
- Decreased level of consciousness: disorientation, restlessness
- Tachypnoea: >15 breaths per minute
- Pyrexia: temperature > 38 °C
- Systolic pressure: < 90 mmHg
- Central venous pressure: < 10 mmHg
- Tachycardia

▶ *Clinical findings:*
- Warm and dry skin
- Decreased peripheral perfusion
- Decreased urine output: < 0.5 to 1 ml/kg/hour or 30 ml/hour.

▶ *Additional findings:*
- Serum-C-reactive protein (CRP): > 12 mg/ℓ
- WBC count: > 12 000 or < 4 000 10⁹/ℓ
- Lactate: > 2 mmol/ℓ

- Arterial blood gas indicates metabolic acidosis (pH, HCO_3 and BE).

Diagnosis, management, intervention and care

Goal-directed therapy in the management of sepsis is often focused on supporting failing organs. Interventions include airway management, fluid replacement, antibiotic therapy and the use of vasopressors. To prevent sepsis progression, it is important to identify the infection source and target the specific source, for example debridement of an abscess.

With the aim of promoting evidence-based sepsis treatment, the Surviving Sepsis Campaign developed specific management guidelines to decrease the mortality of patients with sepsis (see the box on the next page). Initiate these actions and simultaneously call for assistance.

The specific difference and/or special considerations pertaining to septic shock are highlighted in Table 35.7. The principles used during the ABC approach remain the same as shown in Table 35.2.

Table 35.7

Specific considerations in the structured approach to managing septic shock

Key principles	Interventions	Clinical notes
History	Focus on past medical history, specifically pertaining to 'infection'.	
Breathing	*Look:* Observe the respiratory rate, depth and difficulty. *Listen:* Briefly auscultate breath sounds bilaterally. Initiate pulse oximetry, if available.	
Circulation	Turn the woman on her left side or elevate her right hip to prevent supine hypotension. Promptly place one or two large-bore (14 or 16 gauge) IV lines and simultaneously draw blood (lactate, FBC, CRP and procalcitonin [PCT]). Use a 10-drops-per-minute administration set. Administer 20 ml/kg bolus of crystalloid solution (ie Ringer's lactate) as a volume expander. Repeat bolus if systolic BP remains < 90 mmHg.	Monitor and interpret vital signs vigilantly and frequently (every 15 minutes until patient is stabilised). Monitor urinary output using an indwelling urinary catheter (normal = 0.5 to 1 ml/kg/hour).
Drugs	Administer a broad-spectrum antibiotic. Dopamine is the drug of choice (alternatively use phenylephrine or adrenaline).	The woman must receive the first dose of broad-spectrum antibiotic within three hours from diagnosing sepsis. This may decrease mortality by as much as 30–50%. Do not give inotropic drugs before fluid boluses. Inotropic drugs are used to increase the afterload (BP).

Surviving Sepsis Campaign: Resuscitation bundle

The sepsis resuscitation bundle consists of the following:

▶ Perform a serum lactate measurement (draw an arterial blood gas).

▶ Draw blood cultures prior to antibiotic administration.

▶ Administer a broad-spectrum antibiotic within three hours after diagnosing sepsis.

In the event of hypotension and/or lactate being greater than 4 mmol/ℓ:

▶ Give a bolus of minimum 20 ml/kg of crystalloids (eg Ringer's lactate).

▶ Administer vasopressors for hypotension not responding to fluid resuscitation to maintain MAP > 65 mmHg (eg dopamine).

Refer to the following websites for additional reading:

▶ www.alsg.org

▶ www.survivingsepsis.org

▶ https://www.resus.org.uk/resuscitation-guidelines/

35.7   Anaphylactic shock

Anaphylaxis is a life-threatening event that can occur at any point during pregnancy. It has been reported following administration of various substances, with adverse maternal and neonatal consequences. It should be considered in the differential diagnosis of intrapartum collapse. It is important to highlight anaphylaxis as a cause of collapse in pregnancy and birth in relation to a variety of substances that may be given to a woman.

Anaphylactic shock can be severe, can occur within minutes after initial exposure to the offending agent, and can occur with no history of known allergy.

The risk for anaphylaxis in the USA is 1–15 per cent, but it varies between countries and is not well researched (Mustafa, 2017).

The outcomes depend on the age, parity, gestational age (GA), co-morbidities, aetiological trigger, coagulopathy, causing agent and clinical picture. Anaphylaxis can result in significant long-term morbidity, mainly related to cerebral hypoxia after an ineffective resuscitation.

History (patients at risk)

Any person may be at risk for anaphylaxis (drug hypersensitivity) by a known or unknown agent. An anaphylactic reaction is usually precipitated by food (eg nuts or fish), blood products, vaccines, insect bites, latex rubber, plasters, skin antiseptics and certain drugs such as opioid analgesics, neuromuscular blocking agents as well as oxytocin, antibiotics and ranitidine.

A colloid solution is a commonly used plasma expander in clinical practice and anaphylaxis has been reported in the use of some of the colloids. Colloid solutions are used very frequently for PPH and sometimes antenatally for severe haemorrhage. They can trigger an allergic reaction (see Table 35.8 on the next page).

In addition, women with asthma may have a reaction to prostaglandins.

This type of shock is more likely to occur after parenteral administration in atopic individuals who are particularly susceptible because of their (often unknown) hereditary predisposition to anaphylactic reactions.

Pathophysiology

Anaphylaxis is a rapid, systemic hypersensitivity reaction to a substance in a sensitised individual, with potentially life-threatening consequences. IgE antibodies, which can cause histamine and other vasoactive mediators, are released from mast cells and basophils. IgE immunoglobulins are found in plasma and are the only antibodies in humans to produce anaphylactic reactions, for example immediate hypersensitivity. These mast cells are wandering cells that are found in most tissues but are most abundant in connective tissue. The antibodies are generated on exposure to a specific stimulus. The cells release histamine in the tissues as part of the inflammatory reaction. These histamines produce respiratory, circulatory, cutaneous and GI effects. Increased vascular permeability and peripheral vasodilatation reduce venous return and cardiac output.

Clinical picture

A mild reaction is manifested as flushing, urticaria, itching, redness and localised oedema. A more serious reaction is manifested as shock, bronchospasm, laryngeal oedema and angio-oedema.

The clinical picture may include various degrees of chest pain, dyspnoea, tachycardia, hypotension, cyanosis and DIC (as demonstrated by laboratory findings). Cardiac or respiratory arrest may result.

Based on the clinical picture and laboratory findings, amniotic fluid embolism or trophoblastic embolism may be suspected and need to be excluded.

Table 35.8

Comparison of IV crystalloids and colloids

Crystalloids	Plasma substitutes and colloids
Substances from crystals (sodium and chloride) that break down in water	Particles that do not break down in water
The particles are small and weigh 30 kilodaltons (kDa) and can easily pass through compartments.	Most of the particles are larger than 30 kDa.
The particles are available in three tonicities (osmolarity).	The particles cannot fit through most capillary pores and stay in the capillary bed.
Crystalloids are isotonic (same number of particles as plasma).	These are used for volume expansion: 250 ml will give the same effect as 4 ℓ of crystalloids.
Crystalloids will not allow shift of fluid in or out of cells. They should not cause oedema.	A disadvantage is that the pressure in the capillaries stretches so that the pores and the colloids move through. The oedema that results takes longer to resolve than with crystalloids.
Examples: Ringer's lactate and normal saline 0.9%	Examples: Human albumin, dextran, polygeline (Haemaccel®) tetrastarch (Voluven®), pentastarch (HAES-steril®)
This is currently the fluid of choice with resuscitation or electrolyte replacement.	Plasma substitutes are widely used for the treatment of hypervolaemia.
Current evidence suggests that Ringer's lactate may cause pro-inflammatory responses that may trigger acute respiratory distress syndrome (ARDS).	Problems include fluid overload, pulmonary oedema and anaphylaxis.
5% dextrose is not used for resuscitation. The glucose is rapidly metabolised and fluid becomes hypotonic. Water swiftly shifts from the vascular bed into the cells through osmosis. This may correct cellular dehydration and hypernatraemia but will worsen hypotension.	A pre-dosage of 10–20 ml is given and the patient's reaction is monitored for anaphylactic shock.
Hypertonic fluid will pull water from cells and interstitial spaces, shrinking the cells. Hypertonic saline, 0.45%, assists with electrolyte imbalances and suppresses inflammatory responses. It is gaining popularity as the fluid of choice in resuscitation.	

Diagnosis, management, intervention and care

There is no valid predictor of drug anaphylaxis. A history of family occurrences, disease profiles, previous allergies, current medication and the use of natural substances is important when a woman is admitted for interventions in pregnancy and birth, particularly for IOL or Caesarean section and anaesthesia.

The clinical recognition of manifestations is very important. Serial serum tryptase estimations are helpful in the diagnosis of anaphylaxis. Tryptase enzyme is released from mast cells, which parallels histamine release. Peak concentrations that are well above 20 mg/ml indicate true anaphylaxis or anaphylactic reaction. The peak value of tryptase in the serum occurs between 30 minutes to six hours after an anaphylactic reaction.

There must be a written emergency action plan for the management of anaphylaxis in obstetric care. A list of known allergens or agents triggering anaphylaxis and the conditions attached needs to be visible and available to alert staff of substances in obstetrics with a potential for anaphylactic reactions.

Since anaphylaxis can occur with any drug, all the members of the perinatal team should be familiar with the recognition of symptoms and signs of anaphylactic reaction. Furthermore, anaphylactic reactions can be unpredictable and severe reactions manifesting in the form of angio-oedema and cardiovascular collapse need immediate and prompt treatment. Severe anaphylactic reactions can also happen during a surgical procedure. Severe reactions require early recognition and aggressive resuscitation. All obstetricians and midwives should be trained to be able to identify and manage this emergency. The management of anaphylaxis should be included in emergency drills on a regular basis so that this uncommon life-threatening event is tackled in the most effective way. It is very important that the members of the perinatal team are aware of the symptoms and signs of anaphylactic reaction and are familiar with the management of anaphylactic shock.

Treatment includes the following:
▶ Immediately discontinue the agent causing the reaction.
▶ First-line treatment is to restore BP; let the patient lie flat and lift the foot of the bed with a lateral tilt if she is still pregnant to lift the uterus from the inferior vena cava.
▶ Give 100 per cent oxygen.
▶ Give adrenaline (1:1 000 ampoule) 0.01 mg/kg IM. Repeat every 5 minutes until stable for those older than 12 years (0.5 ml). Observe for 4 hours after the last dose of adrenaline.

▶ If haemodynamic instability continues, an adrenaline infusion may be required: 1 mg adrenaline diluted in 250 mg normal saline. Start at 15 ml per hour and titrate as per clinical symptoms.
▶ Administer crystalloid for intravascular volume expansion. If colloid was given prior to the reaction, change to crystalloid because the causative agent might have been the colloid substance (500–1 000 ml Ringer's lactate).
▶ Antihistamines can be administered.
▶ Corticosteroids (100–200 mg) are given slowly.
▶ Bronchodilators may be required.
▶ Perform prolonged monitoring in intensive care or intubation.

Adrenaline is the most important drug in anaphylactic reaction and must be readily available. Intramuscular is the best route of administration.

35.8   Conclusion

There are different types of shock that a midwife may encounter in obstetric practice, each of which may be life-threatening. The ability to differentiate between the type of shock, combined with the immediate initiation of appropriate and systematic collaborative management, may enhance patient health outcomes. A patient may suffer from several types of shock simultaneously, which makes intervention very complex.

Section Six

Postnatal care

The physiology and psychology of the normal puerperium

36.1 Introduction

After birth, a woman's body undergoes physiological changes, including healing of the birth canal, involution of the uterus and breastfeeding. During this time, the body gradually returns to a non-pregnant state. The woman is changed by pregnancy – anatomically, physiologically, emotionally, socially and economically. This chapter will consider the events and experiences of the mother, the newborn and the family that occur shortly after birth.

36.2 Description of the puerperium

The word 'puerperium' comes from the Latin *puer*, meaning 'child', and *perus*, meaning 'to bring forth'.

The puerperium is defined as the period from the completion of delivery (end of the third stage of labour) to the end of the first six weeks postpartum, during which time the woman's body returns to the normal non-gravid state.

During pregnancy, physiological and psychological changes take place in the woman's body and mind, which end in the birth of the baby. During the puerperium, the changes in anatomy, physiology and biochemistry that occurred during pregnancy and labour return to the non-gravid state. However, a woman's body never returns to the pre-pregnancy state. Some of the changes that take place during pregnancy are permanent.

In addition, the woman has to adapt psychologically and socially to motherhood and, together with her husband or partner and other members of the family, faces a time of challenges, happiness and adjustments.

36.3 Normal physiological changes in the puerperium

The postnatal period is a time of restoration. The first concern of the midwife is to make sure that the woman experiences a postnatal period without complications.

After the birth, the woman's body begins the process of returning to the non-gravid state. However, at the same time she needs to be able to breastfeed. These physiological changes occur within the first 14 days and the midwife needs to understand these changes and to detect any abnormalities as early as possible. The first 24 hours after birth carry the greatest risk of postpartum haemorrhage (PPH).

Endocrine changes

The endocrine hormones will have an influence on the woman after birth.

Oestrogen and progesterone

Oestrogen and progesterone levels drop after the delivery of the placenta. By 24 hours after birth, oestradiol has dropped to 2 per cent of the pregnancy level. Progesterone levels do not fall as rapidly as oestrogen, as there is still secretion from the corpus luteum for the first few days after birth. The levels of these hormones remain low for the first few weeks postpartum.

Human chorionic gonadotrophin (hCG), human placental lactogen (HPL), oestrogen and progesterone fall rapidly. Normally, after seven days, hCG is no longer detectable in the woman's urine. After two days, HPL is no longer detectable in the plasma.

Follicle-stimulating hormone (FSH) and luteinising hormone (LH) start to rise slowly over four to six weeks after birth.

Prolactin

Prolactin decreases when labour starts and increases immediately after birth, with a peak three hours postpartum. The release of prolactin is triggered by the suckling of the baby. Prolactin levels also increase with anaesthesia, surgery, exercise, nipple stimulation and sexual intercourse. The more the baby suckles, the higher the levels of prolactin. In women who do not breastfeed, prolactin levels gradually decrease over 14 days.

Oxytocin

Nipple stimulation during suckling also causes the release of oxytocin, which contracts the myoepithelial cells lining the lactiferous ducts and causes the 'let-down' of milk. Oxytocin also causes contraction of the uterine muscle and therefore, at the same time, assists in the involution of the uterus (see Chapter 37).

Restoration of ovulation and menstruation

Ovulation and menstruation are the last major functions to return to normal. In women who breastfeed their babies, ovulation seldom occurs before 20 weeks. It may not occur for up to 28 weeks in women who continue breastfeeding for six months. In most instances, the more frequently the baby suckles, the less chance there is of ovulation occurring. However, ovulation may occur earlier than 20 weeks, particularly if the woman is only partially breastfeeding. In non-lactating women, ovulation and menstruation usually start again within seven to 10 weeks.

Involution of the reproductive organs

Involution is the return of the reproductive tract to the non-gravid state.

The uterus

The uterus is the organ that has to undergo the greatest amount of involution, because it has had to undergo the greatest changes during pregnancy and labour. The enlarged uterus is no longer needed to carry the fetus; therefore, tissues developed in pregnancy break down through the following mechanisms:

▶ *Ischaemia of the myometrium.* This is caused by the continuous contraction and retraction of the uterus after the expulsion of the placenta, making the uterus relatively anaemic and causing atrophy of the muscle fibres. The blood that was contained within the uterine vessels is released into the bloodstream. This greatly increased volume of fluid in the circulation has to be removed by the kidneys, and results in a major diuresis in the early puerperium.

▶ *Autolysis.* With the withdrawal of the placental oestrogens, protein synthesis is no longer stimulated. Instead, proteolytic enzymes break down proteins, which are finally excreted by the kidneys, increasing the diuresis. Simultaneously, phagocytes invade the collagen fibres between the myometrial cells and fat is removed, while thrombosed blood vessels are also broken down and absorbed.

A cellular barrier forms over the placental site and all tissue superficial to this barrier is shed. A new epithelium develops and covers the area.

The following has happened by the end of about the first six weeks after delivery:

▶ The weight of the uterus is diminished from approximately 1 000 g to about 60 g.

▶ The size of the uterus is diminished from approximately 15 × 12 × 8 cm to about 8 × 6 × 4 cm.

The uterus never completely returns to its pre-pregnant size and weight. On the contrary, with each pregnancy the muscle weight and collagen content of the uterus are slightly increased and elastin is deposited around the blood vessels. This means that with each successive pregnancy, the collagen and elastin content increases, causing the uterine muscles to become less elastic and resulting in the uterus becoming a progressively less efficient organ for pregnancy and labour.

After birth, the uterus is below the umbilicus. The ligaments are loose and the uterus can move freely in the abdomen. A well-contracted uterus can be palpated and feels like a tennis ball. Within 24 hours, the uterus is approximately at the level of the umbilicus, because of the increased tone of the pelvic floor. The fundus of the uterus decreases between 1 cm to 1.5 cm or about a finger's breadth per day in a primigravida and 2 cm in a multigravida. This means that by about 10–12 days after delivery, the fundus can no longer be palpated abdominally, because it has sunk below the level of the symphysis pubis (pelvic brim) and is a pelvic organ again.

Involution of the uterine ligaments is gradual and at first the uterus tends to tilt backwards. However, the uterus has usually returned to its normal anteflexed and anteverted position by the end of six weeks. The uterus will never again retain its pre-pregnant size and the size of the uterus will always indicate a previous pregnancy.

After-pains

Intermittent uterine contractions continue for the first few days after delivery, but often go unnoticed by the primipara. However, multiparae experience uterine cramps and after-pains, probably when the uterus has to expel blood clots and particularly when the baby suckles (the release of oxytocin into the blood circulation causing stronger contraction of the myometrium). The pain is likened to that of dysmenorrhoea and can be so distressing that analgesia is required.

The placental site

Once the placenta is expelled and the uterus contracts and retracts normally, the placental site diminishes rapidly. By the day after delivery, it has shrunk to a diameter of about 7.5 cm, from its diameter of 20 cm during pregnancy. By about the 10th day after delivery, the diameter of the placental site is about 2.5 cm. By the end of five to six weeks, the epithelial covering has completely regenerated, leaving only a small depression but no scar tissue.

The endometrium

The epithelial layer of the endometrium, except for the placental site, has regenerated by the end of two weeks.

Lochia

The living ligatures of uterine muscle and the blood clotting at the placental site prevent excessive bleeding, but a slowly diminishing discharge from the placental site continues to take place for up to six weeks. This discharge is known as the lochia. Normal lochia has a characteristically strong, but not offensive, smell.

The amount of lochia varies in different women. Over time it diminishes from slightly more than the usual menstrual flow to mere spotting on the perineal pad towards the end of the puerperium. The quantity will also vary from day to day, for instance when the woman first spends more time walking around. After breastfeeding, the amount of lochia may increase for a while. Where the placental site was larger than normal, as in a multiple pregnancy, an increased quantity of lochia will be noted.

The lochia is differentiated as follows:
- *Lochia rubra.* For the first two to four days after delivery, the lochia is red and consists mainly of blood, dissolved blood clots from the placental site and trophoblastic debris. From three to seven days after delivery, the lochia becomes reddish-brown as the bleeding is controlled.
- *Lochia serosa.* From five to 10 days after delivery, the lochia consists mainly of serum, lymph and leucocytes and varies from pinkish to a yellowish-brown.
- *Lochia alba.* From one week up to four to six weeks after delivery, the lochia contains lymph, leucocytes, cervical mucus, organisms and other debris from the healing process. It is now creamy-yellowish.

A persistent red or heavy lochia for more than 10 days or the continuous passing of clots should receive attention and be reported to the medical practitioner, as this would indicate that the placental site is not involuting as it should. It may suggest the presence of retained products, with the danger of secondary PPH and infection.

For the first four to five days postpartum, the lochia in the uterine cavity is sterile (if there was no prior chorioamnionitis), but it becomes contaminated by microorganisms as it passes down the vagina, and this gives the lochia its characteristically strong but not offensive odour. These microorganisms multiply in the vagina and, after four to five days, invade the uterine cavity. The cellular barrier has formed by this time and normally prevents infection of the placental site.

However, if there has been a delay in the healing process, if the woman's resistance is low, if the woman has been subjected to a particularly traumatic delivery, or if the aseptic technique has broken down and virulent organisms have been introduced into the vagina, cervix or uterus, then the barrier can be penetrated and puerperal infection can occur. A lochia with an offensive smell would indicate infection.

The cervix

The cervix is soft and flabby and reddish-blue after delivery and often has small lateral lacerations. The cervix can often be seen at the introitus after birth. As the pelvic floor regains its tone, the cervix is pulled back into the vagina. The involution of the cervix occurs together with that of the uterus and by two to three weeks, the cervical os is a mere slit. (After the first vaginal delivery, the cervical os never returns to the initial non-gravid size and shape.)

The vagina

The vaginal wall has been extensively stretched during the delivery and is therefore swollen, reddish-blue and flabby after the delivery. The vagina regains most of its tone by the end of the puerperium. The vaginal epithelium (mucosa) and submucosa may be lacerated or may have been incised with an episiotomy. The mucosa takes two to three weeks to heal, but the submucosa requires suturing and remains delicate for four to six weeks after delivery, or even longer.

The vulva

Any superficial lacerations that may have occurred heal relatively quickly. Remnants of the hymen are known as carunculae myrtiformes.

The perineum

Owing to the liberal blood supply to the area, sutured perineal tears and episiotomies should have healed after seven days. However, severe lacerations may remain sensitive or even painful for weeks.

The perineal muscles regain their tone after five to six weeks. This process is speeded up and maintained by exercising after the birth of the baby.

The abdomen

The skin of the abdomen, which has been greatly stretched during pregnancy, appears loose and flabby for weeks or even months. The stretch marks gradually fade, but often do not disappear altogether and instead become silvery-white streaks (stretch marks).

With the aid of postnatal exercises the muscles of the abdominal wall should regain their tone within a few weeks. The rectus abdominis muscles remain separated in the midline, although they do also respond to abdominal exercises. In grand

multiparae, in older women or when a multiple pregnancy has occurred, skin and muscles take longer to regain their tone. These women in particular should be encouraged to do exercises (see Chapter 19).

The pelvic girdle

During the puerperium, the pelvis gradually regains its former stability as the joint ligaments regain their tone. The process takes several weeks and until it is complete, it is common for the woman to experience backache, particularly related to the region of the sacroiliac joints.

The breasts

During pregnancy, the increased amounts of oestrogen and progesterone in the woman's circulation prepare the breast tissues for lactation, but the high levels of oestrogen inhibit the secretion of prolactin by the anterior pituitary gland. This suppresses the production of milk until the puerperium, when levels of oestrogen fall dramatically after the expulsion of the placenta.

Lactation

In the first two to three days, colostrum is secreted by the breasts. This is an important component in the nourishment of the newborn baby (see chapters 9 and 39).

The secretion of milk usually begins on the third day after delivery. The secretion of prolactin is stimulated by the neurohormonal reflex mechanism, which is activated when the baby suckles. Therefore, the more the baby suckles, the more milk is produced by the breasts. Rest and sleep are also an important part of this process.

Lactation can reduce the incidence of pregnancy through suppression of ovulation, but is not a reliable method of contraception.

If a woman wishes not to breastfeed, it is advisable to suppress lactation before the neurohormonal reflex is initiated.

The cardiovascular system

The heart

The cardiac output increases during labour and rises even further after the third stage, when a large volume of blood is squeezed into circulation as the uterus contracts to prevent haemorrhage. The cardiac output gradually decreases during the first few days of the puerperium and, in women without cardiac disease, has returned to the normal pre-pregnant output by the end of the third week.

The vital signs of a woman post-delivery are usually physiologically low.

The BP should be normal in relation to the values before or during labour. A diastolic BP of 90 or above is a danger sign for eclampsia. A drop or rise in the BP of 15 mmHg diastolic and 30 mmHg systolic needs to be monitored. Consider a history of infections, surgical interventions or epidural. Manual removal of the placenta and Caesarean section also alter the vital signs.

A woman's temperature is physiologically low after birth. Any raised temperature needs to be noted. (An epidural can cause an increase in the temperature.)

The pulse rate of a woman (without cardiac disease) is physiologically low after birth. Any pulse rate of 90 beats and higher needs to be noted and monitored until stable.

Respiration returns to normal after birth, at 16–20 breaths per minute.

The blood

With each 250 ml of blood loss, Hb drops by 1 g/dl and the haematocrit drops by four points. A woman who had a haematocrit of 37 per cent and an Hb of 12 g/dl may experience a drop in her haematocrit to 33 per cent and in her Hb to 11 g/dl. A woman who started labour with a borderline haematocrit or Hb may become compromised by moderate blood loss.

Although there is a decrease in the blood flow to the organs after the first few days, the blood flow to the breasts is increased in order to establish lactation. There is a gradual return to normal of the number of red and white blood cells by the end of the puerperium.

During the last few weeks of pregnancy, the levels of fibrinogen, plasminogen and clotting factors increase significantly. In the first few days after delivery, these levels fall fairly rapidly, but the blood is more coagulable, with increased viscosity. This results in an increased risk of thrombosis. The clotting factors of the body are activated in the early postpartum period with a particularly high level of fibrinogen. This may increase the risk of thrombophlebitis and embolism.

The white blood cell (WBC) count increases to 30 000, particularly the granulocytes, to protect the body against infections.

The renal tract

There is major diuresis in the first few days of the puerperium, resulting in a substantial loss of fluid, and the woman is often very thirsty in the first week and after. The midwife needs to be cautioned that diuresis may be inhibited by the use of rectal anti-inflammatory agents. However, at the same time, the neck of the bladder and the urethra may be oedematous and bruised after delivery and this could cause difficulty in passing urine.

The result could be extensive bladder distension, requiring catheterisation.

The physiological dilatation of the urinary system decreases slowly and only returns to normal by the end of the puerperium. Small amounts of protein may be found in the urine during the first few days after delivery.

The woman is at high risk of urinary tract infection (UTI) after catheterisation in labour and during procedures such as epidural or Caesarean section.

The gastrointestinal tract

Women are naturally hungry and thirsty after natural birth. Women who have interventions such as epidural or Caesarean are either kept nil per mouth or on restricted intake. All other women are offered a high-calorie drink or a meal after birth.

There is a very gradual return to normal mobility of the gut, and this may be delayed further by the use of analgesics and possible dehydration after labour and birth and the postpartum diuresis. The woman may not feel like eating (not have a normal appetite) for the first few days and the perineum may be painful, preventing defecation. All these factors contribute to constipation in the first week of the puerperium. Laxatives, suppositories or even an enema may be required to promote elimination within three days.

Breastfeeding requires energy and the energy requirements in a breastfeeding woman's diet thus increases. After the initial birth period, women may experience hunger and thirst associated with breastfeeding. The breastfeeding woman therefore needs to adjust her food intake to meet the needs of lactation.

Weight decrease

About 5 kg is lost as a result of the delivery of the baby, the amniotic fluid and the placenta. As a result of involution and diuresis, a further 2.5 kg is lost. The changes to the breasts and breastfeeding may add another 2 kg onto the weight of the mother. By the end of the puerperium, her weight should have almost returned to the pre-pregnancy weight, although increased weight may persist for some months after delivery.

36.4 General recuperation and the psychological state in the puerperium

Mood swings and depression

Mood swings or emotional instability are common in the puerperium, and even the most easy-going women are likely to suffer from some transient mood changes. The great joy, even ecstasy and the sense of achievement and fulfilment that the woman felt at and immediately after the birth of the baby give way to tiredness, anxiety and a dawning sense of her responsibilities, which, together with the physical changes taking place in her body, often cause an overwhelming sadness or even depression, giving rise to involuntary spells of crying. The woman may not know why she is crying; she just feels very sad and cannot help crying. These postpartum 'blues' (or 'third or fourth day blues') as they are commonly called, alternate with feelings of great happiness and the pride of motherhood. In the first two to three days, the woman is occupied with the baby, with visitors and congratulations, but when the milk comes in, the breasts become full and painful and if the baby will not suckle, the woman becomes upset and depressed. This occurs in about 85 per cent of women (Joy, 2017).

Normally, when the baby is feeding well and the woman is feeling rested and less anxious, her emotions stabilise as her body and mind recover and return to the non-gravid state. However, in about 10–15 per cent of women, a deeper depression may occur and continue for some time after the puerperium, while in about 0.1–0.2 per cent of postpartum women, a frank psychosis occurs (Joy, 2017). It is important to be aware of this and to know the danger signs (also see Chapter 13).

The need for rest and sleep

Directly after birth, the woman may experience alertness and an inability to sleep even though she is tired. It is thus extremely important that the woman has sufficient rest and sleep in the puerperium. This helps to build up her psychological and physical stamina. It also helps to promote lactation and gives the woman time to get to know her baby. If she is mentally under pressure or physically in pain, she will be unable to cope and the general healing process will be slowed down. The return to normal will take longer and complications are more likely to arise.

Sexual function and activity

The postpartum period is characterised by a change in the sexual function of the woman and her partner. Sexual function is modified by:
- trauma to the reproductive organs
- anatomical and physiological problems
- lochia and vaginal discharge
- the presence of the baby and the stress caused by that
- leaking and engorged breasts
- altered lubrication of the vagina for six months
- fatigue
- psychological factors.

Orgasm for women postpartum is shorter and less intense for the first few months due to less vasocongestion of the labia. This, along with painful perineal muscles and episiotomy, may make sexual intercourse less enjoyable for women for the four to six months it takes for complete healing of a perineal wound. Twenty per cent of women report discomfort with sexual intercourse after vaginal birth, and no difference was found between women with or without an episiotomy (Kalis, Rusavy & Prka, 2016). The resumption of sexual intercourse depends on the woman's restoration and varies from a few weeks to several months. In addition, many cultures have a taboo on sexual intercourse after birth. Counselling may be needed.

36.5   The experience of birth

Reactions after birth

A woman's reaction immediately after birth can vary widely, from enthusiastic excitement to dejection and even rejection of the newborn. While it is easy to participate in the joy and pleasure of a mother or couple whose birth experience has been a good one, it is more difficult to remain encouraging and supportive of the woman who appears not to enjoy the initial moments after delivery. Any inner feelings of irritation, disappointment and anger on the part of the midwife need to be carefully managed while the parents' points of view are considered. Sometimes disappointment or a lack of enthusiasm may be an appropriate response, for example following a long, difficult labour that did not go as hoped. This less-than-positive experience needs to be accepted by the midwife, who should build the woman's self-confidence by, for example, praising her for managing a difficult situation well.

Even joyous mothers can respond to their babies in different ways. Some mothers bubble verbally, while others are quieter, preferring to touch rather than talk. Both responses are acceptable. Getting to know a baby takes time. For some mothers, their own baby may be the first they have ever held.

If fathers are present, they often hold their babies soon after birth, as many mothers are quite willing to hand the baby over fairly quickly, particularly if the birth was difficult or if they do not feel too sure of themselves. Research indicates that fathers who were present at the birth and who had the chance to see and hold their babies at this time become more involved with their babies in the early months than do fathers who were not present at the birth. However, cultural differences may mean that fathers are rarely, if ever, present at the birth. African men are not expected to be present, particularly in rural areas. These cultural differences must be respected.

Most maternity units allow parents to spend time together during the first few hours after birth and encourage the father and the family to be involved. Visiting times may be flexible. This allows couples to relive the birth and to incorporate the transition to parenthood into their self-image.

The transition to parenthood, especially for first-time parents, requires adaptation and skills that need to be developed. Talking about the events of the birth together, with the baby present, can assist parents to come to terms with their new experiences.

During this time the midwife should be particularly alert to questions such as: 'How well did I cope?' This question, which may occur in the hours or days after delivery, may come from a woman's self-doubt. It is important that the woman be encouraged to think about her achievements rather than her disappointments, because a negative self-image may predispose her to even more difficulties in the ensuing weeks and months.

Feelings of failure are common and are aggravated by romanticised images of childbearing or by nurturing overly high expectations of the birth 'performance'. Often the expectation that is created is that birth should be unassisted by medical practitioners or drugs and should be exhilarating, exciting, joyous and perhaps painful, but tolerably so. Many mothers regard birth that deviates from this goal as a failure on their part.

Bonding

Bonding should start before conception, as the parents plan the pregnancy. If the pregnancy is unplanned, bonding may be delayed. The parents start to become aware of the baby once there are fetal movements, or earlier if there is an ultrasound. This makes the baby real and can enhance bonding. By the end of the third trimester, most women have positive feelings towards the baby and accept the pregnancy. A percentage of mothers will say that they only 'fell in love' with the baby after birth, while some women say that they learned to love the baby over time and did not feel a bond with the baby immediately after birth.

Bonding is promoted after birth through early mother-to-infant skin-to-skin contact, also called kangaroo-mother-care (KMC), putting the baby on the mother's breast soon after birth, breastfeeding and rooming-in if the baby is not ill and separated from the mother in a neonatal unit (see Chapter 42). Baby-friendly care (BFC) promotes parent and infant bonding. Institutions can apply for baby-friendly status, a process that takes about five years to complete, during which time the institute develops an environment that keeps mother and baby together.

A good birth experience (be it a Caesarean section or a vaginal delivery without any assistance or intervention)

will facilitate the growth of love. Difficult or disappointing deliveries may make this more difficult. Hence the importance of dealing with psychologically difficult birth experiences in the early days after delivery, to release the mother from her emotional constraints.

The birth environment

Family-centred maternity care provides the woman with antenatal care and delivery in a home-like environment in the hospital where she may be accompanied by as many family members as she and the midwives allow. This concept attempts to combine the supportive environment of birth offered by home deliveries with the security of available hospital facilities should things go wrong. There are private midwifery units in South Africa that allow the family to stay with the mother after birth.

Siblings may wish to be present at the birth and, providing there is someone available to care for them during the process and they have been adequately prepared, some institutions allow this.

Baby care

For the first-time mother in particular, starting to care for her new baby is often a nerve-wracking experience. With little prior exposure to babies, as is often the case today, this may be even more difficult. Most pregnant women today will attend antenatal preparation classes or will prepare themselves for parenthood by getting information from their caregivers, midwives or medical practitioners or by reading magazines, books, articles on the internet and talking with their mothers, sisters or friends. A supportive network is valuable during pregnancy and after birth.

The midwife should help the woman to gain the knowledge and skills required to confidently care for herself and her baby during and after the pregnancy. If there is to be early discharge, the midwife should ensure that continuing support is available for the new mother at home, either from family members or from a home nursing care service.

Hospitals and clinics provide toll-free 24-hour support lines for new mothers to consult after discharge.

Common issues in early parenthood

Most young or first-time mothers encounter certain common problems, such as the ones discussed in the following subsections.

Crying babies

Some babies cry a lot. Mothers often find this disconcerting and think that 'good' mothers should be able to calm their babies. The concept of a *good-enough mother* applies. Some distance between the parent and baby can be created by having someone else look after the baby.

Activity

Reread Chapter 10 and explain the different reasons why babies cry and the sleep–wake cycle.

Rooming-in and nursing care

Mothers are often concerned about keeping their babies with them all the time after delivery, or about nursery care. This should be flexible. If a mother still cannot look after herself after the birth, she may be reluctant to have the baby with her, as she may fear she will not be able to care for the child adequately.

If a mother is allowed up and can move around freely, she may opt to keep the baby with her. Having her baby with her will allow a new mother to become more familiar with her baby's routines, needs, sounds and presence than if the child was in a nursery. This will help the new mother to gain confidence and will also help the midwife, who wants to discharge a confident and capable new mother. Learning to care for the new baby herself, while still having the resources of midwives to call on whenever needed, is the best system to follow if possible.

A nursery care system is best for women who have had complicated births. There must be a written policy on the application of BFC.

Responsibility and postnatal 'blues'

Mothers often only come to realise the full responsibility of parenthood in the days following delivery. Full realisation of these demands may result in what are called 'baby blues' or postnatal 'blues'.

Mild emotional disturbances in the days, weeks and months following birth can be classified as baby blues and are transient. This must be distinguished from postnatal depression, which is potentially a very serious condition. The care of a woman experiencing an episode of baby blues includes the following:

- Reassure the woman that the feelings she is experiencing are normal.
- Explain that hormonal disturbances cause the feelings and that it will pass.
- Ask how it can be made better. Offer to take the baby to the nursery, offer a cup of tea, give a painkiller if needed, give privacy, offer her a shower or Sitz bath and make her comfortable or allow her to sleep.
- Give tender loving care and support.

- Try to continue with a normal routine as soon as possible and give support.
- Record the episode and make sure that it is resolved by discharge.
- Observe for signs of psychosis presenting within the first week after birth. These include symptoms of insomnia, suspicion, abnormal behaviour, neglect or overprotection of the baby and the loss of a sense of reality.

The baby blues can also present at home. Postnatal depression and psychosis are more serious problems and are discussed in Chapter 13.

Care after discharge

Unless the midwife is actively involved in district nursing, she will probably have little contact with the new mother after discharge and during most of the puerperium. It is therefore essential that the hospital or clinic-based midwife makes an effort to discharge a confident and capable mother.

The early discharge of women after birth and the lack of supportive postnatal services leave a gap in the care of women postpartum. Support services are needed to help women, particularly very young women, adapt to the demands of motherhood.

A new mother should be provided with a list of resources she can call on, including telephone numbers of support groups or available midwives. Midwives should also provide books and brochures if available.

In addition, if the midwife is concerned about a new mother who is being discharged, she should take particular care to refer her for help or to notify district nursing services to take particular care of her in the ensuing weeks. If necessary, daily home visits could be provided until the district midwife is sure the woman is satisfactorily launched in her new role as a mother.

It is important to consider psychological risk factors during pregnancy that may lead to mental health risks and disorders. The website Babytalk (https://www.babytalk.co.za) provides useful information for the new mother on this topic.

36.6   Conclusion

Although the postnatal period is a period of restoration for the woman, modern demands on women and changed lifestyle patterns do not favour rest, sleep and restoration. The transition to motherhood is dependent on psychological and cultural factors. Pregnancy and birth are considered to be a stress situation that can be normal or can put both the woman's and her partner's mental health at risk.

The lack of a support system, the absence of an extended family and a poor healthcare system with early discharge may put a mother and infant at risk after birth. Most women are discharged within 24 hours and are unsupported at home. The midwife needs to identify potential risks upfront and make allowance for these. Upon discharge, women need to be well informed of what to expect and what to do if things are not normal.

Assessment, diagnosis and care in the puerperium

LEARNING OBJECTIVES
On completion of this chapter, you must be able to:
▶ assess the needs of mother and baby in postnatal care
▶ provide optimum evidence-based immediate, intermediate and follow-up care, comfort and education to women after birth in all healthcare settings, following all kinds of births
▶ educate the mother or parents in the care of the infant and in self-care
▶ assess the woman on discharge and design a discharge care plan.

KNOWLEDGE ASSUMED TO BE IN PLACE
Principles of reproductive healthcare and health education
Anatomy and physiology of pregnancy, birth and the puerperium, including lactation
Fundamentals of general midwifery care, paediatrics, gynaecology and surgery
Fundamentals of emergency care

KEYWORDS
Evidence-based postnatal care

37.1   Introduction

The postnatal period is a critical phase in the mother and baby's life, because if this period is not handled correctly, the mother and baby could die. This period can range from less than 24 hours to a week or more, depending on the place of birth (public or private); the maternal diagnosis, circumstances and co-morbidities; and the policies of the unit. During this time, the mother and baby should remain under direct care and supervision in a hospital, clinic or the community.

37.2   General needs and policies regarding care of the mother and newborn

While the midwife has the mother and baby under direct supervision, the following must be considered:
▶ Assess the individual needs of the mother and the baby, based on the antenatal and birth history as well as risk factors.

▶ Compile a care plan and set goals to meet the needs and resolve as many problems as possible while under supervision.
▶ Include the physical and emotional aspects of care, breastfeeding and child spacing in the assessment.
▶ Consider the mother's and baby's specific needs and compile an appropriate discharge and referral plan.
▶ Assess the woman's need for education and support in terms of self-care activities and childcare.
▶ Consider the effects of early discharge and the adaptations of the mother post-delivery.
▶ Tailor care to meet the woman's particular needs within the boundaries of the policies on baby-and woman-friendly care.
▶ Create a positive, supportive environment.

The postnatal period is a period of adaptation that makes high demands on the mother, psychologically and physiologically.

Each woman's unique environment needs to be considered in the following ways:

- *Philosophy of care.* Each unit should have a philosophy of care that is in line with the principles of best practice while following institutional policies. This philosophy should include some form of community involvement.
- *Staff ratios and allocation.* It is important to develop a system where the entire team has the skills necessary to take care of mothers and babies after birth. Women need to see the same staff consistently. Different people may give conflicting advice and confuse the mother.
- *Policies and procedures.* The policies and procedures in a postnatal unit should be evidence-based. The unit should be working towards obtaining baby-friendly status if it has not already done so.
- *Safety and security.* Most postnatal units have security measures in place to prevent babies from being stolen or abducted. Access control places a burden on a unit, but safeguards mothers and babies and puts them at ease.
- *Scientific care.* A scientific method of care allows for the identification of the individual needs of the mother and for quality care.
- *Supportive care.* It is important that a postnatal unit is a place where women feel welcome and supported by a group of midwives that they trust. The midwife should be sensitive to each individual woman's needs during the puerperium; she should be kind and understanding at all times and must not be critical or judgemental. The midwife should be calm, cheerful, helpful and sensitive to any problems the woman may have. She must listen to what the woman has to say and work out what her problems are. She should help the mother to become independent. The midwife should ensure that the woman gets plenty of rest and sleep and a good, balanced diet.
- *Breastfeeding support.* Midwives should help to establish breastfeeding or, if this is not possible, give advice on artificial feeding. (See Chapter 9 for more on lactation.) First-time mothers who want to breastfeed need supervised support with each feed until they are confident. Ideally, a first-time mother should have support until breastfeeding is well established, usually for about 10 days. Many maternity units have a lactation consultant or clinic.

37.3 Standard procedures for postnatal care

The birth plan (if in use) should include the following:

- *Rooming-in.* One of the principles of baby-friendly care is rooming-in. The mother and baby should not be separated unless special or intensive care is needed. Nursery care is preferable if there has been a complicated birth and the mother needs more time to recover or needs intensive care.
- *Baby care.* Specific requirements for baby care need to be discussed with the midwife. Different cultural approaches should be respected, as long as they are safe.
- *Baby feeding.* Feeding should have been discussed antenatally and the woman's preferences should be respected. If the mother wants to breastfeed, but is separated from the baby, breastmilk can be expressed.
- *Visitors.* Units have different policies, but most allow the partner and siblings to visit soon after birth. Bear in mind, however, that too many visitors can be tiring.
- *Discharge planning.* This depends on the condition of the woman and baby and, in the private sector, on the medical aid scheme. Early discharge is allowed if it is safe and requested. Different units have different discharge policies. The mother will usually have discussed this before the birth and may even choose a unit based on its discharge policy.

37.4 Assessment and diagnosis on admission

On admission to a postnatal unit, the midwife plans care. All records and documentation should be available. The assessment should include:

- the woman's previous and current obstetric history
- the type of antenatal care received
- all prenatal tests done, such as Hb and HIV status.

Specific labour information

The following needs to be recorded:

- Type of delivery: natural, normal, assisted or Caesarean section
- Duration of birth (all stages)
- Mode of pain relief
- Any complications of birth
- Blood loss
- Condition of the pelvic floor.

Information on the baby

Information about the baby or babies should include:

- the date and time of birth
- the gender (check name bands and genitalia)
- the Apgar score
- breast or bottle feeding

- the gestational age (GA) and mass of the baby
- the baby's temperature
- the glucose level
- whether the baby is with the mother or in the neonatal unit, and why
- whether Konakion (vitamin K injection) has been given and eye prophylaxis done
- a visual check to see if the cord clamp is secure and not bleeding
- if urine or meconium has been passed.

Risk factors

Checking for risk factors should include:
- postpartum haemorrhage (PPH)
- pre-eclampsia or eclampsia
- infections
- thromboembolism
- puerperal depression or psychosis.

Assessment of the mother should include:
- the amount of vaginal bleeding
- uterine contraction and fundal height
- vital signs, including temperature, heart rate and BP
- the passing of urine.

Aspects of care include:
- specific individualised care, including the medical practitioner's orders for postnatal care, removal of drips, urinary catheter and pain relief
- individualised care, which depends on specific medical conditions such as anaemia, infection, high BP or diabetes mellitus.

37.5 Assessment and care

The aim of care is to manage the normal physiological and psychological changes in the postnatal period to make the woman comfortable, able to rest and establish bonding and breastfeeding. In the first six to 12 hours after birth, the woman may find it difficult to sleep even though she is tired, and she may still be in pain and discomfort.

Care is based around:
- the physical condition of the mother and baby
- the anticipated length of stay, related to the presence of risk factors and complications
- the availability of a support system (including the father) and their involvement in teaching and care activities.

Routine nursing interventions for postpartum care

During the postpartum period, a full physical examination is done daily, in order to:
- monitor and support physiological status
- assist with the restoration of bodily functions
- promote rest and comfort
- facilitate parent caretaking activities
- promote successful breastfeeding
- teach effective self-care
- plan for appropriate discharge.

Vital signs

The vital signs, temperature, pulse and BP are compared with the pre-delivery findings and are done four-hourly until stable, and thereafter according to the condition of the mother. In case of a Caesarean section, vital signs should be taken with shorter intervals until normal.

The temperature is observed to screen for infection. An epidural and dehydration are possible causes of a mild raised temperature. Cases at risk for infection (PPH, Caesarean section, manual removal of the placenta, amniotic fluid infections, prolonged rupture of membranes and urinary tract infections [UTIs]) usually receive prophylactic antibiotic treatment.

Fluctuations in the BP are common. Hypotension may be due to blood loss and lead to weakness and syncope. When a lower than normal BP for the mother is accompanied by a raised pulse (more than 90 bpm), look for uterine bleeding. Hypertension and eclampsia may develop within 72 hours without previous signs and symptoms.

Bladder function

The mother should pass urine within six hours after birth or after removal of the catheter. Make sure that the bladder is empty. Continued difficulty in passing urine is reported to the medical practitioner. Swelling or trauma of the vulva after vaginal birth may cause difficulty in passing urine.

After Caesarean section, epidural, surgical interventions or complications, a Foley catheter may be in place. Check that the urine is not bloodstained and be alert for possible UTIs. In these cases, the catheter should be removed after six hours unless there are complications.

Care of the uterus

The involution of the uterus is observed on a regular basis for the first 24 hours and daily thereafter if the uterus is well contracted and there is no evidence of active vaginal bleeding (see Figure 37.1).

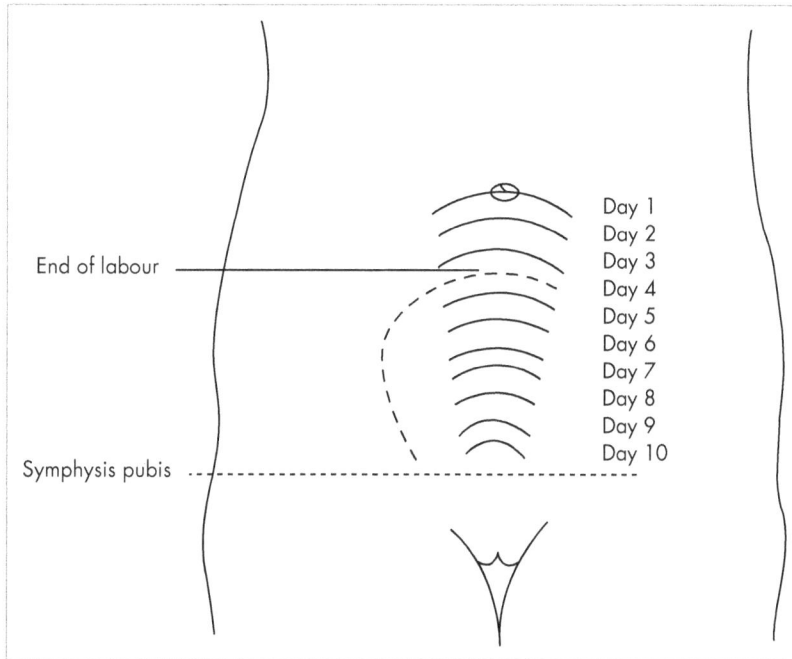

Figure 37.1 Involution of the uterus after delivery

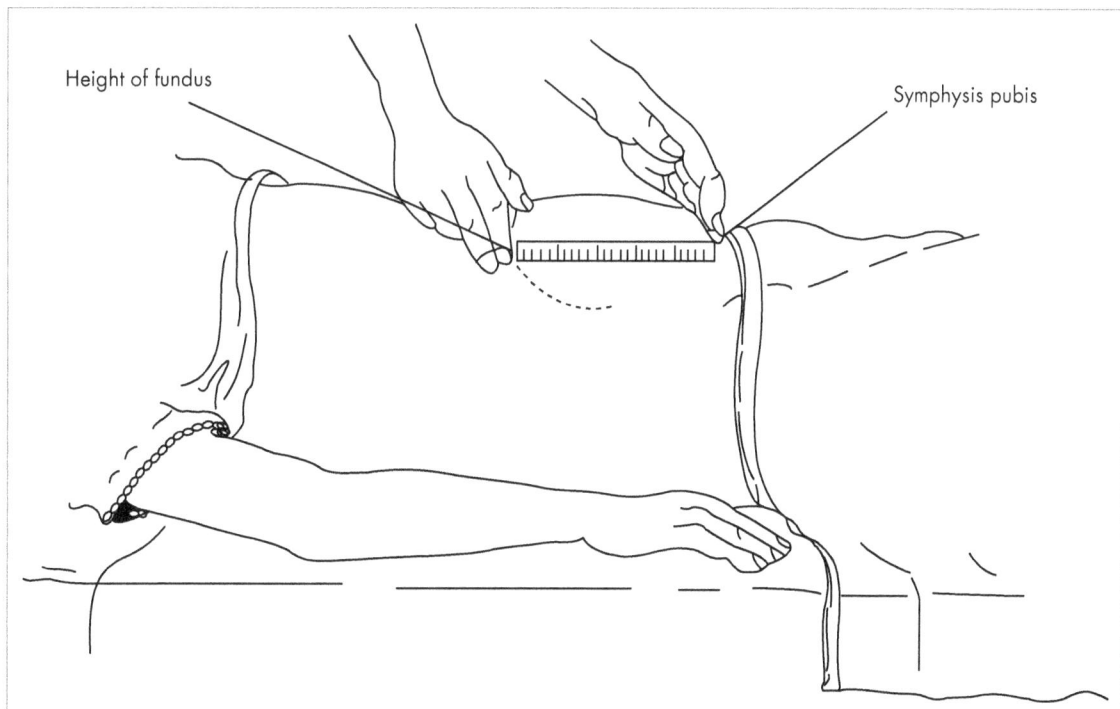

Figure 37.2 Measuring the height of the fundus in the puerperium

Sub-involution of the uterus after vaginal birth may be caused by an overstretched uterus (due to multiple pregnancy, polyhydramnios, multigravidity, abnormalities of the uterus such as bicornuate uterus or myomata, retained products of conception and infections). If a woman is discharged within a short period she may be asked to return on day 3 for assessment. The uterus involutes by 1.5–2.5 cm per day (see Figure 37.1).

Assess vaginal blood loss and Hb level (more than one soaked pad in 20 minutes is considered high blood loss).

The IV infusion and Foley or epidural catheter are removed according to medical prescription or the policies of the unit, based on the condition of the woman. After a Caesarean section, or if high-risk factors for haemorrhage are present, the woman will remain on an oxytocin infusion for 24 hours.

Cases at risk for haemorrhage are women who have undergone Caesarean section or manual removal of the products of conception and those with incomplete placenta and membranes, other pathological placental conditions or infections.

Monitoring the lochia

Check for offensive clots and the amount of lochia. The mother should be taught about changes to the lochia after birth. She should report any foul-smelling lochia, heavy lochia with fragments of placenta, clots, and red lochia after day 3, which suggests infection. Normal lochia is described in Chapter 36.

Breastfeeding

Encourage and promote breastfeeding. Mothers should be offered support to acquire the skills of correct positioning and latching of the baby to the breasts. Explain the required techniques and help the mother to be competent to breastfeed.

If a mother decides not to breastfeed after counselling and education, the necessary information about specific types of formula feed should be given. Start lactation suppression for those women before the hormonal initiation of lactation.

Evaluate the breasts to detect potential problems such as cracked nipples and engorged breasts in women who want to breastfeed. Interventions include cabbage leaves and breast emptying by regular suckling.

Care of the perineum and rectum

Assess the healing of the perineal wound, including swelling, oedema and bruising of the cervix and labia as well as perineal pain. Minimise discomfort in the perineum after vaginal birth. Ice packs may be used for the first 12 hours to reduce oedema and discomfort.

Self-care perineal hygiene should be maintained by changing pads as well as cleansing the perineum regularly to prevent infection in the vagina, which may track to the uterus. Saline Sitz baths with coarse salt twice a day are very effective in ambulant women, who can kneel in the bath or over a bidet to wash the perineum after each bowel movement. To minimise discomfort, the woman can use a ring pillow and should be instructed to tighten her buttocks before sitting. Analgesia can be prescribed.

Any sign of infection needs to be addressed before discharge. If there is severe pain after an episiotomy, the stitches may be removed after five days. Check for infection. A third-degree tear requires bed rest for three to four days and a special diet to soften stools.

Haemorrhoids

Women with a history of haemorrhoids in pregnancy may find that these are worse after a vaginal birth. Some women will develop haemorrhoids for the first time after birth. Treatment is prescribed by the medical practitioner. A ring pillow and laxative may be useful. In extreme cases, surgery may be needed.

Monitoring extremities

After normal delivery (no epidural), women are allowed to be ambulant as soon as possible. The first time the woman gets out of bed, a midwife should be present to make sure that the woman does not faint due to the cardiovascular changes.

Early ambulation after birth significantly reduces the incidence of thrombosis and is encouraged. Examine the calves daily to check for tenderness.

Thrombophlebitis

Women are prone to blood clotting problems post-delivery, specifically if there was trauma to the pelvic floor (forceps and ventouse) and legs (stirrups). The legs are examined daily for tenderness and swelling. The legs can be measured with a tape measure to determine the difference in the size of an affected leg. If thrombosis is suspected, the medical practitioner is informed.

Restoring gastrointestinal function

Immediately after birth, a woman may be nauseous and even vomit. Women are thirsty and often hungry after birth. After a Caesarean section, a woman is allowed to start with oral fluids and light meals as soon as she is hungry, depending on the type of anaesthesia. After general anaesthesia, this can start once bowel sounds are present.

A laxative or suppository is given on day 2–3 to stimulate bowel action and prevent constipation. A high-fibre diet and lots of fluid are given to stimulate peristalsis. If bowel action is not present by day 3–4, an enema may be given.

The mother needs a wholesome, well-balanced diet, rich in protein, with plenty of roughage. Fruit, salads and vegetables provide roughage and vitamins. Extra fluids, vitamin A and mineral supplements, particularly vitamin B and iron, may be given if the woman's general condition is poor.

Emotional well-being

Evaluate the mother's emotional well-being as well as that of her family and social support. Assess their usual coping strategies regarding day-to-day matters. Encourage the woman and her family or partner to mention any changes in mood, emotional state or behaviour that are different to the woman's normal pattern.

Counsel her about the symptoms of mild, transitory postpartum depression ('maternal blues' or 'baby blues') as well as postnatal depression. If symptoms persist, the woman should be evaluated.

Any risks, signs and symptoms of domestic abuse should be observed. Women should be advised to contact the midwife at the clinic and management should this occur.

Body image

Women often have body image concerns after birth. They may be disappointed that they cannot fit into their pre-pregnant clothes. However, breastfeeding women need to eat enough to support lactation and should be discouraged from dieting too stringently. A dietician should be consulted where necessary.

Postnatal exercises are encouraged. Pelvic floor or Kegel's exercises and Pilates are useful. Exercise helps to tone and strengthen the body, improve sleep patterns and lift mood.

Pain

The woman should be kept pain-free. Any pain needs to be assessed and monitored.

Pain is associated with after-pains (multigravidae), thrombosis, inflammation, Caesarean section, episiotomy and haematomas after birth. Occasionally, a woman may suffer from a complication after a spinal tap, causing severe headache. Pain may also be caused by retention of urine associated with trauma of the bladder or swelling of the labia and meatus. Perineal pain and/or bladder infection may occur as a result of catheterisation during labour and birth.

Pain relief starts in the theatre, with the first dosage administered. Post-operative women are offered pain relief for 48 hours. Analgesia is given regularly, according to a medical practitioner's prescription, and the woman's pain level is checked 15–20 minutes after the analgesic is given. If pain

relief is not effective, assess the reason and call the medical practitioner for a change in the regimen.

The mother's position can influence her experience of pain. Prevent stress on the wound by nursing in the Fowler's or semi-Fowler's position, using pillows to support the body, and make sure the woman is warm enough after returning from theatre. Women with catheters and IV lines are assisted with baby care and breastfeeding.

Prevention and care of previous and potential complications

Potential complications in the mother in the puerperium should be prevented.

Anaemia

Check for anaemia. Check the Hb immediately after labour, after three days and again at the six-week visit. After blood loss of more than 500–2 000 ml, check the Hb and haematocrit.

Oedema

Some women may have extensive oedema post-delivery in spite of diuresis. Rest and a normal diet should help this to resolve. Oedema in only one leg should be investigated. Do a Homans' test.

Rh blood factor

Check cord blood and do a Coomb's test within 72 hours in Rh-negative (Rh–) women. Anti-D or Rhogam must be given to the mother within 72 hours if the baby is Rh-positive (Rh+) and the Coomb's test is negative.

HIV status

A woman with an unknown HIV status is counselled before discharge for testing and referral (see Chapter 50).

IV and oral antibiotic therapy is given prophylactically for all HIV-positive women who have had surgical interventions, premature and prolonged rupture of membranes and previous infections in pregnancy, or antepartum haemorrhage (APH) or PPH. Any raised temperature post-delivery is assessed and antibiotic therapy started, if appropriate.

Caesarean section

A Caesarean section is a major surgical intervention. Assessment and specific care for a Caesarean mother includes the following:
▶ The mother and baby should not be separated, unless necessary according to the condition of one or the other.
▶ Check and follow the prescription of the medical practitioner and anaesthetist.

▶ Check the vital signs and pads half-hourly for two hours; then hourly for four hours; then two-hourly for six hours and thereafter four-hourly until discharged. Check temperature and urine output every four hours. If the heart rate is more than 100 bpm and respiration is more than 20, the patient is not discharged.

▶ The catheter is removed six hours after the Caesarean section.

▶ Start the mother with oral fluids and a light diet when she feels hungry.

Specific needs

Women with specific needs include adolescents, who may need special attention with infant and self-care. Older first-time mothers may also need support and individual care planning. Women with physical disabilities, sight and hearing impairments, psychiatric conditions, those who have adopted and surrogate mothers have specific needs and require support beyond the routine.

Women who were bedridden for long periods antenatally or those with multiple pregnancy, APH, cardiac conditions and diabetes mellitus have additional health and emotional needs and may experience pregnancy and birth negatively.

Teaching checklist

Ensure that the mother is instructed in:
▶ hygiene: perineal care and bathing, douching
▶ involution: lochia rate, amount, massage of uterus and after-pains
▶ exercise
▶ contraception
▶ nutrition
▶ how to handle her emotions: 'baby blues'
▶ the care of siblings
▶ self-care after discharge: sleep, rest, assistance and activity
▶ parent classes
▶ sexual activity
▶ bladder and bowel action
▶ immunisation
▶ infant feeding
▶ medication.

37.6   Discharge of mother and baby

The mother and baby should be informed and prepared for discharge to ensure a healthy family.

Preparation for discharge

During the post-delivery period, the whole family is continuously being prepared for discharge. This includes managing the baby's needs and educating the mother or parents on common problems and how to deal with these, including providing them with contact details for specific help. This is particularly important for first-time mothers and for women being discharged within 24 hours of birth.

Discharge within six hours after delivery

Discharge of the mother and baby after six hours depends on the following:

▶ There are no surgical, medical or obstetric problems needing attention.
▶ The mother feels well.
▶ The mother is not anaemic.
▶ The mother's vital signs are within the normal perimeters.
▶ The uterus is well contracted, soft and not tender.
▶ There is no active bleeding.
▶ The mother has passed urine.
▶ The mother is ambulant.
▶ There is no excessive pain in the abdomen and the perineum has been observed.
▶ Infant feeding has been explained and demonstrated and the mother has understood the principles.
▶ Information regarding the necessary support systems has been given.
▶ The mother has been informed about family planning, birth spacing and different contraception options and methods.
▶ The necessary blood results, eg Hb, Rh group, HIV and syphilis, have been discussed and appropriate actions taken.
▶ The mother has been informed about personal hygiene, particularly handwashing.

Common discharge problems

Some of the common problems that the mother may experience in the puerperium and the management of these are discussed below.

Tiredness

Many women feel tired after returning home with the newborn baby. This is mainly due to the demands of pregnancy and labour and to anxiety and concern for the new baby and for the family as a whole. The mother should get sufficient rest and sleep, specifically if she is breastfeeding, otherwise her milk supply may diminish and even dry up. The husband or partner can help the mother to get adequate rest and sleep. In addition, the woman should eat a good, balanced diet and she should get plenty of fresh air and take a walk each day.

Backache

Backache is usually experienced in the puerperium because the mother's joints, particularly the sacroiliac joints, remain pliant for some weeks after delivery. She should therefore be careful to lift the baby correctly and should be advised not to pick up heavy objects. She should not wear high heels for a few months after delivery or while the backache persists. She should conscientiously carry out her programme of postnatal exercises.

If the backache is severe or persists, she should see her medical practitioner or go to the local clinic. The medical practitioner may order a pelvic corset to be worn, in order to give support to the joints.

Dyspareunia

In most cases, sexual intercourse is painful after birth and the body should be given six weeks to recover. If pain persists, women are encouraged to discuss it with a medical practitioner. The mother should be counselled about safe sex and contraception.

Handling visitors

While visitors are likely to make the woman feel happy and wanted, they can also be very tiring. The mother should be assisted to 'manage' visitors. They should be asked to understand if the woman wishes to be excused either to feed the baby or to rest if she feels tired. Visitors should help relieve the burden of the mother and the family rather than add to it, but unfortunately people can sometimes be thoughtless and selfish.

Returning to work

A new mother should ideally not have to go out to work while the child is small, but should be free to stay at home to care for her infant. If the woman has to return to work, she must make adequate preparations for the care of the baby. If the mother has not made adequate arrangements by the time she needs to return to work, this will have an adverse effect on her psychologically and physically, which will in turn affect her relationship with the baby and with the rest of the family. The midwife should enquire about this at discharge, and if there are any problems, she should advise the woman on where she should seek help.

If the woman is working and the baby is established on bottle feeds, adequate feeds should be made up and refrigerated for the alternative caretaker to give to the baby. If the mother is breastfeeding, she can express and store enough breast milk for the alternative caretaker to give to the baby in a bottle while she is away.

Breastfeeding problems

Certain breastfeeding problems may arise later in pregnancy and the midwife should advise the woman and her family about these and tell them how to manage them.

Leaking breasts

The amount of milk that leaks from the breasts varies, from a few drops to a steady stream, any of which may be normal for a particular woman. The parents must be reassured that the condition is normal. It is usually when the breasts are full and the next feed is imminent, or actually during breastfeeding, that the greatest amount of leaking occurs. However, heat, such as on a hot day, or a hot bath or shower, may cause the breasts to leak. Other conditions that are likely to stimulate the milk supply are hearing the baby cry, playing with and loving the baby, watching the baby sleeping or even just thinking of him or her. Love expressed by the husband or partner or by the other children, or any stirring of enjoyable emotions can stimulate the 'let-down' of the milk.

If milk starts to leak, the woman should apply firm pressure to the leaking nipple with the heel of her hand, or if she is in company, she can inconspicuously cross her arms and apply pressure. If milk leaks from the nipple not being used during breastfeeding, the woman can place a thick towelling cloth beneath the nipple. If the milk streams from the other nipple during breastfeeding, the woman can place a container under the nipple and if the container is sterile, this milk could be retained, refrigerated and used within 24 hours, or frozen. It is important, however, to reassure the woman that leaking breasts are a normal occurrence.

The milk supply

The woman should be given written information on how to maintain her milk supply. She should also be given contact details of a support group in the community to assist when needed.

Breast and nipple care

If the woman is discharged early in the puerperium, she should be given some advice on how to care for full and engorged breasts and nipple care (see Chapter 39).

Anxiety

If the mother feels anxious and worries about how she is going to cope on her own, it can cause many problems. The woman who seems anxious and is not managing to cope well with baby care and feeding while under supervision should preferably not be discharged until she has gained confidence in herself and in her ability to care for her infant, or until suitable support is secured. Discharging a woman too early in these circumstances could lead to depression, poor interfamily relationships and, possibly, child abuse.

Every woman and her husband or partner should be told that if they are worried about how they are managing, or if they have any feelings that upset or frighten them, they should not hesitate to speak to their medical practitioner or to the midwife, or to go to the nearest health clinic, where arrangements will be made for someone with specialised knowledge to see them.

Infection

During labour and the puerperium, the woman is particularly susceptible to infections, because of the trauma that occurs during delivery and the open placental site after delivery. Consequently, the woman should be advised to be very careful with her personal hygiene, in order to prevent infection.

More serious problems

The parents must be advised to seek help immediately if there are any problems that are not resolved easily and quickly. In most instances, the longer a problem is left, the more serious it becomes.

The mother or parents must seek help immediately if they notice any signs and symptoms of:
- *postpartum bleeding:* sudden and large amounts of bleeding, an increased amount of blood loss, fainting, dizziness, palpitations or tachycardia
- *infections:* fever, shivering, abdominal pain or an offensive vaginal odour
- *pre-eclampsia or eclampsia:* headaches, visual disturbances, nausea, vomiting, epigastric pain or convulsions
- *thromboembolism:* unilateral calf pain, swelling or redness of the calves, chest pain or shortness of breath.

Guidelines for effective teaching

- Determine each woman's individual learning needs.
- Set priorities.
- Provide a comfortable environment.
- Allow the mother to absorb information, ask questions and review the information provided.
- Use simple terminology.
- Reinforce with visual aids or let the mother carry out care under supervision.
- Include the family and/or friends.
- Document all teaching.

Postnatal check-up

The postnatal check-up and an examination three to six days after delivery are important to:
- go over any concerns regarding the discharge notes
- check the vital signs
- check the contraction of the uterus
- examine the legs for thromboembolism
- check for vaginal bleeding
- check the breasts for possible problems
- assess the baby's condition
- counsel the mother about self-care problems.

The woman should attend a postnatal clinic at six weeks or see her medical practitioner specifically for any problems regarding the baby. However, it is stressed that if any problem should arise, particularly excessive or recurring bleeding, the woman should seek help immediately.

Baby care

The following aspects of baby care should be included in a discharge plan:
- *Physical care of the infant.* Show the mother – and the father, if he wishes – how to change a nappy, how to give the baby a bath and how to care for the umbilical cord. All this should be practised under supervision, particularly for a first baby.
- *Feeding the baby.* Breastfeeding should either be well established or a suitable alternative bottle-feeding regimen should be in place by discharge. Instruct the parents on how to prepare the feed, how to store the feed and how to clean the utensils, all of which should be practical and pertinent to their home and economic situation. It is no good instructing parents on how to care for the baby if, when they return home, they have neither the means nor the facilities to care for the baby in the manner shown to them while in hospital. (Written information is useful.)
- *Nappy rash.* Many babies get nappy rash. This can vary, from a mild, red, non-raised rash over the nappy area to a severe rash with bright red papules that erupt and form ulcers, which can become infected. The urine and faeces cause skin irritation and therefore the parents should be instructed to change the baby's nappy as soon as possible after the baby has passed urine or had a stool and not to leave the baby lying in a wet or soiled napkin. The baby will usually cry when the nappy is wet or soiled. Barrier creams can be used on the buttocks to protect the skin from the urine and to prevent the faeces from sticking to the skin.

▶ *The crying baby.* The parents should be reassured that it is good for the baby to cry, as this helps to expand the lungs and provides exercise for the baby. However, there is normal and abnormal crying. As the parents become used to the baby, they should be able to tell, to some extent, what the baby is trying to convey to them. If they are at all worried about the baby crying or not crying, they should speak to their medical practitioner, the midwife or the local health clinic midwives. Studying the Brazelton's scale will assist midwives to teach women about their baby's behaviour (see Chapter 10).

▶ *Constipation and unusual stools.* Constipation is seldom seen in the breastfed baby, unless the baby is being underfed. However, in the bottlefed baby, constipation may be problematic. It can usually be remedied by adjusting the feed – increasing the sugar and water content of the feed or giving extra water or pure fruit juice to the baby. Any very loose, watery or green stools, particularly if they are frequent and/or explosive, should be reported to a medical practitioner immediately, as they could be due to an alimentary tract infection.

▶ *Vomiting.* The woman and her husband or partner should be told about the differences between milk (which is regurgitated with winds), posseting and abnormal vomiting. Any infant with abnormal vomiting, with or without diarrhoea, should be seen by a medical practitioner immediately. Any vomiting that results in loss of weight should also be referred to a medical practitioner.

▶ *Infections.* Any infection of the newborn, with or without pyrexia, is serious, as the newborn has little resistance to infection. The infant should be seen by a medical practitioner as soon as possible.

▶ *Persistent jaundice.* Breast milk jaundice is a rare condition that occasionally affects breastfed babies. Some factor in the mother's milk prevents the baby's liver from functioning fully and this may prolong physiological jaundice in the newborn. Usually, no treatment is necessary. If jaundice persists or increases after discharge, the baby should be seen by a medical practitioner. The medical practitioner will screen the baby to ensure that the jaundice is not pathological. Pathological jaundice may be caused by obstruction of the hepatic ducts or infection, such as hepatitis or omphalitis.

The parents should be reminded that it is their responsibility to register the birth of the baby, and that this should be done within 30 days of the birth with the Registrar of Births, Department of Home Affairs, according to the Births and Deaths Registration Act 51 of 1992, as amended. Registration of a child within 30 days of birth is free of charge. Early registration helps the parents to access child support grants if the family qualifies. In some hospitals, facilities are provided for the registration of the birth immediately after the delivery.

Depending on the risks and problems, a mother is asked to bring her baby to the well-baby clinic. The '333 programme' of 3 days, 3 weeks and 3 months is followed if discharge took place within 24 hours of birth. A mother who remained in hospital longer is advised to take the baby to the nearest baby clinic at her earliest convenience (but not later than three weeks postpartum) or if she is at all anxious about the baby's condition.

Children under the age of 5 must be immunised against common childhood diseases in South Africa. No child should leave the hospital without the immunisation programme being started and explained to the mother. The parents are given an immunisation card and each vaccine is recorded on the card and in the hospital or satellite clinic records. This card is taken to the baby clinic by the mother at each visit and all further immunisations are recorded on the card.

Maternal help and support

The parents are advised to have some sort of help and support for the mother after discharge. The father or partner can be of great assistance in this early postpartum period. He should be aware of this and should look for ways in which he can help. If the couple do not have domestic help and if the father or partner is unable to be at home to help, then arrangements should be made for either a member of the family or a friend to give the woman support and help in the first few weeks after delivery. This is particularly necessary after the birth of a first baby, if the woman has a heavy home work load (two or more children at home in addition to the new baby) or if the woman is physically or mentally debilitated in any way. Refer to community support or support in the form of online forums, articles, and so on (see Chapter 19).

37.7 Discharge practices in the public and private sector

In the public sector, mothers and babies are generally discharged as soon as possible. After a normal birth, women may leave the healthcare setting within six to 24 hours. This may place new mothers at a disadvantage, because of the lack of support in the community and from healthcare services.

In the private sector, mothers and babies are normally discharged two days after a normal birth and three to four days after a Caesarean section. If a woman experiences complications or the baby has problems, the one may be discharged without the other. Women in the private sector have usually arranged a postnatal follow-up.

In the public sector, women are followed up using the '333 strategy': on day 3, week 3 and month 3 they return to see a midwife or medical practitioner. They are then referred to a specialist clinic if necessary.

37.8   Conclusion

The postnatal period is an exciting time, and the midwife's contact with the mother or couple may be short. The midwife must be skilled to determine the specific needs of the mother and baby, give the best possible care in the time available and, finally, refer the woman to a support system.

38

Complications of the puerperium

LEARNING OBJECTIVES
On completion of this chapter, you must be able to:
▶ demonstrate the knowledge, competency and skill to identify possible postpartum complications
▶ plan and give appropriate nursing care interventions (preventive, curative and emergency) to meet the needs of women with complications postpartum in all healthcare settings
▶ evaluate a woman's understanding of the complications she should report and her ability to manage the condition herself
▶ prevent further complications.

KNOWLEDGE ASSUMED TO BE IN PLACE
The anatomical, physiological and psychological adaptations of the normal puerperium (see Chapter 36)

KEYWORDS
secondary postpartum haemorrhage (PPH) • puerperal infection • stress urinary incontinence (SUI) • incontinence severity index (ISI) • vesicovaginal fistula • rectovaginal fistula • acute urine retention • thromboembolic disease • puerperal sepsis

38.1 Introduction

Complications of the postnatal period range from mild to moderate to severe. The two most common complications of the postnatal period that are life-threatening are haemorrhage and puerperal sepsis.

The risk of maternal death is highest in the first 24 hours postpartum. The main cause is primary postpartum haemorrhage (PPH) (see chapters 22, 33 and 35). This chapter will consider the risk of secondary PPH, urinary tract infections (UTIs) and problems such as thrombosis and pelvic floor complications.

38.2 Secondary postpartum haemorrhage

Secondary PPH is bleeding from the genital tract that occurs any time after the first 24 hours up to six weeks after birth.

Causes

Secondary PPH can be caused by:
▶ retained products of conception, such as cotyledon and fragments; these may become necrotic, resulting in the formation of a polyp
▶ bleeding from the site
▶ tearing of the uterus
▶ poor coagulation of blood
▶ wound breakdown or haematomas
▶ abnormal involution of the placental site.

Predisposing conditions

A woman may be predisposed to secondary PPH by:
▶ antepartum haemorrhage (APH) (placenta praevia, placenta abruptio)
▶ anaemia
▶ obesity
▶ being older than 40 years
▶ being of Asian ethnicity

- primary PPH
- chorioamnionitis
- atony of the uterus; clots may accumulate in the uterus if there is atony of the uterine muscle. The clots formed at the placental site after delivery, which controlled the bleeding from maternal blood vessels and sinuses (between the living ligatures), may become dislodged or dissolve. This may be a result of oxytocin treatment which is not followed up
- pieces of placenta and/or membrane which prevent the uterine muscles from contracting and retracting fully, causing sub-involution of the uterus. Any of the retained products, especially if there has been interference during labour, eg Caesarean section or an episiotomy, could become septic and cause a breakdown in the healing of the placental site, resulting in a large haemorrhage and endo- or myometritis
- any trauma to the genital tract, which the patient may have sustained during delivery; the site could become septic, break down and bleed
- fibroids, carcinoma of the cervix and choriocarcinoma (a rare condition); the latter may manifest towards the end of the puerperium and is known as gestational trophoblastic disease
- abnormalities of the uterus, such as a bicornuate uterus, which may lead to shedding of the decidua (endometrium) that was thickened in pregnancy into the uterine sections that were not used during pregnancy. This usually occurs around 14–21 days postpartum.

Incidence

The incidence of secondary PPH ranges from 0.5 to 1.5 per cent of all vaginal deliveries (Belfort, 2017) and will depend on the standard of care given to the woman before, during and immediately after delivery, and on the length of time the patient spent in hospital after delivery. In midwife obstetrics units (MOUs) with post-delivery services, patients are observed for signs of sub-involution of the uterus and heavy vaginal loss, especially if the placenta and the membranes were ragged and possibly not complete, or if the patient had any conditions predisposing her to PPH.

The early warning signs of possible secondary PPH may be missed with early discharge of the woman. The incidence will be higher in women who live far from obstetric healthcare centres; the maternal mortality rate will also increase accordingly.

Clinical diagnostic signs and symptoms

History is taken, with an emphasis on early warning signs of the risk factors, which include:

- predisposing causes (as listed above)
- a previous history of PPH
- a history of complications of the second and third stage of labour (manipulations, forceps delivery and other interference in this pregnancy)
- placental pathology such as placenta accreta, retained placenta or incomplete placenta and/or ragged membranes after the third stage of labour (retained cotyledon, succenturiate lobe or part of the chorionic membrane).

Early warning signs and symptoms include:

- sub-involution of the uterus
- persistent red vaginal loss
- heavy vaginal loss
- vaginal loss with an offensive smell
- the passing of clots and/or pieces of placenta and/or membrane with the vaginal loss
- severe uterine contractions and after-pains
- uterine tenderness on rubbing up of the fundus
- puerperal pyrexia (infection)
- signs of hypovolaemic shock.

Vaginal blood loss occurs between the fourth to fifteenth day post-delivery and can, at first, be small amounts on successive days (rather like a menstrual period) or can be a sudden deluge of blood. Haemorrhage can be so severe that the patient may die before treatment is available.

Care and management

Preventative measures include the following actions:

- After birth, examine the placenta and membranes under running water, even after Caesarean section and manual removal of the placenta.
- Report any potential defects in the placenta and membranes.
- The uterus must remain well contracted to control haemorrhage. The uterus is stimulated to remain contracted by rubbing it abdominally or placing the baby to the breast. The woman is observed for 12–24 hours post-delivery to make sure that the uterus is well contracted.
- The bladder must be empty at birth and must remain empty for two to six hours after birth and regularly in the postnatal period.

▶ After Caesarean section, after manual removal of the placenta, with atony of the uterus (if the uterus tends to relax), in the case of an overstretched uterus (due to polyhydramnios, multiple pregnancy and grand multiparity) or after APH and PPH, give an IV infusion of 20 U oxytocin in 1 ℓ Ringer's lactate at 120 ml per hour for 24 hours, or misoprostol, until stable.

▶ The amount, colour and consistency of the vaginal blood loss is assessed two-hourly. More than one soaked pad every 20 minutes is considered heavy blood loss and needs to be followed up. Blood clots in the lochia are abnormal. Painful uterine contractions are also abnormal.

On discharge, check for:
▶ any history of placental pathology (Was the placenta complete?)
▶ painful uterine contractions
▶ continuous red lochia.

District midwifery post-delivery services in outlying areas should be set up for the early detection of warning signs of secondary PPH and for admitting patients to a clinic or hospital for immediate treatment.

Specific nursing care and interventions

The midwife must keep calm and start treatment similar to the management of primary atonic PPH (see Chapter 22):
▶ Take a brief history of possible causes.
▶ Call for assistance urgently (if in hospital, call for a medical practitioner; if in a clinic, stabilise the woman and refer).
▶ Assess the physical well-being and status of the woman (temperature, pulse, respiration rate, BP, consciousness, colour, full blood count [FBC] and cross-match, Hb and haematocrit).
▶ The main aim of care is to stop haemorrhage by stimulating the uterus to expel clots and induce uterine contractions.
▶ Give a single dose of oxytocin 10 U IM. Insert an IV line, giving 20 IU oxytocin into a second line of Ringer's lactate at 125 ml/hour.
▶ Give an IM injection of ergometrine 0.5 mg or syntometrine 1 amp to contract the uterus. Alternatively, administer misoprostol 600 μg rectally or orally to contract the uterus.
▶ If the bleeding continues, the midwife must do bimanual compression of the uterus and continue with this until a medical practitioner is available.
▶ Pain relief is administered as per the medical practitioner's prescription.

▶ If the woman is compromised or hypovolaemic, emergency intervention, as presented in Chapter 35, becomes applicable.
▶ If the woman is in hypovolaemic shock, lift the foot of the bed, give oxygen and start fluid resuscitation.
▶ Insert a urinary catheter.
▶ The woman must be transferred to a Level 2 or 3 hospital for further management, accompanied by a midwife or medical practitioner until stabilised.

Obstetric management

If the bleeding is moderate – or, in the case of more severe bleeding, after the woman is stable – the medical practitioner will make a diagnosis using ultrasound. The most common cause is retained products of conception and interstitial endometritis. Sub-involution with an open cervix is diagnostic.

Potential further intervention depends on the cause and clinical picture and may include any of the following:
▶ Exploration and possible curettage may be performed in theatre if bleeding continues, if there are retained products of conception or if a laceration needs to be debrided and sutured. A specimen of the products of conception is sent to a laboratory to exclude choriocarcinoma. If the bleeding is severe, a hysterectomy may be done.
▶ If the bleeding has been moderate to severe, or if the patient shows signs of shock, the medical practitioner may give the patient a blood transfusion.
▶ In case of infection, IV antibiotic therapy is given and the discharge sent for culture and sensitivity.
▶ The woman is on bed rest and remains on an IV infusion until the results are back from the laboratory.

Specific nursing care after stabilisation

▶ The baby is admitted as a lodger and can continue to be breastfed.
▶ The patient is kept in hospital until there is no further bleeding.
▶ Routine care includes vital signs, four-hourly temperature, Hb and bed rest.
▶ On discharge, the patient is told to see the medical practitioner or attend a clinic in two weeks' time (or immediately if there is any further bleeding).

Complications

▶ Lactation may cease if hypovolaemic shock occurred.
▶ Hypovolaemia may cause necrosis of the pituitary gland, leading to Sheehan's syndrome.
▶ Diarrhoea may result in the breastfed baby if misoprostol is given.

- Asherman's syndrome (adhesions within the uterus) may be caused by dilatation and curettage if too much endometrium is removed.
- Perforation of the uterus can occur, because the gravid uterus is soft and can easily be perforated.
- Puerperal infections, peritonitis or septic shock may occur.
- A hysterectomy may be necessary if bleeding cannot be controlled.
- Maternal death may occur.

38.3   Infections

Puerperal sepsis

Puerperal sepsis is an infection of the female reproductive tract after birth in the first 2–10 days postpartum (excluding the first 24 hours). It is indicated by a temperature of 38 °C or more, chills, lower abdominal pain and, possibly, bad-smelling vaginal discharge for at least two days of the first 14 days post-delivery (see Chapter 49). This condition may be life-threatening.

A differential diagnosis is based on the following:
- If amnionitis was present prior to delivery, an infection may occur within 24 hours.
- Endomyometritis may present, without a fever.
- Breast infections may present, with a fever.
- There may be other causes, such as UTI.

Causes

Puerperal sepsis is usually caused by:
- *Streptococcus haemolyticus, Streptococcus faecalis, Streptococcus pyogenes or Staphylococcus aureus*, which lead to septicaemia
- anaerobic *Streptococcus* species, causing thrombophlebitis
- *Escherichia coli*, leading to local infection of the uterus
- *Clostridium welchii*, occurring after septic abortion where there is damage to tissues.

Organisms that are rarely involved are *Gonococcus, Pneumococcus, Pseudomonas* and *Proteus*.

The organisms gain entry from the placental site due to the loss of the epithelial cover at the placental site, from retained products of conception, which serve as a site for infection, and/or from trauma, for example bruising and/or lacerations of the genital tract.

The mode of spread can be as follows:
- Exogenous spread occurs through contamination as a result of poor hygiene of attendants, poor ward cleaning and dirty bed linen.
- Endogenous spread occurs from organisms already present in the vagina that gain entry through torn, bruised and necrotic tissue.
- Autogenous spread occurs from the patient via organisms present in the respiratory tract, skin or any other septic focus.

Predisposing conditions

The woman may have lowered immunity as a result of diabetes mellitus, anaemia, malnutrition, debility from exhaustion or from haemorrhage. The presence of infections such as HIV will also predispose her to infection.

The following are some of the risk factors with regard to the postpartum day (PPD) on which the condition generally occurs:
- *On day 1.* Atelectasis risk factors: general anaesthesia, cigarette smoking and obstructive lung disease
- *Between days 1 and 2.* UTI as a result of multiple catheterisation during labour; interference, such as too many vaginal examinations; untreated local infections
- *Between days 2 and 3.* Endometritis (the most common cause), prolonged rupture of the membranes, prolonged labour, multiple vaginal examinations during labour, bruising, lacerations, vulval oedema, manual removal of the placenta, internal versions, Caesarean section and instrument deliveries
- *Between days 4 and 5.* Wound infection risk factors: emergency Caesarean section, prolonged labour, multiple vaginal examinations during labour and prolonged rupture of membranes
- *Between days 5 and 6.* Septic pelvic thrombophlebitis risk factors: emergency Caesarean section, prolonged membrane rupture, prolonged labour, diffuse difficult vaginal childbirth, retained products of conception or an untreated local infection
- *Between days 7 and 21.* Mastitis risk factors: nipple trauma from breastfeeding.

Pathology

Local infection includes the genital tract, but widespread infection leads to:
- cervicitis
- endometritis
- myometritis
- parametritis
- salpingitis
- peritonitis
- septicaemia
- thrombophlebitis
- breast infections.

Infection of the perineum, vulva and cervix

The causal organism is *Staphylococcus aureus*.

Clinical features

▶ Tachycardia – on the third day
▶ Hyperpyrexia – on the third day
▶ Redness
▶ Tenderness, discomfort and pain
▶ Swelling of the vulva and perineum
▶ Sloughing of the tissues.

Signs and symptoms usually include a fever greater than 38 °C (100.4 °F), chills, lower abdominal pain and, possibly, a bad-smelling vaginal discharge.

Vaginal loss may initially be normal, but if the infection spreads upwards to the uterus, then the vaginal loss will become brownish and offensive.

Endometritis

Endometritis is an infection of the endometrium.

Clinical features

▶ Moderate hyperpyrexia
▶ Tachycardia
▶ Profuse, offensive vaginal discharge
▶ Possible presence of products of conception
▶ A uterus that is tender, soft and bulky
▶ Sub-involution of the uterus with minimal abdominal findings
▶ General signs of malaise
▶ Headache
▶ Anorexia.

Parametritis and pelvic cellulitis

This is an infection of the parametrium and the pelvis.

Clinical features

▶ Hyperpyrexia
▶ Tachycardia
▶ Profuse, offensive vaginal loss
▶ Sub-involution of the uterus.

As the infection spreads to the surrounding tissues, the patient may complain of:
▶ lower abdominal pain
▶ vomiting
▶ general malaise.

Salpingitis

This is an infection that involves the Fallopian tubes.

Clinical features

▶ Lower backache
▶ Lower abdominal pain
▶ Hyperpyrexia
▶ Tachycardia.

Peritonitis

In this condition, the infection has reached the pelvic cavity and involves the peritoneum.

Clinical features

▶ Tachycardia of more than 120 bpm
▶ Rigors
▶ Hyperpyrexia (fifth to seventh day)
▶ Distended, painful and rigid abdomen causing lower abdominal pain with rebound tenderness
▶ Persistent effortless vomiting, dark in colour
▶ Diarrhoea
▶ Restlessness, apprehension
▶ Paralytic ileus with abdominal distention and lack of bowel sounds.

Septicaemia

This is a generalised bloodstream infection that develops from the lower genital tract. With septicaemia the infection has become puerperal sepsis, discussed in chapters 35 and 49.

Management and prevention of puerperal sepsis

The prevention of infections in the postnatal period starts in the antenatal period. Women are educated during antenatal care. Universal infection control must be practised during the intrapartum and postpartum periods.

During pregnancy

Good antenatal care is required during pregnancy:
▶ Provide health education regarding personal hygiene as a life-change attitude, sanitation and hygienic conditions in the home.
▶ Treat any infection and any minor disorders of pregnancy.
▶ Give the woman adequate instructions regarding diet and nutrition and ensure the woman has an adequate intake of vitamins while pregnant.
▶ Treat any diseases in pregnancy, such as TB, diabetes, anaemia and so on.

▶ Prevent and treat any complications in pregnancy, especially haemorrhage.
▶ Offer advice regarding sleep, exercise, adequate rest, etc.

During labour

▶ Aseptic technique must be followed for all procedures.
▶ Reduce the number of unnecessary vaginal examinations.
▶ Recognise and treat complications.
▶ Screen all staff for infection.
▶ Limit traffic through the labour ward.
▶ Prevent prolonged and/or obstructed labour.
▶ Give women who need a Caesarean section a preventive dose of antibiotics.

During the puerperium

▶ Isolate patients who are contagious.
▶ Provide quality care that allows for adequate staffing, prompt observation, accurate recording of vital signs and treatment of complications.
▶ Update staff and do skill drills.
▶ Display posters of the major complications and interventions to keep staff updated so that they are able to manage common and rare complications of the postnatal period.
▶ Ensure a caring environment.

Management of mild to moderate conditions

In mild and moderate conditions, retained products should be excluded. If the products are retained, uterine evacuation should be done. In addition, do the following:
▶ Encourage the woman to take in an adequate amount of oral fluids.
▶ Give an oral antibiotic.
▶ Follow up for reassessment and if there is no improvement, transfer to a higher level of care.
▶ Give analgesics, iron, multivitamins, laxatives and sedatives, as prescribed.
▶ Give oxygen if necessary.

Do a septic work-up, including a high vaginal swab, a nose or throat swab, blood cultures, a midstream urine specimen and a wound swab if needed, or a milk specimen from the breast. In some cases, throat swabs from the nursing staff may be required by infection control.

Special examinations may be requested for typhoid, malaria, viral hepatitis, appendicitis and HIV.

Managing severe conditions

▶ Take a full history of pregnancy and delivery as well as a full physical examination.

▶ Pay special attention to the woman's consciousness, temperature, heart rate, respiratory rate, colour, chest, abdomen and the findings of the vaginal examination.
▶ Be aware of signs of septic shock.
▶ Evaluate organ systems (cerebral, cardiovascular, respiratory, liver and kidney).
▶ Give IV antibiotics – broad spectrum initially and then according to culture and sensitivity results – and oxytocin according to the medical practitioner's prescription for persistent wide fever swings despite antibiotics (Wikipedia, 2017).
▶ Do an FBC and blood transfusion if necessary.
▶ Provide management of IV heparin for 7–10 days at rates sufficient to prolong the partial thromboplastin time (PTT) to double the baseline values.
▶ Take vital signs and symptoms half-hourly in severe cases.
▶ Give IV therapy for hydration for 24–48 hours in severe cases if the woman is nil per mouth and nauseous.
▶ Evaluate the organ systems for possible failures.
▶ Encourage pulmonary (deep breathing) exercises and ambulation (walking).
▶ Note any UTI, indicated by high temperature, malaise and costovertebral tenderness. A positive urine culture requires antibiotics as per culture sensitivity.
▶ Management for wound infections is antibiotics for cellulitis. Thereafter, open and drain the wound and give saline-soaked packing twice a day, with secondary closure.
▶ Manage mastitis (unilateral, localised erythema, oedema and tenderness) with antibiotics.

Complications

▶ Infertility
▶ Hysterectomy
▶ Abscesses
▶ Poor wound healing or secondary suturing
▶ Fistulas
▶ Death.

38.4   Thromboembolic disease

Thromboembolic disease can occur in pregnancy, but is more common in the puerperium.

There are two main types of thrombosis:
1. *Superficial thrombosis* is the most common form of thrombosis. It is called thrombophlebitis, a condition in which a thrombus is formed in a varicose vein with inflammation of the vein wall due to a primary infection.
2. *Deep vein thrombosis* (DVT) is a less common but more serious condition in which there is an obstruction of a

vein by a blood clot without preceding inflammation of its wall. Minor damage of the vessels in labour is aggravated by circulatory stasis and sepsis, which can cause clotting. It can include veins in the pelvis. A pulmonary thrombosis can occur as a result of a whole clot or a part of a large clot entering the cardiovascular system and obstructing the pulmonary circulation. This will cause chest pain, dyspnoea and shock and can end in maternal death.

Incidence

Thromboembolic disease occurs in 0.01 to 0.02 per cent of pregnancies (Pettker & Lockwood, 2008). Many thromboembolic diseases occur in the antenatal period, but the risks are much higher during the postpartum period.

In cases where DVT is not treated, the woman will develop pulmonary embolism in 25 per cent of cases and the mortality rate is 15 per cent (Pettker & Lockwood, 2008).

Risk factors for thromboembolism in the puerperium

The physiological risk for a thrombosis is increased after birth due to the following:

▶ High progesterone levels in pregnancy cause relaxation of the smooth muscles, resulting in stasis of blood and slow venous return in the lower limbs with uterine compression of the inferior vena cava. If varicose veins are already present, they will predispose the woman to stasis. Thus the likelihood of clot formation, hypercoagulation and vascular trauma during pregnancy is increased.

▶ Changes in the blood persist in the puerperium. The increase in the number of platelets that tend to clump together more readily, especially after tissue trauma, as well as an increase in the prothrombin levels, which peak on days 10–12 post-delivery, increase the risk for thrombosis. Several clotting factors, for example fibrinogen and factors VII, VIII, IX and X, also increase the clotting tendency after birth.

A history of previous thromboembolism is a risk factor, and re-occurrence is about 12 per cent (Pettker & Lockwood, 2008). If thromboembolism is present in this pregnancy, the risk of complications is increased and the woman would be on anticlotting treatment.

Other factors that may contribute include:

▶ obesity or forced immobilisation in cases of bedrest over a long time in the antenatal period, epidural in labour and/or following Caesarean section. Patients tend to fear

movement because of pain, which will in fact be reduced by movement

▶ use of the combined oral contraceptive (COC) pill before becoming pregnant

▶ therapy to suppress lactation

▶ heavy smoking

▶ testing positive for lupus anticoagulant

▶ hereditary conditions (eg antithrombin III deficiency)

▶ increasing age; women over 35 are five times more likely to develop thromboembolism than are younger women

▶ any pre-existing inflammatory process

▶ group A blood type

▶ medical conditions such as cardiac disease, diabetes mellitus and anaemia, in particular sickle-cell anaemia syndromes.

Other obstetric factors which may make women more prone to thromboembolism are:

▶ dehydration after prolonged labour

▶ assisted delivery

▶ surgical interventions such as Caesarean section

▶ trauma to the legs as a result of prolonged time spent in the lithotomy position.

General prevention of thromboembolic disease

During pregnancy

The risk of thrombosis is assessed during pregnancy. General prevention measures include the following:

▶ Anaemia is identified and treated with prophylactic oral iron, vitamin A and folic acid. If anaemia persists, the woman is referred to a medical practitioner.

▶ Infections are identified and are prevented or treated immediately.

▶ A pregnant woman must avoid stasis of blood in the legs as a result of long periods of standing or sitting, for example when working with computers for long periods. She should avoid sitting on her legs and also crossing one leg over the other while sitting. This will help to prevent pressure on the veins.

▶ The woman should be encouraged to seek additional advice from a physiotherapist or attend antenatal classes and exercises.

▶ Dieting should be avoided, as weight loss causes ketosis. However, obese women should be helped to control their weight.

▶ A woman with a history of thrombosis or who has had thrombosis in a previous or current pregnancy may require prophylactic anticoagulant therapy during pregnancy and for six weeks after delivery. This woman will be under medical supervision. Regular clotting profiles must be done if this medication is given. The patient will require health education, supervision in hospital and adequate supervision and control once discharged.

▶ The woman's legs are examined during each antenatal visit. Any complaint of leg pain and tenderness must be treated as very serious and the patient must immediately be referred to the medical practitioner.

During labour

Prevention measures include the following points:

▶ Exhaustion, dehydration and haemorrhage must be avoided. IV therapy must be given and the hydration of the patient maintained throughout labour, particularly if labour is prolonged or complicated.

▶ Aortocaval compression (inferior vena cava syndrome [IVCS], which reduces cardiac output) or the supine hypotensive syndrome (preventing venous return to the heart and causing pooling and stasis of blood in the lower limbs) must be avoided.

▶ Over-distension of the bladder must be avoided, because an enlarged bladder, together with the enlarged uterus, can cause pressure on the iliofemoral venous segments.

▶ Avoid trauma to the limbs when moving or transporting an unconscious patient or a patient under epidural analgesia.

▶ Avoid prolonging the use of the lithotomy position, which causes pressure and stasis of blood in the legs. The correct use of the lithotomy position requires two people to lift the legs simultaneously and place them correctly inside and not outside the poles.

In the puerperium

General measures include:

▶ avoiding anaemia
▶ preventing dehydration
▶ encouraging early ambulation from two to four hours after normal delivery, if possible. If this is not possible, the midwife or physiotherapist should teach the woman leg movements and encourage her to do them every two hours. In post-epidural and post-Caesarean section patients, ambulation starts as soon as possible and within 24 hours
▶ encouraging physiotherapy and deep breathing exercises, which facilitate venous flow.

Women who are at risk for thrombosis or who develop symptoms that present in the puerperium:

▶ are prescribed anti-embolism stockings at all times during the day and night, which will limit the pooling and stasis of blood in the legs
▶ will receive anticoagulation therapy as prescribed (regular medical supervision is necessary).

Oestrogen-containing lactation suppressants or contraception are avoided postpartum.

Superficial thrombophlebitis

Thrombophlebitis of the superficial veins occurs in about 1 per cent of patients (Pettker & Lockwood, 2008).

Clinical features

The condition may be asymptomatic, with a low-grade temperature. The clinical features include:

▶ redness over the affected area, with distended superficial veins (phlebitis)
▶ calf and leg vein tenderness
▶ hotness in the limb
▶ slight oedema of the leg
▶ mild tachycardia
▶ tingling in the legs
▶ a positive Homans' sign – a sharp dorsiflexion of the foot by the examiner will cause pain behind the knee or in the calf or affected area.

Medical management

▶ Diagnosis is confirmed by the clinical picture, sensitivity over the affected area and ultrasound or Doppler studies.
▶ The foot of the bed is elevated to reduce swelling. The leg circumference may be measured.
▶ Specific anti-embolism stockings for the affected leg are provided.
▶ Analgesics are prescribed.

Midwifery management

▶ Initially, the patient is nursed in bed.
▶ The foot of the bed is elevated, as well as the affected limb.
▶ Deep breathing exercises are encouraged.
▶ Encourage full activity as soon as possible, with good leg exercises.
▶ Analgesics are given as prescribed.
▶ The patient is given a bed cradle to support the bed clothes and keep the pressure off the affected limb.

▶ Local anti-inflammatories are sometimes used, such as an anti-inflammatory gel, which can be applied to the affected area.

▶ Give health education on the use of the medication and its side effects.

Deep vein thrombosis

DVT is suspected when there is pain on movement of the limb, accompanied by oedema. It occurs 7–10 days after delivery. The incidence varies greatly, from about 0.3–12 women in every 1 000 deliveries (Pettker & Lockwood, 2008). There is a 12 per cent increase in the incidence among women who have had previous DVT postpartum, with an increased risk of pulmonary thrombosis (Pettker & Lockwood, 2008).

A condition known as phlegmasia alba dolens (or milk-white leg) is associated with ileofemoral thrombosis, and clots may occur in the pelvis, the thigh and the calf.

Woman at risk for DVT will be on Clexane® injections prophylactically.

Clinical features

▶ Pain and discomfort of the leg that restricts movement; inability to walk due to spasms and pain

▶ Positive Homans' sign with severe pain

▶ Increased pulse and raised temperature

▶ Exaggerated oedema (a late sign): an increase in the leg girth measurement by as much as 2.5–5 cm

▶ Tenderness in the groin

▶ A leg that feels heavy and painful.

Diagnosis

It is important to correctly diagnose DVT. The clinical signs are not a good guide to the diagnosis and do not give any indication as to whether the clot is stationary, lysing (dissolving) or progressing (enlarging). It must be remembered that it is possible for the clinical signs to be absent. Therefore, investigations must be carried out routinely.

Investigations

▶ *Doppler ultrasound* is used to detect the blood flow through the underlying vein. It is a primary means of differentiating leg thrombosis from normal blood flow. Normal blood flow is characterised by a low-pitched surging sound in the vein.

▶ *Ultrasound* will show the clot and the lack of venous expansion of the affected vein.

▶ *A lung scan (scintigram)* may be required if there is a suspicion of pulmonary embolism.

▶ *Impedance plethysmography* is a method of measuring blood volume changes in the lower calf. The changes are produced by inflation and deflation of a pneumatic thigh cuff. Blood flow changes decrease in patients with thrombi.

▶ The *venogram* is still used in some centres where no other diagnostic means are available.

Medical management

The aim of treatment is to relieve pain and to prevent both extensive thrombi and pulmonary embolism. Curative treatments include:

▶ anticoagulant therapy

▶ heparin

▶ warfarin (not used in pregnancy)

▶ analgesia for pain

▶ IV fluid therapy

▶ pulmonary embolectomy (may be required)

▶ surgery (thrombectomy) (may be necessary in severe cases).

Heparin is given initially in the first 48 hours. It is given intravenously in a saline drip and thereafter subcutaneously. This is followed by oral warfarin for three to six months after birth. The anticoagulant medication is given according to the daily blood prothrombin index.

The advantages of heparin (dosages of which should be determined by the medical practitioner) in pregnancy are the following:

▶ It does not cross the placenta during pregnancy.

▶ It does not enter breast milk.

▶ It can be continued at home.

▶ It has a short life span and disappears from the circulation in six hours.

▶ It gives pain relief.

▶ It is rapidly reversed with protamine sulphate.

The disadvantages of heparin are that it is not easy to control the degree of coagulability and it is very expensive.

The side effects of heparin are:

▶ preterm labour

▶ fetal loss

▶ bleeding tendencies

▶ osteoporosis (long-term use)

▶ thrombocytopaenia.

Warfarin is not used during pregnancy, because it causes congenital defects in the fetus, such as:

▶ optic atrophy

▶ chondrodystrophy

▶ mental retardation
▶ neonatal haemorrhage
▶ nasal septal defects.

The following advice should be given to the patient on anticoagulant therapy:
▶ Report any bleeding immediately.
▶ Avoid trauma while on treatment.
▶ Wear a 'Medic Alert' bracelet at all times.
▶ Avoid salicylates, as they potentiate the effect of the anticoagulants.
▶ Warn the medical practitioner and nursing staff if you are on anticoagulant treatment.
▶ Avoid amniocentesis and epidural analgesia.
▶ Report regularly for prothrombin index or international normalised ratio (INR).
▶ Avoid fish oil supplements.

Midwifery care

▶ Bed rest, with the foot of the bed elevated
▶ Support for the affected limb
▶ A bed cradle to support the bedclothes
▶ Analgesia for pain, as prescribed
▶ Psychological support, reassurance and encouragement
▶ Physiotherapy and exercises – when the patient is able to do them – according to the medical practitioner's orders
▶ Anti-embolism stockings and medication.

The use of oestrogen for contraception is contraindicated. If the family is completed, a vasectomy or a tubal ligation is a possibility, as is an intrauterine contraceptive device (IUCD). Depo-provera or Nuristerate are suitable contraceptives.

Complications of deep vein thrombosis

Pulmonary embolism is the most common acute complication and may result in death.

Pulmonary embolism associated with deep vein thrombosis

This is a condition that can have a silent onset, with catastrophic consequences. It is a common cause of maternal death. Warning signs include:
▶ unexplained pyrexia
▶ syncope
▶ haemoptysis
▶ tachycardia
▶ coughing
▶ painful and difficult breathing.

Major pulmonary embolism results in:
▶ collapse
▶ cyanosis
▶ acute pleural chest pain
▶ dyspnoea
▶ anxiety and restlessness
▶ hypotension
▶ death.

Diagnosis is made by:
▶ pulmonary angiogram, to identify the clot
▶ lung scan (scintigram) – both ventilation and perfusion scan, to show ischaemia
▶ chest X-ray (not used often)
▶ electrocardiogram, which shows specific changes associated with pulmonary embolism.

Immediate intervention consists of the following:
▶ This is a medical emergency: call for help.
▶ Give the patient oxygen and start an IV therapy line.
▶ Nurse the patient in the semi-Fowler's position.
▶ Reassure, support and encourage the patient.
▶ The woman will be transferred to the ICU for further treatment.

Also see the discussion on obstetric shock in Chapter 35.

38.5 Urinary tract complications in the puerperium

Trauma to the urinary tract is common in prolonged labour due to big babies, assisted deliveries and Caesarean sections. Blood in the urine on a catheter specimen after Caesarean section indicates bladder trauma (a nick). Other problems of the urinary tract are detailed below.

Acute retention of urine

Predisposing conditions

▶ *Reduced tone in the bladder.* This occurs with prolonged labour and obstructed labour and is aggravated by the dominant effect of progesterone, particularly after the decrease in oestrogen, when the placenta is expelled. Lack of tone allows the bladder to become over-distended; this may occur during or after labour.
▶ *Trauma.* Oedema of the bladder occurs with an over-distended bladder during labour. The tissue at the base of the bladder becomes oedematous due to pressure of the fetal head. Bruising of the bladder neck and the urethra occurs, especially if the second stage is prolonged.

Postpartum vulval haematoma is also responsible for acute retention.

▶ *Pain.* Discomfort and pain in the vulva may be caused by lacerations, oedema and suturing of the perineum, inhibiting relaxation of the urethral sphincter.

▶ *Spasm.* Urethral spasm following catheterisation causes acute retention of urine.

▶ *UTI.* This might occur due to catheterisation.

Psychological factors that influence micturition include:
▶ the fear of pain and using a bedpan
▶ the woman's position in bed while using a bedpan
▶ a lack of privacy
▶ a reduction in intra-abdominal pressure
▶ weak abdominal muscles
▶ loss of sensation, which usually occurs after epidural anaesthesia.

Medical management

A woman should pass urine within two hours post-delivery. If a woman cannot or has not passed urine after six hours, consult a medical practitioner. The following interventions are helpful in encouraging micturition:

▶ Encourage the woman to void frequently to avoid bladder distention.
▶ Use a natural position.
▶ If available, a warm bedpan or a bidet may be helpful.
▶ A dripping tap or running water within hearing may stimulate micturition.
▶ Pour warm water over the vulva.
▶ Give extra fluids. If the woman drinks a glass of water, it may evoke a reflex contraction.
▶ Give analgesia on medical prescription for the pain.
▶ Use heat or ice packs on the vulval area and the perineum.
▶ If all the above fail, catheterisation may have to be carried out, as requested by a medical practitioner.

Retention with overflow

Acute or chronic over-distension leads to a rise in pressure in the bladder. This forces the internal sphincter to open, so that small quantities of urine escape repeatedly, without, however, relieving the bladder of the large amount it contains. The rise in pressure is due to the excretory force of the kidneys. The urinary overflow to the exterior takes place quite involuntarily.

Bruising of the urethra, pain and temporary paralysis from an epidural analgesia will also cause retention with overflow.

Medical management

The patient is given encouragement, support and reassurance. Consult the medical practitioner. On prescription, the following may be done:

▶ A self-retaining catheter can be inserted for 48 hours. Clamping and opening of the catheter can be done to develop bladder tone.
▶ On the second day, a midstream specimen of urine is sent to the laboratory.

Complications

The dangers of prolonged urine retention include:
▶ atony of the bladder, which results in retention with overflow and residual urine
▶ hypertrophy of the bladder, with the formation of diverticula
▶ urethral reflux as a result of atonicity of the bladder musculature. The valve at the urethrovesical junction becomes incompetent, allowing the reflux of urine into the ureters. This in turn may cause pyelonephritis, hydronephritis, renal atrophy and renal failure.

38.6 Pelvic floor complications

Trauma to the pelvic floor occurs in pregnancy and birth. If the pelvic floor is damaged in pregnancy and birth, it may lead to morbidity and severe loss of quality of life in both the short and long term. Prolapse of the uterus and abdominal organs can occur. Other complications, such as vesicovaginal fistula, also arise.

Vesicovaginal fistula

This is the presence of an unnatural opening between the bladder or the urethra and the vagina. It is a common condition in developing countries.

Necrosis occurs about five to seven days post-delivery, due to the prolonged pressure of the presenting part on the soft tissues of the bladder or urethra and vagina during prolonged or obstructed labour. This pressure causes the tissues to become necrotised and to slough off, thereby causing an artificial opening between the bladder and the vagina. Mechanical trauma from difficult instrumental deliveries can also cause this condition. Vesicovaginal fistula results in incontinence of urine.

Predisposing conditions

▶ Neglected, prolonged and/or obstructed labour
▶ Inadequate or unavailable transport delaying arrival at hospital

- A lack of skilled attendance (failure of a woman to come to a hospital or refusal of permission for hospital treatment from the husband)
- Female genital mutilation (FGM).

Prevention

- Basic education
- The provision of maternal clinics
- The provision of midwifery services
- The availability of referral centres
- Community education programmes
- Skilled attendance.

Medical management

- The woman is hospitalised.
- A urologist is consulted.
- The patient is given extra fluids and kept on a strict intake and output chart.
- A self-retaining catheter is kept in place for two to three weeks to encourage the fistula to close spontaneously. It may be necessary to wait two to three months to repair the fistula, to allow infection to clear and to allow healthy tissue to form.
- The patient's nutritional status must be improved, with added vitamins and minerals.
- Surgical repair is undertaken if no spontaneous healing occurs in 8–10 weeks. The repair is performed, using a support graft, and the vaginal wall is closed. An indwelling catheter is inserted for 14 days.
- Coitus is avoided for three months.

Complications

Vesicovaginal fistula causes severe scarring of the vaginal and bladder walls. The patient must be counselled regarding future pregnancies. Future deliveries should be by Caesarean section if the patient has had a successful vesicovaginal repair.

The cure rate is 80 per cent, with a 10 per cent failure rate and a 10 per cent stress urinary incontinence (SUI) rate (Kumar, Kekre & Gopalakrishnan, 2007).

Rectovaginal fistula

Cystocele

A cystocele is the prolapse of the anterior vaginal wall beneath the bladder due to damage to the pelvic floor. This may be present after birth, but usually develops later in life. (Involus is the prolapse of the upper part of the anterior vaginal wall and the bladder muscular wall, leading to herniation of the bladder.)

Cystocele is a common condition. It can be symptomless, but it often presents with:

- SUI
- a bearing-down sensation
- a vaginal protrusion
- urethral angulation and hypertrophy of the muscular walls of the bladder (if the cystocele is present for a long period)
- bladder irritation
- frequency of micturition
- dysuria
- at a later stage, pyelonephritis and recurrent episodes of UTI.

Rectocele

A rectocele is the prolapse or herniation of the middle portion of the posterior vaginal wall over the perineal body. The supports are weakened or torn by childbirth.

Occasionally there are no symptoms, but if sacculation of the vaginal wall occurs, defecation is only accomplished by digital pressure vaginally.

Predisposing conditions for rectovaginal fistula

- Trauma to the pelvic floor in labour
- Assisted labour
- A large baby.

Prevention of rectovaginal fistula

- Prevent trauma to the pelvic floor in the second stage of labour.
- Prevent prolonged labour.
- Forceps should be used by skilled practitioners only.
- Large babies should be delivered by Caesarean section.

Medical management of rectovaginal fistula

Both cystocele and rectocele can only be rectified through surgery, although this is often not successful.

38.7 Conclusion

For every woman who dies in childbirth, five will have a problem that results in long-term health consequences that affect their quality of life. It is important that the midwife is able to identify potential problems, advise and refer women appropriately. The midwife must be skilled in emergency care to prevent morbidity and mortality.

Infant feeding

LEARNING OBJECTIVES

On completion of this chapter, you must be able to:

▶ assist the mother with finding a comfortable breastfeeding position of her choice

▶ guide and support the mother to establish breastfeeding following baby-friendly principles

▶ demonstrate knowledge, skill and competency in educating and assisting families on infant feeding choices

▶ use a problem-solving approach to identify and manage infant feeding issues (breast milk and formula).

KNOWLEDGE ASSUMED TO BE IN PLACE

Anatomy and physiology of the breasts (see Chapter 9)
The physiology of lactation
Infant and Young Child Feeding Policy (DoH, 2013)
Newborn Care Charts, paragraphs 2.1.3, 2.1.4, 3.1–7 and 5.8 (DoH, 2014)

KEYWORDS

Baby-Friendly Hospital Initiative (BFHI) • formula/replacement feeding • donor milk • supplementary and complementary feeds

39.1   Introduction

This chapter should be studied in conjunction with Chapter 9. This chapter provides the best practice standards developed and proposed by the baby-friendly initiative of the United Nations Children's Fund (UNICEF). (For more information on this initiative, go to https://www.unicef.org.uk/babyfriendly/).

The global initiative to promote breastfeeding coincides with the HIV pandemic, which has a particularly high incidence in sub-Saharan Africa. Newborn care for HIV-positive mothers – as well as a procedure on flash pasteurisation of mother's milk – is discussed in Chapter 50.

39.2   The BFHI

The Baby-Friendly Hospital Initiative (BFHI) is a global initiative aimed at the protection, promotion and support of breastfeeding. Its main focus is to encourage and facilitate the transformation of birthing centres in accordance with the ten steps for successful breastfeeding, to improve the quality of life for both mothers and babies. In South Africa, the BFHI was officially launched in 1994 and there are ongoing efforts to accredit all public healthcare facilities as baby-friendly.

Although breastfeeding is a natural process, it is also learned behaviour and is influenced by the social environment and practices (see Chapter 9). Breastfeeding needs to be actively supported and promoted.

South African authorities are eager to develop and implement a strategy of 'baby-friendly communities', which will entail growth monitoring and promotion, and increased advocacy for exclusive breastfeeding. To help with this, UNICEF has provided technical assistance in the development of a draft document entitled the South African Code of Ethics for the Marketing of Breast-milk Substitutes (1986) (see Behr, 2013). (See the box below for the criteria for baby-friendly accreditation.)

Ten steps to the BFHI

1   Have a written policy that is routinely communicated to all healthcare staff.

2   Train all healthcare staff in skills necessary to implement this policy.

3   Inform all pregnant women about the benefits and management of breastfeeding.

continued

4   Initiate breastfeeding. Help mothers initiate breastfeeding within half an hour after birth.

5   Show mothers how to breastfeed and maintain lactation, even if they should be separated from their infants.

6   Give newborn infants no food or drink other than breast milk – not even sips of water – unless medically indicated.

7   Practice rooming-in: allow mothers and infants to remain together 24 hours a day.

8   Encourage breastfeeding on demand.

9   Do not give artificial teats or pacifiers (also called dummies or soothers) to breastfeeding infants.

10 Foster the establishment of breastfeeding support groups and refer mothers to them on discharge from the hospital or clinic.

Rooming-in and demand feeding

Rooming-in, where the infant remains in the same room as the mother, is important to establish the mother–baby relationship as early as possible. It is also a requirement of the BFHI. In addition, rooming-in creates the opportunity for the new father and the newborn to get to know one another and is thus beneficial to family relationships as a whole. Women are educated on the benefits of rooming-in during antenatal care and many choose to have their babies in their rooms, even when such a policy does not exist.

Women who are sick, who have had a traumatic delivery or who suffer from any adverse conditions may not be well enough to keep the baby with them all the time. However, if a mother who had a normal, uncomplicated pregnancy and birth is reluctant to participate in rooming-in, the midwife should assess the mother's emotional and psychological needs and determine why she is hesitant to keep the baby at her bedside. Referral to a psychologist or social worker can be suggested if the midwife is concerned about the bonding between mother and child.

A compromised or sick newborn is usually admitted to higher levels of care (high-risk unit or intensive care) and is separated from the mother. Breastfeeding will then only be attempted when the maternal or neonatal conditions have changed and kangaroo-mother-care (KMC) can be instituted.

In most South African hospitals, babies receiving phototherapy are seldom treated at the mother's bedside, because of early discharge policies. For instance, the mother might be discharged before breastfeeding is fully established and before jaundice is detected. However, many medical aids provide for home phototherapy care by authorised home-visiting midwives.

The benefit of this includes the reduction of the mother's anxiety by involving her in the care and especially the feeding of the baby.

The principles of rooming-in should be clearly stipulated in a policy and need to be explained to mothers before and on admission. Where rooming-in is practised, the midwife cares for the mother and baby as a unit, has the opportunity to teach the mother and family about baby care and can observe for gaps in mother–child bonding and care, which allows for early intervention. The care of the mother and baby as a unit remains the responsibility of the midwife as long as the mother is under the midwife's care in hospital.

Some medical insurances have embraced a system of midwives who conduct home visits; the midwife visits the new mother at home for at least five days after discharge, to help and support her, especially with breastfeeding. However, these services are not available to mothers in state-funded facilities.

39.3   Promoting breastfeeding

The WHO promotes exclusive breastfeeding for the first six months of life for all babies, with the exception of those women with certain medical conditions.

A woman needs to be prepared for breastfeeding. Midwives competent in breastfeeding must advocate and support women for breastfeeding using counselling and printed and electronic information. They must encourage the woman to attend antenatal preparation classes and also display a positive attitude. All these factors then need to be reinforced by adequate support for breastfeeding. Having skilled assistance at the first feed and in the days afterwards can make all the difference in the initial adjustment to breastfeeding. In many communities there are postnatal support groups that assist with breastfeeding. Finally, some valuable assistance can come from friends. Some research has in fact suggested that a concerned layperson may be just as good a source of support for breastfeeding as a professional adviser.

The South African Department of Health (DoH) ascribes to the WHO's guidelines to promote exclusive breastfeeding for the first six months of life for all babies, with the exception of women with severe medical conditions (eg active, untreated TB) (see Behr, 2013). The midwife is furthermore guided by the South African Nursing Council (SANC) and its regulations (R2488) (see www.sanc.org.za) in this regard.

To create the necessary change in our society, in order to encourage women to breastfeed their babies, the following must happen:

▶ More women need to breastfeed in public so that people become desensitised to it.

▶ Television shows and movies need to feature more breastfeeding.

- Public service announcements about how breastfeeding protects the health of the baby and of the mother should become the norm.
- Laws that protect the rights of breastfeeding mothers should be promulgated.

Principles to observe in the promotion of breastfeeding

- Refer to breastfeeding as 'normal' rather than 'best'.
- Refer to 'the risks of not breastfeeding' rather than 'the advantages of breastfeeding'.
- Make the neurological development benefits of breast milk known.
- Infant formula was developed as an emergency feed and needs to be viewed as such.
- Infant formula is a poor alternative to human milk.
- Adverse health outcomes related to infant formula feeding need to be pointed out.
- The economic implications of infant feeding methods should be discussed.
- Clarify the cost savings of breastfeeding.

Factors that may affect initial breastfeeding

The following are some of the aspects that may interfere with a mother initiating breastfeeding:

- *Psychological factors.* The mother may feel embarrassed and shy about exposing her breasts, especially in a general ward. Adequate screening must be provided to give her privacy.
- *The husband and/or other family members.* The woman may be experiencing relationship problems with her partner, her mother or her mother-in-law, or family members may be trying to discourage her from breastfeeding. The new mother may be worried about other children at home and wondering if she will cope once she gets home.
- *Other patients in the ward.* The atmosphere in the ward and the attitude of other mothers or patients in the ward towards breastfeeding can affect the progress of breastfeeding. In addition, a very ill patient in the ward, or a woman who has lost her baby, can cause anxiety and distress.

Understanding breastfeeding

During the antenatal period, the midwife prepares the expectant couple for successful breastfeeding and lactation. Knowing the anatomy of the breast and how milk is produced can help the mother and midwife to understand some of the initial problems the mother may be faced with. The following information will be helpful.

Milk production and the anatomy of the breast

The basic structure within the breasts develops during puberty. Inside each breast are about 20 lobes, each with its own duct system. During pregnancy, the ducts and milk-producing cells grow and multiply. The main duct branches out into smaller ducts that end in clusters of milk-producing cells called alveoli. Muscle cells surround the alveoli. The ducts widen into tiny reservoirs that hold a small amount of milk, then converge on the nipple. See figures 9.1 and 9.2 on pages 146 and 147 in Chapter 9 for the anatomy of the breast.

The blood flow to the breasts increases during pregnancy, increasing the size of the breasts. The breasts and nipples also change during pregnancy. They become larger and the area surrounding the nipple (the areola) darkens.

The process by which the breast produces milk after pregnancy is called lactation. Early skin-to-skin contact between mother and baby has been shown to promote breastfeeding. The establishment and maintenance of lactation after delivery depends on early suckling by the baby, the physiological neurohormonal processes that are started (see Figure 39.1 on the next page) and the support provided by the maternity unit. (Also see Chapter 9 for a discussion of the physiological processes of lactation, including colostrum, milk production and the let-down reflex.)

Questions the mother may ask about breastfeeding

Q: Does the size of the breast influence the milk supply?

A: Size has little to do with the ability to make milk; small breasts may contain as many milk glands as large ones. The fatty and connective tissue determines the size of the breast. Women with small or large breasts are equally capable of producing sufficient milk for the needs of their babies.

Q: How do I prepare my breasts for feeding?

A: The aim of breast care is to improve suppleness, not toughness, of the nipple. The following measures may help achieve this:

- Each day late in pregnancy, gently draw out the nipples. Where the nipple joins the areola, roll it gently between the thumb and forefinger to make it easier to stretch.
- Wear a supportive bra to reduce the risk of stretch marks and sagging.
- Avoid soaps and drying agents on the nipples.
- Do not scrub nipples with hard brushes and rough towels (it removes the natural oils and causes damage to the skin of the nipple).
- Expose the breasts to fresh air and sunlight, but limit the time and expose them gradually.

A. The production of breast milk

2. The **anterior** pituitary gland releases **prolactin** into the bloodstream.

3. This causes the cells of the alveoli to secrete milk which then distends the alveoli.

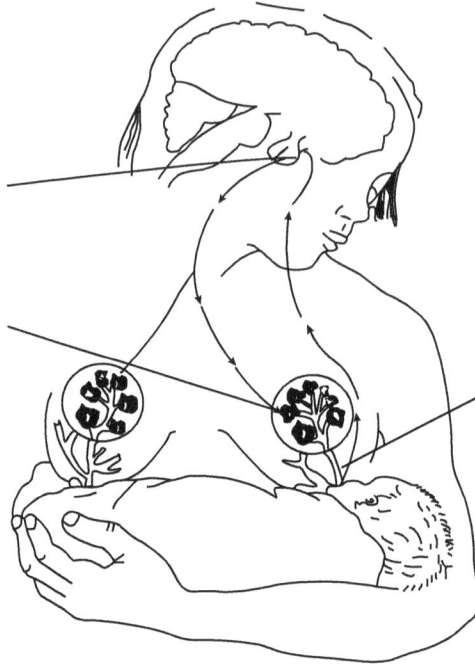

1. Nerve impulses from sucking

B. The release of breast milk

2. The **posterior** pituitary gland releases **oxytocin** into the bloodstream.

1. Nerve impulses from sucking

3. This causes the minute muscles around the alveoli to squeeze milk into the lactiferous ducts, and brings about the 'let-down' of milk.

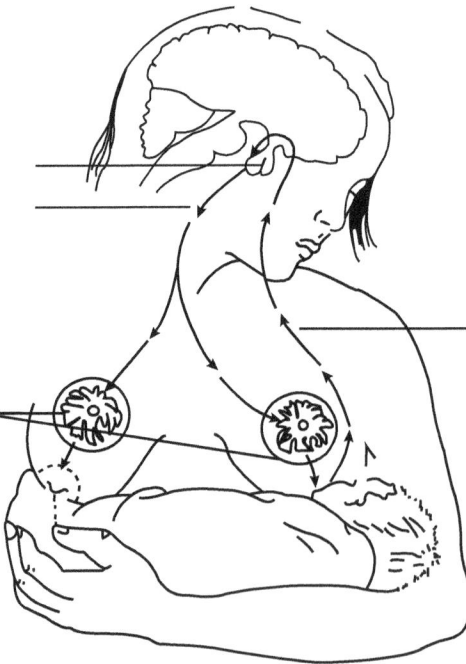

Note: The oxytocin also causes further erection of the nipple, as well as uterine contractions.

Figure 39.1 Sucking and the hormonal cycle of milk production

Q: Will flat or inverted nipples affect my ability to breastfeed?

A: According to Du Plessis (2008), a nipple that is truly inverted, may hinder the woman from establishing breastfeeding. However, inverted nipples are a rare occurrence. Nipples that appear flat often become normal when the baby starts suckling. The woman can do the following to test whether her nipples are inverted (Du Plessis, 2008):

▶ Press the areola using the forefinger and thumb, behind the nipple base, as in Figure 39.2.
▶ If the nipple protrudes, the flatness is likely to self-correct.
▶ If the nipple stays flat or retracts, it is truly inverted and latching may be more difficult.

During pregnancy, the woman may try wearing breast shells or commercial devices (Nipplettes) designed to help the nipples stand out. A flat or inverted nipple may be also drawn out by the sucking action of the baby. After feeding, the nipple may stay erect or it may return to its previous state.

Assisting the mother to breastfeed

Any mother, regardless of how many children she has previously breastfed, will need help and assistance, especially with the first feed. Learning to breastfeed, often when the mother is exhausted after a long labour, can be a real struggle. Many breastfeeding problems start because the baby did not latch properly to the breast.

The high rates of Caesarean sections in private healthcare may also make breastfeeding more stressful because of the experience of pain related to the surgery.

Teenage mothers are especially vulnerable and may need continued assistance and supervision.

Bearing the above points in mind, the midwife should remember the following when she assists the mother in her breastfeeding attempts:

▶ Although a number of automatic reflexes are involved in breastfeeding (meaning that it usually happens without a person having to think about it), it generally takes time to perfect the breastfeeding technique.
▶ The baby is alert during the first hour after birth and should be breastfed as soon as possible after birth. This might be difficult to achieve if the mother had surgery, but many hospitals encourage midwives to assist mothers in the recovery area of the surgical suite.
▶ Early breastfeeding (even if the baby is merely licking the nipple) helps to establish the bond between mother and baby and encourages the baby's sucking response.
▶ The removal of milk from the breast is an important factor in the continued production of milk.
▶ Babies need to feed frequently in the early weeks to stimulate the production of milk.
▶ When giving the first feed, the action of gently brushing the nipple against the baby's lips will cause him or her to automatically open the mouth (the rooting reflex).
▶ Once the nipple is inside the baby's mouth, a second reflex occurs: the baby automatically sucks upon the nipple. (This action stimulates nerve endings and activates the pituitary gland in the brain to release oxytocin into the bloodstream as shown in Figure 39.1).
▶ The mother's breast milk will be different from other mothers' milk, but 'different' does not imply 'not as good'. Each mother's milk differs due to her particular diet and may contain more or less fat or antibodies.
▶ The breasts will produce as much milk as the baby requires (the demand–supply principle [see Figure 39.1]).

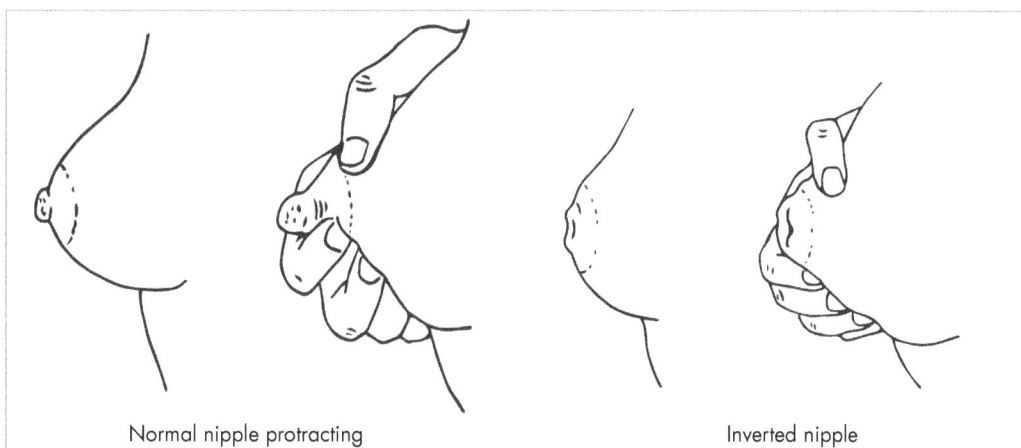

Normal nipple protracting   Inverted nipple

Figure 39.2 An inverted nipple

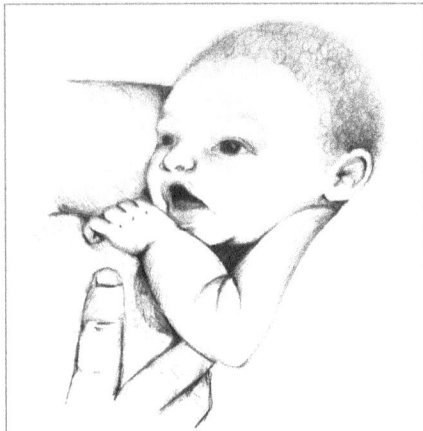

Figure 39.3 The seeking reflex

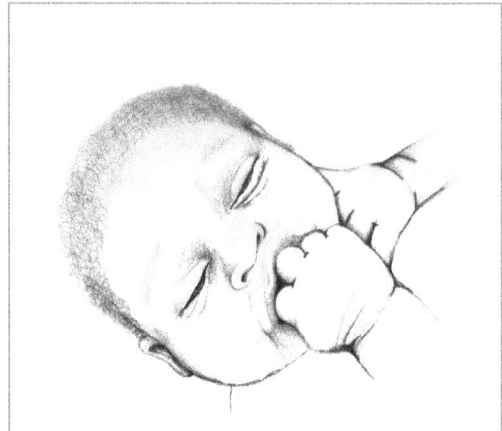

Figure 39.4 The sucking reflex

- If the baby is content and sleeps for a few hours between feeds, the mother will have enough milk.
- There is always milk in the breasts, but 80 per cent of the milk is produced when the baby sucks. The milk in the breasts is foremilk and the milk that is produced during a feed is hindmilk. The hindmilk contains more fat and protein.
- The oxytocin stimulates the cells surrounding the alveoli to contract, squeezing the milk into the ducts and reservoirs, where the milk is released into the baby's mouth.
- When the baby suckles, prolactin levels are stimulated in order to produce more milk for the next feed. The more the baby suckles, the more milk is produced: thus, a simple case of supply and demand.
- It is normal for a newborn to be fed frequently, sometimes every two to three hours during the day and the night.
- Frequent feeds will increase the maternal milk production, improve the mother's confidence, reduce breast discomfort associated with engorgement and reduce the possibility of the development of sore nipples.

The first feed: Readiness to start

The mother and the baby must be ready for feeding. A baby may be affected if the mother is not willing or ready and in these cases often refuses to take the nipple. If given the opportunity to be with her baby and talk to her or him, the mother will relax enough to try the baby at the breast. When she relaxes or when the baby starts to suckle, the let-down reflex may kick in.

The baby, given time to adjust to extrauterine life, will give the mother the following clues, indicating his or her readiness for a feed (see also Figure 39.1):

- The baby makes eye contact.

- The baby roots and drools, making lip movements. The baby may be searching for the nipple. However, if not, the baby's attention can be attracted by touching the lips or stroking the cheek with the nipple (see Figure 39.3).
- The baby tries to get his or her hands into the mouth and sucks vigorously (see Figure 39.4).
- The baby says the word 'Neh' (see the discussion on Dunstan baby language in the box below).

Dunstan classification of infant cries (Lester & La Gasse, 2004)

Priscilla Dunstan tested her theory about baby 'language' on over a thousand infants in different countries. She concluded that there are five sounds with similar meaning for all cultures that all babies – regardless what race and culture they belong to – from birth to three months make to communicate what they want to say. Although not clinically and scientifically verified, many women use this as a guide to learn to know their babies and to respond appropriately:
- Neh = 'I am hungry.'
- Owh = 'I am sleepy.'
- Heh = 'I am experiencing discomfort.'
- Eair = 'I have lower gas.'
- Eh = 'I need to burp.'

Parents should listen for these 'clues' in their baby's pre-cry, before the baby starts crying hysterically. You can view a fascinating video clip on YouTube at https://www.youtube.com/watch?v=PgkZf6jVdVg to assist you in identifying the pre-cry reflex.

| **PROCEDURE** | Breastfeeding techniques |

Positioning the mother and baby correctly is essential in establishing a pain-free breastfeeding experience. There are many positions the mother can try, but it is recommended that the midwife assists the mother in one particular position until she gets comfortable with it before she attempts a new position. Here, especially, the maternity unit should have a standard procedure or protocol to avoid confusing the new mother.

Position

▶ Position the mother upright with her back straight, her lap flat and her feet on a flat surface. Choose a comfortable chair which gives the woman's back firm support. She needs to be upright, not leaning back or tipping forward. Sitting in bed is best avoided, as it is difficult to get upright without slipping and if the mother crosses her legs, the circulation is impaired and she will experience pins-and-needles.

▶ If a mother is ambulant, this position might be difficult if the mother had a Caesarean section or an epidural, where her sensation has not yet fully returned. Put plenty of cushions behind her back to bring her slightly forward. If she is still in bed, another position is used for feeding.

▶ Use a pillow on the mother's lap or use a breastfeeding cushion to raise the baby to below the level of the breast. This will support the baby's weight so there will be less strain on the mother's back. The mother must move the baby to the breast and not the breast to the baby; otherwise, the position will be awkward and uncomfortable.

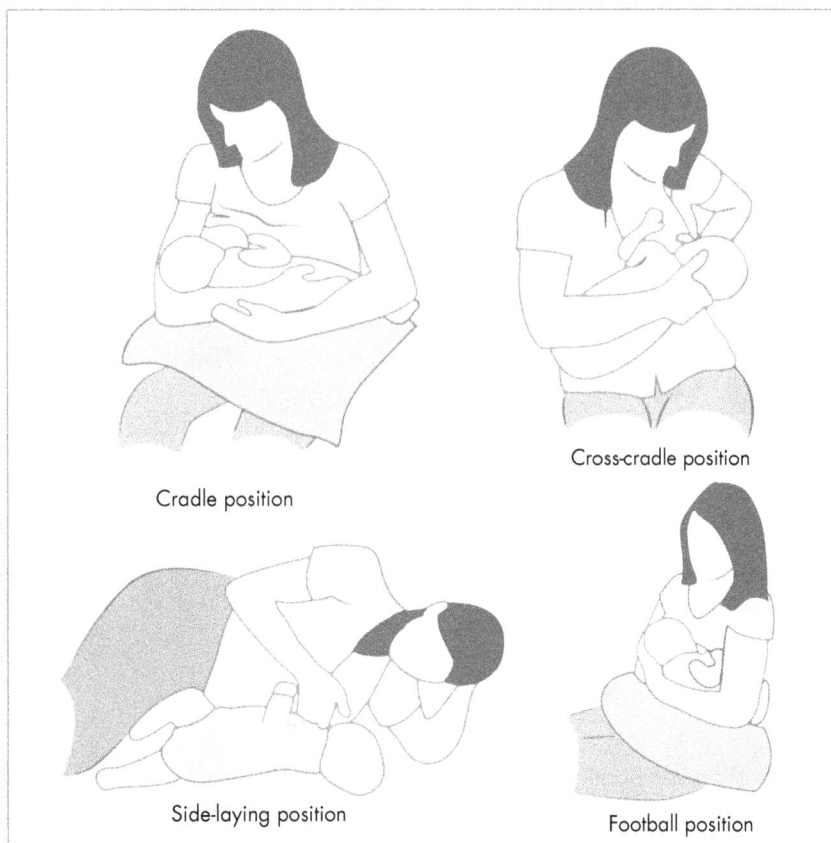

Cradle position

Cross-cradle position

Side-laying position

Football position

Figure 39A Positions for breastfeeding: 1 = cradle hold; 2 = modified football hold; 3 = lying down to breastfeed; 4 = football hold

continued

If a woman has twins, she can feed them simultaneously, using the positions shown below.

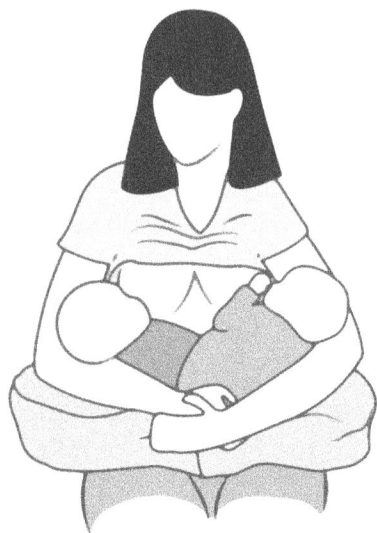

Front cross position

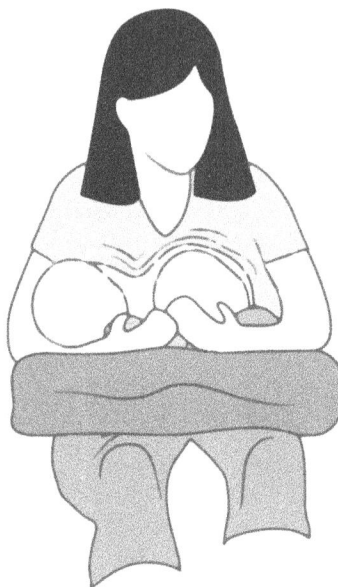

Football and cradle position

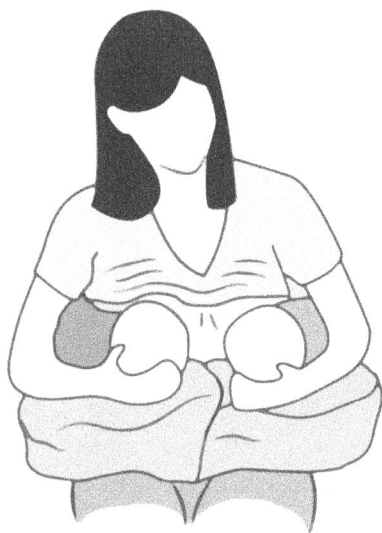

Double football position

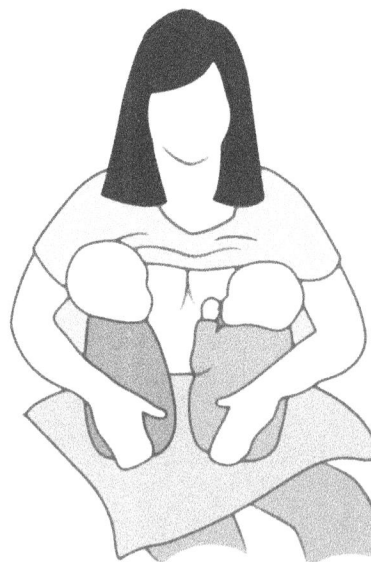

Upright latch position

Figure 39B Positions for breastfeeding with twins

continued

Breastfed baby suckling **correctly**

1a. Commencing suckling

1b. Suckling

Tongue below the nipple but back behind the gums

Gums pressing behind the nipple, with the nipple well back into the baby's mouth

2. Bottle feeding

Tongue forward and wrapped around teat

Breastfed baby sucking **incorrectly**

3. Chewing the nipple

4. Nipple confusion

Tongue forward as in bottle feeding

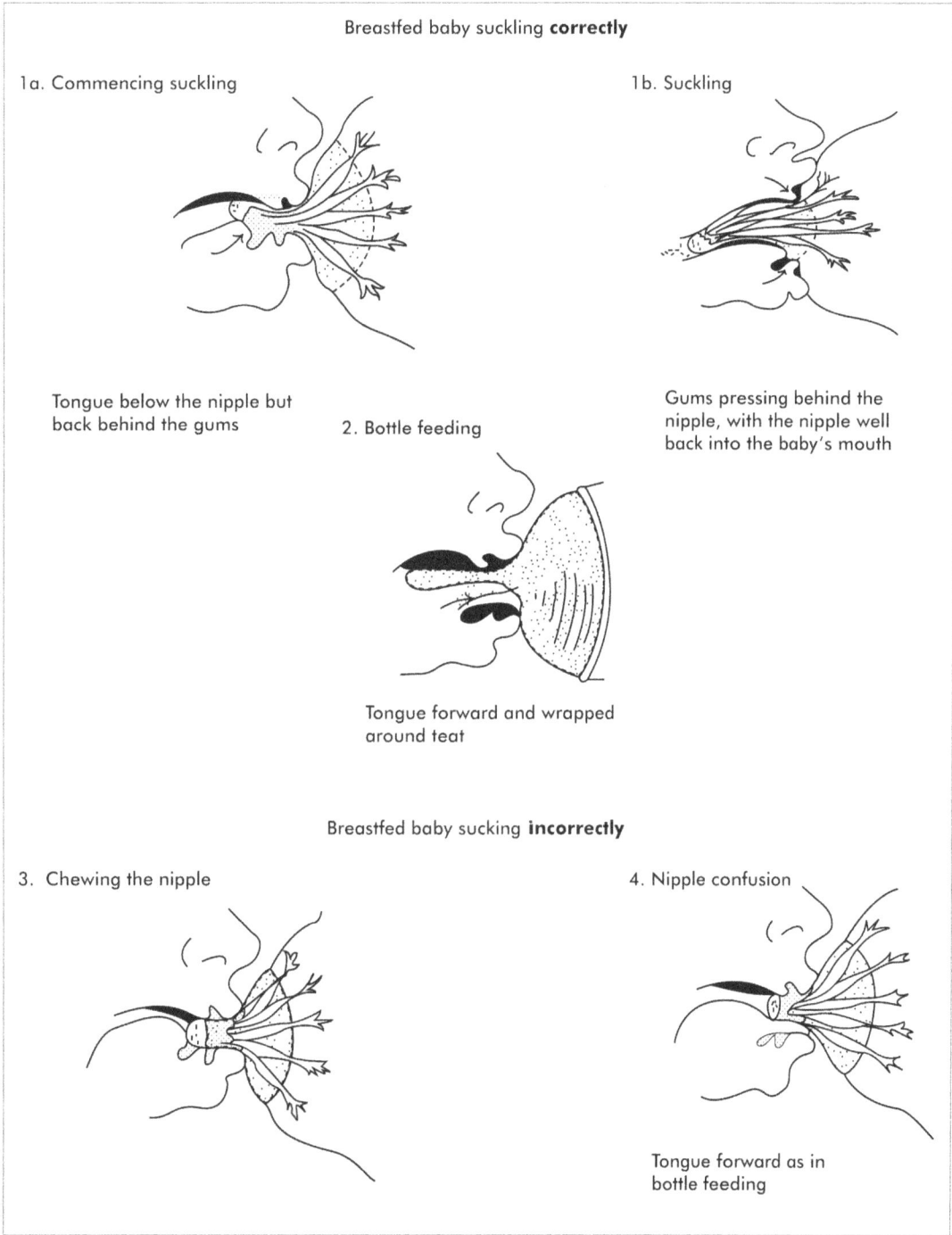

Figure 39C Latching

continued

▶ It may not be necessary to support the breast at all, but for the mother with fuller breasts, Figure 39A will be helpful.

▶ The mother holds the baby with the right arm when feeding from the left breast (and vice versa). The baby should lie on the forearm, not in the crook of the arm, as this will tilt the head forward.

▶ The baby should be facing the mother, with the head, neck and back in a straight line and the head tilted back slightly. If the baby has to turn his or her head to reach the nipple, swallowing will be difficult.

▶ The mother supports the base of the baby's neck and head with an open hand so that the baby's neck is free to tip backwards as he or she moves the chin upwards. Never hold the baby by the head, as this will flex the head forward, making it difficult to open the mouth wide enough.

▶ If the mother has to press under the nose for the baby to breathe, the head is too straight or too tilted forward.

Correct and incorrect latching

The correct latching of the baby to the breast (see Figure 39C) is the key to successful and prolonged breastfeeding. The midwife supports women and teaches them the correct way to latch a baby, to take the baby off the breast and how to care for the nipples.

Follow these steps:

▶ Bring the baby's body towards the mother and position the baby so that his or her nose is roughly in line with the nipple, the body tucked in close to the mother's.

▶ Gently touch the baby's mouth against the breast while waiting for him or her to open the mouth really wide, like a yawn. This ensures that the baby takes more of the breast tissue into the mouth from below the nipple. Not all of the areola needs to be in the baby's mouth. In this position, the nipple touches the baby's soft palate and latching will then not be painful.

▶ If the baby hasn't latched on properly, gently slip your little finger in-between the breast and mouth to break the suction.

▶ The mother should feed from one breast for as long as the baby wants and until the baby lets go of the nipple.

Burping

The mother burps the baby gently between feeds and then allows the baby to feed from the other breast as well. If the baby has swallowed air, he or she may not be willing to suck. This can be determined by looking in to the mouth and checking that the baby places the tongue against the palate. The baby may not be ready to feed until the air has come out.

Continuing with the second breast

The baby will not suckle as long or as strong on the second breast as on the first breast. With the following feed, the mother should simply offer the second breast first.

▶ When the baby is feeding well, change the supporting arm if necessary.

▶ If the baby seems calm and contented and the mother feels comfortable, the baby is probably well latched on.

After the baby has fed from the second breast, the mother must burp the baby well to avoid discomfort and winds.

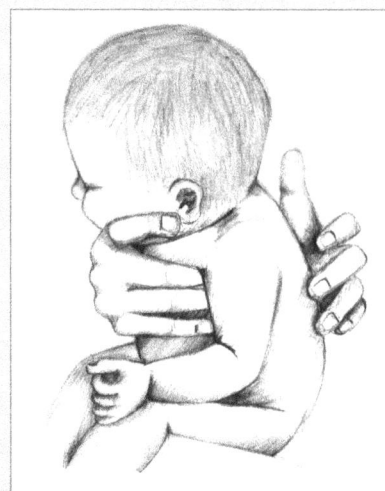

Figure 39D Burping the baby

Milk banks

Donor milk banking (DMB) is a service that screens, collects, processes and dispenses human milk donated by volunteer nursing mothers who are not related to the recipient infants. Donors of human milk must be healthy, lactating women who have had X-rays and a Tyne test done and are free of venereal diseases and hepatitis.

DMB plays an important role in reducing mortality and morbidity in a small population of critically ill or premature infants and is only available for such in South Africa. Some indications for donor milk are:

▶ prematurity
▶ malabsorption syndrome
▶ renal failure

▶ inborn errors of metabolism
▶ cardiac problems
▶ paediatric burns cases
▶ failure to thrive
▶ short gut syndrome
▶ feeding intolerance
▶ post-surgical nutrition
▶ bronchopulmonary dysplasia (BPD).

This milk is only used when the mother's own milk is not available for her infant.

Expressing breast milk

A Cochrane systematic review (Becker, Cooney & Smith, 2011) concluded that 'the most suitable method for milk expression may depend on the time since birth, purpose of expression and the individual mother and infant.'

Low-cost interventions, including early initiation when not feeding at the breast, relaxation, hand expression and lower-cost pumps may be as effective, or more effective, than large electric pumps for some outcomes.

Breast milk can be expressed for healthy infants, but is more often required to feed low-birth-weight (LBW) or premature infants. If a mother is not able to provide expressed milk, premature babies in some hospitals will receive donor breastmilk. If a mother is separated from her baby, it is essential that she maintains the milk flow by regular expression (see figures 39.5 and 39.6).

Some mothers express milk as donor milk for the breast milk banks, following the set processes.

Guidelines for expressing breast milk
▶ Maintain hygienic principles by always washing your hands thoroughly and using a sterile container to receive the milk.
▶ Create a safe and comfortable environment.
▶ Apply heat before starting and drink a cup of tea to relax.
▶ Massage the breast with gentle strokes from the axilla to the nipple.
▶ When the milk flows, express the milk with gentle rhythmic movements that mimic the baby's sucking.

Maintaining lactation

The following interdependent factors are responsible for maintaining lactation:

▶ *Suckling and nipple stimulation.* Without suckling and emptying the breasts, there will be no stimulus for the breasts to produce more milk, hence the importance of continued suckling (and/or expression of milk), particularly when there is an apparently insufficient milk supply.

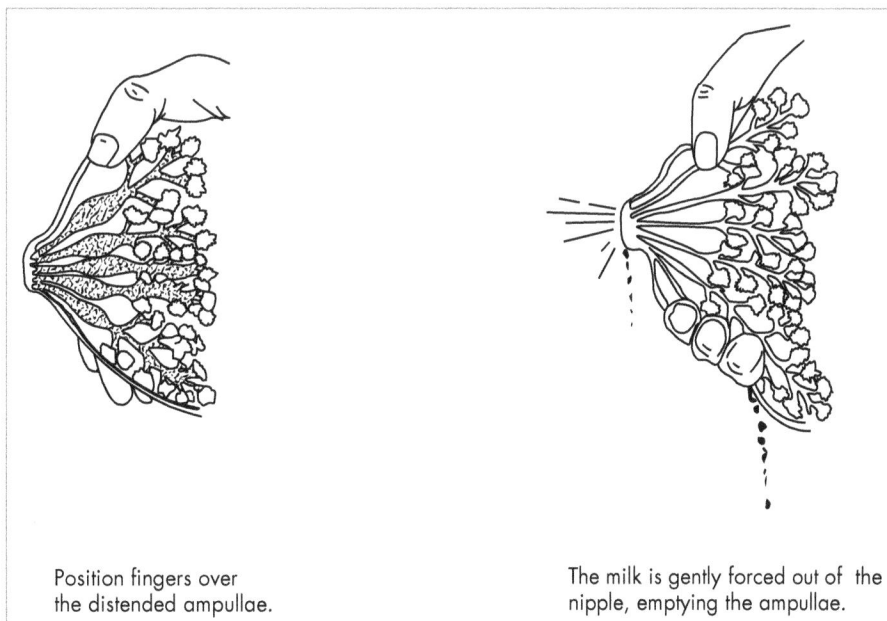

Position fingers over
the distended ampullae.

The milk is gently forced out of the
nipple, emptying the ampullae.

Figure 39.5 Guidelines for expressing milk

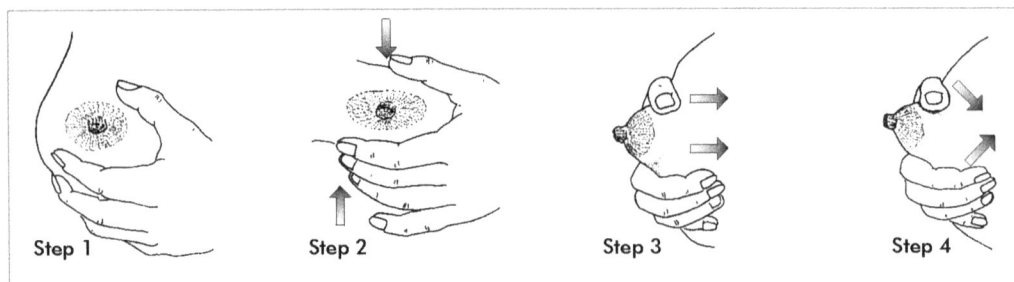

Figure 39.6 Stages in manual expression

Therefore, if the baby is unable to suckle or to suckle properly – which could be caused by a problem with the nipples or some adverse condition of the baby or the mother – milk production will decrease.

▶ *The mother's emotional state.* Milk secretion is influenced, via the hypothalamus, by the mother's emotional state, which affects the release of oxytocin and the let-down of the milk. Sleep deprivation, anxiety and stress will interfere with milk production, as prolactin secretion and milk production take place during rest and sleep.

▶ *An adequate and balanced maternal diet.* The lactating woman needs a balanced and nutritious diet to sustain her milk supply. This may be difficult if there are financial constraints or if the mother wants to lose weight.

The most important assessment of the quality of a mother's milk is whether the baby gains enough weight (150–299 g per week) after the first 10 days post-birth.

Questions the mother may ask about maintaining lactation

Q: Must I top-up breastfeeding with formula?

A: No formula or glucose water should be given, as it reduces the number of feeds and interferes with the establishment of breastfeeding. Women whose babies are given extra fluids are more likely to discontinue breastfeeding. Top-up feeds have been associated with:

▶ nipple confusion
▶ reducing milk supply
▶ undermining maternal confidence
▶ the development of reactive hypoglycaemia.

Q: Will I be able to produce enough milk for my baby/twins?

A: The production of milk works on a demand–supply principle; the more the baby feeds, the more the milk supply will increase. No matter what the size of the baby, the mother can produce enough milk. If the baby is thriving and gaining weight after the first ten days of life, he or she is getting enough milk.

Q: Can breasts be empty? I was told my milk had not 'come in' yet.

A: Breasts are never empty, because they are filled with colostrum, which will satisfy the baby's needs for the first few days after birth.

Q: How long should each feed last? My doctor says I must take the baby off after 10 minutes.

Some babies need short, fast feeds; others want to suck for 20–30 minutes. The baby should feed on the first breast when and for as long as he or she wants, until the baby releases the nipple. If the baby is switched from the first breast too soon, before receiving the fatty high-calorie hindmilk, he or she will experience poor satiety and may take time to settle down. The second breast should be offered as well.

Q: Must I wake my baby up for a feed?

A: Opinions differ in this area. If the baby is healthy, the important thing is that he or she is allowed to suck at the breast without restriction. If the newborn sleeps for long periods (five hours or longer), the nappy can be changed to allow the baby to wake up. If the baby's weight is low, or if the baby is premature or sickly or does not gain sufficient weight (150–200 g per week), it may be necessary to wake the baby for a feed.

Q: How should I wake my baby?

A: Waking should be done gently: first release the wrappings and nappy and then stroke the baby's body lightly. A cold cloth should not be used, as this may cause hypothermia.

Q: Should I be concerned if my baby, who normally feeds three-hourly, suddenly starts to sleep for four hours or longer?

A: If the baby is in good health, he or she will wake when hungry. A long sleep indicates that the baby is still satisfied from the last feed.

Q: Why is my baby fussing at the breast?

A: The following are possible reasons:

▶ *Fussiness from birth to one week.* The baby may experience problems in latching, or the let-down reflex may be delayed.

▶ *Fussiness between the second and fourth day.* The mother may experience engorgement or forceful or inhibited let-down reflexes. If the let-down reflex is forceful, the baby may choke and pull away from the breast.

▶ *Fussiness between one and four weeks in a baby who previously breastfed well.* Nipple confusion may be a reason if the baby is supplemented with bottles. Alternatively, the mother's milk may taste different, the baby's temperament may be developing, or there may be competing stimuli from the environment that make it difficult for the baby to settle down.

Q: How do I breastfeed twins?

A: In practice, many mothers of multiples use a mixture of bottles and breast, often putting formula milk in the bottle, but the mother may use expressed breast milk as well. The following are helpful guidelines:

▶ Breastfeed early and often. If you are separated from your babies, express milk to sustain the milk supply.

▶ Avoid bottles and dummies, to encourage the babies to suck effectively.

▶ Breastfeed simultaneously or separately.

▶ Try a variety of breastfeeding positions.

▶ If one twin is less effective at the breast, simultaneous nursing will increase the milk flow and may help encourage the baby to suck more effectively. See Figure 39B on page 618.

Q: Is breastfeeding possible if the baby was born prematurely?

A: Yes. The baby tolerates colostrum well and the mother's own fresh milk is generally better for the baby than formula. In addition, do the following:

▶ Express milk with an electric breast pump, especially when the baby needs to be hospitalised for a long time.

▶ Express early and frequently to establish and maintain a full milk supply over time.

▶ Continue with expressing after and even between feeds if the baby feeds for short periods only. This milk may be given by cup or syringe, or expressed directly into the baby's mouth (see Figure 39.7).

▶ If the premature baby is healthy, commence breastfeeding within the first hour or two after birth.

▶ Finger feeding is a great option if the baby is fed intravenously or by tube.

▶ It is normal for a mother's milk supply to temporarily decrease while her baby is going through a crisis.

Note that KMC provides opportunities for early breastfeeding, enhances the let-down reflex and increases the duration and frequency of breastfeeding.

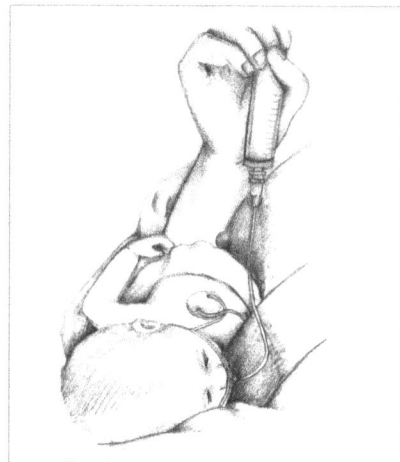

Figure 39.7 Tube feeding

39.4 Coping with breastfeeding: Breastfeeding difficulties

Breastfeeding is not always an easy process for mother or baby, often because of lack of knowledge, help and support during the first few days while the mother is still in hospital. Du Plessis (2008) found that although many mothers want to breastfeed their babies, only 69 per cent of them still continue to do so when discharged on day 3 or day 4.

Mothers need a sensitive midwife who guides them to breastfeed with confidence. Some mothers object to midwives touching their breasts. Others may feel incompetent and doubt their mothering ability or may be reluctant to bother the busy midwives when feeding their babies. Midwives need to understand they are in the maternity unit not only to provide physical assistance, but to coach mothers on succeeding with breastfeeding after discharge. If the midwife is unable or unwilling to provide the necessary assistance, the mother should be referred to a lactation consultant (usually an independent practitioner).

Ideally, all staff should follow the breastfeeding policy of the particular unit to avoid conflicting advice. This might be difficult when new or temporary staff are on duty. All efforts should be made to inform new staff members of the breastfeeding protocol to ensure continuity of care. Du Plessis (2008) found that midwives are harshly criticised for the lack of consistent breastfeeding advice and mothers give up breastfeeding because of this, sometimes with deep-seated regret or even feelings of guilt.

Psychological factors for successful breastfeeding

Research shows that the duration of breastfeeding is more associated with psychological factors than socioeconomic ones. Psychological factors include an optimistic outlook, feeling comfortable with breastfeeding, faith in breast milk as a food, expectations of breastfeeding, anxiety and the planned duration of breastfeeding.

Breast refusal

Some babies simply refuse to breastfeed. They do this by arching the back, screaming and fighting with the hands as soon as they go near the nipple. This may be caused by a slow let-down reflex, which frustrates the baby. To stimulate the let-down reflex, the midwife should encourage the mother to:

▶ take deep breaths to relax, as the constant screaming of the baby will upset her

▶ apply warmth in the form of a hot shower, wheat bag or face cloth

▶ express a little milk before attempting to feed, to get the milk flowing

▶ put a droplet of milk on the baby's tongue to calm him or her down before putting the baby back on the breast

▶ calm the baby down with gentle rocking motions

▶ express some milk which can be given in a feeding cup if the situation is desperate and the baby hasn't fed for four to six hours.

Breast refusal may also be caused by a forceful let-down reflex, where the milk gushes out. To regulate the let-down reflex, the midwife should encourage the mother to attempt breastfeeding while lying back (against gravity) to slow the flow of milk. Alternatively, press the nipple inward toward the chest with the palm of the hand.

Refusal may also be the result of incorrect positioning of the baby, with the head flexed forward and the nose pressed into the breast tissue.

Managing breast refusal

The following points will help the mother to manage breast refusal:

1. *Position the baby:*
   ▶ Tilt the baby's head slightly backwards, to free the nose from the breast.

▶ Check that the nose is clear, as it may be clogged with mucus. Put a saline nasal drop in each nostril and clear with a nose cleaner.

▶ If it appears that the baby does not 'like' a particular breast, allow the baby to feed on the easy side first; it might be that the mother feels clumsy with a particular hand.

2. *Reduce the mother's anxiety:*
   ▶ The mother should take deep breaths to help her to stay calm. Sometimes this will be hard to do and she may feel frightened or angry at the baby.
   ▶ If this happens, ask another caring adult to help the mother regain her composure.
   ▶ Calm the baby down and do not attempt breastfeeding while the baby is screaming.

3. *Re-latching the baby:*
   ▶ Try and feed the baby while he or she is still half-asleep.
   ▶ Allow the baby to suck on the mother's little finger and then try and shift him or her onto the breast.
   ▶ Experiment with different feeding positions.
   ▶ Express a few drops of milk onto the nipple to tempt the baby.

If the above does not work, express milk and cup-feed the baby (see the box below).

Cup feeding

Newborn babies are able to drink milk from a small feeding cup. The baby thus receives expressed breast milk in the early days without confusing the bottle teat with the nipple.

Using a cup takes no longer than using a bottle. Milk can also be given to the baby using a feeding syringe, spoon or dropper. (For more information on this topic, see Torrance, 2014.)

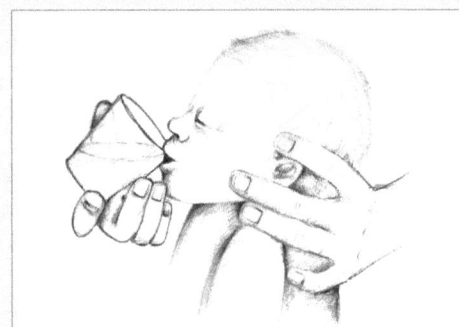

Figure 39.8 Cup feeding

Engorged breasts

Engorgement of the breasts occurs as a result of venous and lymphatic engorgement and not necessarily as a result of overproduction of milk. The milk flow is obstructed, resulting in stasis of milk and increased pressure in the tissues.

Engorgement of the breasts usually occurs between the third and fifth days post-delivery and may vary from minor to severe.

Signs and symptoms

▶ The breasts are full, heavy and painful.
▶ The breast may feel lumpy and hot.
▶ Oedema of the overlying skin is present; the skin is red and the veins are prominent.
▶ The baby cannot latch properly.

Causes

▶ The time between feedings is too long.
▶ The baby has a poor suck.
▶ Tension, insecurity and pain inhibit the let-down reflex.
▶ A tight-fitting bra blocks the ducts.
▶ The nipple opening is clogged with dried milk.
▶ The use of breast shells or breast shields can cause engorgement.
▶ A poor feeding position can lead to engorgement.

Managing engorged breasts

▶ If the mother is breastfeeding and the baby is unable to suckle, encourage her to express milk by hand or with a pump (manual or electric) just before a feed.
▶ If the mother is breastfeeding and the baby is able to suckle, encourage her to stay calm and feed frequently, for as long as the baby wants, using both breasts at each feeding.
▶ Eliminate external obstacles (such as a tight bra or badly adjusted straps from a baby carrier) that may prevent milk from flowing in certain spots.
▶ Apply warm compresses or encourage the woman to take a warm shower for approximately 10 minutes before a feed to promote milk flow.
▶ Massage the mother's neck and back to reduce the pain and to help her to relax.
▶ Have her express some milk manually before breastfeeding and wet the nipple area to enable the baby to latch on.
▶ Soften the area of high pressure surrounding the nipple by placing the thumb and first finger on the areola and gently squeezing inward. Express only enough milk to assist with the latching.

▶ Support the breasts with a bra to reduce the pressure.
▶ Apply a cold compress (gel pads) or refrigerated green cabbage leaves for 15–20 minutes to the breasts between feeds to reduce swelling and pain.
▶ The mother may take paracetamol 500 mg every six hours for pain.
▶ Homeopathic remedies may be used under supervision to reduce the amount of milk (eg two to four cups of peppermint or sage tea daily).
▶ If engorgement is not relieved in 24 hours, seek medical advice.

The mother can avoid recurrence of the problem by feeding frequently, feeding for long enough and positioning the baby well enough to drain the breast efficiently.

Mastitis

Mastitis means inflammation (not necessarily infection) of the breast. It occurs usually only in one breast (often in the left) and in one area (often the upper outer quadrant). See Chapter 49 for more on mastitis.

Assisting with mastitis

The midwife should check the positioning of the baby at the breast (see Figure 39A on page 617) and latching (see Figure 39C on page 619). Advise the breastfeeding mother as follows:
▶ Use the suggestions for treating a blocked duct.
▶ Continue with breastfeeding.
▶ Feed the baby more frequently, and use a breast pump if the baby is not taking all the milk available. Frequent feeding without restriction will improve the condition.
▶ Feed from the side which is sore first. The milk from the affected breast is not harmful and breastfeeding is still safe for the baby.
▶ Support the breasts with a supportive bra without an underwire.
▶ Perform arm-swinging exercises to boost circulation.
▶ Rest as much as possible.
▶ Treat alternatively with warmth and cold.
▶ Take paracetamol 500 mg or ibuprofen by mouth as needed.
▶ Seek medical treatment if self-help techniques produce no improvement in 12–24 hours, or if mastitis recurs.

A doctor may prescribe an antibiotic that is safe during lactation if any of the following applies:
▶ Symptoms do not improve after 12–24 hours of improved milk removal.
▶ Cell and bacterial colony counts and culture are available and indicate infection.

▶ Symptoms have been present for a day or more and are increasing in severity.

The non-breastfeeding mother should do the following:
▶ Support breasts with a supportive brassiere without an underwire.
▶ Rest as much as possible.
▶ Apply cold compresses to the breasts to reduce swelling and pain.
▶ Avoid stimulating the nipples.
▶ Take paracetamol 500 mg or ibuprofen by mouth as needed.
▶ Seek medical treatment if self-help techniques produce no improvement within 12–24 hours or if mastitis recurs.

Breast abscesses

Occasionally, the process of mastitis continues and a breast abscess develops, usually after a few weeks. An abscess can be deep in the breast and invisible or a soft swelling may be seen nearer the surface. The symptoms are similar to those of a blocked duct or mastitis. Blood or pus may be present in breast milk.

Managing breast abscesses

▶ The woman should see a medical practitioner.
▶ Antibiotic therapy may be recommended.
▶ The breast abscess will need incision and drainage.
▶ The wound will be packed with sterile gauze which is gradually decreased to allow the affected area to heal properly.
▶ The mother may continue with breastfeeding on the unaffected breast or she may express the milk with a pump if feeding is too painful.

Painful nipples

Breastfeeding should not be painful, but the nipples may become very sensitive in the first few weeks. Severe pain is often the result of improper latching.

If the nipple cracks, it may bleed every time the mother feeds or form scabs between feeds. Cracked nipples usually happen because the baby is sucking on the nipple rather than sucking on the nipple and the biggest part of the areola as well.

In the first few days of breastfeeding, painful nipples at the start of the feed is normal, but if the soreness continuous throughout the feed or if the nipple skin is red, bumpy, blistered, itchy or flaky, it indicates that the baby is not latching properly and does not open the mouth wide enough. If the baby has thrush (white waxy coating of the tongue and gums)

or if the mother is sensitive to soaps, nipple creams and lotions, painful nipples may result.

Managing sore, cracked or bleeding nipples

The midwife should check:
▶ the positioning of the baby at the breast (see Figure 39A on page 617)
▶ latching (see Figure 39C on page 619)
▶ the baby's mouth for signs of thrush.

In addition, suggest the following:
▶ Change the feeding position – tuck the baby under the arm rather than lying him or her across the lap.
▶ Before putting the baby to the breast, express some milk, gently rub it round the nipples and allow to dry. Breast milk is sterile and antiseptic.
▶ Offer the unaffected, or less affected, side first – the pain subsides once the milk is flowing.
▶ It might be necessary to feed from one breast at a time only. Express the second breast slightly to reduce discomfort and offer this breast to the baby for the second feed.
▶ Apply ice wrapped in a cloth to the nipples before feeding, as this will numb them.
▶ Keep the nipples dry between feeds; use a proper breast pad to absorb excess milk and change this regularly.
▶ Apply purified anhydrous lanolin ointment after every feed until the nipples have healed.
▶ Air the nipples as much as possible (expose to sunlight if possible).
▶ Treat with crushed cucumber or lemon juice to aid healing.
▶ Take the homeopathic remedy Calendula.

Nipple shields

A nipple shield is made from thin latex and fits over the nipple. It may be used to protect sore nipples. The baby sucks the milk through the nipple shield.

Nipple shields can make feeds take longer and restrict efficient emptying of the breast. In addition, they may lead to a conditional rejection of the breast by the baby.

Advise the mother to use a nipple shield only as a last resort, as they can reduce the milk supply and lead to bad suckling habits.

Silicone implants or breast reduction surgery

If a woman has had breast augmentation or reduction, her ability to breastfeed thereafter depends on whether any milk ducts or glands were cut or damaged.

Silicone implants are inserted under the chest muscle and thus do not interfere with breastfeeding. If the polyurethane coating breaks down, this may release potentially harmful chemicals; however, this is extremely rare and the benefits of breastfeeding may still outweigh the risks.

If the breasts were reduced, the type of surgery done may interfere with the amount of milk being produced. It is, however, not a contraindication to breastfeeding and the mother will be able to produce milk. The amount of milk that will be produced is unknown and these babies need to be weighed more frequently.

Overfeeding

Overfeeding seldom occurs in breastfed babies; the baby usually takes only what he or she requires. Occasionally, when there is an over-supply, vomiting may occur. This may happen towards the end of the first or second week after birth. Because the infant is vomiting and also losing fluids with the stools, he or she may be both hungry and thirsty and may cry and suck his or her fists. The infant who started by gaining weight well may have a static weight or may even start to lose weight.

Intervention and care

▶ Demand feeding is started, if this is not already being carried out.
▶ The amount of time on each breast is reduced slightly.
▶ The mother is encouraged to express a little milk before the feed, to reduce the first rush of milk at the let-down.
▶ The baby can be fed from one breast only, offering alternate breasts at each feed and expressing some milk from the breast that is not taken. However, the mother should be careful that the milk supply does not decrease too much if only one breast is offered at each feed.
▶ The baby usually settles down and takes the required amount if demand feeding is carried out.

Underfeeding

Underfeeding can be due to either maternal or newborn causes, or both:

▶ *Maternal.* An inadequate milk supply, inverted or retracted nipples or inadequate maternal nutrition can contribute to underfeeding.
▶ *Newborn.* The infant could be unable to take sufficient milk for normal growth and development. This could be caused by a number of factors, such as weakness, vomiting, diarrhoea, immaturity, congenital abnormalities, digestion and absorption problems, infections and other disorders (most high-risk and LBW babies).

Signs of underfeeding

▶ Weight loss
▶ A baby that is often hungry and crying, with winds and colic that cannot be pacified
▶ A very lethargic baby
▶ Small, greenish-brown stools, which are more formed than the usual stool of the breastfed baby and may contain mucus
▶ Reduced urinary output and concentrated urine
▶ Hypoglycaemia.

If not noticed and/or not treated, underfeeding could lead to dehydration and to starvation, with the risk of marasmus and deficiency disorders such as kwashiorkor, scurvy, pellagra, beri-beri, rickets, etc. However, these conditions are more often found in infants who are artificially fed, during the transition from breastfeeding to solids (weaning) and in late infancy.

Intervention and care

The mother's breasts should be inspected and all feeds carefully supervised. If the milk supply is insufficient, the breasts should be stimulated by applying a little heat to them before feeds, for example by a hot shower and warm clothes, followed by a breast massage.

The baby is encouraged to suckle on the breast. If the baby is not suckling well, the mother is encouraged to express milk after each feed. In addition, the mother's nutritional state, Hb level and diet should be checked.

The midwife should carefully observe the baby in the following manner:

▶ Assess the gestational age (GA) of the baby, because an LBW baby may have suckling problems.
▶ Inspect the baby's mouth for thrush or any abnormality of the tongue or palate.
▶ Note any vomiting.
▶ Assess and observe the stools.
▶ Assess and observe the urine.
▶ Observe for excessive crying or lethargy.
▶ Check the temperature – is it raised or subnormal?
▶ Look for any other abnormality.

Any serious problem should be reported to a medical practitioner immediately and the condition treated. If the baby still does not manage to take in enough after all possible problems have been excluded, alternative feeding should be started. This could take the form of an alternative method, such as cup feeding, syringe feeding or IV feeding. The preferred feed is expressed breast milk or formula feed.

39.5 Weaning

Weaning starts when the baby begins to take nourishment other than mother's milk. This does not only refer to introducing solid foods, but also when replacing breast milk with formula milk. Many mothers are hesitant to ask about weaning and may feel vulnerable to criticism. However, weaning is a natural stage in the baby's development.

There is no right time to wean; it is an entirely personal decision. Some babies decide to wean themselves before their mothers have even considered it, while other babies and their mothers go on happily breastfeeding for years.

The decision to give up breastfeeding

A woman may decide to stop breastfeeding for a variety of reasons, such as the following:

▶ The mother is feeling overwhelmed by caring for her baby.
▶ The baby is teething.
▶ The mother is going back to work.
▶ The mother develops breast problems (mastitis), gets sick or is hospitalised or is prescribed medications that may be excreted in breast milk.
▶ There is a lack of support or the woman is pressured by family members or her spouse or partner.
▶ The mother has had enough.

Once a decision has been made to stop breastfeeding, the following principles are applicable:

▶ Minimise stimulation of the nipple (to avoid stimulation of the oxytocin reflex).
▶ Minimise expressing milk (it may be necessary for a few days if the mother is producing a lot of milk and experiences discomfort).
▶ The mother must wear a firm, supporting bra, but should not bind the breasts, as this may result in mastitis.
▶ Medication may be necessary if a mother's milk has been established and milk is then suppressed.
▶ It will take a few days before the milk is suppressed.

Approaches to weaning

There are various different ways in which to wean a baby:

▶ *Gradual weaning.* Eliminating one feed daily will allow the mother's milk supply to gradually decrease, without fullness and discomfort. The mother makes a slow and careful transition from breast to bottle or cup.
▶ *Partial weaning* is an alternative to total weaning. The mother may decide to go back to exclusive breastfeeding at a later stage, or to stop it completely.

▶ *Abrupt weaning* is when there is a sudden, planned or unplanned stop to breastfeeding. This type of weaning is most difficult for both baby and mother, and she will continue to produce milk for a period of time. The baby may experience difficulty in adapting to formula feeds or taking the bottle.
▶ *Natural weaning* is when the process is led by the child. The mother continues with breastfeeding until the child decides to stop.
▶ *Planned weaning* is when the mother decides to stop breastfeeding.

Questions the mother may ask about weaning

Q: The doctor said I should not express any milk, but I am really very sore, my breasts ache and I could not sleep at all last night. What must I do?

A: The mother should express some milk, just enough to relieve the fullness. The following principles apply:

▶ The frequency of expressing will depend on the mother's level of discomfort.
▶ A hot shower or bath prior to expressing may help the mother to relax and stimulate the let-down reflex.
▶ She must wear a nursing pad if she experiences leaking milk.
▶ There is no need for the mother to restrict her fluid intake, but she should restrict her intake of salt to prevent fluid retention.
▶ Parlodel® (bromocriptine) is no longer sanctioned for use, due to adverse drug reactions.

Q: I'm still breastfeeding my one-year-old, but my family are making nasty comments. Should I wean him?

A. It's a great shame if friends and family interfere with the mother's privilege to breastfeed. Exclusive breastfeeding should be encouraged for the first six months and continued for the first two years if possible. The baby is receiving nourishment and comfort and will wean when he or she is ready.

Making the transition from breast to bottle

Some breast-fed babies are reluctant to take a bottle and it may take time for the mother and baby to make a smooth transition from breast to bottle. The following may be helpful:

▶ Try moistening the bottle teat with a few drops of expressed breast milk to tempt the baby to suck.
▶ Do not offer a bottle when the baby is very hungry, as it will be very frustrating for the baby. Instead, offer the bottle when the baby is half-asleep or alert and inquisitive.

- If the mother has a special place where she breastfeeds, she must not offer the bottle feed there, as the situation may trigger the baby's desire for the breast.
- Put breast milk in the bottle so that the milk at least tastes the same.
- Do it slowly, one feed at a time.
- Offer small amounts of milk from a sterilised spoon so the baby gets used to the new taste of formula milk.
- If possible, ask someone else to give the first few formula feeds, as it may be confusing or upsetting for the baby to see, feel and smell the mother's breasts but not be offered them.

Introduction of solids

Babies should not take solids until five or six months. They do not have the necessary enzymes in their saliva and cannot roll food in the mouth. It is thus advisable not to start with solids before five months.

39.6 Replacement feeding (formula)

The choice of whether to bottle-feed or breastfeed the baby is one which all new parents will have to make at some time. Even if pressure is placed on the mother to breastfeed her baby, she may decide during pregnancy to bottle-feed. Other women experience breastfeeding difficulties and then decide to give it up. The introduction of a bottle and the move to formula feed does not necessarily mean the end of breastfeeding.

Midwives need to know about formula feeds. It remains the mother's choice how and what she wants to feed her baby, but it is the midwife's responsibility to provide her with enough information to enable her to make the best possible decision in the interests of the baby's well-being and growth and development.

Different types of formula milk

Formula milk is designed to mimic breast milk as closely as possible. Breast milk contains two different proteins: whey (60 per cent) and casein (40 per cent). The whey, which is watery, quenches the baby's thirst. The casein, also called curd, contains more solids that satisfy the baby's hunger.

Formula milk comes in a number of different forms, namely:

- infant formula (whey-dominant) (0–6 months)
- follow-on formula (6–12 months)
- soya-based formula
- goat's milk infant formula
- heavy (casein-dominant) formula
- special formula.

Infant formula (starter feeds)

This formula contains whey (60 per cent) and casein (40 per cent). It resembles breast milk and should be the first choice for a healthy full-term baby. (An infant that weighs 2.5 kg or more at birth is considered a full-term infant.) Starter feeds may be given from 0 to 6 months but can be continued for longer if the baby is satisfied and growing well according to the road to wellness growth chart (Tarwa & De Villiers, 2007).

The whey-based formulas are highly modified and result in a softer curd, resembling breast milk. Most infant formulas are derived and modified from cow's milk and have the extra advantages of added vitamins and minerals. They are low in sodium. Starter formulas have added long-chain polyunsaturated fatty acids, similar to breast milk. This is necessary for the development of the brain, eyes and nervous system. The formula contains lactose and thus no sugar, honey or syrup should be added. The formula mixes easily: add one scoop to 25 or 30 ml pre-boiled, cooled water.

Note: There are several nutritional differences between formula and human milk. The types of fats in human milk are more easily digested than those in formula and may contribute to better neurological development.

Examples of starter infant formula include S26, S26 Gold, Nan 1 Nestle, Similac 60/40 Ross and Novolac (stage 1). The major difference between starter formulas is that they are produced by different companies. The compositional differences are minor, but there may be a slight taste variance.

Note the following points:

- Follow instructions carefully and do not dilute or add extra powder to the water.
- Sterilise all bottles, teats and equipment for at least the first year.
- Be scrupulous about hygiene and discard left-over milk.
- Write the date that the tin was opened on it.

Formulas should never be changed unnecessarily. Switching formulas too often can cause rather than resolve problems. Specialised formulas such as the lactose-free and anti-reflux formulas should be used only under medical supervision.

Babies do not have the enzymes to digest cow's or goat's milk. The kidneys of a newborn are also too immature to excrete the high sodium and minerals contained in cow's milk. Cow's milk is low in vitamin D and iron and should not be used as infant feeding before 12 months.

Follow-up formula should only be given when the baby is six months or older, as it contains more protein, iron and vitamin D.

Follow-on formula (6–12 months)

Follow-on feeds are for babies older than six months and are to be taken together with solids during the weaning phase. These formulas have a higher protein and sodium content and are casein-based (resembling cow's milk). They contain extra iron, vitamin C and vitamin D.

Examples of follow-on infant formula include Lactogen 2, Infacare 2, Nan 2, Nan 2 Probiotic, Nan HA, S26 Promil 2 and S26 Promil Gold.

Soya-based formula

Soya formula contains protein obtained from soy beans (vegetable protein). This is suitable for a baby with cow's milk intolerance or for a mother who cannot breastfeed but wants to bring her baby up on a vegan diet.

Soya feeds are not safer, cheaper or better than other formulas and should not be given to a baby unnecessarily, as this may lead to dietary intolerance later. They do not contain the milk sugar lactose, but are sweetened with glucose syrup (sucrose and maltose). Soya-based formulas are not suitable for premature babies or babies with kidney problems, as they contain traces of aluminium. They are also not suitable for babies with a family history of allergy to soya products.

Goat's milk infant formula

This formula can be less allergenic than cow's milk, as it does not contain the enzyme gamma-casein. However, goat's milk infant formula is not regarded as nutritionally suitable for babies and should only be given after getting medical advice.

Heavy or casein-dominant infant formula

Casein-dominant formulas contain less whey (which is watery and quenches thirst) than casein (which contains solids and satisfies hunger). These feeds should be offered to the slightly bigger, hungrier or older baby.

Examples of casein-dominant formulas are SMA, Similac, Lactogen 1 and Nan Pelargon. The following products should only be given on medical advice:

- Lactogen 1 is an infant formula designed for use from birth, for the bigger, hungrier baby (with a weight of more than 3.6 kg at birth)
- Nan Pelargon is pre-digested, has a lower pH and is antimicrobial. It is used in babies with diarrhoea or who suffer from colic or for the infant in hygienically compromised conditions.

Choosing a formula

Mothers may choose a formula based on information from family and friends. People may have preferences for particular formula feeds, based on their experience. Factors that influence the choice of formula milk are:

- the type of milk available
- socioeconomic conditions
- literacy level
- the prevalence of breastfeeding in a community
- the gestational age of the baby
- the health condition of the baby (intrauterine growth restriction [IUGR] or galactosaemia)
- allergies
- the availability of clean running water and hygienic conditions.

Complications

Complications associated with replacement or formula feeding include:

- an associated risk of infections, including *Candida albicans* infections from poorly cleaned teats
- increased perinatal and neonatal death
- allergies and eczema
- malnutrition because of incorrect mixing of the milk to make it last longer (resulting in kwashiorkor, marasmus and vitamin deficiency)
- cramps because of milk that was mixed incorrectly
- colic
- lactase deficiency
- constipation or diarrhoea, because the feed is not well suited for the baby
- over- or under-feeding
- more posseting and sour smell, rumination and habitual vomiting and regurgitation
- a higher incidence of grommets due to ear infections related to feeding positions
- upset of the baby's gastrointestinal (GI) system due to changing the types of milk given.

The International Code of Marketing of Breastmilk Substitutes

The midwife should take note of the International Code of Marketing of Breastmilk Substitutes. This code requires (see Behr, 2013):

- that no faces or baby pictures be used when formula is advertised
- that advertisements only be placed in medical journals and not in social publications.

Principles of bottle feeding

The following is important when bottle feeding:

▶ Maintain asepsis and ensure that all bottles and utensils are kept clean or sterile to prevent infections.

▶ Babies should not be propped up and left on their own when drinking. The baby is held in the arms when fed.

▶ The preparation of the milk must be as instructed on the formula tin. Use only cooled boiled water, which prevents the destruction of vitamins. Also ensure accuracy when measuring the powder.

▶ Use only bottles that have been approved as safe for babies.

▶ The amount of food is determined by the age and weight of the baby. Preterm babies require more per kilogram than term babies (see Table 39.1 below and Chapter 42).

Bottle safety

BPA (Bishenol-A) is a chemical used in the manufacture of baby bottles that has been found to be unsafe for babies. These bottles are banned in Canada and the Cancer Association of South Africa (CANSA) has warned against their use.

Table 39.1

Guidelines for volumes for formula feeding

	Term babies: > 2 500g	LBW: < 2 500g
Day 1	60 ml/kg/24 hrs	90 ml/kg/24 hrs
Day 2	90 ml/kg/24 hrs	120 ml/kg/24 hrs
Day 3	120 ml/kg/24 hrs	150 ml/kg/24 hrs
Day 4	150 ml/kg/24 hrs	180 ml/kg/24 hrs

The daily requirements indicated in Table 39.1 can be divided up between five to six feeds in 24 hours. Premature babies and babies that are small for gestational age (SGA) use different formulas because they need more energy for growth. They are fed smaller volumes every three hours (eight feeds a day).

After this, a term baby will be offered 150 ml/kg in 24 hrs. A baby needs 600 ml of milk a day until the age of nine months. Milk remains the main source of nutrition up to the age of three.

39.7 Growth and development

The full-term baby is getting enough food if it gains 25–30 g per day in the first weeks after birth. This is about 170–200 g per week. Babies that are SGA are expected to gain more weight, normally 50–60 g per day. (See Chapter 42 for food requirements for LBW babies.) In addition, a baby with eight wet nappies a day is well fed. If a baby is on formula feeds, the baby must have a bowel movement every day.

The DoH's new growth development chart (DoH, nd) is an essential tool to assess a baby's growth. Note that there are different charts for boys and girls and different charts (see CDC, 2010) for breastfed infants.

39.8 Conclusion

A common feeling among mothers who experience problems with breastfeeding is guilt. While feelings of disappointment on the part of mothers who want to breastfeed but find they cannot is only human, feelings of guilt are frequently unjustified and may be caused by the expectations of healthcare professionals and the community. The midwife plays an essential role in helping the mother with infant feeding, assisting with problems and referring the mother and baby to a paediatrician where necessary.

Section Seven

Newborn care

The physiology, abilities, characteristics and needs of the newborn

40.1 Introduction

Under normal circumstances, all the needs of the fetus are perfectly catered for *in utero*. The placenta supplies nutrition and oxygen and removes waste products. The environment is safe and insulated from shock, trauma, infection and changes in temperature by the placenta, membranes and amniotic fluid.

At birth, the baby is projected out of the warmth and security of the mother's body, into a new, challenging environment. The baby needs to make major physiological adaptations in the new environment to become independent. The main adjustments involve:
- initiating and maintaining pulmonary respiration
- initiating circulatory changes, in order to ensure adequate oxygenation of the whole body
- regulating body temperature
- ingesting, retaining, digesting and absorbing nourishment via the alimentary tract
- eliminating all waste products
- maintaining the full functioning of all the body systems
- protecting the body against infection.

40.2 The respiratory system: Initiation and maintenance of respiration

The initiation of respiration at birth is the most important physiological adjustment to occur. *In utero*, the respiratory tract produces fetal fluid that enlarges the alveoli. Near term, the production of this fluid decreases. There is approximately 40 ml of fluid in the uninflated lungs at birth. During labour, some of the fluid is lost through the nose and mouth. The rest moves into the interstitial spaces, where it is absorbed and removed by lymphatic channels to allow for air to replace the fluid in the respiratory tract.

With the first breath, considerable negative intra-thoracic pressure develops and about half of the air that is drawn in will remain as residual pulmonary air with negative pressure to keep the lungs open. Although considerable trans-thoracic pressure is needed to expand the alveoli, which still contain fluid, this expansion is normally achieved with only a few initial breaths. The negative pressure is brought about by the elastic recoil of the compressed chest wall at birth, the downward movement of the diaphragm and the contraction of the intercostal muscles. With the onset of respiration, there is reduced pulmonary vascular resistance. Once the alveoli have expanded, breathing requires less pressure because surfactant then lines the alveoli, reducing the surface tension, and a functional residual capacity (FRC) is maintained.

Respiration at birth can be divided into two stages: initiation and maintenance.

The initiation of respiration

This process is characterised by sharp intake of air and loud crying and normally should occur within 60 seconds. The newborn experiences mild asphyxia *in utero* as a result of interruption in placental blood flow during uterine contractions. This sets the responses for extrauterine life in motion. Chemo-receptors in the carotid artery and aorta are stimulated by the lowered arterial oxygen tension (PaO_2) and the decrease in arterial pH and rise in carbon dioxide as a result of the cold air and harder surfaces outside the uterus.

The negative pressure created in the thorax required to take the first breath to expand and fill the alveoli is greater than the pressure needed for normal respiration. This pressure is usually 20–30 cmH_2O, but can sometimes be as high as 60 cmH_2O. Phospholipid substances (surfactant) lining the alveoli reduce this tension and prevent the alveoli from collapsing between each expansion. The negative pressure required for breathing after the first few minutes is smaller and is in the region of 5 cmH_2O.

The maintenance of respiration

The initiation of respiration is followed by the maintenance of respiration. This is characterised by quiet, shallow, more rhythmical breathing that is often irregular with short periods of apnoea and ranges between 30–60 breaths per minute. This normally occurs within the first 90 seconds after birth.

Premature infants may adapt well at the initiation of respiration but fail to maintain respiration. In this case the negative pressure in the lungs is not enough (due to a lack of surfactant) to prevent the alveoli from collapsing. Babies born by Caesarean section may have retention of fluid in the lungs, causing transient respiratory problems. Babies with meconium aspiration will have great difficulty in establishing and maintaining breathing until the meconium is removed.

A respiration rate of 80 breaths per minute and above indicates respiratory distress. Grunting (audible sounds) and the use of the intercostal muscles are signs of breathing difficulties.

40.3   The cardiovascular system

From fetal status to newborn, essential changes take place in the cardiovascular system.

Circulatory changes

In the uterus, oxygen exchange takes place from the mother's blood via the placenta to the fetal blood (see colour illustration C12 on page 79). The umbilical vein transports this oxygenated blood to the inferior vena cava and to the right atrium of the heart, where the pressure is greater than in the left atrium. The heart contracts and acts as a pump to distribute the blood, with its oxygen and nutrients, to all the fetal tissues.

At birth, with the maternal link severed, the heart continues to beat, but the pulsations will gradually decrease and cease if oxygen does not continue to reach the brain and the heart muscles. The following paragraphs describe the essential changes that take place during and immediately after birth in the cardiovascular system (also see colour illustration C13 on page 80).

With the first breath at birth and the subsequent inflation of the lungs, the pulmonary vascular resistance is markedly reduced. The fluid that is forced through the alveolar walls into the circulation increases the volume of fluid in the pulmonary circulation and this in turn helps to increase the pressure in the left atrium, making it greater than the pressure in the right atrium and so forcing the valve of the foramen ovale to close by pressing it against the atrial septum.

With the initiation and maintenance of respiration, the oxygen tension in the blood rises, causing the release of prostaglandins which, in turn, cause contraction of the smooth muscle in the wall of the ductus arteriosus. There is a gradual closure of this temporary blood vessel which, after about two months, becomes the ligamentum arteriosum.

When the umbilical cord ceases to pulsate or when the cord is clamped and severed, no blood enters the ductus venosus, which further reduces the pressure on the right side of the heart. The ductus venosus constricts several hours after birth. After about a week it becomes permanently closed and forms the ligamentum venosum, which is attached to the left branch of the portal vein, and the ligamentum teres, which is attached to the liver. The hypogastric or umbilical arteries (which convey blood from the fetal internal iliac arteries to the placenta) also constrict and become the umbilical ligaments.

The normal BP of a term newborn is 60/30 to 80/40 mmHg. The normal pulse of a newborn varies between 110 and 140 bpm.

The haematopoietic system

Normally, the average Hb (18–22 g/dl) and red blood cell (RBC) values are high at birth, but they fall to normal levels by the end of the first month of life. The body breaks down the extra red blood cells and in this normal breaking down process, there is often an accumulation of (unconjugated) bilirubin in the neonatal blood stream, resulting in what is known as physiological jaundice.

40.4 Thermogenesis: Temperature regulation and requirements

At birth, the temperature of the newborn is more or less the same as that of the mother, at 37.2 °C. Within seconds, however, there is a sharp drop in body temperature, brought about by convection, evaporation, conduction and radiation. Although in the newborn – as in an adult – heat is constantly being produced as a result of metabolic reactions, there is greater heat loss from the skin to the environment. This happens because the baby is naked and wet, has a larger body surface area in relation to body weight and has blood vessels that lie closer to the surface of the skin. A newborn does not have the mechanisms for shivering and heating up. Under normal circumstances a full-term baby can usually maintain a normal core body temperature by producing sufficient heat to balance the amount of heat lost; however, there is always the danger of hypothermia at birth – a very serious condition in the newborn baby.

The heat produced by the newborn is mainly through non-shivering thermogenesis, accomplished by increased metabolic activity in the brain, heart and liver from brown fat around these organs. Brown fat is very vascular and is present only in a newborn baby. This unique source of heat (the reserves of brown fat) is laid down in the body during the last few weeks *in utero* and these reserves can be used for several weeks after birth. (Premature infants have fewer reserves of brown fat than term babies and are prone to neonatal hypothermia and cold stress or injury through the rapid metabolisation of these reserves.)

The increased metabolic activity necessary to use brown fat increases heat production by as much as 100 per cent, but at the same time uses up large quantities of oxygen and glucose. Therefore, hypothermia can lead to cyanosis and hypoglycaemia. If the baby is already compromised, the use of large quantities of oxygen and glucose will cause further compromise. In addition, oxygen and energy are diverted from normal functions such as brain cell activity, heart function and growth towards maintaining body temperature (thermogenesis). If neonatal hypothermia is allowed to continue for any length of time, depleting the oxygen in the blood, anaerobic glycosis occurs, which leads to metabolic acidosis.

The baby's temperature can drop to 36.5 °C. The baby must not be bathed until the temperature is stabilised at 36.5 °C. A temperature of less than 35 °C needs immediate intervention.

40.5 The digestive system: Starting oral feeding

The newborn baby needs to suck and swallow in order to obtain food, which has to be retained, digested and absorbed in order to supply the nourishment required for growth and development.

In the uterus, the fetus begins to swallow liquor from about 17 weeks' gestation. At term the baby swallows the same amount of fluid that it will drink after birth, ie 360–400 ml per day in a term infant. If there is an obstruction in the upper digestive tract, there is often an excessive amount of liquor present in the mother (polyhydramnios).

The liquor plays a part in the formation of the meconium. Meconium is made up of mucosal epithelial cells and embryonic secretions, enzymes, bile pigments, urea, mucopolysaccharides and hair. The baby swallows these and the cells accumulate in the digestive system. At birth, the bowel contains about 200 ml of meconium, which is a black, sticky substance. Although peristaltic bowel movements are present in the fetus from about 16 weeks, meconium is usually only passed *in utero* if the fetus is subjected to hypoxia.

The first stool (meconium) of the neonate is a greenish black, viscid, semi-solid substance which is characteristically odourless and sterile at birth. Meconium has a smooth and tenacious consistency. Normally, meconium is first passed within 24 hours after birth.

Once feeding has started, defecation often takes place during or soon after feeds. Feeding stimulates the production of hormones and enzymes in the gut, which are necessary for the digestion of food, and also promotes bacterial colonisation. The normal intestinal flora are essential for digestion and for the synthesis of vitamin K.

As the gut is colonised and the infant starts to feed on milk, the stools change from about the third to the fifth day. This occurs when the last amounts of meconium are passed and when the bowel becomes colonised by bacteria. The type of milk given to the infant will determine the change in the stools. The colour changes to a greenish-brown at first and then a yellowish-brown. Within four to five days, the stool is much softer and looser than that of meconium.

The breastfed newborn has a typical stool from the fourth or fifth day onward, when the gut is colonised by lactobacillus, which protects the gut by preventing the growth of pathogenic organisms. This colonisation is dependent on the first feed being human colostrum. The colour is a rich yellow to orange, but may even be bright green in the transition period. The consistency is soft and possibly semifluid. The number of stools passed varies, from three to five in 24 hours to once in three to five days – whatever is consistent in that particular infant. The stool has a non-offensive odour and the pH of the stool is acidic. As the infant is established on breast milk, the pattern of stools will change. Some babies can go 10 days without a stool (provided they are on breast milk only). Some babies will have 20 stools a day. Both are considered normal for exclusively breastfed infants.

Newborns on formula feeds also pass stools from the fourth or fifth day onward. The colour is a pale yellow, which may acquire a greenish tinge when exposed to air. The consistency is semi-formed to formed. The number of stools is one to two per day, but constipation may be a problem. The stool has a rather strong and offensive odour and the pH of the stool is more alkaline. Small amounts of mucus may be present in any normal stool. When an infant is formula-fed, he or she must have at least one stool a day. A common problem of formula-fed babies is constipation and sore buttocks due to the stools.

The breathing, suckling and swallowing mechanism necessary for oral feeding in the newborn consists of specially co-ordinated movements. The suckling reflex is present *in utero* from 36 weeks. Babies born before 36 weeks often have poor sucking abilities. The newborn baby is unable to move food from the lips to the pharynx (if these passages developed normally) and therefore it is essential for the nipple to be placed well back inside the infant's mouth. Sucking takes place in small bursts of three or four sucks at a time, between breaths. Swallowing and peristaltic activity in the oesophagus moves the food down the oesophagus and into the stomach through the cardio-oesophageal sphincter. This whole mechanism, although not fully co-ordinated at birth, soon becomes efficient in the normal newborn. Persistent lack of co-ordination of sucking and swallowing could indicate brain damage or some anomaly of the upper digestive tract.

The normal baby swallows a variable quantity of air during feeds, most of which is expelled afterwards through burping. Air that is stuck in the stomach and digestive system can cause discomfort and cramps.

Babies have limited enzymes for digestion. The food is partly digested in the stomach and digestion is completed in the small intestine, followed by absorption. These processes are made possible by secretions, hormones and enzymes from the stomach, pancreas, liver and duodenum. Simple carbohydrates and proteins are more easily digested and assimilated than are fats.

The emptying time of the stomach varies greatly in the newborn (from one to 24 hours) and depends upon the time, spacing and volume of the feeds, the type and temperature of the food, as well as other factors such as the infant's size, weight, gestational age (GA), physical well-being and the amount of stress incurred before, during and after labour.

40.6   The renal system

During intrauterine life, the fetal renal system assists in regulating the volume of amniotic fluid. The products of metabolism are transferred from the fetal circulation to the maternal circulation via the umbilical arteries and the placenta.

At birth, the kidneys have to become functional in order to cope with the products of metabolism, but they do not usually reach an adult level of maturity and function before 12 months of age. Therefore, if the kidneys are subjected to any extra load, as may occur with infection, incorrect feeding, vomiting and diarrhoea, this can rapidly lead to acidosis and fluid imbalance, with dehydration or oedema.

A small amount of urine is often voided at birth, but it is quite normal for the neonate not to pass urine in the first 12 hours after birth. A newborn should pass urine within 24 hours. After this, with correct feeding, the infant should pass urine frequently and should wet 6–10 napkins with dilute urine every 24 hours. This will indicate an adequate fluid intake.

40.7   The reproductive system

In the normal full-term female newborn, the ovaries contain thousands of primitive germ cells. The labia majora are well developed and cover the labia minora. The uterus is proportionally the largest organ in the body in a newborn, because of the high levels of oestrogen in the mother. The uterus involutes and becomes more proportional at puberty.

The high levels of oestrogens present during pregnancy often also cause a swelling of the breast tissue in both males and females and a drop or two of a whitish liquid may even be seen exuding from the nipples. This condition (called 'witch milk') will subside as the oestrogen is eliminated from the infant's body; it requires no treatment and is best left completely alone. The drop in the levels of oestrogen in the infant's body after delivery may cause a thick, white mucoid vaginal discharge and slight blood-spotting in baby girls. Vaginal tags are often noted; these gradually shrink and disappear.

In male infants, the testes have usually descended into the scrotum by the end of 36 weeks. The foreskin of the penis adheres to the glans penis and cannot be fully retracted for the first few weeks of life. Undescended testes need to be reported.

40.8   The hepatic system

In the newborn baby, the liver is large and occupies about 40 per cent of the abdominal cavity. Some of the functions performed by the placenta in fetal life, such as the excretion of bilirubin, must now be undertaken by the liver.

In the full-term infant, the hepatic system has normally attained the state of physiological maturity that is necessary for normal body function. Immaturity of the liver could have a number of consequences. The liver may not produce sufficient amounts of the enzyme glucuronyl transferase and the unconjugated bilirubin produced by the breakdown of fetal red blood cells will not be conjugated by the liver. The build-up of unconjugated bilirubin in the bloodstream will cause physiological jaundice and may reach levels that could cause kernicterus (yellow staining of the basal ganglia of the brain), resulting in athetoid paralysis. However, this is more usual in the preterm (immature) infant.

Any obstruction in the hepatic duct system will result in the accumulation of (conjugated) bilirubin, also causing jaundice, which is referred to as pathological jaundice (see Chapter 44).

During fetal life, the liver plays an important part in blood coagulation. This is continued after birth for the first few months of life. In the presence of vitamin K, certain substances necessary for blood coagulation are synthesised in the liver. If the normal gut flora is absent, vitamin K is not synthesised in the gut and is therefore lacking in the liver. This can result in a transient blood coagulation deficiency during the first week of life. To compensate for this, an injection of vitamin K is given to the newborn infant soon after birth.

The liver of the newborn also stores iron for the production of Hb. If the mother has had a diet containing adequate iron, the stores should last for the first five months of life. After this, an iron supplement should be given to the infant if the diet does not contain enough iron for daily needs.

40.9   Immunity

The normal newborn is protected against infection through passive immunity, but is nevertheless highly susceptible to invading organisms. Septicaemia is more common in the neonate than at any other age. It is therefore extremely important that the management and nursing care of the neonate at delivery and after birth are aimed at the prevention of infection.

There is always the danger of cross-infection in the midwifery unit and neonatal nursery. Therefore, the staff must adopt strict anti-infection practices, such as frequent handwashing; cleanliness of cots, linen, feeding equipment, drains, etc; the isolation of infants (and mothers) with suspected or proven infections; and no overcrowding in nurseries.

Immunoglobulins

Immunoglobulins enhance the immunity of the fetus and the neonate. They are a type of antibody secreted by the lymphocytes and the plasma cells and found in the body fluids. The immunoglobulins found in the infant are the antibody fractions IgG, IgM and IgA, acquired from the mother.

Immunoglobulin G (IgG)

The fetus receives IgG *in utero*, as the small molecules of IgG are able to pass through the placenta from the mother's system to the fetus. The type and amount of IgG that the fetus receives depends upon which infections the mother has built up immunity against, the quantity in the mother's system and the GA of the fetus. A preterm baby has less protection than a full-term baby. The length of the acquired immunity is variable and can last from one to four months, depending upon the quantity of IgG received. This antibody fraction is present in all body fluids, both intravascular and extravascular. This type of immunity is called acquired passive immunity.

Soon after birth, the infant's own immunological system begins to manufacture IgG. However, the active antibody synthesis which should take place after immunisation procedures in the first few months of life may be interfered with by the passively acquired IgG antibodies.

IgG antibody fractions with a good transplacental transfer are:

▶ viruses, including rubella, measles, mumps, variola and poliomyelitis
▶ bacteria, including diphtheria and tetanus, and the anti-staphylococcal antibody.

The antibody fraction of *Escherichia coli* appears to have no passive transfer.

IgG antibody fractions that have a poor transplacental transfer are viruses, bacteria and other organisms including *Haemophilus influenzae*, *Bordetella pertussis* (whooping cough), *Streptococci* and the causal organisms of dysentery.

Immunoglobulin M (IgM)

The antibodies of IgM have a larger molecular weight and are therefore unable to cross from the mother to the fetus via the placenta. The infant normally manufactures IgM after birth.

IgM may be found in the cord blood if the mother was subjected to an infection during pregnancy and the fetus also contracts the condition. IgM antibodies are then manufactured by the fetal immunological system. This is a very useful test, because cord blood that contains IgM for a specific organism indicates that the fetus has acquired that infection *in utero* and must therefore be treated accordingly. Some conditions that the fetus can contract *in utero* and which cause the fetus to produce IgM are:

▶ the TORCH diseases: toxoplasmosis, others (such as syphilis), rubella, cytomegalovirus and herpes.

▶ conditions such as maternal measles, chickenpox and hepatitis. These affect the newborn and the baby may be born with the condition.

This type of antibody is confined mainly to the bloodstream and the type of immunity is called active immunity.

Immunoglobulin A (IgA)

IgA is unable to pass through the placenta and is only produced by the infant after the first few weeks of life. The antibody is found in the bloodstream and also in the secretions of the intestines and respiratory tract. This secretory function is active against some viruses, such as poliomyelitis, and also against some strains of *E. coli*. This type of immunity is known as naturally acquired active immunity.

Immunity through breast milk

All three types of immunoglobulins are found in breast milk. Breast milk also contains lactoferrin and transferrin that promote the growth of the bowel flora (lactobacillus).

Cell-mediated immunity

Other means of immunity in the newborn are the T- and B-lymphocytes, which are derived from the thymus gland and which protect against many viral, fungal and bacillus infections. These T- and B-lymphocytes do not become fully functional until two weeks after delivery.

The inflammatory response

The inflammatory response is not well developed in the newborn infant and is poor in the preterm infant.

General genetic make-up

Immunoglobulin synthesis is related to the gene locus on the X chromosome. This therefore favours the female, who has two X chromosomes, one from each parent, rather than the male who has only the one X chromosome from the mother.

The skin

The skin offers a barrier to microorganisms and toxins, protects against infection and plays a vital role in fluid and electrolyte homeostasis. It also helps with thermoregulation. Movement of the limbs and body will be accommodated by the elasticity of the skin. The subcutaneous fatty layers serve as an energy store.

The umbilical cord

At birth, the umbilicus is an open wound and is therefore a very significant place of entry for infection in the newborn baby.

In the first 24 hours, the Wharton's jelly (the gelatinous substance within the umbilical cord) starts to dry up. This causes cord shrinkage, which is greater in a thick cord. It should be carefully checked, as the ligature may become loose, allowing bleeding to take place.

The cord usually sloughs off between the sixth and the tenth day. A delay in cord separation could be due to a low-grade infection. A thick cord takes longer to separate and may be moist, predisposing the infant to the development of omphalitis.

The hepatic system and immunology

The hepatic system was discussed in Section 40.8. In cases of intrauterine infection, the baby may be born with hepatosplenomegaly, which is an enlargement of the liver and spleen due to systemic infections. Infections in the newborn can also present with jaundice.

40.10 The neurological system

The nervous system in the newborn is very immature anatomically and differs from the adult nervous system both chemically and physiologically.

Neuromuscular development

Newborn babies have poorly myelinated nerves (white matter) and 80 per cent of myelination occurs within the first nine months after birth. In the average, normal infant, the post-delivery growth of the brain follows a set pattern. The brain grows very rapidly during infancy and early childhood and then the growth rate begins to slow down.

Because of this pattern of brain growth, the newborn interacts with the environment in a fairly predictable way. However, only a trained and experienced person can readily interpret deviations from the normal pattern. Monitoring of the development of a baby is used to determine normal growth and development after birth. Deviations in an infant's reactions may result from a variety of conditions, both normal and abnormal, namely:

▶ *intrauterine causes* such as intrauterine growth restriction (IUGR), which may be due to placental insufficiency, maternal nutritional deprivation, intrauterine hypoxia, intrauterine infections or congenital disorders

▶ *intrapartum causes* such as hypoxia or anoxia during labour or delivery, birth injuries such as intracranial haemorrhage or oedema or muscular-skeletal injury, etc

▶ *postpartum causes* such as congenital metabolic disorders (for example phenylketonuria [PKU] and cretinism), chromosomal disorders (for example Down's syndrome), neonatal infections (for example meningitis), poor nutrition leading to retarded brain growth, or many other causes such as GA, state of arousal, surrounding temperature, direct medication or medication via the breast milk, etc.

Brain growth affects not only the child's physical growth and sensory capabilities, but also motor function, reflexes and behaviour. Various authorities have been able to draw up assessment charts to assess an infant's neurological and neuromuscular states at birth in order to arrive at the infant's GA, and also to assess progress in infancy and childhood by assessing the child's milestones.

Enzymes

In the neonate, enzymatic activity is not fully operational, as this has been performed to a large extent by the placenta during intrauterine life. Some enzymes are activated before and at birth, but others are only gradually activated as the infant matures. More research needs to be done in this area.

40.11 Conclusion

This chapter focused on the physiological changes from fetal to neonatal life and the adaptations the neonate has to make. The midwife needs to know the normal to identify the abnormal.

41

Assessment and care of the newborn

41.1 Introduction

All newborn babies are assessed at birth and have a full examination and assessment within 24 hours to ensure that they have adapted to extrauterine life and that there are no physical or genetic abnormalities.

The early diagnosis of abnormalities, such as an imperforated anus, greatly increase the chances of successful surgery and frequently make the difference between survival and death. In other cases, such as congenital dislocation of the hips, early detection and treatment prevents or greatly reduces life-long health problems.

41.2 Assessment of the newborn

The assessment of the newborn follows a systematic process that includes assessment and triage at birth, full assessment within 24 hours and daily assessment as indicated in the *Newborn Care Charts* (DoH, 2014a) and discussed in this chapter.

Assessment includes the screening, prioritising, classifying and referral of newborns for routine care, observation, treatment, counselling or follow-up. The following systematic steps form part of the assessment:
1. Taking a history
2. Doing a physical examination
3. Carrying out special examinations.

History

The risk for abnormalities may be present in the history of the family or mother, or may develop in pregnancy or during labour. They may present at birth without any warning. The history of the parents and the obstetric history give information to indicate if the baby is at risk.

If the mother attended antenatal care, risk factors from the antenatal period are reviewed, highlighted and explored before and during labour to prevent serious complications. Where necessary, the mother and fetus are referred for medical care, preferably before the baby is born.

If the woman is admitted without having attended any antenatal care, a full history is taken as soon as possible to identify risk factors. Risk factors are highlighted from the history (see the box below).

History needed for newborn assessment and care after birth

The history of the current pregnancy includes:
- the social history, eg risk factors for drug, medication and alcohol abuse
- the gestational age (GA) of the pregnancy;
- medical and obstetric problems: screening tests for HIV, Rh and ABO blood factors; sepsis; serious problems such as antepartum haemorrhage (APH), pre-eclampsia, preterm labour, fetal growth abnormalities and amniotic fluid abnormalities (polyhydramnios or oligohydramnios)
- fetal warning incidents, such as poor movement
- current medication
- a history of the labour and delivery, including any fetal distress, progress and duration of labour, type of delivery, condition of amniotic fluid (premature rupture of membranes [PROM] or pre-premature rupture of membranes [pPROM]), old or new meconium. See *Guidelines for Maternity Care in South Africa* (DoH, 2015: 52)
- past pregnancies, including history of abnormal babies or genetic conditions such as blood disorders, cleft lip or palate, haemophilia, cystic fibrosis, albinism
- a history of family conditions, such as mental disorders, diabetes, cardiac disease or hypertension
- a history of the fourth stage, including the Apgar score, Silverman-Anderson score and Helping Babies Breathe (HBB) interventions if the newborn was distressed (see the box below and Chapter 46). Note any medication administered. Record the outcome: Was the baby referred for medical care?
- whether the baby was breastfed
- the baby's blood sugar and temperature.

The Apgar score, HBB and the Silverman-Anderson score

The Apgar score (see Chapter 29) is taken at birth and repeated within five and 10 minutes after birth. This gives a good indication of the baby's ability to adapt to extrauterine life. A baby with a low Apgar score, of 6/10 or less, needs to be monitored.

continued

HBB is an approved resuscitation education technique designed to up-skill birth attendants. The HBB training programme and its principles are explained in Chapter 46 and will give birth attendants skills to assist all newborns to breathe at birth and continue with routine care or give specialised care as needed, do triage and refer for medical care.

Babies should breathe independently after 60 seconds and maintain respiration at 60 breaths per minute. While an Apgar score of four indicates asphyxia, at which time the skilled birth attendant takes remedial steps to care for the newborn, the HBB mainly focuses on breathing and correcting the breathing as soon as possible using a learned technique (see Chapter 46).

The Silverman-Anderson score assists the birth attendant to identify respiratory distress in newborns after resuscitation.

Table 41.1

The Silverman-Anderson score

Score	0	1	2
Upper chest retractions	Synchronised	Lag on inspiration	See-saw movement
Lower chest retractions	None	Just visible	Marked
Xiphoid retractions	None	Just visible	Marked
Nasal flaring	None	Minimal	Marked
Expiratory grunting	None	Stethoscope only	Naked eye and ear

Premature babies may have a normal Apgar score at birth (8/10) and deteriorate over the next few hours. The Silverman-Anderson score is used to indicate respiratory distress in the neonate.

Physical examination

The first examination of the newborn is undertaken in the hospital or community setting by competent and suitably qualified professionals.

The purpose of the newborn physical examination is to assess:
▶ the transition of the newborn from intrauterine to extrauterine existence directly after birth
▶ gestational age
▶ physical aspects for identification, such as gender, mass, length and head circumference
▶ any physical or neurological abnormalities present
▶ physiological status.

Principles

▶ The attending midwife is responsible for assessing the newborn directly after birth to determine the need for interventions, resuscitation and referral, especially in the absence of medical assistance during labour.
▶ The presence of a paediatrician during birth does not absolve the midwife from the responsibility of newborn assessment.
▶ The initial assessment must be followed up with a full physical and neurological examination before 24 hours after birth by the postnatal midwife.
▶ It remains the responsibility of the midwife to perform the follow-up assessment if the paediatrician is unavailable to do so.
▶ At discharge, a physical examination must be completed and recorded by the midwife when the mother leaves the health facility.

▶ Referral notes should accompany the mother during transfer and in case of suspected abnormalities, with all relevant details pertaining to the pregnancy, labour, birth, management of the newborn and findings of the physical assessment.
▶ Documentation of all findings must be completed in full in the neonatal assessment document.
▶ The physical examination is only done when the newborn is stable and in a warm environment, both immediately after birth and in 24 hours. The newborn's temperature should be 36.5 °C and above.

Identification of the newborn

The weight, length and head circumference measurement form part of the identification of the newborn and are performed in the presence of the mother or father to prevent errors such as babies being swopped soon after birth. In many institutions, parents sign to indicate the accuracy of the gender and other details of weight and lengths as well as a footprint of the baby, which is imprinted on the documents for identification.

The midwife carefully plots the information on the documents and the baby's growth chart and puts two name bands on the newborn's ankles, as per protocol.

PROCEDURE	The physical examination of the newborn

Action	Physical examination process and rationale
Birth weight (see Chapter 29)	The average weight for term babies (born between 37–41 weeks' gestation) is 3.2 kg, which lies between the 10th and 90th percentile on the growth chart. The baby scale is calibrated and a paper towel placed on it to prevent the baby touching a cold surface. Precautions: The scale is placed on a safe surface. Safety: The baby is in a crib near the scale and the process is done quickly to prevent coldness. The room temperature is 26 °C. The baby is weighed. The weight is checked by a colleague or the father and recorded. The scale is disinfected between use.
Head circumference	The head circumference is measured from the occiput with a tape measure. A term baby's head circumference is 32–34 cm. An abnormally large head may be caused by hydrocephaly. A head smaller than 32 cm after 32 weeks may be caused by microcephaly. A caput succedaneum, haematoma or severe moulding may make readings inaccurate. In the case of a small-for-gestational-age (SGA) baby, a smaller head is symmetrical with a smaller body.

continued

Action	Physical examination process and rationale
Measuring length	Measure the length from the occiput to the heel of the foot. The normal length of a term baby varies between 49 to 52 cm. The method of measurement makes a difference. Best practice is to use a measure board. There are differences between males and females. Male infants tend to be taller, but length is genetically determined and the parent's height is a factor. Short parents may produce short babies.
The vital signs	Temperature is taken to determine if the newborn is able to maintain a stable body temperature in a normal room environment. Normal temperature is 36.5 °C and measures are taken to keep the baby warm and prevent hypothermia. Temperature is measured in the axilla of the arm for two minutes if a low-reading thermometer is used. The pulse is normally 120–160 bpm in the newborn period. The breathing rate is normally 40–60 breaths per minute in the newborn period. Observe the rhythm and synchronicity of chest and abdominal movements. The heart rate and respiration are observed using a stethoscope.
The head	*The head.* Check the shape, size and symmetry in relation to the face and the rest of the body. Check the size and shape of fontanelles. The sutures must be moveable and not too wide and both fontanelles must be present and not bulging. *The eyes.* Check the eyes' position, the presence of epicanthic folds (indicating Down's syndrome), colour, spacing or conjunctiva haemorrhages. Check for the presence of the eye ball and possible cataracts and/or infections. *The ears.* Check that both ears are present and normal. Abnormalities of the ear are associated with abnormal development of internal organs, such as kidneys, and syndromes. *The nose.* Note the shape, patency and presence of discharge or flaring. *The mouth.* Check for patency, presence of teeth and the size of the jaw. A cleft lip is obvious but a cleft palate may be missed. *The tongue.* A protruding tongue may indicate Down's syndrome or hypothyroidism. Tongue ties are common and may need attention.
The neck	The newborn has a short neck. Observations are made for a webbed neck (Turner's syndrome in females). Note an enlarged thyroid.
The chest	*Nipples.* The presence and position of the nipples on the chest is observed. Note any absence of nipples, abnormal positions or extra nipples. *Chest.* The form and shape of the chest is observed as well as the presence of ribs in the rib cage. Babies are abdominal breathers; chest movement in breathing is not normal. Breast engorgement is normal in newborns. This is called 'witch milk' and is due to maternal hormones.
Arms, elbows and hands	Check both clavicles and the ability of the baby to move both arms to exclude birth injuries. Check the rotation ability of every joint. Check for the presence of the normal number of digits. Check for webbing of fingers and tags. The presence of a single palmar line across the palm of both hands suggest Down's syndrome.
Legs, knees and feet	The legs are checked to ensure that they are the same length. The toes are counted for normality. Check and note webbing between toes. The knees and ankles are moved to make sure there is normal function. Talipes or club feet may be present in one or both feet and may be of varying degrees.

continued

Action	Physical examination process and rationale
Hip observations	All midwives need to be able to do Ortolani's test to check for hip dislocation: 1. The long finger is placed on the hip joint. 2. The legs are abducted with the finger as splint. 3. The knee is bent and held in the palm of the hand. 4. A hip click is reported to the medical practitioner.
Genitalia	The following are abnormalities that may be present at birth: • Girls: Fused labia or vaginal bleeding • Boys: Hypospadias, hydrocele or undescended testes.
Back and spine	The fingers of the examiner are run alongside the spine to make sure there is no gap in the spinal column that is not visible or occult. Obvious abnormalities include spina bifida.
Anus	The patency of the rectum is checked if the baby has not passed meconium by the time of the examination. Not passing meconium with 24 hours may be a sign of an imperforated anus.
Skin observations	Observations of the skin are noted and abnormalities are recorded and referred. Normal skin lesions include vernix caseosa, milia and lanugo. Erythema toxicum neonatorum is a rash found in newborns that must be distinguished from skin infections. Abnormalities include: • *Injuries:* Common injuries include skin cuts on the head due to Caesarean section and on the chignon due to vacuum delivery. • *Birth marks:* These may be benign (Mongolian spots, usually on the back) or more severe, such as a strawberry haemangioma, epidermal naevi or malignant conditions such as neuroblastoma. • *Infections:* These include herpes simplex, congenital syphilis, infections from amnionities or bullous impetigo caused by *Staphylococcus aureus*.

The physical examination can be done immediately after birth and does not take more than 5–10 minutes. The neurological observations (demonstrated in the procedure box that follows) are done simultaneously with the physical examination. The neurological observation includes the following reflexes: moro, sucking, grasping, walking, rooting, clenching fists and toes and the sitting position.

Recording and interpretation
Accurately and carefully record all actions and findings.

PROCEDURE Neurological assessment of the newborn (done simultaneously with the physical examination)

Reflex/other: Procedure	Normal characteristics of the term infant	Abnormality
Moro reflex (Figure 41.1):		
The supine position:		
1. Grasp the infant's hands, extend the arms, and release suddenly.	Gives a startled response. Arms fling out in embracing movement, fingers fan out, symmetrically.	Abnormal if absent, asymmetric, weak or incomplete, or exaggerated.
2. Lift the infant's head off a surface into the palm of the hand, then allow head to fall back about 2cm.	Legs may extend and eyes may open wide. Slow return to normal flexed position. Full reflex present from birth, to about 8 weeks.	
Grasp reflex (Figure 41.2):		
1.Palmar: place finger in the palm of the infant's hand.	Finger is firmly grasped by infant's fingers.	Abnormal if absent, asymmetric, weak or incomplete, or exaggerated.
2. Plantar: place finger at base of toes.	Toes curl downward. Present from birth, to 2–3 months.	
Walking reflex (Figure 41.3):		
Hold baby around upper thorax, under arms, in a standing position with feet on a flat surface.	When head and shoulders lean forward, infant simulates walking, by lifting and placing one foot in front of the other (very unsteadily). Present from birth, to 3–6 week. Term infants walk on soles of feet.	Preterm infants walk on toes.
Rooting and sucking reflex (figures 41.4 and 41.5):		
Touch infant's cheek, corner of mouth or lip, with nipple or finger. Must be done before feeds.	Infant turns head toward stimulus, seeking nipple. Opens mouth, accepts nipple and sucks strongly. Both present from birth, rooting goes after 6 months.	Weak suck at birth (preterm, sedation, jaundice, infection, breathing problems, cerebral injury, mental retardation, cleft lip/palate)
Swallowing:		
Offer nipple or bottle.	Sucking co-ordinated with swallowing without gagging, coughing or vomiting.	Weak, absent or not co-ordinated (brain injury or preterm).
Posture and movement (figures 41.6 and 41.7):		
Lying in supine or prone position	Limbs semiflexed, head to one side. Can yawn, sneeze, cough, burp, hiccup. Active.	Abnormal posture. Weak (floppy), asymmetric or absent movement, twitches, fits or convulsions, coma, (preterm, fractures, sedation, brain or nerve injury, congenital and other disorders)
	1. Stretches limbs and curves back. Intermittent clenching of fists and thumb abduction, also of toes. 2. Head turned to one side and lifted momentarily. Hips flexed and tucked under pelvis, which is held up. (Voluntary movements start at about 3 months, when flex or tone recedes.)	

continued

Reflex/other: Procedure	Normal characteristics of the term infant	Abnormality
Muscle tone:		
1. Prone: suspended with palm of hand/s under mid-trunk	1. Spine and limbs keep the semi-flexed position. The neck may extend briefly.	Hypotonia, hypertonia, or asymmetric tone.
2. Supine, lying	2. Arms and legs spring back to flexion, when extended and suddenly released.	
3. Pull up to sitting position with gentle traction, holding wrists.	3. Head lags at first, then is briefly held upright before rolling forward for the chin to meet the chest.	
4. Supported sitting position (Figure 41.8)	4. Back curved, head forward with chin on chest.	
Behaviour: sleeping and wakefulness		
Deep sleep: intermittent sleep, interspersed with waking and feeding. Sleeps for ± 20 hours out of every 24 hours.	Closed eyes, shallow breathing, abdomen rises and falls with breathing, very little limb movement. During dreaming periods: eyelids flicker, face moves, limbs jerk and breathing changes.	Lethargic or over active. Not waking to take sufficient food or not getting sufficient sleep.
Awake	Eyes open, alert and responsive. Limbs, head and trunk move. May cry. Many infants can smile in first 24 hours.	
Crying	Lusty, sustained cry. Eyes close tightly during crying.	Weak cry. High-pitched or hoarse cry. Grunting when asleep.
Vision:		
Supine, lying or sitting	Limited vision. Can follow bright light or object, ie face or hand or red object, up to ± 20 cm away.	Absent or poor following (blindness, dim vision, cataract)
Hearing:		
Voice, shout, bang, music. (Clap hands at side of cot and baby turns head toward sound.)	Moves eyes in direction of sound. Startled by loud noise, may cry. Soon able to distinguish mother's voice.	No response to noise. Deafness.
Touch, taste and smell:		
Touch	Soothed by gentle massage, warmth and cuddling. May be less sensitive to pain in first few days.	Will not be comforted (drug-dependency withdrawal)
Taste	Sensitivity to sweet and bitter tastes is present at birth, but reactions to salty foods don't come until about 5 months.	
Smell	Will try to avoid unpleasant smells. Can soon distinguish 'mother's smell' (breasts).	

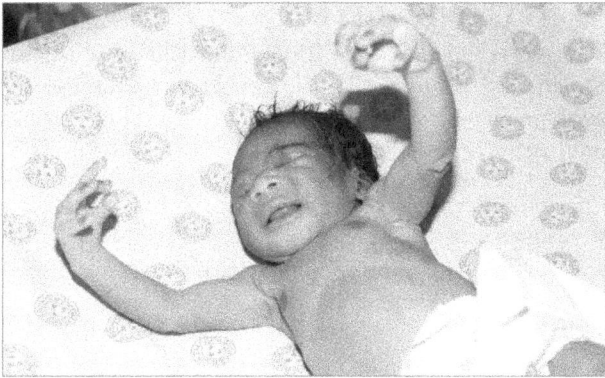

Figure 41.1 The Moro reflex

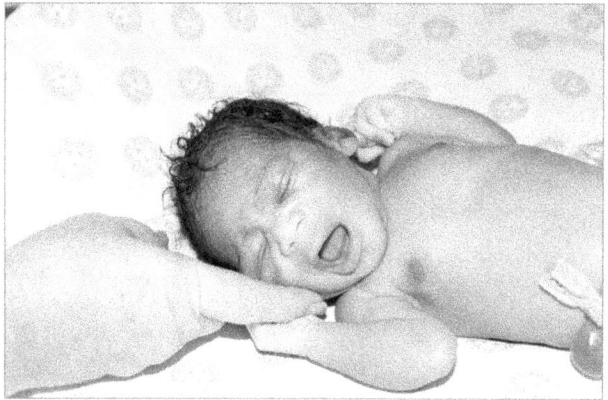

Figure 41.2 The grasp reflex

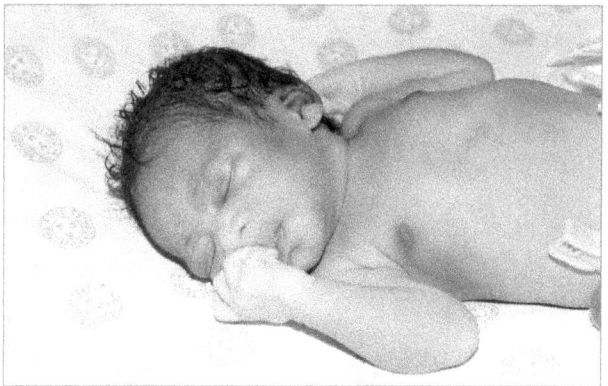

Figure 41.3 The walking reflex

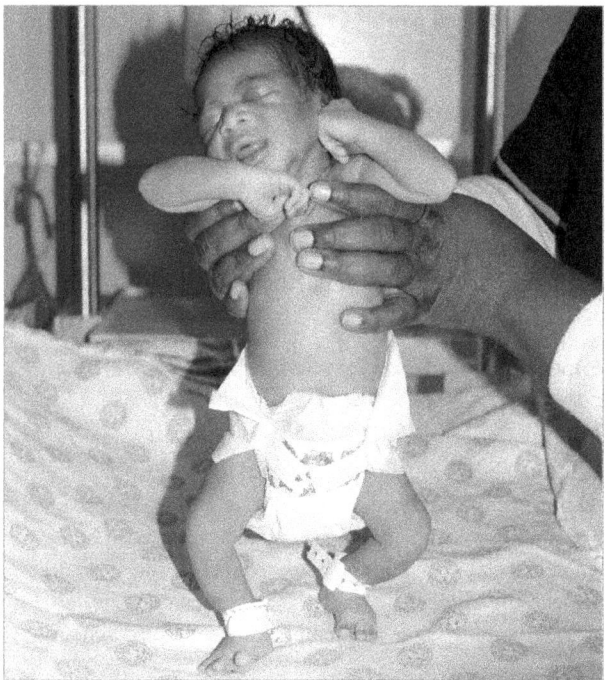

Figure 41.4 The rooting reflex

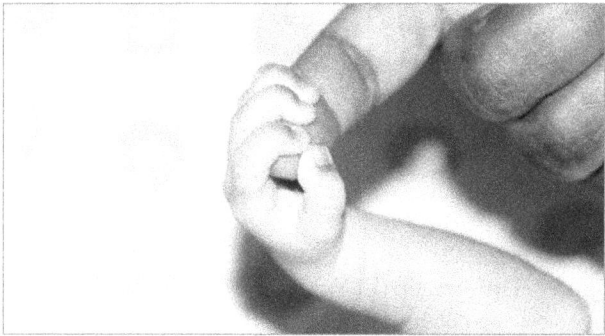

Figure 41.5 The sucking reflex

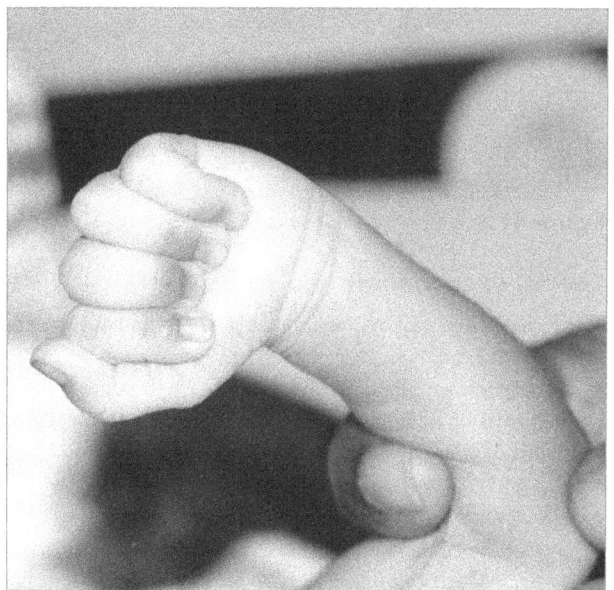

Figure 41.6 Intermittent clenching of fists

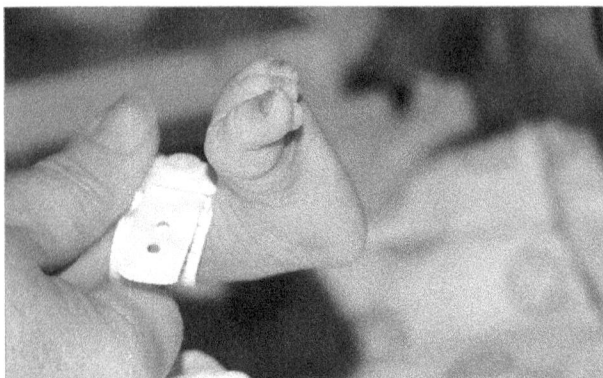

Figure 41.7 Intermittent clenching of toes

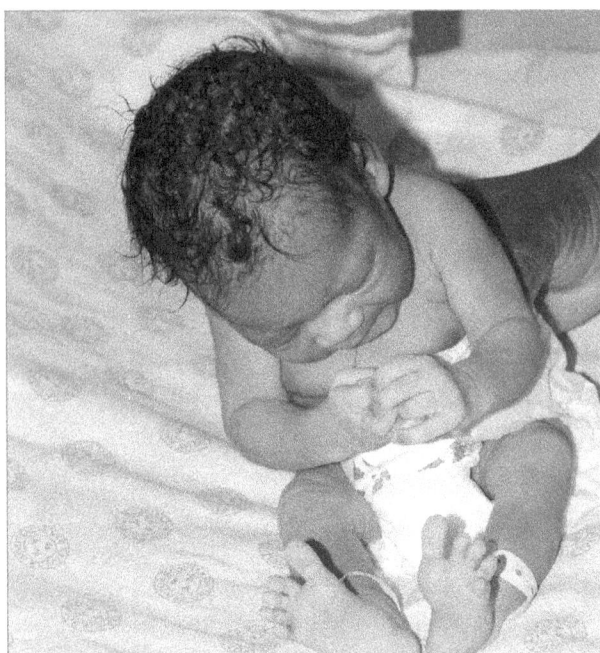

Figure 41.8 Supported sitting position

Special examinations

The following special examinations may be carried out as part of the assessment:

▶ *Gestational age.* The determination of GA through Dubowitz or Ballard scoring is the task of the medical practitioner or advanced midwife (see Figure 42.2 on page 655).
▶ *Blood glucose.* Heel-prick blood can be done for blood glucose. Normal blood sugar is 2.5 mmol/ℓ (45 mg/dl).
▶ *Jaundice.* Cord and maternal blood is gathered and sent to the laboratory in cases where the Rh factor is not known and for all known Rh-negative mothers.

41.3   Newborn care

The *Newborn Care Charts* (DoH, 2014a) are the national Department of Health's (DoH) strategy and guidelines for newborn care in South Africa, particularly for the district and primary healthcare (PHC) setting.

Principles of newborn care include:
▶ maintenance of body temperature
▶ maintenance of respiration and oxygen therapy
▶ maintenance of energy and normal glucose levels
▶ maintenance of fluid balance and feeds for growth
▶ prevention of infections
▶ identification and classification of problems
▶ referral and transfer.

The *Newborn Care Charts* (DoH, 2014a) propose that after assessment at birth, the healthcare professional classify (triage) the newborn as follows:

▶ Babies who are well may continue to be with the mother and receive routine newborn care. They can be discharged within 24 hours and should have follow-up services within three days and six weeks, based on the birth weight.
▶ Low-birth-weight (LBW) babies (< 2.5 kg) who are stable and not critical can be discharged. They must be brought back within three days, then every two weeks, then at four months and finally at nine months.
▶ Sick and small newborns are referred for medical care or to the next level of care and treated as needed.

Immediate and transitional care

After birth and after the physical and neurological assessment of the newborn, the midwife institutes care according to the findings and classification (see above). Regardless of the history and risk factors, each baby is observed through looking, listening and feeling, asking questions, checking and recording data.

Emergency care for immediate life-threatening conditions

All babies are assessed for the need for emergency care immediately after birth and on arrival in the ward. Babies who do not breathe well, are lethargic, have a heart rate of greater than 160 bpm or are hypoglycaemic are prioritised and given emergency care. They are admitted for observation in the nursery. Breathing, respiratory rate, colour, heart rate, lethargy or tone, blood glucose and temperature are monitored.

Actions include the following:

▶ *Hypothermia:* Prevent hypothermia and keep the baby warm.
▶ *Respiration:* Give oxygen (DoH, 2014a: 17–20).
▶ *Cardiovascular:* Call for medical help; establish an IV line with 10 per cent neonatalyte.
▶ *Hypoglycaemia:* Give 10 per cent glucose as per guidelines for volume per age and weight (DoH, 2014a).

Priority care for life-threatening situations

All newborns are observed for priority care in the transitional period. Observe for any of the following:

▶ Observe for apnoea or no breathing for 60 seconds. Stimulate breathing:
  • Babies with signs of severe respiratory distress and a respiration rate of 60 breaths per minute are started on oxygen.
  • Preterm babies are started on continuous positive airway pressure (CPAP), sent for a chest X-ray, have hourly observations, are nil per mouth (NPM) for 24 hours and are started on antibiotics.
  • Babies with central cyanosis but no chest recession and grunting are potentially having cardiac problems; therefore, start oxygen and refer for medical care.
  • LBW babies are treated in accordance with the *Newborn Care Charts* (DoH, 2014a).
▶ Abnormal signs and symptoms, high or low temperature, not feeding, low tonus, lethargy, jerky movements, abdominal distension, vomiting and jaundice within 24 hours are cared for as per the *Newborn Care Charts* (DoH, 2014a).
▶ Babies with abnormal conditions such as neural tube defects (NTD) or gastrointestinal (GI) defects are cared for by covering the lesions with Opsite and referring for tertiary care.
▶ In cases of hydrocephaly, microcephaly, clubfeet or cleft lip or palate, start feeding, support the mother and refer for medical care.
▶ For care of HIV-positive mothers, see Chapter 50.

Routine postnatal care

Babies who are low risk can safely be cared for with the mother. The following specific actions are recommended:

▶ On transfer, identify the newborn and keep him or her with the mother at all times, allowing demand feeding.
▶ Weigh the newborn daily and record the weight.
▶ Record routine observations, including 12-hourly temperature, respiration, heart rate, colour and activity.
▶ Newborns are 'topped and tailed' and the vernix is left to be absorbed.

▶ Surgical spirits are applied to the cord six-hourly.
▶ If the mother tests positive on the rapid plasma reagin (RPR) test, examine the baby for congenital syphilis and follow guidelines.
▶ If the mother's RPR status is unknown, take blood from the mother and baby and treat according to results.
▶ For mothers who have had TB within the last six months, observe the newborn for respiratory distress and follow protocol (see Chapter 50).
▶ If the mother is HIV positive, follow treatment protocols (see Chapter 50).
▶ If the mother's HIV status is unknown, counsel and test for HIV and manage according to protocol.
▶ If the mother's blood group is O negative, then check total serum bilirubin (TSB) at six hours. Start or refer for phototherapy if TSB is more than 80 µmol/ℓ. (If unknown, check the mother's Rh factor.)
▶ Do daily observations of the baby in the presence of the mother, using the examination chart. Check for jaundice, the eyes, the umbilical cord and the buttocks. Check whether the baby has passed urine and meconium. Ask the mother if she has any concerns.
▶ Assist with breastfeeding or replacement feeding.
▶ Give routine preventative care, including polio drops and the Bacilli Calmetti-Guérin (BCG) vaccine within five days.
▶ Before discharge, give vitamin K and eye prophylaxis.

Discharge

In the PHC setting, after normal birth and if the baby is not at risk, the mother and baby will be discharged within 24 hours. Under these circumstances there is limited contact with the mother and midwives need to follow strict guidelines to ensure that the mother receives the needed care and information.

The midwife develops a discharge plan, checks all the risk factors and makes sure that the preventative treatments have been done before discharge. The midwife also provides:

▶ a follow-up appointment date to visit the nearest clinic within three days and at six weeks
▶ emergency contact details
▶ information on danger signs and symptoms for the baby.

The following are noted and recorded on discharge:

▶ Does the baby suck well? How often?
▶ Is the baby satisfied?
▶ Are the nipples and breasts normal?
▶ Has the baby passed meconium?
▶ Has the baby passed urine?
▶ Is the temperature normal?

▶ How is the baby's behaviour? Is the baby alert? How is the sleep–wake cycle?

▶ What is the skin colour? Is there any jaundice or risk of jaundice?

▶ Is there any discharge from the eyes?

▶ How is the cord? Is it drying and clean?

▶ Were any vaccines given?

▶ Is blood sugar normal?

▶ Is the HIV status known?

▶ Are there any maternal risks present?

41.4   Conclusion

The assessment of the newborn starts before birth in the antenatal period and continues during labour, immediately at birth, in the transitional period and daily thereafter. The skilled midwife will identify problems early and intervene appropriately and on time to prevent morbidity and mortality. Education of the parents is a very important aspect of care.

Disorders of maturation, growth and development in the newborn

LEARNING OBJECTIVES

On completion of this chapter, you must be able to:
▶ demonstrate competency in the care of specific categories of newborns
▶ demonstrate competency in kangaroo-mother-care (KMC)
▶ demonstrate competency in incubator care.

KNOWLEDGE ASSUMED TO BE IN PLACE

Fetal development *in utero*

The anatomical, physiological and psychological adaptation of a neonate after birth (see Chapter 40). *Newborn Care Charts:* paragraphs 2.1.1 to 2.1.4, 2.2.2 (DoH, 2014a)

KEYWORDS

extreme low-birth-weight (LBW) neonate • LBW neonate • preterm neonate • small for gestational age (SGA) • post-term • large for gestational age (LGA) • intrauterine growth restriction (IUGR)

42.1 Introduction

The last few weeks of pregnancy are a period of maturing, with physiological processes such as the addition of subcutaneous fat; maturing of the liver, lungs and gastrointestinal (GI) system; and the increased production of glycogen in the liver. Most babies are born between 38 and 42 weeks.

Babies born before 37 weeks' gestation are considered premature, with immature organs. Those born after 42 weeks are post-mature and have reduced body fat, as fat was used to sustain them *in utero* (placental function is reduced after 36 weeks; hence the need to use up fat stores). Mortality and morbidity are increased in babies born under 37 weeks or after 42 weeks.

42.2 Definitions

▶ The *preterm infant* is a baby born before 37 completed weeks of gestation.
▶ The *small-for-gestational-age (SGA) infant* – or the 'light-for-dates baby' – has a weight below the 10th percentile for GA standards. These babies may or may not also be preterm.

▶ The *large-for-gestational-age (LGA) infant* has a weight above the 90th percentile for GA standards. Although the birth weight is high, these babies may also be preterm. These babies are usually born of mothers with diabetes mellitus (latent or clinical).

42.3 Assessment of gestational age and maturity

As shown in Figure 42.1 on the next page, babies can be categorised based on birth weight:
▶ SGA babies are under the 10th percentile.
▶ Appropriate-for-gestational age (AGA) babies are between the 10th and 90th percentile.
▶ LGA babies are above the 90th percentile.

Although Figure 42.1 is a useful guide, it is not an accurate reflection of GA or maturity. After birth, GA and maturity can be accurately gauged by using the Dubowitz or Ballard scores (see Figure 42.2 on page 655) or the simpler SPLEN method (see Figure 42.3 on page 656). The SPLEN method is very useful for the initial assessment of all babies born at outlying clinics. In this way, any high-risk baby can be quickly identified and transferred to hospital. Scoring should be done within the first 72 hours of birth for accurate results. (See the discussion on page 657.)

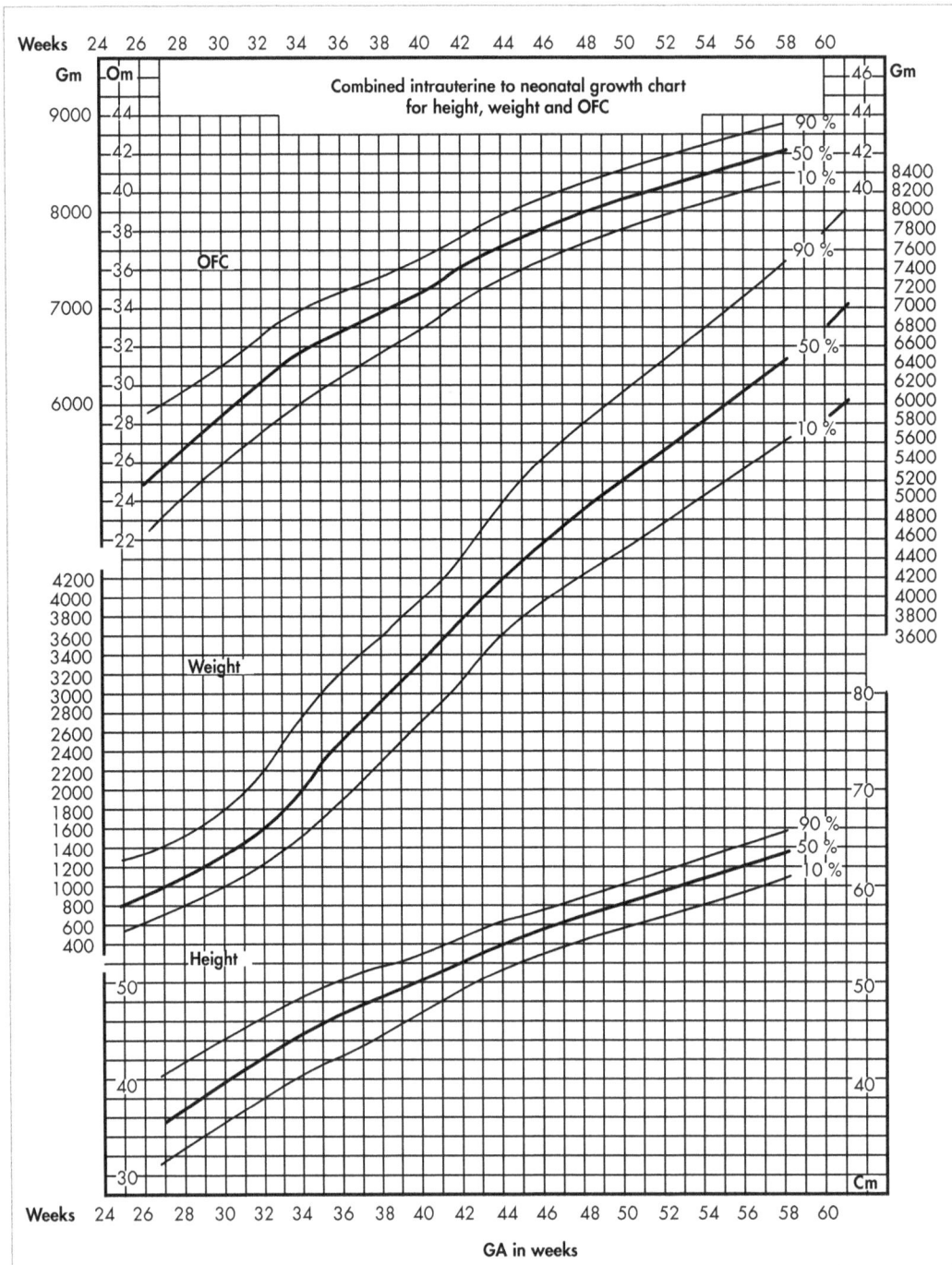

Figure 42.1 The standards of weight, length and head circumference for assessing GA, according to percentiles (adapted from Riddle et al, 2006)

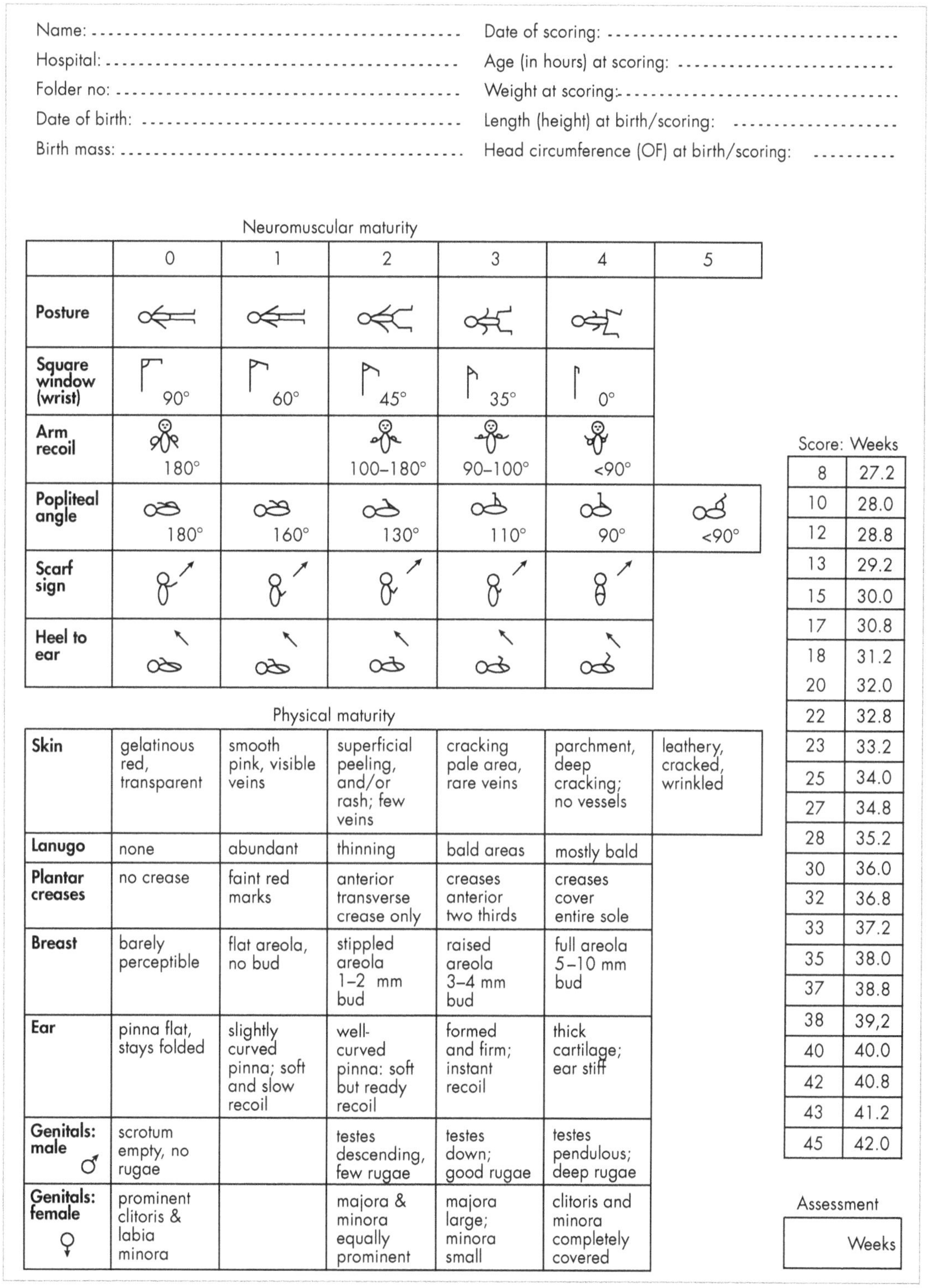

Name: --

Hospital: ---

Folder no: ---------------------------------------

Date of birth: ------------------------------------

Birth mass: --------------------------------------

Date of scoring: ----------------------------------

Age (in hours) at scoring: ------------------------

Weight at scoring: --------------------------------

Length (height) at birth/scoring: ------------------

Head circumference (OF) at birth/scoring: ----------

Neuromuscular maturity

	0	1	2	3	4	5
Posture						
Square window (wrist)	90°	60°	45°	35°	0°	
Arm recoil	180°		100–180°	90–100°	<90°	
Popliteal angle	180°	160°	130°	110°	90°	<90°
Scarf sign						
Heel to ear						

Physical maturity

Skin	gelatinous red, transparent	smooth pink, visible veins	superficial peeling, and/or rash; few veins	cracking pale area, rare veins	parchment, deep cracking; no vessels	leathery, cracked, wrinkled
Lanugo	none	abundant	thinning	bald areas	mostly bald	
Plantar creases	no crease	faint red marks	anterior transverse crease only	creases anterior two thirds	creases cover entire sole	
Breast	barely perceptible	flat areola, no bud	stippled areola 1–2 mm bud	raised areola 3–4 mm bud	full areola 5–10 mm bud	
Ear	pinna flat, stays folded	slightly curved pinna; soft and slow recoil	well-curved pinna: soft but ready recoil	formed and firm; instant recoil	thick cartilage; ear stiff	
Genitals: male ♂	scrotum empty, no rugae		testes descending, few rugae	testes down; good rugae	testes pendulous; deep rugae	
Genitals: female ♀	prominent clitoris & labia minora		majora & minora equally prominent	majora large; minora small	clitoris and minora completely covered	

Score:	Weeks
8	27.2
10	28.0
12	28.8
13	29.2
15	30.0
17	30.8
18	31.2
20	32.0
22	32.8
23	33.2
25	34.0
27	34.8
28	35.2
30	36.0
32	36.8
33	37.2
35	38.0
37	38.8
38	39,2
40	40.0
42	40.8
43	41.2
45	42.0

Assessment
Weeks

Figure 42.2 Scoring system for simplified clinical assessment of maturation in newborn infants (adapted from Hall et al, 2014)

Signs of physical maturity	Score			
	0	**1**	**2**	**3**
Skin	Smooth, pink, visible veins.	Superficial peeling or rash. Few veins.	Cracking, pale areas of skin.	Leathery, deep cracking, and wrinkled.
Plantar creases	Anterior transverse crease only.	Creases on anterior two-thirds of sole.	Creases over whole sole.	Creases over whole sole.
Labia or male genitals	Clitoris and labia minor are prominent. No testes in scrotum.	Labia majora and minora equally prominent. Testes high in scrotum.	Labia majora cover minora. Testes low in scrotum. Rugae seen.	Labia majora deeply pigmented. Deep rugae.
Ear	Slightly curved pinna. Slow recoil.	Well-curved pinna. Soft with ready recoil.	Ear formed and firm with instant recoil.	→
Nipples	Flat areola. No bud.	Raised areola. Bud larger than 5 mm.	→	→
1. The score obtained from examining the infant as above is added to 30 in order to arrive at the number of weeks gestation.				
2. The infant's birth weight (and head circumference and length) is compared to the **Number Of Weeks Gestation** on the **'Percentile Chart'** (Figure 42.1) and the examiner is then able to assess whether the infant is small, average or large for the GA. (Average for GA: between 10th and 90th percentiles.)				

Figure 42.3 The SPLEN method of rapid gestational ageing

Physical maturity characteristics of the newborn are assessed as well as neuromuscular characteristics. These are plotted on a scale that will indicate the GA.

In order to ascertain whether the neonate is within the average age standards for weight, as well as for overall length and head circumference, the score obtained by using the methods above should be plotted on a graph that has been specifically devised for this purpose.

In this way, the examiner can work out whether the neonate falls within the average standards for his or her GA. For example, if the weight of a neonate of a certain GA falls below the 10th percentile, the neonate is below weight for GA. The neonate is thus SGA and has intrauterine growth restriction (IUGR). The same applies to the length and the head circumference.

Table 42.1

Classification of newborns based on birth weight

Classification	**Percentile**	**Weight**
Low birth weight (LBW): SGA	Below 10th percentile	Premature or IUGR 1.5–2.5 kg at birth
Very LBW (VLBW)		1–1.5 kg
Extreme LBW (ELBW)		Less than 1 kg
AGA	Between 10th and 90th percentile	Within normal range for GA or 2.5–3.5 kg at term
LGA	Above 90th percentile	More than 3.5 kg at term or higher than for GA

On the other hand, if the weight of a neonate is above the 90th percentile for GA, then the neonate is LGA, and is probably the neonate of a mother with either latent or clinical diabetes mellitus.

42.4 Classification of maturity

The classification of the maturity of a fetus at birth depends on the history of the pregnancy, the first day of the last menstrual period (LMP) (if accurate), the time of the first visit, the physical and/or special examination findings before 20 weeks (whichever is more accurate) and serial physical and/or ultrasound examinations in the second and third trimesters.

At birth, the birth mass, length and head circumference, physical characteristics and neurological observations and behaviour give an indication of the GA. All these measures can be determined against set scientific charts that assist to determine the GA (regardless of other factors). The estimation of GA in pregnancy is indirect, while the determination of GA after birth is direct and more real and accurate.

Characteristics of the preterm baby

▶ *Weight.* This depends on the GA, but less than 2 500 g is considered LBW.
▶ *Length.* The length of the preterm baby is 49 cm or less.

▶ *Head circumference.* The head circumference is 34 cm with soft skull bones and sutures and fontanelles that are relatively wide for the small head. The ears are small and the cartilage soft and pliable.
▶ *Skin and subcutaneous tissue.* The skin is thin, red and smooth and is easily broken. There is little subcutaneous fat and the bony structure is easily seen. The blood vessels are clearly visible under the thin skin and are fragile. The skin creases are poorly developed. Lanugo is plentiful and vernix caseosa is sparse. The nails are short and soft.
▶ *Respiratory system.* Respiration is abdominal and the soft rib cage may indent between the ribs and at the sternum – called rib retraction and sternal retraction. If there is a lack of surfactant, the lungs collapse and the baby makes a noise on exhaling, called expiratory grunting. The respiration is faster than 60 breaths per minute. The Silverman-Anderson score can be used to identify the presence of respiratory distress and/or the development of hyaline membrane disease (HMD).
▶ *The reflexes.* The sucking reflex is weak but present at 34 weeks. The sucking reflex is strong after 36 weeks.

General appearance

▶ In a preterm female infant, the clitoris and labia minora are prominent while the labia majora are underdeveloped. In a male infant, the testes may not have descended into the scrotum before 36 weeks.

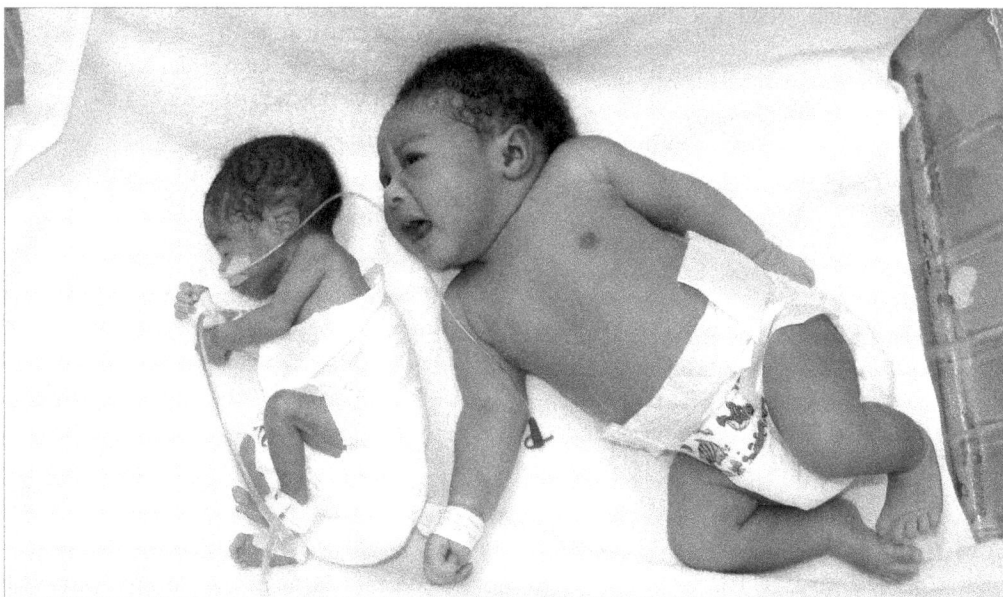

Figure 42.4 Differences between a term and a preterm baby

- The hair is soft and silky.
- The breast nodules are small or absent.
- The hands and feet are often oedematous.
- The abdomen is relatively large and easily distended.
- The posture of the baby after birth is a very good indicator of GA. The legs and arms are extended before 32 weeks. The legs are flexed by about 32 weeks and the arms by 34 weeks. A term baby lying supine will take up a normal position, with the head turned to one side, lying slightly on one side with the arms and the legs flexed.
- The baby sleeps most of the day, but often stretches and yawns from 32 weeks' gestation.

Characteristics of the immature or small-for-gestational-age baby

- *Weight.* The weight is low for GA and below the 10th percentile.
- *Length.* The length is below the 10th percentile.
- Head circumference. In asymmetric growth restriction, the head is larger than the body (out of proportion) because the brain was given preference in development. In symmetric growth restriction, both the head and the body are smaller than usual. The skull bones are firm and the head circumference is below the 10th percentile.
- *Hair.* The hair is sparse, coarse and straight.
- *Ears.* The ear cartilage is well developed.
- *Skin and subcutaneous tissue.* Loose, peeling, meconium-stained skin is present, with creases on the soles of the feet, indicating the gestational period. The skin may be dry and scaly. There is a lack of subcutaneous tissue. Meconium staining is present on the skin, nails and umbilical cord.
- *General appearance.* The baby has a wasted, dehydrated look. The baby appears to be thin, long, wasted and wizened. Some babies appear to be dwarfed, with a reduced weight (below the 10th percentile). The baby is active and hungry at birth. The infant has a scaphoid (boat-shaped) abdomen.
- *Respiratory system.* The thoracic cage is relatively small, with the rib cage easily seen. Breathing is usually irregular in rate and depth and there may be periods of apnoea. The breathing is abdominal. The nostrils are small and easily blocked. The crying is often weak and may be high-pitched. The cough reflex is weak or absent.

LBW or SGA babies can be preterm, term or post-term. It is thus important to plot the findings on the percentile chart to make the right decision. A preterm or post-term infant that is also growth restricted has a higher risk of morbidity. Often babies that were growth restricted *in utero* have more mature organs and are more able to adapt after birth.

Characteristics of the large-for-gestational-age or post-term baby

- *Weight.* An LGA baby is above 3 500–4 000 g at term or on the 90th percentile for GA, regardless of weight.
- *Length.* The baby's length is more than 52–58 cm.
- *Head circumference.* The baby has a head circumference of 35 cm and more. The skull is hard, with narrow sutures and small fontanelles.
- *Skin and subcutaneous tissue.* The toe- and fingernails are well developed. The ear cartilage and the nipples are well developed. The skin is often loose, and may be dry and peeling. The skin may be meconium-stained. If the baby is post-mature, the subcutaneous fat may be diminished, giving the baby the appearance of an old person.
- *General.* The genitalia are well developed.
- *Respiratory system.* Respiratory distress may be present if there was meconium in the amniotic liquor.

A baby may be LGA due to the overproduction of insulin *in utero* in diabetic mothers. These babies may be completely normal, or may be macrosomic and at risk.

42.5   The low-birth-weight baby

LBW newborns can either be premature or have IUGR. It is important to be able to differentiate so as to give the best care for the situation. Each case has its own set of risks and problems. Some newborn babies are premature and also growth restricted, and as such may be more at risk.

Causes

There are maternal, obstetric, fetal and other causes of LBW. Some of the causes include:

- premature birth
- accidents and trauma that may cause early or premature birth
- infections or disease of the mother that may threaten the growth and development of the fetus *in utero*
- IUGR
- multiple pregnancy
- maternal health issues such as using drugs, alcohol and smoking
- poor maternal nutrition, which could be due to lower socioeconomic status
- inadequate prenatal care
- pregnancy complications, such as pre-eclampsia

- perinatal infections
- HIV
- congenital abnormalities.

African women are twice as likely as Caucasian women to have LBW babies, and teen mothers also have a greater likelihood.

Common problems

The basic problem of the LBW baby is immaturity of the organs:

- An immature respiratory system may lead to HMD or respiratory distress and/or apnoeic attacks (see Chapter 46).
- An immature GI system with poor sucking leads to an inability to breastfeed, digestive problems, low capacity for food and the risk of necrotising enterocolitis (NEC) associated with shock and tissue necrosis of the gut (see Chapter 43).
- An immature liver may predispose the infant to blood clotting problems (intraventricular haemorrhage due to vitamin K deficiency), hypoglycaemia and jaundice (see Chapter 44).
- A lack of brown fat may cause hypothermia and hypoglycaemia (see Chapter 40).
- An immature immune system and responses predispose the baby to infections (see Chapter 44).
- Iatrogenic problems (pneumothorax) can occur due to the high pressure of oxygen. Chronic lung disease (bronchopulmonary dysplasia [BPD]) can occur due to high levels of oxygen (toxicity) and the pressures of ventilators (barotraumas).
- Retrolental fibroplasia (see the box below) is damage to the retina that leads to blindness. It is associated with high levels of oxygen during ventilation.

Retinopathy in newborns

The blood vessels in the inner retina begin to grow halfway through pregnancy and are only fully developed by term. They are thus incompletely developed in the preterm infant. The more immature the infant is, the less vascular development has taken place. Out of babies of less than 1 kg at birth, about 80 per cent develop retrolental fibroplasia (also called retinopathy of prematurity, or ROP). The continuous administration of high dosages of oxygen after birth increases the risk of ROP.

High-quality care is the key to survival and positive outcomes for premature and LBW babies. Babies above 1 500 g are less at risk of ROP. Intervention starts with the prevention of LBW in infants.

Other complications may include impaired bonding caused by separation from the mother for long periods, tissue damage due to intubation and the pressure caused by tubes, and thrombosis due to arterial lines that may cause a loss of a limb.

The prevention of low birth weight in infants

The high incidence of LBW in babies necessitates early intervention and prevention. The following principles must be observed:

- Identify high-risk mothers at early antenatal visits.
- Suppress preterm labour for long enough to transfer the patient to a Level 2 or 3 facility or until corticosteroids have been administered (see the box below).
- Where possible, the mother is transferred to the best level of care before the baby is born.
- Prepare for complications before the baby is born.

Prophylaxis against HMD

The IM administration of corticosteroids to the mother in two dosages 12 hours apart between 32 and 34 weeks of gestation greatly reduces the incidence of HMD (see Chapter 23).

Immediate care of the low-birth-weight baby

If the baby is born before referral takes place, the following steps should be taken:

- The baby with a low Apgar score should be resuscitated immediately after birth. (See the information on Helping Babies Breathe [HBB] in Chapter 46.)
- Provide medical care as soon as possible.
- Conduct a full physical and neurological assessment (see Chapter 41).

Standard care for low-birth-weight infants

The care of an LBW or SGA infant, whether premature or growth restricted, is aimed at the provision of an optimal environment and support for the immature organs, in order to ensure survival. All preterm and LBW babies are admitted to high-care units and given hourly observations.

The physical immaturity of the baby is the basis of the care and includes all of the items discussed below.

Maintain respiration

See the *Newborn Care Charts*, para 2.2.1 (DoH, 2014a):

- Keep the airways clear.
- Suction secretions hourly and when needed.
- Administer oxygen by funnel. Oxygen is humidified and warmed.

▶ Measure oxygen saturation through a pulse oximeter and maintain between 89 and 92 per cent.

Maintain oxygenation

See the *Newborn Care Charts*, para 2.2.1 (DoH, 2014a). Oxygenation is achieved by continuous positive airway pressure (CPAP). A nosepiece that fits into the nostrils is effective (nCPAP, or nasal CPAP), as it increases the residual capacity and reduces respiratory effort significantly. All babies at risk of developing HMD should be started on CPAP.

Prevent hyaline membrane disease

The paediatrician may prescribe surfactant for babies over 750 g. It is injected into the trachea in divided doses (100–200 mg/kg). It is given soon after birth and reduces mortality and morbidity in 70 per cent of cases. A second dose may be needed for 30 per cent of cases (Wikipedia, 2017).

Maintain a thermo-neutral environment of 36.5 °C

See the *Newborn Care Charts*, para 2.2.1 (DoH, 2014a):
▶ All precautions are taken to maintain the baby's temperature at 36.5 °C. (The room temperature in a neonatal unit is 22–26 °C.)
▶ The baby is not bathed but dried.
▶ The baby is nursed in an incubator or open crib. The normal temperature of an incubator is 32 °C.
▶ The baby's temperature is recorded hourly if stable.
▶ If the baby weighs less than 1 kg, the incubator temperature is set to 38 °C and the baby is covered with cling wrap or space blankets.
▶ Extra interventions to prevent heat loss include covering the baby's head (most heat is lost from the head) and kangaroo-mother-care (KMC) (if the baby's condition is stable).

Maintain fluid balance

See the *Newborn Care Charts*, para 2.2.2 (DoH, 2014a). Start an IV line and give fluids. Keep a record of intake and output. A baby with a weight of less than 1 500 g should be given IV neonatalyte (without potassium) or 10 per cent dextrose water, 60 ml/kg/day. If the baby can suck, he or she can be breastfed or can take expressed breast milk (EBM) per cup, which is given for babies over 1 500 g.

Maintain the blood glucose

Test the blood glucose four-hourly and maintain through IV fluid and milk feeds if allowed. A blood glucose of less than 2.5 mmol/ℓ is treated as an emergency.

Maintain energy and feed

See the *Newborn Care Charts*, para 2.2.2 (DoH, 2014a). Newborn babies of less than 1 000 g with respiratory distress, or extremely small newborns, are started on EBM from the mother or from the milk bank if stable from day 2, given three-hourly through a nasogastric tube. The fluid is administered intravenously for newborn premature babies weighing 1.5–2 kg, the total fluid requirements being determined based on scientific guidelines.

The total fluid requirements for preterm newborns depend on their weight and condition. The smaller the preterm, the higher the fluid requirements. The average fluid is calculated as follows:
▶ Day 1: 90 ml/kg/24 hrs (< 1 kg/100 ml and 1/2 ml EBM 2-hourly)
▶ Day 2: 120 ml/kg/24 hrs
▶ Day 3: 150 ml/kg/24 hrs.

Note: If the baby is extremely small or sick (with infection) or receiving phototherapy, the fluid intake is increased by 10–20 per cent.

A special dummy is available to help the baby to develop the sucking reflex. A nasogastric tube is inserted (size 6–8) to drain the stomach contents and feeds may be started within two to three days. EBM is the milk of choice. There is a reduced incidence of NEC when breast milk feeds are given.

Prevent and treat infections

▶ The baby is cared for in its own micro-environment and the use of communal surfaces is avoided. Each baby has his or her own thermometer and utensils.
▶ Washing hands before and after handling the baby is a principle of care. Parents are encouraged to wash their hands when entering the unit and before touching the baby.
▶ Antibiotic treatment is given according to prescription. The guidelines for antibiotic therapy are found in paragraph 2.2.2 of the *Newborn Care Charts* (DoH, 2014a).
▶ The incubator is cleaned daily.
▶ Only sterile utensils are used.
▶ Drip packs and tubes are changed daily.
▶ The eyes are cleaned with normal saline.
▶ The cord is treated daily with alcohol.

Encourage bonding

Keep the parents and the baby together if possible to encourage bonding. If the baby is out of danger, KMC can be instituted.

Observations

Half-hourly observation is essential when caring for sick or SGA babies. The following actions are strictly done, observed and recorded:

- Body temperature: every four to six hours
- Heart rate, BP, respiration and colour
- Incubator temperature
- Oxygen concentration and saturation target, which must be 88–93 per cent
- Blood glucose: every three to four hours
- Intake and output: continuously
- Serum bilirubin: daily
- IV drips and other device sites on the baby
- Routine care of lips, buttocks, eyes and cord
- Stool, urine, vomit and aspiration
- Feeding instructions and daily intake
- Medical prescription(s), including feeds
- Education and support of parents
- Supporting and positioning the neonate to promote developmental care and comfort
- Vitamins
- Immunisation
- Skin integrity.

Quality improvement in the care of low-birth-weight infants

High-quality nursing care of a premature baby is recognised as the most important aspect in the survival of small babies. Caring for LBW babies requires special skills. The ratio of staff to babies is 1:1 in intensive care and 1:2 in high care. Certain types of care are particularly effective, such as KMC, developmental supportive care (DSC) and baby-friendly care (BFC) principles.

PROCEDURE Providing kangaroo-mother-care

Definition

KMC is a form of care that promotes skin-to-skin contact between mother and baby. KMC is a low-cost, effective intervention to stabilise LBW infants and improve mortality by 30 per cent. It is easy to do, inexpensive and highly rated by parents.

Very small babies with major health issues or on a mechanical ventilator can benefit from *intermittent* KMC (done only for periods when the mother or father visits the baby). Continuous KMC is care given 24 hours by the mother, day and night.

Guidelines for instituting KMC
- There must be a written unit policy on KMC.
- Written guidelines must be available for staff and mothers.
- All staff should receive training on KMC.

Benefits for mother and babies
KMC babies:
- stabilise faster, with a more stable heart rate, breathing, temperature, oxygenation and brain development
- cry less
- sleep better
- gain more weight, thus reducing the length of hospital stay
- have better self-regulation abilities and more stable organ function.

The following are further benefits of KMC:
- Breastfeeding is facilitated by increasing the let-down response.
- There is a lower incidence of infections.
- There is less apnoea; babies sleep better with less bradycardia and improved oxygen saturation and consumption.
- It is a safe and effective way to transport babies.
- It increases the volume of breast milk in the mother; babies as small as 30 weeks can be breastfed.
- The rooting instinct develops more rapidly.
- Bonding between baby and parent is promoted.

continued

Contraindications

Unstable and critically sick newborns requiring intensive medical care and treatment are not candidates for KMC.

Prerequisites

▶ Health education on the benefits of KMC should be given.
▶ The mother should provide informed consent.
▶ The mother must have fully recovered from childbirth or any related complications.
▶ There must be family support available.

Preparation

KMC care requires a comfortable place to sit, with several pillows for support and to help position the baby. (KMC is also possible in a standing position.)

Parents may be offered a wrap or a stretchy shirt with a large neck opening with space for the baby to be tucked inside for privacy.

Position

▶ During KMC, the baby is undressed down to the diaper. The baby also wears a woolen cap and socks.
▶ The baby is placed directly on the mother's or father's chest, in a frog-like position. The head is turned slightly to the side.
▶ Any wires or tubes are carefully positioned.
▶ The parent and baby are covered with a lightweight blanket or wrap to stay warm and for privacy.
▶ The baby's temperature is taken several times to make sure it is maintained.
▶ Initially, the monitors must be observed closely to determine the neonatal response.
▶ Two-hourly breastfeeding or giving breast milk by cup or by nasogastric tube is encouraged, using manually expressed breast milk or donor milk.

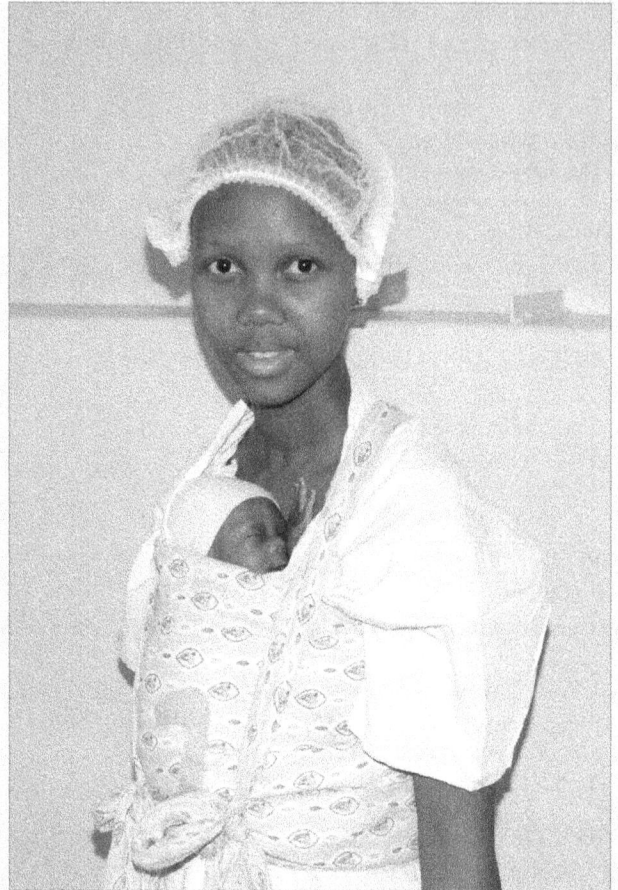

Figure 42A Kangaroo-mother-care

The mother or father practises KMC for 30 minutes once a day, gradually increasing to two to three hours per day, as tolerated. Eventually, the aim is 24 hours a day.

The parents are educated on the recognition of danger signs such as apnoea, decreased movement, lethargy or poor feeding and abnormal breathing patterns. The parents are trained and given skills in managing problems.
For example, in the case of apnoea, parents are shown how to stimulate the baby by rubbing its back for 10 seconds.

There must be trained staff support on hand and encouragement to breastfeed.

Recording and interpretation

▶ Observations (vital data) are done at regular intervals, as per protocol, and recorded.
▶ Weight is assessed daily and recorded.
▶ Sleep and feeding patterns are documented.
▶ Positive parent–child interaction is assessed, enhanced and recorded.

Developmental supportive care

If the newborn is not ready for KMC, care is modified for stress reduction. This care is referred to as DSC. It seeks to manipulate the environment to reduce complications for the newborn. DSC was developed in 1980 and is defined by the National Association of Neonatal Nurses (NANN) in the USA as care of the neonate to support positive growth and development (Symington & Pinelli, 2006). Infant responses are monitored and care is modified to the needs of the infant.

As indicated earlier, the ideal situation is for the baby to remain with the mother. When separated, the baby becomes stressed. It is the task of the midwife to protect the baby as far as possible and minimise the effects of the unfamiliar extrauterine environment. The DSC principles must be applied to all neonates.

Neonatal stress

The short- and long-term effects of incubator care or separation from the mother in the care of the LBW baby are both physical and psychological, and are referred to as iatrogenic stressors. Iatrogenic stressors and the care environment can affect the baby and cause stress. They include:

- bright lights
- sleep interruptions
- position, routine and excessive handling
- loud sounds
- unattended crying
- reduced suckling
- social isolation and separation from the mother
- medical interactions and painful procedures.

The effects of these stressors on small babies include:

- disorientation of the sensory system
- increased cortisol and sensory overload
- increased morbidity
- hypoglycaemia
- anaemia
- hypothermia
- hypoxia
- pain and discomfort.

The short- and long-term outcomes of stress on the baby include:

- physiological instability
- cognitive impairment
- attention deficit disorders
- visiomotor and spatial orientation impairment
- language, comprehension and speech difficulties
- posture pathology (supine positions)
- impeded developmental milestones.

The baby communicates positive or negative observable behaviour and responses through autonomic, motor and behavioural indicators, as summarised in Table 42.2.

Table 42.2

Neonatal stress cues

Autonomic	Motor	Behaviour
Colour change	Generalised hypotonia	Irritable behaviour
Hiccupping and sneezing	Floppiness	Sleep disturbances
Gagging and spitting up	Hyperextension of extremities	Inappropriate behaviour
Increased or decreased heart rate	Splaying of fingers and toes	
BP fluctuations	Facial expression: grim and frowning	
Changes in respiration rate		
Unstable temperature		
Apnoea		
Pallor and vasoconstriction		
Decreased gastric mobility		
Increased secretion of cortisol, adrenaline and catecholamines (inhibiting the repair of tissue)		

Principles of developmental supportive care

DSC includes the following principles, which are in line with BFC principles:

▶ Baby care is individualised, based on the needs of the baby, as communicated by the baby's cues and physiological and behavioural responses.
▶ The approach is family-centred and the family is involved in all decision-making processes.
▶ External environmental manipulation includes adaptation of noise, light and odour in the environment. For example, no radios are allowed, and midwives and parents do not use strong perfume, as this can irritate the infant.
▶ Minimal handling and touching is allowed. The flat surface of the palm of the hand is used to calm the infant. Hard touching and tickling is prohibited. Pain management procedures need to be stipulated for a unit. Swaddle-bathing and -weighing are used to minimise the shock of cold surfaces.
▶ Non-nutritive sucking is allowed, using a pacifier. This calms the infant down.
▶ Developmental supportive positioning (flexion, three-dimensional containment, midline orientation) is aimed at the simulation of the position *in utero*. The infant is positioned to be oriented in the mid-line (hand-to-mouth) or in the contained fetal position. Self-regulation and soothing behaviour are promoted and linen and soft toys are used to position the infant so that the hands are in front, the knees are flexed and the head is in a neutral position, supine or lateral.
▶ Cluster care is used. This is the arrangement of activities based on the cues of the infant, with longer periods of rest and fewer interruptions.

Outcomes of developmental supportive care

▶ Improved respiration
▶ Earlier transition from nasogastric feeding
▶ Increase in self-regulatory abilities and physiological stability
▶ Reduced morbidity
▶ Improved neurological organisation
▶ Improved growth and mass gain
▶ Decreased length of stay in hospital
▶ Decreased costs
▶ Improved neurological development at 24 months
▶ Improved mother–child bonding

42.6   Hypoglycaemia

An adequate supply of glucose is essential for normal body function and an insufficiency can lead to severe brain damage.

Clinical features and diagnosis

Normal blood glucose in a neonate is 2.5 mmol/ℓ (45 mg/dl). Hypoglycaemia occurs if this drops to less than 1.1 mmol/ℓ. Brain damage occurs at this level.

Non-specific signs and symptoms include tremors, seizures or hypotonia, apnoea and cyanosis, lethargy, poor feeding and tachycardia.

Causes

Hypoglycaemia may be due to:

▶ inadequate or depleted glycogen stores in the placenta before delivery
▶ inadequate or depleted glycogen stores in the liver after delivery (preterm, LBW, late feeding)
▶ an increased demand for glucose (respiratory distress, hypothermia, infection)
▶ hyperinsulinism (a diabetic mother, Rh disease)
▶ liver damage.

The predisposing causes of hypoglycaemia are therefore very similar to those of hypothermia. Less common causes are post-exchange transfusion, Rh disease and galactosaemia.

Management and care

All infants are routinely observed for hypoglycaemia. However, prevention by early feeding is the best course. If the baby is very small or very ill and unable to suck, tube feeds (and, if necessary, IV feeding) are commenced as soon as possible after birth. In addition, the following is done:

▶ The baby is kept warm.
▶ Blood glucose levels in high-risk babies are tested by means of test strips (Dextrostix) every 1–4 hours for 24–48 hours until the condition is stable. High-risk babies include those who are preterm, LGA (especially those whose mothers are diabetics) or growth restricted and those who suffer from prolonged asphyxia, intracranial injury, hypothermia, haemolytic disease or infections.
▶ Blood sugar levels are maintained through regular milk feeds and are monitored.
▶ Energy needs are reduced by correcting acidosis, preventing hypothermia and infection and treating sepsis early.

Specific care

If the blood sugar drops to less than 1.4 mmol/ℓ (25 mg/dl), urgent intervention is needed (DoH 2014a: 2.1.3, page 21):

▶ The baby is immediately given a 50 ml breastmilk feed.
▶ Check glucose in 15 minutes.
▶ If the blood glucose does not show improvement, give 10 per cent glucose (Neonatelyte) 5 ml/kg IV and continue at the recommended rate for the age and weight. Repeat blood glucose in 15 minutes. Continue with the IV infusion until the blood sugar is stable and milk feeds are introduced. This may take 48–72 hours after birth.
▶ The blood glucose levels are monitored at least every hour until the baby's condition is stable. It is advisable to maintain the blood sugar readings at or above 2.2 mmol/ℓ.
▶ Glucagon in a dose of 0.2 mg/kg IM is effective in an emergency for the treatment of babies who have no glycogen stores with which to respond. Discuss with a paediatrician if hydrocortisone is needed.
▶ Hydrocortisone 5 mg/kg is given IV as prescribed if the blood sugar remains low.
▶ Babies of diabetic mothers are routinely on a dextrose IV infusion after birth for a 24-hour period or until stable.

Complications

Hypoglycaemia may result in brain damage of varying severity, ranging from learning problems to severe intellectual retardation. Whatever the cause, the first step in the treatment of hypoglycaemia is to recognise its presence as early as possible. The permanent neurological effects of hypoglycaemia correlate with the duration of time the cerebral tissues are deprived of glucose.

42.7   Large-for-gestational-age infants

An LGA baby is one that falls above the 90th percentile for length and weight for GA.

Causes

The most common cause of LGA is macrosomia associated with diabetes in the mother. Other causes may include obesity in the mother, prolonged labour, obstructed labour, a large infant, Caesarean section, assisted deliveries and placental pathology such as antepartum haemorrhage (APH), erythroblastosis fetalis and family trends.

Common problems

▶ There is a fivefold increased risk of mortality for LGA infants.

▶ The large size and head often result in these infants having traumatic births and they are exposed to birth injury.
▶ If the infant is born to a diabetic mother, the risk of hypoglycaemia is increased, because the fetal pancreas hypertrophies and continues to secrete insulin.
▶ Of LGA infants, 70 per cent are polycythemic, with a risk of jaundice.
▶ Infants of diabetic mothers are immature and are at risk for HMD and infections.
▶ Large infants are hungry and tend to require larger feeds than normal.
▶ There is an increased risk of congenital abnormalities associated with diabetes in the mother.

Care of the large-for-gestational-age infant

The LGA infant is identified in pregnancy or during labour. If the mother is prediabetic or diabetic and on treatment, the midwife should anticipate the potential problems of the newborn.

Care in these cases include the following principles:

▶ Resuscitation of the newborn is done by skilled staff.
▶ A full examination is done to exclude birth injuries and congenital abnormalities.
▶ The baby is kept under observation for hypoglycaemia and hypothermia for 24 hours.
▶ If the blood sugar drops to 2.5 mmol/ℓ, a 10 per cent or 5 per cent dextrose/water infusion may be used to maintain the blood sugar (not higher than 7 mm/ℓ). Early feeding (breastfeeding or EBM) is essential for maintenance of blood sugar.
▶ To prevent hypothermia, the baby is nursed in an incubator for 24 hours and KMC is instituted thereafter if the baby drinks well and is stable.
▶ The mother is taught how to ensure that the baby's feeding requirements are met.
▶ The standard routine care and observations for a neonate are given.

42.8   The post-mature infant

A post-mature infant is any infant born after 42 weeks of gestation. This baby may be LGA, but can also be SGA.

Causes

The cause of post-maturity is unknown. Abnormalities of the fetus (the pituitary–adrenal axis in neural tube abnormalities such as anencephaly) may play a role. Maternal causes are unknown. The mother, placenta and baby all play a role in the onset of labour and the mechanism is not well understood.

Diagnosis of post-maturity

The duration of pregnancy must be determined accurately. The history of the pregnancy, if accurate (early assessment before 20 weeks, including an ultrasound before or at 20–22 weeks), will indicate a post-mature pregnancy.

The function of the placenta decreases after 36 weeks and the fetus will start to metabolise subcutaneous fat for energy. The amniotic fluid will decrease and the fetal skull ossifies, losing the ability to mould. An ultrasound after 36 weeks will indicate the maturity and function of the placenta. Placental function tests may be performed.

Care of the post-term baby

When a pregnancy is prolonged (see Chapter 23), the baby is at risk. The function of the placenta starts to diminish after 36 weeks to prepare the fetus for extrauterine life. After 40 weeks, the baby may not receive sufficient oxygen and nutrients and after 42 weeks, the skull starts to ossify and is less flexible.

Before birth

The growth and development of the fetus is monitored using:
- maternal weight gain
- the mid-upper-arm circumference (MUAC) measurement
- the symphysis fundal height (SFH) measurement between 20 and 35 weeks
- amniotic liquor volume, as observed on palpation and measured by ultrasound
- fetal movement, as determined by a kick chart
- the assessment of the fetus by a non-stress test (NST), biophysical profile and Doppler studies.

During labour

The pregnancy is not allowed to continue after term, in case of a compromised fetus. Labour is induced by the medical practitioner or, if the baby is severely compromised, a Caesarean section may be performed.

A woman who has had a prolonged pregnancy is monitored for the duration of labour and for signs of fetal distress during labour. Meconium-stained liquor in a vertex presentation and abnormal fetal heart rate (FHR) patterns in labour indicate fetal distress.

The physical appearance of the baby at birth is diagnostic:
- The post-term infant is alert and mature.
- A decrease in subcutaneous fat and soft tissue mass is observed.
- The skin may hang loose and is dry and peeling. The baby has the appearance of an old person.
- The finger- and toenails are long.
- The skin and cord may be meconium-stained.
- The head is hard and mature and the fontanelles may be smaller and closed.

After birth

There is an increased morbidity and mortality associated with post-term infants. The main problem of post-mature infants is intrauterine growth impairment due to placental insufficiency syndrome (caused by infarcts and villous degeneration).

Asphyxia *in utero* and after birth is common in post-term infants. Meconium aspiration syndrome (MAS) is anticipated and prevented by suctioning the airways. This is done by a skilled medical practitioner or midwife before the first breath and under direct supervision, using a laryngoscope. If respiratory distress is present, a medical practitioner is consulted and the baby is admitted to a neonatal care unit.

The risk of hypoglycaemia and hypothermia is increased in post-term babies (DoH, 2014a, paragraph 2.1.3).

Care includes the following points:
- The temperature of the baby is carefully observed and maintained.
- Blood sugar is checked after birth. Early feeding is started to maintain the blood sugar if the baby is not distressed. A regular breastfeeding regimen with complementary feeding is followed to meet the energy needs of the baby.
- A full examination is done to exclude congenital abnormalities.

42.9 Conclusion

Midwives should be skilled in the assessment and care of preterm, immature and post-mature infants. It is important that the midwife knows how to assess intrauterine status as well as neonatal status, to ensure adequate, appropriate and effective interventions.

Common disorders
of the newborn

LEARNING OBJECTIVES
On completion of this chapter, you must be able to:
▶ identify common disorders of the newborn
▶ demonstrate competency in the care of a newborn, including diagnosis, treatment, health education and referral of common disorders (gastrointestinal, temperature, infections and jaundice).

KNOWLEDGE ASSUMED TO BE IN PLACE
Normal anatomy and physiology of newborns
Newborn Care Charts, paragraphs 2.1.1, 2.1.5, 2.2.4 and 2.2.6 (DoH, 2014a)

KEYWORDS
gastroenteritis • necrotising enterocolitis (NEC) • hernia • hypothermia • Hirschsprung's disease • neonatal cold injury • omphalitis • ophthalmia neonatorum

43.1   Introduction

Some of the most common minor and serious disorders that affect the newborn are briefly presented in this chapter. The remaining common respiratory and metabolic conditions are presented in following chapters.

In order to get a full understanding of these disorders and the care required, the midwife needs to regularly update her knowledge. Only basic principles are presented in this chapter.

43.2   Complications of the alimentary tract: Stools

It is important to know the difference between normal and abnormal stools in the newborn infant. Any abnormality in the stools can be very significant in the early diagnosis and treatment of an abnormal condition.

The first stool: Meconium

Meconium is the first stool passed by the newborn. It is black and sticky. It is passed at birth or within 24 hours after birth and remains sticky and black during the first two days after birth. It is made up of material ingested *in utero*, such as epithelial cells, lanugo, mucus, amniotic fluid, bile and water. Colostrum acts as a laxative and facilitates the passing of meconium.

It is not usual for the fetus to pass meconium *in utero*. This is associated with fetal distress. It may indicate that the fetus is compromised by a lack of oxygen due to one of various causes, such as:
▶ maternal disease: pregnancy-induced hypertension (PIH), diabetes, etc
▶ perinatal infections and placental pathology: placental insufficiency, retroplacental bleeding, detachment or abruption, infarct and ageing
▶ cord conditions: cord prolapse, a short cord or velamentous implantation, or vasa praevia
▶ abnormalities of the fetus: intrauterine growth restriction (IUGR), twin pregnancy with twin transfusion syndrome or congenital abnormalities.

After birth, a newborn will usually pass meconium within 24 hours. This is noted. If meconium is not passed, it needs to be reported (see the discussion on the next page). The patency of the rectum is confirmed at birth as a part of the first physical examination. Other birth abnormalities may be present.

During a breech delivery, the infant may pass meconium as the body is squeezed through the birth canal.

The changing stool

After the passing of meconium and the initiation of breastfeeding, the gut is colonised with bifidobacteria, causing the stools passed from about the third to the fifth day after birth to change. The type of milk given to the infant will determine the change in the stools. The colour changes to a greenish-brown at first and then a yellowish-brown. Within four to five days, the stool is much softer and looser than the sticky, black meconium.

The normal stool of the breastfed newborn

The breastfed newborn has a typical stool from the fourth or fifth day onward. The colour is a rich yellow to orange, but may even be bright green in the transitional period. The consistency is soft and possibly semi-fluid. The number of stools passed varies from three to five in 24 hours, to whatever is consistent in that particular infant. The stool has a non-offensive odour and the pH of the stool is acidic.

An infant's stool patterns will change as breastfeeding is established. Some exclusively breastfed babies will not have any stools in 10 days, while others can have up to 20 a day.

The normal stool of the formula-fed or bottle-fed newborn

A newborn fed on formula also passes stools after the fourth or fifth day. The stools are semi-formed to formed, and a pale yellow with possibly a greenish tinge if exposed to air. The odour is quite offensive and the stool is more alkaline than in breastfed infants. Normal stool may also contain small amounts of mucus. An infant on formula feeds must pass at least one stool a day, and may pass two. Formula-fed babies often have constipation and sore buttocks.

Constipation

The fully breastfed infant is not usually constipated if the volume of feed is sufficient. The vast difference in the number of stools a breastfed infant may have often causes unnecessary concern.

The formula-fed infant has a much firmer stool than the breastfed infant and the mother may be concerned that the infant is constipated. The formula-fed infant should have one or two stools per day and may have to strain more than the breastfed infant in order to pass the stool. In true constipation, the anal region may be red and abraded from passing hard faeces.

Babies on iron supplements will present with black, sticky stools, often causing constipation that may require management.

Constipation may be a sign that the infant is underfed or requires more fluid, or that the feed is too rich. The feed is reassessed and if it is of the correct proportions, the mother may be instructed to give water after feeds, or to give fruit juices or pureed fruit as the infant grows.

Constipation may be a sign of an abnormal condition such as cretinism (congenital hypothyroidism) or Down's syndrome (Trisomy 21).

Types of abnormal stools

Abnormal stools in the newborn are indicative of an abnormal condition. It may simply be due to incorrect feeding, but it could also be extremely serious. Abnormal stools are frequently associated with abdominal distension, and vomiting may also be a clinical feature. The midwife should investigate every abnormal stool and immediately report any stool that is not caused by incorrect feeding: the sooner an abnormality is treated, the greater are the chances of a full recovery.

In order to be able to differentiate between types of abnormal stools, the midwife must be familiar with all the abnormal stools that can occur in the neonatal period. Table 43.1 summaries the types of abnormal stools.

Failure to pass meconium within 24 hours

This condition needs to be reported for medical attention. All newborns are examined for a patent anal opening. If there is no meconium after 24 hours, it may be accompanied by abdominal distension and later by the vomiting of foul-smelling, bile-stained vomitus if the condition has not been diagnosed and treated. The causes may be atresia of the lower bowel, or other causes of obstruction to the bowel such as meconium ileus or an imperforate anus.

In preterm babies with respiratory distress syndrome (RDS), there may be a delayed passage of meconium with no bowel sounds. Other clinical features will be present.

The medical practitioner is notified if the newborn has not passed meconium in the first 24 hours and if the abdomen is distended. Investigation is required and surgical intervention is usually indicated in obstruction of the bowels.

Table 43.1

Abnormal stools of newborns

Types of abnormality	Clinical picture and possible causes	Intervention
Large, loose, greenish-yellow stools	This is usually due to overfeeding of the infant, specifically the breastfed baby.	Observe and determine the baby's intake. Observe the growth card to determine the pattern of weight gain. Reduce the length of time of feeding until the stool is normal if the infant is also vomiting and/or losing weight.
Small, fairly frequent, loose, green-brown stools with mucus	This denotes underfeeding and starvation in breastfed newborns. These stools are often semi-transparent and have a faint musty but not offensive odour. (This stool must not be confused with infective diarrhoea, as this infant requires extra milk feeds and should not be taken off milk.) The newborn is losing weight, crying a lot, is lethargic and has a reduced urinary output.	The use of the growth card will indicate if the baby is growing. The midwife should show how the mother's milk supply can be increased and the infant should suckle more frequently. If, despite all efforts, the infant still does not receive sufficient nutrition, alternative feeding will have to be started.
Small, hard, pasty, infrequent stools	This is an indication of the formula-fed infant not obtaining sufficient nutrition. The infant will be underweight and will appear undernourished.	Investigate the socioeconomic background and the mental ability of the parents so that they can get help to provide the infant with sufficient nutrition and care. The feed should be reassessed, and strength and quantity increased gradually until the correct nutrition is achieved. The condition and progress of this infant should be carefully followed up.
Frothy, loose, greenish-yellow stools with a sour odour	This may indicate lactose intolerance.	Special feeds may be necessary. Refer to the medical practitioner.
Pale, greasy, bulky, very offensive smelling stools (steatorrhoea)	This may be accompanied by vomiting and is caused by undigested fat in cow's milk feeds. The fat curds are either not being digested or there is too much fat in the feed. The cause may be cystic fibrosis, but this is not usually seen in the newborn. These newborns will present instead with a meconium ileus.	Refer to the medical practitioner.
Large, pasty, smelly, infrequent stools with curds	This type of stool is usually accompanied by colic with constipation. It may indicate that casein in the milk is not being digested. Appropriate infant feeds need to be given. The mineral content is adapted for babies. Feeds not suitable for babies, such as undiluted cow's milk, could result in hypernatraemia.	Reassessment of the feed is necessary, with boiling and dilution of liquid cow's milk, or the correct proportions used for making up powdered milk. The parents should be given careful explanations about how to make up feeds. The progress of the infant should be carefully followed up.

continued

Types of abnormality	Clinical picture and possible causes	Intervention
Large, pasty, smelly, infrequent stools with curds (continued)	Feed not suited for babies predisposes an infant to necrotising enterocolitis (NEC) and could also lead to intestinal obstruction from the inspissated milk syndrome (lactobezoar).	
Loose, frequent, greenish-yellow stools (diarrhoea)	This stool usually indicates the onset of an infection, such as Rotavirus, bacteria or a parasite. However, this must not be confused with the normal stool or the underfeeding or overfeeding stool of the breastfed infant. Diarrhoea is rare in the breastfed newborn, but is a frequent and dangerous occurrence in the formula-fed newborn, particularly in communities with poor socioeconomic conditions. Diarrhoea is also a feature of middle-ear infection, NEC, congenital adrenal hyperplasia, a sensitivity to cow's milk protein, lactose intolerance and food intolerance or sensitivity.	The cause must be determined. Make sure the baby is getting enough fluids to prevent dehydration. If the cause is intolerance for food or lactose, remove the cause. All mothers in rural areas should be given the instruction (see the box on the next page) for an electrolyte solution which can be given to a child with diarrhoea. Refer to the medical practitioner.
Frequent, watery, green, offensive smelling and possibly explosive stools (advanced infective diarrhoea)	Advanced diarrhoea, caused by an infection of the GI tract, is an extremely serious condition in the newborn. The main organisms causing diarrhoea are *Escherichia coli*, Salmonellae, Shigella, Staphylococcus, *Candida albicans*, Coxsackie virus, Rotavirus and *Vibrio cholera*.	Refer to a medical practitioner. The newborn is usually admitted to a clinic or a hospital and isolated from other newborns. IV fluids are commenced immediately and the infant is given no oral feeding. Stool and blood specimens are taken and sent to a laboratory immediately in an attempt to isolate the infecting organism. Broad-spectrum antibiotics or specific medication is commenced as soon as possible. When the stools begin to normalise, gradual oral feeding is introduced, starting with an electrolyte solution and gradually progressing to a normal milk feed.
Melaena (black, tarry stools) which stain the napkin pink and contain blood	The blood could be maternal blood swallowed during delivery or from cracked and bleeding nipples in breastfed newborns. Alternatively, it could be the newborn's blood caused by trauma to some part of the alimentary tract, or due to bleeding into the alimentary tract in haemorrhagic disease of the newborn (hypoprothrombinaemia). In the latter condition, the melaena stool often also contains fresh blood from the lower intestinal tract (colon and rectum). On careful inspection, the white napkin assumes a pinkish tinge at the edges of the stool, due to the blood (Hb) in the stool.	Refer to a medical practitioner. An injection of vitamin K1 should be given, if not already given at birth. The medical practitioner may order further vitamin K1 and vitamin C to be given. If the haemorrhage is severe, a blood transfusion may be necessary. The newborn is nursed in high care. This stool must not be confused with the black stool which results from the administration of iron to the newborn.
Pale, putty-coloured stools	This can be a sign of jaundice, liver conditions or an obstruction that prevents bile from entering the alimentary canal. It can also be caused by congenital atresia or obliteration of the bile ducts (intra- or extra-hepatic), or inspissated bile syndrome in cystic fibrosis infections or metabolic conditions that affect the liver.	The medical practitioner is informed immediately. The appropriate management is started.

Life-saving electrolyte solution for rehydration of newborns and infants in cases of diarrhoea
1   Pour one litre of clean water in a clean container.
2   Add to this eight level teaspoons of sugar and half a level teaspoon of salt.
3   Stir well.
4   Pour into a clean mug.
5   Give plenty of the mixture to the child by spoon while the diarrhoea lasts and continue breastfeeding.
6   Take the infant for medical attention.

No further stools after the passage of meconium

This condition is usually accompanied by vomiting. There may be distension of the upper abdomen but not the lower abdomen, or distension of the whole abdomen. The condition is suggestive of either a high obstruction of the bowel or a partial obstruction of the bowel, such as in Hirschsprung's disease.

The medical practitioner is informed if no further stools or very infrequent stools are passed. Immediate investigations are started.

43.3   Gastrointestinal abnormalities

Common gastrointestinal (GI) conditions that present in infants are briefly explained in this section. If detected early and referred, these can be treated in time.

Abdominal distension

Abnormal abdominal distension is usually accompanied by some vomiting and may also be associated with either a delay in passing stools (the absence of stools) or with diarrhoea.

Any excessive distension and/or hardness of the abdominal wall may be abnormal. Abdominal distension in the upper abdomen with marked peristalsis could indicate a pyloric stenosis or an obstruction in the duodenum. Gross abdominal distension without peristalsis could indicate lower intestinal obstruction.

Causes of abdominal distension

There are many causes of abdominal distension. If this condition is present, the midwife should note any other clinical signs that may assist in a diagnosis, such as the size and gestational age (GA) of the infant, vomiting, any delay in passing stools, diarrhoea, pyrexia, weight loss, dehydration and/or malnutrition, or bleeding.

The following are potential causes of abdominal distension:

▶ *Poor feeding techniques.* Abdominal distension – and, possibly, vomiting – can be caused by the swallowing of air during feeding. It can thus be due to the infant feeding too rapidly from an over-abundant milk supply, an excessive 'let-down' when breastfeeding or an excessively large hole in the teat when bottle feeding. Difficulty with or neglecting to wind or burp the infant after feeds may also result in abdominal distension and vomiting. The management of this condition consists of changing the feeding technique as well as the teat in the case of bottle feeding.

▶ *Infection.* Gastroenteritis, peritonitis and generalised infections such as septicaemia can cause abdominal distension. Treat the cause and refer to the medical practitioner.

Intestinal obstruction

Intestinal obstruction may be high or low:

▶ *High obstruction.* In conditions such as pyloric stenosis, duodenal atresia or stenosis, abdominal distension may not be noticed at first, as only the stomach and the duodenum will distend. No further stools are passed after the passage of meconium. This condition is usually accompanied by projectile vomiting in the case of stenosis. The medical practitioner is informed if no further stools or very infrequent stools are passed and immediate investigations are started.

▶ *Low obstruction.* In conditions such as intestinal atresia of the lower bowel, malrotation of the gut with volvulus and periduodenal bands (Meckel's diverticulum), incarcerated inguinal hernia, meconium ileus, rectal agenesis and imperforate anus, and Hirschsprung's disease (a congenital condition of the colon where nerves have not developed), the abdominal distension is prominent. The abdominal wall becomes stretched and veins may be seen beneath the skin. Lower intestinal obstruction could be indicated by gross abdominal distension without peristalsis. If the infant does not pass meconium within 24 hours, abdominal distension is usually found; if the condition is not treated, this will be followed by vomiting (foul-smelling, bile-stained vomitus). Preterm babies with RDS may present with a delayed passage of meconium with no bowel sounds.

The management of intestinal obstruction includes checking that the anus is patent at the first physical examination. The medical practitioner is notified if the newborn has not passed meconium in the first 24 hours and if the abdomen is distended. Investigation is required and surgical intervention is possible.

Perforation of the bowel

Perforation of the bowel will lead to abdominal distension and may be due to conditions such as sepsis, Meckel's diverticulum, spontaneous perforation – which may occur after an exchange blood transfusion – or NEC. Refer to the medical practitioner.

Herniation or enlargement of an intra-abdominal organ

Localised distension can occur in an umbilical hernia, enlarged kidneys, hepatosplenomegaly and bladder neck obstruction.

Ascites

Gross abdominal distension (ascites) may be found in haemolytic disease due to Rh incompatability in nephrotic syndrome, in cardiac failure and in other unknown conditions.

Necrotising enterocolitis

NEC is a common acquired condition of GI obstruction that occurs most commonly in low birth weight (LBW) babies who are not breastfed or given breast milk. The cause is not known, but predisposing factors appear to be birth asphyxia and shock, umbilical catheterisation, cow's milk feeds and certain antibiotics, any of which result in ischaemic necrosis of portions of the gut, mainly the terminal part of the ileum and the colon.

Clinical signs

The condition is characterised by necrotic areas of the small and/or large intestines, with bacterial growth. The clinical signs are abdominal distension three to five days after oral feeding has started, with the outline of distended loops of bowel visible beneath the abdominal wall, ileus or diminished bowel sounds, vomiting (bile-stained), GI bleeding (blood in the stools), apnea, irregular temperature (hypothermia), lethargy, possibly peritonitis and shock.

Initial symptoms include feeding intolerance, increased gastric residuals, abdominal distension and/or tenderness and bloody stools. Symptoms may progress rapidly to abdominal discolouration with intestinal perforation and peritonitis and systemic hypotension, requiring intensive medical support.

Diagnosis

The diagnosis is usually made on the basis of:
- a physical examination
- radiographic results, which include an abnormal gas pattern, dilated loops and thickened bowel walls

- ultrasound investigation, which can identify areas of location and/or abscess and ascites consistent with a walled-off perforation
- laboratory reports, including:
  - haematocrit and Hb – if there was blood loss
  - platelet count, to diagnose thrombocytopaenia
  - blood culture, which is usually negative
  - hyponatremia
  - low serum bicarbonate (< 20) in babies with poor tissue perfusion, sepsis and bowel necrosis
  - arterial blood gas levels, to evaluate the acid–base status.

Prevention

The prevention of NEC is an important measure. After birth, prevention includes using only breast milk for feeds. If the mother cannot give breast milk, mother's milk from the milk bank is used. This greatly reduces the incidence of NEC.

Treatment

Oral feedings should be stopped. The newborn is kept nil per os. Antibiotics should be given. Perform nasogastric decompression and start IV fluid therapy, including total parenteral nutrition (TPN).

In serious conditions, the neonate is nursed on a ventilator. Surgery may be required.

This condition is associated with a high neonatal mortality rate (NMR), but the outcome is better when the condition is diagnosed and treated early.

43.4 Vomiting in the newborn

Any fluid coming from the mouth of the infant constitutes vomiting. This fluid may ooze gently from the mouth, spill out of the mouth in small or large amounts, or spurt out of the mouth (precipitate vomiting). The quantity of fluid may vary from small amounts to the regurgitation of a whole feed. The vomitus may consist of watery mucus, frothy mucus, plain or curdled milk, or milk or mucus containing blood or bile. Projectile vomiting is associated with pyloric stenosis.

Types of vomiting

- *Bile-stained* vomitus can be caused by any obstruction of the bile ductus.
- *Blood-stained* vomitus may be caused by:
  - swallowed maternal blood at birth
  - swallowed maternal blood during breastfeeding, due to cracked nipples

- trauma to the pharynx or to any other part of the upper respiratory or alimentary tract
- haemorrhagic disease of the newborn (hypoprothrombinaemia) or any other haemorrhagic condition.

▶ *Vomited mucus* is usually caused by liquor or blood that was swallowed during birth. This irritates the gastric mucosa, resulting in expulsion of mucus and liquor soon after birth, possibly with some stomach juices. Swallowed liquor may also contain swallowed blood and/or meconium. If the infant appears to have swallowed a lot of liquor, a stomach wash-out is indicated.

▶ *Frothy mucus* may be present soon after birth and could be a sign of the very serious conditions of tracheo-oesophageal fistula or oesophageal atresia, where the saliva is not swallowed but is directed into the trachea or pharynx and mixed with expired gases. If the mother had polyhydramnios in pregnancy, care is taken to make sure the GI tract is intact. The midwife can pass a number six feeding tube and use litmus paper to test that it is in the stomach (litmus paper turns pink in the presence of acid). This condition should be reported immediately and no feed should be given to the newborn until further examination and tests have been carried out.

▶ *Vomiting of milk*, with or without mucus, is the most frequent type of vomitus seen in the newborn. It could be due to a variety of causes:

- *Posseting and ruminating* is caused by overfeeding, especially in LBW babies who have very small stomachs and a low stomach emptying time due to immaturity and difficulty in digesting feeds.
- *Congenital abnormalities* such as chalasia or lax cardiac sphincter of the oesophagus cause feeds to be regurgitated. The infant needs to be propped up on pillows, especially after feeds, to prevent the feed from flowing back out of the stomach.

Causes of vomiting

In the early days after birth, babies vomit due to blood or meconium swallowed. In the early weeks after birth it is not unusual for babies to vomit as they adjust to feeding. However, most types of vomiting are abnormal and may be extremely serious. Any persistent or unusual vomiting should be reported and investigated immediately, because the sooner after birth a newborn is treated for an abnormality, the greater are the chances of complete recovery.

Vomiting in the newborn may originate from low or high intestinal obstruction, caused by several factors, or metabolic, biochemical, endocrine and other disorders, as mentioned further down below.

Low intestinal obstruction below the entry of the bile duct will lead to bile-stained vomiting within the first 24 hours of birth, caused by:

▶ atresia of the bowel
▶ an imperforated anus
▶ meconium ileus
▶ volvulus
▶ Meckel's diverticulum
▶ A strangulated hernia
▶ Hirschsprung's disease.

High intestinal obstruction or partial obstruction that will lead to vomiting may be caused by:

▶ pylorospasm, which is a spasm of the pyloric sphincter of the stomach
▶ pyloric stenosis, which is a congenital hypertrophic closure of the pyloric sphincter of the stomach
▶ hiatus hernia
▶ oesophageal atresia or fistula, which causes drooling and frothy mucus.

Metabolic, biochemical, endocrine and other disorders that may cause vomiting are:

▶ galactosaemia
▶ congenital adrenal hypoplasia
▶ infective gastritis: non-infective gastritis is caused by the swallowing of liquor and possibly blood and/or meconium. Infective gastritis is caused by *E. coli* or *Candida albicans* (thrush) or the Coxsackie virus
▶ urinary tract infection (UTI)
▶ neonatal hepatitis
▶ septicaemia
▶ meningitis
▶ raised intracranial pressure causing cerebral trauma, resulting in oedema, bleeding meningitis and hydrocephaly.

In addition, incorrect techniques and the incorrect strength of feed (for example if the mixture is too rich for the newborn), as well as rough handling of an infant after a feed or not burping an infant, can lead to vomiting.

Diagnosis

The midwife reviews the history of the pregnancy and birth (amniotic fluid and placental pathology, Apgar score, first examination of the newborn, and any factor in the history that my cause concern, such as Rh factor of the mother or perinatal infections). The midwife does a full examination to exclude congenital abnormalities.

Any vomiting is a cause for concern, because the infant is losing fluids and nourishment, which could be extremely serious in a newborn. The midwife should observe the infant very carefully in order to assess whether the vomiting is caused by faulty feeding techniques, which merely require adjusting, or whether the vomiting is due to an abnormality, which requires immediate attention.

There are specific points relating to vomiting that the midwife should observe and report on in order to assist the medical practitioner in making a diagnosis. These points are:
▶ the time of vomiting in relation to feeds
▶ if the vomiting has any relation to feeding
▶ the amount of fluid vomited; the actual amount cannot be measured, but the midwife should be able to gauge whether the whole or half or only a small portion of the feed is returned.

Further points to note include the following:
▶ Most vomiting occurs during or soon after feeds.
▶ If the vomiting is delayed after feeds, it is important to note the time lapse between the end of the feed and the vomiting.
▶ A large vomit before a feed is suggestive of delayed emptying of the stomach.
▶ The vomiting may have no relation to feeding.
▶ If the vomiting is related to feeds, the midwife should note whether it occurs at or after every feed or only occasionally.
▶ The force of the vomiting is important to consider, as it gives clues to the cause.
▶ The appearance of the vomitus must be considered: is it blood-stained, yellow or frothy?
▶ The odour of the vomitus should be noted. The vomiting of any feed results in an unpleasant, sour odour. If the feed has been retained for any length of time, the vomitus has an unpleasant stale smell. Foul-smelling vomitus is found in obstruction of the lower intestine and has an unmistakable faecal odour.

General condition and appearance of the infant

If any vomiting occurs, the infant should be very carefully monitored. The temperature, respiration and pulse must be taken and recorded at least every four hours. Any abnormalities should be reported immediately.

The general appearance of the infant should also be noted. Check whether the infant is losing or gaining mass (weight), the number of wet nappies, the colour of the urine and whether the infant has sunken eyes and a sunken fontanelle.

Do a Dextrostix and alert a medical practitioner. Without alarming the mother, the baby is kept in the nursery and, if needed, is given IV fluid.

43.5   Hypothermia and neonatal cold injury

Hypothermia

Hypothermia is a condition where the axillary temperature is less than 36 °C.

Causes

All newborns have a tendency to hypothermia, for the following reasons:
▶ A newborn's temperature-regulating mechanism is not as efficient as that of an older child.
▶ Body heat is very easily lost, because the newborn has a large body surface area in relation to the body mass and often less subcutaneous fat.
▶ The infant is naked and wet at birth.
▶ The blood vessels are closer to the skin's surface.

Risk factors

The following newborns are more likely to develop hypothermia:
▶ Newborns born outside the facilities, or born before arrival (BBA), and those who needed to be transferred to a higher-level hospital
▶ A wet newborn who is not dried immediately after birth
▶ LBW newborns
▶ Sick newborns, especially those with infections
▶ Newborns born in a cold environment and undergoing medical procedures such as resuscitation
▶ Newborns who are not fed in time and who have a low blood glucose level.

It is very important, therefore, that great care is taken at birth to prevent heat loss and to maintain the body temperature. Hypothermia is easier to prevent than to cure and serious side effects may arise. Hypothermia leads to hypoglycaemia and to respiratory distress, causing metabolic derangement and tissue damage.

Management and prevention of hypothermia

▶ Dry the infant as soon as possible after delivery to prevent loss of heat by evaporation.
▶ Cover the baby's head.
▶ Wrap the baby in warm blankets immediately after drying and keep him or her out of draughts.

▶ For the normal newborn, the room temperature should be above 22 °C, in order to prevent heat loss by convection.
▶ Perform frequent observations, particularly if the infant is at risk. At-risk babies should be placed in a warmed incubator as soon as respiration has been established.

Care of a hypothermic infant

▶ *Recognise early.* Observe the infant's temperature with care.
▶ *Control the environment.* The infant is placed in a pre-warmed incubator. The temperature of the incubator may range between 32 °C for a near-term newborn, and 36 °C for an extremely LBW newborn.
▶ *Protect from heat loss.* If the infant is already in an incubator, the temperature can be increased, a perspex heat shield can be placed over the infant and the infant can be dressed in a woolen cap, gloves and socks.
▶ *Kangaroo-mother-care (KMC).* If no incubator is available, the infant can be placed on the mother's chest and an aluminum or silver swaddler and blankets placed over them both. This is very useful for transporting the newborn.
▶ *Prevent hypoglycaemia.* Feed the newborn early and regularly.
▶ *Perform continuous observations.* Observe for colour, respiration and pulse frequently or continuously and check blood sugar levels.

Neonatal cold injury

The attribution of neonatal hypothermia to indirect or direct causes of newborn death is complex and difficult for several reasons (Lunze et al, 2013). Although hypothermia is a direct cause of death only in a small proportion of newborn mortality, it is closely associated with mortality from common causes of newborn deaths such as severe infections, prematurity and asphyxia. Neonatal cold injury, or severe hypothermia, mainly affects LBW babies. Everything possible should be done to prevent this condition. The brown fat that is metabolised for heat production becomes hard and the condition can be fatal. Neonatal cold injury has a mortality rate of about 25 per cent and many of the newborns who do survive, suffer brain damage due to hypoxaemia, hypoglycaemia or hyperbilirubinaemia (Culic, 2005).

Clinical features

The baby presents with:
▶ cold skin – the temperature may be below 32 °C
▶ lethargy – the infant does not feed well
▶ a feeble cry
▶ bradycardia (below 100 bpm)
▶ oliguria
▶ depressed or absent reflexes
▶ oedema, which may lead to sclerema (a non-pitting swelling of the skin and subcutaneous tissues which, if it develops around the thorax, can cause splinting of the thorax and further respiratory impairment)
▶ possibly a ruddy face and extremities, which is called pink hypoxia (due to oxygenated red blood cells being trapped in skin capillaries).

Management and care of cold injury

▶ The medical practitioner is notified.
▶ The infant is warmed in an incubator.
▶ Hourly temperature is done until stable.
▶ On the medical practitioner's prescription, an IV infusion of 10 per cent dextrose water is given to prevent hypoglycaemia.
▶ Antibiotics may be prescribed.
▶ Oxygen is given by a headbox.

Complications

▶ Hypoxaemia may occur due to bronchopneumonia and result in cyanosis.
▶ Metabolic acidosis or acidaemia may occur as a result of hypoxaemia.
▶ Hyperbilirubinaemia, leading to kernicterus, may occur in very small babies.
▶ Intrapulmonary haemorrhage may occur, which usually results in death.

43.6   Conclusion

The midwife must have the knowledge and skill to identify abnormalities in the physical and metabolic function of the newborn and refer the infant for medical attention. In some cases, the mother needs to be educated to change the way she cares for the baby.

Jaundice and infections in the newborn

LEARNING OBJECTIVES
On completion of this chapter, you must be able to:
▶ explain the physiological basis of neonatal jaundice
▶ demonstrate competence in the care of a newborn with jaundice
▶ demonstrate competence in the care of a newborn with neonatal infections
▶ demonstrate competence in phototherapy
▶ demonstrate competence in educating parents on jaundice and phototherapy.

KNOWLEDGE ASSUMED TO BE IN PLACE
The physiological abilities and adaptation of the newborn (see Chapter 40)
Newborn Care Charts (DoH, 2014a: 2.2.6, page 39)

KEYWORDS
physiological jaundice • hyperbilirubinaemia • phototherapy • Rh incompatibility • ABO incompatibility • kernicterus • omphalitis • conjunctivitis • ophthalmia neonatorum

44.1   Introduction

This chapter covers neonatal jaundice and common infections in newborns (DoH, 2014a, para 2.2.6). It is important for the midwife to know how to diagnose and manage these conditions.

44.2   Types of hyperbilirubinaemia in newborns

About 50 per cent of newborns develop what is called physiological jaundice of the newborn and a small percentage develop *pathological jaundice*, which is more serious (Hansen, 2016). The differentiation between physiological and pathological jaundice is detailed in Table 44.1.

Neonatal physiological jaundice is one of the most common conditions that need medical attention.

Pathophysiology of neonatal jaundice

The newborn has more red blood cells (RBCs) (fetal Hb) than children and adults (between 18–22 g/dl). After birth, the excess RBCs are broken down and removed from the circulation in large numbers. There is degradation of the haem component of haemoglobin to form bilirubin, which needs to be changed through conjugation and excreted from the system. The enzyme system that conjugates bilirubin in the liver into a water-soluble state is enzyme beta diglucuronide, which converts bilirubin into conjugated bilirubin by binding it to a protein. Glucose is needed in this process. Conjugated bilirubin is carried in the bile to the small intestine and is excreted in the stool.

44.3   Physiological jaundice in the newborn

The immature liver of the newborn lacks glucose availability and is dysfunctional in the first week of life. The amount of unconjugated bilirubin in the serum thus increases, the unconjugated bilirubin binds to the fat in the tissue and the baby becomes jaundiced.

Jaundice in the newborn appears first in the face and upper body and progresses downward toward the toes. Preterm newborns are more likely to develop jaundice than full-term newborns.

Table 44.1

Differences between physiological and pathological jaundice

	Physiological jaundice	**Pathological jaundice**
Onset	Seldom present before the third day after birth Clears within a week	Can be present from birth or within 24 hours Continues for long periods
Cause	Breakdown of RBCs Liver too immature to metabolise breakdown of products	Infant: metabolic congenital abnormalities (eg cystic fibrosis) Obstructive: liver conditions and bile obstruction Birth trauma: eg cephalohaematoma Infections: result in jaundice Maternal: Rh and ABO incompatibility Breast milk jaundice
Blood levels	Safe levels seldom exceeded	High bilirubin levels
Treatment	Phototherapy	Phototherapy and other medical interventions such as antenatal intrauterine exchange infusion and postpartum exchange transfusion
Outcomes	Clear; baby is normal	Prolonged jaundice (> 10 days) and neurotoxicity (kernicterus)

The brain barrier that protects the brain from high bilirubin levels is not developed and when the blood values of unconjugated bilirubin reach a level of 250 µmol/ℓ (15 mg%) in a preterm infant and 350 µmol/ℓ (20 mg%) in a term infant, the bilirubin binds to the fat in the brain and can cause permanent damage. Unconjugated bilirubin is neurotoxic and can cause death or kernicterus.

Incidence

About 50 per cent of normal newborns may develop a degree of physiological jaundice, which appears on about the third day after birth. About 5–10 per cent of newborns may develop bilirubin levels of more than 165 µmol (10 mg%) (Hansen, 2016). Newborns of 37 weeks' gestation and lower are four times more likely than term newborns to have a serum bilirubin of over 220 µmol/ℓ (13 mg%).

In babies who nurse poorly, the likelihood of becoming jaundiced is even greater. It must also be remembered that babies of 36–37 weeks' gestation (or less) do not nurse as well as more mature babies.

Causes

The reason for the high bilirubin levels may be to increase the number of RBCs that need to be replaced in the body, because of factors such as:

▶ abnormal blood cell shapes

▶ a difference in blood type between the mother and newborn
▶ cephalohaematoma, as a result of a difficult delivery
▶ higher levels of RBCs, which is more common in small-for-gestational-age (SGA) babies and some twins
▶ infection
▶ lack of (deficiency of) certain important proteins, called enzymes.

Raised conjugated hyperbilirubinaemia in the newborn of about 38 µmol (2 mg%) is rare and abnormal. In this situation, obstruction to biliary outflow, for example biliary atresia, may be a possibility. Uncommon enzyme deficiencies (such as alpha-1 antitrypsin deficiency) and other metabolic abnormalities, sepsis, certain medication, infections present at birth, cystic fibrosis, hepatitis and parenteral nutrition may also cause high levels of conjugated bilirubin in the newborn.

Signs and symptoms

Jaundice starts with a yellow discolouration of the sclera of the eyes and then spreads progressively over the body. If the trunk of the baby is affected, the bilirubin levels will be higher. Jaundice of the palms of the hands and feet indicates extreme levels in the blood. Some newborns will be tired and feed poorly.

The yellow colour of the skin and other tissues of the newborn are caused by the accumulation of indirect unconjugated bilirubin due to an overall increase in the total bilirubin in the blood.

Note the following about the presentation and duration of neonatal jaundice:

▶ Physiological jaundice normally presents on the second or third day of life.

▶ If jaundice is visible during the first 24 hours of life, further evaluation is suggested.

▶ If severe jaundice continues after the first two weeks of life, the newborn should be observed for galactosaemia, congenital hypothyroidism and other conditions associated with pathological jaundice.

Diagnosis

A history predisposing an infant to jaundice includes:

▶ siblings with jaundice

▶ a known family history of Gilbert's syndrome or other family members with jaundice

▶ known heritable haemolytic disorders, eg thalassaemia in babies of Asian mothers

▶ liver disease

▶ maternal illnesses such as diabetes mellitus or infections

▶ Rh and ABO incompatibility

▶ any birth trauma (eg bruising or haematoma).

The postnatal history includes the following:

▶ The stool is dark yellow or green.

▶ The baby is lethargic, sleepy and does not want to drink.

▶ The baby turns jaundiced.

The diagnosis is made on the history and clinical picture. Risk factors are considered and the condition is confirmed by the blood values of bilirubin in the baby. (The blood values are expressed in µmol/ℓ or mg%; 1 mg% = 17 µmol/ℓ. Only total bilirubin is reported.)

Three criteria are important in the diagnosis:

1 *Gestational age (GA) and birth mass.* The levels of jaundice are considered against the infant's weight. A preterm infant is treated earlier than a term infant.

2 *Days after birth.* If the jaundice starts before day 3, the cause is considered and treatment begins.

3 *Levels of unconjugated bilirubin.* The levels for treatment and other interventions depend on the blood levels of unconjugated bilirubin against the age and mass of the infant.

Many institutions check total bilirubin levels on all newborns at 24 hours after birth. Hospitals use probes that can estimate the bilirubin level just by touching the skin. High readings need to be confirmed with blood tests.

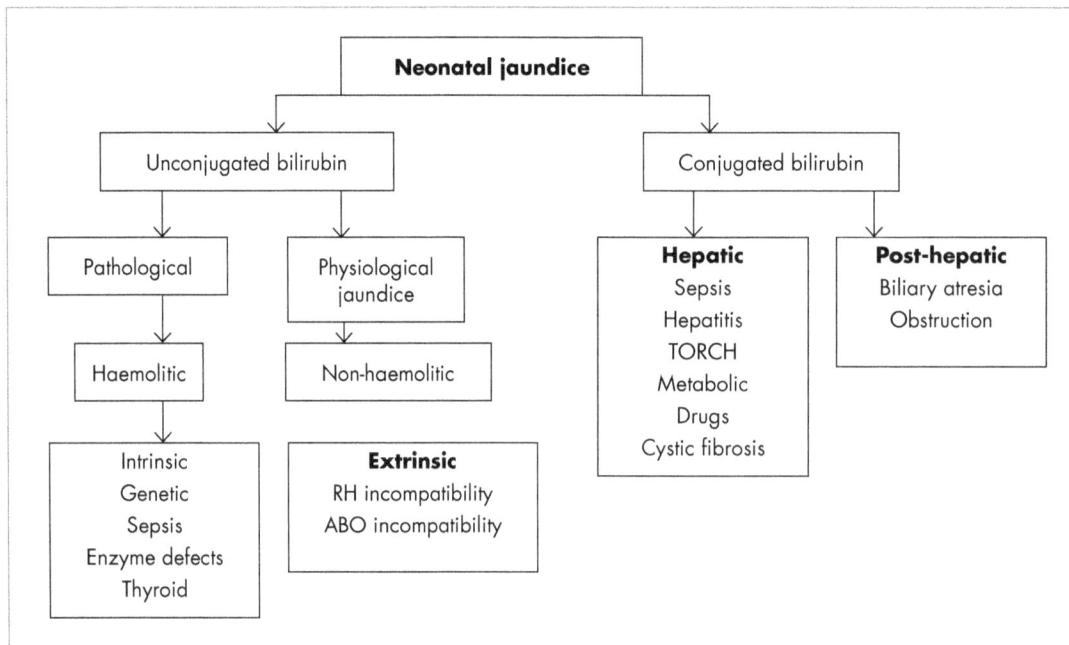

Figure 44.1 Diagram for classification of physiological and pathological neonatal jaundice

If jaundice does not clear up with phototherapy, other causes must be considered (see Table 44.1 and Figure 44.1).

Care of a baby with jaundice

All newborns are examined daily for jaundice. The examination is done in natural light. The midwife starts by looking at the face, continues to the arms and legs and then examines the body. However, it is not accurate to only go on the colour of the skin; a blood serum test is a more accurate way of determining the severity.

Finally, most authorities agree that if a newborn is discharged early from hospital, he or she must be checked for jaundice by a competent practitioner on day 2 or 3 postpartum. (See DoH, 2014a: 67.)

Prevention, management and treatment

Early discharge has resulted in fewer opportunities to teach new mothers how to breastfeed or to detect medical conditions that don't become evident until 24–72 hours after birth. This has resulted in a doubling of readmission to hospital within one to two weeks of birth, mainly due to jaundice and dehydration.

The early feeding of a newborn with colostrum can stimulate peristalsis and meconium stools. There seems to be a lower risk of neonatal jaundice with early feeding. Mothers are thus encouraged to start breastfeeding soon after birth.

In most cases treatment is not necessary, but this will depend on the blood bilirubin level, the GA of the newborn and the development of the condition.

Jaundice in the newborn, whether physiological or pathological, is always referred for medical care. The medical practitioner will choose the intervention required based on existing guidelines and clinical judgement.

The first line of treatment is phototherapy. The aim of phototherapy is to change the bilirubin that is bound to the fat in the skin to a water-soluble state. When the newborn is exposed to fluorescent light of 400–500 nm, unconjugated bilirubin becomes water-soluble and is excreted in the urine and stools.

PROCEDURE Phototherapy

Indications for phototherapy
The following are the serum bilirubin levels and individual conditions of the newborn (DoH, 2014a, para 2.2.6: 67):

- Preterm newborn of < 1 500 g: 85–140 µmol/ℓ (5–8 mg%)
- Preterm newborn of > 1 500 g, sick infants and those with haemolysis: 140–165 µmol/ℓ (8–10 mg%)
- Healthy term newborns jaundiced after 48 hours: 280–365 µmol/ℓ (17–22 mg%)

Note that values of µmol/ℓ are divided by 17 to get mg%.

Care of the newborn receiving phototherapy
A newborn can be cared for at home, next to a mother in a maternity ward or in a nursery or neonatal unit. The choice of care depends on the condition of the infant and the type of jaundice. The newborn can be in a crib or in an incubator.

Devices
Different devices exist for phototherapy, including phototherapy fluorescent lights, the Bilibed and the Wallaby (a fibre-optic blanket with tiny bright lights placed around the infant's chest). It is important to use the device according to its specifications.

General principles
- Phototherapy is prescribed by a medical practitioner based on blood values.

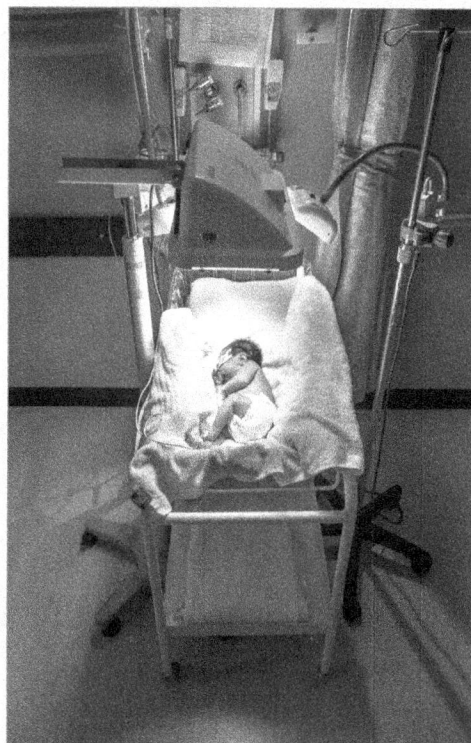

Figure 44A A phototherapy unit

continued

> ❱ Total serum bilirubin (TSB) levels are measured daily.
> ❱ Careful monitoring of the newborn is essential. This includes the baby's temperature, fluid intake and general well-being.
> ❱ The baby is nursed naked under the lights, with his or her eyes covered for protection when using fluorescent lights or a fibre-optic blanket with bright lights.
> ❱ The lights are 30–50 cm above the infant regardless of the bed used.
> ❱ If fluorescent lights are used, they need to be replaced every 1 000 hours. Effectiveness measuring depends on the type of treatment (see the device manual).
> ❱ Continue with breastfeeding or bottle feeding to prevent dehydration.
> ❱ The baby must be removed from under the lights for feeds, but should remain under the lights for most of 24 hours without a nappy for better exposure time.
> ❱ Observe the eyes, cord and buttocks.
> ❱ If the mother and baby are discharged, phototherapy can be done at home by accredited providers approved by the medical practitioner. If the service is not available, the mother is admitted in the hospital as a lodger.

Potential complications of phototherapy include:
❱ dehydration – babies do not drink and are lethargic
❱ interruption of feeds, with slower weight gain
❱ trauma to the eyes from the eye pads (infection)
❱ mother–infant separation and emotional upset
❱ overheating caused by a lack of temperature control
❱ a bronze discolouration of the skin in babies who are under the lights for long periods
❱ skin rashes – these are common due to the heat
❱ diarrhoea – babies tend to have loose stools when excreting the bilirubin.

Complications of jaundice

Serious complications in severe or untreated jaundice include cerebral palsy, deafness and kernicterus (the staining of the basal ganglia of the brain with unconjugated bilirubin, causing irreversible brain damage). As per age and birth mass: in term babies 375 µmol/ℓ and preterm babies 190–200 µmol/ℓ.

Maternal milk jaundice

There is a low incidence of breast milk jaundice. If a baby presents with jaundice that develops from four to seven days after birth and is continuous (longer than normal), maternal milk jaundice is suspected – provided that all other pathological causes are excluded. There is no specific explanation for this condition, but the maternal hormones through the breast milk interfere with the breakdown of bilirubin.

When breast milk jaundice is suspected, the baby may be taken off the breast for 24 hours. If the bilirubin falls, then it is likely to be caused by breast milk. The mother and medical practitioner decide the risk if the baby remains on the breast and make a decision accordingly. It is not always necessary to stop breast milk.

44.4 Pathological jaundice in the newborn

Pathological jaundice in the newborn generally appears within 24 hours after birth, reaches levels of 275 µmol/ℓ and persists beyond 10 days.

Causes

Rh incompatibility

Before the problem of Rh incompatibility was recognised and addressed, this was a relatively common cause of fetal morbidity and mortality. Mothers who are Rh negative become sensitised to the Rh antigen when small amounts of fetal (Rh positive) blood leak into the Rh negative maternal circulation. With the next pregnancy, the mother produces immunoglobulin G (IgG), which crosses the placenta to cause massive haemolysis in the fetus (see Chapter 24). The newborn is often severely anaemic, grossly jaundiced and critically ill, with serious neurological consequences.

ABO incompatibility

Some Group O mothers will produce IgG antibodies to the A or B blood group antigens (commonly A) and these may cause a situation similar to Rh incompatibility, but often milder.

Other causes

❱ *Enzyme deficiencies.* Glucose 6-phosphate dehydrogenase (G6PD) deficiency and other uncommon hereditary enzyme deficiencies, such as RBC abnormalities, hereditary spherocytosis, polycythaemia, bleeding into tissues, including cephalohaematomas related to application of a ventouse (vacuum extraction)
❱ *Inborn errors of metabolism.* Galactosaemia, tyrosinosis, hypermethionaemia, alpha-1-antitrypsin deficiency, etc

▶ *Obstructive jaundice.* Atresia of bile ducts, inspissated bile syndrome and choledocal cyst
▶ *Infections.* Syphilis, toxoplasmosis, cytomegalovirus and rubella
▶ *Congenital abnormalities.* Cystic fibrosis.

Clinical signs and symptoms

If untreated, the pathway of the disease leads to severe complications and death. Early diagnosis and treatment is thus essential. Any baby with jaundice that presents within 24 hours or continues after 10 days needs referral. Signs and symptoms include the following:

▶ The first phase includes lethargy, hypotonia and poor sucking.
▶ The second phase includes hypertonia, opisthotonos and fever.
▶ The third phase – after about a week – includes hypertonia, an abnormal Moro reflex (exaggerated or reduced), cerebral irritation, convulsions and seizures.
▶ The long-term sequelae are devastating delayed motor skills, abnormalities of tone and reflexes, athetoid cerebral palsy and deafness.

With severe haemolysis, there is kernicterus.

Care of pathological jaundice

The cause of the condition should be determined; this is done by taking a thorough history from the mother and examining the infant. The newborn's blood group can be determined if ABO incompatibility is suspected. Make sure that a sample of cord blood is available after birth for a Coomb's test.

Besides levels of conjugated and unconjugated bilirubin, it may be appropriate to do a full blood count (FBC) with a blood smear for red cell morphology. Other tests may be required, depending on ethnicity and clinical suspicion of red cell haemolytic disorders. Remember that with ABO incompatibility, a negative Coomb's test does not exclude haemolysis, as this test is infrequently positive, although a positive result may suggest more severe haemolysis.

The clinical assessment of the degree of jaundice is often poorly correlated with serum levels. However, it is well recognised that as the severity increases, yellow pigmentation spreads from the face to the trunk and eventually the extremities. If there is staining of the feet, a serum bilirubin is most advisable.

In severe cases of jaundice, it may be necessary to perform one or more exchange transfusions on the infant to prevent kernicterus from occurring. Depending on the age and mass of the infant, an exchange transfusion is done when the total bilirubin is 20 mg/dl (340 μmol/ℓ) in a term infant and 15 mg/dl (255 μmol/ℓ) in a preterm infant.

Complications of Rh haemolytic disease

If Rh haemolytic disease is not prevented, it results in serious consequences for the fetus or newborn, such as:

▶ intrauterine death (IUD)
▶ hydrops fetalis (oedema of the fetus)
▶ icterus gravis neonatorum (grave jaundice of the newborn), which manifests within 24 hours of birth and can result in kernicterus and death if untreated
▶ haemolytic anaemia (see Chapter 22).

44.5 Infections

Newborns are more at risk of certain infections, as their immune systems have a limited ability to prevent and fight infectious diseases. Special care – sometimes in the neonatal care unit – may be needed for the newborn who develops an infection before, during or after birth (see Chapter 49).

Causes of infection

Most infections in newborns are caused by bacteria, but some are caused by viruses. The newborn can be infected by the mother during pregnancy if the causal organism passes through the placenta to the fetus. Examples of those infections include rubella, syphilis, toxoplasmosis, cytomegalovirus (CMV) and HIV.

The newborn can also catch infections, particularly respiratory conditions and septicaemia, via infected amniotic fluid if the membranes have ruptured early. This condition is known as amniotic fluid infection syndrome (AFIS), but it is very difficult to distinguish between intrauterine or intrapartum infection and an infection acquired after birth.

Herpes infection can be acquired by the newborn from a labial lesion during vaginal delivery. These newborns are therefore ideally delivered by Caesarean section.

Hepatitis B is acquired at or shortly after birth. The exact mode of transmission is not known. A high percentage of newborns born to mothers who are Hepatitis B 'e' antigen (HBeAg) positive become infected with the virus and become carriers.

General infections that the newborn may acquire and which could have serious consequences are septicaemia, meningitis, pneumonia, tuberculosis and tetanus. Immunisation of the mother against tetanus in the last trimester produces antibodies in her blood, which reach the fetus in sufficient quantities to protect the infant from neonatal tetanus.

Signs and symptoms

Signs and symptoms of infections include:

▶ a decreased or elevated temperature: below 36.6 °C or above 37.7 °C (newborns tend to have a subnormal temperature with infections)

- poor feeding and difficulty waking to feed
- breathing difficulties
- listlessness
- an unusual skin rash or changes in skin colour
- persistent crying
- unusual irritability
- excessive sleepiness
- changes in behaviour
- hepatosplenomegaly (enlarged liver and spleen).

Systemic and local infections

Infections can be systemic or local. A number of these are discussed below.

Omphalitis

Omphalitis is an infection of the umbilical cord that can lead to septicaemia. The usual causal organisms are *Staphylococci aureus*, *Streptococcus* and *Escherichia coli*. A mixed Gram-positive and Gram-negative as well as anaerobic bacteria can also cause omphalitis.

Signs and symptoms include:
- a moist cord
- redness and swelling of skin
- an offensive smell
- bleeding
- a purulent discharge.

Preventive measures include keeping the cord clean and dry by using full-strength alcohol or surgical spirits after bathing, and at each nappy change.

The management and care of omphalitis includes the following:
- A swab is taken for Gram stain and culture.
- The cord is cleaned with surgical spirits every three hours.
- In mild infections, the appropriate antibiotic is prescribed.
- In severe infections, an IM antibiotic is given, as prescribed by the medical practitioner, and the infant is referred to the medical practitioner.

Conjunctivitis

Conjunctivitis is an inflammation of the conjunctiva within the first month of life, often caused by *Staphylococcus aureus*, *Neisseria gonorrhoeae*, *Streptococcus pneumoniae*, *Haemophilus influenzae*, *Escherichia coli*, *Klebsiella*, *Pseudomonas* and *Chlamydia trachomatis*.

Ophthalmia neonatorum

Ophthalmia neonatorum is caused by the gonococcus bacteria. It is a very serious notifiable condition that can lead to scarring and blindness, septicaemia, meningitis and endocarditis.

The signs and symptoms include the following:
- Between the second to third day of life, there is a purulent discharge from the eyes.
- The eyes become red and puffy, with a purulent green discharge.
- The progress of the infection is rapid and severe conjunctivitis results.

It is best to take routine preventive precautions by instilling Chloromycetin® or Erythromycin® eye ointment into each eye at birth.

If the condition has presented, do the following in order to manage and treat the infant:
- The baby's eyes should be cleaned with sterile swabs and normal saline at bath time and before each feed for 24 hours.
- The medical practitioner must be informed immediately.
- Take a swab before treatment is commenced.
- Apply antibiotic eye ointment or drops.
- Carefully wash the hands before and after handling the baby.
- The baby should lie on the affected side for drainage, unless both eyes are affected.
- Follow up on the progress of the infant.
- Provide health education to the mother with regard to the future care of the infant.

Skin infections

Skin infections may vary from infected pustules or vesicles to abscesses, and from impetigo to cellulitis.

A serious skin infection can be caused by *Staphylococcus aureus*, which presents with pus in blisters on the skin. The blisters rupture to reveal dry, reddish skin. In severe cases the skin looks burnt. Medical care is instituted.

Treatment for newborns (under 6 days) with limited pustules consists of cleaning the area with an antiseptic lotion and prescribing an appropriate antibiotic such as flucloxacillin 10–25 mg/kg twice a day or cloxacillin 25–50 mg/kg twice daily. For serious infections, ceftriaxone is given intramuscularly and the newborn is transferred to a Level 2 hospital.

44.6 Conclusion

The prevention of complications in newborns starts in the antenatal period and continues during labour and in the postnatal period. Many of the postnatal complications discussed in this chapter originate in the antenatal period.

Congenital abnormalities

LEARNING OBJECTIVES

On completion of this chapter, you must be able to:

- define a congenital abnormality, birth defect and inborn error
- give the prevalence of priority problems in South Africa
- explain the causes of birth defects
- differentiate between genetic and congenital disorders
- institute measures to prevent congenital abnormalities and related complications in pregnancy, birth and in the newborn, related to the specific abnormality
- identify the most common types of congenital abnormalities of newborns
- demonstrate the skills required to care for mothers and newborns with a specific congenital abnormality.

KNOWLEDGE ASSUMED TO BE IN PLACE

Basic knowledge of genetics, diagnosis of genetic diseases and their prevention (see Chapter 7)

KEYWORDS

congenital • genetic birth defect • inborn errors

45.1   Introduction

One of the most stressful situations in midwifery practice is the birth of a newborn with a birth defect. Because of the debilitating effects of a congenital abnormality and the effects of this on the individual, the family, the healthcare system and society, primary prevention programmes such as screening for defects should be developed to identify mothers at risk.

The prospect of a child with a congenital abnormality places extra stress on the parents, especially when the question of termination of the pregnancy becomes relevant. The midwife is in the unique position to identify abnormalities early and to refer the pregnant mother for management and care.

A number of defects may occur in the newborn. This chapter will discuss the most common conditions and the priority conditions as identified by the national Department of Health (DoH). Some of these conditions are structural abnormalities that can be seen in the womb using sonar or are visible after birth, whereas some conditions are not so visible and are only identified when signs and symptoms or functional errors present. This chapter needs to be studied in conjunction with Chapter 7.

45.2   Birth defects

Definitions

A *birth defect* is an abnormality of structure or function in a newborn that is present at birth. The abnormality may be diagnosed at birth or later in life. Birth defects can occur as an abnormal appearance or as failure to grow and develop normally.

An anomaly may or may not be perceived as a problem condition. Many, if not most, people have one or more minor physical anomalies if examined carefully. Examples of minor anomalies can include curvature of the fifth finger (clinodactyly), a third nipple, tiny indentations of the skin near the ears (preauricular pits), shortness of the fourth metacarpal or metatarsal bones, or dimples over the lower spine (sacral dimples). Some minor anomalies may be clues to more significant internal abnormalities.

Table 45.1

Common birth defects in newborns

Mouth	Cleft lip and palate, ankyloglossia, Pierre Robin syndrome
Eyes	Anophthalmia, microphthalmia, cataracts, glaucoma, ptosis, strabismus
Ears	Microtia, auricular tags
Face	Micrognathia
Central nervous system	Anencephaly (three times more likely in girls than boys), spina bifida (occulta or aperta), hydrocephaly, microcephaly, cranial meningocele, encephalocele
Respiratory system	Diaphragmatic hernia, choanal atresia
Gastrointestinal (GI) system	Cystic fibrosis, oesophageal atresia, duodenal atresia, pyloric stenosis, Hirschsprung's disease, meconium ileus, exomphalos, gastroschisis, umbilical hernia, imperforated anus, prune belly syndrome, malrotation of the gut, volvulus
Genito-renal system	Extrophy of the bladder, ectopic kidney, hydronephrosis, hypospadia, hypoplasia (double), horseshoe kidney, hermaphroditism, polycystic kidneys, cryptorchidism (undescended testes), renal agenesis, hydrocele, torsion of testes, fused labia, hymenal tag
Cardiovascular system	Dextrocardia, univentricular heart Acyanotic conditions: coarctation of the aorta, atrial/ventricular septal defects (VSD), patent ductus arteriosus (PDA) Cyanotic conditions: total anomalous pulmonal veins, transposition of the great vessels, under-perfused lungs, tricuspid atresia, tetralogy of Fallot, pulmonary atresia
Skin	Aplasia cutis, cutis lax, Ehlers-Danlos, incontinentia pigmenti, bullous impetigo Lesions: vascular naevi, haemangiomata, simple naevi, portwine stains, spider naevi, strawberry spots, pigmented naevi, Mongolian spots, hairy mole, non-vascular naevi
Musculoskeletal system	Osteogenesis imperfecta, dislocation of the hip (dysplasia), achondroplasia, limb reduction anomalies, amniotic bands, talipes equinovarus (club foot), syndactyly, webbing, polydactyly, microdactyly, arachnodactyly, macrodactyly, symbrachydactyly, amelia, hammer toe, hemimelia, phocomelia, micromelia, craniotabes, cleidocranial dystosis, mermaid infant, Vater syndrome, craniostenosis

Congenital abnormalities are abnormalities that are present at birth.

Inborn errors are genetic defects that may be inherited, chromosomal or multifactorial.

Incidence

Congenital abnormalities are the cause of an estimated 1 538 babies dying within four weeks of birth per year in South Africa (NaPeMMCo, 2014; Lui et al, 2015). The *Saving Babies 2012–2013* report (Pattinson & Rhoda, 2014) indicates fetal abnormalities as the second highest cause of perinatal deaths in primary obstetrics for fresh and macerated stillbirths in South Africa. Globally, congenital malformations are rapidly emerging as a major worldwide problem, and are important causes of childhood death, chronic illness and disability in many countries (Agarwal et al, 2017).

Congenital anomalies of the heart carry the highest risk of death in infancy, followed by chromosomal and respiratory anomalies.

Causes of birth defects

The cause of 40–60 per cent of congenital anomalies is unknown (Bale, 2003; Quizlet, 2017); these are random occurrences with a low recurrence risk for future children.

Congenital abnormality may be the result of a physical, metabolic or anatomic deviation from the normal development of the fetus, which in the most cases appears at birth or in the first year of life. There are some known causes or risk factors, some of which are discussed below.

Socioeconomic, demographic and environmental factors

Countries with a low and middle income may have a 94 per cent greater chance of severe congenital abnormalities (WHO, 2016). The causes may include:

▶ inadequate nutrition, leading to nutritional inadequacies of iodine, folate or vitamin A

▶ maternal age: advanced maternal age increases the risk of chromosomal abnormalities, including Down's syndrome, while young maternal age increases the risk of some congenital anomalies

▶ environmental factors such as drug abuse in the mother, certain medications such as tetracycline, streptomycin, anti-cancer drugs (eg methotrexate), warfarin (an anticoagulant), some anticonvulsants (eg phenytoin, valproic acid), lithium (an antidepressant) and environmental pollutants such as methyl mercury

▶ maternal exposure to pesticides and chemicals

▶ maternal use of alcohol or tobacco.

Genetic factors

Some anomalies have a purely genetic cause. The majority of these are chromosomal anomalies. Table 45.2 lists the most common genetic and chromosomal disorders.

Many chromosomal disorders are caused when the DNA structure is altered, resulting in trisomy or monosomy of different chromosomes. Most fetuses with trisomy and monosomy are not capable of living and result in early spontaneous abortions.

Chromosomal defects include trisomy 13, 18, 21, X and Y. Chromosome X and Y mutations are as follows:

▶ Extra X chromosome mutations are associated with mental retardation, for example XXY.

▶ Extra Y chromosomes are associated with aggression, for example YYX.

▶ The lack of an X chromosome in the female results in Turner's syndrome (ie 45 XO).

▶ A mutation of YO is not viable.

▶ The most common birth mutation is Trisomy 21 or Down's syndrome.

Table 45.2

Common genetic and chromosomal disorders

Autosomal	Trisomy 21 (Down's syndrome) Trisomy 8 (Warkany's syndrome) Trisomy 18 (Edwards' syndrome) Trisomy 13 (Patau's syndrome) 5p minus syndrome (cri du chat)
Sex chromosomes	Klinefelter's syndrome (XYY) Turner's syndrome (XO)
Endocrine	Congenital hypo-/hyperthyroidism Congenital adrenal hyperplasia Gigantism Cushing's syndrome
Single gene (autosomal dominant)	Arachnodactyly (Marfan's syndrome)
Autosomal recessive	Albinism Ichthyosis (scaling) Osteogenesis imperfecta
Metabolic	Phenylketonuria (PKU) Galactosaemia Cystic fibrosis

The most common autosomal recessive conditions originate from tropical countries. Some single-gene disorders are more common in particular populations or regions, including:

▶ sickle cell disease (SCD) in West Africa

▶ thalassaemia in Mediterranean countries

▶ oculocutaneous albinism, in African people across the world

▶ polydactyly in black South Africans

▶ cystic fibrosis in people of European descent.

The most common X-linked recessive conditions are:

▶ red–green colour blindness

▶ haemophilia.

Some conditions, such as polycystic kidneys, osteogenesis imperfecta and retinitis pigmentosa, may be inherited by more than one mode of inheritance. For example, in some families it is a dominant trait while in other families it is a recessive trait.

Multifactorial birth defects

These are birth defects that have a combined genetic and environmental cause. The environmental factor is often not known. The person affected with a multifactorial birth defect inherits a combination of genes from his or her parents that places him or her at an increased risk for a birth defect. If that individual then experiences certain environmental factors, the result will be a multifactorial birth defect. Multifactorial birth defects therefore require both genetic and environmental factors before they present. Neither the genetic factor nor the environmental factor alone will cause the birth defect. (This is different from teratogens, which cause birth defects without an obvious genetic factor.) The risk that another child of the same parents will be affected by a multifactorial birth defect is small.

Multifactorial birth defects are the most common form of birth defect and usually affect a single structure, organ or system. They often present in infancy or childhood as malformations such as:

- neural tube defects (NTDs)
- isolated hydrocephalus
- clubfoot
- cleft lip and/or palate
- congenital heart defects.

45.3 Prevention

Because the cause of birth defects is often unknown, it is not always possible to prevent them. Health services should deliver preventative public health measures to decrease the frequency of certain congenital anomalies; such services should include genetic counselling, reproductive health services, early screening, assessment and diagnosis, and nutritional advice and support.

Ultrasound can be used during the first trimester to screen for abnormalities such as Down's syndrome. Other fetal anomalies are visible with ultrasound during the second trimester. Amniocentesis may be used in the detection of NTD and chromosomal abnormalities during the first and second trimesters.

Preconception assessment

A pre-pregnancy evaluation is done to identify any risk factors that may complicate the pregnancy, including family history, genetic tests, personal history and conditions. This includes:

- a family history of both biological parents to exclude medical problems such as hypertension and diabetes
- a full medical and obstetric history to determine any medical conditions such as anaemia, epilepsy, diabetes and hypertension as well as information of previous pregnancy outcomes and abnormal babies
- prevention by immunisation of diseases such as rubella; if the woman did not have this during childhood, then she

must be immunised at least one month before becoming pregnant to prevent congenital rubella syndrome
- screening for infections such as sexually transmitted infections (STIs) and urinary tract infection (UTI), which can be harmful to the woman or fetus.

The steps that can be taken to minimise the chances of congenital defects include:

- following a healthy lifestyle
- stopping smoking to prevent a low birth weight (LBW) baby
- eating a balanced diet, including an adequate intake of vitamins and minerals and an increased folic acid intake; the diet should include foods such as wheat or maize flour to lower the risk of birth defects
- maintaining a well-balanced weight
- avoiding exposure to alcohol and drugs during pregnancy
- avoiding exposure to X-rays and other harmful substances during pregnancy
- lowering the risk for infections by avoiding eating undercooked meat, raw eggs and avoiding contact and exposure to cat faeces
- managing pre-existing medical problems, such as diabetes or high BP.

In addition, it is important to educate healthcare professionals and others who are involved in promoting the prevention of congenital anomalies. Screening the profile of the woman, including screening for teenage mothers or advanced maternal age, alcohol use, tobacco or other psychoactive drugs, must be done. Early screening for the neonate includes a clinical physical examination, screening for abnormalities of the blood, metabolism and hormone production, as well as early detection of congenital anomalies. These can be life-saving treatments.

45.4 Priority genetic conditions in South Africa

This section discusses the conditions that are prioritised in South Africa for screening, prevention and treatment.

Down's syndrome (Trisomy 21)

This abnormality occurs in 1:600 births (Permezel, Walker & Kyprianou, 2015). It is associated with increased maternal age (1:60 mothers over 35 years) but can occur with a mother of any age; the risk is increased with parity in younger women after the third child and in older women after the fourth child (95% confidence interval) (Doria-Rose et al, 2003). It is caused by a pair of 21 chromosomes that fail to separate during meiosis.

Screening is done through blood tests at 15–18 weeks for alpha-fetoprotein (AFP) as part of the triple test. The results take four weeks. If the woman comes late for antenatal care – at or after 20 weeks – she can have the fluorescent *in situ* hybridisation (FISH) test done, which is also available in the public sector. The results can be available in 36 hours.

The nuchal fold ultrasound scan is done at 12 weeks and repeated after 20 weeks (Glick & Gaillard, 2017). It measures the fluid content at the back of the baby's neck. Diagnosis is possible through amniocentesis at 16–20 weeks. A positive blood test is followed up with an amniocentesis, usually after counseling, if the parents are considering a therapeutic abortion.

Clinical features

The clinical picture (Figure 45.1) can be detected after birth:
▶ Hypotonia is the most common feature (a floppy baby).
▶ The skin and hair are smooth.
▶ The head may be small and under the third percentile.
▶ Epicanthic folds are prominent and the eyes slant upwards. The iris can be speckled (Brushfield's spots).
▶ The tongue looks big and protrudes and the nose may be flat. The ears may be malformed and placed low.
▶ The neck is short, with a thick ridge posteriorly.
▶ The hands and feet are broad, with short digits. A wide gap may be present between the first and second digit and there is one palmar crease which stretches across the hand.
▶ In the male, the testes are not descended.

▶ Associated abnormalities include cardiac defects, which are common, as well as GI defects such as duodenal atresia.

Management and care

If no antenatal tests were done, the diagnosis is made after birth on the clinical picture and confirmed by chromosomal tests of blood taken from the baby.

If co-morbidities such as cardiac defects are present, the child mortality is higher. Most children survive and are happy children. The prognosis depends on the level of retardation and care they receive. The milestones are delayed. Walking is at 25 months. Normal schooling is unlikely and repetitive work is more suitable. Some well-trained children are able to function in the open market. Males cannot reproduce and females have lower rates of conception than normal. Common problems are respiratory infections and an increased risk of leukaemia.

Central nervous system malformation: Hydrocephalus

Hydrocephalus (see Figure 45.2 on the next page) is the excessive accumulation of fluid in the ventricles due to an obstruction in or outside the ventricular draining system.

The enlarged lateral ventricles are noted, along with thinning of the white matter. This is characteristic of hydrocephalus due to obstruction of cerebrospinal fluid (CSF) pathways. The increase in CSF pressure in the ventricles causes distension of the ventricles and pressure atrophy of the brain.

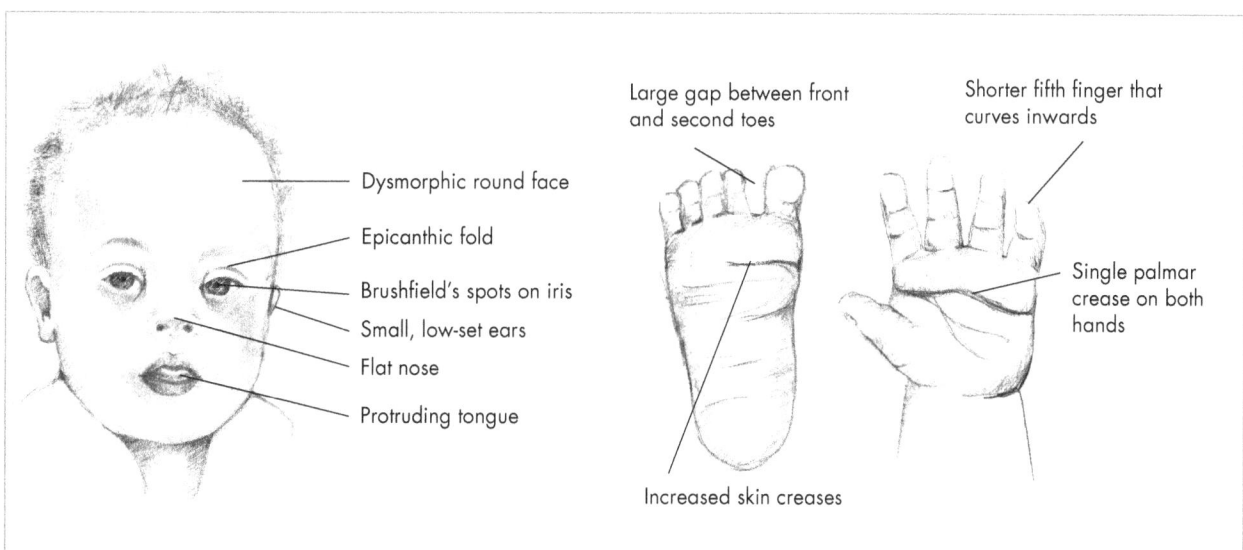

Dysmorphic round face
Epicanthic fold
Brushfield's spots on iris
Small, low-set ears
Flat nose
Protruding tongue

Large gap between front and second toes
Increased skin creases

Shorter fifth finger that curves inwards
Single palmar crease on both hands

Figure 45.1 Signs and symptoms of Down's syndrome

There are two types of hydrocephalus: communicating and non-communicating. In communicating hydrocephalus, CSF can expand into the subarachnoid space, but fibrosis of the meninges or arachnoid granulations prevents it from draining into the superior sagittal sinus. In non-communicating hydrocephalus, CSF cannot get to the subarachnoid space because its flow is blocked by gliosis of the aqueduct, fibrosis of the foramina of Luschka and Magendie or a colloid cyst of the third ventricle. In spite of the fact that CSF pathways are blocked, CSF is formed at a normal rate, so the ventricles have to dilate, particularly at the expense of the white matter.

Hydrocephalus is often an accompaniment of meningomyelocele. It can also be caused by isolated stenosis of the Aqueduct of Sylvius due to *in utero* viral infection. Meningitis can cause communicating hydrocephalus.

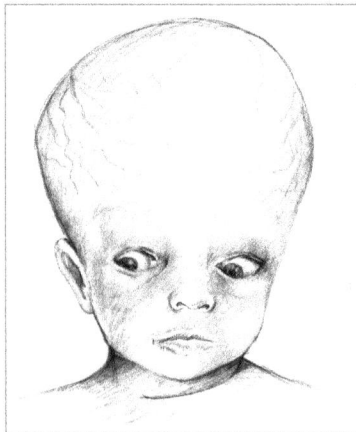

Figure 45.2 Hydrocephalus

Clinical features

▶ In hydrocephalus, there is a blockage of the flow of CSF, with enlargement of ventricles at the expense of the white and grey matter.
▶ The head is enlarged above the 97th percentile.
▶ The sutures are wide open.
▶ The newborn may present with poor sucking, vomiting, irritability, eyes that appear to gaze downwards and a failure to thrive.

Diagnosis, treatment and care

The condition is detected in pregnancy; for this, ultrasound is useful. After birth, an ultrasound confirms the enlargement of the ventricles.

If diagnosed in pregnancy, intrauterine surgery may be possible in specialised units. The alleviation of the pressure on the brain is essential to prevent mental retardation. A shunt is placed in position to drain the fluid.

Neural tube defects

These abnormalities occur during the second and fourth weeks of gestation. Vitamin deficiency and nutritional factors play a role in the aetiology, particularly folic acid insufficiency. AFP accumulates in the amniotic fluid and is suggestive of a variety of defects.

A blood test at 14 weeks or an amniocentesis is offered for women with diabetes mellitus, women who have given birth to a previously abnormal baby and women on medications that are folic acid antagonists.

Types of defects include encephalocele, spina bifida, meningomyelocele and anencephaly.

Encephalocele

There is no accurate data on NTDs globally. NTDs are an important global burden, causing neonatal mortality and morbidity worldwide (Zaganjor et al, 2016).

Encephalocele, where the brain is outside the skull in a skin-covered sac, is less common than anencephaly. Occipital encephaloceles are much more common than parietal or frontal ones. The disorganised brain in the sac is usually attached to the remainder of the brain and may contain CSF.

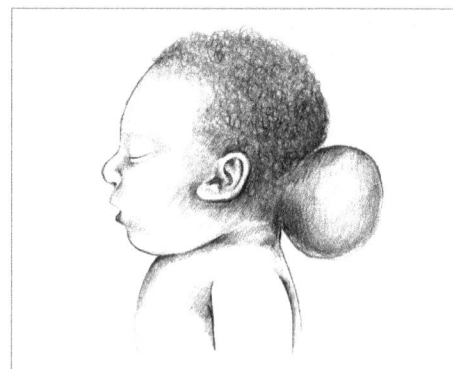

Figure 45.3 Occipital encephalocele

If the encephalocele is large and there is a large volume of abnormal brain in the sac, then the baby may be profoundly mentally retarded. If it is very small, then the child may be normal mentally. In either case, the sac must be excised so that the skin does not erode and cause meningitis.

Spina bifida

This is a defect of the vertebral column with or without protrusion of spinal cord content.

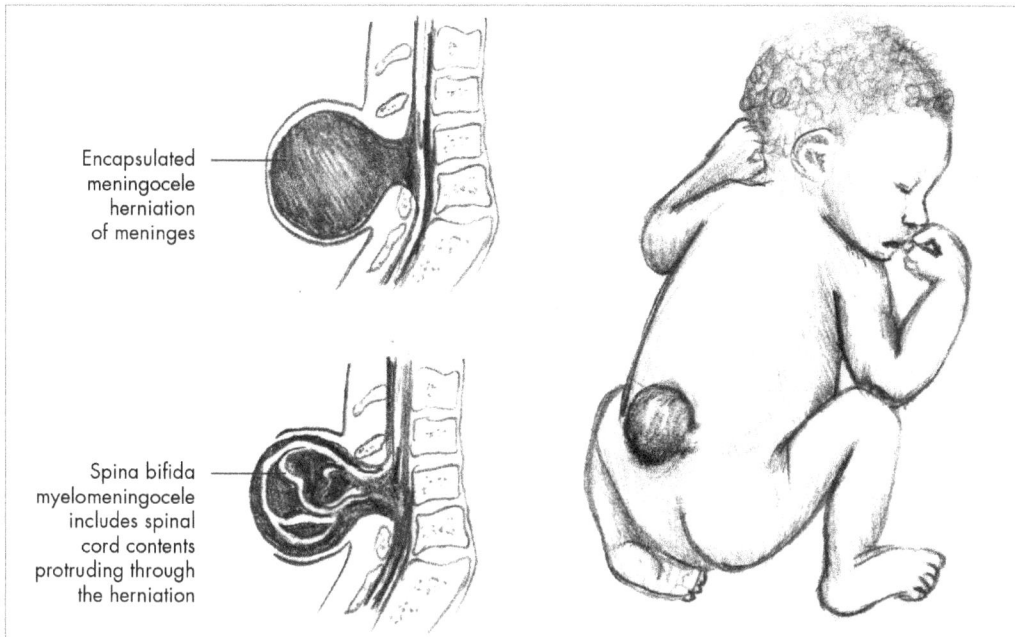

Figure 45.4 Spina bifida, meningocele and myelomeningocele

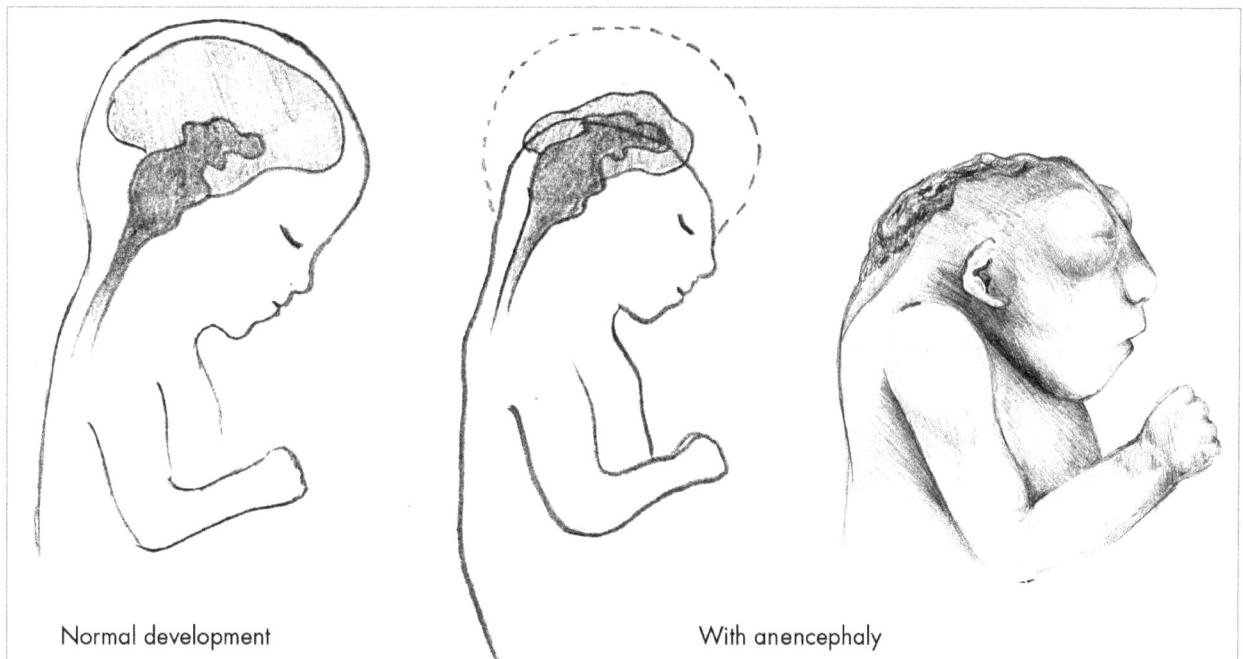

Normal development

With anencephaly

Figure 45.5 Anencephaly

Spina bifida occulta refers to a condition where a birth mark in the lower back may be the only sign of the malformation and an X-ray is needed to make a diagnosis. Treatment may not be needed.

Spina bifidia cystic is the protrusion of meninges or spinal content through the laminar arches of the spinal column that did not close:

▶ A *meningocele* is a protrusion of meninges and CSF, often covered with skin. It occurs in the lower back. Motor function may be normal. Surgical correction is done soon after birth, with a good prognosis.

▶ *Meningomyelocele* is a serious malformation that occurs ten times more commonly and includes a spinal cord that may or may not be in a sac. Motor and sensory loss of the lower limbs and bladder is present in varying degrees depending on the level of the lesion. Mental retardation, hydrocephalus and fecal and urinary incontinence are common problems associated with the condition.

A full neurological examination is needed for every NTD that presents at birth. Care of these children is long term, and although they may be of normal intelligence, they are often paralysed in the lower body and need a wheelchair and long-term care.

Anencephaly

This condition is characterised by the absence of the vault of the cranium, with a partial or total absence of the cerebrum and cerebellum (see Figure 45.5 on the previous page). Most infants are stillborn or die within hours. It is three times more common in girls than boys.

Fetal alcohol syndrome

This syndrome is dealt with in detail in Chapter 51.

Albinism

Albinism is hypopigmentation of the skin, hair and eyes. It occurs in partial or complete form. The features are photophobia, nystagmus and impaired vision. There is no prenatal test available.

These children experience a great deal of social discomfort. Mothers need to be supported and educated about the risk of sunburn and the need to protect the eyes from radiation and the sun. The children need to wear sunscreen due to the risk of skin cancer later in life.

Cleft lip and palate

The face, lip, tongue, jaws and palate develop during the fourth and sixth weeks *in utero* up to the twelfth week. The condition can be diagnosed with ultrasound during the antenatal period.

Genetic factors can play a role in the development of cleft lip or palate. It may be hereditary, but may also be a spontaneous defect. More boys (60 per cent) than girls (40 per cent) are affected. Babies born with a cleft lip or palate are also more likely to have other associated birth defects than babies not born with a cleft palate. The risks of giving birth to a child with a cleft palate are highest when both parents have clefts themselves. If only one parent has a cleft palate, the risk of having a baby with a cleft palate is 1 in 20 (5 per cent). If a set of parents, neither of whom have a cleft, gives birth to a child with a cleft, the chances of them giving birth to a second child with a cleft palate is between 2 to 4 percent (University of Virginia, 2017).

Cleft lip

The chances of having a baby with a cleft palate (without a cleft lip) is thought to be 1 in every 3 000 live births (University of Virginia, 2017).

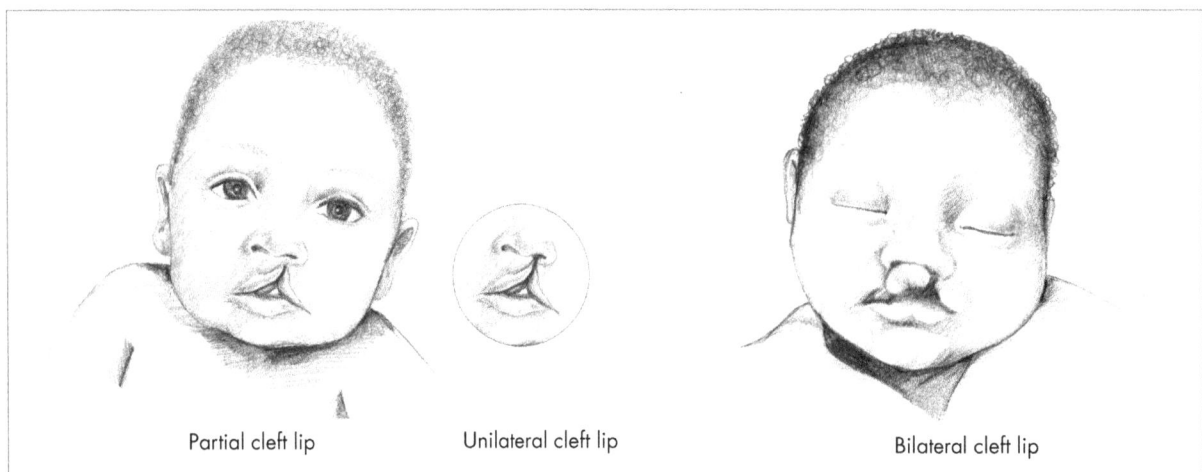

Partial cleft lip   Unilateral cleft lip   Bilateral cleft lip

Figure 45.6 Cleft lip

A cleft lip is more commonly left-sided and more common in boys than girls. The severity can vary, from a small notch in the upper lip to a complete split. Although a cleft lip is disfiguring, it can be corrected by plastic surgery with minimal effects. The parent needs reassurance and referral to a specialist. A cleft lip is corrected at three months of age.

Cleft palate

This condition is more common in girls than boys, with an incidence of 1:700 live births (Mossey & Castilla, 2003). The condition can be diagnosed with ultrasound.

A cleft palate is more serious than a cleft lip and has implications for eating and speech development. The baby will be able to breastfeed; an orthodontic device soon after birth can assist the mother with feeding difficulties. The device remains in the mouth and is only removed to be cleaned after feeds. Pictures of before and after the procedures can help to educate parents about care.

Corrective surgery is done before 12 months, but more operations may follow, depending on the extent of the condition.

Speech therapy is required and teeth may need to be aligned. The child will need orthodontic consultation and intervention.

Club feet (talipes equinovaris)

According to the WHO (2017), 100 000 babies worldwide are born with a clubfoot annually. Clubfoot is an inborn deformity of the foot, where either or both feet are twisted inward, causing the child to walk on his or her ankles. Left untreated, the condition causes severe lifelong disability. Eighty per cent of untreated clubfoot cases are found in developing countries (WHO, 2017). It is twice as common in boys as girls. It can be isolated or associated with other congenital abnormalities, such as spina bifida, hydrocephaly and other conditions. It can affect only one foot or both feet.

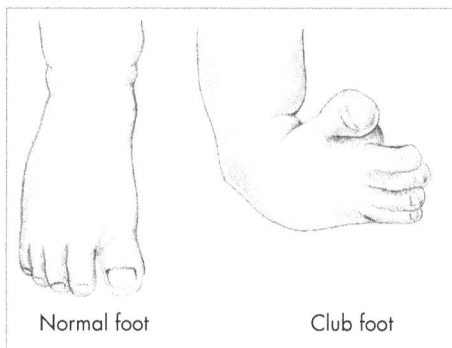

Normal foot   Club foot

Figure 45.7 Right club foot

The foot is plantar flexed (equinus) (sole of the foot turned in and upwards) and medially deviated (varus) (turned inwards at the ankle). Wasting of the calf muscle may be present, with a small heel.

Immediate orthopaedic intervention is required. Mild cases can be treated with extension strapping that needs to stay on day and night. The Ponseti method can be used to correct clubfoot by aligning the feet using a series of casts. It is non-invasive and inexpensive. The success rate is 98 per cent, and success can be achieved with as little as five casts and 20 days of treatment (WHO, 2017).

In severe cases, surgery is needed. In most cases, the condition can be corrected. The affected person will require two to three surgeries over his or her lifetime to have a high quality of life.

45.5 Cardiac disorders of the newborn

The heart is the first organ that is formed and functions in the fetus as early as the third week *in utero*.

The incidence of congenital heart disease at birth depends on how a population is studied. The introduction of echocardiography and improved early diagnosis provides an opportunity for greater detection. The incidence is five to eight per 1 000 live births for milder conditions up to eight to 12 per 1 000 live births (Hoffman, 2013).

Cardiac abnormalities are associated with Down's and Turner's syndromes, arachnodactyly and rubella syndrome.

Congenital cardiac defects are divided in to cyanotic and acyanotic conditions.

Cyanotic cardiac conditions

Transposition of the vessels

This occurs twice as often in boys compared to girls and should be suspected in babies that are cyanotic. The great vessels open incorrectly into the wrong atrium and normal circulation cannot be maintained (see Figure 45.8 on the next page). Oxygen-rich blood will go to the lungs and oxygen-poor blood to the body. Heart murmurs may not be audible. If the ductus arteriosus and foramen ovale close, severe cyanosis occurs.

A shunt is created between the atria and the condition is corrected later in infancy.

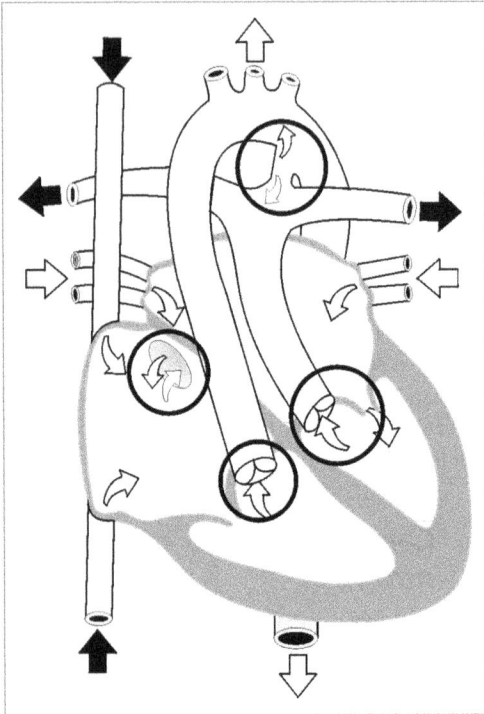

Figure 45.8 Transposition of the vessels

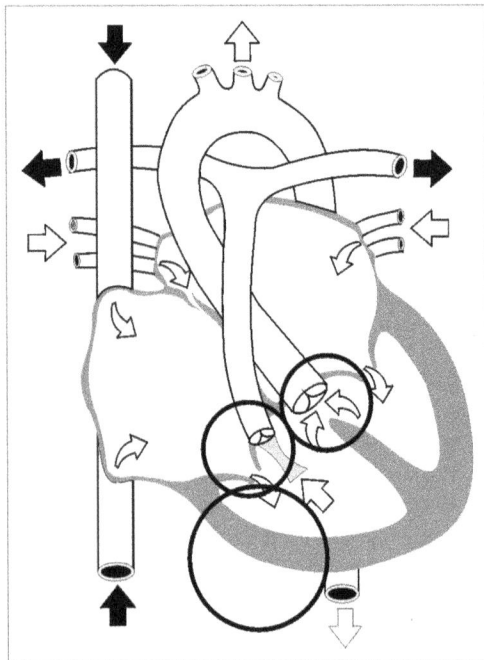

Figure 45.9 Tetralogy of Fallot

Tetralogy of Fallot

This is a fairly common abnormality with pulmonary stenosis, overriding aorta and right ventricular hypertrophy (see Figure 45.9). Cyanosis develops over months. It is more difficult to diagnose. A murmur may be present.

The condition can be corrected with surgery by four years of age.

Pulmonary atresia

This is a rare abnormality. If the pulmonary valve cannot function, blood can only reach the lungs through the ductus arteriosus. If the ductus arteriosus closes, severe cyanosis occurs. This presents soon after birth, with signs of cardiac failure. Death will occur if the obstruction is not reversed.

Acyanotic cardiac conditions

Hypoplastic left heart

Hypoplastic left heart is a common disorder, causing cardiac failure due to an underdeveloped left ventricle. The BP is low and the blood is shunted to the right atrium and ventricle through the atrial defect. If the ductus arteriosis closes prematurely, shock and death may occur.

Ventricular septal defects

These are the most common cardiac defects, varying in size and position. There is left-to-right shunting of blood. A harsh murmur is present down the left sternal border.

Larger defects may cause cardiac failure within weeks. Studies from 1969 to 2014 indicated that a varied number of small VSDs (5–80 per cent) may close spontaneously by the age of 10 years (Zhang et al, 2015). Surgery is needed for larger defects (see Figure 45.10).

Coarctation of the aorta

The narrowing of the aorta at any point will impair the flow of oxygenated blood to the body (see Figure 45.11). Blood will bypass the obstruction through other vessels. A PDA is maintained. Cardiac failure may present within days or weeks after birth. Murmurs are present. Weak femoral pulses are diagnostic, with the BP in the upper body higher than in the lower extremities. Surgery is recommended later in life.

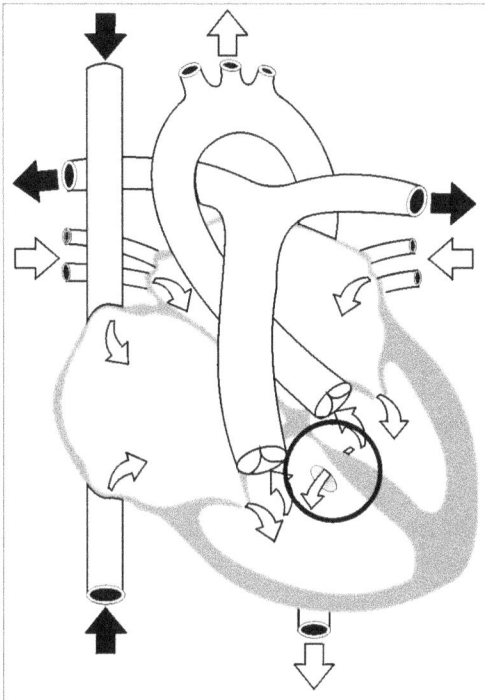

Figure 45.10 Ventricular septal defect

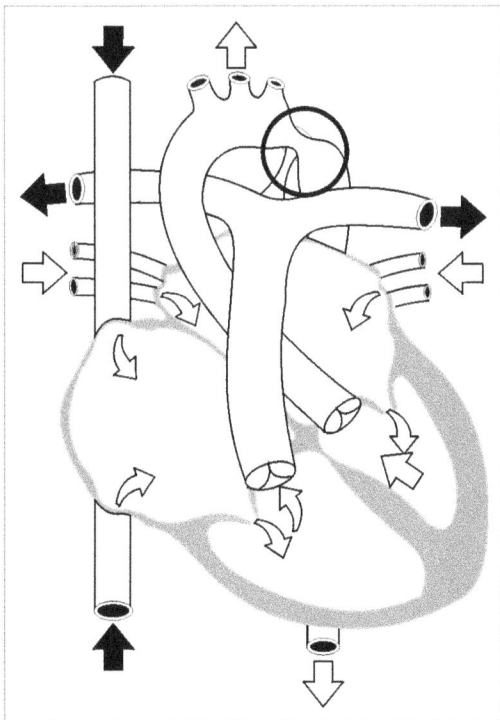

Figure 45.11 Coarctation of the aorta

Patent ductus arteriosus

The ductus arteriosus is between the aortic arch and the left pulmonary artery, and is vital *in utero* to direct blood away from the lungs before birth. The mechanism that causes the ductus to close has not been determined, but it seems to be related to oxygen.

The ductus fails to close in premature babies and in some children born at term. It should be suspected when the oxygen requirements in the baby increase or respiratory support is needed for more than 24 hours.

The ductus can be closed with the administration of indomethacin (an inhibitor of prostaglandins) in 40–60 per cent of cases of LBW babies and 80 per cent of cases in term babies, or it can be corrected surgically (Gal, 2009).

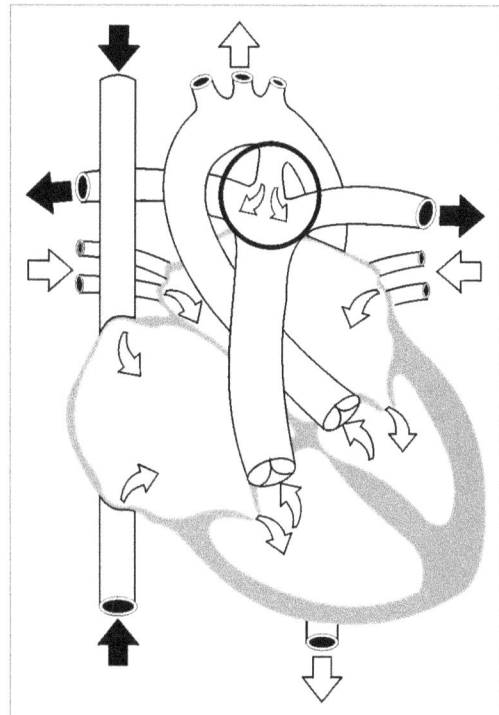

Figure 45.12 Patent ductus arteriosus

A newborn with the following clinical signs should be referred for immediate care:

▶ Cyanosis
▶ Cardiac failure
▶ Hypotension.

A midwife may be the first to notice an episode of cyanosis and hypotonia or floppiness. These newborns may appear normal but are often poor feeders, may vomit and have episodes of cyanosis. (See Figure 45.12.)

693

45.6 Gastrointestinal abnormalities

Tongue

A tongue tie is a common disorder where the cells have grown into the underlying mesenchyme of the mouth. Treatment is seldom required, as the tongue will grow forward in infancy. If it affects breastfeeding (latching), surgical intervention may be needed.

Teeth

Natal teeth may be present at birth. These may be covered by gums. If loose, they may be removed to prevent inhalation.

Epignathus

Various tumours may be present on the jaw; these are usually benign. They may be removed if they interfere with respiration.

Oesophageal atresia or tracheo-oesophageal fistula

Changes to the oesophagus occur from three to six weeks *in utero*. Five varieties of defects occur in 1:2 500–4 500 live births (Pinheiro, Simões e Silva & Pereira, 2012). Polyhydramnios is usually present in the pregnancy, because the baby cannot swallow the fluid. At birth, the baby has excessive fluid draining from the mouth. Later, the baby chokes when fed (see Figure 45.13).

The diagnosis can be made by passing a nasogastric tube. The tube will not advance or come out through the mouth. The litmus test remains alkaline.

Aspiration of milk may cause pneumonia. This is a surgical emergency. The baby is kept nil per mouth. An IV infusion of 10 per cent dextrose is given and the baby is suctioned to remove the fluid. An improvement in survival has been observed over the most recent decades, with a 95 per cent survival rate in centres offering the best neonatal care (Pinheiro, Simões e Silva & Pereira, 2012).

Pyloric stenosis

This occurs in 3.2–3.4 per 1 000 live births (Kuma, 2012: 306) and it is more common in boys than girls.

The baby presents with vomiting, visible peristalsis, constipation and weight loss. Vomiting may be projectile. The baby is referred to a surgeon.

Hirschsprung's disease

This is a condition where the rectum and lower bowel are affected by the absence of ganglion cells. There are no nerve cells in the affected areas and obstruction results. The passing of meconium may be delayed. A colostomy is required.

Meconium ileus

This is the first sign of cystic fibrosis. Sticky meconium blocks the bowel and abdominal distension occurs. An enema may unblock the meconium, but an enterostomy may be needed.

Imperforated anus

Malformation of the anus can be divided into low and high defects. Rectal agenesis is the absence of the rectum. An imperforated anus (see Figure 45.14) is when the anal opening is obstructed by skin; this occurs in 1:5 000 live births and affects boys and girls (Levitt & Peña, 2007). The defects can be corrected surgically.

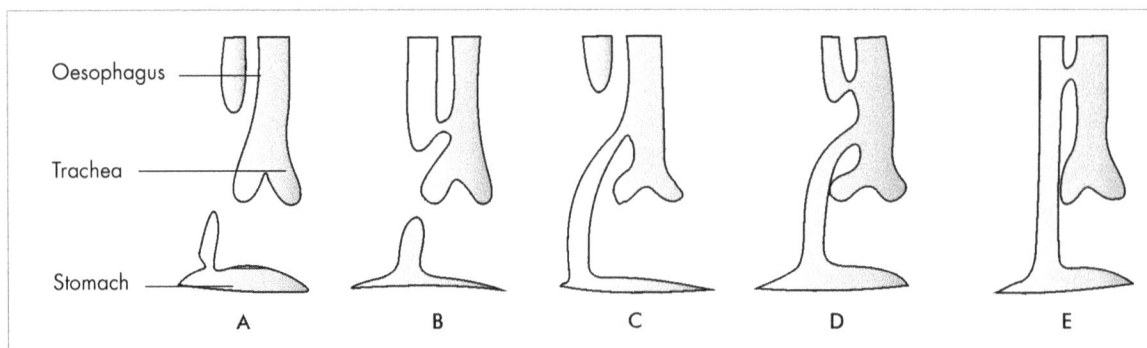

Figure 45.13 Different types of tracheo-oesophageal fistula (TEF) and tracheo-oesophageal atresia. A = oesophageal atresia; B = oesophageal atresia and upper TEF; C = proximal oesophageal atresia and TEF to the distal pouch; D and E = examples of TEF without atresia

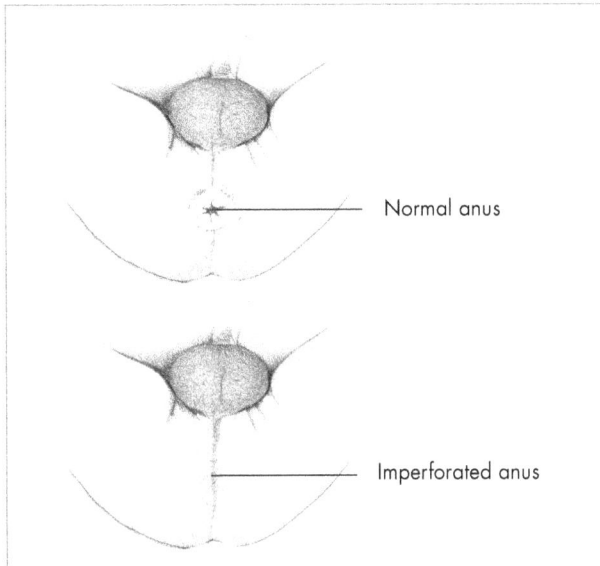

Figure 45.14 An imperforated anus

Exomphalos

Examphalos is a birth defect where the abdominal wall does not close and the contents (intestines and sometimes organs) protrude through the herniation in the abdominal wall, surrounded by a sac. There are often associated congenital abnormalities as well (see the box below).

There is not sufficient documented information for South Africa, but in New Zealand, the incidence of exomphalos has increased between 1996 and 2004 from 0.69 per 10 000 live births to 3.27 per 10 000 live births (Srivastava et al, 2009).

South African case study of omphalocele and associated defects (Singh & Madaree, 2016)

During the retrospective study period of ten years, 154 patients were diagnosed with an omphalocoele. There were various associated abnormalities and complications, namely:

▶ associated congenital abnormalities: 117 (75.9 per cent)
▶ minor omphalocoeles (defined as 5 cm): 64 (41.5 per cent)
▶ ruptured omphalocoeles: 11 (7.1 per cent)
▶ Beckwith-Wiedemann syndrome (the most commonly associated abnormality): 37.6 per cent
▶ cardiac defects: 34.4 per cent.

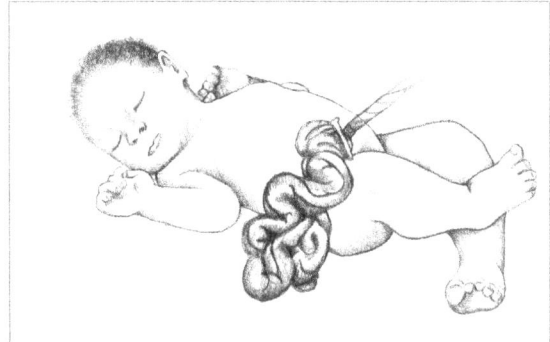

Figure 45.15 Exomphalos (omphalocele)

Small hernias can be repaired surgically. Conservative treatment of larger defects is given, because the bowel cannot be accommodated in the cavity. The sac is treated to prevent it from becoming fibrotic. The contents should be retracted into the abdomen by five to eight weeks.

Gastroschisis

Gastroschisis is a congenital defect of the anterior abdominal wall. Abdominal contents protrude through this wall, without a covering amniotic sac (Wright, Zani & Ade-Ajayi, 2015). The incidence is 1:2 000–4 000 live births in the West (Arnold, 2004). In New Zealand the incidence of gastroschisis has increased from 2.96 per 10 000 live births to 5.16 per 10 000 live births between 1996 and 2004 (Srivastava et al, 2009). There is also evidence of an increase in the incidence in South Africa from 1981 to 2001 (Arnold, 2004).

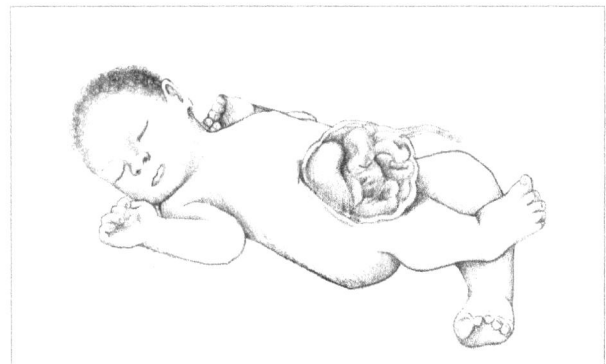

Figure 45.16 Gastroschisis (omphalocele)

Immediately after birth, the intestines are covered with a warm sterile saline dressing. A silastic bag is placed over the intestines and stitched to the abdomen. It is gradually reduced until the intestines are in the abdomen.

45.7   Renal abnormalities

Renal agenesis is usually unilateral, and more common in males. The prevalence is 1 in 1 500–3 200 live births (Natarajan et al, 2013). The presence of one congenital anomaly is an indirect indicator of abnormalities in the other systems. Early diagnosis and treatment of urological anomalies are important to improve the long-term renal prognosis. In these cases, there is a history of oligohydramnios in pregnancy. The newborn has wide-set eyes, epicanthic folds, low-set ears or other abnormalities of the ears.

Other abnormalities of the renal system include hypoplastic or underdeveloped kidneys and polycystic kidneys (the kidney is filled with cysts). Many of the babies affected by these conditions are stillborn and survivors have continuous health problems in life.

45.8   Genital abnormalities

Various problems may occur with the genitalia. The most common of these are detailed below.

Undescended testes

The testes are present in the inguinal canal by 28 weeks and descend into the scrotum by 36 weeks. The scrotal temperature is 4 °C lower than the body temperature. The testes may descend spontaneously after birth. If this has not occurred by six weeks, the undescended testes may atrophy or become malignant. In uncomplicated cases, the testes may be relocated at two years of age.

Hydrocele

The scrotum contains a soft cystic swelling. In most cases, it will disappear spontaneously.

Hermaphroditism

A true hermaphrodite has testes and ovarian tissue in the gonads. The external organs show a phallus and fused labia. Diagnosis requires a laparotomy and biopsy. Virilised females are reared as girls and need lifelong therapy.

45.9   The musculoskeletal system

Various limb malformations may occur in newborns.

Syndactyly

This is the fusion of two digits, which is the most common form of this congenital anomaly.

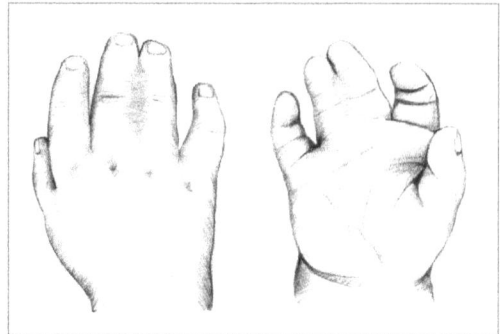

Figure 45.17 Syndactyly

Polydactyly

Extra digits are present. The extra digit may be tied off in infancy.

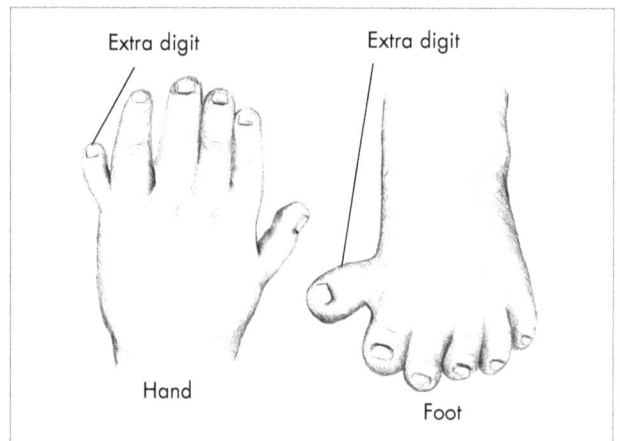

Figure 45.18 Polydactyly

Osteogenesis imperfecta

Brittle bone disease is a mutation of the genes for collagen. Four varieties – I, II, III and IV – are found. Type II is incompatible with life; fractures occur *in utero* and the baby is stillborn. Babies with other forms will develop bone deformities. There is no treatment for this condition.

Hip dysplasia

Hip dysplasia is congenital hip dislocation. One or both hips may be affected. The diagnosis is made using Ortolani's test, where a hip 'click' is present after birth. A splint or harness (see Figure 45.19) will be applied for several months until the acetabellum has developed normally.

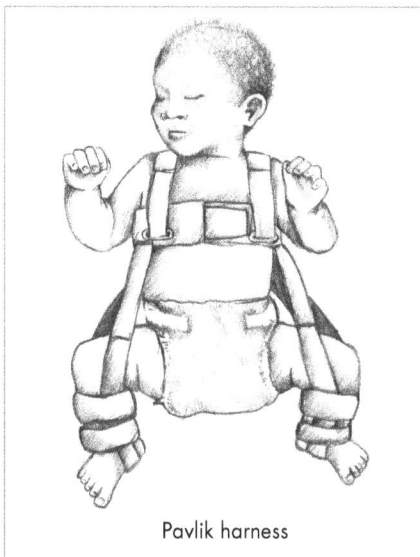

Pavlik harness

Figure 45.19 A splint for hip dysplasia

45.10 Genetic and inborn errors

Congenital hypothyroidism (cretinism)

Congenital hypothyroidism is an insufficiency of thyroid hormone and it is present at birth. This may be an inborn error. Early detection of this disease can be treated with oral doses of thyroid hormone to permit normal development. According to worldwide data obtained from neonatal thyroid screening programmes, congenital hypothyroidism occurs with an incidence of 1:3 000 to 1:4 000 (Klett, 1997).

Causes

- Iodine insufficiency in the mother in pregnancy
- Genetic defects
- Unknown causes

Signs and symptoms

- Post-dates birth
- Decreased activity and hypotonia
- Poor feeding and weight gain
- Jaundice
- Decreased stooling and constipation
- Hoarse cry or no crying

Physical features

- Macroglossia
- Umbilical hernia
- Goitre
- Pallor
- Myxoedema

Diagnosis

This is a disorder that is easy to identify by means of a simple newborn screening test, done from a few drops of heel blood. Decreased levels of serum thyroid hormones (TSH or T4) are present. X-rays of the legs are needed to check the bone ends at the knee for immaturity.

Management

Early diagnosis and thyroid hormone replacement are required.

Observe for cretinism. The child will have regular checks and blood tests to monitor his or her development (personal behaviour, language, adaptiveness and motor ability).

Complications

The prognosis is poor if the condition is not treated within two weeks after birth. The condition may lead to retardation in growth and brain development.

Galactosaemia

Galactosaemia, caused by the lack of an enzyme called galactose-1-phosphate uridyl transferase (GALT), is a rare autosomal recessive metabolic disorder. It is not the same as lactose intolerance. Newborns with galactosaemia lack the enzyme that converts galactose (one of two sugars found in lactose) into glucose, a sugar the body is able to use.

There are 30 types of galactosaemia. Classic galactosaemia is diagnosed in 1:16 000 to 1:48 000 births through newborn screening programmes around the world, depending on the diagnostic criteria used (Zupan & Berry, 2015).

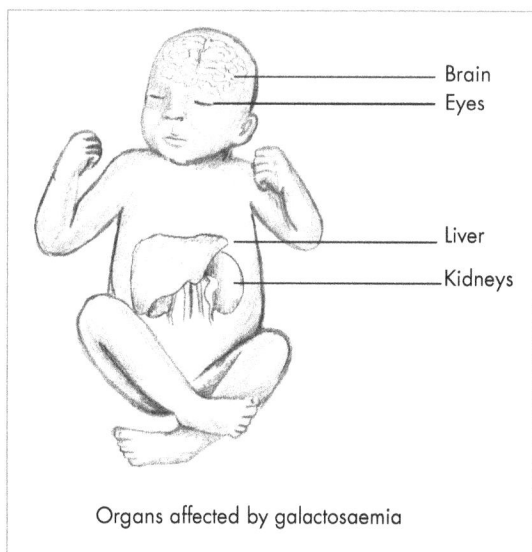

Organs affected by galactosaemia

Figure 45.20 Complications of galactosaemia

Signs and symptoms

These babies are normal until milk feeds are introduced. Liver disease develops. Within weeks they start vomiting, become jaundiced and listless. They fail to gain weight. Classic galactosaemia can result in life-threatening complications, including feeding problems, failure to thrive, hepatocellular damage, bleeding, and *E. coli* sepsis in untreated infants.

Diagnosis

Clinical diagnosis with urine screening will show reduced sugar and albumin. The levels of the enzyme GALT in the body are measured. At birth, a heel-prick blood test can be done. Genetic testing to look for mutation in the GALT gene may be useful.

Management

Milk (including breast milk) and other dairy products (galactose-free) must be eliminated from the diet. The baby will be on a lifelong galactose-free diet. If this diet is not observed, galactose can build up in the system and damage the body's cells and organs, leading to blindness, severe mental retardation, growth deficiency and even death.

There are several less severe forms of galactosaemia that may be detected by newborn screening and that may not require any intervention. The prognosis is good if the diet is maintained.

Complications

If not treated, cataracts, liver disease with jaundice, delayed speech and language, sepsis and developmental delays result.

Sickle cell disease

SCD is an inherited blood disease where red blood cells have an abnormal shape, like a sickle. This can cause episodes of pain, damage to vital organs such as the lungs and kidneys, and even death. The incidence in South Africa is low. However, the demographics are changing due to immigration from sub-Saharan Africa, where there is a higher prevalence.

Sign and symptoms

Newborns are asymptomatic, but a family history may alert the midwife to the need for testing.

Management

Newborns at risk can have a screening test (blood, hearing and heart). This allows for early detection and treatment. With early screening of the newborn, a diagnosis can be made and antibiotic treatment can be started before infections occur. The screening test can also detect other disorders affecting Hb.

Young children with SCD are especially prone to certain dangerous bacterial infections. Common problems include anaemia, acute chest syndrome (infection and blocked blood flow to the lungs) and pain. More rarely, splenic crisis, vision problems and strokes occur.

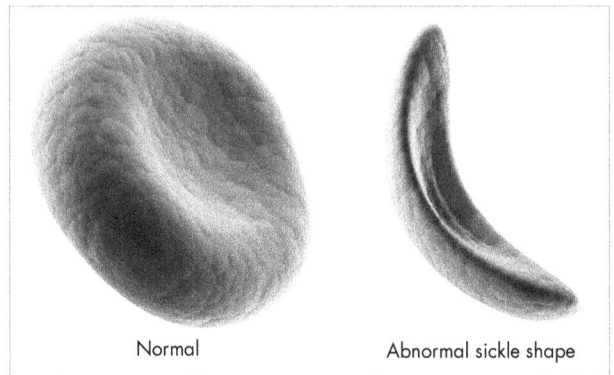

Normal   Abnormal sickle shape

Figure 45.21 Sickle cell anaemia: Normal and abnormal cells in the blood vessels

Cystic fibrosis

Cystic fibrosis is an inherited disorder that causes severe damage to the lungs and digestive system. The cells of these organs produce thick mucus, sweat and digestive juices that block and obstruct the passageways.

Signs and symptoms

The signs vary, depending on the severity of the condition. There is a higher level of salt in the sweat. Symptoms may develop within a month or later in life. These include a persistent cough, thick mucus, breathing difficulties, lung infections, a stuffy nose, greasy stools, poor weight gain and meconium ileus constipation.

Diagnosis

The screening of newborns includes a sweat test (see Figure 45.22) and genetic tests as well as a blood test for pancreatic chemical levels.

Complications

Depending on the severity, this is a lifelong condition with a limiting life span. The newborn will be exposed to repeated lung infections.

There is no known cure. The management is complex. Options include antibiotics, mucus-thinning drugs, bronchodilators and oral pancreatic enzymes. The condition can be treated by trying to prevent serious lung infections and providing adequate nutrition. Early detection helps medical practitioners reduce the problems associated with cystic fibrosis.

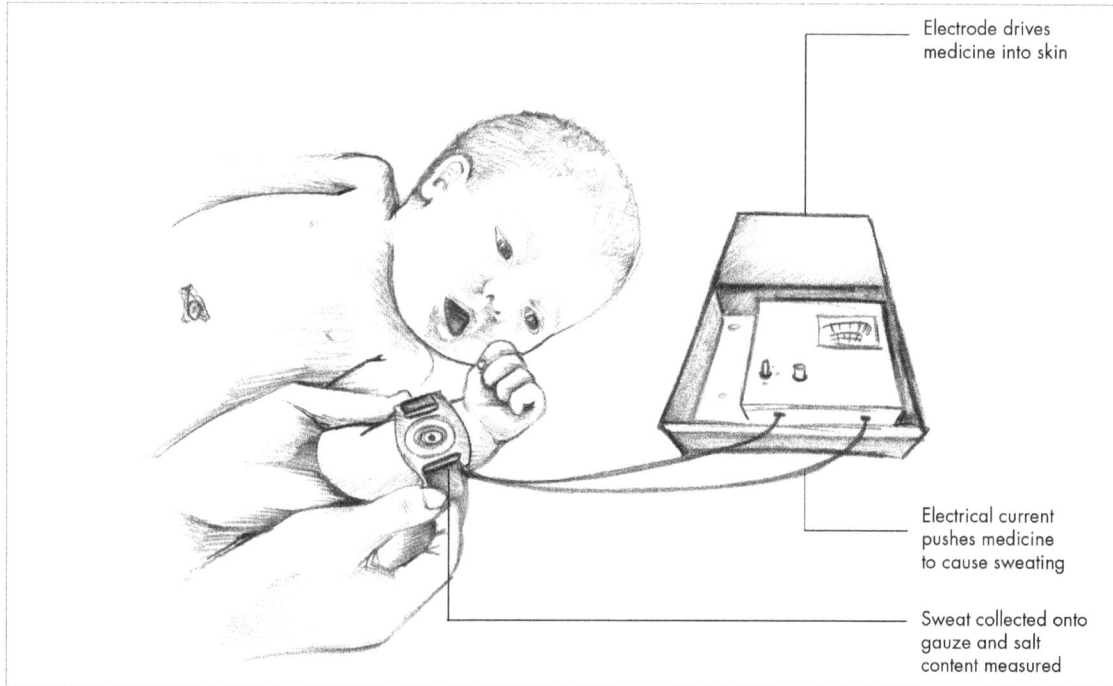

Electrode drives
medicine into skin

Electrical current
pushes medicine
to cause sweating

Sweat collected onto
gauze and salt
content measured

Figure 45.22 Sweat tests

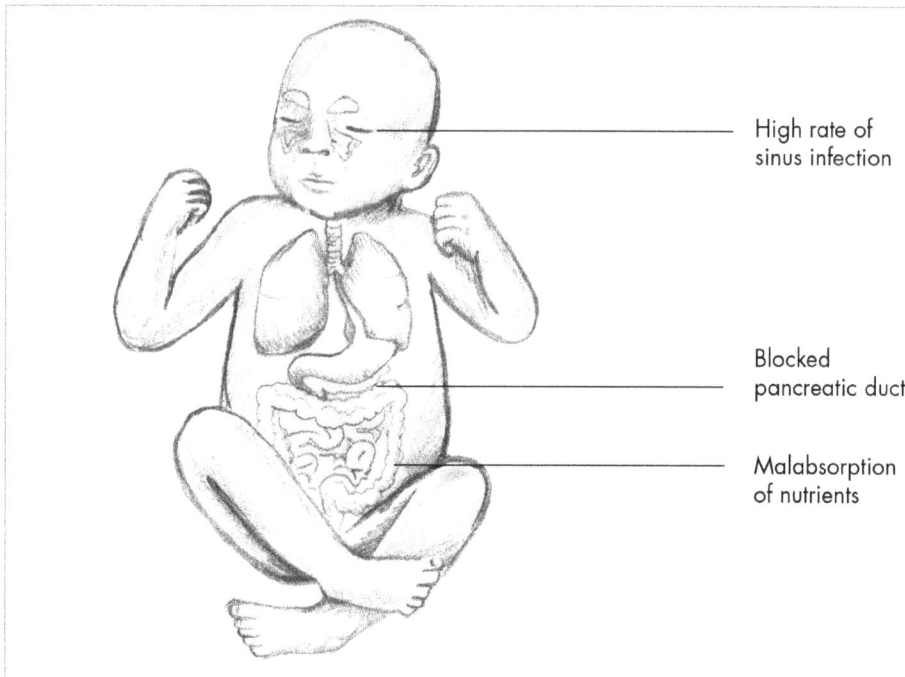

High rate of
sinus infection

Blocked
pancreatic duct

Malabsorption
of nutrients

Figure 45.23 Organs affected by cystic fibrosis

Phenylketonuria

PKU is an autosomal recessive disorder. Phenylalanine is an essential amino acid present in food. Normally, it is changed by the enzyme phenylalanine hydroxylase to tyrosine. When this enzyme is absent, phenylalanine accumulates in the body, and can poison the brain and cause mental retardation.

The incidence of PKU has not been well researched. In 1995 the incidence in South Africa was 1 in 20 000 newborns (Hitzeroth, Niehaus & Brill, 1995).

Signs and symptoms

Infants may present with vomiting, eczema and a 'mouse-like' smell to their urine. Convulsions may occur. Most children are blonde with blue eyes, due to a lack of melanin.

Management

Care is mostly preventive:
- Children are screened for phenylalanine using the Guthrie test on a drop of blood from the heel. The optimal time is five to seven days after birth.
- A phenylalanine-free diet is prescribed.
- Breastfeeding continues in the early months.
- The blood levels of phenylalanine should be kept between 0.24 and 0.48 mmol/ℓ.
- Mental retardation can be avoided.

Complications

Early detection is important. Performing a urine test of a newborn is possible but not routinely done in South Africa.

Varied degrees of retardation are present and children may be hyperactive, have microcephaly and show growth retardation.

Congenital lactose intolerance

Disaccharides in the diet are changed into monosaccharides by the enzymes in the gut before absorption. Congenital lactose intolerance is caused by the lack of the enzyme lactase. The presence of lactose in the gut causes fermentation of sugar by intestinal bacteria, with the release of carbon dioxide and lactic acid.

Signs and symptoms

The infant has frothy and sour-smelling stools with a low pH, which test positive for reducing substances. The infant develops diarrhoea in the first week of life and fails to gain weight.

Management

Withdrawal of lactose in the diet will stop the condition within 24 hours. A lactose-free diet is prescribed for the first two years.

45.11 Conclusion

This chapter presented some of the more common abnormalities and disorders that may be encountered in the newborn, some which may be life-threatening or, if not identified, lead to mental retardation. Midwives need the knowledge to identify conditions; they need to be skilled to act if needed and refer the mother and baby for consultation to a paediatrician.

Infant respiratory disorders and neonatal resuscitation

LEARNING OBJECTIVES

On completion of this chapter, you must be able to:
- demonstrate the ability to maintain the temperature of a newborn
- compare methods of maintaining an adequate oxygen supply
- outline the emergency procedure for the Helping Babies Breathe (HBB) resuscitation protocol
- review anticipatory guidance for parents.

KNOWLEDGE ASSUMED TO BE IN PLACE

Anatomy and physiological changes of the neonate after birth

KEYWORDS

infant respiratory distress syndrome (IRDS) • respiratory distress syndrome (RDS) • meconium aspiration syndrome (MAS) • transient tachypnoea of the newborn (TTN) • resuscitation of the neonate: Helping Babies Breathe (HBB)

46.1   Introduction

Infant respiratory distress remains one of the major causes of neonatal morbidity and mortality. Respiratory distress in the newborn is an overarching term for several conditions with various causes, as presented in this chapter.

Successful management of the newborn who has respiratory distress is based on obtaining a complete maternal and neonatal history, performing a thorough physical examination, recognising the common respiratory disorders, differentiating among various diagnostic entities, identifying those that are life-threatening and implementing the appropriate treatment.

46.2   Definition and classification of respiratory distress

Infant respiratory distress is an emergency condition where a newborn has difficulty in breathing. It also includes hyaline membrane disease (HMD), surfactant deficiency disorder (SDD), transient tachypnoea of the newborn (TTN), genetic disorders and malformations such as pulmonary dysplasia.

Midwives should be competent in the management of respiratory conditions and resuscitation of the newborn.

> **Activity: Neonatal lung pathology**
>
> Watch the Kalamazoo Valley Community College's slide show on neonatal respiratory pathology, available from http://classes.kvcc.edu/ralbrecht/NEOpaho.ppt.

46.3   Neonatal respiratory distress syndrome

Neonatal respiratory distress syndrome (RDS), also known as HMD, is one of the most common complications. It is seen almost always in premature newborns of less than 37 weeks' gestation.

Predisposing conditions

Preterm (immature) babies are mostly affected and the condition is aggravated by asphyxia of the newborn. The synthesis of surfactant is inhibited by hypoxia, acidosis, hypothermia and hypoglycaemia.

Babies who are large for gestational age (LGA) – as babies born to mothers with diabetes mellitus often are – are also prone to RDS.

Causes

The cause of RDS is pulmonary surfactant deficiency in the lungs of newborns, most commonly in those born before 37 weeks' gestation and babies of diabetic mothers. The risk of this condition increases with the degree of prematurity and is higher in babies born before 28 weeks, because of underdeveloped lungs.

The risk decreases in fetal growth restriction, pre-eclampsia or eclampsia, maternal hypertension, prolonged rupture of membranes and maternal corticosteroid use; the reason for this is that the stress of these situations causes the newborn's lungs to mature sooner.

Pathophysiology

Pulmonary surfactant diminishes the surface tension of the water film that lines the alveoli, thereby decreasing the tendency of alveoli to collapse and the energy required to inflate them.

With surfactant deficiency, the lungs present with diffuse atelectasis (collapsing), triggering inflammation which results in pulmonary oedema. Because blood passing through the portions of the lung where atelectasis has taken place is not oxygenated, the infant becomes hypoxaemic. Lung compliance is decreased, and breathing effort is increased. In severe cases, the diaphragm and intercostal muscles fatigue, and carbon dioxide retention and respiratory acidosis develop.

Signs and symptoms

Symptoms and signs include rapid, laboured, grunting respiration appearing immediately or within a few hours after delivery, with suprasternal and substernal retractions and flaring of the nasal alae, cyanosis of the skin and mucous membranes, decreased urine output, decreased peripheral pulses and, possibly, oedema of the peripheries. As atelectasis and respiratory failure progress, the symptoms worsen, with cyanosis, lethargy, irregular breathing and apnoea.

Newborns who weigh less than 1 000 g may have lungs so stiff that they are unable to initiate or sustain respiration after birth. Many of these babies are asphyxiated at birth and require resuscitation. The lungs offer resistance to inflation due to the raised surface tension of the alveoli. The condition is progressive, with the development of:

▶ tachypnoea
▶ sternal and rib recession
▶ expiratory grunting
▶ cyanosis.

(See the discussion on the Silverman-Anderson score in Chapter 41.)

In addition, the following will be observed:

▶ The infant is lethargic and usually lies in the 'frog' position (see the discussion on the Ballard score in Chapter 42).
▶ Air entry is diminished and crepitations may be noted.
▶ Very preterm babies have irregular, slow breathing and apnoeic spells.
▶ Bowel sounds may be absent and the passage of meconium delayed for a few days.
▶ Generalised oedema is usually present within 24 hours.

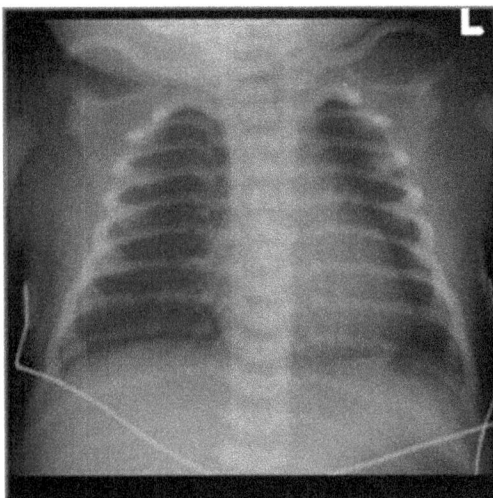

Figure 46.1 X-ray of a normal newborn

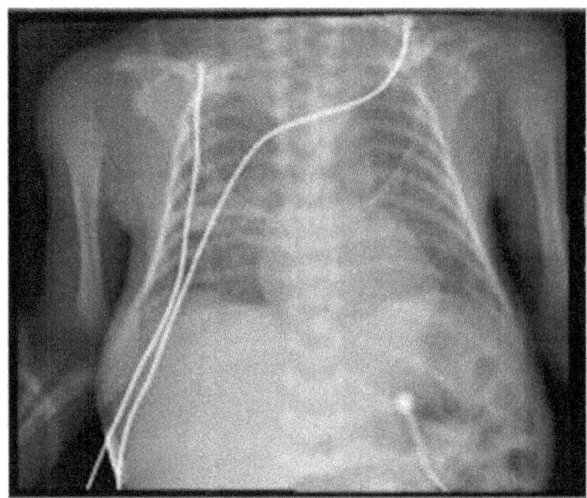

Figure 46.2 X-ray of a newborn with HMD rice grain (matt glass) appearance

Diagnosis

Diagnosis is made by clinical presentation, including recognition of risk factors such as hypoxaemia and hypercapnia. Chest X-rays show diffuse atelectasis, classically described as an under-expanded chest with a fine reticulogranular (rice grain) or ground-glass appearance, with visible air bronchograms over both lung fields (see Figure 46.2). The appearance correlates loosely with clinical severity.

The differential diagnosis includes group B streptococcal pneumonia and sepsis, TTN, persistent pulmonary hypertension, aspiration, pulmonary oedema and congenital cardiopulmonary anomalies. The clinical diagnosis of group B streptococcal pneumonia is extremely difficult; thus, antibiotics are usually started pending culture results.

Management and care

The management and care of RDS of the newborn starts with the anticipation of a risky situation and taking evidence-based steps to prevent such a situation. If prevention is not possible, the knowledge, skill and competency to manage RDS, particularly in an emergency, are essential.

Prevention

Preventing prematurity is the most important way to prevent neonatal RDS. Good prenatal care results in larger, healthier babies and fewer preterm births.

Elective Caesarean sections should not be done before 39 completed weeks, unless there is a sound clinical indication or reason.

If the test of amniotic liquor does not contain sufficient surfactant, Caesarean section or induction of labour (IOL) can be delayed, or the newborn can be managed for RDS immediately after birth. The best practice is the prevention of HMD by ensuring the lungs are mature or the administration of corticosteroids to the mother after 32 weeks to stimulate lung maturity.

Neonatal continuous positive airway pressure

Neonatal continuous positive airway pressure (CPAP) is a non-invasive ventilation strategy for newborns. Nasal CPAP (nCPAP) is widely used for a range of neonatal respiratory conditions and can be used at any level of care, from the primary healthcare (PHC) level to the ICU. Newborns with RDS respond well if the therapy is started soon after birth.

A protocol for use needs to be in place and staff must be trained on the effective use of the apparatus.

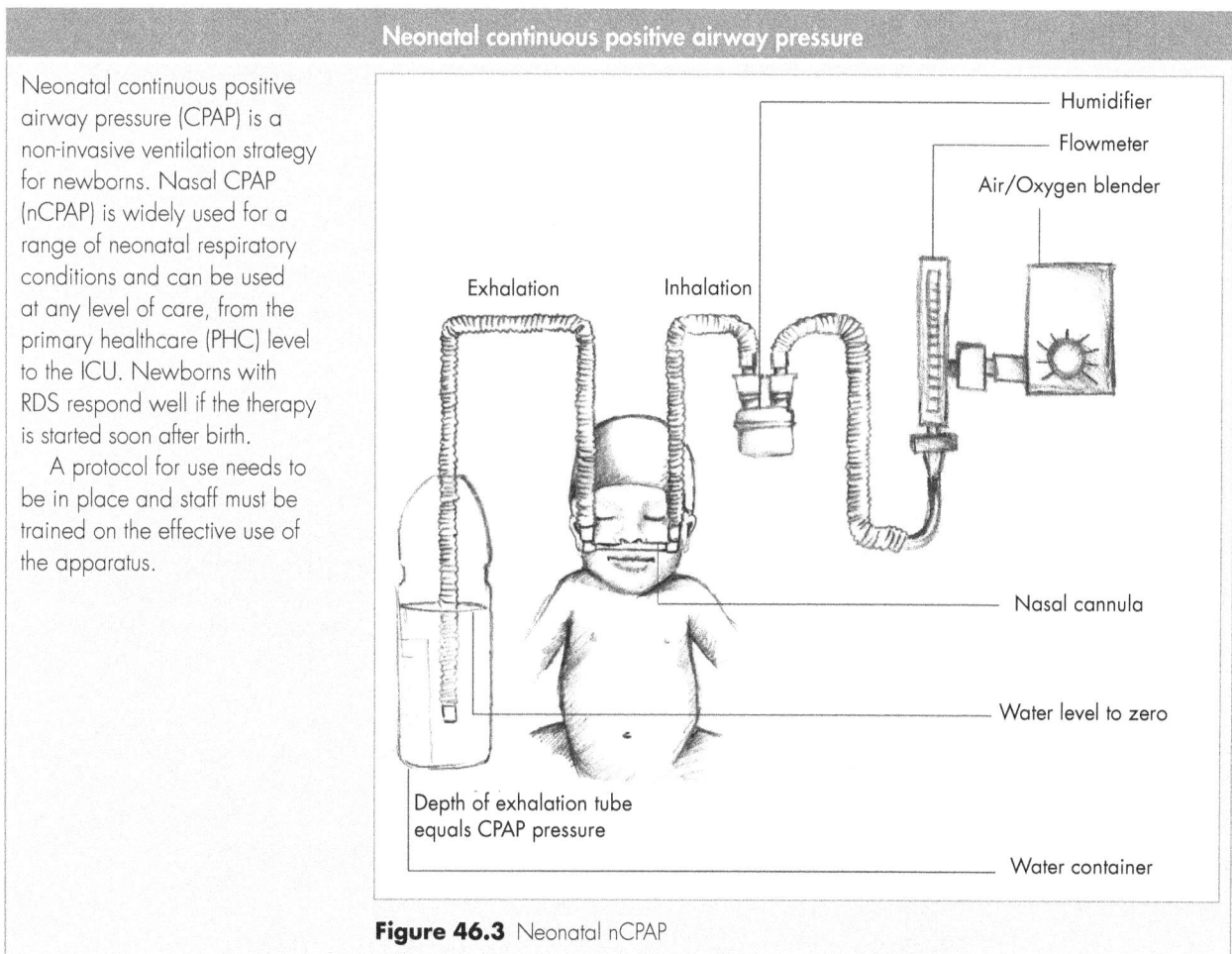

Figure 46.3 Neonatal nCPAP

In the case of preterm labour between 24 and 34 weeks, a laboratory test to determine the lung maturity (surfactant) of the fetus is essential. Fetal lung maturity can be determined in the antenatal period through amniocentesis. The lecithin sphingomyelin (LS) ratio indicates lung maturity (see Chapter 42). This can help determine the optimal timing of delivery in elective cases where gestational age (GA) cannot be confirmed. The risk of RDS is low when the LS ratio is 2:1, but this ratio is different in diabetic women.

The administration of corticosteroids to the mother 24 hours before delivery may also help speed up lung maturity in the fetus.

Immediate care

Lung maturity is greatly advanced after birth if the baby receives immediate endotracheal administration of surfactant (see the information on Curosurf® in Table 53.5 on page 857).

Premature newborns require prompt attention by a neonatal resuscitation team. Newborns will be given warm, moist oxygen. Although this is very important, care must be taken to reduce the side effects associated with too much oxygen.

Most of these newborns are nursed on a ventilator, which can be life-saving, especially for babies with:

- high levels of carbon dioxide in the arteries
- low blood oxygen in the arteries
- a low blood pH (acidosis)
- apnoea.

Neonatal continuous positive airway pressure therapy

CPAP, which delivers slightly pressurised air through the nose, can help keep the airways open and may prevent the need for a ventilator for many newborns (see Figure 46.3). Even with CPAP, oxygen and pressure will be reduced as soon as possible to prevent the side effects associated with excessive oxygen or pressure.

Newborns with RDS should receive developmental supportive care (DSC), which includes little disturbance, gentle handling, the maintenance of optimum body temperature, careful fluid management and close attention to other situations such as infections, if they develop (see Chapter 42).

In very severe respiratory distress and cyanosis, artificial ventilation is necessary. The baby may need CPAP or intubation and intensive care. The medical practitioner must be informed immediately.

Acidosis and hypoglycaemia must be prevented or treated immediately.

The infant is usually fed parenterally at first, because of the danger of vomiting and the inability to digest feeds, and by umbilical catheter or via a peripheral vein. Later, nasogastric tube feeds of expressed breast milk are given as per the medical practitioner's prescription.

In a study performed in a South African public hospital, early use of CPAP in extremely low-birth-weight (ELBW) infants was associated with survival rates similar to those seen in developed countries (Kirsten et al, 2012). The administration of surfactant hastens recovery and decreases the risk of complications, thereby improving mortality rates for the neonate and babies under 12 months (see Figure 46.4).

With adequate ventilator support alone, natural surfactant production eventually begins. Once this happens, RDS can resolve within four or five days. In most cases, the condition worsens for two to four days after birth and thereafter a slow improvement occurs.

Surfactant replacement therapy

Exogenous surfactant therapy is a well-established practice in newborn infants with RDS. It is administered prophylactically straight into the lungs of newborns at risk for RDS via endotracheal tube and intubation. The clinical protocol and guidelines for use are followed as per unit policy.

Complications

The complications of RDS include intracranial complications, tension pneumothorax, sepsis, iatrogenic insults, bronchopulmonary dysplasia (BPD), retinopathy and neonatal death:

- Neurological impairment: Intracranial and intraventicular haemorrhage complications have been linked to hypoxaemia, hypercarbia, hypotension, fluctuation in arterial BP and low cerebral perfusion. This may lead to long-term complications, including neurological damage, delayed mental development and mental retardation associated with brain damage or bleeding, and cerebral palsy.
- Tension pneumothorax is a complication of the newborn that is a rare but life-threatening condition. It occurs when air escapes out of the lung between the chest wall and lung, causing the lung to collapse. It may follow meconium aspiration syndrome (MAS), the use of ventilators or resuscitation, and is more common in premature infants. With appropriate diagnosis and treatment, the prognosis is good.
- Sepsis is a type of bacterial infection, such as meningitis, pneumonia, pyelonephritis or gastroenteritis, in the blood of the newborn. It is a serious condition.

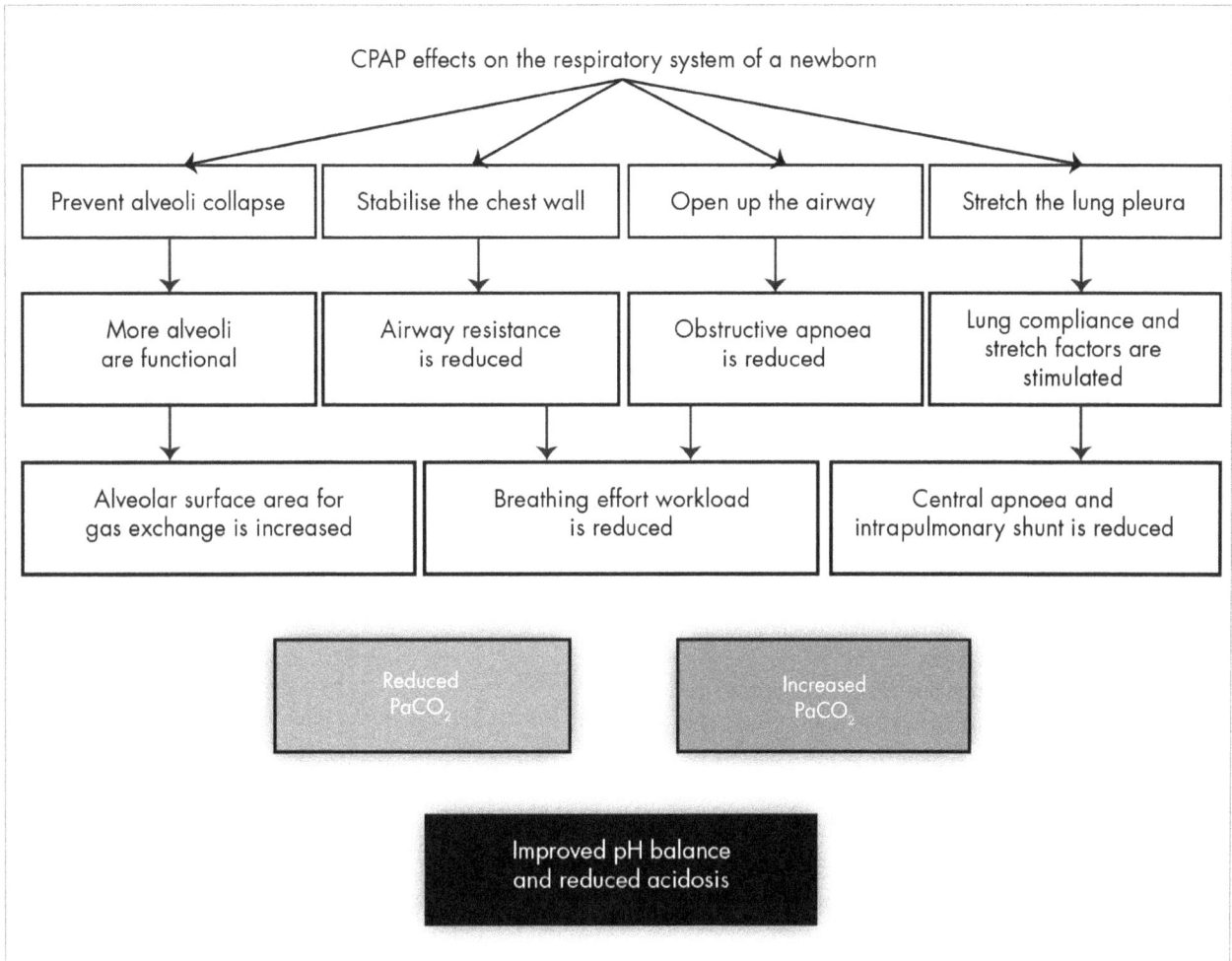

Figure 46.4 nCPAP effects

▶ Iatrogenic damage: An example of an iatrogenic insult is blood clots (due to an umbilical arterial catheter) that may spread into the body and cause an arterial blockage, leading to the loss of a limb. BPD is a chronic lung disease of low-birth-weight (LBW) infants caused by prolonged mechanical ventilation in the treatment of RDS. Long-term complications may develop as a result of oxygen toxicity and the high pressures delivered to the lungs, the severity of the condition itself, or periods when the brain or other organs did not receive enough oxygen.

▶ Retinopathy of prematurity (ROP) is caused by abnormal blood vessels growing in the retina, leading to blindness. It is caused by high levels (100 per cent) or high concentrations of oxygen in LBW premature babies.

▶ RDS is the leading cause of death in premature babies. It is frequent in infants of diabetic mothers and in the second-born of twins.

46.4 Transient tachypnoea (wet lung syndrome)

TTN is a self-limiting condition in newborns. The newborn presents with tachypnoea within hours after birth.

Predisposing conditions

The clinical picture of this condition is very similar to RDS in the early stage, but it affects full-term or near-term newborns who are born by Caesarean section, particularly those of mothers with diabetes mellitus. Newborns subjected to hypoxia immediately prior to or at birth (for example, in placenta praevia, prolapse of the cord and intrauterine or intrapartum asphyxia or depression) can also be affected. The condition is also associated with heavy maternal sedation and/or general anaesthesia.

All newborns who are at risk of this condition but who do not show immediate signs should be observed in the high-care or intensive care nursery.

Causes

The condition is probably due to the retention of lung fluid or a delay in the absorption of lung fluid, causing a temporary decrease in lung compliance due to hyperinflation of the lungs.

Signs and symptoms

There may be respiratory distress at birth or the newborn may appear normal at birth with the condition usually presenting within the first two to four hours after birth:

▶ Tachypnoea (more than 60 breaths per minute) is always one of the first signs. It may reach extreme rates of 100–140 breaths per minute.

▶ The signs of over-sedation due to medication used during birth may be the cause of depression of the cough, gag and swallowing reflexes. It predispose the newborn to the risk of aspiration. If left unstimulated, the baby may become lethargic, hypoventilate and become distressed.

The diagnosis is confirmed by a chest X-ray showing hyperinflation of the lungs with fluid patches, a peripheral streaky pattern and fuzzy vessels, as in Figure 46.5 below.

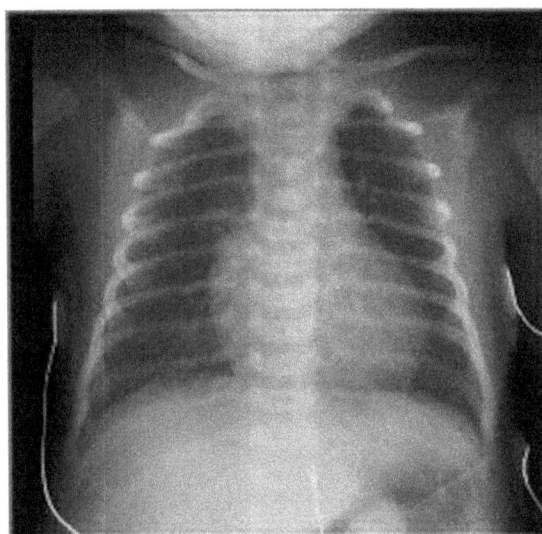

Figure 46.5 X-ray image for wet lung syndrome

Management and care

Care is aimed at supplying the newborn with sufficient oxygen to prevent deterioration of the condition leading to distress (preventing hypothermia, acidosis and hypoglycaemia). The newborn rarely requires ventilation and when the lung fluid clears, the clinical signs disappear and respiration becomes normal. This condition usually resolves within 24 hours and the prognosis is excellent if the condition is treated immediately.

The avoidance of excessive maternal sedation and anaesthesia in labour or during Caesarean section, especially in high-risk conditions, is essential.

46.5 Meconium aspiration syndrome

MAS occurs when a newborn aspirates meconium. It may occur *in utero* or at birth. The greater the amount of meconium passed *in utero*, the greater the respiratory distress. Airway obstruction (of the glottis and/or the trachea and the smaller airways) results if large amounts of meconium are aspirated due to deep gasping movements at birth.

Causes

Physiological stress at the time of labour and delivery (eg due to hypoxia caused by umbilical cord compression or placental insufficiency or infection) may cause the fetus to pass meconium into the amniotic fluid before delivery. This triggers lung injury and respiratory distress, which is termed MAS. Post-term newborns delivered through reduced amniotic fluid volume are at risk of more severe disease, as the meconium is less diluted and thus more likely to cause airway obstruction.

Pathophysiology

The mechanism by which aspiration induces the clinical syndrome is complex and controversial. It starts with fetal gasping and mechanical airway obstruction by meconium, causing non-specific cytokine release and surfactant inactivation that lead to chemical pneumonitis (Figure 46.6).

Underlying physiological stressors may also contribute. If complete bronchial obstruction occurs, atelectasis results; partial blockage leads to air trapping on expiration, resulting in hyper-expansion of the lungs and possible pulmonary air leaks with pneumomediastinum or pneumothorax. Persistent pulmonary hypertension can be associated with meconium aspiration as a comorbid condition or because of continuing hypoxia.

During delivery, newborns may also aspirate vernix caseosa, amniotic fluid or blood of maternal or fetal origin. This can lead to respiratory distress and signs of aspiration pneumonia on chest X-ray. Treatment is supportive. If a bacterial infection is suspected, cultures are taken and antibiotics are started.

The grading of meconium

Meconium-stained liquor in pregnancy and labour are graded in the following way:
- *Grade 1:* A good volume of liquor lightly stained with meconium
- *Grade 2:* A reasonable volume of liquor with a heavy suspension of meconium
- *Grade 3:* Thick meconium which is undiluted and resembles spinach. Overall mortality is slightly increased.

Signs and symptoms

Some, most, or all of the following clinical features may be present at birth.

The skin

- The skin is covered in a yellow-green pigment from the meconium.
- The fingernails and umbilical cord are stained with meconium.
- The skin is cracked and peeling.

General

- Decreased muscle tone
- Decreased respiration at birth, with poor respiratory effort and asphyxia being common
- Marked tachypnoea, cyanosis and grunting
- Chest wall retraction, which may be intercostal and/or sternal
- Hypotonia
- Squinting as a result of cerebral hypoxia and/or oedema
- Nasal flaring
- Hyper-inflation of the chest, with anterior bowing of the sternum
- Extreme pallor
- Irregular gasping attempts
- Apnoea
- Bradycardia
- A low Apgar rating

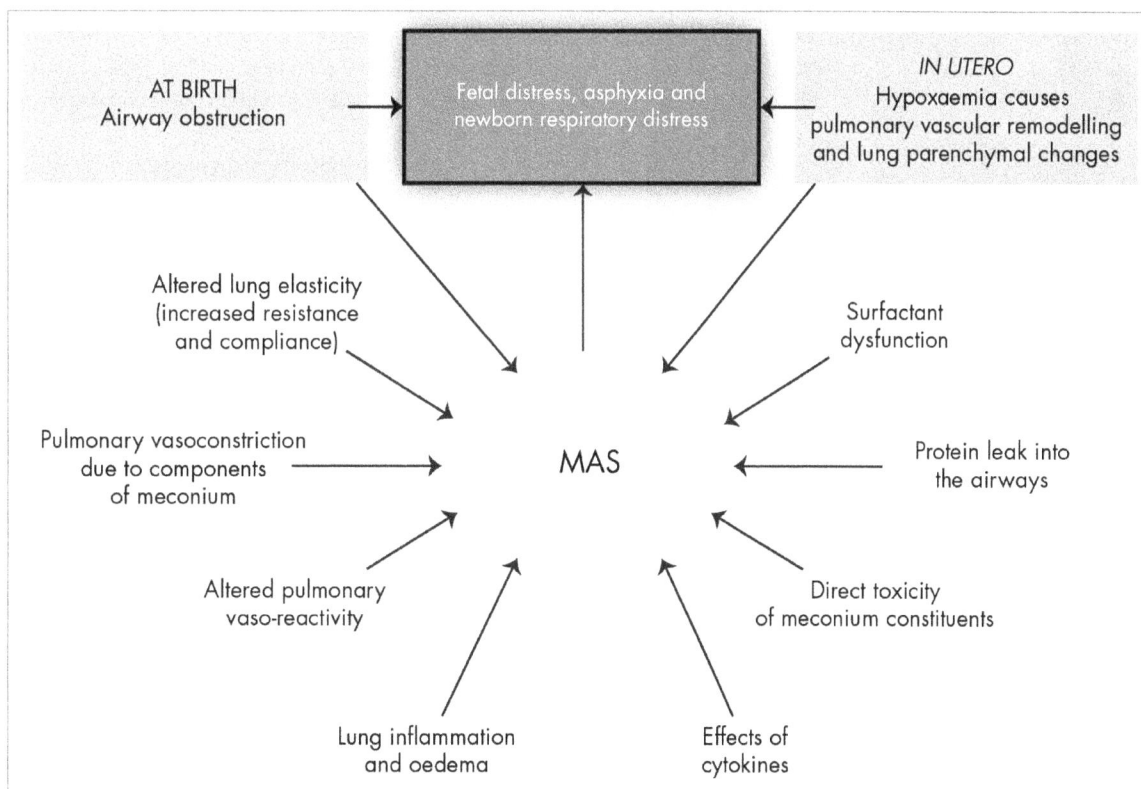

Figure 46.6 The pathophysiology of MAS

▶ Growth restriction, or a baby who is small for gestational age (SGA) due to fetal hypoxia (in many cases).

The chest

▶ There are rales and wheezing.
▶ There may be rhonchi (a musical noise produced by air passing through narrowed bronchi during respiration).
▶ There may be no signs of respiratory distress for several hours, and then sudden, severe respiratory distress occurs, with tachypnoea, cyanosis, rales and rhonchi, a hyper-expanded chest, congestive cardiac failure and irregular, gasping respiration and desaturation.
▶ Meconium staining may be visible in the oropharynx and (on intubation) in the larynx and trachea.
▶ A newborn with air trapping may have a barrel-shaped chest and also symptoms and signs of pneumothorax, pulmonary interstitial emphysema and pneumomediastinum.

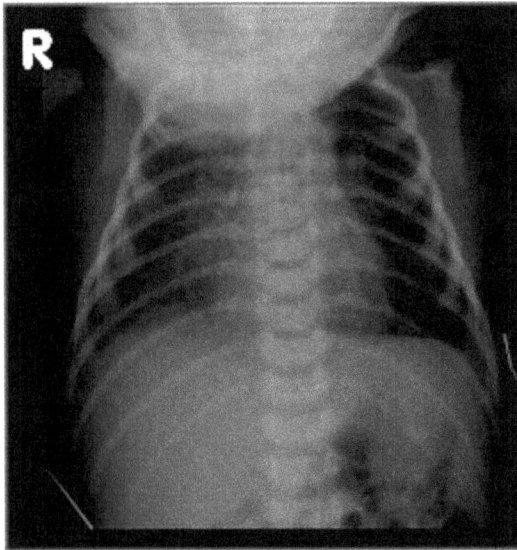

Figure 46.7 X-ray image of MAS

Diagnosis

The condition is suspected if a newborn shows respiratory distress in the context of meconium-tinged amniotic fluid. The diagnosis is confirmed by chest X-ray (see Figure 46.7) showing hyper-inflation with variable areas of atelectasis and flattening of the diaphragm. Initial X-ray findings can be confused with the findings of TTN. Fluid may be seen in the lung fissures or pleural spaces and air may be seen in the soft tissues or mediastinum. Because meconium may enhance bacterial growth and MAS is difficult to distinguish from bacterial pneumonia, cultures of blood and tracheal aspirate should also be taken.

Management and care

Meconium aspiration is an extremely dangerous condition for the baby and therefore everything possible must be done to avoid the passing of meconium by the fetus *in utero*. Management includes the principles discussed in the following subsections.

Antenatal prevention

▶ Encourage all women to attend an antenatal clinic early in pregnancy.
▶ All pregnant women at the antenatal clinic must be screened for risk factors.
▶ Refer all high-risk women to a tertiary hospital so that any problem can be dealt with when it arises.
▶ In the following cases, transfer to hospital is required:
  • Meconium staining during labour
  • A mother with pre-eclampsia, hypertension, prolonged pregnancy (post-maturity) or diabetes mellitus
  • Decreased fetal movements
  • A fetus with intrauterine growth restriction (IUGR).

During labour

Careful observations should be done throughout labour.

During the first stage, the observations and preparations include the following:

▶ Fetal compromise must be recognised early.
▶ Any case of fetal compromise should be referred to a medical practitioner immediately.
▶ Appropriate intervention should be undertaken immediately.
▶ The nursery staff should be informed beforehand of the possible transfer of an infant suffering from MAS and asphyxia.
▶ A paediatrician should be notified of the impending delivery.
▶ Resuscitation equipment must be available and in perfect working order.
▶ A large suction catheter – the larger the better – should be available (see Figure 46.8).

During the second and third stage, the observations and preparations include the following:

▶ Note the procedure for Helping Babies Breathe (HBB).
▶ The paediatrician is notified.
▶ After delivery of the head, an assistant to the person delivering holds back the newborn's shoulders to prevent immediate delivery.

▶ The newborn's mouth and then the nose are thoroughly aspirated, using a large suction catheter.

▶ The newborn is then delivered. The cord is clamped and cut as quickly as possible.

▶ The newborn is removed to the resuscitative area and dried quickly. It is essential that the newborn is kept warm.

Follow best practice guidelines for the management of meconium-exposed newborns, as follows:

▶ If the baby is not vigorous (depressed respiratory efforts, poor muscle tone and a heartbeat of less than 100 bpm), a skilled professional uses direct laryngoscope intubation to suction the trachea for no longer than five seconds. This can be repeated if meconium is retrieved and there is no bradycardia. If there is bradycardia, positive pressure ventilation should be considered and suctioning later.

▶ If the baby is vigorous (normal respiration with a heartbeat above 100 bpm), clear the secretions with a bulb syringe from the nose and the mouth or a meconium aspirator (a control port for intermittent suctioning of the mouth).

After intubation

Observations and preparations in this stage include the following:

▶ As much of the meconium as possible is cleaned off the skin and the newborn is kept dry.

▶ The newborn is transported to the nursery as soon as possible (when in a stable condition) and ventilated if necessary.

▶ The newborn should be placed in a pre-warmed incubator if available.

The prognosis is generally good, although it varies with the underlying physiological stressors.

Complications

Meconium is toxic in the lungs and sets up an intense inflammatory reaction, which causes severe respiratory distress, resulting in interstitial chemical pneumonitis. This leads to bronchiolar oedema and narrowing of the small airways.

There is uneven ventilation, due to areas of partial obstruction, and superimposed pneumonitis causing severe carbon dioxide retention and hypoxaemia.

There may be rupture of the alveoli, with air entry into the mediastinum and/or into the pleural cavity.

Pulmonary vascular resistance is increased as a result of hypoxia, acidosis and hyper-inflation of the lungs. This leads to atrial or digital right-to-left shunting through the foramen ovale and the ductus arteriosus, due to persistently high pulmonary arterial hypertension. The newborn therefore suffers from extreme metabolic acidosis as a result of cardiopulmonary shunting and hypoperfusion, and also from extreme respiratory acidosis due to shunting and alveolar hypoventilation.

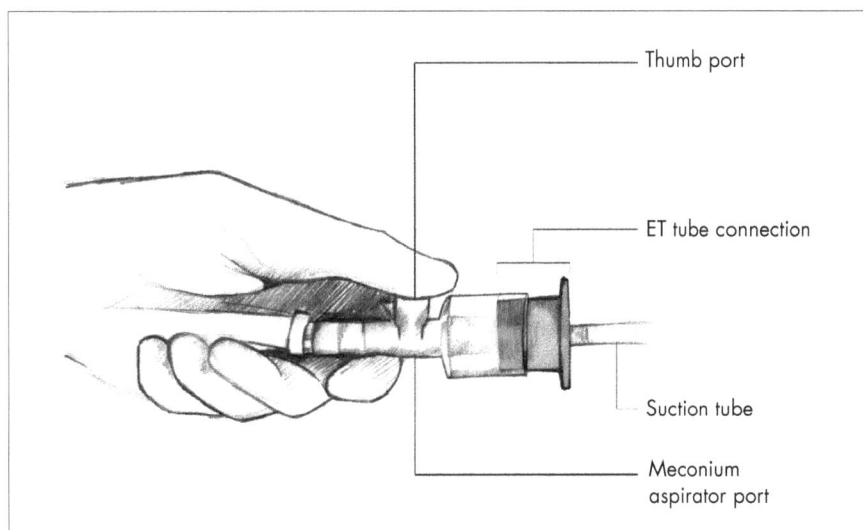

Figure 46.8 A meconium aspirator port for intermittent suctioning

46.6   Asphyxia neonatorum

Asphyxia means 'pulseless'. It is diagnosed in a newborn who fails to breathe within 60 seconds of birth. The risk of asphyxia is anticipated from the antenatal and birth history. (See the sequelae of asphyxia in Figure 46.10 on page 712 and the consequences of asphyxia in Figure 46.11 on page 713.)

Rarely, an asphyxiated infant presents unexpectedly. The most common tool of evaluation is the Apgar score. The fetus may already have experienced primary apnoea *in utero* (see Figure 46.9).

Causes

▶ Prematurity
▶ Birth trauma
▶ Fetal distress
▶ Meconium
▶ Antepartum haemorrhage (APH) or abruption
▶ Congenital abnormalities
▶ IUGR
▶ Post-maturity
▶ Maternal diseases such as pregnancy-induced hypertension (PIH)
▶ A difficult delivery and/or a prolonged second stage
▶ Caesarean section and/or general anaesthesia.

Signs and symptoms

Table 46.1 compares the signs and symptoms of moderate and severe asphyxia. Figure 46.9 details the original research into the pathophysiology.

If a baby is born with a low Apgar score, it is not possible to know if the baby has primary or secondary apnoea. The following criteria are important:

▶ The heartbeat is less than 100 bpm.

▶ There is no response to stimuli.
▶ The baby is pale (central cyanosis is better than a pale grey colour, indicating the baby is in shock with a low BP and vasoconstriction).
▶ There is poor muscle tone.
▶ The baby does not respond.
▶ The baby is not breathing and needs to be intubated.

Complications of asphyxia

Asphyxia can lead to complications such as:

▶ neonatal hypoxic-ischaemic encephalopathy (HIE) (see Chapter 47)
▶ hypoxaemia, which damages the neurological system (brain) and can lead to brain damage, deafness and eye movement problems
▶ hypercapnia, which can cause vasodilatation of the cerebral vessels leading to brain oedema and increased intracranial pressure and haemorrhage
▶ ischaemia due to poor blood supply when the BP drops, which is more devastating than hypoxia because the baby becomes acidotic
▶ respiratory acidosis, which causes a rise in carbon dioxide and a fall in oxygen, with an effect on the pH balance of the cerebrospinal fluid (CSF)
▶ metabolic acidosis, which is the accumulation of lactic acid and pyruvic acid
▶ a fall in the BP, causing multiple organ damage
▶ necrosis of tissue caused by deep vein thrombosis (DVT), renal shutdown, congestive heart failure and lack of blood to the gut
▶ clotting defects.

Table 46.1

A comparison between moderate and severe asphyxia

Criterion	Moderate asphyxia: 4–6/10*	Severe asphyxia: 0–3/10*
Muscle tone	Poor	Placid
Colour: cyanotic/pale	Central cyanosis	Pale
Respiratory rate	Poor efforts	No efforts
Heart rate	100 bpm	< 100 bpm
Reflex irritability	Grimacing	No response

* Based on Apgar scores after birth and within 10 minutes of birth.

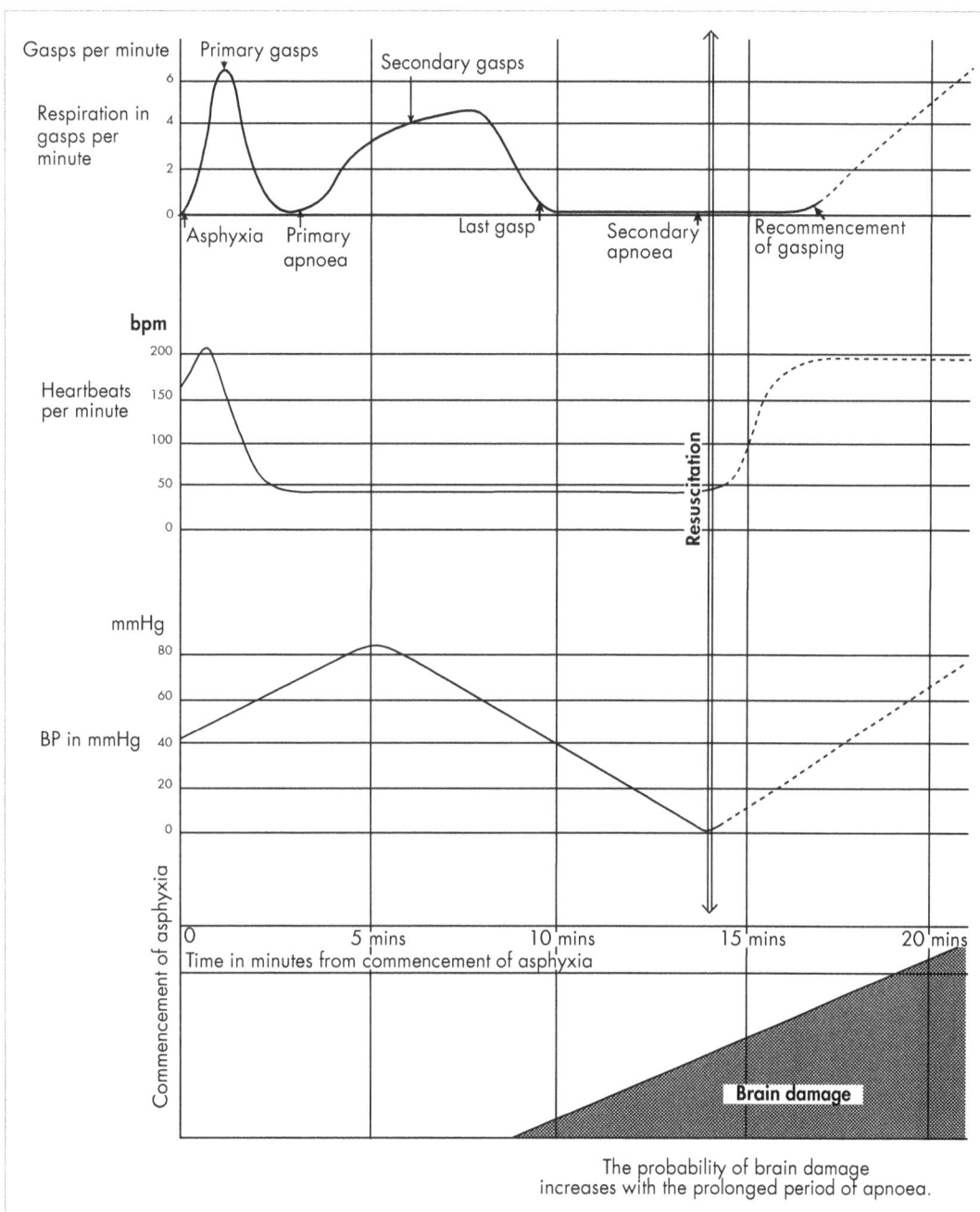

Figure 46.9 Primary and secondary apnoea. Changes which have been noted in the Rhesus monkey during asphyxia (adapted from Shore, Keet & Harrison, 1978)

Immediate management and care

Neonatal resuscitation constitutes a series of actions that are taken in order to revive a newborn infant so that normal respiration may be initiated and maintained. The objective is to obtain a normal respiratory rate and pattern, heart rate, BP, colour and general activity level. If these objectives can be achieved within seven minutes of birth, cerebral damage – leading to cerebral palsy, long-term handicap and even death – can be avoided (see the discussion on neonatal HIE in Chapter 47).

The Apgar score is used to determine if the infant needs resuscitation. The Apgar score at one minute after birth shows the immediate situation and is an index of asphyxia and the need for intervention and resuscitation.

The Apgar score obtained at five minutes after birth gives a good indication of the infant's response to resuscitative measures and of the infant's ability to withstand hypoxaemia.

This score correlates best with the long-term prognosis for mental development and/or neonatal death.

All babies need assessment and basic care at birth:
- 5–10 per cent of babies need stimulation.
- 3–6 per cent need bag-and-mask ventilation.
- 1 per cent require advanced resuscitation.
- 0.1 per cent require chest compression.
- 0.05 per cent require drugs.

The HBB programme was developed to safely manage the 99 per cent of cases that can be managed by skilled staff during birth. The timely identification of the cases that may form part of the 1 per cent of babies who need advanced care is an essential part of quality care (HNN, 2017; Kak et al, 2015). These cases should be referred to be delivered under the supervision of an obstetrician and a paediatrician.

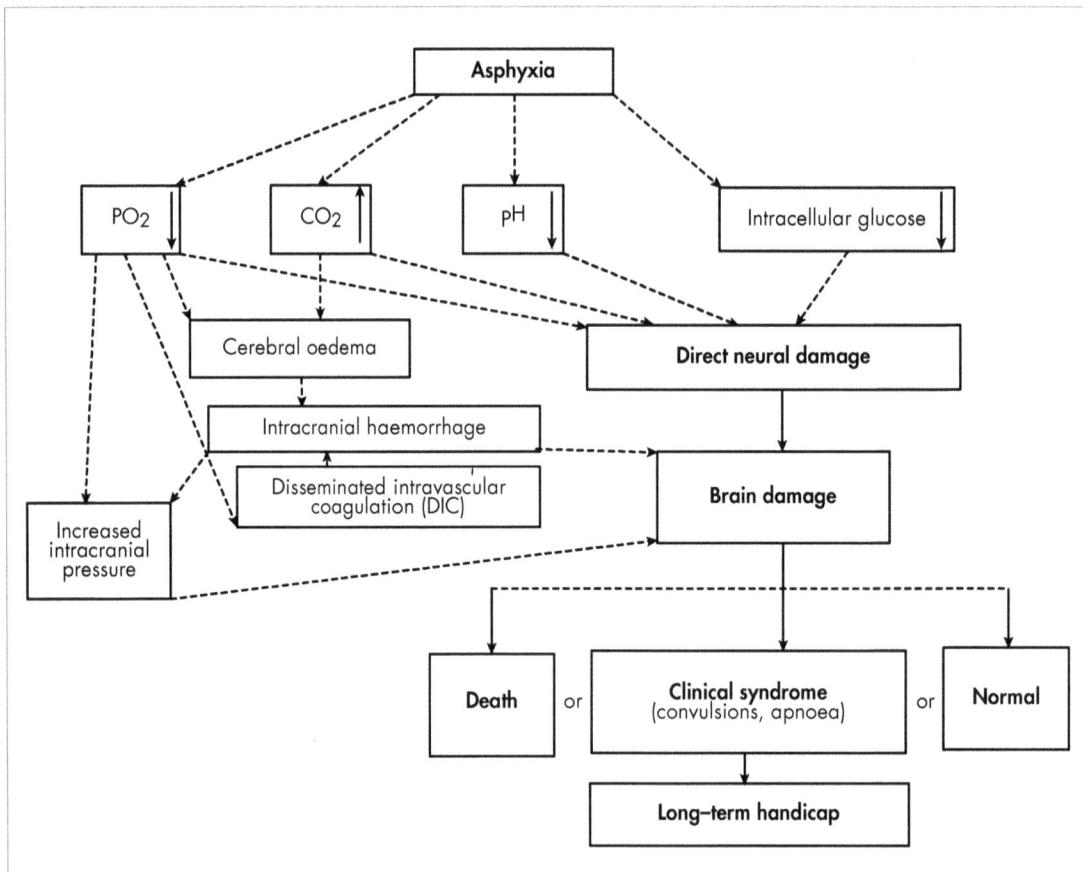

Figure 46.10 The sequelae of asphyxia

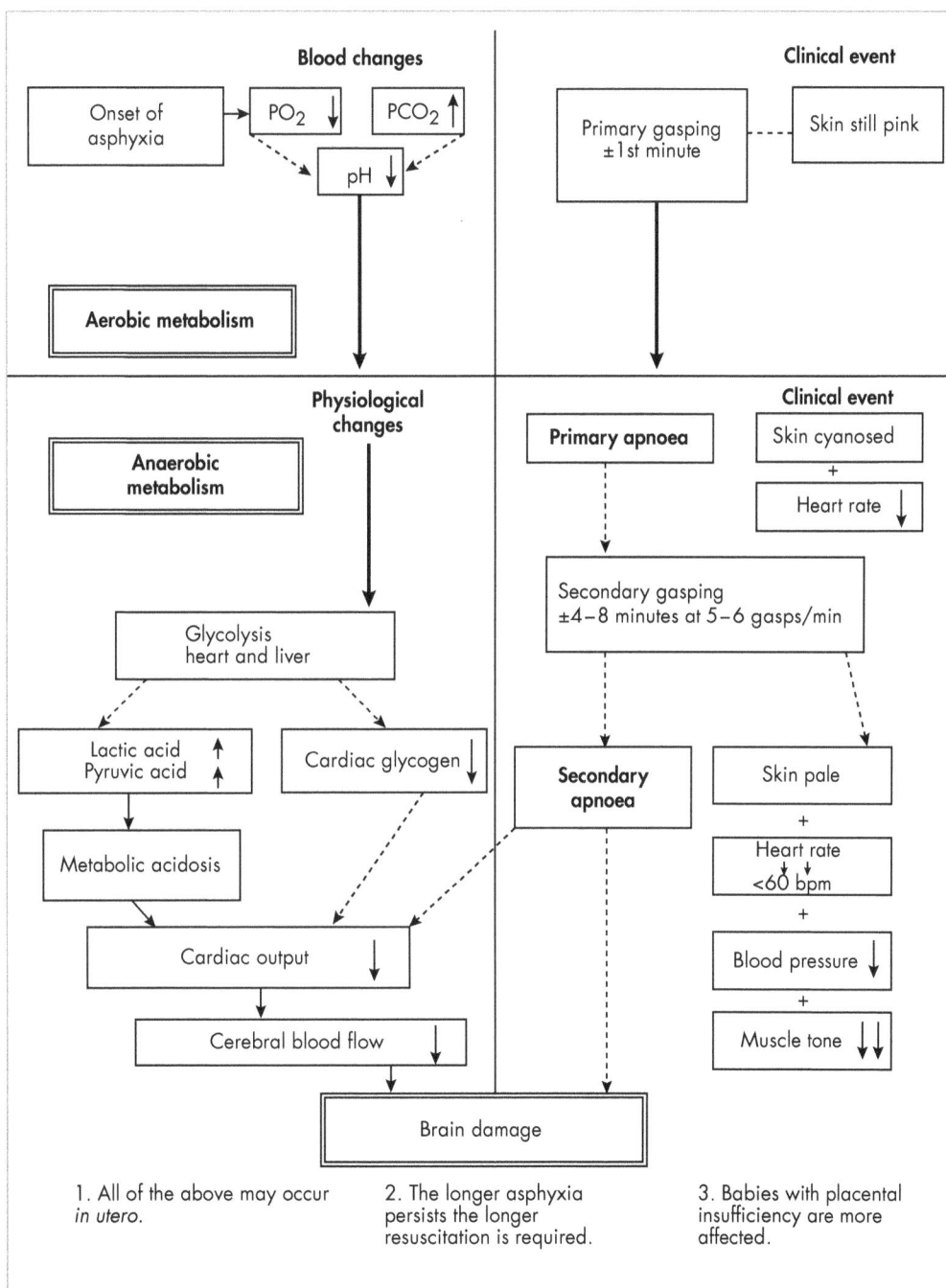

Figure 46.11 Important changes associated with asphyxia

Resuscitation management

The latest evidence-based procedure to resuscitate newborn babies is called the HBB programme. It is part of the essential newborn care guidelines for South Africa and focuses on the 'golden minute' – a time period when stimulation and ventilation with a bag and mask can save the life of the baby (DoH, 2013b).

713

The Helping Babies Breathe programme

The HBB programme is a global initiative and is part of the *Guidelines for Maternity Care in South Africa* (DoH, 2015). Information on the programme is available from: https://www.aap.org/en-us/advocacy-and-policy/aap-health-initiatives/helping-babies-survive/Pages/Implementation-Guide.aspx.

All staff working in the maternity section and casualties should have formal training in this method and the workplace should be appropriately equipped.

PROCEDURE Neonatal resuscitation

Definition

HBB is a sustainable, effective, low-cost neonatal resuscitation programme that is easy to integrate. It has been accepted as the best practice for birth attendants in South Africa through the national programme implemented by the Department of Health (DoH). The procedure is effective with room air and no piped oxygen is needed.

Principles

This procedure is based on the principles of the HBB training programme and is in line with WHO expert review:

▶ The necessary equipment should be procured for the birthing unit.
▶ All students and birth attendants should complete HBB training, presented at an HBB centre by master trainers, to gain competency as skilled birth attendants.
▶ HBB skills must be renewed every five years.
▶ At least one person skilled in HBB should be present at every birth. However, more than one person is needed for the resuscitation (see Figure 46A) and another is required to take care of the mother. Every person working in the unit should therefore be given the opportunity to be trained in HBB, preferably during orientation.
▶ Birthing units should keep a register of staff members skilled in HBB and of the functional equipment.
▶ To retain skills, clinical mentoring, refresher training, supervision and self-assessment should be an ongoing process.
▶ Planning starts in the antenatal period, when women are educated and advised to have a skilled birth attendant present at birth (meaning delivering in an institution in South Africa).

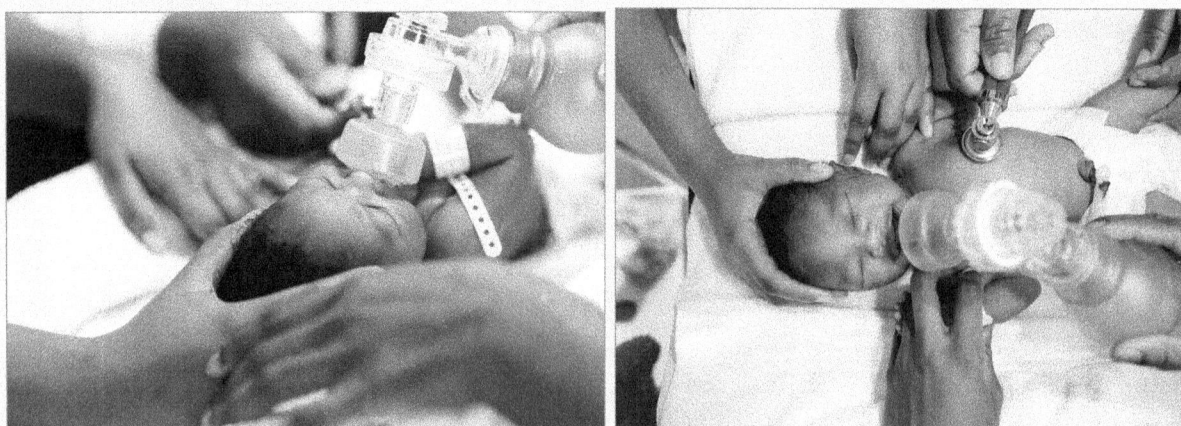

Figure 46A Team effort in neonatal resuscitation

continued

The following aspects are covered in HBB training.

Preparation

The principles of preparation include:
- a written emergency plan for communication and transport for advanced care
- a helper on stand-by
- the preparation of an area for delivery and baby care
- handwashing facilities
- equipment that has been checked and is in working order.

Equipment and staff

- Gloves
- A cloth or warm towel
- A head covering
- A cord clamp
- Cord scissors
- A bulb for suction
- A ventilation mask and bag
- A stethoscope
- A timer (clock or watch)
- Two to three staff members.

Principles of routine neonatal care at birth (for 98.4 per cent of births)

1. Dry the baby to stimulate breathing.
2. Clear the airway before drying if meconium is present in the liquor.
3. Observe if the baby gasps, cries or breathes spontaneously.
4. Keep the baby warm.
5. If the baby breathes, clamp and cut the cord (after one minute) and give routine care.
6. If the baby is not breathing after drying, exercise the golden minute principles of emergency care.

The golden minute principles of care

Drying, clearing the airway and stimulation should take less than one minute. Two staff members are needed; one competent staff member stays with the mother and continues with the third stage, while one staff member takes care of the baby.

1. Call for assistance.
2. Clear the airway and stimulate breathing.
3. Dry the head, body, arms and legs by gently rubbing with a cloth and wipe the face clean.

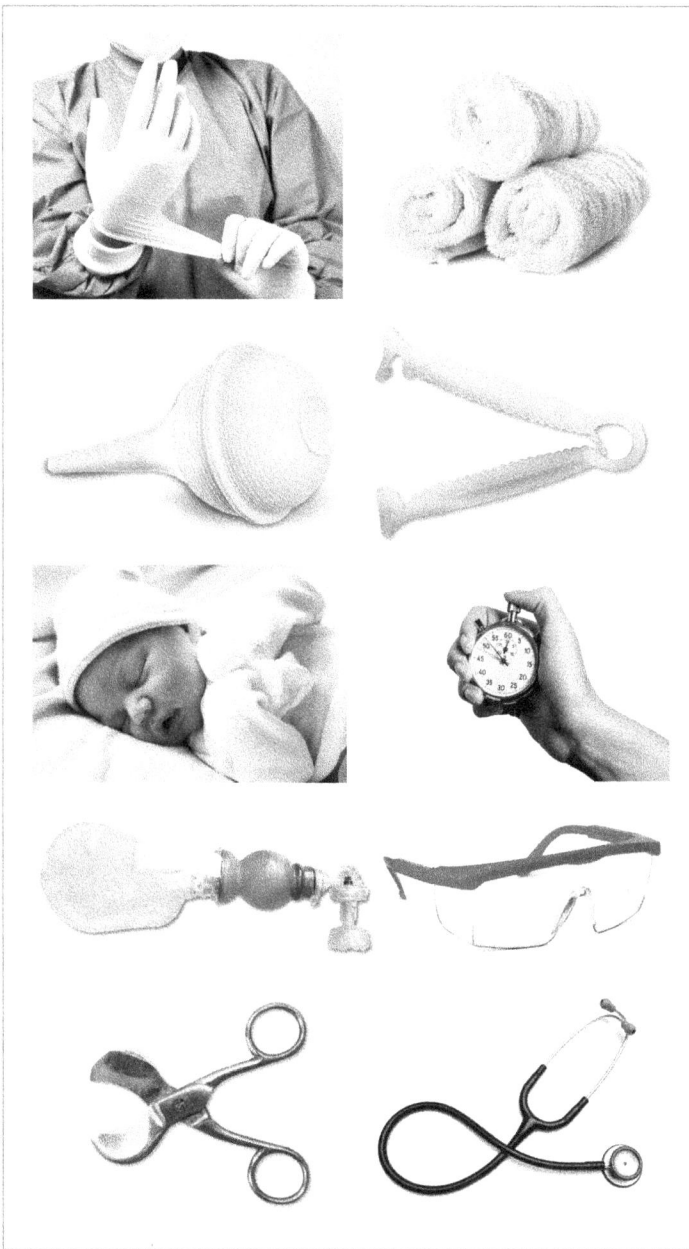

Figure 46B Equipment needed for HBB

continued

4   Remove the wet cloth.
5   Place the baby skin-to-skin on the mother's chest or abdomen if possible. If not possible, place the baby on a warm, dry blanket beside the mother or on the warm resuscitation surface.
6   Position the baby with the neck slightly extended to help keep the airway open.
7   Clear the mouth and nose with a clean suction device.
8   Gently but deliberately rub the back once or twice.
9   Do not delay or stimulate longer. Move quickly to evaluate breathing and decide if intervention with the ambubag is needed.

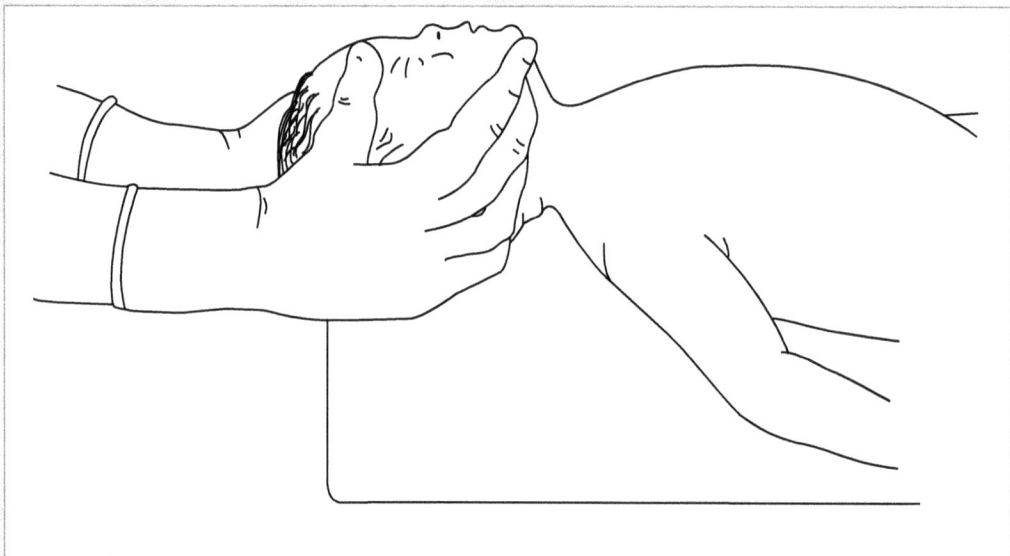

Figure 46C The 'sniffing' position

Ambubag ventilation during the golden minute
1   Clamp and cut the cord about two fingerbreadths from the abdomen.
2   Position the baby with the neck slightly extended to help keep the airway open, as shown in Figure 46C.
3   Select the correct bag and mask.
4   Position the mask on the face. Ensure there is a seal between the face and mask.
5   Squeeze the bag to produce gentle chest movements at 40 breaths per minute. As the chest moves, count one, two, three, one, two, three, etc.
6   Evaluate the baby during the procedure.
7   Keep the baby warm.
8   Stop the procedure when the baby breathes spontaneously.
9   If the baby is not breathing, continue with ventilation.

Recording and interpretation
Keep a record of routine care, resuscitation or advanced interventions. Record:
▶ the time of birth
▶ the Apgar score
▶ breathing
▶ duration of resuscitation

continued

716

> ◗ the baby's response to the interventions
> ◗ outcomes
> ◗ referral.
>
> **Actions**
> If there is no spontaneous breathing after one minute, check the heart rate. If is is under 100 bpm, call for help, refer for advanced care and mobilise appropriate trained staff for assistance.

Drugs needed for newborns

In some cases where medical assistance is not easily available, midwives may be trained to administer drugs. To this end, the following drugs should be available:

◗ Naloxone (Narcan®)
◗ Adrenaline ampules 1:10 000 (1ml = 100 μg)
◗ Vacolitre of 10 per cent dextrose water (200 ml)
◗ Sodium bicarbonate ampules 4.2 per cent strength or solution
◗ 50 per cent dextrose water 20 ml ampules.

ALERT: Naloxone administration to newborns

Naloxone (0.1 mg/kg IV/IM) should only be given to infants who are receiving adequate ventilatory support and whose respiratory depression has resulted from maternal opiate administration.

Care of the parents

Care of the parents is extremely important and yet is often neglected while the midwife attends to the immediate needs of the asphyxiated newborn and his or her subsequent transfer to the nursery for further management. Once the newborn is stable, explain the whole procedure to the parents. Alternatively, if there are enough staff, ask another midwife to do so while the resuscitation is taking place.

46.7   Conclusion

All midwives need to develop a safe level of competency in the resuscitation of a newborn at birth. Besides the ability to intubate the newborn, this includes the ability to recognise dangerous conditions and to perform resuscitation correctly if needed.

47

Birth trauma

LEARNING OBJECTIVES

On completion of this chapter, you must be able to:

▶ identify factors that can cause birth trauma

▶ demonstrate competence to implement measures to prevent birth trauma

▶ demonstrate skill in the early assessment and diagnosis of birth trauma

▶ demonstrate skill and competency in the facilitation of care of the neonate and the family.

KNOWLEDGE ASSUMED TO BE IN PLACE

Standard care during birth

KEYWORDS

caput succedaneum • cephalohaematoma • intracranial haemorrhage • neonatal hypoxic-ischaemic encephalopathy (HIE) • vacuum haematoma • cranial nerve injury • brachial palsy • Erb's palsy • spinal cord injury • *Saving Mothers* report (DoH, 2014b) • *Saving Babies* report (Pattinson & Rhoda, 2014) • confidence interval (CI) • *Newborn Care Charts* (DoH 2014a: 2.2.5, page 37)

47.1 Introduction

There are many conditions that cause birth trauma to the neonate, which can be either minor or serious. This chapter presents the most important aspects that a midwife should be able to prevent, identify and treat. Trauma may be physical, mechanical or due to a lack of oxygen.

47.2 Mortality, morbidity and birth injury

Although some birth injuries are mild and will heal, other injuries are severely debilitating and irreversible. These may lead to death or result in life-long disability.

It is the intention of maternal services and healthcare professionals to prevent birth injuries by setting standards of care and practice. Some birth injuries can be prevented, whereas others cannot be prevented or predicted. Maintaining best practices and keeping clear records are key factors to all actions and interventions during care.

Litigation in healthcare – and particularly in birth injury – has increased in South Africa. (See Chapter 3 for a discussion on litigation.)

Causes of birth injury

The five Hs recommended in the *Saving Mothers 2011–2013* report (DoH, 2014b) addresses the risks of HIV, hypertension, haemorrhage, health worker training and health system factors as causative of fetal morbidity and mortality. Birth injury should be viewed in terms of these reports.

The forces of labour and delivery interventions (or malpractice) occasionally cause physical injury to the newborn. During labour, compression, contraction, torque and traction takes place. When complications such as abnormal fetal size, presentation or neurologic immaturity occurs, the intrapartum forces may lead to tissue damage, anoxia, oedema, haemorrhage or fractures in the neonate. The use of obstetric instrumentation may further increase the risk of birth injuries.

A traumatic delivery is anticipated if the mother has a small pelvic capacity, if the infant seems large for gestational age

(LGA) (often the case with diabetic mothers), or with a breech or other abnormal presentation, especially in a primigravida. In those cases, labour and the fetal condition should be monitored closely. If fetal distress is detected, the mother should be positioned on her side and given oxygen. If fetal distress persists, an immediate Caesarean section should be done. All babies are at risk of anoxia, but smaller and immature babies are more at risk for haemorrhage resulting from anoxia.

Factors predisposing to injury include those detailed below.

Obstetric factors

Obstetric factors often present from the pregnancy and birth, such as:

▶ the mother being a primigravida
▶ cephalopelvic disproportion (CPD) due to small maternal stature or maternal pelvic anomalies
▶ prolonged labour
▶ deep transverse arrest of the descent of the presenting part
▶ oligohydramnios
▶ abnormal presentation (breech)
▶ anaemia
▶ antepartum haemorrhage (APH)
▶ a very low-birth-weight (LBW) infant
▶ extreme prematurity
▶ fetal macrosomia and a large head, leading to CPD and prolonged labour
▶ placental factors
▶ fetal anomalies
▶ maternal infections
▶ fetal distress.

Any condition that puts the baby at risk in the womb or during and after birth and that causes a lack of oxygen to the fetal brain is serious. The most important factors here include intrauterine acute and chronic fetal distress in pregnancy and during birth (with or without meconium), APH and pregnancy-induced hypertension (PIH) complications.

All patient factors identified in the *Saving Mothers* (DoH, 2014b) and *Saving Babies* reports (Pattinson & Rhoda, 2014) are considered, such as late bookings, poverty and transport issues.

Healthcare professionals

▶ *Staff factors.* These factors include substandard care related to a delayed diagnosis of prolonged first and second stages of birth. Common factors include poor monitoring of labour by the midwife through poor use of the partogram as well as poor recording generally. Some of these factors cannot be prevented, but it is essential that all health

professionals are able to practise life-saving techniques when assigned to work in obstetrics, such as the Helping Babies Breathe (HBB) programme for resuscitation of the newborn (see Chapter 46).

▶ *Interventions.* There is an increased risk of trauma associated with assisted deliveries and obstetric emergencies. The incidence of neonatal injury from difficult or traumatic deliveries still exists, in spite of Caesarean section replacing difficult versions, vacuum extractions or mid- or high-forceps deliveries. The average was found in 2002 to be 6,92 injuries per 1 000 live births in South Africa (Pattinson, 2003).

▶ *Skills.* All health workers need to have been trained in the Essential Steps in the Management of Obstetric Emergencies (ESMOE) programme and must be regularly updated on Essential Obstetric Simulation Training (EOST). Certain procedures are only performed by experienced obstetricians, such as the use of mid-cavity forceps or vacuum extraction, versions and extractions (vaginal or during Caesarean section), and anaesthetics.

Health system factors

Chapter 2 discussed the signal functions for essential clinical and health system interventions needed to reduce the incidence of trauma and complications for mothers and babies, as per the *Saving Mothers* (DoH, 2014b) and *Saving Babies* reports (Pattinson & Rhoda, 2014). Healthcare managers and clinical care managers will follow the guidelines, as these are updated and published regularly. The *Guidelines for Maternity Care in South Africa* (DoH, 2015) also give regular guidance on clinical practice standards.

47.3 Life-threatening conditions

Neonatal hypoxic-ischaemic encephalopathy

Perinatal asphyxia (see Chapter 32, which discusses fetal distress, and Chapter 46, which discusses neonatal asphyxia) is associated with neonatal hypoxic-ischaemic encephalopathy (HIE).

Lack of universal agreed definitions of neonatal encephalopathy (NE) and the subgroup with hypoxic-ischaemia (HIE) makes the estimation of incidence and the identification of risk factors problematic. For this reason, we refer to both conditions.

NE is the clinical manifestation of disordered neonatal brain function. HIE refers to brain injury due to a hypoxic event.

Incidence

The incidence of NE is estimated as 3:1 000 live births (95% CI 2.7 to 3.3) and the incidence of HIE as 1.5 (95% CI 1.3 to 1.7) (Kurinczuk, White-Koning & Badawi, 2010). It is estimated that 30 per cent of cases of NE in developed populations and 60 per cent in developing populations have some evidence of intrapartum hypoxic ischaemia.

In South Africa, the *Saving Babies* report (Pattinson & Rhoda, 2014) does not reflect directly on HIE, but indirectly on fetal distress and hypoxia in labour. A 2015 study of neonates weighing less than 2 kg in a public academic hospital found an incidence of 8.5–13/1 000 live births. Sixty per cent were moderate to severe (Bruckmann & Velaphi, 2015).

Definitions

▶ *HIE:* Acute or sub-acute brain injury caused by asphyxia, based on clinical or laboratory evidence; abnormal neurological behaviour in the neonatal period may result
▶ *Hypoxia or anoxia:* A lack of oxygen in the brain or blood; hypoxia is partial whereas anoxia is complete
▶ *Asphyxia:* A state in which placental or pulmonary gas exchange is compromised or ceases altogether
▶ *Ischaemia:* The reduction or cessation of blood flow to an organ, which compromises both oxygen and substrate delivery to the tissue.

Risks and causes

The risk factors for NE vary. Potentially modifiable risk factors include:
▶ maternal thyroid disease
▶ antenatal care
▶ infection
▶ aspects of the treatment of labour and delivery
▶ a response to fetal compromise.

Maternal causes include:
▶ cardiac arrest and asphyxia
▶ severe anaphylaxis
▶ eclampsia or status epilepticus
▶ hypovolaemic shock (APH).

Uteroplacental causes include:
▶ placental abruption
▶ cord prolapse
▶ uterine rupture
▶ hyperstimulation with oxytocic agents.

Fetal causes include:
▶ feto-maternal haemorrhage
▶ twin-to-twin transfusion
▶ severe isoimmune (Rh) haemolytic disease

▶ hydrops fetalis
▶ intrauterine growth restriction (IUGR).

Pathophysiology

When anoxia occurs, there is redistribution of blood flow to vital organs. If this episode is prolonged or compensatory mechanisms fail, cerebral blood flow falls or is reduced and ischaemic brain injury occurs (Zanelli, 2016). Also see figures 46.10 and 46.11 on pages 712–713.

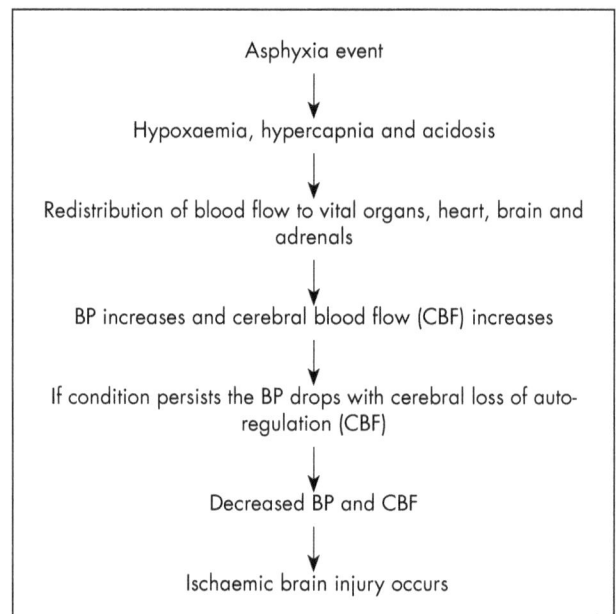

Asphyxia event
↓
Hypoxaemia, hypercapnia and acidosis
↓
Redistribution of blood flow to vital organs, heart, brain and adrenals
↓
BP increases and cerebral blood flow (CBF) increases
↓
If condition persists the BP drops with cerebral loss of auto-regulation (CBF)
↓
Decreased BP and CBF
↓
Ischaemic brain injury occurs

Figure 47.1 The pathophysiology sequelae of HIE

Diagnosis

The clinical diagnosis is based on:
▶ an Apgar score of 3 or lower that persists for more than five minutes
▶ neonatal neurological sequelae (eg seizures, coma or hypotonia)
▶ multiple organ involvement: heart (< 100 bpm), kidneys, liver and intestines.

The tests performed include:
▶ laboratory studies: serum electrolyte, renal function, cardiac and liver enzymes, coagulation and arterial blood gas for acid–base status
▶ imaging: MRI scan, ultrasound and ego-grams as well as electroencephalography (EEG) at a later stage
▶ hearing and eye tests.
▶ HIE scorecard (DoH 2014a: 2.2.5, page 38)

Management

▶ Perform immediate and effective resuscitation, intubation and ventilation.
▶ Refer the baby for medical care in NICU.
▶ BP management is essential to improve blood flow to the brain.
▶ Manage fluid carefully in order not to overload.
▶ Avoid hypo- and hyperglycaemia.
▶ Treat seizures.
▶ Perform hypothermia therapy.

Outcomes

The short-term outcome is death. The long-term outcomes include (Allan & Sobel, 2004):
▶ multiple disabilities
▶ a mild to moderate form of palsy
▶ developmental delay, considered similar to the control population who did not have a known incident of hypoxia.

Short-term outcomes

▶ *Mild HIE* typically resolves within 24 hours. The baby may exhibit slightly increased tendon reflexes, poor sucking, irritability, excessive crying or sleepiness.
▶ *Moderate HIE* may resolve within one to two weeks, with better long-term outcomes. The baby's grasping, Moro and deep-tendon reflexes may be diminished, with occasional episodes of apnoea and seizures occurring within 24 hours after birth.

▶ *Severe HIE* is characterised by seizures that are resistant to conventional treatment and increase within the first 48 hours. After this, the seizures subside, but wakefulness deteriorates due to cerebral oedema, with a potential for bulging fontanelles. The baby may be in a coma and unresponsive, with irregular respiration and an irregular heart rate. The baby may exhibit hypotonia and poor sucking, grasping or Moro reflexes. The eyes may be skewed or deviate and nystagmus may present. The pupils may be dilated, fixed or not reactive to light.

Hypothermia therapy

Hypothermia has become standard care for infants of 35 weeks or more.
▶ Treatment must be started within six hours of birth to be effective.
▶ The Apgar score must be 5 or less at 10 minutes, with an arterial pH of less than 7 within one hour after birth.
▶ Cooling therapy may include the whole body, the head or both.
▶ The aim is to get the core (rectal) temperature to 33–35 °C for 72 hours.
▶ This reduces the extent of brain damage, and death or disability at 18 months is significantly reduced.

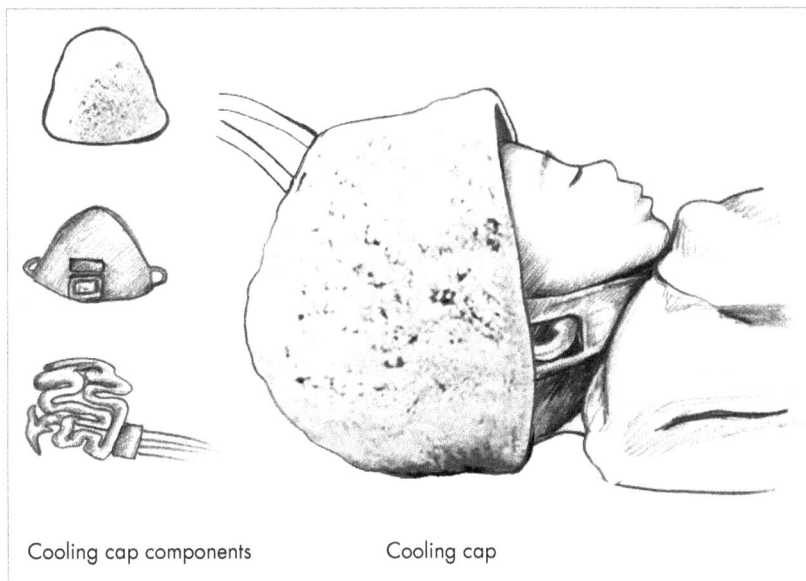

Cooling cap components   Cooling cap

Figure 47.2 Hypothermia therapy

Long-term outcomes

HIE can cause long-term physical, mental and cognitive problems, including:

▶ cerebral palsy
▶ epilepsy
▶ hearing impairment
▶ blindness
▶ cognitive learning problems
▶ speech difficulties
▶ physical disability – low psychomotor development index (PDI).

Brain haemorrhage

Haemorrhage in or around the brain can occur in any neonate, but is particularly common in those born prematurely; about 20 per cent of premature infants weighing less than 1 500 g (or born before 32 weeks) have intraventicular haemorrhage (IVH) (Szpecht et al, 2016).

Intraventricular and/or intraparenchymal haemorrhage is usually present during the first three days of life and is the most serious type of intracranial bleeding. It occurs most often in premature neonates, is often bilateral and usually arises in the germinal matrix. Mostly, small amounts of sub-ependymal or intraventricular blood are involved (see Figure 47.3).

Intraventricular haemorrhage

IVH is bleeding into the cerebrospinal fluid (ventricles) inside the brain, most often in babies that are born prematurely:

▶ *Signs and symptoms.* Neonates may present with apnoea, seizures and lethargy. The signs and symptoms may include a rapidly enlarging head or an abnormal neurological examination with hypotonia, a poor Moro reflex, or extensive retinal haemorrhages.
▶ *Diagnosis.* Either cranial ultrasound or CT scanning is done. For screening of very premature infants (eg under 30 weeks' gestation), ultrasound is used. If the diagnosis is in doubt, the cerebrospinal fluid (CSF) can be examined for red blood cells (RBCs): it usually contains gross blood.
▶ *Complications.* In severe haemorrhage, there may be bleeding into the parenchyma or a cast of the ventricular system, with large amounts of blood in the cisterna magna and basal cisterns. With large haemorrhages, the associated meningeal inflammation may lead to a communicating hydrocephalus as the infant grows.
▶ *Prognosis.* Most neonates who present with small IVHs survive the acute bleeding episode and do well. Neonates who present with large IVHs have a poor prognosis, especially if the haemorrhage extends into the parenchyma.

▶ *Management.* Careful monitoring of preterm neonates with a history of severe IVH must be done, as they are at risk of developing post-haemorrhagic hydrocephalus. Neonates with progressive hydrocephalus require neurosurgical evaluation. Because many neonates will be left with neurological deficits, careful follow-up and referral for early intervention services are important.

Prevention and management of all types of brain haemorrhage

The prevention of prolonged labour, respiratory distress and asphyxia in the newborn can reduce the incidence of brain haemorrhage and poor outcomes. Prevention includes:

▶ early and accurate diagnosis in premature birth
▶ early diagnosis after assisted deliveries or complicated births
▶ referring the baby for medical care
▶ giving vitamin K, if not previously given
▶ giving platelets or clotting factors, if deficient.

47.4   Non-life-threatening head injuries

Moulding of the fetal head is common in vaginal delivery due to the high pressure exerted by uterine contractions on the neonate's malleable cranium as it passes through the birth canal. This rarely causes problems or requires treatment.

Caput succedaneum

The caput succedaneum is an oedema of the fetal scalp due to prolonged pressure of the fetal head on the pelvis and cervix.

A caput succedaneum is present at birth. It usually enlarges and can cross a suture line, starts to reduce in size soon after birth and has disappeared within 24 hours. If, however, the labour has been prolonged and difficult, the caput will be excessive and may persist for up to 36 hours.

Cephalohaematoma

A cephalohaematoma is an effusion of blood under the periosteum. The periosteum is torn off the cranial bone and there is a slow oozing of blood underneath it, eventually causing a large swelling. The swelling can be present at birth or develop between 12 and 24 hours after birth. It does not cross a suture (see Figure 47.3).

This condition occurs in a prolonged second stage of labour, as a result of CPD, usually affecting the presenting parietal bone.

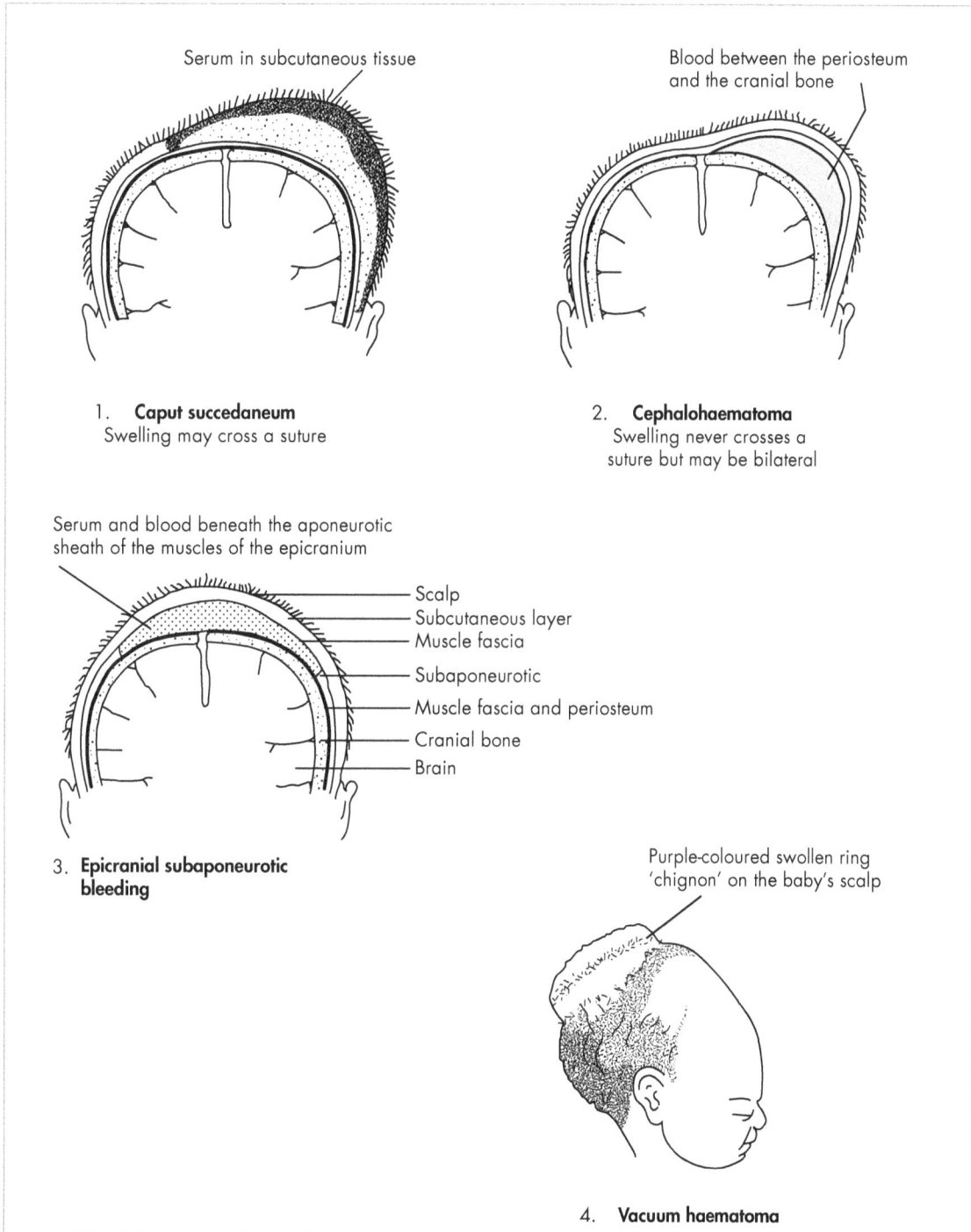

Serum in subcutaneous tissue

Blood between the periosteum and the cranial bone

1. **Caput succedaneum**
Swelling may cross a suture

2. **Cephalohaematoma**
Swelling never crosses a suture but may be bilateral

Serum and blood beneath the aponeurotic sheath of the muscles of the epicranium

Scalp
Subcutaneous layer
Muscle fascia
Subaponeurotic
Muscle fascia and periosteum
Cranial bone
Brain

3. **Epicranial subaponeurotic bleeding**

Purple-coloured swollen ring 'chignon' on the baby's scalp

4. **Vacuum haematoma**

Figure 47.3 Injuries to the scalp and skull

Cephalohaematoma can be differentiated from subaponeurotic haemorrhage (which is a rupture of the emissary veins between the dural sinuses and scalp veins) because it is sharply limited to the area overlying a single bone, the periosteum being adherent at the sutures. Subaponeurotic haemorrhage (Figure 47.3) can be lethal when blood accumulates from the veins. Cephalohaematoma does not pose any risk to the brain cells.

Signs and symptoms

Cephalohaematomas are commonly unilateral and parietal. In a small percentage, there is a linear fracture of the underlying bone. It can be bilateral.

Complications

Usually the haematoma is gradually re-absorbed into the circulation over six to eight weeks. The neonate may develop hyperbilirubinaemia, jaundice, anaemia or hypotension in severe cases. Occasionally, the haematoma persists as a hard lump on the head, as calcium is laid down. In some cases, it may be an indication of a linear skull fracture or that the baby is at risk of an infection leading to osteomyelitis or meningitis.

Management

No active treatment is necessary, but extra observation and care must be taken with the infant. Vitamin C has been reported to hurry the absorption of the haematoma. In severe cases, the baby may need a blood transfusion.

Vacuum haematoma

Vacuum haematoma (see Figure 47.3 on the previous page) is bleeding of the soft tissues in the area where the vacuum was attached during a vacuum extraction.

Sign and symptoms

The suction of the vacuum extractor can cause a purple-coloured swollen ring, called a 'chignon', on the baby's scalp. The edge of the swelling may be excoriated and the scalp torn, which may cause the tissues to slough off. When excessive suction is produced in the vacuum, a part or even the whole circle of scalp can be torn off the head.

Management and care

The lesion normally heals within a few days, but there is always the danger of infection where there is a laceration and an antiseptic agent must be applied.

Other injuries to the scalp and skull

Abrasions and lacerations sometimes occur from scalpel cuts during Caesarean delivery or during instrumental delivery (eg vacuum or forceps). Infection remains a risk, but most heal uneventfully.

Any laceration is dangerous, because if the mother is HIV positive, her blood may enter the abrasion at birth, transferring the virus to the infant. Because of this danger, scalp electrodes for cardiotocograph (CTG) tracings are no longer used in high-risk conditions.

Management and care

With any scalp injury, there may also be an underlying injury to the skull and brain. The neonate will therefore require frequent observation and specialised nursing care. Management consists of careful cleaning, the application of antibiotic ointment and observation. Bring the edges of the injury together using steri-strips. Lacerations occasionally require suturing.

47.5   Injury to the neurological system

Cranial nerve and spinal cord injuries result from hyperextension, traction and overstretching with simultaneous rotation. They may range from localised neurapraxia to complete nerve or cord transection.

Cranial nerve injury

The facial palsy is a muscle limitation of one side of the face due to injury of the facial nerve, which results in temporary or permanent paralysis. This may occur as a result of forceps pressure on the facial nerve in front of the ear. Most injuries probably result from pressure on the nerve *in utero*, which may be due to fetal positioning (eg from the head lying against the shoulder, the sacral promontory or a uterine fibroid). The compression appears to occur as the head passes by the sacrum.

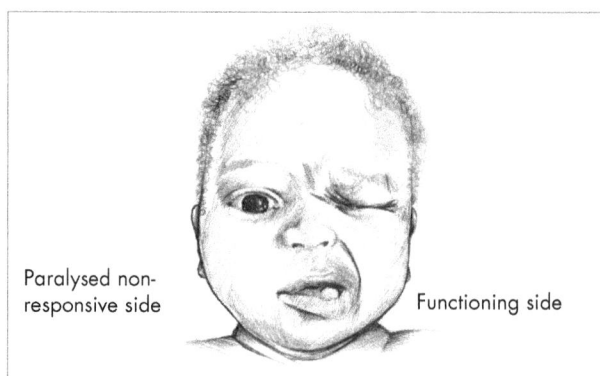

Paralysed non-responsive side

Functioning side

Figure 47.4 Facial paralysis

Signs and symptoms

The sign of a cranial nerve injury is an asymmetric face during crying (see Figure 47.4). The mouth is drawn towards the normal side, wrinkles are deeper on the normal side, and movement of the forehead and eyelid on that side is unaffected. The paralysed side is smooth, with a swollen appearance. On this side the nasolabial fold is absent and the corner of the mouth droops. With peripheral nerve branch injury, the paralysis is limited to the forehead, eye or mouth.

No evidence of trauma is usually present on the face. In the case of a forceps delivery, forceps marks may be present.

The condition starts to recover within the first week, but full resolution may take several months. Palsy caused by trauma usually resolves or improves, whereas palsy that persists is often due to the absence of the nerve.

Management and care

Management consists of the careful surveillance of respiratory status. Intervention, when appropriate, is critical. Protect the affected eye – which cannot blink and remains open – with patches and synthetic tears (methylcellulose drops) every four hours. If there is no improvement in 7–10 days, consult a neurologist and a surgeon.

Most patients recover in the first 6–12 months. The outcome for bilateral lesions is poorer.

Brachial plexus injuries (brachial palsy)

Brachial plexus injuries follow stretching caused by excessive traction on the head and neck. This may occur spontaneously *in utero* due to a difficult position or during a difficult cephalic delivery, for example in the case of shoulder dystocia, breech extraction or hyperadduction of the neck in cephalic presentations. Injuries can be due to simple stretching, haemorrhage within a nerve, tearing of the nerve or root, or avulsion of the roots with accompanying cervical cord injury. The prognosis depends on the site and type of nerve root injury.

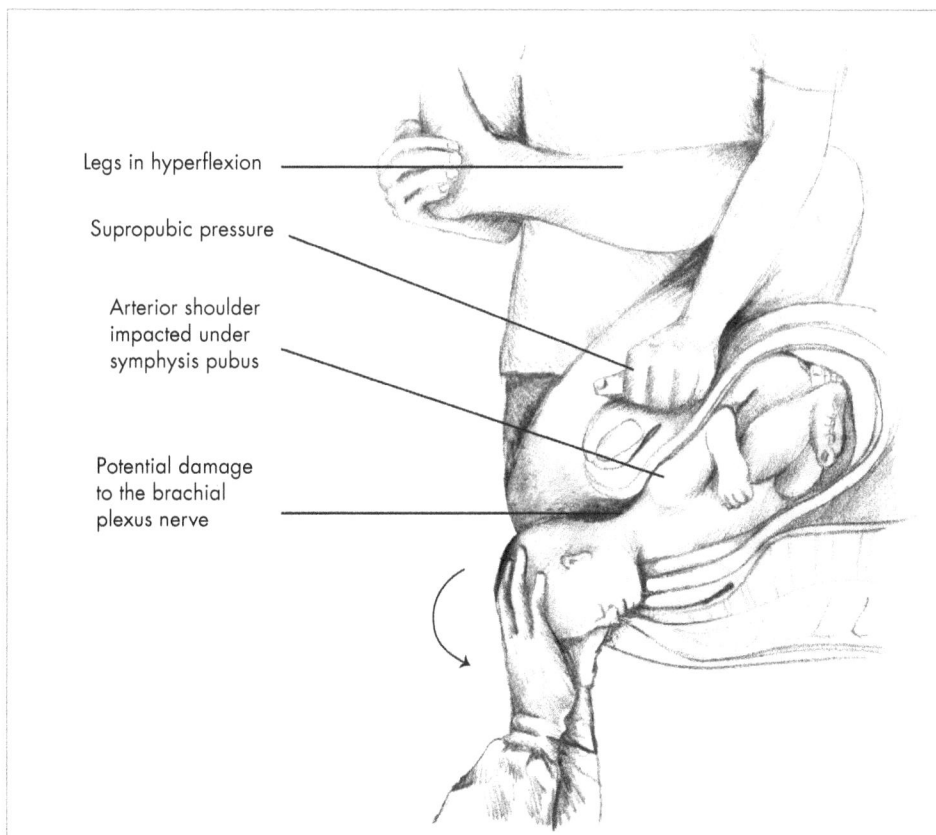

Legs in hyperflexion

Supropubic pressure

Arterior shoulder impacted under symphysis pubus

Potential damage to the brachial plexus nerve

Figure 47.5 Brachial plexus injury due to traction

Signs and symptoms

Erb's palsy is an upper brachial plexus injury causing adduction and internal rotation of the shoulder with pronation of the forearm. The arm is fully extended, with rotation inwards. The movement of the fingers and hand is normal, but the Moro reflex is asymmetrical. There is no tenderness, pain or swelling of the arm if there is no fracture.

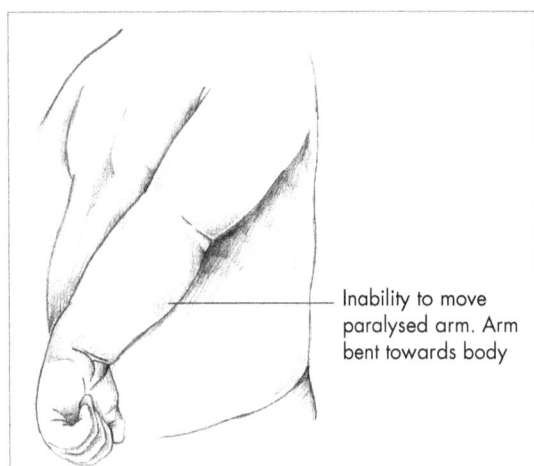

Inability to move paralysed arm. Arm bent towards body

Figure 47.6 Erb's palsy

Prevention, management and care

Protect the shoulder from excessive motion by immobilising the arm across the upper abdomen. Prevent contractures by doing passive range-of-motion exercises with the involved joints. This must be done gently every day, starting at one week of age. If there is no improvement after six weeks, the baby must be referred to a Level 3 hospital for evaluation and possible surgery.

Klumpke's palsy is a lower plexus injury resulting in paralysis of the hand and wrist, often with ipsilateral Horner's syndrome (miosis, ptosis, facial anhidrosis). Passive range-of-motion exercises are the only treatment needed.

Spinal cord injury

Spinal cord injury is rare. It involves variable degrees of cord disruption, often with haemorrhage. Complete disruption of the cord is very rare. Spinal cord injury incurred during delivery results from excessive traction or rotation. Traction is more important in breech deliveries (the minority of cases), and torsion is more significant in vertex deliveries. The true incidence is difficult to determine.

In breech delivery, the lower cervical and upper thoracic regions are the major sites of injury, while in a vertex delivery these are the upper and mid-cervical regions. When the injury is higher, lesions are usually fatal, because respiration is completely compromised. Sometimes a click or snap is heard at delivery.

Major neuropathological changes which consist of acute lesions such as haemorrhages, especially epidural, intraspinal and oedema, may develop or present. Haemorrhagic lesions are associated with varying degrees of stretching, laceration and disruption or total transaction. Occasionally, the dura may be torn. Rarely, vertebral fractures or dislocations may be observed.

Signs and symptoms

▶ Initially, spinal shock with flaccidity below the level of injury occurs, with irregular retention of sensation or movement below the lesion.
▶ Spasticity develops within days or weeks.
▶ Diaphragmatic breathing occurs, because the phrenic nerve remains intact as its origin is higher (at C3 to C5) than the typical cord lesion.
▶ The intercostal and abdominal muscles become paralysed.
▶ The rectal and bladder sphincters cannot develop voluntary control if the spinal cord lesion is complete.
▶ Sensation and sweating are lost below the involved level, which can cause fluctuations of body temperature with environmental changes.

Diagnosis

The diagnosis is made using MRI or CT myelography.

Prevention, management and care

Prevention is the most important aspect of medical care. The obstetric management of breech deliveries, instrumental deliveries and the pharmacologic augmentation of labour must be appropriate. (Occasionally, injury may be sustained *in utero*.)

With appropriate care, most infants survive for many years. The usual causes of death are recurring pneumonia and progressive loss of renal function. Treatment includes nursing care to prevent skin ulcerations, the prompt treatment of urinary and respiratory infections and regular evaluations to identify obstructive uropathy early.

47.6   Fractures

Fractures occur mainly because of traction during delivery – and even during a Caesarean section – either because of a complicated delivery or a lack of skill on the part of the professional. Fractures vary, from skull fractures related to forceps to fractures of the spine, ribs, clavicles, humerus and femur.

Clavicular fracture

One of the most common fractures during birth, mid-clavicular fracture, may occur with shoulder dystocia and with normal, non-traumatic deliveries.

Initially, the neonate is irritable and does not move the arm on the involved side either spontaneously or when the Moro reflex is elicited.

Healing is usually rapid (7–10 days) and uneventful, as most clavicular fractures are greenstick. A large lump forms at the fracture site within a week, and re-modelling is completed within a month. The condition is treated by making a sling by pinning the shirt sleeve of the involved side to the opposite side of the newborn's shirt.

Long-bone fractures

Loss of spontaneous arm or leg movement is an early sign of long-bone fracture, followed by swelling and pain on passive movement. The obstetrician may feel or hear a snap at the time of delivery. Radiographic studies of the limb confirm the diagnosis.

Femoral and humeral shaft fractures are treated with splinting. Closed reduction and casting are necessary only when displacement is present. Watch for evidence of radial nerve injury with humeral fracture. Callus formation occurs, and complete recovery is expected in two to four weeks. In 8–10 days, the callus formation is sufficient to discontinue immobilisation. Orthopaedic consultation is recommended.

Radiographic studies distinguish this condition from septic arthritis.

47.7   Soft tissue and organ damage

Intra-abdominal injury

Intra-abdominal injury is relatively uncommon and can sometimes be overlooked as a cause of death in the newborn. Haemorrhage is the most serious acute complication, and the liver is the most commonly damaged internal organ. This is related to abdominal pressure from using the hands for delivering a breech delivery.

Intraperitoneal bleeding

In the absence of bleeding disorders, intra-abdominal bleeding is caused by rough handling during birth.

Signs and symptoms

Bleeding may be fulminant or insidious, but infants ultimately present with circulatory collapse. Intra-abdominal bleeding should be considered for every infant who presents with shock, pallor, unexplained anaemia and abdominal distension. The overlying abdominal skin may show a bluish discolouration. Radiographic findings are not diagnostic, but may suggest free peritoneal fluid. Paracentesis is the procedure of choice.

Hepatic or organ rupture

Predisposing factors include prematurity, post-maturity, coagulation disorders and asphyxia. In cases associated with asphyxia, vigorous resuscitative efforts (often by unusual methods) is the cause.

Splenic rupture is at least a fifth as common as liver laceration. Predisposing factors and mechanisms of injury are similar.

The most common lesion is sub-capsular haematoma, which increases to 4–5 cm before rupturing.

Lacerations are less common, often caused by abnormal pull on the peritoneal support ligaments or the effect of excessive pressure by the costal margin. Infants with hepatomegaly may be at higher risk.

Signs and symptoms

Symptoms of shock may be delayed. Patients usually present immediately following birth, or rupture becomes obvious within the first few hours or days.

Management and care

The rapid identification of the condition and the stabilisation of the infant are the keys to management, along with the assessment of coagulation defect.

Blood transfusion is the most urgent initial step. Persistent coagulopathy may be treated with fresh frozen plasma, transfusion of platelets and other measures.

47.8   Conclusion

The recognition of trauma necessitates a careful physical and neurological evaluation of the infant to establish whether additional injuries are present. Occasionally, injury may result from resuscitation. Symmetry of structure and function should be assessed as well as specifics such as cranial nerve examination, individual joint range of motion and the integrity of the scalp or skull.

Midwives should be skilled in the full examination of the newborn and able to identify any abnormality.

Daily examinations during nappy changes will also give clues if something is not in order. Listening to the concerns of the mother and family is useful and should not be ignored. On discharge, all babies should have a full examination.

Section Eight
Family planning

48

Contraception and fertility planning

LEARNING OBJECTIVES

On completion of this chapter, you must be able to:

▶ develop competencies in counselling and healthcare screening in reproductive healthcare

▶ assess women and give guidance regarding an appropriate method for contraception

▶ demonstrate knowledge of the appropriate use of all available contraceptive methods used after childbirth

▶ demonstrate knowledge, health education and advocacy skills on termination of pregnancy (TOP).

KNOWLEDGE ASSUMED TO BE IN PLACE

Basic anatomy and physiology of human reproduction and pregnancy

KEYWORDS

contraception • termination of pregnancy (TOP) • medical termination of pregnancy (MTOP) • emergency contraception (EC) • combined oral contraceptive (COC) • progesterone-only oral contraceptive (POC) (also known as the progesterone-only pill, or POP) • lactational amenorrhoea method (LAM) • copper-bearing/-containing intrauterine contraceptive device (CuIUCD) • intrauterine contraceptive device (IUCD)

48.1 Introduction

This chapter focuses on the role of the midwife in reproductive healthcare. Pregnancy is an ideal time to assist women to make appropriate choices to space pregnancies and plan their children.

The contact visit 12 weeks after birth for infant care creates an opportunity to assist families with contraceptive choices and give attention to cervical cancer screening, in line with the WHO's *Statement of Collective Action for Postpartum Family Planning* (2016b). Support of the client and the management of problems relating to reproductive health are important during this period.

48.2 Reproductive healthcare and fertility planning

Health is defined by the WHO as 'a state of complete physical, mental and social well-being and not merely the absence of disease or infirmity. Reproductive health addresses the reproductive processes, functions and system to ensure the well-being of women, families and communities at all stages of life including fertility planning' (WHO, 2016c).

Family planning therefore allows individuals and couples to anticipate and attain their desired number of children and the spacing and timing of their births. This is achieved by using contraceptive methods. A woman's ability to space and limit her pregnancies has a direct impact on her health and well-being as well as on the outcome of each pregnancy (WHO, 2017).

Reproductive health rights

Reproductive healthcare gives couples the right to be informed of and to have access to safe, effective, affordable and acceptable methods of fertility regulation of choice, and the right of access to appropriate healthcare services that will enable women to go safely through pregnancy and childbirth and provide couples with the best chance of having a healthy infant (WHO, 2013b). In South Africa, the Choice on Termination of Pregnancy Act 92 of 1996, as amended by Act 1 of 2008, extends the right to women to choose to terminate a pregnancy within the boundaries of the Act.

Reproductive healthcare

On a global level, the world's population has become potentially unsustainable, at 7.4 billion in 2016. However, in the developed world, the number of children born has declined to levels where some countries are facing declining population growth, which has implications in terms of their ability to care for the elderly and ultimately the decline of the population.

In the developing world, however, this is not the case. Many countries still see rising populations. Educating women is known to be the single most important way of ensuring that pregnancies are planned and children do not grow up in poverty.

Statistics South Africa assists the government to plan healthcare through annual statistical data. In 2015, Statistics South Africa indicated a South African population of 54.96 million, of which 51 per cent (28.07 million) is female, with a crude birth rate that dropped from 24:1 000 in 2005 to 22.7:1 000 in 2015 (Stats SA, 2015). Simultaneously, the crude mortality rate decreased from 14.4:1 000 in 2005 to 9.6:1 000 in 2015. This decline in mortality rate could be related to improved HIV care and is a contributing factor to the increase in life expectancy in 2015, estimated at 60.6 years for males and 64.3 years for females. The fertility rate has declined between 2005 and 2015, from an average of 2.79 children per woman to 2.55 children per woman, suggesting improved access and use of contraception (Stats SA, 2015).

The national Department of Health (DoH) monitors health indicators. These indicated in 2016 that sexual behaviour among young South Africans remains risky and teenage pregnancy remains a problem. The use of contraceptives is low in Africa (at 33 per cent) and South Africa (at 64 per cent). The rate is 77 per cent in northern Europe, 75 per cent in North America, 82 per cent in East Asia and 84 per cent in China. In South America (including Latin America and the Caribbean), the prevalence of use of any method is 75 per cent (UN, 2015). In South Africa, the prevalence of contraception use (of any method) among young women of 18–24 years was 89.1 per cent in 2012 (Seutalwadi, 2012). In spite of the high prevalence of contraceptive use, the couple year protection rate (CYPR) remained suboptimal. The CYPR indicates the percentage of women aged 15–49 who are protected against unplanned pregnancies using modern contraceptive methods, including sterilisation, male and female condoms

and subdermal implants. The CYPR target is 55 per cent but averaged at 46.8 per cent in 2015 (see Table 48.1).

Public health reproductive indicators
In South Africa, the District Health Information System (DHIS) monitors the indicators for health and healthcare performance. Trends are updated annually from the District Health Barometer (DHB).

Table 48.1

South African reproductive health indicators 2014–2015 (Massyn et al, 2015)

Indicator	Target	Average
Cervical screening coverage (women 30+)	60%	54.5%
CYPR	55%	46.8%

Cervical cancer screening

One in 41 women in South Africa will get cervical cancer, the second most common female cancer in South Africa. Papanicolaou smears (Pap smears) are the current method of screening. The main cause of cervical cancer is certain strains of a sexually transmitted virus, the human papillomavirus (HPV).

Screening with HPV testing will replace traditional cervical cytology in future years. The possibility of patient-collected (self-sampling) specimens will cater for a large number of women who may not have access to healthcare facilities (SASOG, 2015). The advantage of liquid-based samples, as will be used in the future, is that they can be used for the primary HPV test and cervical cancer triage testing.

The current guidelines published in the *National Guideline for Cervical Screening Programme* (DoH, nd) for South Africa aims at an adequate coverage of 70 per cent in 10 years, gives referral criteria for atypical smear results, follow-up criteria and infection control related to HPV. The guidelines state the following (DoH, nd):

▶ The target group is women 30 years and older.
▶ Women aged 30 years or older will be screened three times at 10-year intervals (at the approximate ages of 30, 40 and 50), with follow-up and treatment for abnormal tests also free of charge.
▶ The aim is three Pap smears per woman in a lifetime.

- In the case of an HIV-positive status, the woman must have a diagnostic Pap smear after the age of 20 years. If normal, the HIV-positive woman will then have a Pap smear every three years. If the Pap smear is abnormal, it is repeated after six months.
- The pregnant woman's Pap smear needs to be done before 28–30 weeks of pregnancy due to cervical hormonal changes in pregnancy.
- If the woman is more than 30 weeks pregnant and needs a screening smear, a Pap smear is done three months postpartum.

All women attending family planning who are 30 years or over should be advised to have a Pap smear. **Alert:** The HPV Advisory Board suggested new guidelines for South Africa that will be put in place in the next few years (SASOG, 2015). HIV-positive women need to be tested every year until normal results are reported.

Termination of pregnancy

All healthcare professionals need to have the knowledge and skill to assist women to make appropriate choices in a crisis situation of pregnancy to ensure long-term health outcomes. When family planning has failed or when there is an unwanted or unplanned pregnancy, termination of pregnancy (TOP) is a potential outcome. The midwife will encounter this situation at all levels of healthcare.

The Choice on Termination of Pregnancy Act 92 of 1996, as amended by Act 1 of 2008, guides the legal conditions for TOP in South Africa (see the box on this page) and came into effect from 1 February 1997. The legalisation of TOP has resulted in a reduction in maternal morbidity and mortality caused by illegal abortions. Women do sometimes still resort to these practices through ignorance of their legal rights or because of a variety of reasons.

It is of the utmost importance that contraception options are discussed with every client and that information is provided on how to delay the start of a family, the best methods of spacing children and the right time to stop having children. TOP by choice is not considered a form of contraception or population control, but it affords the pregnant woman the freedom of choice to decide if she wants an early, safe and legal TOP, according to her individual beliefs.

The role of the healthcare professional

Healthcare professionals should be able to counsel and provide pre -and post-termination care irrespective of any conscientious objection (Truter, 2011) (see the box on this page). The woman has a right to pre- and post-TOP counselling. This counselling is and should be available at all facilities that offer TOP. At state hospitals or clinics TOP is free of charge.

Registered nurses are under no obligation to perform or take an active part in TOP if they do not wish to. However, if the termination becomes life-threatening, healthcare professionals are ethically obliged to assist and deliver pre- and post-TOP care. In a non-emergency situation, healthcare professionals who do not wish to be involved in TOP are ethically obliged to refer a woman to a practitioner and facility that will help her.

Choice on Termination of Pregnancy Act 92 of 1996, as amended by Act 1 of 2008

Section 2(1a). Until 12 weeks of gestation, a medical practitioner or registered nurse, trained in the procedure, can end a pregnancy at the request of the pregnant woman.

Section 2(1b). Between 13 and 20 weeks of gestation, only a medical practitioner, after consultation with the pregnant woman, can perform the procedure. A pregnancy can only be terminated during this period if the medical practitioner is of the opinion that:

- there is a risk to the woman's mental or physical health
- there is a substantial risk that the fetus would have a severe physical or mental abnormality
- the pregnancy resulted from rape or incest
- the pregnancy would severely affect the social and economic status of the woman.

Section 2(1c). After 20 weeks of gestation, termination is allowed by a medical practitioner, after consultation with another medical practitioner or registered nurse, only if the woman's life is in danger, in case of severe malformation of the fetus or if a continued pregnancy would pose a risk of injury to the fetus.

The state promotes the provision of non-mandatory and non-directive counselling before and after termination. Spousal or partner consent is not required. Minors will not be forced to get consent from their parents, but should be advised by a medical practitioner or registered nurse to consult with their next of kin before the pregnancy is terminated.

All terminations must be recorded by the medical practitioner or registered nurse who performed the procedure. Information must remain confidential.

continued

The Director General (relevant Head of Department) must be notified of all terminations performed at health facilities within one month of the termination.

A person guilty of the following will be fined or sentenced for maximum 10 years:
- Performing a TOP contrary to the rules set out by the Act
- Preventing TOP or obstructing access to services for TOP
- Failing to notify the Director General of terminations performed at health facilities.

National trends

Table 48.2

National trends in TOP in South Africa 2011–2015 (Massyn et al, 2015: 142)

Data element	2011/12	2012/13	2013/14	2014/15
TOP	77 693	82 910	90 160	89 125

The national figures for TOP reflect an upward trend. However, it is known that there are not sufficient accredited legal service points available in the districts and professionals are obliged to refer for assistance when the need arrives. Any case of illegal abortion should be reported.

Methods used to terminate pregnancy

In the first trimester, the following options are available:
- *Medical.* During the first nine weeks (63 days) of pregnancy, oral mifepristone followed by a single dose of misoprostol is used for termination. Patients first take mifepristone to reduce the body's level of progesterone, which sustains an early pregnancy, and later take misoprostol, which makes the uterus contract and expel its contents. There is a risk of complications and death; women need to be informed of the risk and when and where to refer to if needed.
- *Surgical.* Manual or electrical vacuum aspiration is the recommended technique of surgical abortion for pregnancies of 12–14 weeks' gestation. A syringe or pump is used to remove the contents of the uterus. This does not need to be completed by dilation and curettage (D&C). There is a risk of haemorrhage and infection.

If the gestational age (GA) is more than 14 weeks, the following options are available:
- *Medical.* Mifepristone is given, followed by repeated doses of misoprostol. If mifepristone is not available, give

misoprostol alone in repeated doses. The risks and side effects should be considered and women should be well informed.
- *Surgical.* Dilatation and evacuation (D&E) is performed, using vacuum aspiration and forceps. This will mainly be done by a medical practitioner and preferably under general anaesthetic in a hospital.

The lack of medical practitioners at primary healthcare (PHC) level and/or the lack of skills hamper processes and services. However, the appointment of the district clinical specialist teams (DCSTs) in 2012 has served to strengthen health services at district level and has improved services for male and female sterilisation and TOP.

The benefits of contraception and fertility planning

According to international human right treaties (Cook, 1993), everyone has the right to decide freely and responsibly the number and spacing of their children and to have the information, education and means to exercise this right. The Constitution of the Republic of South Africa, 1996, enshrines reproductive health rights through access to reproductive health services.

There is evidence that the health and survival of children can be improved by:
- ensuring an adequate inter-pregnancy interval
- ensuring childbearing within certain age limits
- limiting the number of children in the family.

Fewer children mean that the mother can care for each baby adequately, because she has the time and the energy to do so. This prevents poor child care and the high morbidity and mortality associated with repeated pregnancies.

Benefits to the health and life expectancy of the mother

- Fertility planning ensures that the mother has the time to recover completely after delivery before falling pregnant again.
- The mother is able to continue breastfeeding as long as she wishes, with benefits for both herself and her baby.
- Maternal mortality rates are reduced.
- TOPs will be avoided.
- Teenage pregnancy rates drop.
- Health screening tests can be provided during family planning consultation.

▶ Fertility planning helps to reduce the rate of HIV-positive women falling pregnant, with the result that there are fewer infected babies and orphans.

▶ Fertility planning reduces infant mortality.

Benefits to the family

▶ Fertility planning promotes a stable and harmonious relationship within the family, as couples can enjoy their sexual relationship free from the anxiety of an unwanted pregnancy.

▶ Families can plan childbirth and childrearing for the time when they have the resources to cope with the increased responsibility.

▶ Families can limit the number of children to the number that they are able to care for adequately, including proper education, food, clothing, shelter and medical care.

▶ Children are brought up in a stable family, where mother and father can devote more time to each child.

Benefits to the community

▶ Stable families form a strong foundation for stable communities, with less family disorganisation and socially deviant behaviour such as crime, substance abuse etc.

▶ Planning prevents the population rising above the carrying capacity of the environment, thus improving food security; preventing shortages of water, housing and healthcare services; and improving job security.

▶ Environmental problems such as air pollution and illnesses caused by overcrowding are prevented.

▶ Fertility planning empowers people and enhances education, giving women the opportunity to pursue additional education and to participate in public life, including the formal employment system.

48.3 Counselling, screening and assessment

Decisions on sexual and reproductive health are made daily. Healthcare professionals are trained to counsel individuals and couples in a non-judgemental and effective way, for the best possible results for the well-being and health of the individual or couple. Taking a detailed, focused history also allows the healthcare professional to screen for problems and infections, treat conditions or refer.

Counselling

Reproductive healthcare counsellors should be comfortable with their own sexuality and have an understanding of cultural differences in this regard. They should be able to give advice to clients who have problems in their sexual relationships or should refer them to the psychologist who visits the PHC clinic. Counsellors should be aware of their own attitude, especially how their own perceptions influence their client care. Effective, open communication is important and counsellors should be aware of their non-verbal communication. It is important to respect the rights of the client, especially regarding the choice of contraceptive method. Complex problems will require referral, but information or simple advice may solve many difficulties.

All women or couples requesting contraception should be given adequate counselling to help them to make an informed and voluntary choice about the methods available and the correct way to use them. Counselling should be provided in a comfortable, private room with confidentiality ensured throughout. Counselling starts with the first contact in pregnancy and is followed up throughout pregnancy, birth and the postnatal period.

Women generally fall into the following groups:
▶ Those who know exactly what they want
▶ Those who have little idea about what is available or have problems explaining their wishes
▶ Those who, because of previous experience or advice from friends, know the method(s) they do not want to use
▶ Those with special needs due to breastfeeding, contraindications or HIV/AIDS.

Screening

All women who visit antenatal or PHC services – for whatever reason – should be screened and assisted to choose the most appropriate contraceptive method. This can be done by:
▶ establishing a rapport with the woman or couple by ensuring privacy and making her or them feel comfortable
▶ using language that is understood by both healthcare professional and the woman or couple
▶ engaging in interactive communication
▶ creating a trusting, caring relationship
▶ assisting clients to choose a contraceptive method that is appropriate to their personal circumstances and is medically safe, taking into consideration the risk of exposure to sexually transmitted infections (STIs) and HIV, and possible drug interactions with antiretrovirals (ARVs), TB medication and other medications.
▶ providing complete information on the method of choice: composition, effectiveness, advantages, disadvantages, contraindications, side effects, mechanism, how to use the method and complications.

All women should be provided with information on emergency contraception (EC) and TOP. In addition, do the following:

▶ Encourage the dual method of contraception – a combination of a condom and a non-barrier contraceptive method – to prevent HIV and STIs.
▶ Encourage self-examination of breasts. Explain the purpose and value of this procedure.
▶ Encourage cervical screening, according to policy.
▶ Encourage a healthy diet (some progesterone increases appetite).
▶ Encourage the client to keep appointments.

Assessment

The woman's needs are assessed by the following steps.

History taking

The history should include the following:

▶ *Personal history.* Name, address, age, occupation and marital status
▶ *Social history.* Habits such as smoking and alcohol intake
▶ *Contraceptive history.* Present and previous methods, complications and reasons for discontinuation of the method
▶ *Menstrual history.* Age of menarche, regularity of cycle, amount and length of bleeding
▶ *Obstetric history.* Number of pregnancies
▶ *Birth intervals.* Number, ages and health of children
▶ *Problems.* Any problems experienced during pregnancy, labour or after childbirth
▶ *TOPs.* Any miscarriages, abortions or TOPs
▶ *Gynaecological history.* Any STIs, pelvic inflammatory disease (PID), vaginal discharge, ectopic pregnancies, pain during sexual intercourse (dyspareunia)
▶ *Medical history.* History of any serious illnesses or operations, any chronic illnesses such as diabetes mellitus, hypertension, etc
▶ *Family history.* History of anyone in the family suffering from any of the chronic conditions (diabetes mellitus, hypertension, asthma, etc)
▶ *Risk assessment.* Assess risk for exposure to STIs and HIV; do this by asking questions about sexual relationships in a positive, confidential and supportive manner
▶ *Drug history.* Always take a drug history as an essential part of prescribing oral contraceptives, due to possible interactions with other substances.

The physical examination

A full physical examination should be done on all women requesting contraceptive methods. This should include the following aspects:

▶ *General attitude.* Observe how the woman walks into the consulting room.
▶ *General physical state.* Observe the woman's general physical state. Does she look sick? Does she look upset? What is her weight? What is her BP and pulse?
▶ *Pallor.* Check for signs of illness such as jaundice.
▶ *ACCOL.* Using the acronym ACCOL, look for:
  • A: anaemia
  • C: cyanosis
  • C: clubbing
  • O: oedema
  • L: lymphadenopathy.
▶ *Chest examination*
  • Check for abnormal heart sounds.
  • Check for abnormal lung sounds.
▶ *Abdominal examination.* Check for masses, distension or tenderness.
▶ *Breast examination.* Palpate for masses. Check nipple discharge and discolouration. Check the axillae for lumps or enlarged lymph nodes.
▶ *Screening.* Screen for HIV and TB. Also do breast screening.
▶ *Pelvic examination.* Check for signs of infection in the external and internal genitalia.

Special investigations

▶ Exclude pregnancy by doing a pregnancy test if in doubt.
▶ Do a cervical smear if the woman is over 30 years of age and under 30 weeks pregnant.
▶ Do all routine tests, such as HIV, TB and anaemia.

48.4 Contraceptive methods

Table 48.3 gives a summary of the types of contraception methods available. Provide information about the available contraceptive methods and dual protection. Briefly discuss each available method, the effectiveness and benefits of the method, common side effects and how to deal with them. Also recommend protection against STIs and HIV. Help the woman make an informed choice (see also Table 48.4 on page 738).

Check with your local clinic for the types of oral contraceptives prescribed in the PHC service. These will differ from those prescribed by private medical practitioners.

Table 48.3

Types of contraceptives

Types of contraceptives available for non-pregnant women	Postpartum contraceptives for breastfeeding mothers up to six months after birth
Oral contraceptives: Combined oral contraceptive (COC) Progestin-only pill (POPs or POC)	POPs/POCs can be used. COCs: Oestrogen in the combined oral tablets carry the risk of suppressing milk production and can pose a risk for thrombosis postpartum.
Progestin-only injectable: Depot medroxyprogesterone acetate (DMPA): 12-weekly NET-EN (progesterone injection): 8-weekly	Injectables can be used because they are mainly progesterone and will not interfere with breast milk production.
Subdermal implants: Implanon NXT® for three years, one rod, containing etonorgestrel Jadelle® for five years, containing levonorgestrel, a synthetic hormone	Implants can be used.
Intrauterine contraceptive devices (IUCDs): Progesterone-releasing Mirena: five years Copper-bearing intrauterine contraceptive device (CuIUCD) – Nova-T380: five years	An IUCD can be inserted up to 48 hours postpartum or after four weeks postpartum.
Voluntary surgical contraceptive method: Female sterilisation Vasectomy (male)	Women can be sterilised after birth, before discharge or at six weeks.
Barrier methods: Male condoms Female condoms	Barrier methods can be used.
Natural methods: Lactational amenorrhea method (LAM) Abstinence Fertility awareness methods (FAM)	LAM consists in exclusive breastfeeding for the first six months of the baby's life.
EC: Oral IUCD	Emergency oral contraception can be used when needed. An emergency IUCD can be inserted.

Guidelines on choosing a method

The final choice of the method must always be made by the woman, based on the following:

▶ *Suitability.* The method must be medically appropriate and suitable for the woman's social habits. It must be in accordance with the standardised clinical practice guidelines for contraceptive method provision.
▶ *Effectiveness.* The efficacy of a contraceptive method depends on a number of factors that have to be considered and thoroughly explained when giving advice (see Table 48.4 on the next page).
▶ *Access to services.* Contraceptive service delivery must be accessible geographically (within reasonable distance), financially (what the woman can afford) and functionally (the service must be available for the community to meet their needs).
▶ *Acceptability.* The method must be acceptable to the client.
▶ *Confidentiality:* Privacy and confidentiality must always be ensured during consultation.
▶ *Cultural and religious factors.* The method must be acceptable for the woman and her family in terms of religious or cultural norms.

▶ *Previous contraceptive use or current fertility.* The woman who has previously used a method successfully will generally want to continue this method, unless she is breastfeeding or has developed contraindications to the method.

▶ *Breastfeeding.* Women who wish to breastfeed have a limited number of methods available that are compatible with breastfeeding. POP/POC is the method of choice if a hormonal method is preferred.

▶ *Protocols.* Follow the standard protocols for the provision of contraception methods.

▶ *Drug interactions.* Drug interactions may reduce the effectiveness of oral contraceptives and lead to an unwanted pregnancy, or the oral contraceptive may interfere with other medication.

Table 48.4

The Pearl index for contraceptive effectiveness (adapted from Trussel, 2014)

Method	Percentage of women experiencing an unintended pregnancy within the first year of use		Percentage of women continuing use at one year
	As commonly used	**Used correctly and consistently**	
FAM	24		47
Female condom	21	5	41
Male condom	18	2	43
COC	9	0.3	67
Evra patch	9	0.3	67
NuvaRing	9	0.3	67
POP/POC During breastfeeding Not breastfeeding	9	0.3	67
Progestin injectables: Depo Provera 150 mg; Nur-Isterate 200 mg	6	0.2	56
Copper-T: CuIUCD	0.8	0.6	78
Mirena (LNg IUS)	0.2	0.2	80
Subdermal implant: Implanon NXT®	0.05	0.05	84
Female sterilisation	0.5	0.5	100
Male sterilisation	0.15	0.10	100
EC: The insertion of an IUCD within five days of unprotected intercourse or taking EC pills after unprotected intercourse substantially reduces the risk of pregnancy.			
LAM is a highly effective, *temporary* method of contraception.			

The basic information on common essential contraceptive methods is briefly explained in the rest of this section. Table 48.5 on pages 746–752 provides a comparison of the various methods, their disadvantages, side effects, contraindications and so forth.

Combined oral contraceptives

COCs contain oestrogen and cannot be used during lactation, as this suppresses breast milk and there is concern for the infant's safety.

Starting the method

Non-breastfeeding women may start COCs at three weeks postpartum, unless there is an additional risk for venous thromboembolism; if there is, they may start COCs after six weeks.

In general, the following applies for non-pregnant and non-lactating women:

▶ Start within the first five days of the onset of menses. If the cycle is normal, the treatment can start and there is safety immediately.

▶ If the treatment is started at another time in the cycle or if the woman has an irregular cycle and is reasonably sure she is not pregnant, the woman is advised to avoid sex or use condoms for the next seven days.

▶ The pill must be taken daily at more or less the same time.

Drug interactions

A wide range of drugs increase the rate of metabolism of contraceptive steroids in the liver, thereby reducing the effectiveness of the contraceptive. The effect may take several weeks to develop and to wear off. These drugs include:

▶ anti-tuberculous drugs, eg rifampicin
▶ anticonvulsants, eg phenytoin, phenobarbitone, primidone, carbamazepine
▶ hypnotics, sedatives or other central nervous system (CNS) depressants
▶ some antibiotics, eg tetracyclines
▶ some diuretics, eg spironolactone
▶ some ARVs (see Chapter 50)
▶ St John's wort.

Additional contraceptive cover is advised during treatment with broad-spectrum antibiotics and for seven days afterwards. If the client is on any other of the abovementioned drugs, the best possible hormonal method will be DMPA (three-monthly injection).

In addition, always ask a woman whether or not she is taking an oral contraceptive before prescribing therapy likely to interfere with drug action.

Efficacy

Some conditions, such as gastrointestinal (GI) disorders, diarrhoea and vomiting may decrease the efficacy of oral contraceptives, so women should be advised to use additional contraception during such an illness and for seven days after the illness is finished. If the problem arises late in the cycle, the pill-free week should be omitted and the next pack started immediately.

Missed pills

▶ The woman should take any missed hormonal pill as soon as possible. If one pill is missed by less than 48 hours, she must take it as soon as possible and complete the pack. There is little or no risk of pregnancy.

▶ If two or more pills are missed by more than 48 hours, the woman must take them as soon as she remembers. She must take the next pill at the usual time. However, advise the woman to avoid sex or use condoms for the next seven days.

▶ If two or more pills of the last seven active pills in the pack are skipped, the woman must take one pill as soon as she is aware of the mistake and then take the rest of the active pills, one per day. When the active pills are finished, she must not take the inactive pills, but start on a new pack. Advise the woman to avoid sex or use condoms for the next seven days.

▶ If any non-hormonal pills are missed, the woman must keep taking one pill a day and start on a new pack as usual.

Progestin-only oral contraceptive

The POC, or the mini-pill, (eg Microvil®) is the contraceptive of choice during breastfeeding or for those who cannot use oestrogen for some reason.

Starting the method

▶ The woman can start any time after birth and continue daily during lactation.
▶ Precautions must be taken for the first 48 hours after the first dosage.
▶ If it is started after childbirth and breastfeeding, there is immediate protection and no back-up is needed.

Efficacy

The eligibility criteria indicate that POCs are more than 99 per cent effective in preventing pregnancy if used consistently (Dhont & Verhaeghe, 2013). When the tablets are discontinued, fertility is restored.

Missed pills

These must be taken as soon as possible. Intercourse is unsafe for 48 hours, and therefore a back-up method must be used or the woman must abstain from intercourse.

Drug interactions

The contraceptive effect is reduced with enzyme-inducing drugs such as anticonvulsants, rifampicin, griseofulvin and some ARVs. An additional back-up method should be used during treatment with griseofulvin and for two days afterwards. If clients are on any other of the abovementioned drugs, the best possible hormonal method will be DMPA (three-monthly injection).

DMPA (progestin-only injectable)

Injectables are popular because they are highly effective, easy to comply with, require only periodic clinic visits and do not required the woman to keep a supply at home. Missing a dose due to forgetfulness is therefore minimised. The method is fully reversible and has no oestrogen-related side effects. There is also no risk of interfering with lactation in the postpartum woman. There is less dysmenorrhoea, endometrial cancer, uterine fibroids and symptoms of endometriosis. It is also a preferred method in HIV-positive women.

Starting the method

The treatment is started within the first seven days of the onset of menses and the woman is immediately safe. If it is given later in the cycle, she is unsafe for seven days and should use a back-up method or abstain from intercourse.

Repeat injections may be given two weeks early for NET-EN and DMPA, or two weeks late for NET-EN and four weeks late for DMPA.

Drug interaction

The contraceptive effect of NET-EN is reduced when enzyme-inducing drugs such as rifampicin is used. The woman must be warned of the effect of rifampicin, which may last up to two months after the treatment is stopped. If she is on any of these drugs, the best possible hormonal method will be DMPA (three-monthly injection).

Abstinence

Abstinence is one of the pillars of HIV prevention and is also presented to young girls as a method to prevent teenage pregnancy and early motherhood.

Sexual abstinence is when somebody refrains from sexual activity (Mandal, 2014). Abstinence from vaginal intercourse is the safest method of preventing pregnancy. The reasons could be religious, philosophical or for the prevention of pregnancy, STIs and HIV. Support for the person choosing this lifestyle is important and the choice should not be judged negatively (Mandal, 2014).

Fertility awareness methods

FAM can be used as a 'natural' contraceptive method or a method to plan a pregnancy, as no synthetic hormones or methods are involved. This means that the woman must know when she is fertile and the couple must abstain or use other methods during this period. With both Billing's ovulation method and the Sympto-thermal method, fertility is never suppressed. Clients should be referred to trained FAM teachers for intensive counselling if they are interested in these methods. (See http://www.fertaware.com/ for further information.)

Subdermal implants

The subdermal implant is a hormone-releasing, flexible plastic rod the size of a matchstick, which is implanted under the skin, usually in the woman's upper non-dominant arm (see the procedure on the following pages). The hormone (etonogestrel 68 mg) is released slowly over three years in the case of the Implanon NXT®.

This is a long-term method. The woman does not need to attend a clinic regularly and there are no oestrogen-related side effects, as the implant does not contain oestrogen. It does not suppress ovulation totally, which means that there is more endogenous oestrogen, fewer cardiovascular risks and less suppression of calcium. It does not have an effect on bone density.

It is rapidly reversible, within seven days after removal.

Risks of pregnancy

Implanon has the highest efficacy among available contraceptives. The Pearl Index was 0.38 pregnancies per 100 woment in a clinical trial of 923 women (ARHP, 2008). It has not been tested in overweight women and efficacy in this group cannot be guaranteed. It may assist in protecting against iron-deficiency anaemia and has a minimal metabolic effect, and no effect on BP.

PROCEDURE	Insertion of a subdermal contraceptive implant

The subdermal contraceptive implant Implanon NXT® (etonogestrel 68 mg) used in South Africa is inserted with a special applicator. The implant is a semi-rigid plastic rod 4 cm x 2 mm.

Contraindications
See Table 48.5 on pages 746–752.

Principles
▶ This procedure is performed only by trained professionals.
▶ Exclude allergies for antiseptics and anaesthetics.
▶ Schedule the procedure at a specific time of the woman's menstrual cycle (for example, within the first six days of a regular menstrual bleeding).
▶ Perform a pregnancy test before inserting Implanon NXT®. If the woman has had unprotected intercourse in the last three weeks, pregnancy is not excluded even if the pregnancy test is negative.

Instruments
▶ An Implanon NXT® applicator in an unopened, undamaged sterile package
▶ A dressing pack with 5 ml syringe and needles
▶ A pressure bandage
▶ Iodine or antiseptic
▶ Sterile gauze
▶ Clear adhesive dressing
▶ Local anaesthetic: 1 per cent lignocaine 5 ml.

Procedure
Implanon NXT® should be inserted at the inner side of the non-dominant arm, 8–10 cm above the medial epicondyle of the humerus, overlying the triceps muscle (see Figure 48A). The subdermal insertion therefore avoids the large blood vessels. Vital signs, weight and height are important for body mass index (BMI).

1 The woman signs consent.
2 Observe aseptic technique.
3 The healthcare professional is seated for clear vision and control of insertion of the needle.
4 Position the woman on her back.
5 Make two marks. For the first one, draw a circle with a sterile marker on the insertion site and draw the second mark 4–6 cm on a parallel line to the groove separating the biceps and the triceps. This is the guidance dot and is used to guide insertion.
6 Clean the insertion site with antiseptic solution.
7 Anaesthetise the insertion site area with 5 ml of 1 per cent lignocaine to make it pain-free.

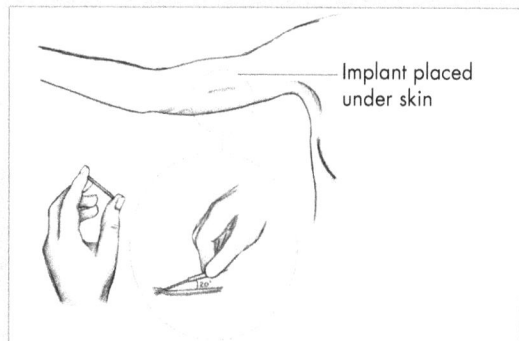

Figure 48A Insertion of a subdermal implant

8 Remove the Implanon NXT® introducer and insert it very carefully under the skin. An aseptic process is observed.
9 When the introducer is in place, unlock it, allowing the implant to be left behind under the skin.
10 Check the implant to ensure it is in place by palpating both ends. The implant should be palpable. If not, it may have failed to insert or been inserted too deep.
11 Cover the site with a small dressing.
12 Ask the woman to palpate the rod.

continued

13 Remind the woman that the implant is effective for three years and that it can be removed at any time if necessary.

14 Apply a pressure bandage. Tell the woman that this should be left in place for 24 hours to minimise bruising.

15 Remind the woman that the first seven days after implantation are unsafe and she should use a back-up method or abstain from intercourse.

16 Remove the small dressing three to five days later.

Learn more

YouTube has a worthwhile video demonstrating this procedure. Visit https://www.youtube.com/watch?v=Ir2MHzq9RYA to view this clip.

Drug interactions

There can be drug interactions with barbiturates, carbamazepine, oxcarbazepine, phenytoin, primidone, topiramate or rifampicin, St John's wort and ARVs. Backup contraception should be used if any of these drugs are prescribed, because they reduce the effectiveness of the implants (DoH, 2014).

Recording and interpretation

The woman will receive a user card to keep at home. On the user card will be the insertion date and the date the implant is to be removed. The woman must attend one follow-up visit during the first menses after implantation.

Copper-containing intrauterine contraceptive devices

The Copper T or coil is the CuIUCD most commonly available at public health facilities. There are different types of CuIUCDs, with varied efficacy. It is a long-acting, reversible contraception method and is very effective. The Copper T 380A compares with sterilisation with a failure rate of 1.9 per 100 women (Kaneshiro & Aeby, 2010).

The CuIUCD should be inserted by a qualified medical practitioner or midwife trained in the procedure. The best time for insertion is any time within the first 12 days after the start of menses. It can also be inserted at any other time during the menstrual cycle, if it is reasonably certain that the woman is not pregnant. Should the woman fall pregnant, some medical practitioners prefer that the IUCD is removed, as there is a risk of antepartum haemorrhage (APH) later in the pregnancy. It can also be inserted after birth within 48 hours or four weeks post-delivery, or at the six-week follow-up visit.

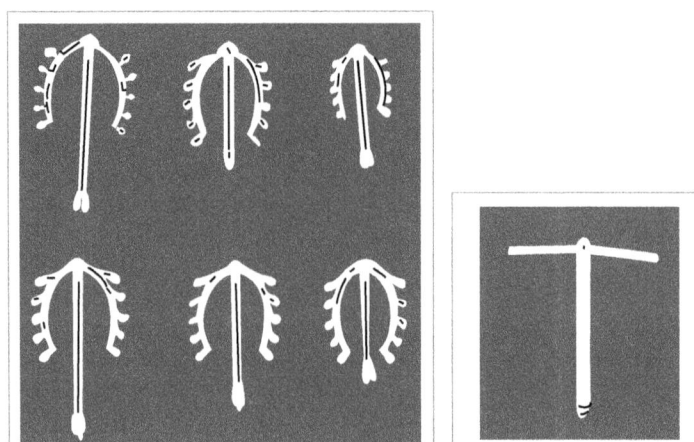

Figure 48.1 Intrauterine contraceptive devices

PROCEDURE	Insertion of an intrauterine contraceptive device

Indication
An IUCD is inserted to prevent pregnancy.

Contraindications
See Table 48.5 on pages 746–752.

Principles
▶ Insertion is done preferably during menstruation, but if pregnancy is excluded, the IUCD may be inserted at any time during the cycle.
▶ The IUCD should be inserted under aseptic conditions and sterile gloves should be used.

Equipment
▶ Speculum
▶ Tenaculum
▶ Uterine sound
▶ Scissors
▶ Forceps
▶ Light, to enable the healthcare professional to see the cervix
▶ A bowl with cotton wool
▶ A drape or cloth to cover the table and the woman's pelvic area
▶ An IUCD in an unopened, undamaged sterile package.

Procedure
IUCD insertion requires special training and practice under direct supervision. What follows is therefore only a brief explanation of the procedure:

1 Wash your hands.
2 Do a bimanual examination. Establish the position of the uterus.
3 Cleanse the vagina with an appropriate antiseptic.
4 Gently insert the speculum with the screw facing sideways (blades closed, angled downwards and backwards).
5 Rotate the speculum back 90 degrees (so that the screw is facing upwards).
6 Open the speculum blades until the optimal view of the cervix is achieved.
7 Screw the bolt to fix the blades of the speculum.
8 Check the cervix for abnormalities.
9 Clean the cervix with an appropriate antiseptic.
10 Slowly insert the tenaculum through the speculum and close it enough to gently hold the cervix and uterus steady.
11 Slowly and gently pass the uterine sound through the cervix to measure the depth and position of the uterus (the size of the uterine cavity).
12 Load the IUCD within the sterile package, observing aseptic technique.
13 Insert the IUCD using the directions for the type of IUCD.
14 Set the IUCD for the measurements taken for the uterus.
15 Slowly and gently insert the IUCD in the fundus of the uterus, without touching the speculum blades or vaginal wall.
16 When in place, pull back one centimetre and count 10 for the IUCD's arms to open.
17 Remove the inserter and cut the strings so that about 3 cm hang out of the cervix.
18 Remove the tenaculum and the speculum. Dispose of these with contaminated waste according to institutional policy.
19 Let the woman rest after the insertion. She remains on the examination table until she feels ready to get dressed.
20 Provide post-insertion information.

continued

Lactational amenorrhoea method

LAM is where breastfeeding provides natural protection against pregnancy by suppressing ovulation. A study in Italy (in 1996) by 24 specialists found that LAM is 98 per cent effective when the following three criteria have been met (Finger, 1996):
1. The woman must be amenorrhaeic from delivery.
2. Breastfeeding must be practised fully and exclusively.
3. The period includes the first six months postpartum.

Women practising LAM should change to another contraceptive method by nine months.

Advantages

LAM is effective for the first six months after birth. There are no direct costs involved and it can be used directly after birth. There is no need for supplies or procedures and it has no hormonal side effects, which is advantageous for the baby.

Disadvantages

Frequent breastfeeding is challenging and LAM does not protect against STIs and HIV. There is still a risk (20–35 per cent) of HIV passing through breast milk (see Chapter 50).

Emergency contraception

EC is a method that can be used just before or up to 120 hours after unprotected sexual intercourse to reduce the risk of pregnancy. Unprotected intercourse also includes instances of default or potential risk of pregnancy, such as in the following cases:
- The contraceptive method was used incorrectly, eg missed pills or medication interactions such as antibiotics and COCs.
- The woman defaulted on a method, eg late injections, condom slips or breaks.
- An IUCD was expelled.
- No contraceptive method was used (also in cases of rape).

Take note that EC is not the same as TOP.

Forms of emergency contraception

- *EC pills* (ECPs) can be used any time in the menstrual cycle within five days (120 hours) after the first episode of unprotected intercourse, but it is most effective when used within the first 24 hours following unprotected intercourse. The tablets are COCs (containing progesterone and oestrogen) or progesterone-only tablets. They contain hormones that prevent or delay ovulation and possibly prevent implantation of a fertilised ovum. ECPs are distinct from medical abortion methods that act after implantation; they have no effect on an already established pregnancy.
- The *progestin-only method* (levonorgestrel, or LNG) can be taken as a single (stat) dose or as two doses 12 hours apart. A Cochrane study reviewed 115 randomised controlled trials with 60 479 women for efficacy, safety and convenience of EC and concluded that LNG (2.4/100) is less effective than mifepristone (1.0/100), but more effective than the estradiol-levonorgestrel combination (2.9/100). LNG users had fewer side effects, and appeared to find it more convenient and liked having a menstrual period return before the expected date (Shen et al, 2017).
- The *COC* consists of two tablets taken 12 hours apart.

Note that the progestin-only method (LNG) is always the first choice for EC.

If the client is using enzyme-inducing drugs, the CuIUCD is the method of choice if possible. If not, the dosage is increased to LNG 3 mg stat dose or COC, 3 tablets orally, followed by 3 tablets 12 hours later.

Side effects of emergency contraception

The most common side effects reported by users of ECPs are nausea and vomiting. If a woman vomits within two hours of taking an ECP, she should take a further dose as soon as possible. Less common side effects include abdominal pain, fatigue, headache, dizziness and breast tenderness.

The side effects usually do not last for more than a few days after treatment, and they generally resolve within 24 hours.

Emergency contraception and copper-containing intrauterine contraceptive devices

CuIUCDs are usually used as a primary contraception method. However, they can be used as EC at any time of the cycle within five days (120 hours) after the first episode of unprotected intercourse, if it is certain that the client is not pregnant. This method is close to 100 per cent effective as EC. A CuIUCD may be left in place following the subsequent menstruation to provide ongoing contraception (3–10 years depending upon the type of device).

Summary and comparison of methods

Table 48.5 on the following pages gives a summary of aspects to consider in terms of contraceptives, such as the method or mechanism, the disadvantages, side effects, contraindications and usage after birth.

48.5   Conclusion

The role of the midwife in maternity care includes assessing the woman's health status, informing her about contraception, counselling her and empowering her to make appropriate choices. The education of young women to delay pregnancy also forms a part of the midwife's role. TOP care has become incorporated into the function of the midwife.

The midwife is often the primary caregiver in public healthcare facilities in South Africa; she or he should therefore have the knowledge, skill and competency to deliver effective reproductive healthcare services and care.

Table 48.5

Summary of contraceptive methods, disadvantages, side effects, contraindications and use in pregnancy and lactation

Hormonal contraceptives

Hormonal contraceptives consist of manufactured (synthetic) steroids, which are very similar to the hormones produced by the female body to control the menstrual cycle. These steroids are very effective when taken regularly every day and most can be prepared cheaply and very easily. The following methods are available: oral, injectable, intravaginal, subdermal and transdermal.

Oral contraceptives

Method	Mode of action	Disadvantages	Side effects	Contraindications	Use after birth
Low-dose COCs contain oestrogen and one of the progesterones. The only oestrogen now in common use is ethinyl oestradiol. They are very effective in preventing pregnancy when taken regularly every day and are safe for most women.	Ovulation is inhibited. The endometrium becomes unsuitable for implantation.	COCs do not protect against STIs or HIV.	*Life-threatening factors:* Altered clotting factors, raised BP. *Related to menstrual cycle:* Interferes with menstrual cycle. *Other side effects:* depression, reduction in libido in some women, headache, may worsen migraine, nausea and vomiting, weight gain, breast tenderness, skin changes, reduces the quantity of breast milk and may shorten the duration of lactation.	Undiagnosed vaginal bleeding Pregnancy Migraine Liver disease Malignancy Diabetes Smoking Age > 45 years Porphyria Do not use four weeks before and after surgery Severe depression Cardiovascular disorders	*If breastfeeding:* After the woman stops breastfeeding or when the baby is six months old *If not breastfeeding:* Three weeks postpartum, unless there is an additional risk for venous thromboembolism; if there is, the woman may start COCs after six weeks, after a pregnancy test indicates that she is not pregnant *After TOP:* Immediately after an uncomplicated first- or second-trimester TOP
POPs, or the mini-pill, are oestrogen-free oral contraceptives containing a very low dose of progesterone. *Advantages:* They are appropriate for breastfeeding women and women who experience oestrogen-related side effects.	The effect on ovulation varies, from complete suppression of ovulation to normal ovarian activity. The cervical mucus thickens, thus preventing penetration by sperm.	POPs are less effective in protecting against ectopic pregnancy. The woman must take a pill every day. The woman must get a new packet of pills monthly. It offers no protection against STIs or HIV.	*Bleeding problems:* irregular bleeding, spotting, amenorrhoea Headache Breast tenderness Weight gain Nausea and vomiting Depression	Pregnancy Undiagnosed irregular vaginal bleeding Previous ectopic pregnancy Liver disease Severe arterial disease Forgetful clients	*If breastfeeding:* Immediately after birth, if requested. Can be used at six weeks postpartum or at any later time if it is confirmed that the woman is not pregnant.

Method	Mode of action	Disadvantages	Side effects	Contraindications	Use after birth
	The endometrium becomes unreceptive to implantation of the fertilised ovum. There may be interference with ovum transportation in the Fallopian tube.				*If not breastfeeding:* Can be used immediately, although it would be most beneficial to wait until after three weeks post-delivery to reduce the possibility of bleeding disturbances. *After TOP:* Can be used immediately after first- or second-trimester TOP and later if confirmed not pregnant.

Injectable contraceptives

Method	Mode of action	Disadvantages	Side effects	Contraindications	Use after birth
Two progestin-only injectables are available: DMPA is usually given in a dose of 150 mg every 12 weeks. Norethisterone enanthate (Nur-Isterate, or NET-EN) is given every 8 weeks in a dose of 200 mg. *Advantages:* They are safe and effective methods which contain synthetic progesterone and are administered by deep IM injection.	*Inhibition of ovulation:* When the serum level of progesterone reaches a maximum at about seven days, it reduces the pituitary output of follicle-stimulating hormone (FSH) and luteinising hormone (LH). Ovulation does not occur. *Suppression of endometrium:* Inhibition of proliferation of the endometrium makes the endometrium unfavourable for implantation.	There is a delayed return to fertility. It offers no protection against STIs and HIV.	*Bleeding problems:* Irregular bleeding, spotting and amenorrhoea Lassitude Headache Nausea Breast tenderness Possible risk of postpartum depression in DMPA Loss of libido Weight gain Abdominal bloating Mood changes	Hypertension with vascular disease or severe hypertension Pregnancy Thromboplastic disease Undiagnosed abnormal uterine bleeding Secondary amenorrhoea Suspected hormone-dependent breast and genital organ malignancies Trophoblastic disease Psychiatric problems Liver disease Migraine Diabetes mellitus Porphyria	Breastfeeding mothers Suitable for older women not wanting sterilisation HIV-positive women

continued

Method	Mode of action	Disadvantages	Side effects	Contraindications	Use after birth
	Effects on cervical mucus: Alteration of cervical mucus makes sperm penetration difficult. *Alteration of tubal function:* Abolishes cyclical changes in the tubal mucosa, making it unfavourable for sperm and ovum transport and sperm nutrition. It has anti-oestrogen properties.				

Intravaginal contraceptives

Method	Mode of action	Disadvantages	Side effects	Contraindications	Use after birth
Combined contraceptive vaginal ring: A ring containing LNG (1 mg) and natural oestrogen (50 mg) is inserted by the woman herself in the upper vagina. It remains in the vagina for about three months, during which the hormone is released slowly. *Advantages:* (Same as for COCs.) The method is well accepted. Women have control over the method. It is effective.	All action is local. Ovulation is suppressed.	Some women object to examining themselves. It offers no protection against STIs and HIV. The woman must remember to start each new ring on time to prevent pregnancy.	May cause irregular uterine bleeding Headaches Vaginitis White vaginal discharge (Same as for COCs)	Same as for COCs	Breastfeeding (same as for COCs)

continued

748

Method	Mode of action	Disadvantages	Side effects	Contraindications	Use after birth
Subdermal implant contraceptives					
Progesterone implants: Implants consist of flexible tubes containing progesterone. They are placed under the skin on the inside of the woman's upper arm. The hormone is released slowly over several years (levonorgestrel in Jadelle® and etnogestrel in Implanon NXT®).	The contraceptive effect of the implant is similar to that of POPs. Like other hormonal methods, implants thicken the cervical mucus. This prevents sperm from getting into the uterus and makes fertilisation of the egg unlikely. The changes in the cervical mucus are more consistent compared with POPs.	It offers no protection against STIs and HIV. The woman cannot remove or insert the implant on her own; it must be done by a healthcare professional.	*Changes in bleeding patterns:* Lighter and less bleeding for the first several months. Irregular bleeding that lasts more than eight days, amenorrhoea Headaches Abdominal pain Acne (can improve or worsen) Weight changes Breast tenderness Dizziness Mood changes Nausea	Current blood clot in deep veins of legs or lungs Unexplained vaginal bleeding before evaluation for possible serious underlying condition Breast cancer more than five years ago which has not returned Severe liver disease, infection or tumour	No effect on breastfeeding
Transdermal contraceptives					
The combined patch releases progesterone and oestrogen. The skin patch is applied once a week for three weeks. The fourth week is patch-free. Advantages: (Same as for COCs.) The method is well accepted. Women have control over the method. It is effective.	Ovulation is stopped.	It offers no protection against STIs and HIV. The woman *must* remember to start each new patch on time to prevent pregnancy.	May cause irregular uterine bleeding Headaches Vaginitis Abdominal pain Flu symptoms (Same as for COCs)	Same as for COCs	Same as for COCs

continued

749

Method	Mode of action	Disadvantages	Side effects	Contraindications	Use after birth
IUCDs (see Figure 48.1 on page 742)					
Numerous devices (over 200) have been developed, and experimentation continues. IUCDs can be classified as inert or bioactive, the latter being either copper-containing or steroid-containing. The basic core is made of polyethylene and comes in a variety of shapes. IUCDs are now easier to insert than they used to be, are more effective and may have fewer complications, but the penalty for these changes has been an increase in cost and somewhat more frequent replacement. However, they are still more effective than non-medicated IUCDs.					
CuIUCDs *Copper T:* Each different device contains different levels of copper. Some recent innovations include a silver core to the copper wire, such as Nova T380 (used for five years) and the Cu-380A (for 10 years). Progesterone-containing IUCDs *LNG:* This releases a low dose each day. An example is Mirena® (can stay in for five years).	IUCDs with progesterone cause the cervical mucus to thicken and also interfere with the development of the decidua, thereby inhibiting implantation. IUCDs prevent implantation of the ovum and make the endometrium unreceptive for the ovum. CuIUCDs have an effect on sperm activity and motility and transport. Increased macrophage activity affects ova and sperm.	It offers no protection against STIs and HIV. A medical procedure is required for insertion. There is a risk of expulsion. The woman cannot stop using an IUCD on her own.	Menstrual changes Dysmenorrhoea Risk of perforation Risk of expulsion Death due to sepsis: very low risk Four times more likely for PID Perforated uterus Ectopic pregnancy	Postpartum: Do not insert an IUCD if the woman had ruptured membranes for 24 hours or longer, if the woman had postpartum haemorrhage (PPH) or if there is sepsis present. Undiagnosed vaginal bleeding Current PID Pelvic TB Suspected cervical or uterine carcinoma AIDS not controlled with ARVs Previous ectopic pregnancy Uterine abnormalities Pregnancy	No effect on breastfeeding
Surgical methods					
Male and female sterilisation can be performed to permanently prevent reproduction.					
Female: Female sterilisation is the most popular contraceptive method worldwide (Lawrie, Kulier & Nardin, 2016). The Fallopian tubes are cut or blocked. Sterility is immediate.	The Fallopian tubes are blocked to prevent the ovum and sperm from uniting.	It is permanent and irreversible. Therefore, women under 30 without children are advised to wait. It is 99% effective (CDC, 2017).	*Post-surgery:* No sex for one week (until the pain is gone). The woman must see a doctor in case of post-surgery complications, eg fever, bleeding, abdominal pain,	Young women who have not completed their families are advised to wait. It is a major surgical procedure that requires anaesthesia and a short hospital stay.	No effect on breastfeeding

continued

Method	Mode of action	Disadvantages	Side effects	Contraindications	Use after birth
In South Africa, the proportion of women who want to stop childbearing or are sterilised increases rapidly with the number of living children, from 24% of women with one child to 61% of women with two living children, and 88% of women with four or more children (Stats SA, 2016).		It offers no protection against STIs and HIV.	swelling and redness of the wound. Diarrhoea, fainting or extreme dizziness.		
Male: *Vasectomy* is a minor surgical procedure where the vas deferens is severed and then tied or sealed so as to prevent sperm from entering the seminal stream (ejaculate).	The vas deferens is blocked to prevent sperm being released in the ejaculate. A vasectomy is not immediately effective. Safety is determined after 20 ejaculations or three months.	It offers no protection against STIs and HIV.	*Post-surgery:* No sex for three to four days (until the pain is gone). The man must see a doctor in case of post-surgery complications, such as fever, bleeding, abdominal pain, swelling and redness of the wound. Diarrhoea, fainting or extreme dizziness	A varicocele A large hydrocele A local scar An inguinal hernia Genital tract infection Diabetes Recent coronary heart disease Filariasis	Most medical practitioners who perform vasectomies recommend one (sometimes two) post-procedural semen specimens to verify if the vasectomy was successful. The procedure can be done whenever a couple requires it.

Natural methods (non-hormonal)

There are natural contraceptive methods for women or men, but they are not very effective.

Method	Mode of action	Disadvantages	Side effects	Contraindications	Use after birth
Coitus interruptus involves withdrawal of the entire penis from the vagina before ejaculation.	Fertilisation is prevented by lack of contact between spermatozoa and the ovum.	The effectiveness of this method of natural contraception is *really* low and depends largely on the man's ability to withdraw prior to ejaculation.	None	No effect on breastfeeding	

continued

751

Method	Mode of action	Disadvantages	Side effects	Contraindications	Use after birth
Advantages: Immediate availability, no devices, no cost, no chemical involvement, and a theoretical reduced risk of transmission of STIs.		Unreliable. In typical use of this natural method of contraception, the unwanted pregnancy rate is approximately 24% during the first year of use (CDC, 2017).			
Condom (barrier methods) There are barrier methods available for use by men and women.					
Female condom: The female condom is a pouch with flexible rings at each end. *Advantages:* Protection against pregnancy, STIs and HIV; no hormonal side effects; temporary backup method; not tight and constricting like male condoms	Before intercourse, the ring inside the pouch is inserted deep into the vagina while holding the condom in the vagina. The penis is directed into the pouch through the ring at the open end, which stays outside the vaginal opening during intercourse.	Expensive Sound and visibility during use may be a problem for users Risk of pregnancy: about 21% (CDC, 2017)	None	None	Use as soon as sexual intercourse is started after birth, usually after six weeks.
Male condom: The male condom is a latex sheath that is placed over the penis. *Advantages:* Protection against pregnancy, STIs and HIV; no hormonal side effects; temporary backup method; easy to obtain, available at most shops	It prevents sperm from entering the vagina.	The possibility of breaking or slipping The possibility of defective products Risk of pregnancy: 12% failure rate (CDC, 2017)		Risk of latex allergy	If used correctly every time, it is effective protection against pregnancy, HIV and other STIs.

Section Nine

Perinatal and other infections in obstetrics

Infections in obstetrics

LEARNING OBJECTIVES
On completion of this chapter, you must be able to:
- identify and explain infections that complicate obstetrics
- differentiate between infections that are life-threatening to the fetus and newborn, and infections that are life-threatening to the mother
- explain perinatal infections
- discuss measures to prevent infections and their related complications in pregnancy, birth and the newborn period.

KNOWLEDGE ASSUMED TO BE IN PLACE
Basic knowledge of infections, their prevention and treatment, immunity and antimicrobial treatment
Policy guidelines by the national Department of Health (DoH) (as regularly updated)

KEYWORDS
perinatal infections • TORCH (toxoplasmosis, other agents, rubella, cytomegalovirus, herpes simplex) • sexually transmitted infections (STIs) • communicable diseases • puerperal infection • mastitis • chorioamnionitis • polymerase chain reaction (PCR) • C-reactive protein (CRP) • rapid plasma reagin (RPR)

49.1 Introduction

Infections and sepsis have been identified as one of the major causes of maternal mortality in pregnancy and birth in South Africa. Pregnancy can predispose women to some infections because of anatomical and physiological changes, relative anaemia, the altered pH of the vagina and masked symptoms of infection.

The infections presented in this chapter focus on the South African situation. HIV and TB are presented in Chapter 50. Infections may co-exist with HIV. (Co-infections are complicating factors and compromise maternal and infant health outcomes negatively.) Drug therapy in pregnancy is restricted due to the risks to the fetus; in co-infections, drug interactions or other HIV-related factors must be taken into account during care and management.

The focus in this chapter is on the basic information on infections and the associated health risks in obstetrics in South African health. This is discussed in terms of:
- the pathogen and the disease, with reference to viruses, bacteria, fungi or parasites
- the risks and problems associated with the condition in general and in obstetrics in particular
- the diagnosis, including clinical signs and symptoms for mother and fetus or newborn (acute or chronic status [malaria or HIV]), and the basic on-site screening or laboratory systemic tests
- comprehensive preventive strategies and treatment during all stages of care (pre-conception, ante- and perinatal, postpartum and newborn care).

This chapter presents selected infections commonly known to threaten the well-being of the mother and that are often also life-threatening to the fetus or newborn. These are:
- *perinatal infections* which, when vertically transmitted from the mother to the fetus, are known to cause severe damage to fetal development and health *in utero* and may cause abortion, intrauterine death (IUD), stillbirth or life-long disability when contracted
- *sexually transmitted infections* (STIs), which put the health and life of both mother and fetus at risk (excluding HIV, which is presented in Chapter 50)
- selected common *communicable conditions* (excluding TB, which is presented in Chapter 50) which, if contracted, complicate pregnancy or affect the fetus or newborn,

including environmental conditions from vectors such as insects (malaria) and food and water-borne diseases

▶ infections from non-pathological *colonised organisms* that can flare up (overgrow) and become pathological in pregnancy due to the relative changes in pregnancy

▶ life-threatening perinatal and postnatal *obstetric infections*, including chorioamnionitis, puerperal sepsis and mastitis.

49.2 Managing infections in obstetrics

The role of the midwife

The role of the healthcare professional and midwife is to have knowledge and skills of all clinical guidelines and policies related to infection control and care. The monitoring and evaluation of infections should adhere to quality improvement policies for improved service delivery and health outcomes. The strategies and protocols discussed in the following subsections guide roles and functions in this regard.

Policy

▶ Standard evidence-based clinical protocols for antenatal, intrapartum and postpartum care must be in place to guide clinical practice, which must be updated and maintained at all times. Essential treatment follows guidelines.

▶ Protocols for the diagnosis and treatment of infections should be known and visible in all clinics and units.

▶ Improving the nutritional status of women through health education and supplementation, as guided by policy, is a primary function of the healthcare professional.

▶ Special attention is needed for the screening of anaemia, vaginal infections and STIs, as per the current *Guidelines for Maternity Care in South Africa* (DoH, 2015a).

Practice

▶ The midwife must have knowledge of the infective conditions complicating obstetrics (all stages and levels of care) and the treatment thereof to advise and support women and care for babies during therapy.

▶ History taking and identifying risk factors are important in all the stages of childbirth (see Table 49.1).

▶ A high level of alert and constant awareness is needed in practice to identify the risk of infections to the mother and fetus or baby as well as to practise universal precautions for self-protection.

▶ Adherence to a high level of antiseptic care is required during prenatal care, labour and care of the newborn.

▶ The midwife must observe, listen, advise and support the woman and family as advocate, motivator and healthcare professional.

Immunology

Antibodies react to antigens or organisms and viruses. All immunoglobulins work together, although each has its own function. Immunoglobulins are glycoprotein molecules produced by plasma cells (white blood cells [WBCs]) for defence of the body. When a person is tested for immunoglobulin, all types are included. Antibodies belong to immunoglobulin. Different immunoglobulins have specific functions in the body:

▶ IgG is the most common antibody found in the circulation. It works effectively to coat microbes. IgG without raised IgM indicates a previous infection and is often indicative of passive immunity. IgG is the only immunoglobulin that can cross the placenta and give passive immunity to the baby. Maternal IgG can inhibit the induction of protective vaccine responses throughout the first year of life.

▶ IgM is physically the largest antibody in the circulation. It is the first antibody to respond in an infection and is very effective in killing bacteria. When elevated levels are present, it is indicative of a recent infection.

▶ IgA plays a role in the immunity of mucous membranes and is present in body fluids, tears, saliva and the digestive tract. IgA is also secreted in breast milk and gives passive immunity to the baby.

▶ IgE protects against parasites and is involved in allergic reactions.

▶ IgD signals IgM in B-lymphocytes to initiate an early immune response to infections.

In pregnancy, the woman's body lowers the immune response to prevent the body from reacting to the fetus as a foreign body. The following has been determined:

▶ IgG is small enough to go through the placenta and is transferred from the mother to the fetus and gives immunity against certain viruses.

▶ IgA and IgM cannot cross the placenta, but can be manufactured by the fetus.

▶ Elevated IgM at birth indicates that the fetus was exposed to an infection.

▶ IgA protects the respiratory tract, gastrointestinal (GI) system and eyes, and although the levels are low after birth, the levels improve within two months.

▶ IgA is present in breast milk, in particular in colostrum.

Table 49.1

Universal preventative measures and precautions for infections in pregnancy (PAHO & WHO, 2008)

Aspect/risk factor		Education on measures to be taken to prevent infections
Contact with adults	Respiratory	Practise hygienic precautions of frequent handwashing and using disinfectant hand rub in high-risk conditions, such as during flu seasons. Avoid contact with others with symptoms of communicable conditions (no kissing, handshaking or sharing of food utensils or drinking cups).
	Sexual activity	Avoid casual sexual relations and all kinds of sexual intercourse if the HIV status of the person is not known. Use condoms consistently and correctly. In the third trimester, avoid oral and other sex with herpes-infected persons.
	Blood	Do not use IV drugs. Do not share personal items such as razors and toothbrushes.
Children < 3 years of age	Flu or respiratory issues	Careful handwashing with soap and running water for 15–20 seconds; if available at home, use alcohol gel rub after the following situations have occurred or use protective gloves: ▶ during exposure to an infected child's bodily fluids and diaper changes ▶ during exposure to saliva during feeding or sharing utensils (spoons) ▶ when bathing the child in the tub ▶ when handling dirty laundry or nappies ▶ when touching the child's toys and other objects. Avoid close or intimate contact, such as kissing on the mouth or cheek or sleeping together, with an infected child. (Kiss the child on the head or give him or her a hug.)
Food and water	Handling and processing of food	*Water:* Drink only water certified for human consumption or water which has been filtered or cooked. *Meat, chicken and fish:* Avoid consumption of raw or undercooked lamb, pork, beef or poultry. Do not eat pre-cooked chicken, as it may contain bacteria. Sushi can be taken in moderation; make sure it was frozen first. Wash hands, knives and cutting boards thoroughly after handling raw meat, uncooked foods or fluids from their packages. *Ready-to-eat foods:* Check for hygienic warranties and freshness in refrigerated perishable and ready-to-eat food (eg cold meats, hotdogs, deli meat, pâté and salads). Pâtés, meat spreads and smoked seafood may only be eaten if they are canned or shelf-stable. *Dairy.* Eat only pasteurised dairy products. *Fruit and vegetables:* Peel or wash raw fruit and vegetables thoroughly to remove contaminated soil.
Environmental factors	Soil and animal litter	*Gardening:* Wear gloves when gardening or working in soil. *Cats:* Avoid handling cat litter, but if you must do it, use gloves and wash your hands immediately after. Change cat litter daily. If possible, do not feed cats uncooked meat. Cover children's sandboxes when not in use (cats like to use them as litter boxes).
	Insects	*Malaria:* If in an endemic or high-risk area, use precautions or repellent and bed nets.
Work	Crèches and healthcare professionals	If possible, avoid working with children younger than three years. Healthcare professionals must always adhere to universal precautions by protecting clothing, using goggles when handling blood, body fluids, needles or sharps.

Health system factors

The prevention and treatment of infections is not the exclusive function of the midwife. A functional multidisciplinary team and care for the mother and baby requires effective co-ordination of care and activities, and input from specialities and laboratories. An important function for the midwife is to link care between various members of the multidisciplinary team and also support women by referring effectively. This can save lives.

A functional referral system to diagnose and treat infections appropriately should be established. HIV, TB and many infections need to be referred to a medical practitioner and, in many cases, a specialist obstetrician, physician or paediatrician.

Monitoring and evaluation of the quality of care at all points of care using Quality Improvement Plans (QIP) as measures for improvement are necessary.

Perinatal infections

Perinatal infections are communicable diseases in obstetrics. Communicable diseases are infectious diseases transmitted through a variety of ways, including direct person-to-person contact, through body fluids, by breathing an airborne virus, being bitten by an insect, or environmental exposure such as contaminated food, water or contact with animals that carry the disease. There are many conditions that a pregnant woman can contract. Selected common conditions, relevant to South African healthcare, are presented in this chapter (see Table 49.2 on the following pages).

49.3 Perinatal vertical transmission of conditions damaging to the fetus (TORCH)

The specific group of perinatal infections vertically transferred from mother to fetus during pregnancy with a high risk of fetal damage or that are teratogenic are referred to by the acronym TORCH:

▶ Toxoplasmosis
▶ Other agents
▶ Rubella
▶ Cytomegalovirus (CMV)
▶ Herpes simplex virus (HSV) Type 2.

Although these are not the only infections with risk, they are known to be damaging. However, they are often asymptomatic in the pregnant woman.

The TORCH screening test is a group of blood tests. These tests check for several different infections in a newborn.

Toxoplasmosis

Pathogen

The condition is caused by a protozoa parasite called *Toxoplasma gondii*.

Risks and problems

Toxoplasmosis infection comes from cat faeces and/or the contaminated soil of cats or raw meat. The infection affects one-third of the world's population. The parasite invades and multiplies asexually in the cytoplasm of the nuclei of the host and increases the immunity in the host. Tissue cysts form. Primary infection in pregnancy can be acute or subacute. The incubation period is two weeks.

Early maternal infection (first or second trimester) has a 4–15 per cent risk of being transferred over the placenta (Palansanthiran et al, 2014). If this happens, it may result in severe congenital toxoplasmosis, leading to spontaneous abortion or IUD. Late infection (third trimester) may result in infection of the fetus in 30–75 per cent of cases and is less severe (Palansanthiran et al, 2014: 71).

Diagnosis

▶ *Maternal.* This is mainly asymptomatic.
▶ *Neonate.* In congenital toxoplasmosis, the baby has a poor prognosis. The clinical manifestation of congenital toxoplasmosis includes hydrocephaly, intracranial calcifications, chorioretinitis, strabismus, blindness, epilepsy, psychomotor or mental retardation and anaemia.
▶ *Laboratory.* Polymerase chain reaction (PCR) or serology test. Maternal antibodies peak after eight weeks of infection and remain high for months. There is a four-fold rise in IgG.

Prevention

There is no effective vaccine. Avoid handling cat litter and wash hands if it cannot be avoided. Avoid the consumption of undercooked meat. Women can check if they are protected – an IgG test pre-pregnancy indicates if a woman has antibodies against toxoplasmosis.

Treatment

▶ *Maternal.* There is no evidence that antenatal or neonatal screening and treatment affect neonatal infection rates. Women need to be aware and take preventative action in pregnancy. Treatment may not be effective.
▶ *Neonatal.* Current treatment regimens for congenital infections stretch over a year.

Table 49.2

Perinatal infections transferred from mother to infant (*in utero*, during birth and postpartum) (PAHO & WHO, 2008)

Type	Pathogen	Route	Clinical signs and symptoms	Prevention, treatment and complications				
				Pre-conception	Antenatal	Postnatal	Neonate
TORCH	*Toxoplasma gondii*	Intrauterine	Flu-like IgG	Prevent infection from cat litter or soil	Abortion or premature labour	Treat	Congenital syndrome
	Rubella virus	Intrauterine	Rash or arthritis IgG	Maternal measles, mumps and rubella (MMR) vaccine before pregnancy	Avoid contact		Congenital syndrome
	CMV	Intrauterine	Flu-like or asymptomatic	Avoid children < 3 years			Congenital CMV
	HSV 1 and 2	Perinatal and birth	Genital and oral lesions	Safe sex (eg condoms)	Acyclovir if severe C-section if active	Acyclovir if severe	Neonatal herpes
STIs	Syphilis: *Treponema pallidum*	Intrauterine Perinatal	Genital ulcer Asymptomatic or rash-like illness Routine rapid plasma reagin (RPR) syphilis serology at < 20 weeks, repeat at 32–34 weeks	Safe sex Penicillin G: 2.4 million units to be given in 3 dosages over 3 weeks	RPR/venereal disease research laboratory (VDRL) Treat 4 weeks before delivery	Penicillin G	Test for virus in cases where the mother is positive Identify Congenital syphilis syndrome present
	HIV (see Chapter 50)	All stages of pregnancy	Flu-like symptoms HIV antibodies	Safe sex (eg using condoms); no IV drugs; voluntary counselling and testing (VCT) for HIV; antiretrovirals (ARVs)	Test and ARVs Deliver the baby following guidelines	Continue with ARVs Infant feeding to be decided as per the case	Infant: PCR and test at 18 months
	Neisseria gonorrhoeae	Perinatal	Cervicitis, vaginal discharge or culture	Safe sex (eg condoms)	Penicillin	Penicillin	Opthalmia or blindness if not treated

continued

Type	Pathogen	Route	Clinical signs and symptoms	Prevention, treatment and complications			
				Pre-conception	Antenatal	Postnatal	Neonate
Common communicable diseases	Hepatitis B	All stages	Test HBsAg: surface antigen of the hepatitis B virus (HBV) indicating current infection	Vaccinate if at risk	Treat if acute	Treat mother	Test if born to positive mothers
	Chickenpox: Varicella zoster virus (VZV)	Intrauterine Perinatal	Maternal symptoms and rash	Varicella vaccination pre-pregnancy or postpartum is an option for sero-negative women	Avoid contact IgG if in contact Acyclovir if severe Caesarean section if active	Immunoglobulin Acyclovir if recently infected Isolate mother and baby	Congenital varicella syndrome Neonatal varicella
	Parvo virus	Intrauterine	Flu-like symptoms is common; can also affect the joints (arthritis)	Nil	Fetal blood transfusion	Blood transfusion	Hydrops fetalis
	Malaria: Plasmodium falciparum (There are many types.)	Intrauterine	Fever, headache, impaired consciousness, convulsions Microscopic blood smears needed for diagnosis	Bed-nets Antimalarials	Admit Artemether-lumefantrine Quinine		Miscarriage, stillbirth or preterm labour Congenital malaria (very rare)
	Listeria monocytogenes	Intrauterine Perinatal	Diarrhoea and fever	Avoid unpasteurised dairy	Penicillin	Penicillin	Sepsis
Common infections	Escherichia coli: asymptomatic urinary tract infection (UTI)	Vagina and bladder	Urine culture	Urine culture	Antibiotics	Antibiotics	Neonatal sepsis
	Group B Streptococci (GBS)	From vagina	Vaginal and rectal swabs for cases at risk	Rectal and vaginal culture	Treat in labour or 4 hours before birth		Neonatal sepsis
	Gardnerella vaginalis: bacterial vaginosis (BV)	From vagina and cervix	Screen for infectious conditions and vaginal pH	Safe sex	Treat vaginal discharge in pregnancy Antibiotics		Neonatal sepsis (uncommon)

Rubella (German measles)

Pathogen

The rubella virus was isolated in the USA in 1961 and was the first virus identified to be a teratogen.

Risks and problems

Rubella is endemic in South Africa and immunity is life-long after being infected. The incidence of congenital rubella in South Africa is not known, but was estimated at 660 cases annually in 2012 (Boshoff & Tooke, 2012).

Rubella is spread by droplet infection. If a woman contracts the condition before 18 weeks of pregnancy, it poses a serious risk to the developing fetus. Viremia occurs five to seven days after the contact period, during which the virus may be transmitted from the mother to the fetus transplacentally.

Malformations occur due to the invasion of fetal cells by the virus at rapid organogenesis. Those organs forming at the time of infection are the most affected. The risk of congenital infection and defects is highest during the first 12 weeks of gestation and decreases after the 12th week, with defects rare after the 20th week (McLean et al, 2014).

Common congenital defects of congenital rubella syndrome (CRS) include:
▶ cataracts
▶ congenital heart disease
▶ hearing impairment
▶ developmental delay.

Congenital rubella infection usually presents with more than one sign or symptom. However, a single defect may present, most commonly hearing impairment.

Diagnosis

▶ *Maternal.* The woman may experience a low-grade fever for one to five days, malaise and mild conjunctivitis. Swollen, tender lymph nodes, usually in the back of the neck and behind the ears, and a rash occur by day 5–10. The rash is maculopapular and usually starts on the face and then spreads down the body, which lasts about three days and is occasionally itchy. In 70 per cent of adults, painful joints or arthritis may develop (McLean et al, 2014). A serological test for IgG and IgM is done. The titres will indicate the risk to the fetus for damage. The medical practitioner and parents will make a decision regarding a possible abortion if severe damage is indicated.
▶ *Neonate.* CRS may present in the neonate, with a range of problems depending on the stage of pregnancy when the condition was contracted.

▶ *Laboratory.* Pregnant women with a rubella-like illness or exposed to a person with rubella-like illness should be tested for both IgG and IgM. Recent infection may be confirmed by either rising IgG antibody titre or rubella-specific IgM. If the initial rubella-specific IgM is negative and a rash develops, a repeat serology is needed.

Prevention

Vaccination has been available since 1969. A single dose of vaccine is part of the immunisation programme (MMR) and is 95 per cent effective life-long (CDC, 2016). All young women should be vaccinated. Women of childbearing age should be tested for immunity before they fall pregnant. Should a pregnant woman be exposed to rubella, a medical doctor is consulted. Rubella antibody testing is not offered routinely in South Africa in the public sector during antenatal care.

Treatment

Rubella vaccination is contraindicated in pregnancy. Women who remain sero-negative should receive vaccination after giving birth. There are no contraindications during breastfeeding.

If exposed to rubella in pregnancy, a woman should seek medical care.

Cytomegalic inclusion disease or mononucleosis

Pathogen

CMV is part of the herpes group. It infects cells and causes them to enlarge.

Risk and problems

The prevalence of CMV infections ranges between 60 per cent in developed countries to 70–100 per cent in developing countries (Gardella, 2008). CMV spreads through human contact, by the infected person's saliva, blood, urine, semen, cervical/vaginal secretions or breast milk. CMV survives on fomites, including diapers, toys and on the hands. There is a high risk of infection in daycare centres. In urban settings, up to 78 per cent of children will acquire the infection in daycare centres through saliva and urine contact (Boppana & Fowler, 2007). Children will shed the virus for up to 42 months in their saliva and urine after being infected and can infect the mother when pregnant again.

Most CMV-infected people have not been clinically diagnosed or treated. CMV primary infections happen in 1–5 per cent of pregnancies, with a 40 per cent risk of transferring the infection (Boppana & Fowler, 2007). CMV-seropositive mothers in reactivation of a previous infection have less than 1 per cent risk of transferring it to the fetus (Manicklai et al, 2013). During pregnancy, the virus can be transferred across the placenta. It can be transferred at birth or via the breast milk, saliva or blood transfusions. CMV is the most common congenital viral infection; it may affect up to 1 per cent of all live births (Carlson, Norwitz & Stiller, 2010).

Most CMV-infected newborns appear normal. Of these, 10–20 per cent will be symptomatic at birth, of which 8–15 per cent will later develop complications, principally hearing loss (Carlson, Norwitz & Stiller, 2010).

CMV is the most common cause of congenital infection and non-hereditary deafness. Other central nervous system (CNS) sequelae include mental retardation, cerebral palsy, seizures, or chorioretinitis.

Diagnosis

▶ *Maternal.* A primary CMV infection may be asymptomatic, subclinical or atypical (symptoms of mild hepatitis and lymphocytosis). The virus then becomes latent, but is reactivated periodically without clinical signs or symptoms. Seropositive individuals can also be re-infected with different strains of CMV. It is therefore a condition that is often not clinically diagnosed until fertility or perinatal mortality and morbidity presents.

▶ *Neonate.* Symptoms of infection are similar to other conditions, but neonates that present with hepatosplenomegaly and severe thrombocytopaenia are most likely CMV-infected (Diar & Velaphi, 2014). The neonate may appear normal, or have mild to severe disseminated life-threatening disease, intrauterine growth restriction (IUGR), pneumonia, jaundice, encephalitis and hydrops. CMV sequelae such as mental retardation, cerebral palsy, seizures, visual defects and sensory-neural hearing loss may follow.

▶ *Laboratory blood test.* Maternal viral load testing can be done. If an amniocentesis after 22 weeks is positive for CMV DNA C-reactive protein (CRP) in the amniotic fluid, it is indicative of fetal infection. However, this is rarely done. PCR detection of the CMV DNA in urine or saliva of the neonate within three weeks is a reliable indication that the neonate has congenital CMV infection. CRP and serology antibodies can also be done.

Prevention

CMV is the single most important cause of birth defects and developmental disabilities that needs to be addressed for improved outcomes in children. Education and awareness is important, especially in crèches and daycare centres.

Treatment

▶ *Maternal.* If an acute infection is diagnosed and proven in the mother, antiviral therapy can be given orally or intravenously as per regimen. CMV hyper-immunoglobulin may prevent transfer from mother to fetus.

▶ *Neonate.* If confirmed, the neonate should receive the same antiviral therapy as the mother.

Genital herpes simplex virus

Pathogen

The majority of genital herpes infections are caused by HSV-2. It is a sexually acquired condition.

Risks and problems

A viral genital herpes infection (HSV 1 and 2) is a very demoralising condition that cannot be cured. Both clinical and subclinical reactivations can occur for many years, with HSV-2-infected persons shedding the virus intermittently in the genital tract during asymptomatic periods. The virus remains dormant in nerves to be reactivated later in life or under conditions of stress, pregnancy or lower immune responses.

The risks are as follows:

▶ *First trimester.* An acute HSV-2 infection in the first trimester is associated with an increased risk of early miscarriage, but the chance transplacental infection to the fetus is less than 1 per cent (Straface et al, 2012).

▶ *Late third trimester acute infection.* The risk for transmission to the neonate from an infected mother is high (30–50 per cent) in acute or reactivated infections among women near the time of delivery (Straface et al, 2012).

Diagnosis

▶ *Mother.* HSV-2 infections are mostly asymptomatic, with painful vesico-ulcerative lesions. When symptomatic, this is referred to as a 'breakout'. This is painful and takes weeks to heal.

▶ *Neonate.* Among mothers of infants who acquire neonatal herpes, the majority lack a history of clinical genital infection. The vast majority of neonatal herpes cases occur as a result of contact with HSV in the maternal birth canal during delivery. Although rare, neonatal HSV infection may lead to severe disseminated neonatal HSV syndrome and/or encephalitis.

▶ *Laboratory.* Genital herpes screening can be done through blood antibody (IgG and IgM) serology, but can give false positives. A culture of a blister is the preferred testing method.

Prevention

Women should inform their caretakers in pregnancy about their herpes status (if known) to prevent the infection being transferred to the baby. If the genital herpes infection is active, a Caesarean section is indicated to prevent the baby being infected in the birth canal.

In active genital herpes infection and premature rupture of membranes (PROM), a Caesarean section needs to be performed within four hours.

Treatment

▶ *Maternal.* There are no best practice guidelines. Suppressive antiviral therapy is advised from 36 weeks for women with reoccurring lesions.
▶ *Neonate.* Swabs are collected from the eye, throat, umbilicus and rectum for HSV 1 & 2 PCR. Urine is collected. Lumbar puncture can be done. IV antiviral therapy may be needed.

49.4 Sexually transmitted conditions

Sexual transmitted conditions are those conditions that are mainly contracted through sexual contact. They may pose a health threat for the mother and the unborn fetus and may lead to life-long disability.

During the clinical assessment, it is important to take a good sexual history and undertake a thorough anogenital examination for diagnosis. The history should include questions concerning:
▶ symptoms
▶ recent sexual history
▶ sexual orientation
▶ type of sexual activity (eg oral, vaginal and anal sex)
▶ the possibility of pregnancy
▶ the use of contraceptives, including condoms
▶ recent antibiotic history
▶ any drug allergies.

The most common infections are briefly discussed below. However, it must be kept in mind that national guidelines change on a regular basis.

Syphilis

Pathogen

Syphilis is a chronic condition caused by a bacterium called *Treponema pallidum* (a corkscrew-shaped spirochaete), contracted primarily through vaginal, anal or oral sexual intercourse. It is also vertically transmitted from mother to infant in pregnancy.

Risks and problems

In 2007, the WHO estimated that there were 2 million syphilis infections among pregnant women annually. Of these, 65 per cent led to adverse pregnancy outcomes, fetal death, stillbirth, neonatal death or the birth of an infected baby (Newman et al, 2013). Babies born with syphilis often have a low birth weight (LBW). They may develop problems such as blindness, deafness and seizures if the infection is not treated.

In 2007, the WHO launched a programme for the global elimination of congenital syphilis by 2015. The goal was to test 90 per cent of pregnant women for syphilis and treat 90 per cent of sero-positive women adequately (Newman et al, 2013).

Treatment may be inadequate because of patient factors, including late booking, the first visit only taking place at birth or failure to complete treatment. Staff issues such as inadequate staff training, suboptimal records and inadequate client counselling, as well as system issues, including laboratory result delays and stock shortages, may also hamper treatment efforts.

Vertical transmission can occur at any stage of pregnancy if untreated.

Transplacental transmission can occur as early as six weeks in utero. The transmission risk depends on the stage of the disease and the stage of pregnancy. The risk is almost 100 per cent if the woman has a primary infection. The probability of transmission to the fetus up to four years after acquiring the disease is 70 per cent if untreated (Berman, 2004).

Intense inflammatory responses and prostaglandins induced by fetal infection may be responsible for fetal death or preterm delivery and severe growth retardation. The placenta is severely affected and a large and oedematous placenta with chronic villitis and acute chorioamnionitis develops.

On 22 February 1991, in Regulation 328, congenital syphilis became a notifiable medical condition in South Africa.

Diagnosis

This is based on clinical symptoms and blood tests.

Maternal clinical signs include the following:
▶ *Primary infection.* The signs are often missed because the infection is asymptomatic. The first clinical manifestation of syphilis is not noted, because it is a single, local, painless red sore (chancre) in the vagina, cervix or oropharynx, appearing two to six weeks after infection. There are also enlarged local lymph nodes (swollen glands) on the area affected. This highly infective stage heals by four to six weeks.

▶ *Secondary syphilis.* If untreated, a typical skin rash appears on the body, including the palms of the hands and feet. The rash is not itchy or painful. Hypertrophic papular growths (condyloma lata) may develop around the vagina and anus. These can be confused with the condyloma acuminata caused by papillomavirus infection. Other symptoms include generalised lymphadenopathy, malaise, fever, splenomegaly, joint pain, sore throat and headache. The symptoms may disappear spontaneously and if untreated the infection remains latent for years.

▶ *Latent syphilis.* If untreated, an infected person will progress to the latent (hidden) stage of syphilis. After the rash of the secondary stage goes away, the person will not have any symptoms for a time (latent period). The latent period may be as brief as one year or range from five to 20 years.

▶ *Tertiary syphilis.* The infection of the brain, nerves, eyes, large blood vessels, heart, skin, joints and bones persists throughout life. If left untreated, the disease affects the brain and neurological systems, which is called neurosyphilis. HIV-infected people are at increased risk.

Neonates may be asymptomatic even if the mother tests RPR positive, she delivers within four weeks after starting treatment or she has not completed her three doses of treatment.

Vertical transmission can occur at any time and stage of syphilis. The risk of transmission correlates with the extent of spirochaetes present in the blood circulation. Thus, primary and secondary syphilis carry a higher risk of transmission than latent and tertiary syphilis. Most pregnant women have latent syphilis (asymptomatic but antibody-positive).

All neonates of syphilis-positive mothers must be examined at birth for signs of congenital syphilis. These include a characteristic rash, purpura, pallor, anaemia, jaundice, nasal muco-purulent discharge (which is highly infectious), enlarged liver and spleen, IUGR or LBW and respiratory distress.

In untreated, the symptoms of congenital syphilis may only present in later childhood. Early signs and symptoms that may indicate congenital syphilis include poor feeding; snuffles (syphilitic rhinitis); chronic saddle nose; failure to thrive; pneumonia; rash on the palms of the hands, feet and anus; bullous skin and a copper-coloured rash.

Laboratory screening includes the following

▶ *Maternal.* The RPR test, which detects syphilis antibodies, is routinely done on all pregnant women in all stages of care when encountered for the first time. Some conditions may give false positive results, such as malaria and tuberculosis, as may some drugs. The RPR test is similar to the VDRL serology laboratory test. If the RPR test for the virus is positive, it may be followed up with a more specific laboratory test for syphilis titres.

▶ *Newborn.* Testing is problematic and all newborns of positive mothers are referred for medical care.

Prevention

The screening of women during pregnancy is essential to eradicate congenital syphilis. At the first visit, all pregnant women have a full history taken as well as a physical examination done according to the current *Guidelines for Maternity Care in South Africa* (DoH, 2015a). This includes routine blood test screening for syphilis serology, which is recorded. Appropriate treatment is started where necessary.

If the test is negative, it is repeated at 32 weeks. If the test is positive, the titre is determined and the appropriate flowchart is used for management – see the management guidelines for sexually transmitted infections (DoH, 2015b).

In addition, all women are educated on the risk of vertical transmission treatment and compliance. Couple counselling is promoted, if applicable, as well as consistent condom use, particularly during pregnancy. Condoms are provided and usage is demonstrated. The importance of partner treatment is stressed.

Issue one notification slip for each sexual partner. HIV counselling and testing is also done.

Treatment

▶ *Maternal.* If a woman is syphilis RPR-positive, treatment is commenced. The appropriate flowchart for treatment is followed. If she is HIV positive as well, the guidelines for treatment are as follows (DoH, 2015b): Benzathine benzylpenicillin IMI 2.4 MU once weekly for three weeks. Dissolve benzathine benzylpenicillin IM, 2.4 MU in 6 ml lignocaine 1 per cent without epinephrine (adrenaline). If penicillin-allergic, refer for penicillin desensitisation.

▶ *Asymptomatic newborns.* Newborns may be asymptomatic. All exposed babies are treated with benzathine benzylpenicillin (depot formulation), 50 000 units/kg IM as a single dose into the lateral thigh (*never to be given IV*) in cases where:
  • the mother has a positive syphilis result and was not treated
  • the mother received less than three doses of benzathine benzylpenicillin
  • the mother delivered within four weeks of commencing treatment.

▶ *Symptomatic newborns.* All newborns that are symptomatic are referred for medical care. The baby is followed up at three months after the last injection to confirm a fourfold (ie 2 dilution) reduction in RPR titres, provided the initial titre was greater than 1.8. If the initial titre was less than 1.8, further reduction may not occur.

Hepatitis B virus

Pathogen

HBV is a deoxyribonucleic acid (DNA) virus that is transmitted by percutaneous or mucosal exposure to blood or body fluids (vaginal secretions, semen, saliva, sweat, urine, faeces and menstrual blood). It is a life-long chronic condition.

Risks and problems

Globally, approximately 70 per cent of persons with chronic HBV infection are believed to have acquired the infection as a result of perinatal or early childhood transmission (Alexander & Kowdley, 2006).

In pregnancy, the risk of HBV vertical transmission is high without prophylaxis. The HBV is readily transmitted to the infant in 10–40 per cent of infants born to infected mothers (Gentile & Borgia, 2014).

Infection in the first trimester can cause fetal anomalies, fetal and/or neonatal hepatitis, premature labour or IUD. Children who are not infected at birth are at risk for infection from the mother after birth. The majority of infants who become positive after maternal exposure are clinically healthy, show no signs of acute clinical hepatitis and remain HBsAg positive for an extended period. A low percentage will have liver function changes.

Chronic hepatitis (leading to hepatic carcinoma) occurs in 85 per cent of infants who acquire chronic HBV infection *in utero* (Eke et al, 2017), in 90 per cent of babies who acquire it during the first year of life and in 5–10 per cent of children six years and older (Gentile & Borgia, 2014).

Fulminating disease of the newborn, leading to death after birth, is more common in mothers who are chronic HBV carriers.

Diagnosis

▶ *Maternal.* Maternal manifestations may be more severe and prolonged when the primary or acute disease occurs in advanced pregnancy. Signs and symptoms include a low-grade fever, flu-like symptoms with general malaise and fatigue, marked anorexia, abdominal pain due to an enlarged liver, nausea, vomiting, jaundice and dark urine or pale stools. The onset is abrupt and of short duration, with the early appearance of antibodies.

▶ *Newborn.* Most babies born to HBV-positive mothers are asymptomatic but develop subclinical elevated transaminases. Some develop acute hepatitis, jaundice, lethargy, failure to thrive, abdominal distension and clay-coloured stools. In severe cases, symptoms include hepatomegaly, ascites and hyperbilirubinaemia and the condition could be fatal.

▶ *Laboratory.* A diagnosis of acute or chronic HBV infection requires serologic testing. HBsAg is present in both acute and chronic infection. All HBsAg-positive persons should be considered infectious.

Prevention

▶ *Primary.* The primary strategy to prevent HBV infection is universal vaccination of infants, beginning at birth, with subsequent hepatitis B vaccine doses integrated into the routine childhood immunisation schedule.

▶ *Before and during pregnancy.* Women should be educated on avoiding high-risk behaviour (eg unprotected intercourse with multiple partners, or the use of unclean injection needles). Pregnant women who are identified as current injection-drug users, or having had an HBsAg-positive sex partner, should be vaccinated. All pregnant women should be tested for HBsAg if laboratory services are available. If the HBsAg test result is positive, appropriate treatment should be given to the baby at birth.

▶ *Perinatal.* A paediatrician should be present at the birth. Passive–active post-exposure (postpartum) prophylaxis (PEP) with hepatitis B vaccine and hepatitis B immunoglobulin (HBIG) administered 12–24 hours after birth, followed by completion of a three-dose vaccine series, has been demonstrated to be over 70 per cent effective in acute and chronic infections in the newborn (DoH, 2015b).

Treatment

▶ *Maternal.* There is no specific therapy available for persons with acute HBV. Treatment of chronic HBV with antiviral drugs can achieve sustained suppression of HBV replication and remission of liver disease in some people.

▶ *Newborn.* The serological markers for the different stages of the disease are complex and treatment is dependent on these markers. Treatment for the newborn should be given within 12–24 hours. In mothers with an HBsAg-positive test result, the baby should receive treatment in the first 12 hours with the recommended dose of HBIG (0.5 ml), which is able to decrease infection rates from over 90 per cent to less than 25 per cent (CDC, 2017a; Nguyet-Cam, Gotsch & Langan, 2010).

Vaccination for healthcare professionals

The hepatitis B vaccine 1.0 ml IMI is the vaccination for health workers. The dose is repeated at one and six months. No boosters are necessary after the initial series of successful vaccinations. About 10 per cent of vaccinated persons do not obtain sufficient immunity (CDC, 2017b). If the risk of exposure to the virus is high and long-lasting (eg healthcare professionals with ongoing exposures to blood), the presence of immunity should be confirmed serologically about two months after the third dose.

Human papilloma virus

Pathogen

The human papilloma virus (HPV) is mainly sexually acquired.

There are 150 types of papilloma viruses. Some are mucosal (infecting cells of the moist surfaces in cavities in the body) and some are cutaneous (causing general warts of the skin, hands and feet). Some types are more common and some have a high risk for carcinoma. (Table 49.3 gives a summary of the mucosal conditions and risks associated with sexual transmission.)

There are 40 types that affect the genital area. Each is given a number to indicate its type.

Risks and problems

The infection is mainly asymptomatic and transferred during oral or vaginal sexual contact. The virus may remain in the system and become dormant but manifest as genital warts or (many years later) as cervical or vulval cancer. The type of HPV that causes warts is not the same as the type that causes cancer. When the immune system is weakened, as in HIV, the immune system cannot fight off HPV.

HPV does not have a direct effect on the fetus *in utero*.

Diagnosis

- *Maternal clinical.* Asymptomatic until a woman develops warts or cancer.
- *Newborn.* Asymptomatic.
- *Laboratory testing.* A Pap smear or a swab can be done to detect the cell changes of the cervix to identify precancerous lesions. A swab of the cervix can detect the DNA of the cancer-causing virus (HPV subtypes 16, 18 and others).

Prevention

The groups at risk for cervical cancer include those engaging in sexual intercourse before 26 years of age and those engaging in unsafe sexual practices with many sexual partners.

It is recommended that young women of 11–12 years receive two doses of the HBV vaccine at least six months apart. Teens and young people (15–26 years) will need three dosages.

According to South African guidelines, women aged 30 years and older should have at least three Pap smears, with intervals of 10 years. The rules for HIV-positive women are different (see Chapter 50).

Treatment

The treatment of warts is mainly by surgery or diathermy. Local application of imiquimod or podophyllin may be preferred. Warts are generally not treated during pregnancy. If cervical cancer develops, treatment is given as per oncology protocols.

Table 49.3

Common mucosal HP viruses and the risk in sexual health (adapted from Braaten & Laufer, 2008)

Genotypes: mucosal	Sexual health risk	Clinical manifestation
Most common types: 6 and 11	Low risk	General warts (no cancer) Condylomata acuminata Respiratory and laryngeal papillomata
40, 42, 43, 44, 54, 61, 70, 72, 81 and CP6108	Low risk	Condylomata acuminata
23, 53 and 66	Moderate risks	Pre-cancerous lesions
Most common types: 16 and 18	High risk	Low-grade abnormalities Cause 70% of cervical cancers
31, 33, 35, 39, 45, 51 ,52, 56, 58, 59, 68, 73 and 82	High risk	Pre-cancerous abnormalities Cancerous

Vaginal discharge syndrome

All women complaining of abnormal vaginal discharge, itching or burning should be examined, diagnosed and treated in pregnancy. Vaginal discharge syndrome (VDS) refers to vaginal infections, symptoms and lower abdominal pain (LAP) presenting in sexually active adults.

Vaginal infections may also be due to changes in the vaginal pH and are referred to as BV, discussed later in this chapter.

The diagnosis of a vaginal infection requires a history from the woman. An experienced clinician can examine the woman and make a diagnosis that may need to be confirmed by a laboratory test. This chapter refers to these conditions, as they may complicate pregnancy. Table 49.4 lists various conditions – chlamydia, gonococcal infection and trichomoniasis – and discusses their risks, diagnosis and treatment.

Table 49.4

Vaginal discharge syndrome

Chlamydia	
Pathogen	*Chlamydia trachomatis* is a bacterium that can live and reproduce inside human cells without actually damaging them. It can cause prolonged infection with minimal or no symptoms. Ninety per cent of infected men and about 80% of infected women have no symptoms (Kaneel, 2007: 243).
Risks and problems	Chlamydia is sexually acquired in adults and is asymptomatic in most adults. Chlamydia may cause those infected to be more susceptible to a number of other STIs. Chlamydia ophthalmia neonatorum conjunctivitis is recognised in babies born of infected mothers one to two weeks after birth. Pneumonitis may develop in 5–30% of newborns of one to three months of age (Mishra et al, 2011).
Diagnosis	*Maternal.* In pregnant women, a yellow muco-purulent discharge with a swollen inflamed cervix with erosion is noted. Other symptoms may include dysuria or swelling of the Bartholin's gland. Inguinal lymphadenopathy is uncommon. If left untreated, chlamydial infection in the non-pregnant woman can spread from the uterus to the Fallopian tubes, scarring them, causing severe LAP, ectopic pregnancy and sterility. It is a major cause of pelvic inflammatory disease (PID). However, many women can be carriers and asymptomatic. *Newborn.* Conjunctivitis 5–12 days after birth. *Laboratory:* *Maternal.* A urine or vaginal swab specimen is taken for culture. *Newborn.* Eye swab for *Chlamydia* and *Neisseria gonorrhoeae*.
Prevention	*Maternal.* Practise safe sex with a known and tested partner or use a condom when not sure. *Newborn.* Ocular antibiotic ointments or drops can be used prophylactically to prevent congenital Chlamydia ophthalmia neonatorum, but they do not prevent perinatal pneumonitis caused by *C trachomatis*.
Treatment	*Maternal.* Both sexual partners and the baby need to be treated when diagnosed. The treatment is Azithromycin 1 g orally in a single dose or Doxycycline 100 mg orally twice a day for 7 days (CDC, 2015). *Newborn.* Erythromycin opthalmic ointment.
Gonococcal infection	
Pathogen	*Neisseria gonorrhoeae* is a bacterium found only in humans and is acquired through sexual intercourse.
Risks and problems	In South Africa, a study by Mhlongo et al (2010) indicated that gonorrhoea and BV were confirmed as the most frequent causes of male urethral discharge syndrome (MUDS) and VDS. The infection rate is higher in males than females. It is an asymptomatic condition and is a major cause of chronic cervicitis in women in spite of repeated antibiotic treatments. If a baby is infected when moving through the birth canal, it can lead to infection in the newborn, including ophthalmia neonatorum. If it results in the perforation of the globe of the eye, it may lead to blindness, sepsis, arthritis and meningitis.

continued

Diagnosis	*Maternal clinical.* A purulent, offensive, profuse, greenish and watery discharge is noted, or persistent cervical bleeding. The discharge comes from the cervix, and there is no vaginal infection, as the organism cannot invade the squamous epithelium. The patient complains of LAP and backache, which comes from the cervix. Other symptoms may include frequency of urination and dysuria caused by gonococcal urethritis. Bartholinitis may occur, leading to abscess formation. *Newborn.* Severe conjunctival purulent secretions occur two to five days after birth. Palpebral oedema may present. *Laboratory:* *Maternal.* A urine sample or a microscopic examination of a specimen from the cervix or vagina. *Newborn.* A positive eye swab.
Prevention	*Maternal.* Women must engage only in safe sexual practices with a partner who is not infected, or use a condom if unsure. *Newborn.* The antenatal diagnosis and treatment of gonococcal and chlamydial infections in pregnant women is the best method for preventing neonatal gonococcal disease.
Treatment	*Maternal.* The condition is cured with the correct treatment within two weeks, which is ceftriaxone 250 mg IMI as a single dose. The partner must also be treated. *Newborn.* Ceftriaxone 25–50 mg/kg IV or IM in a single dose, not to exceed 125 mg. Infants who have gonococcal ophthalmia should be hospitalised and evaluated for signs of disseminated infection (eg sepsis, arthritis and meningitis).

Trichomoniasis

Pathogen	*Trichomonas vaginalis* is a unicellular, anaerobic, oval or pear-shaped four-flagellate protozoan (parasite) with an undulating lateral membrane. It is a sexually transmitted condition.
Risks and problems	*T vaginalis* is likely the most common non-viral STI worldwide. In 2005 it was estimated that 284 million people, of which 180 million are women, worldwide were infected with Trichomoniasis, 90% of them in developing countries (Kissinger, 2016). Risk factors include increased age, concomitant STIs, incarceration, IV drug use, commercial sex work, BV and smoking cigarettes. Infections are asymptomatic in 80% of cases and often goes undetected (Kissinger, 2016). *Trichomonas* infection is associated with a two- or three-fold increased risk for HIV infection. Repeat infections are common, ranging from 5 to 31% (Kissinger, 2016). The infection is often asymptomatic and may therefore remain untreated for years. In pregnancy, trichomoniasis infection is associated with adverse pregnancy outcomes, such as PROM, preterm labour and LBW babies.
Diagnosis	*Signs and symptoms.* In women, the condition manifests in vaginal discharge that can vary greatly, from a mild, watery discharge to a profuse, white, greenish-yellow, frothy and offensive discharge. Pruritus may be troublesome; severe dysuria and cystitis can occur; dyspareunia is common. Severe vaginitis may result, which is associated with a 'strawberry cervix' – cervicitis with occasional bleeding from the cervix, especially during pregnancy. *Laboratory and screening.* Direct microscopy may identify the organism. A culture of the vaginal fluid should be considered. A rapid diagnostic kit is available (90% sensitive and 99.8% specificity) (Gaydos & Hardick, 2014).
Treatment	*Medication.* A single dosage of metronidazole (Flagyl) 2 g given orally is effective therapy, and is safe in pregnancy. The sexual partner should also be treated and coitus is avoided for seven days after treatment. The use of alcohol is avoided for three days after treatment. Educate the woman on the side effects of the medication: gastrointestinal (GI) tract disturbance, furred tongue, dizziness and hallucinations. Instruct her to use a condom for future sexual activity, as re-infection is possible.

49.5 Common communicable infections, vectors and diseases from environmental contamination and food

The following sections discuss various viral infections (chickenpox and parvovirus B19), malaria (an infection caused by vectors) and infections caused by bacteria (tetanus and listeriosis).

Viral infections

Table 49.5 details two viral infections, namely chickenpox and parvovirus B19.

Table 49.5

Viral infections

Chickenpox: VZV	
Pathogen	VZV is highly contagious. After the primary infection (droplet), lesions develop within 10–20 days and skin lesions appear in varied patterns after three to seven days on the trunk, face, scalp and extremities. Lesions progress through macular, papular, vesicular and pustular stages, with scabs at the end stage. The condition is highly contagious and is spread by the airborne route from the skin lesions and oropharynx of infected individuals.
Risks and problems	*Maternal.* About 90% of childbearing women may be immune against VZV (Lamont et al, 2011). The infection may be more severe in pregnant women than in other adults, with maternal pneumonia developing one week after the onset of the rash. *Fetus.* The effect on the fetus will depend on the stage of the pregnancy. In the first two trimesters, VZV intrauterine infection occurs in 25% of cases and in 12% of cases congenital abnormalities are present (Lamont et al, 2011). The onset of VZV in pregnant women in the period from five days before birth to two days after birth can result in severe neonatal varicella in 17–30% of newborn infants. These infants are exposed to VZV without sufficient maternal antibodies, which lessen the severity of disease (PAHO & WHO, 2008).
Diagnosis	*Maternal.* The mother may present with a sore throat, fever, malaise and a rash or blisters. *Newborn.* Congenital varicella syndrome may be present if the infection occurred between 13 and 24 weeks. Signs and symptoms of this include LBW, skin scarring, limb hypoplasia, microcephaly, cortical atrophy (brain cell), cerebral ventriculomegaly and eye problems such as chorioretinitis, cataracts and eye abnormalities. *Laboratory and systematic screening:* • *Maternal.* A rapid PCR or blood test for IgG antibodies can be done. • *Newborn.* Take a history of maternal infection around the time of delivery, and observe for clinical signs in the baby. The baby should be followed up, as babies can develop herpes zoster infections until one year after birth. At seven months, if the baby is healthy and normal, a blood test of IgM and a persistent increase in IgG may indicate a risk for later infection.
Prevention	*Maternal.* Women should be vaccinated before pregnancy. Infected persons should be avoided. If contact occurs, a blood test is done; if this is negative the woman should be offered zoster immunoglobulin (ZIG) within 72 hours of contact to prevent or attenuate the disease: 0.1 ml/kg stat is given once only IMI. *Newborn.* If the mother became infected five days before or directly after birth, the baby should be given immunoglobulin as soon as possible after birth.

continued

Treatment	*Maternal.* Oral acyclovir treatment should be initiated within 24 hours of the onset of the rash of varicella infection during pregnancy, due to the risk of complications and severe outcomes. Hospitalisation and early treatment with IV acyclovir is required and life-saving at any stage of pregnancy if varicella pneumonia occurs, or in the presence of other signs of dissemination. *Newborn.* Infants with signs and symptoms of congenital varicella do not require treatment. Newborn infants with severe or rapidly progressing varicella should be treated with IV acyclovir at a dose of 30–45 mg/kg in 3 divided daily doses (Wilson et al, 2016: 694). VZV immunoglobulin should be administered to neonates whenever the onset of maternal disease is between five days before and two days after delivery (III-C) (Shrim et al, 2012).
Parvovirus B19	
Pathogen	Parvovirus B19, also known as fifth disease or erythema infectiosum, is a small virus that causes a mild rash, referred to as 'slapped cheek' rash because of the red cheeks.
Risks and problems	Twenty per cent of infections are asymptomatic. It is transmitted through respiratory droplets. An infected person is infective four to seven days before the rash appears and two weeks after (PAHO & WHO, 2008). An estimated 1.5% of women of childbearing age seroconvert with a parvo B19 infection (PAHO & WHO, 2008). After infection, the person has life-long immunity. Transplacental vertical transfer of the parvovirus B19 infection occurs in 30–50% of acute maternal parvovirus B19 infections (PAHO & WHO, 2008). Most babies are normal and the risk of adverse fetal outcomes is low. If the infection occurs during the first and second trimesters, the risk is highest between 9–16 weeks' gestation. Fetal disease may manifest as severe fetal anaemia, non-immune hydrops fetalis, IUGR, IUD or fetal death.
Diagnosis	*Maternal.* The woman may be asymptomatic, or she may have mild malaise, cold-like symptoms with a typical rash, inflammation of joints and anaemia. *Newborn.* A mild rash appears, mainly on the face, trunk and limbs, for 7–10 days, with malaise, a low-grade fever, anaemia and hydrops fetalis. *Laboratory and systematic screening.* A blood test for antiparvovirus B19 IgM indicates acute maternal parvovirus B19 infection. Antiparvovirus B19 IgG antibodies indicate previous infection and immunity. Cord blood or amniotic fluid with PCR assays can detect fetal infection antiparvovirus B19 IgM.
Prevention	There is no vaccine against the virus. Basic precautionary measures should be taken, such as washing hands with soap, covering the nose and mouth when sneezing and coughing, not touching the eyes, nose and mouth, avoiding sick people and staying at home, particularly in pregnancy. Healthcare professionals must follow the 'clean hands save lives' principle.
Treatment	*Maternal.* There is no specific treatment for the virus. Symptoms of anaemia and painful joints can be treated. *Newborn.* Ultrasound scanning is important for fetal surveillance. With early signs of hydrops, intrauterine transfusion may be performed to correct the anaemia of the baby to prevent cardiac failure. The baby is delivered as soon as it reaches viability.

Infections caused by vectors: Malaria

Pathogen

Malaria is caused by a parasite, plasmodium, carried by the Anopheles mosquito. Only four of the 100 species of plasmodium are infectious to humans. Most deaths are caused by *Plasmodium falciparum*.

Risks and problems

Malaria is endemic in 21 countries and is an enormous global burden. In pregnancy, malaria results in a wide range of adverse complications and outcomes. HIV infection also lowers the immunity against malaria.

The mother may experience headache, very high fever, hypoglycaemia, severe haemolytic anaemia and pulmonary oedema. It may also present after delivery with postpartum bacterial infection. Severe infections, which manifest with cerebral malaria or pulmonary oedema, may be fatal.

The parasite is sequestered (cloistered, hidden and hard to find) in the placenta and affects the placenta; it may lead to spontaneous abortion, stillbirth and LBW, congenital defects, premature birth, congenital infection and neonatal death. Rarely, congenital infection is transmitted vertically.

Diagnosis

In terms of maternal diagnosis, a high level of clinical suspicion based on the history and clinical manifestation is needed for rapid diagnosis and treatment for a good outcome. Malaria is a medical emergency – see the current *Guidelines for Maternity Care in South Africa* (DoH, 2015a). If one of the signs, as mentioned below, is present, and it is confirmed with a laboratory test, immediate treatment is indicated. Test any patient with unexplained fever for malaria, even in the absence of a travel history.

Uncomplicated malaria is a symptomatic infection without signs of severity or evidence of vital organ dysfunction. Persistent vomiting, clinical jaundice, a change in mental state or an increase in respiratory rate constitute severe malaria.

Diagnostic clinical signs and symptoms include (DoH, 2015a):
- impaired consciousness or convulsions
- the inability to sit
- hypotensive systolic BP < 80 mmHg
- respiratory distress > 30 breaths per minute
- visible jaundice or hyperbilirubinaemia
- macroscopic haematuria
- abnormal bleeding: disseminated intravascular coagulation (DIC)
- renal impairment.

Laboratory (DoH, 2015a):
- Hyperparasitemia > 4 per cent parasites
- Severe anaemia Hb < 5 mg/dl
- Hypoglycaemia < 2.2 mmol/ℓ
- Acidosis pH < 7.25 or plasma bicarbonates < 15 mmol/ℓ
- Serum creatinine > 250 µmol/ℓ
- Hyperlactatemia (venous lactate > 4 mmol/ℓ
- Bilirubin > 50 µmol/ℓ.

In terms of the newborn, the perinatal outcomes depend on the maternal condition, anaemia, stage of pregnancy, diagnosis and treatment.

For the purposes of laboratory and screening, blood smears remain the standard for diagnosis. Malaria is only excluded after three negative blood smears in 12–24 hours. The malaria rapid diagnostic test (RDT) needs minimal skill and can be done with a finger prick. It can be falsely negative in the case of low viral concentrations.

Prevention

The use of mosquito nets and pesticides is standard in malarial areas. When travelling, pregnant women are advised to avoid malarial areas. Should a trip to a malarial area be taken, prophylaxis is advised. Current guidelines should be followed.

Stray malaria must be considered when a woman presents with clinically suggestive symptoms and signs, even if she has not visited a malaria area.

Treatment

Saving the life of the mother is the main goal of care. Treatment protocols for pregnant women are different from those for non-pregnant adults.

If uncomplicated (in South Africa), the following applies:
- *First trimester:* Supervised 7-day course of oral quinine plus clindamycin (Blumberg, 2015).
- *Second and third trimesters:* Artemether-lumefantrine is considered safe and efficacious.

Regime:
- Four tablets: 80 mg artemether and 480 mg lumefantrine immediately (if > 35 kg). Repeat after 8 hours on day 1.
- Repeat 12-hourly on following 2 days.
- Give a total of 5 doses.
- Give each dosage with food containing fat.

If artemether-lumefantrine is not available:
- Give oral quinine as for first trimester. Two to three days after quinine, start oral Clindamycin 10 mg/kg 12-hourly for 7 days (DoH, 2015a: 128).
- Monitor blood sugar.
- Keep hydrated (avoid overload).
- Control pyrexia.
- Anaemia should be suspected in all women diagnosed with malaria and treated.
- If acute and complicated, admit in ICU.
- IV treatment is commenced.
- Reduce high body temperature.
- Good nursing care is vital.

Infections caused by environmental and food contamination

Table 49.6

Infections caused by bacteria

Tetanus neonatorum
If a baby has not received passive immunity from the mother, the baby is at risk for neonatal tetanus through the umbilical stump if unhygienic cord practices are followed.

Pathogen	Tetanus develops from *Clostridium tetani*, an anaerobic, Gram-positive rod.
Risks and problems	Infections occur when the bacteria enter a wound in a non-immunised individual. In the newborn this happens mainly through the umbilical stump, often due to poor hygiene. Most body organs, as well as the nervous system, are severely affected by tetanus toxins. Tetanospasmin (exotoxin) is taken up by the neuronal end plates and prevents neurotransmitter release at the synaptic junction. This leads to irreversible muscle spasms. It is a major cause of neonatal death. Recovery requires the formation of new neurons and may take months.
Diagnosis	Diagnosis is based on the history and clinical picture. The clinical picture is rigid muscles and the newborn's head being pulled back. *Laboratory test.* C tetani can sometimes be cultured from the wound, but the culture is not sensitive.
Prevention	Immunisation of all pregnant women with tetanus toxoid should be performed. Two or three doses must be given in pregnancy. Hygienic practices must be observed when cutting the umbilical cord and during care. The use of traditional dressings and ointments on the cut umbilical cord should be avoided.
Treatment	The treatment of an infected newborn includes adequate ventilation, IV antibiotics, human tetanus immunoglobulin and antitoxin, and medication to control seizures. This must all take place in an ICU.

Listeriosis (monocytogenes)	
Pathogen	Listeriosis is caused by food contaminated with the Gram-positive bacterium *Listeria monocytogenes*, which grows on food stored in refrigerators if the food has not been thoroughly cooked.
Risks and problems	*Listeria monocytogenes* is found in uncooked meat, vegetables, seafood, unpasteurised milk and soft cheeses. The disease primarily affects pregnant women, newborns and people with weakened immune systems. Fetal infection occurs through vertical transplacental transmission following maternal infection. Vertical transmission can cause abortion, stillbirth, premature birth, severe CNS infection of the newborn, sepsis and meningitis, with high mortality.
Diagnosis	*Maternal.* Mild flu-like symptoms, fever and muscle aches, nausea and diarrhoea. In severe cases, listeriosis can cause encephalitis, leading to death. *Newborn.* In early neonatal onset, during the first week of life, infected babies may present with respiratory distress, fever and neurological abnormalities. Severe cases present with a rash. Late onset develops after seven days, most frequently with meningitis. *Laboratory and systematic screening.* Blood cultures are done in women with a high fever.
Prevention	Take care to cook food thoroughly. Women are advised not to drink unpasteurised milk in pregnancy.
Treatment	*Maternal.* Antibiotics are given as soon as the disease is identified. Ampicillin 4–6 gr/day in 4 equal doses for 14 days. This will protect the fetus. *Newborn.* Ampicillin 200 mg/kg/day divided in 4 to 6 dosages adjusted for age and weight intravenously for 14 days.

49.6   Other infections

The human body hosts many organisms that become part of the normal bioflora in the body, even playing a role in the normal physiology. This is called colonisation. Organisms enter through the skin, mouth, oropharynx, nasopharynx, ear, eye, stomach, intestines, urethra and vagina. They are hosted by the body throughout life; they are not pathological and do not cause disease. Common organisms that inhabit most humans are *Escherichia coli*, *Candida albicans*, *Gardnerella*, *Streptococci*, *Lactobacilli*, *Mycobacterium*, *Staphylococcus*, *Pseudomonas* and others.

When the environment in the host changes, such as the weakening of a person's immune system, these organisms may overgrow and become pathological. This is referred to as an opportunistic infection. In pregnancy, the immune system is relatively diminished to protect the fetus *in utero*; coupled with the relative anaemia, this predisposes the woman to infections. The endocrine changes affect the pH of the vagina and predispose the woman to vaginal infections. These common conditions are briefly discussed.

Bacterial vaginosis

Description

BV is a polymicrobial clinical syndrome caused by the replacement of normal *lactobacilli* in the vagina with bacteria that change the normal balance of the vagina. It is not an STI. The normal pH of the vagina is acidic, at 3.8–4, and 5. The neutral pH of water is 7. An elevated pH of more than 4.5 causes non-lactobacillus micro-organisms to flourish. Factors that may influence the pH are diet, hormonal fluctuations, blood (pH 7.4), semen (pH 7.1) and body soap (pH 7–14).

Pathogen

In BV, the vaginal flora are replaced by an overgrowth of anaerobic bacteria such as *Gardnerella vaginalis*.

Risks and problems

BV is the most prevalent cause of vaginal discharge, pruritus and malodour and is mostly asymptomatic. BV is a strong independent risk factor in adverse outcomes in pregnancy.

Asymptomatic BV is implicated in the incidence of preterm birth. Ascending infections from the vagina through the cervix into the uterus give rise to chorioamnionitis. This condition is strongly correlated with intra-amniotic infections and preterm birth. Women with BV are more likely to have *Gardnerella vaginalis* and *Mycoplasma hominis* in the amniotic fluid.

BV also puts women at risk for other infections, such as HIV.

Diagnosis

There is no value in routine screening of women in pregnancy. Where needed, BV can be diagnosed by the clinical criteria. If available, a laboratory test can determine the concentration of *lactobacilli*, Gram-negative rods and cocci in a vaginal fluid sample. The findings can be used to correlate the signs and symptoms with the laboratory test. Signs and symptoms include:

▶ a thin white discharge that smoothly coats the vaginal wall
▶ the presence of clue cells under microscope
▶ a vaginal pH of more than 4.5
▶ a fishy odour when potassium hydroxide is added to the discharge.

Prevention

Safe sexual practices and a healthy diet with fresh fruit and vegetables are required. The woman should avoid using douches and soaps that affect the vaginal flora. She should use probiotics when on antibiotics.

Treatment

Common treatment includes metronidazole and clindamycin oral and vaginal creams and gels. Follow-up is needed, as the infection repeats.

Group B Streptococcus infection

Pathogen

GBS, also known as *Streptococcus agalactiae*, is an encapsulated Gram-positive bacterium that is a common inhabitant or coloniser of the human GI and genito-urinary tracts. Colonisation refers to a state where the host does not show symptoms.

GBS was identified as a cause of puerperal sepsis in 1935, but since 1960 the association between neonatal infection and GBS has been determined.

Risks and problems

The overgrowth of GBS in a percentage of women in the vagina or rectum may be transient or chronic. Most women will be colonised at some point in their lifetime. About 20–30 per cent of pregnant women are colonised by GBS (PAHO & WHO, 2008). This may lead to UTIs that may complicate pregnancy and result in amnionitis, endometritis or sepsis. There is a risk of the transfer of the organism to the fetus during pregnancy and birth. Globally, the incidence has been reported from 0.6–2.5 cases per 1 000 live births in untreated mothers (PAHO & WHO, 2008).

Early-onset GBS infection can be severe in newborns, causing sepsis, pneumonia, meningitis and sometimes arthritis. It usually starts within 24 hours or the first week after birth. Late onset disease happens within three months after birth, when the infant comes in contact with an infected person or a carrier. It can be life-threatening to the infant if not treated promptly.

Diagnosis

▶ *Maternal:* Women may be asymptomatic. They may have a history of chorioamnionitis or GBS UTI in pregnancy, or a previous baby who had GBS infection. Clinical risk factors for the condition include women less than 35 years of age with ruptured membranes for 18 hours or more, a temperature of 38 °C and a history of GSB UTI in pregnancy.
▶ *Newborn.* The condition presents within 24 hours, with cyanosis, respiratory distress, abnormal heartbeat, lethargy, paleness or coldness (shock), poor feeding and unstable temperature.
▶ *Laboratory and systematic screening.* In the newborn, cultures are done for blood, urine and cerebrospinal fluid (CSF).

Prevention

There is no vaccine for GBS.

Screening includes culture of the vagina and rectum in pregnancy between 35 and 37 weeks to diagnose the infection. In women who test positive, antibiotic treatment is given during labour to prevent early-onset neonatal infection. If a screening programme is not available (as in South African public health facilities), antibiotic treatment is given.

In terms of *prophylaxis*, the treatment of choice is IV penicillin or ampicillin. Treatment is given in cases of:
▶ premature birth
▶ mothers with a history of previous babies infected with GBS
▶ mothers with a temperature of 38 °C
▶ PROM
▶ prolonged rupture of membranes of more than 18 hours.

Treatment

Newborns exposed to GBS should be under the supervision of a medical practitioner and receive IV antibiotics even before the laboratory confirmation has been received. CRP has a high negative predictive value in low-risk cases and treatment can be postponed until symptomatic.

Candidiasis

Pathogen

This infection is caused by a fungus (yeast-like organism) called *Candida albicans* in 80–90 per cent of cases (Soong & Einarson, 2009). Other less common organisms are *Candida glabrata* and *Candida tropicalis*. It is not sexually transmitted.

Risks and problems

Candida albicans is a yeast that is normally present in the body but that overgrows under certain conditions. Vulvovaginitis (yeast syndrome) is an ailment that affects three out of four women during their life cycles (Soong & Einarson, 2009). It is the most common infection in women and can particularly occur during pregnancy because of the pregnancy hormones and changes in the pH of the vagina. More than 40 per cent of women will have more than one episode in their lives (Soong & Einarson, 2009). If more than four episodes manifest in a woman, it is considered a reoccurring infection and it may indicate diabetes mellitus, an immune-compromised patient (HIV/AIDS), corticosteroid therapy and the use of broad-spectrum antibiotic therapy. The baby may be infected when passing through the infected birth canal. The breasts and nipples can be infected. The condition can become systemic.

Diagnosis

This is based on the clinical picture and history, and an examination of the white cheese-like layer on the mucous membrane of the affected organ (the mouth or vagina). Bleeding can occur when the layer is removed. The vaginal pH is less than 4.5. The discharge may have a slightly offensive odour and covers the vaginal walls in thick white plaques, with raw areas present. The vulva may be swollen, with pruritis and erythema.

On a vaginal smear, Gram-negative spores (oval-like cells with elongated pseudohyphae) are visible.

Prevention

Douching should be avoided. Hand washing is essential.

Treatment

All women must receive probiotics with any course of antibiotic treatment to prevent overgrowth. Diet and balanced blood sugar is important to maintain the pH balance.

Antifungal therapy is the treatment of choice. Nystatin oral and vaginal treatment is safe in pregnancy, as is intravaginal imidazole antifungal treatment, for example clotrimazole. Effective treatment for at least seven days is needed and in 80 per cent of cases the condition can be resolved (Sweet & Gibbs, 2009: 202).

Urinary tract infection

Pathogen

Bacteria implicated in UTI in pregnancy include *Escherichia coli* and *Staphylococcus saprophyticus*. In pyelonephritis, organisms such as *E coli*, *Enterobacterium*, *Proteus mirabilis*, *Klebsiella* and *Pseudomonas aeruginosa* are implicated.

Risks and problems

UTI is one of the most common medical conditions in pregnancy. It is estimated that the prevalence of asymptomatic bacteriuria (ASB) varies between 2 per cent and 10–13 per cent, similar to non-pregnant women (Matuszkiewicz-Rowińska, Małyszko & Wieliczko, 2015). The urethra, bladder, ureters and renal pelvis are affected, but the infection can also often involve the renal parenchyma.

It is important to understand the changes in the renal system during pregnancy. Progesterone relaxes the smooth muscles and so causes dilatation and atony of the bladder, of the ureters (with kinking) and of the renal pelvis. Women have a short urethra (3.5 cm) in close proximity to the rectum, the perineum and the vagina. The ureters are subjected to pressure from 12 to 20 weeks. At 20 weeks, the uterus dextroverts (turns) to the right, causing extra pressure on the right ureter, which is usually the first to be affected in cases of pyelonephritis. At 38 weeks, engagement of the fetal head will also subject the urethra to pressure when the fetal head pushes down on the bladder.

Trauma can occur during labour, as the bladder base and neck are fixed structures. They become bruised, resulting in damage and atony, leading to urinary stasis and infection.

UTI may be asymptomatic in pregnant women until a substantial bacteriuria is present. The only serious maternal consequence of untreated ASB in pregnant women is a significant risk of acute pyelonephritis in later pregnancy (30–40 per cent vs 3–4 per cent in treated patients (Matuszkiewicz-Rowińska, Małyszko & Wieliczko, 2015). If the UTI complicates to pyelonephritis, the pregnancy is at risk and may lead to premature birth.

Post-delivery, women are more likely to get UTIs due to infections of the urinary tract in pregnancy, anaemia and catheterisation during the second stage of labour and during epidural and Caesarean section.

Diagnosis

Bacteriuria is asymptomatic in pregnancy. Pyelonephritis is a complication and presents with fevers, rigors and pyrexia, tachycardia and pain in one or both loins, leading down to the groin in some cases. There is costovertebral angle tenderness on fist percussion, burning on micturition, frequency and dysuria and hypotension. Oliguria occurs in the first 24–36 hours, which is due to oedema and congestion of the renal parenchyma, the tubules, the renal pelvis and the ureters, and to dehydration as a result of the nausea and vomiting.

On dipstick, albumin is present in the urine and, sometimes, a trace of blood. A clean-catch midstream urine specimen should be sent for microscopy, culture and sensitivity (MC&S). The presence of bacteria (> 100 000 colonies/ml) is a positive test.

Prevention

During pregnancy, 30–40 per cent (vs 3–4 per cent in treated patients) of women with asymptomatic bacteriuria develop clinical renal tract infection (Matuszkiewicz-Rowińska, Małyszko & Wieliczko, 2015).

Women with a history of previous preterm births, postpartum infections, reoccurring uterine and vaginal infections, STIs and/or HIV, diabetes, anaemia and cardiac disease are high-risk patients for UTI. A midstream specimen should be sent for culture and sensitivity. A course of oral antimicrobials is given to woman who are found to have asymptomatic bacteriuria.

Treatment

Women with a history of UTI and previous pyelonephritis may receive prophylactic treatment in pregnancy. In acute pyelonephritis, the woman can become severely ill and be hospitalised and on bed rest and sometimes will require intensive care facilities. Treatment includes the following:

▶ Perform fluid administration of IV therapy Ringer's lactate (125 ml/h).
▶ If the woman is nauseous, give anti-emetics as prescribed.
▶ Start IV antibiotics while awaiting urine results and change to appropriate antibiotics as prescribed.
▶ Observe the fluid balance: strict intake and output of at least 30 ml/hr.
▶ Give symptomatic pain management, as prescribed.
▶ Observe the fetal well-being.
▶ Observe vital signs.
▶ Alert: If the woman's temperature is 38 °C, pulse is 120 bpm and BP is 90/50, notify the medical practitioner.

49.7 Obstetric infections of the female reproductive organs

Infections of the female reproductive organs related to pregnancy and birth are serious life-threatening conditions, resulting in high maternal and perinatal morbidity and mortality. There are endogenous and exogenous bacterial causes of infections.

Endogenous infections are caused by bacteria normally present in the vagina and body that are not pathogenic. These include *E coli*, *Staphylococci*, *Streptococci*, *Clostridium welchii* and others. BV includes the overgrowth of anaerobic organisms. Infections develop when the bacteria move into the uterus through the cervix in pregnancy and become pathogenic. The bacteria may gain entry when the membranes rupture, during birth and through vaginal examinations.

Exogenous infections develop from bacteria introduced to the closed biological system from an external source. Exogenous infections include sexually transmitted conditions but also refer to iatrogenic conditions. This includes vectors such as malaria, or STIs or iatrogenic conditions due to cross-infections and trauma of the tissue in labour or during Caesarean section. In case of the breast, cracked nipples give entry to bacteria to cause infections.

Chorioamnionitis

Description

Chorioamnionitis is the inflammation of the chorion, amnion and amniotic fluid that occurs when bacteria gain access to the amniotic fluid and multiply.

Pathogen

Chorioamnionitis is a bacterial infection, usually from the vagina. *E coli*, GBS and anaerobic bacteria are most commonly the cause. Viruses rarely cause the condition.

Risks and problems

The incidence of chorioamnioitis varies. In a study by Tita & Andrews (2010), it was indicated that chorioamnionitis complicates as many as 40–70 per cent of preterm births with PROM or spontaneous labour, and 1–13 per cent of term births. Twelve per cent of primary Caesarean births at term involve clinical chorioamnionitis (Tita & Andrews, 2010).

It is often subclinical and asymptomatic in the early stages. The main route of infection is through the cervix. Other routes are amniocentesis, intrauterine infusion, cervical cerclage and PROM. Frequent vaginal examinations late in pregnancy can also cause the condition.

Pathogenesis

Inflammation is always present at the membranes near the cervical os. In twins, the first-born twin is most affected. If the organism is of low virulence, the membranes remain intact. The infection reaches the placenta within 12–24 hours after rupture of membranes along the chorionic cell layer and bacteria are shed into the amniotic fluid.

Antimicrobial activity appears in the second trimester and is often asymptomatic. The condition progresses as the pregnancy continues and may worsen and become symptomatic.

In acute amnionitis, the inflammation of the chorionic plate occurs in stages. The leukocytes infiltrate the chorion and spread from the chorion to the amnion. When the leukocytes reach the amnion, it is classified as Stage 3. Figure 49.1 illustrates the progression of infection from the chorion to the amniotic fluid.

PROM is defined as the rupture of membranes before the onset of contractions. The inflammation that occurs with chorioamnionitis can contribute to 50 per cent of cases of PROM and 40–70 per cent of premature births (Tita & Andrews, 2010). If the membranes rupture before 36 weeks, it is classified as pPROM, or pre-premature rupture of membranes. The infection will reach the uterus within 24 hours after the rupture of membranes, exposing the baby to organisms from the vagina through the infected amniotic fluid, even when delivered through Caesarean section.

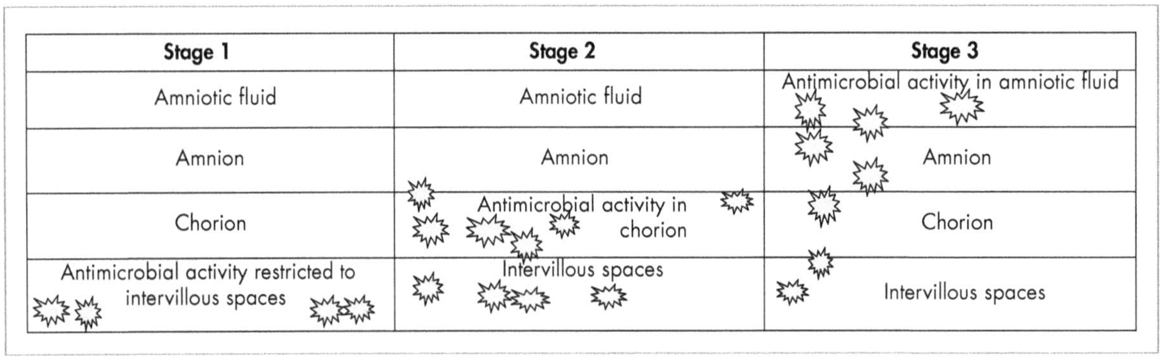

Stage 1	Stage 2	Stage 3
Amniotic fluid	Amniotic fluid	Antimicrobial activity in amniotic fluid
Amnion	Amnion	Amnion
Chorion	Antimicrobial activity in chorion	Chorion
Antimicrobial activity restricted to intervillous spaces	Intervillous spaces	Intervillous spaces

Figure 49.1 The progression of infection from the chorion to the amniotic fluid

The newborn can be infected by any of the organisms, with the risk of serious infections such as sepsis, pneumonia and meningitis. The fetal gut is exposed to the organism and the cord is at risk for infection after birth. There is also a risk of puerperal sepsis.

The mother is also at risk for postpartum haemorrhage (PPH) and embolism.

Diagnosis

Diagnosis is based on the level of antimicrobial activity of the amnion and chorion and the presence of leukocytes in the amniotic fluid. The leukocytes come from the mother and the fetus.

- *Maternal clinical diagnosis.* Chorioamnionitis is mostly subclinical and asymptomatic. One of the signs of the condition is preterm labour. The signs and symptoms of chorioamnionitis include:
  - maternal tachycardia > 100 bpm
  - pyrexia (> 38 °C)
  - fetal tachycardia (160 bpm)
  - a tender uterus
  - foul-smelling amniotic fluid
  - an elevated white blood cell count.
- *Newborn.* The newborn can present with fetal distress *in utero* and neonatal infections depending on the duration of the pregnancy, the duration of the inflammatory responses *in utero*, the type of organisms in the amniotic fluid and prophylaxis therapies given. Respiratory distress, pneumonia, sepsis and bronchopulmonary dysplasia (BPD) are common in the premature baby if the cause of the preterm birth was chorioamnionitis, whether diagnosed or undiagnosed.

Prevention

A history of previous chorioamnionitis, preterm births and infections is important to identify risks, as is the identification of any current infection present during pregnancy. Screen the mother in pregnancy for any infection that can cross the placenta. Identify and treat vaginal infections, particularly BV and GBS. In labour, vaginal examinations need to be minimised, as the risk of amnionitis increases after four internal examinations.

Treatment

- *Delivery of the baby.* Once the diagnosis is made, birth is facilitated. If the patient is in premature labour, the delivery will proceed. A Caesarean section is not desirable, unless there is an obstetric reason due to the risk of infection. The mother and fetus need close observation

during labour using hourly vital signs and electronic monitoring of the baby. It is advisable to start Ringer's lactate IV infusion at 125 ml/hr and to notify the paediatrician of the risk. If labour does not commence, induction is needed if 24 hours are exceeded.

- *Antibiotic prophylaxis.* If birth is anticipated within two hours, antibiotic therapy is delayed until after the birth. This gives the paediatrician time to identify the organism so that treatment can be more effective. The mother receives a broad-spectrum IV antibiotic, depending on the situation, before birth or during the third stage of labour and after birth.
- *Identification of the pathogen.* The amniotic fluid is cultured and cultures from the maternal and fetal side of the placenta and the cord are taken.
- *Further treatment.* Antibiotic therapy continues until the temperature is normal, within 24–48 hours. The baby is transferred to high care and as soon as the organism is identified, specific treatment is started. Care is given according to the baby's gestational age (GA), weight and Apgar score.

Puerperal sepsis

(See Johnson & Buchmann, 2012; RCOG, 2012)

Pathogens

Puerperal sepsis is caused by Group A streptococci (GAS) commonly found in the throat, also known as *Streptococcus pyogenes*, *E coli*, *Staphylococcus aureus*, *Streptococcus pneumoniae* and *Clostridium* species. Other organisms include *Neisseria gonorrhoeae*, *Bacteroides* species, *Chlamydia*, *Gardnerella vaginalis*, *Streptococcus agalactiae*, *Trichomonas*, *Klebsiella*, *Enterobacter* and *Proteus*.

Risks and problems

The WHO defines puerperal sepsis as infection of the genital tract, occurring anytime between the onset of rupture of membranes and the 42nd day postpartum, in which fever manifests with pelvic pain, abnormal vaginal discharge and sub-involution (WHO, 2008).

Risk factors for puerperal sepsis include poor socioeconomic conditions, poor nutrition, anaemia, prolonged rupture of membranes, more than five vaginal examinations in labour, Caesarean section, instrumental deliveries, retained products of conception, PPH, diabetes and infections such as HIV, malaria, STIs and conditions such as BV.

Infection pathway

The infection usually spreads from the vagina into the uterus and involves the endometrium, parametrium and Fallopian tubes. It then spreads into the pelvis or into the bloodstream, causing septicaemia. Figure 49.2 shows the spread of infections after birth.

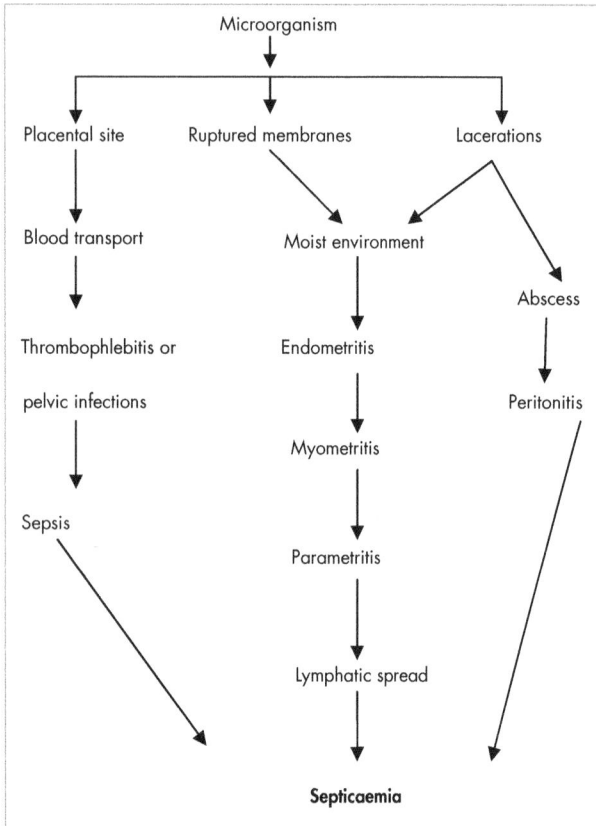

Figure 49.2 The spread of infection postpartum

Diagnosis

Any temperature of 37.8 °C in 24 hours or a rise in temperature to 38 °C in two days following birth indicates puerperal infection. Other symptoms are:
- offensive lochia and sub-involution (2.5 cm a day)
- pelvic or other pain in the abdomen, legs or genitalia
- malaise
- headaches
- nausea and vomiting.

If untreated, the woman may go into septic shock when the organism enters the bloodstream (see Chapter 35). Irreversible shock with multi-organ failure has an almost 100 per cent mortality rate. The pathology of septic shock is shown in Figure 49.3 and Table 49.7.

Special diagnostic examinations include:
- blood cultures
- full blood count (FBC), Hb and haematocrit
- platelets, fibrinogen, clotting time
- electrolytes
- urea and creatinine
- liver function tests
- serum protein
- arterial blood gasses
- cultures, including swabs from the vagina, wound and breast milk and urine MC&S.

Imaging includes chest X-ray and ultrasound of the uterus and pelvis.

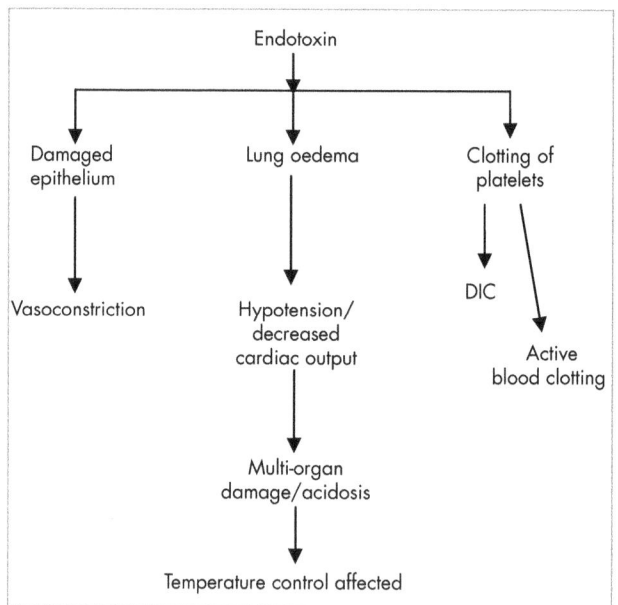

Figure 49.3 The pathology of septic shock

Prevention

Early recognition, treatment and referral of infections are essential.

Women at risk should be under medical care and some will receive prophylactic antibiotics. This includes women identified in the antenatal period as HIV positive or with TB, anaemia, UTI, diabetes mellitus, cardiac disease, chorioamnionitis, BV, STIs or malaria.

Prophylactic antibiotics are recommended for women who have complications of birth, including premature birth, PROM, surgery such as Caesarean section or episiotomy, retained placenta, antepartum haemorrhage (APH) or PPH, eclampsia and urinary catheters (WHO, 2015).

Early discharge puts women at risk. Clear information must therefore be given to ensure that problems are identified and that the woman returns timeously. In some cases, women with high risk factors, such as Caesarean section with chorioamnionitis or APH or PPH, should remain on antibiotic therapy. Make sure that all the medication is provided and understood on discharge. Follow up high-risk cases through the outreach teams.

Treatment

- *Medical care.* Postpartum women are admitted to hospital under the care of a specialist. Some will be transferred to a high-care area or ICU.
- *Antimicrobials.* Early and adequate broad-spectrum IV antibiotic is started immediately until the blood and swab cultures have been reported.
- *Fluid resuscitation.* Volume expanders, isotonic crystalloids.
- *Oxygenation.* Give oxygen. If Hb is less than nine, packed cells may be needed.
- *Pharmacological.* Corticosteroids and alpha/beta adrenergic agonists, as per medical prescription.

The medical management of puerperal fever is indicated in Figure 49.4. (Also see Chapter 35 and Table 49.7 below.)

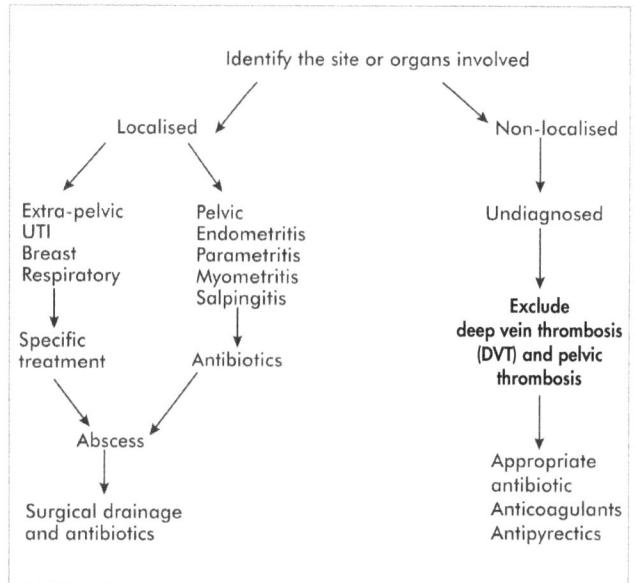

Figure 49.4 The medical management of puerperal fever

Table 49.7

The progression of septic shock

Signs and symptoms	Early or warm phase: 6–72 hrs	Late cold phase: After 72 hrs	Irreversible shock
Pulse	Tachycardia (140 bpm or more)	Tachycardia (140 bpm or more)	Cardiac failure
Respiration	Rapid	Hyperventilating	Respiratory distress
Skin colour	Normal	Cyanotic	Grey, clammy and cold
Clotting	Mottling of the legs	Legs cool and mottled	DIC
Temperature	High fever	High fever Flushed skin Chill Rigors	Rigors
BP	Hypotension	Drop by 25% of normal	Drop by more than 25%
Urine output	Decreased urine output	Oliguria: < 30 ml/hr	Anuria, acidosis
Mental status	Patient orientated and aware	Confusion	No responses

Breast infections (mastitis)

Pathogens

The causative organism in mastitis and breast abscess is usually *Staphylococcus aureus*, but it can also be *Staphylaccocus albus*, *E coli* and *Streptococcus* (non-hemolytic). Infections caused by *Salmonella* and *Mycobacterium tuberculosis* sometimes occur related to maternal infections. Fungal mastitis may be caused by *Candida* and *Cryptococcus*. Organisms from the skin, such as *Staphylococcus epidermidis*, diphtheroids and alpha-haemolytic and non-haemolytic streptococci, may be present in expressed breast milk (EBM) if hygiene is not maintained and contamination occurs. (See WHO, 2000.)

Risks and problems

Lactational or puerperal mastitis is the inflammation of the breast ducts, glands or tissue. Mastitis presents in about 10 per cent of pregnant or postnatal women (lactating and non-lactating) (WHO, 2000). Breast abscess is a severe complication of mastitis.

Mastitis can occur at any time, but is most common within the first two weeks after birth. Breast abscess is more common 12 weeks after birth. The most common cause is stasis of milk and infection. Poor hygiene, cracked nipples, previous and current infections of the mother and baby, poor diet, and hospital-acquired cross-infection are predisposing factors.

Thompson (WHO, 2000) classified mastitis based on the concentration of organisms and leukocytes found in the breast milk. These are the following:

▶ *Milk stasis* occurs due to engorgement and will improve with continued breastfeeding and early interventions.
▶ *Non-infective mastitis* follows after stasis and is the stage where microorganisms colonise the breast and start to multiply ($< 10^3$/ml bacteria and $< 10^6$/ml leukocytes). Colonisation of the breast by organisms is a normal process called *natural interference*. Bacteria are shed from the mother onto the baby's skin and nasopharynx when in contact with the baby after birth. The organisms grow in the baby's gut, respiratory system and skin. The baby then transfers the organisms to the mother's milk ducts. Once the normal flora of organisms is established between the mother and infant, pathogenic bacterial growth is inhibited. The presence of even potential pathological bacteria in breast milk does not indicate infection. Non-infective mastitis needs care such as expression of milk.
▶ *Subclinical infections* are infections where there are no clinical signs or symptoms, but there are inflammatory responses in the breast. This is associated with poor weight gain of the baby due to a lower number of feeds, leading to reduced milk production of 400 ml per day, resulting in milk stasis. This is a risk in HIV-positive mothers, who may transfer the virus from the mother to the baby.
▶ *Infective mastitis* develops when the organisms become pathological ($> 10^3$/ml bacteria and 10^6/ml leukocytes). Infective mastitis requires both milk removal and systemic antibiotics. The condition may develop into cellulitis, where the connective tissue is inflamed (which may lead to abscess formation) or adenitis, which affects the ducts and alveoli (and which may cause puerperal mastitis). If untreated, the condition may complicate or can rarely be fatal.
▶ *Hospital-acquired mastitis* may occur due to women and babies becoming exposed to cross-infections in maternity sections and nurseries.

Diagnosis

Clinical diagnosis by a skilled practitioner remains the principal method for the diagnosis of mastitis. It requires taking a history of previous and current infections of the mother and considering hospital-borne risks.

Signs and symptoms will depend on the stage of the development of the condition. Initially there is localised pain, a hard and swollen breast (usually only one breast is affected). This may be followed by headaches and general malaise. In a number of women, this may manifest with pyrexia of 38–39 °C, tachycardia, enlarged axillary glands, tender breast tissue and red and flushed skin. Rigors indicate more serious systemic effects.

Candida infection is more often found in diabetic women or after antibiotic treatment. It is characterised by a deep burning breast pain occurring during and after feeds.

The WHO (2000) set the standard guidelines for staging and diagnosis. Cell counts and culture of breast milk are useful to distinguish between infective and non-infective mastitis. These tests are rarely done. The WHO (2000) found that 50 per cent of milk cultures may be sterile because of the contamination of the skin organisms. The presence of organisms in breast milk does not necessarily indicate infection. There is no correlation between clinical signs and symptoms and the presence of organisms in the breasts and tissue. (The only way to distinguish if bacteria in milk are due to an infection is to look for organisms covered with IgG and IgM, indicating an immunological response to the bacteria.)

Prevention

All health professionals need to be trained on breastfeeding management so that they understand the principles and can give safe, evidence-based care.

The washing of hands before feeding and after changing the baby remains the most important preventive measure. Practices conducive to prevention of milk stasis are:

▶ the commencement of breastfeeding within one hour post-delivery

▶ education on demand feeding

▶ frequent demand feeding to prevent engorgement and to stimulate neurohormonal reflexes

▶ the prevention of cracked nipples by proper latching and unlatching of the baby on the breast

▶ rooming-in (this carries a lower incidence of breast infections due to early colonisation of bacteria between the mother and baby)

▶ early identification and treatment of cracked nipples.

Treatment

In case of engorgement, take care to promptly identify and treat. Help if there is difficulty with feeding and provide nipple care and supportive counselling and intervene appropriately. Advise the woman to perform manual expression of milk until the engorgement has cleared up. The application of hot or cold packs to the breasts can be very soothing. The woman must continue with breastfeeding, except if she is HIV positive. Consider professional treatment from a physiotherapist with ultrasound on the breast (available in institutions) to open ducts and reduce pain and engorgement.

In case of infection, the woman is referred for medical care. IV or oral antibiotics are prescribed and administered. Symptomatic treatment for pain relief is given, ie heat or sonar. Breastfeeding may be discontinued on the affected breast for 24 hours to give the antibiotic time to work.

If complications are present, refer for medical attention. The woman may be admitted for treatment, such as incision and drainage of the abscess. Suppression of lactation is sometimes prescribed by the medical practitioner.

49.8 Conclusion

The management of infections in obstetrics is in the hands of the professional who makes contact with the mother and baby. Since many infections are symptomatic, midwives should ask the right questions and look for signs and symptoms. There are standing basic care models that assist with the identification of infectious conditions. These are essential tools to assist with diagnosis and treatment in order to save the lives of the mother and the baby.

The midwife should ensure that the woman understands the importance of treatment adherence and how to identify the adverse effects of medication, as well as aspects that will indicate worsening of the condition, with possible complications. The lives of mothers and children depend on good quality care.

50

HIV and TB in pregnancy, birth and the newborn

LEARNING OBJECTIVES
On completion of this chapter, you must be able to:
▶ understand HIV replication and its impact on the immune system
▶ have knowledge of HIV counselling and testing (HCT)
▶ understand the clinical staging of HIV and the identification of opportunistic infections
▶ have knowledge of nurse-initiated management of antiretroviral therapy (NIMART) and prevention of mother-to-child transmission (PMTCT) of HIV
▶ understand care of the HIV-exposed/-affected newborn
▶ understand and manage the health risks of HIV and TB co-infection in obstetrics
▶ educate women on infant feeding in the context of HIV.

KNOWLEDGE ASSUMED TO BE IN PLACE
Basic knowledge of HIV and infection, prevention and treatment
Guidelines for Maternity Care in South Africa (DoH, 2015a)
National Consolidated Guidelines for the Prevention of Mother-to-Child Transmission of HIV (PMTCT) and the Management of HIV in Children, Adolescents and Adults (DoH, 2015d)

KEYWORDS
retrovirus • prevention of mother-to-child transmission (PMTCT) of HIV • perinatally acquired HIV (PAHIV) • antiretroviral therapy (ART) • human immunodeficiency virus (HIV) • tuberculosis (TB) • direct observation treatment short-course (DOTS) • fixed-dose combination (FDC) • multi-drugresistant TB (MDR-TB) • isoniazid preventive therapy (IPT) for those at risk for TB • polymerase chain reaction (PCR) test • *Pneumocystis carinii* pneumonia (PCP), now called *Pneumocystis jiroveci* pneumonia (PJP) • persistent general lymphadenopathy (PGL) • trimethoprim/sulfamethoxazole (TMP/SMX) (co-trimoxazole as Bactrim or Septra) • INH (isoniazid) for active TB • ddI (didanosine) • estimated glomerular filtration rate (eGFR)

STANDARD UNITS OF MEASURE FOR HIV IN SOUTH AFRICA
CD4 count = cells/µl
viral load = copies/ml
serum creatinine = µmol/ℓ

50.1 Introduction

Infection with the human immunodeficiency virus (HIV) is the main cause of maternal mortality in South Africa. Statistics SA indicated that the average HIV prevalence in South Africa is 12.6 per cent. The rate among young adults (15–49 years) is estimated at 18 per cent (Stats SA, 2017: 1).

According to the *Saving Mothers 2011–2013* report, non-pregnancy-related infections (NPRIs), mainly HIV-related, accounted for 34.7 per cent of maternal deaths (DoH, 2014).

When a person is co-infected with both HIV and TB (whichever came first), the co-infection speeds up the progress of the other condition and increases the mortality risk. Untreated TB in pregnancy poses a significant threat to the mother, fetus and family.

HIV is incurable, but TB is curable.

HIV is now viewed as a chronic condition, alongside hypertension and diabetes. The integrated approach to these two conditions is of particular importance in childbirth, as HIV is preventable, particularly for the unborn baby, and TB, with its debilitating effects, can be prevented.

This chapter gives an update of HIV and TB as they impact on the role and function of midwives. Background information on the conditions as well as current prevention and treatment in childbirth and for the newborn are covered, in compliance with current national and international guidelines. This chapter should be studied in collaboration with the applicable policies and guidelines for HIV and TB issued by the national Department of Health (DoH), and the *Guidelines for Maternity Care in South Africa* (DoH, 2015a).

50.2 What is HIV?

There are two types of HIV infections commonly diagnosed in human beings:

▶ HIV1 is the aggressive type and the cause of the epidemic in central and southern Africa.

▶ HIV2 is the less aggressive type. It is absent in South Africa but present in West Africa and in Mozambique.

These two viruses do not show the same sensitivity to antiretroviral (ARV) drugs.

HIV infection in the human body

HIV is a virus that carries its genetic information in the form of RNA (ribonucleic acid). It is a retrovirus that replicates itself in the host cell by using an enzyme to generate complementary DNA, in a process called reverse transcription. To replicate, the viral RNA must be transcribed in DNA and be integrated in the host cell's genome (human DNA that holds all the genetic hereditary information) (see Figure 50.1).

Target cells

HIV can only target and enter cells with CD4 receptors or T-cells with a co-receptor on their membrane. CD4 cells are types of white blood cells (WBCs) that play a role in protecting the body from infection. These cells are the CD4 lymphocytes, the macrophages (fixed in tissue or free-moving in blood) and the Langerhans dendritic cells (found in skin and mucosa) called antigen-presenting cells that attack and fix the foreign antigen. (Also see the box on circumcision on the next page.)

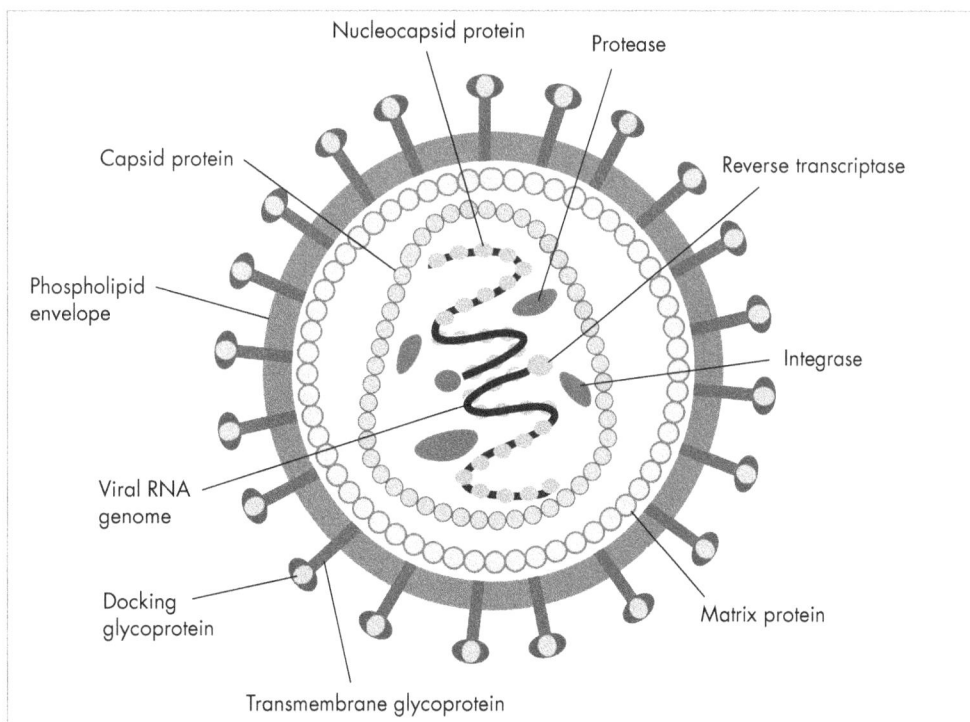

Figure 50.1 The human immunodeficiency virus (HIV)

Immune response

The activated lymphocytes of the immune system start to secrete numerous small protein chemical messengers, called *cytokines*, that will activate the CD8 T-lymphocytes and the B-lymphocytes. Activated CD8 T-lymphocytes (cytotoxic cells) kill infected cells and activated B-lymphocytes produce antibodies.

CD4 lymphocytes (helper cells), CD8 lymphocytes (cytotoxic cells) and B-lymphocytes (producers of antibodies) are all components of the immune system and their activation and actions are closely interlinked.

Circumcision and HIV

The foreskin is particularly rich in Langerhans dendritic cells (targeted by HIV) and is a major route for HIV infection when tiny tears occur in the foreskin.

Circumcision in HIV-negative males can reduce the risk of HIV infection by 60 per cent (WHO, 2017b).

HIV antibodies in HIV-infected persons

In an HIV-infected person, antibodies produced by the B-lymphocytes are detected only after a few weeks. The antibodies are not able to neutralise the virus.

Replication processes

HIV replicates in a six-step process through the three viral enzymes (*reverse transcriptase, integrase* and *protease*), which are the targets of some ARV drugs (*reverse transcriptase inhibitors, anti-integrase* or *anti-protease*):

1. *Attachment:* The virus attaches preferentially to the membrane receptor– co-receptor of activated CD4 lymphocytes and enters the cell.
2. *Fusion:* Viral RNA is transcribed in the cell's DNA by the viral enzyme reverse transcriptase.
3. *Reverse transcription:* The enzyme reverse transcriptase is responsible for the fusion.
4. *Integration:* HIV viral DNA, called provirus, is integrated in the nuclear DNA by the viral enzyme integrase and replicated along with the cell's DNA.
5. *Assembly:* HIV RNA copies are made and the enzyme protease processes proteins for viral assembly.
6. *Maturation:* Newly made HIV buds from the cell and can infect other cells.

See Figure 50.2 below.

Antiretroviral therapy (ART) and HIV viral enzymes

The three ARVs used in HIV treatment – reverse transcriptase inhibitors, anti-integrase and anti-protease – block the activity of the three relevant viral enzymes. In so doing, ARVs block the process of HIV replication. See Table 50.1 on page 787.

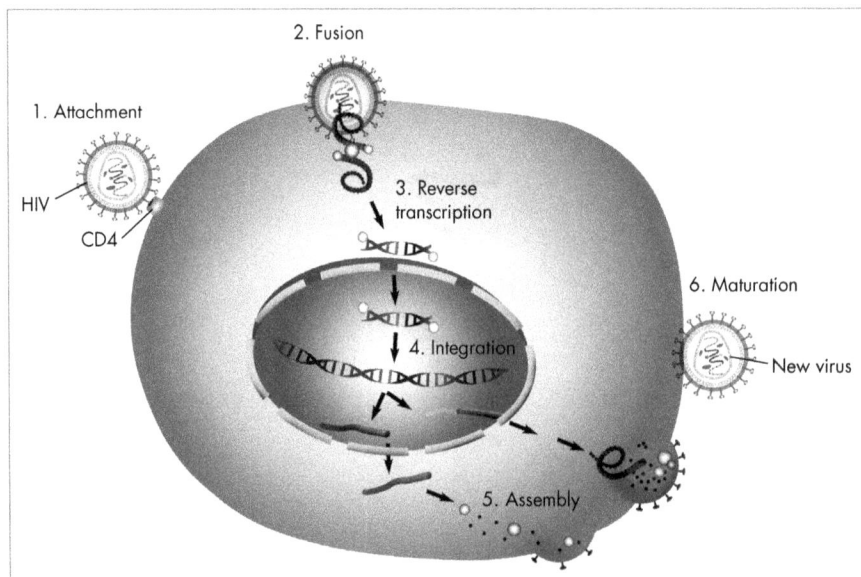

Figure 50.2 HIV replication in a six-step process

HIV infection: Pathological processes or stages

Three clinical, virological and immunological pathological progressions can be identified in HIV-infected persons. This progression may stretch over many years and is described as presented below.

Acute retroviral syndrome

HIV is usually transmitted during unprotected sex through semen and vaginal secretions, which contain a high quantity of the virus in an infected person. The virus can also be transmitted through body fluids such as blood and breast milk. (Tears, urine and saliva do not contain the virus and it cannot be transmitted in that way.)

Symptoms of the infection appear after two to three weeks and are the same as for other viral infections, for example fever, fatigue, headaches, sore throat, nausea and vomiting, swollen lymph nodes and a transient maculopapular rash. The acute syndrome usually goes undiagnosed. The rash is not itchy and disappears.

During the acute period, the HIV RNA viral load is very high, reaching several million copies per ml. This is associated with a marked drop of the CD4 T-lymphocytes and a high level of contagion and risk of transferring the virus.

Antibodies are formed at 8–12 weeks. The cytokines produced by activated CD4 lymphocytes activate the CD8 lymphocytes (cytotoxic cells). This causes a reduction in plasma viraemia. A few weeks after infection, antibodies (anti-HIV) are formed (seroconversion). The HIV1 viral load continues to decrease while the CD4 cells increase without returning to the baseline level.

HIV diagnosis and tests

- *The window period.* The period that precedes detectable anti-HIV antibodies – up to 8–12 weeks after HIV infection – is called the *window period* and the serological tests based on detection of antibodies are negative. During the window period, diagnosis of HIV infection is based on a positive polymerase chain reaction (PCR) HIV RNA test (qualitative–quantitative information: HIV1 viral load) or positive PCR HIV DNA test (qualitative information: positive vs negative).
- After seroconversion, the diagnosis is based on tests showing the presence of anti-HIV antibodies, using the Rapid or ELISA test.
- In babies, because of the transfer of maternal anti-HIV antibodies through the placenta, diagnosis of HIV infection is based on a positive antigen test (PCR DNA). Serological tests (anti-HIV antibodies) become reliable 18 months after delivery.

The latency period: 7–10 years

The infected person remains asymptomatic for a period of time. This can stretch from an average of seven years in developing countries up to 10 years in developed countries. During these years, there is a steady-state viral load, resulting from the virus-specific immune response and a progressive decrease of the CD4 cells.

Over time, the immune system (CD4 cells) is attacked and depleted. The CD4 cell count decline depends on the viral load and is a predictor of the risk of developing acquired immunodeficiency syndrome (AIDS).

AIDS

After a period of 7–10 years, symptomatic AIDS of the late-stage disease develops. This is characterised by the following:
- *Clinically:* The development and presentation of opportunistic infections, selected tumours, wasting and neurologic complications
- *Biologically:* The decline of CD4 cells, usually to below 200 cells/μl
- A high HIV viral load.

Risks of high HIV viral load and a compromised immune system

When the CD4 cell count falls below a threshold, the following risks increase:
- If < 350 cells/μl: active TB, pneumococcal pneumonia, herpes zoster, *Candida albicans* in the mouth and the vagina
- If < 200 cells/μl: *Pneumocystis jiroveci* pneumonia (PJP) (formerly known as *Pneumocystis carinii* pneumonia, or PCP), pleural/extra-pulmonary TB
- If < 100 cells/μl: cerebral toxoplasmosis, cryptococcal meningoencephalitis, non-typhoid salmonella septicaemia, atypical mycobacteria infection, severe intestinal infection due to *Cystoisospora belli* (previously known as *Isospora belli*), cyclospora, giardia, microsporidium and cryptosporidium.

The box above lists some opportunistic infections that may occur. Many of these are not only life-threatening, but they also:
- induce an increase of the HIV1 viral load, with a further drop in the CD4 cells
- show a high trend for relapse after successful treatment.

Therefore, both primary and secondary prophylaxis programmes focus on targeting as many opportunistic infections as possible. Several infections frequently seen in

AIDS patients could have been efficiently prevented with low-cost drugs such as trimethoprim/sulfamethoxazole (TMP-SMX and isoniazid (INH). These drugs include the following:

▶ TMP-SMX (co-trimoxazole) prevents PJP, cerebral toxoplasmosis, pneumococcal pneumonia, non-typhoid salmonella septicaemia and intestinal infection with *Cystoisospora belli* or cyclosporine. **Pregnancy is not a contraindication for co-trimoxazole administration** (the benefits outweigh the small risk for the fetus).

▶ Isoniazid preventive therapy (IPT) is INH 300 mg/d plus pyridoxine 25 mg/d and prevents the development of active TB. **Pregnancy is not a contraindication**.

▶ Fluconazole (200 mg/d) (anti-fungal) is too expensive for primary prophylaxis, but is used as a secondary prophylaxis to prevent a relapse of cryptococcal infection. **This should only be given in pregnancy if the benefits outweigh the risks.**

▶ Dapsone (diaminodiphenyl) is used in case of allergy to TMP-SMX and is effective in the prevention of only PCP (it is a narrow spectrum prophylaxis). **It is considered safe in pregnancy, but is excreted in breast milk and may cause haemolytic anaemia in the neonate.**

WHO classifications and clinical staging of HIV/AIDS infection

The South African HIV programme uses the HIV staging system developed by the WHO (2016a), which is based on clinical manifestations that can be recognised by clinicians working without any laboratory support, such as the CD4 cell count. Staging in adults is categorised from stages 1–4, from primary HIV infection to advanced HIV/AIDS, and is defined by the following specific clinical conditions or symptoms:

▶ *Primary infection.* Asymptomatic, or acute retroviral syndrome

▶ *Stage 1.* Asymptomatic, persistent general lymphadenopathy (PGL)

▶ *Stage 2.* Moderate weight loss (< 10 per cent) with or without re-occurring respiratory infections, herpes zoster, oral ulcerations, seborrheic dermatitis and fungal nail infections

▶ *Stage 3.* Diagnosis can be made on clinical symptoms: severe weight loss (> 10 per cent), unexplained chronic diarrhoea or persistent fever for more than a month, oral candidiasis or oral hairy leukoplakia (oral white patches), TB in the last two years, severe bacterial infections, acute necrotising stomatitis, gingivitis and periodontitis.

▶ *Stage 4.* HIV wasting, PCP, chronic herpes infections, oesophageal candidiasis, pleural/extra-pulmonary TB, Kaposi sarcoma, central nervous system (CNS) toxoplasmosis, cryptococcal meningoencephalitis, HIV encephalopathy, atypical mycobacteria.

CD4 levels and clinical disease

There is often a link between the clinical condition of a person and the level of CD4 cells found. For example, PCP usually develops when the CD4 count is below 200 cells/µl, while cryptococcal meningitis, cerebral toxoplasmosis or atypical mycobacteria infections develop when the CD4 count is below 100 cells/µl. However, the correlation is not absolute: Kaposi sarcoma (WHO stage 4) often develops when the immune depression is not yet severe. Some patients who are extremely immune-compromised (CD4 near zero) are still asymptomatic (stage 1).

People who develop clinical conditions and progress to stage 4 will never recover to stage 1 again, even after successful treatment of the opportunistic infection.

Note: It is important that a clinician record the staging of HIV on the initial assessment of a person and during the ongoing monitoring (according to the abovementioned WHO staging guidelines) and explain the clinical reasons for this decision. This practice is helpful for making future diagnoses in case of relapse of the opportunistic infection and for making treatment decisions.

Antiretroviral therapy

The objective of ART in general (for the non-pregnant person) is to stop viral replication. It is expected that:

▶ the viral load will become undetectable after six months on ART

▶ the viral load will remain undetectable during life-long treatment

▶ progressive normalisation of the CD4 cell level will occur during treatment.

Note: Not all patients show the same response to the treatment, even if they adhere to it.

There are currently six classes of ARV agents, namely:

1. nucleoside/nucleotide reverse transcriptase inhibitors (NRTIs)
2. non-nucleoside/nucleotide reverse transcriptase inhibitors (NNRTIs)
3. protease inhibitors (PIs)
4. integrase strand transfer inhibitors (INSTIs)
5. fusion inhibitors (FIs)
5. chemokine receptor antagonists (CCR5 antagonists).

Integrase inhibitors

INSTIs are a class of ARV drug that have been in use since 2009. They are designed to block the action of integrase, a viral enzyme that inserts the viral genome into the DNA of the host cell. INSTIs were initially developed for the treatment of HIV1 infection, but they can be applied to other retroviruses. In early studies, they were very effective in reducing viral load and were also administered to pregnant women.

ARVs inhibit viral replication but do not kill the virus; if treatment is interrupted, replication restarts (see Table 50.2).

ARV drugs available in the HIV national programme aim to block HIV replication (as shown in Table 50.1) by inhibiting two of the viral enzymes: reverse transcriptase (see Step 2) (NRTIs and NNRTIs) and protease (see Step 4) (PIs).

A combination of a minimum of three anti-HIV drug regimens need to be prescribed to effectively prevent viral resistance developing. The choice of drugs is based on:

⦁ previous exposure to ARVs
⦁ co-morbidities (such as TB).

Table 50.1

Actions of ART on HIV duplication

Steps of viral duplication	Replication process	ARV drug actions
Step 1	The virus attaches preferentially to the membrane receptor–co-receptor of activated CD4 lymphocytes and enters the cell.	No action
Step 2	Viral RNA is transcribed in the cell's DNA by the viral enzyme reverse transcriptase.	NRTIs and NNRTIs block this action.
Step 3	Inside the core of the DNA, the virus releases integrase (HIV enzyme), used to integrate viral DNA into the CD4 cell's DNA.	INSTIs block replication of viral DNA into the CD4 DNA (not in the current SA HIV regime).
Step 4	HIV RNA copies are made and the enzyme protease processes proteins for viral assembly.	PIs inhibit this process.
Step 5	Newly made HIV buds from the cell and can infect other cells.	No action

ARV drugs used in the South African HIV programme belong to three classes, as shown in Table 50.2.

Table 50.2

ARV drugs in the South African HIV programme

ARV drug class	Types of drugs
NRTIs	Tenofovir (TDF), zidovudine (AZT), abacavir (ABC), lamivudine (3TC), emtricitabine (FTC), stavudine (d4T), didanosine (ddI)
NNRTIs	Efavirenz (EFV), nevirapine (NVP)
PIs	Lopinavir/ritonavir (LPV/r)

The short- and long-term efficacy of ART greatly depends on the patient's adherence to the regimen. This, in turn, is highly linked to the involvement of the healthcare professionals, who have to constantly motivate and encourage the patient and explain, in simple words, the 'why, what for, how long' of ART and of chemoprophylaxis.

The first-line regimen combines two NRTIs and one NNRTI. The preferred combinations are based on efficacy, tolerability and the potential side effects. The combinations are:

▶ TDF (300 mg/d) + FTC (200 mg/d) + EFV (600 mg/d in one capsule) fixed-dose combination (FDC) taken in the evening 2 hours after supper to decrease the side effects of EFV

▶ TDF (300 mg/d) + 3TC (300 mg/d) + EFV (600 mg/d), taken 2 hours after supper.

Other valid first-line combinations for adults are:

▶ ABC + 3TC + EFV (in case of renal failure)
▶ AZT + 3TC + EFV (in case of renal failure and allergy to ABC)
▶ d4T + 3TC + EFV (in case of renal failure and allergy to ABC and anaemia or neutropenia).

Second-line ARVs for adolescents and adults combine two NRTIs and an antiprotease (PI). The most usual combinations are:

▶ AZT + 3TC + LPV/r
▶ ABC + 3TC + LPV/r.

The first-line regimen in babies (0–3 years) combines ABC/3TC and an antiprotease (PI): ABC + 3TC + kaletra syrup (LPV/r). See Table 50.3 below and Table 50.4.

Table 50.3

Standard dose of commonly used ARVs and major side effects

Drug	Standard dose	Major side effects
NRTIs	TDF 300 mg daily	Renal failure, proteinuria or glycosuria
	3TC 300 mg daily	Dose adjustment required in case of renal failure
	d4T 200 mg daily	None
	AZT 300 mg twice a day	Macrocytic anaemia/neutropenia
	ABC 300 mg twice a day	Lactic acidosis, vomiting, abdominal pain, itchy rash
	d4T 30 mg twice a day	Peripheral neuropathy or lactic acidosis
NNRTIs	EFV 600 mg nocte if weight > 40 kg 400 mg nocte if weight < 40 kg NVP 200 mg 2 x per day	Headache Nightmares Confusion Acute hepatitis and rash
Anti-protease (PIs)	LPV/r: Aluvia is a combination of lopinavir 200 mg and ritonavir 50 mg: 2 to 4 tablets per day	Diarrhoea or hyperlipidaemia/heart disease
	Atazanavir comes in 150 mg, 200 mg and 300 mg capsules. Use as prescribed under medical supervision.	Benign unconjugated hyperbilirubinaemia Atazanavir can cause serious, life-threatening side effects (contraindicated in pregnancy).

Table 50.4

ARV side effects

Side effect	Notes for therapeutic decisions
Renal failure (estimated glomerular filtration rate [eGFR] < 50 ml/min)	TDF is avoided except if absolutely necessary (chronic hepatitis B). In that case, the dose of TDF must be adjusted according to eGFR. *During pregnancy, the eGFR formula is not valid. Serum creatinine level must be used. (Note that eGFR is based on blood creatinine, but not in all cases.)* **TDF is contraindicated during pregnancy if serum creatinine is > 85 µmol/ℓ.** TDF may cause renal tubular lesions with glucose in urine despite normal glucose levels in blood. In case of renal failure, the dose of ABC, EFV, NVP and LPV/r is unchanged (standard dose) irrespective of creatinine level. In case of renal failure, the dose of AZT, 3TC, TDF, EFV and d4T must be adjusted according to the eGFR.
Active psychiatric disease or EFV intolerance (headache, confusion)	EFV is replaced by NVP if the baseline CD4 cells are below 250 cells/µl in female patients. Above these thresholds, the risk for developing NVP-induced acute hepatitis, sometimes life-threatening, is too high and EFV is replaced by LPV/r.
Co-infection: HIV and hepatitis B virus (HBV) (chronic hepatitis B)	In case of HIV-HBV co-infections, treatment must target HIV and HBV. Only TDF plus 3TC or TDF plus d4T are active against both viruses. Hepatitis B surface antigen (HBsAg) must be tested. If positive, the second-line regimen must still contain TDF and 3TC; it usually is AZT, 3TC, TDF and LPV/r.
Symptomatic hyperlactataemia, lactic acidosis	This life-threatening ARV side effect is limited to NRTIs. It is caused by a toxic effect of the drug on the cellular enzyme polymerase gamma, necessary for replication of the cellular mitochondrial DNA. Functioning of the mitochondria is disturbed and cellular respiration becomes anaerobic, with production of lactic acid. Among the NRTIs, those associated with a high risk are d4T and ddI (Table 50.3). AZT shows moderate risk, while 3TC, ABC and TDF show an extremely low risk. *Since the d4T drug has been removed from the HIV national programme, the incidence of lactic acidosis has been minimal.* However, because the second line is often based on AZT, the syndrome will not disappear and healthcare professionals must know the alarming symptoms: unexplained loss of weight in a patient on AZT, abdominal pain and vomiting. Acidotic respiration develops later and waiting for symptoms puts the patient in danger. Blood must be taken for measuring the lactate level (note *not to use a tourniquet* when drawing blood). Send the blood on ice to the laboratory.
Hypersensitivity reaction to ABC	ABC, a major NRTI drug, particularly for the treatment of babies, children and adolescents, can cause a hypersensitivity reaction. This usually develops between one and six weeks after treatment initiation. It is more frequent in white patients (5.8%) and is associated with an identified genetic predisposition (Hewitt, 2002). Possible symptoms are high fever, nausea, vomiting, abdominal pain, a maculopapular or urticarial rash and arthralgia. Diagnosis is highly suggested by a worsening of the symptoms after each dose. If the drug is interrupted, it must never be re-challenged because of the risk of a life-threatening reaction resembling anaphylaxis.
LPV/r and dyslipidaemia, hyperglycaemia	This combination can cause an increase in blood cholesterol, triglycerides or both. It also causes resistance to insulin and disturbs the control of diabetes. Cholesterol and triglycerides must be checked before starting treatment and again after three months. In case of dyslipidaemia, existing before treatment or appearing during treatment, LPV/r is replaced in adults, associated with an appropriate diet.

Life-threatening opportunistic infections for men and non-pregnant women

Several life-threatening infections may present, as detailed below.

Active TB

The following are four symptoms of active TB (pulmonary and pleural/extra-pulmonary):
1. Loss of weight (> 1.5 kg in 1 month)
2. Coughing for more than one week
3. Drenching night sweats
4. Fever.

Severe headaches

A new, severe headache may present for a few days in the severely immune-compromised patient. This is a very alarming symptom and must be investigated to exclude cryptococcal meningoencephalitis, cerebral toxoplasmosis and TB meningitis. The investigation is done by means of a CT brain scan and a cerebrospinal fluid (CSF) tap.
- At baseline assessment, all patients with CD4 cells below 100/ml must undergo a cryptococcal antigen test (Crag).
- If the test is positive, but the patient is asymptomatic (and not pregnant), she or he is treated at primary healthcare (PHC) level with fluconazole (800 mg/d for 2 weeks, 400 mg/d for 2 months, 200 mg/d as secondary prophylaxis for a minimal duration of 1 year).
- If the test is positive and the patient is symptomatic (most frequently day and night headache) or a woman in the first trimester of pregnancy, the patient must be referred for investigations and treatment. **Alert:** During the first trimester of pregnancy, amphotericin B IV is preferred because of the potential teratogenic effect of fluconazole.

Difficult, painful swallowing

Difficult and painful swallowing, with or without retrosternal discomfort, is commonly caused by candida infection of the mouth and the oesophagus. Oral thrush is not always present in cases of proven candida oesophagitis. Treatment is based on fluconazole (200 mg/d for 2 weeks). If there is no improvement, the patient should be referred for oesophagoscopy and exclusion of other diagnoses.

Persistent watery diarrhoea with massive loss of weight

Intestinal infections caused by different opportunistic agents (*giardia*, *Cystoisospora belli*, *cyclospora*, non-typhoid *salmonella*, *microsporidium* or *cryptosporidium*) can cause persistent watery diarrhoea, sometimes with massive loss of weight.

The clinical presentation of small-bowel infections is not specific and identification of the pathogen may need repeated stool examinations. An empirical syndromic treatment without stool investigation is often successful. It combines metronidazole, active against giardiasis (500 mg 3 times a day [tds] for 7 days), and a high dose of TMP-SMX, active against *Cystoisospora belli*, *cyclospora* and *salmonella*.

Alert: Metronidazole is contraindicated during the first trimester of pregnancy and should be replaced by paromomycin 500 mg orally 4 times a day for 7 days. For some of the pathogens (*microsporidium* and *cryptosporidium*), there is no specific treatment: diarrhoea will be controlled by ART and improvement of the CD4 cell level.

In case of bloody diarrhoea (large-bowel infection with *shigella* or *Clostridium* difficile), loperamide (Imodium) is absolutely contraindicated: this drug causes bacterial stasis with risk of septicaemia.

Coughing with white sputum and progressive, severe dyspnoea on effort

Patients with CD4 cells around or below 200 cells/μl are at risk to develop PCP, especially if they are not on TMP-SMX (also known as Bactrim, cotromoxazole or Septra) prophylaxis.

Symptoms of PCP develop over two to three weeks. They are suggestive, but not specific: miliary TB and atypical pneumonia (caused by *Mycoplasma pneumonia* and *Chlamydia*) may give similar clinical pictures and must be excluded. The patient must be referred.

Patients presenting with a persistent cough and white sputum, progressive dyspnoea on effort and negative gene Xpert test must be referred for chest X-rays, diagnosis and a treatment opinion.

Treatment of PCP includes a high dose of TMP-SMX for three weeks, followed by secondary prophylaxis.

Effectiveness of antiretroviral treatment

HIV can never be cured, but viral suppression is possible. The first six months of treatment may not elicit the same biological response or effect in all patients on ART.

The following outcomes can be observed to guide further therapeutic decisions:
- *Full responders* have an undetectable HIV1 viral load and a significant increase in CD4 cells (above 50 cells/μl). These patients are considered to be virological and immunological responders (full responders).
- *First-line failure* occurs in patients who have a detectable viral load, confirmed at two-month intervals, and no significant increase in CD4 cells. In these patients, the first line has failed, and they must move to the second line.

▶ *Virological-only responders* have an undetectable viral load but no significant increase in CD4 cells. In these cases, the viral load is undetectable and treatment is not modified.

▶ *Immunological-only responders* (a small group) show a significant increase in CD4 cells despite a confirmed, detectable viral load. In these unclear cases, second-line treatment is prescribed.

Very-low-level viremia (VLLV) is a relatively new concept in the realm of HIV care. A delayed increase in CD4 cells in spite of an undetectable viral load at six months is common. The increase may take years. In some patients initiated on ART with an undetectable viral load, the CD4 cells fail to increase, for unknown reasons (Helou et al, 2017). However, the low CD4 status may increase the risk for developing opportunistic infections, cardiac disease, liver problems and cancers.

Although HIV and TB are discussed in the following sections as separate conditions, it is important to consider that a high percentage of pregnant women who are HIV positive have TB as a co-infection and, as such, are at risk for complications.

50.3 HIV in pregnancy, intrapartum and postpartum

The national DoH subscribes to all international programmes to reduce maternal mortality, including the reduction of HIV in pregnancy.

Programmes and interventions to reduce HIV in obstetrics

The national DoH's interventions regarding the Campaign on Accelerated Reduction of Maternal and Child Mortality in Africa (CARMMA), aimed at reducing maternal and infant deaths, focus mainly on PHC at district level (DoH, nd). The interventions include the following indicators:

▶ *Maternal:*
  • An increase in early access of antenatal care, before 20 weeks of pregnancy
  • Universal testing
  • The initiation of ART treatment, without delay, for all pregnant women who have tested HIV positive.

continued

▶ *Neonatal:*
  • 100 per cent first PCR testing at six weeks after birth
  • Increased incidence of six-week uptake of treatment for HIV-positive infants.

These targets are reported on a quarterly basis by all districts.

The 90-90-90 strategy to reduce HIV has been adopted as policy in South Africa (HST, 2016):

▶ 90 per cent of all people should know their HIV status.
▶ 90 per cent of those living with HIV will be on ARV treatment.
▶ 90 per cent of those receiving ARV medication will have viral suppression.

Women in general are physiologically three times more likely to be infected by HIV than men if having unprotected sex. The Langerhans cells of the cervix have the CD4 receptor–co-receptor system on the surface of their membranes and may provide a portal of entry for HIV; it has been suggested that some HIV serotypes may have a higher affinity for these. The main mode of infection in women is unprotected sex.

Potential effects of HIV on the outcomes of pregnancy

Although pregnancy itself does not accelerate the progress of HIV, women who do not know their HIV status are at risk for certain effects that HIV can have on a pregnancy. The reported effects of HIV on pregnancy outcomes include:

▶ a tripled risk of spontaneous abortion (WHO & UNAIDS, 1998)
▶ an affected thymus gland (in 29 per cent of fetuses of HIV-positive mothers who aborted, in a study by Kourtis et al [1996]
▶ an increased risk of ectopic pregnancy
▶ an increased risk of syphilis
▶ an increased risk of all infections, including TB
▶ twice the risk of preterm labour
▶ twice the risk of stillbirth
▶ an increased risk of postpartum infections
▶ an increased risk of placental abruption
▶ an overall 35 per cent risk of transmitting the virus to the baby (mother-to-child transmission, or MTCT) if the mother is not treated or on ART
▶ an increased risk of maternal death.

Mother-to-child transmission of HIV and its prevention

The unborn child of an infected mother has the potential to be the unprotected, silent victim in the HIV pandemic. It is essential to protect the unborn child from contracting the condition.

Prevention

The main method of preventing transmission of the virus to babies is to identify the HIV status of all pregnant women and start treatment for HIV-infected women, according to DoH protocols. ARVs and ART are able to prevent the virus from being transmitted via the placenta to the fetus and to prevent HIV progression in the mother.

Risk factors

Not all babies of HIV-positive mothers (who are not on treatment) are equally at risk during pregnancy and breastfeeding to become HIV infected (see Table 50.5). The transmission periods are divided into early transmission *in utero* and the late transmission period, which includes the labour period and the period of infant feeding. In addition, there are modifiable conditions that may increase or decrease the risk (discussed in the next section).

Table 50.5

Risks for MTCT during the phases of pregnancy and childbirth in untreated women (WHO, 2017a)

Period	Factors increasing the risk for MTCT	Best-practice prevention	Reduced risk with ARV
Early transmission (in pregnancy)			
The risk for transmission is present from eight weeks *in utero*.	The virus is present in the fetus within 48 hours after infection.	Perform universal testing. In South Africa, the fixed-dose treatment is started as soon as diagnosis is made, irrespective of CD4.	Highly effective if compliant with treatment
Late transmission (during labour and breastfeeding)			
In labour 50% of babies are negative at birth if the mother is not treated with ARVs.	The virus is present after 7–90 days in case of vaginal birth if the baby was not infected during pregnancy. Rupture of membranes more than four hours before birth increases the risk of infection from the mother. The first-born twin has twice the risk of acquiring the virus. The risk is increased in premature labour and antepartum haemorrhage (APH).	Caesarean section is an option *only if it is safe* and mainly in private healthcare. Avoid rupture of membranes. Intervene four hours after rupture of membranes. Avoid interventions such as induction of labour (IOL) and performing an episiotomy.	Caesarean section reduces the risk if done under safe conditions.
Breastfeeding Increased risk after three months of breastfeeding. 5% increased risk with mixed feeding for each additional six months of feeding. Double risk after 18 months of breastfeeding.	The virus is present in the cellular and cell-free portions of breast milk. The risk is increased with the volume of breast milk taken by the baby, a high maternal viral load and oral thrush and breast infections. Premature infants have an increased risk for infection.	Exclusive breastfeeding (EBF) for six months with no mixing of feeds prevents HIV in the newborn. Replacement feeding (bottle) is the best practice only where conditions are optimal. A lack of clean water would make breastfeeding a safer option.	100% reduced rist with total replacement feeding.

Modifiable factors

There are a variety of modifiable conditions that can have an influence on the risk of transmitting the virus, or which may reduce the risk. Besides ART, women should also be examined for these risk factors and advised on behaviour and practices to reduce the risk. The risk factors could then be reduced through modifying behaviour or practices, for example a low CD4 count can improve if the woman is on ART and practises good nutrition.

Other modifiable risks and modifying behaviour or practices include the following:

- ART should be given for all HIV-positive women.
- ART should be given to all HIV-positive women who breastfeed.
- Supplement with vitamin A if the woman is deficient, to reduce risks.
- The woman should discontinue smoking or using recreational drugs.
- The woman should practice protected sex even when on ART. An HIV-positive woman can be re-infected through unprotected sex with an HIV-infected person.
- Vaginal infections need to be treated to reduce the risks associated with amnionitis and placental infection.
- The risk of fetal trauma during birth needs to be minimised, as it can cause transmission, mainly in vaginal birth.
- Prematurity carries an increased risk due to the baby's immature skin and defence mechanisms. Refer for specialised paediatric care.

Prevention of mother-to-child transmission: best practice

Global best practices to improve health outcomes of HIV-positive pregnant women in obstetrics have resulted in achieving less than 2 per cent MTCT (Paintsil & Andiman, 2009). This includes:
- universal testing of all pregnant women
- ARV triple therapy when diagnosed, preferably before 14 weeks
- safe delivery practices for HIV-infected women (DoH, 2015d)
- replacement feeding (bottle).

continued

These best practice guidelines are difficult to institute in some settings due to the unavailability of safe Caesarean sections and the lack of clean running water. The 90-90-90 strategy in South Africa will allow for improvement if all women can be identified and treated during pregnancy.

Adherence

Factors that may affect adherence and poor health outcomes when on ART include the following:

- A high prevalence in a community may have a discriminatory effect; communities may deny and hide the condition. Some communities do not acknowledge or talk about HIV. Adherence is affected.
- The local views on testing and subsequent discrimination may influence the choices women make, particularly around infant feeding. Bottle feeding may increase the risk of disclosure of HIV status in the community.
- Services and resources are more available in urban areas than rural areas.
- Rural areas may not have clean running water, putting babies at risk if not breastfed.
- The availability of investigations and laboratories may cause a delay in diagnosis and treatment.
- The unavailability and inconsistent supply of ARVs or stock-outs put women and babies at risk.
- Decisions around feeding will be influenced by the availability of safe water supplies and affordability.
- The side effects of the medication may cause lack of adherence. Also, when a person starts to feel better, he or she may stop adhering to the treatment.

Midwifery, HIV and antiretroviral therapy (prevention of mother-to-child transmission)

Midwives are the first point of contact for many women and are the healthcare professionals who will care for many women during childbirth. This means that a midwife may be the provider to diagnose HIV, initiate and monitor ARVs, and identify complications and comorbidities such as TB.

HIV counselling and testing

All pregnant women should know their status. Pregnant women must be advised to be tested at any point of contact during pregnancy, from the labour ward to the postnatal period and beyond. Those who are counselled and tested for HIV must give informed consent for such testing and be informed of their right to decline testing before the procedure. (Consult the current *Guidelines for Maternity Care in South Africa* [DoH, 2015a]).

It was found in 2012 that 2.4 per cent of women who initially test HIV negative in early pregnancy in South Africa test HIV positive after six to 12 months (Bhowan et al, 2012). This shows the need for regular testing during pregnancy.

Sexual partners of HIV-negative pregnant women should also be tested so that they can be linked to care if found to be positive. This can prevent new infections in pregnancy and realted health risks.

HIV and antiretroviral therapy in obstetrics

Table 50.6 gives a list of ARV drugs used during pregnancy in cases of HIV/AIDS. Not all available ART combination therapies are safe for use in pregnancy (see Table 50.4 on page 789 and Table 50.6).

The triple FDC tablet has been given to pregnant women in South Africa since 2013 to simplify the first-line therapy. It contains 300 mg TDF, 200 mg FTC and 600 mg EFV in one tablet. Occasionally, women may have a contraindication for one of the components; they will then be referred for medical consultation and the regimen changed. Women stable on treatment regimens prior to 2013 may remain on their original regimes used in pregnancy.

Table 50.6

ARV drugs for use in pregnancy in South Africa (see Chapter 53 for classification of risks)

Drug	Health risks
NRTIs	
Zidovudine (ZDV, AZT)	High risk of anaemia neutropenia Moderate risk of symptomatic hyperlactataemia
FTC	Mild or severe headache, diarrhoea, nausea and rash
ABC	Discontinue if there is fever, pruritis, abdominal pain, sore throat after each dose (ABC allergy; never to be re-challenged)
3TC	Rare risks include peripheral neuropathy, gastrointestinal (GI) tract effects, headaches and other
TDF	Nephrotoxic (no TDF if creatinine above 85 µmol/ℓ in pregnant women)
NNRTIs	
NVP	Rash and acute hepatitis that can be life-threatening Contraindicated if the baseline CD4 > 250 cells/µl
EFV	Teratogenic with CNS effects (this potential toxic effect seems to have been overestimated and EFV is now prescribed to pregnant women irrespective of the stage of pregnancy) Other effects: insomnia, dreams, depression, nausea, gynaecomastia, increased liver enzymes
PIs	
LPV/r	GI tract effects (diarrhoea)

HIV, antiretroviral therapy and antenatal management

The FDC policy has improved stock management, adherence, efficacy and health outcomes due to the reduced risk of misunderstanding and dispensing errors.

The following aspects of practice need consideration:

- ▶ *Level of care:* HIV care is not part of basic antenatal care (BANC). Nurses and midwives should be trained in nurse-initiated management of antiretroviral therapy (NIMART) to care for women in pregnancy.
- ▶ *Counselling and testing:* At the first visit, all women are routinely counselled and tested.

Tests to be done at the first antenatal visit
▶ Hb and Rh
▶ Syphilis tests
▶ HIV staging
▶ Clinical screening for TB and STIs
▶ Clinical and laboratory screening for renal disease, including serum creatinine
▶ Screening for active psychiatric illness
▶ Initiation of ARV treatment
▶ Viral load testing if already on ART.

Initiation of treatment for HIV-positive cases

All women who test positive or have previously tested positive and are not on ART are started on FDC *on the same day* at the first antenatal visit, unless contraindicated (history of psychiatric illness or renal disease or symptoms of TB):

▶ *Renal disease.* FDC is contraindicated because TDF is nephrotoxic. Women with renal disease (serum creatinine > 85/µmol/ℓ) are managed by a medical practitioner at a high-risk clinic and delivered in a hospital. HIV-associated nephropathy is related to a low CD4 count and needs special investigations. The medical team will decide on a non-TDF ART regimen.

▶ *Active psychiatric disease.* FDC is contraindicated in active psychiatric cases because EFV has CNS effects. The woman is referred for medical care and placed on a non-EFV ART regime.

▶ *TB.* All pregnant women – regardless of their HIV status – presenting for routine care at clinics and labour wards should be screened for symptoms of active TB and should be asked to provide a sputum specimen for smear microscopy, mycobacterial culture and drug-susceptibility testing (Gounder et al, 2011). See page 790 for the symptoms of TB.

One week follow-up, staging and treatment

HIV-positive women should return one week after their initial antenatal visit for follow-up of their creatinine and CD4 cell count results and be staged and managed accordingly:

▶ *Serum creatinine:*
  • If > 85µmol/ℓ: Refer for change of regimen
  • If < 85µmol/ℓ: Staging and CD4
▶ *CD4 count:* All HIV-positive women are on ART for life, regardless.

Monitoring

▶ *HIV-negative women.* HIV counselling and testing (HCT) is repeated for all pregnant and breastfeeding women whose HIV status is negative. Thereafter it is repeated every three months throughout pregnancy.

▶ *Unbooked women admitted to give birth or who have given birth, with a unknown HIV status:* An HIV test is done on admission or directly after birth.

▶ *HIV-positive women on FDC.* A laboratory test of serum creatinine is done at three months, six months and 12 months. If there is any evidence of renal impairment, refer the patient for investigation to determine the cause, and to change from TDF.

▶ *Women on AZT.* These women will have Hb and full blood count (FBC) tests done at one month, two months, three months and six months.

▶ *TB.* Symptom screening for TB should be performed for both HIV-positive and HIV-negative women at every antenatal visit, and on admission to the labour ward.

▶ Viral load follow-up is important.

▶ Continued adherence to ART is monitored.

Health information

▶ Patients should receive a nutritional assessment and be provided with the appropriate nutritional care and support.

▶ Midwives must also consider the modifiable factors and advise women accordingly.

▶ All women are monitored for the side effects of ARVs. Initially, some who switch over may experience new side effects, but this may settle with reassurance. Those who experience severe side effects may be discontinued to a new regimen (eg EFV-associated CNS effects, and TDF-related renal dysfunction).

Intrapartum care and HIV

All women whose HIV status is unknown or who have tested negative before are tested again during labour. The following guidelines should be followed in case of a first-time HIV positive result at the following points in time:

▶ *In labour.* A single dose of the following drugs is given at the onset of labour:
  • NVP 200 mg stat
  • 3TC 300 mg
  • TDF 300 mg
  • AZT 3-hourly.
▶ *If membranes are ruptured for more than four hours.* Augment labour if not in spontaneous labour and give prophylactic antibiotics.

▶ *In case of Caesarean section.* If the woman undergoes a Caesarean section, the ARV regimen for labour is given before the procedure. Prophylactic antibiotics are given for both elective and emergency Caesarean section: cefazolin 1 g IVI when on the operating table prior to the start of surgery, followed by a broad-spectrum antibiotic for three to five days.

Neonatal care

All newborns should receive standard routine neonatal care. This includes skin-to-skin care and being latched to the breast within one hour if the breastfeeding choices have been determined. Thereafter, newborns should be nursed in their own micro-environment.

A neonate is considered to be HIV exposed if the mother's HIV status is known to be positive, she tests positive at birth, is on ARVs or is newly diagnosed. All babies should be considered exposed unless the mother's status is known.

A newborn born to an HIV-positive mother will have a PCR test at birth, at 10 weeks and at 18 months. PCR tests are the only tests that can diagnose HIV in HIV-exposed babies. Consent is needed from parents or guardians before testing of newborns.

PCR test in newborns: The HIV PCR test (PCR DNA)

Testing for certain **symptomatic HIV-exposed infants** is included in the South African *National Consolidated Guidelines for PMTCT and the Management of HIV in Children, Adolescents and Adults* (DoH, 2015d). It requires all babies to have a PCR at **six weeks** (Sherman, 2015). There is evidence that FDC treatment, if used by the mother, and a daily dose of NVP for the newborn may reduce the effectiveness of the PCR test (Sherman, 2015).

Babies who are **tested at birth** include babies who are:
▶ premature and have a low birth weight (LBW) < 2.5 kg
▶ born from mothers who were on TB treatment in pregnancy
▶ born from mothers who have a viral load of more than 1 000 copies/ml
▶ born from mothers who started ARVs four weeks before birth
▶ born from unbooked mothers
▶ born from mothers who have symptoms at birth.

Criteria for testing of infants for HIV (if under 18 months, use PCR; if over 18 months, use rapid test)

▶ Family and social history
▶ Parental request to test the child
▶ A father or sibling with HIV infection
▶ Death of the mother, father or sibling
▶ If the mother's HIV status is unknown, her whereabouts are unknown, or she is unavailable to be tested
▶ All infants/children with clinical features suggestive of HIV infection
▶ Acute, severe illness
▶ Integrated Management of Childhood Illnesses (IMCI) classification of suspected symptomatic HIV infection
▶ IMCI classification of possible HIV infection
▶ TB diagnosis or history of TB treatment
▶ Risk of sexual assault
▶ If the child was nursed or breastfed by an HIV-positive woman or a woman with unknown or HIV status
▶ Children considered for fostering or adoption.

Any baby with a positive PCR should immediately be referred for medical attention:
▶ *At 6–10 weeks.* All HIV-exposed infants are tested at 6–10 weeks (PCR DNA).
▶ *At 16 weeks.* All infants who received 12 weeks NVP prophylaxis are tested at 16 weeks.
▶ *At 18 months.* All HIV-exposed babies are tested at 18 months for HIV. If this period is missed, the test is done at the next best opportunity.

All breastfed babies should be tested six weeks after discontinuing breastfeeding. If positive, repeat PCR at 18 months. If the breastfed infant tests PCR DNA positive, it can be accepted that the virus was transferred through the breast milk and the infant is considered HIV positive.

The PCR HIV test is highly sensitive (98.8 per cent) and specific (99.4 per cent) at six weeks of age (Feucht, Forsyth & Kruger, 2012). It will detect virtually all infections that have occurred *in utero*, during labour, delivery and breastfeeding in infants younger than 18 months. An HIV-exposed but uninfected child will test PCR negative and an HIV-exposed infected child will test PCR positive. There is a possibility of a false negative or indeterminate result, particularly at the six-week PCR test, as the infant has been on NVP prophylaxis.

A negative antibody detection test at any age excludes HIV infection, provided that the infant was last breastfed six or more weeks before the test and has no clinical signs of HIV infection.

Neonatal HIV prophylaxis

HIV-exposed infants must receive ARV prophylaxis immediately after birth.

The ARV prophylactic treatment against HIV is a daily dose of NVP syrup for six weeks, given within 72 hours after birth. The dose is based on the birth weight:

▶ > 2 500 g: 15 mg (1.5 ml)
▶ 1 000–2 500 g: 10 mg (1 ml)
▶ < 1 000 g: start at 2 mg/kg (0.2 ml/kg).
▶ AZT: Consult an expert.

Treatment guidelines

All infants who test HIV positive at any stage are started on ART regardless of clinical staging or CD4 count. Viral load is no longer used as a baseline assessment for ART in children. The following cases are indicated for ART:

▶ All babies of women on ART more than four weeks before delivery must receive NVP at birth and daily for six weeks, irrespective of feeding practice.
▶ If the mother is diagnosed as HIV positive within 72 hours post-delivery or less than four weeks before delivery and if breastfeeding the baby: Give NVP immediately and daily for 12 weeks. This is to cover the 12 weeks needed for maternal viral suppression. If the baby is not breastfeeding, NVP is given for six weeks.
▶ All babies of women on AZT are given NVP treatment until one week after breastfeeding is discontinued
▶ HIV-exposed newborns are given NVP prophylaxis until six weeks if not breastfed.
▶ NVP should be discontinued only when maternal viral suppression has been reached. If a mother who is breastfeeding an infant has been on ART for 12 weeks, NVP is only discontinued when tests prove that viral suppression has been reached.
▶ For non-breastfeeding mothers that are positive, start maternal ART.

Breastfeeding advice

▶ All breastfeeding, HIV-positive women should be on ART, regardless of their CD4 count.
▶ Initiate breastfeeding immediately after delivery, preferably within one hour.
▶ Intensive counselling should be given on the benefits of EBF, the dangers of mixed feeding and the importance of adherence to ART.
▶ EBF should be practised for the first six months.
▶ Complementary (mixed) feeding can be given from six months onwards only.

continued

▶ Encourage breastfeeding:
  • If the infant is HIV negative: Breastfeed until 12 months old.
  • If the infant is HIV positive: Breastfeed until at least two years old.
▶ Women who plan to breastfeed should be initiated on FDC as soon as possible after birth. Request CD4 count and creatinine for all women starting FDC.
▶ HCT is repeated every three months while the woman is breastfeeding.

Mothers with confirmed second- or third-line ART failure should not breastfeed unless exclusive formula feeding will be unsafe for that infant, for example if there are no facilities to sterilise bottles.

Prophylaxis for other infections

Prophylactic treatment against *Pneumocystis jirovecii* and other bacterial infections is given to all babies born to mothers who have tested HIV positive. Treatment is started at four to six weeks with cotrimoxazole syrup. It can be discontinued at one year of age in infants who are well, infants whose HIV screening test is negative or infants who have a negative PCR test six weeks or more after the last breastfeed. Cotrimoxazole syrup is usually given as a 5 ml dose (10 ml after 3 months) on 3 days of the week (Monday, Wednesday and Friday). PCP prohylaxis, as a suspension, is prescribed by a paediatrician.

Cotrimoxazole prophylaxis

The recommended dose of cotrimoxazole for a newborn is weight-related:

▶ below 5 kg: 5 ml
▶ 5–9.9 kg: 7.5 ml
▶ 10–19.9 kg: 10 ml
▶ from 20 kg: 20 ml.

The treatment is recommended from six to eight weeks of age due to the risk of adverse side effects.

Infant feeding

Infant feeding should be discussed with all mothers; HIV-positive mothers need specific advice on their infant feeding choices. Types of feeding methods for newborns include the following:

▶ *Exclusive breastfeeding for six months*. This is the recommended best practice and means that the infant receives only breast milk from the mother, or expressed breast milk from the mother, and no other liquids.

(Mother's milk can be flash-pasteurised; see the procedure in the box below.) Babies under 2 kg may receive mother's milk from a donor milk bank (DMB).

▶ *Mixed feeding.* Most studies show that non-exclusive (mixed) breastfeeding increases the likelihood of HIV transmission significantly more than in the case of EBF (Coovadia et al, 2007).

▶ *Introduction of solids.* No solids are introduced in the first six months, with the exception of drops or syrups consisting of vitamins, mineral supplements or medicines.

▶ *Additional fluid.* The infant's predominant source of nourishment is breast milk. However, if the infant is also given water or water-based drinks, oral rehydration salts (ORS), drops and syrup forms of vitamins, minerals and medicines and traditional remedies or fluids (in limited quantities), this is referred to as mixed feeding. Giving the baby some breastfeeds and some artificial feeds, such as milk or cereal, is not ideal and puts the baby at risk.

▶ *Replacement feeding.* Replacement or bottle feeding is the process of feeding a child who is not receiving breast milk with other milk suitable for infants. The midwife needs to take the woman's lifestyle and choices into account and respect these while counselling the woman on the best possible options for her and her infant.

▶ *Breast milk substitutes.* These are any substance (infant formula) for partial or total replacement of breast milk. It is essential that midwives are familiar with suitable and safe products for newborns.

PROCEDURE Flash pasteurisation of breast milk

Definition
Flash pasteurisation is a method of pasteurising expressed breast milk. It is an option for safe infant feeding for HIV-positive women and babies. Flash pasteurisation has been tested and is reliable under a range of conditions. The virus is eliminated. This is a cheap and easy way to pasteurise breast milk for the HIV-positive mother if not fully viral-suppressed.

Indication
Women who are HIV positive and:
▶ want to breastfeed
▶ are not in a position to afford artificial feeding
▶ do not have access to safe drinking water – a situation which would put the baby more at risk.

Principles
Without specific interventions, HIV-infected women will pass the virus to their infants during pregnancy or delivery in about 15–25 per cent of cases, and an additional 5–20 per cent of infants may become infected postnatally during breastfeeding, for an overall risk of 30–45 per cent (WHO, 2007).

In South Africa, infants who received both breast milk and other feeds were significantly more likely to be infected by 15 months of age (36 per cent) than those who had been exclusively breastfed (25 per cent) or formula-fed (19 per cent) (WHO, 2004c). EBF carried a significantly lower risk of HIV infection than mixed breastfeeding.

This is a particularly important procedure if mixed feeding is started. The principles of cleanliness must be observed.

Procedure (Chantry et al, 2012)
Written information is provided and the procedure is demonstrated to the mother, helpers and family.
1 Hands are washed.
2 Breast milk is expressed into a clean glass jar.
3 The glass jar containing the milk is placed in a pan with water two finger-widths above the level of the milk.
4 The water is brought to the boil on a high heat source. (It typically reaches a temperature of 72.9 °C.)
5 The milk is cooled and fed to the baby with a syringe or cup.

Bacteriologic, virologic, immunologic and nutritional studies have indicated that this can be a safe feeding method.

Recording and interpretation
Record the intervention and advice given to the mother on the mother-and-baby document for follow-up.

Actions
Refer the mother to the nearest clinic and home-based care team for follow-up.

Immunisation

Newborns of HIV-positive mothers and babies testing positive for HIV should receive all the usual immunisations on the expanded programme on immunisation (EPI). However, the following exceptions apply:

▶ *The Bacilli Calmetti-Guérin vaccine (BCG).* Infants of mothers who have TB do not get the BCG.
▶ *Measles.* If the burden of measles is high, measles vaccination at six months of age is likely to benefit children of HIV-infected women, regardless of the child's HIV infection status.
▶ *HCT* is repeated at the six-week visit for the EPI.

Postpartum care

The routine postpartum care of HIV-positive women should be similar to that of uninfected patients. They do not require separate nursing facilities. However, HIV-positive women are more prone to postpartum infectious complications, including infections of the urinary tract, chest, episiotomy and Caesarean section wounds. Midwives should be aware of this and observe for signs of infection.

Considerations for postpartum care of HIV-positive women

HIV-positive women should receive infection prophylaxis and be discharged with appropriate treatment and advice after birth. Mothers should be given information on the early symptoms of infection at the time of discharge, especially where the postpartum hospital stay is short. Mothers should also be given instructions on strict perineal care and the safe handling of lochia and blood-stained sanitary pads or materials.

Information should be given on how to care for the baby without the risk of exposure to infection, and there should be a detailed discussion on the risks and benefits of infant feeding choices. If, after counselling, the mother chooses not to breastfeed, she should receive full information on suppression of breast milk, adequate replacement feeding up to two years of age and guidance on breast care until lactation stops. Safe bottle feeding must be explained. Mothers who choose to breastfeed should be advised of the possible increased transmission risk in the case of cracked nipples, mastitis, breast abscesses or oral lesions in the child and should be taught how to prevent such problems through adequate breastfeeding techniques. A reduced duration of breastfeeding and early cessation may be encouraged to reduce the risk of transmission, where this can be achieved safely.

The importance of continuing with ART and adhering to the treatment should be emphasised, as well as the necessity for a follow-up of viral load.

Counsel the mother on the need for follow-up care for her and her child, and the available options for testing the child. She should be given information about and referred to a local HIV support group.

Contraceptive advice should be given and early arrangements made to start with an appropriate method. Contraceptive advice is particularly important if the mother does not breastfeed, because of the loss of the contraceptive properties of breastfeeding. Special consideration is given to the interaction between contraceptives and ARVs.

50.4 TB in pregnancy

The WHO reported that, globally, 10.4 million people fell ill and suffered from TB in 2015 (WHO, 2016b). TB is one of the top three causes of death for women between 15 and 44 years of age. The BRICS countries (Brazil, Russia, India, China and South Africa) account for 50 per cent of cases in the world (Cresswell et al, 2014).

TB remains a major health problem in South Africa. TB and MDR-TB are leading causes of premature mortality in South Africa, where TB has the second highest incidence (TBFacts.org, 2017a). The District Health Barometer (DHB) for 2014/15 indicated a variation of 238–1 127 per 100 000 (average 593) of the population diagnosed per annum (Massyn et al, 2015).

When co-infected with HIV, TB causes more than half of the maternal deaths in HIV-positive women in South Africa (DoH, 2014). It is therefore important that all pregnant women be tested and given care for TB in pregnancy alongside HIV care. This chapter provides general information on the causes, care and outcomes of TB as applied to the pregnant woman and her baby. The risks of co-infection with HIV are also considered due to the increased risk of adverse outcomes.

The history of TB

TB dates back as far as ancient Egypt (it has been found in mummies) and spread through epidemics in Europe and North America in the 18th and 19th centuries. The causative bacterium was discovered in 1882 and a vaccine was subsequently developed. In 1993, the WHO declared TB a global emergency.

Causative organism

TB is caused by *Mycobacterium tuberculosis* (Koch's bacillus). This infectious disease is transmitted by sputum and spreads rapidly in congested, unhygienic conditions. It is rarely transferred across the placenta.

Pathology

TB is an extremely debilitating disease. Pregnancy does not adversely affect the course and prognosis of the disease, but if untreated, it poses a threat to the mother's health, her life and the life of the fetus. *If a woman is TB co-infected with HIV, the risk for complications increases even when on treatment.*

Principles of antenatal care

▶ All women are routinely screened for HIV and TB antenatally and referred for high-risk care.
▶ Treatment regimens are prescribed by a medical practitioner.
▶ Treatment adherence is followed up with direct observation treatment short-course (DOTS).
▶ Special care is taken to check and treat for anaemia to reduce the risks associated with anaemia, such as abruption placenta.
▶ A hospital delivery is planned and an assisted delivery is recommended to reduce the risk of the strain of delivery.

Signs and symptoms

The symptoms of TB may include:
▶ weight loss
▶ haemoptysis
▶ a low-grade fever
▶ general malaise
▶ chest pain.

Diagnosis

A history must be taken, including:
▶ any family history of TB cases
▶ any history of HIV-positive status
▶ symptoms (four-system screening)
▶ the clinical picture (pulmonary and extra-pulmonary).

Collect sputum for sputum investigations; collect two samples and send to the laboratory. Meyer et al (2017) found that salivary sputum does not have a lower diagnostic yield (in fact, it may have a higher yield) when testing for TB with Xpert. This may have great clinical importance. In contrast, blood-stained sputum appears less desirable for Xpert testing in smear-negative populations. If the patient is symptomatic, two sputum samples must be sent for culture.

> ### GeneXpert MBT
>
> The GeneXpert was approved by the WHO in 2010, with a recommendation that this test be done at the initial diagnosis of HIV-associated TB and MDR-TB (TBfacts.org, 2017b).
>
> Within two hours, the GeneXpert test performed on a sputum sample gives two pieces of information:
> 1 If the TB mycobacterium gene is present or absent
> 2 If the gene is present, the test can also detect mutations associated with resistance to the drugs rifampicin and INH.
>
> Because the sensitivity of the GeneXpert test is proven in approximately 70 per cent (not 100 per cent) of cases for pulmonary TB affecting HIV-positive patients (TBfacts.org, 2017b), a negative test does not exclude the diagnosis of pulmonary tuberculosis (PTB).

X-rays (of the chest in cases of lung tuberculosis) should only be done if the diagnosis is strongly suspected, and the fetus must be protected by a lead apron during the X-ray. Once diagnosed, the family and immediate household must be fully investigated and treated if they have the disease.

Pleural or extra-pulmonary TB

Pleural/extra-pulmonary TB, with or without associated pulmonary involvement, is frequently present in AIDS patients. Diagnosis is more difficult. Coughing is absent if there is no involvement of the lungs or the pleura. Repeated sputa investigations remain negative if there is no communication between the TB lesions and the air pipe, causing a delayed diagnosis.

The symptoms of pleural/extra-pulmonary TB depend on the structure involved:
▶ Swollen lymph nodes with possible fistulisation (TB of lymph nodes)
▶ Headaches, confusion, fits (TB meningitis)
▶ Exudative lymphocytic ascites (TB of the peritoneum)
▶ Persistent dysuria with sterile pyuria on standard culture (TB of the urinary tract)
▶ Persistent diarrhoea with right iliac fossa mass (TB of the small intestine).

Prevention of TB in HIV-positive women

The importance of effective primary and secondary prophylaxis includes the efficient prevention of infections with low-cost drugs (IPT 300 mg/d plus pyridoxine 25 mg/d) that prevent the development of active TB, and is *not contraindicated in pregnancy* (Salam, Zuberi & Bhutta, 2015).

Guidelines for isoniazid preventive therapy

If the four symptoms of TB screening are negative, the probability of active TB is very low and IPT can be started without further investigation. A regimen of IPT (isoniazid 5 mg/kg daily to a maximum of 300 mg daily and pyridoxine 25 mg daily) for a 12-month period reduces the incidence of TB in all people living with HIV, including those on ART.

All HIV-positive pregnant women who screen negative for TB are eligible for IPT.

If a tuberculin test has been done and is positive for a pregnant woman on lifelong ART, the duration of IPT can be extended for 36 months.

The adverse effects of isoniazid include:
▶ liver injury
▶ jaundice
▶ right upper quadrant pain or tenderness
▶ nausea and vomiting
▶ skin rash
▶ peripheral neuropathy (numbness and/or tingling of the feet); pyridoxine is always given with INH in HIV-positive patients because their risk for developing INH-induced peripheral neuropathy is higher than in HIV-negative patients.

If only one of the four TB screening symptoms is positive, IPT must be postponed and the reason for the symptom(s) must be investigated. Often it will be active TB (pulmonary or pleural/extra-pulmonary), but other causes are possible and must be excluded.

During and after IPT, TB screening must be repeated at each visit and the patient's weight, a sensitive test for early identification of new clinical events, must be accurately recorded.

Treatment for TB in pregnancy

In the *Saving Mothers 2011–2013* report, 92 per cent of women who died from TB were HIV positive, and 55.2 per cent of these were on ART (DoH, 2014: 29).

Untreated TB represents a far greater hazard to a pregnant woman and the fetus than the treatment of the disease. It is important to know if a woman is pregnant before starting ART or TB treatment. The aim of the treatment is to make the sputum negative by the time the baby is born. All the standard first-line TB drugs are safe during pregnancy.

If the diagnosis of active TB is confirmed or probable, TB treatment based on the four standard drugs (rifampicin, INH, pyrazinamide and ethambutol) must be started, given for two

months (intensive phase), followed by four months of the continuation phase based on two drugs (rifampicin plus INH).

For pleural/extra-pulmonary TB and in cases of TB meningitis, TB of the bones or joints or miliary TB, the continuation phase is extended to seven months. The dose of anti-TB drugs is adjusted according to weight when changing to the continuation phase.

The principles of treatment are as follows:
▶ ART is not started if TB symptoms are present.
▶ AZT monotherapy should be started at the same time as TB treatment, and changed to FDC two weeks later.
▶ Steroids should also be given until ART is started.
▶ If a TB diagnosis is delayed, find out from a referral centre when to start FDC in the absence of TB treatment.
▶ The use of streptomycin (a category D substance) is avoided in pregnancy, as it is ototoxic and may damage the eighth cranial nerve, leading to deafness of the fetus. It is only given when the benefits outweigh the risks.
▶ Rifampicin is used in spite of the risks because of its effectiveness in treating TB.

Outcomes of TB infections

In general, almost all cases of TB can be cured with proper treatment, adherence and support. The DOTS or TB-DOTS is a WHO strategy to effectively stop the spread of TB in communities with a high incidence of infection. It includes direct observation by a healthcare worker for six to nine months or observation with support from a community worker for a further two years, which includes drug supply support, record keeping and reporting of the progress and outcomes.

Complications of TB for maternal health outcomes

Maternal complications are debilitating and life-threatening and include:
▶ a high incidence and risk of mortality
▶ the development of drug-resistant TB if treatment is not adhered to.

Obstetric complications of untreated TB include:
▶ miscarriage
▶ stillbirth
▶ rupture of membranes before 32 weeks of pregnancy
▶ intrauterine growth restriction (IUGR)
▶ LBW
▶ maternal and perinatal mortality.

Treatment for the newborn

A baby born to a mother who has been diagnosed with TB in the last two months of pregnancy or who has a documented smear conversion needs to be carefully managed:

▶ The baby should **not** receive BCG at birth.
▶ If the baby is asymptomatic, INH prophylaxis isoniazid (10 mg/kg/day) is given for six months.
▶ If the baby continues to be asymptomatic, the BCG is administered after completion of the preventive treatment to protect the baby against TB meningitis (unless the child is HIV infected or has symptoms suggestive of HIV infection).
▶ If the baby is symptomatic, the baby should be referred to a hospital for evaluation to exclude TB.
▶ If the baby has TB, the baby is referred for medical care and should receive a full course of TB treatment.

Breastfeeding and women with TB

A woman who is breastfeeding and has TB should receive the standard TB treatment regimen. The breast milk is not infected and breastfeeding should be encouraged. Proper and timely applied chemotherapy is the best way to prevent transmission of the tubercle bacilli to the baby. All the TB drugs are compatible with breastfeeding. An HIV-positive mother should be counselled about exclusive feeding options (EBF or exclusive formula feeding). Although anti-TB drugs are secreted in breast milk, the concentrations are very low and do not affect the baby. However, the concentrations are also too low to protect the baby.

Complications for the newborn

Postnatal risks include the following:

▶ Long-term health complications could present in any organ of the body in childhood, for example a brain abscess, which has a high mortality if the mother and baby are not treated.
▶ Newborn congenital TB, which presents 24 days after birth, is a risk. The signs and symptoms include all cases of fever, irritability, failure to thrive, cough and respiratory distress in 90 per cent of cases, hepatosplenomegaly, abdominal distension, lymadenopathy, meningitis, septicaemia, disseminated intravascular coagulation (DIC), abscesses or other symptoms.

Multi-drug-resistant TB

In South Africa, there has been an increase in multi-drup-resistant TB (MDR-TB). In 2012, 1 596 cases were diagnosed and in 2014 there were 11 500 patients on treatment (TBfacts.org, 2017c).

MDR-TB is defined as TB disease caused by strains of *Mycobacterium tuberculosis* that are resistant to both rifampicin and isoniazid, with or without resistance to other drugs. MDR-TB is a laboratory diagnosis made only by TB culture and drug susceptibility in a patient with proven TB who is not improving clinically. One positive culture with resistances to rifampicin and isoniazid is diagnosed as MDR-TB. A laboratory result that is not consistent with the clinical picture should be repeated if necessary.

Extreme drug-resistant TB (XDR-TB) refers to resistance *in vitro* to isoniazid and rifampicin and/or any of the fluoroquinolones and one or more of the second-line injectable drugs (capreomycin, kanamycin, amikacin). The diagnosis of XDR-TB is a laboratory diagnosis made through second-line drug susceptibility testing (DST).

Until recently, patients with MDR-TB were automatically referred to the MDR-TB unit. The new policy is not only to decentralise treatment of drug-resistant TB, involving nursing professionals and doctors at PHC level, but also to promote shorter regimens (9–12 months instead of 18–24). To be eligible for the shorter MDR-TB regimen, patients must fulfil strict criteria (WHO, 2016d):

▶ They have never been exposed to second-line anti-TB drugs.
▶ Resistance to fluoroquinolones is absent or unlikely.
▶ Resistance to second-line injectable anti-TB drugs is absent or unlikely.

Those who develop MDR-TB are referred for medical care and clinicians need to change the therapy, following the guidelines. All the general principles for HIV and TB care as reflected in the guidelines and in sections 50.2 and 50.4 apply.

According to studies done in Malawi and Bangladesh (WHO 2016c), a shorter MDR-TB regimen gives better results (rate of patients cured/rate of loss to follow-up) than the extended standard regimen. It also decreases the pressure on health facilities.

The diagnosis, treatment and monitoring of the different types of drug-resistant TB are outside the scope of this textbook. Practical, useful information can be found about the standard MDR management at PHC level in the new edition of *Adult Primary Care* 2016/2017 (DoH, 2016/17: 60–65). The shorter regimen of MDR is not addressed in that document.

50.5 Conclusion

Midwives in the public sector will be involved in the roll-out of ART for women and their babies and the assessment of women for TB according to the HIV and TB policy guidelines and regulations of the national DoH. Because clinical and health practice guidelines change, healthcare professionals need to remain up to date with new guidelines to ensure improved quality and safety and effective healthcare.

Section Ten

Nutrition

Nutrition in pregnancy, birth and lactation

LEARNING OBJECTIVES

On completion of this chapter, you must be able to:

▶ demonstrate knowledge of the requirements of human nutrition in pregnancy and birth

▶ develop skills to assess nutritional risk factors in pregnancy and birth

▶ demonstrate competence in assessing the nutritional status of a pregnant or lactating woman

▶ give culturally appropriate advice on nutrition to a pregnant or lactating woman.

KNOWLEDGE ASSUMED TO BE IN PLACE

The basic anatomy and physiology of human nutrition

KEY WORDS

nutritional supplementation • micronutrients • vitamins • minerals • basal metabolic rate (BMR) • recommended dietary allowances (RDAs)

51.1   Introduction

Nutrition influences health from the beginning of conception and plays an important role in the reproductive ability, lactation and healthcare outcomes of women and infants. The nutrition received during sensitive and critical growth periods can influence normal growth and childhood development. Nutrition can influence physical and mental status, immunology and general well-being.

Nutrition is regionally and culturally based, carries an emotional value and is associated with satisfaction, love and community. However, food can be non-nutritional and even harmful.

In general, women have specific nutritional needs during pregnancy and lactation, needs which may be aggravated by factors such as teenage pregnancy, anaemia, dietary preference such as a vegetarian diet, and diseases such as hypertension, cardiac disease, diabetes and HIV/AIDS.

This chapter aims to give an overview of the physiological basis for nutrition in pregnancy and lactation from a scientific point of view. The basic nutritional requirements and supplementation during pregnancy are considered, as well as special nutritional concerns in pregnancy.

51.2   Nutrition-related physiology of pregnancy

From the time of conception and throughout pregnancy, anatomical and physiological changes occur in the mother's body to support, protect and nourish the developing fetus and to prepare the mother for delivery and lactation. The growing fetus depends entirely on the mother, not only to meet every need during pregnancy, but also to lay down metabolic stores such as iron, subcutaneous fat and glycogen, which are needed in the early neonatal period.

The assessment of maternal and fetal well-being includes taking a history as well as physically assessing the growth and development of the pregnancy; indirectly, this assessment includes an assessment of the fetus, because by assessing weight gain, fetal growth may be established.

Weight gain in pregnancy

Weight gain during pregnancy results from maternal anatomical and physiological changes and the growth of the fetus. Failure to achieve an adequate weight gain during pregnancy is associated with increased perinatal morbidity and mortality. Fetal growth may be compromised, resulting in preterm delivery and low birth weight (LBW), both of which have long-term consequences for the infant.

Weight gain during pregnancy varies widely. Previously, the recommended weight gain during a healthy term pregnancy was approximately 25 per cent of the pre-pregnancy weight, or 12.5 kg for a normal weight woman. It is now widely accepted that both underweight and overweight mothers are more at risk of complications than mothers who are in the normal weight range. The most recent recommendations for weight gain in pregnancy are based on the mother's pre-pregnancy body mass index (BMI). The BMI is calculated as mass (kg) divided by height (m^2) and is used as an indicator of whether or not a person has a healthy or unhealthy weight. A mother who is underweight (BMI < 18.5 kg/m^2) should gain more weight than a mother whose pre-pregnancy BMI is in the normal range (18.5 to 24.9 kg/m^2). In contrast, a mother who

is overweight (BMI = 25 to 29.9 kg/m^2) or obese (BMI > 30 kg/m^2) should gain less weight than a mother in the normal weight range.

The WHO and the South African Basic Antenatal Care (BANC) programme recommend that weight and height be measured at the first visit, with referral of underweight, overweight and obese women (see Chapter 16). The measurement of mid-upper-arm circumference (MUAC) is recommended as a simple way of monitoring weight gain during pregnancy for mothers of normal weight (see chapters 17 and 18). Since MUAC does not normally change during pregnancy, a decrease or increase could indicate the risk of inadequate or excessive weight gain.

Table 51.1 shows the ranges and rate of weight gain according to the BMI and MUAC classifications. (Also see the discussion on MUAC in chapters 17 and 18.)

Table 51.1

Recommendations for total and rate of weight gain during pregnancy according to pre-pregnancy BMI and MUAC (Rasmussen & Yaktine, 2009)

Pre-pregnancy BMI	Classification	Total weight gain range (kg)	Rate of weight gain: second and third trimester (kg/week)	MUAC (cm)
< 18.5 kg/m^2	Underweight	12.5–18	0.4–0.6	< 23
18.5–24.9 kg/m^2	Normal weight	11.5–16	0.35–0.5	23–33
25.0–29.9 kg/m^2	Overweight	7–11.5	0.2–0.3	> 33
≥ 30 kg/m^2	Obese	5–9	0.2–0.3	

Weight gain during the first trimester is low (1–1.5 kg). The rate of weight gain increases gradually during the second and third trimester to approximately 0.5 kg/m^2 per week, but slows towards term. The critical period of weight gain is the third trimester, when the fetus undergoes accelerated growth.

Weight measurement in pregnancy

In the public sector in South Africa, the BANC programme does weight screening at the first visit and thin or obese women are referred. No further routine weight screening is done except for the MUAC to identify risks.

The distribution of weight gain during pregnancy, as shown in Figure 51.1, are as follows:
- The fetus, placenta and amniotic fluid account for slightly less than half of the total weight gain.

- The deposition of fat and protein stores account for approximately one-third of the weight gain.
- The increase in size of the breasts, uterus and other maternal tissues account for one-fifth of the weight gain.
- The remainder of the weight gain is due to increased blood volume, fluid and electrolyte changes.

The weight gain of under- and overweight or obese mothers must be monitored throughout pregnancy. Weight may be plotted on a chart showing weight gain according to pre-pregnancy weight and month of gestation. Weight gain charts provide a quick way of ascertaining whether the mother's weight gain is optimal (see Figure 51.2 on page 810). Guidelines for monitoring weight gain are given on the next page. (Also see chapters 17 and 18.)

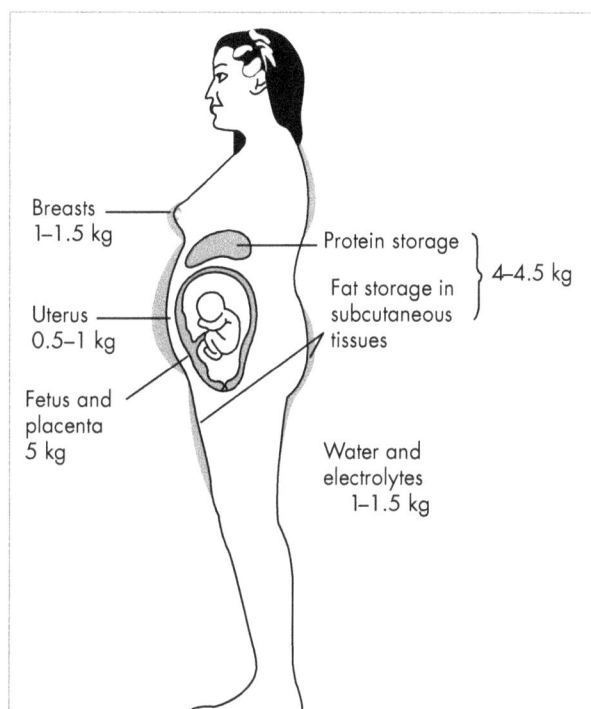

Figure 51.1 Distribution of weight gain during pregnancy (Hanretty, 2010)

Monitoring weight gain during pregnancy

Follow these guidelines during antenatal care to monitor a pregnant woman's weight gain (Rasmussen & Yaktine, 2009):

- Measure the woman's height, without shoes, using a fixed stadiometer (height measure).
- Weigh the woman in light clothing, using an accurate scale and correct procedures, at the first antenatal visit.
- Make sure to use the same equipment and procedures at all subsequent visits.
- Calculate her BMI using the following formula: weight (kg)/height (m²).
- Estimate the gestational age from the onset of her last period.
- If the woman is underweight, overweight or obese, set weight gain goals together with her, taking into account her pre-pregnancy BMI and other considerations.
- Monitor the woman's weight gain at each visit by plotting her weight on a weight-gain chart.
- Identify and investigate any abnormality in the pattern of weight gain.

51.3 Nutritional requirements during pregnancy

As a result of the anatomical, metabolic and physiological changes in the mother and the growth of the fetus, nutritional requirements are increased during pregnancy. Failure to meet these needs can have serious consequences for the mother, fetus and infant.

The Institute of Medicine (IOM) has published recommended dietary allowances (RDAs) for energy and nutrient intakes for different ages, genders and life stages (National Academy of Sciences, 2017). The RDAs are set to meet the needs of almost all individuals of a specific age, life stage and gender group. Thus, a pregnant woman whose energy and nutrient intake meets the RDAs is likely to meet her nutritional requirements.

Since many factors affect nutritional requirements, it is vital that each woman is carefully monitored throughout pregnancy and her diet modified to meet her specific individual needs. Table 51.2 on page 811 compares the RDAs for pregnancy and lactation with those for non-pregnant women and adolescents.

Baseline

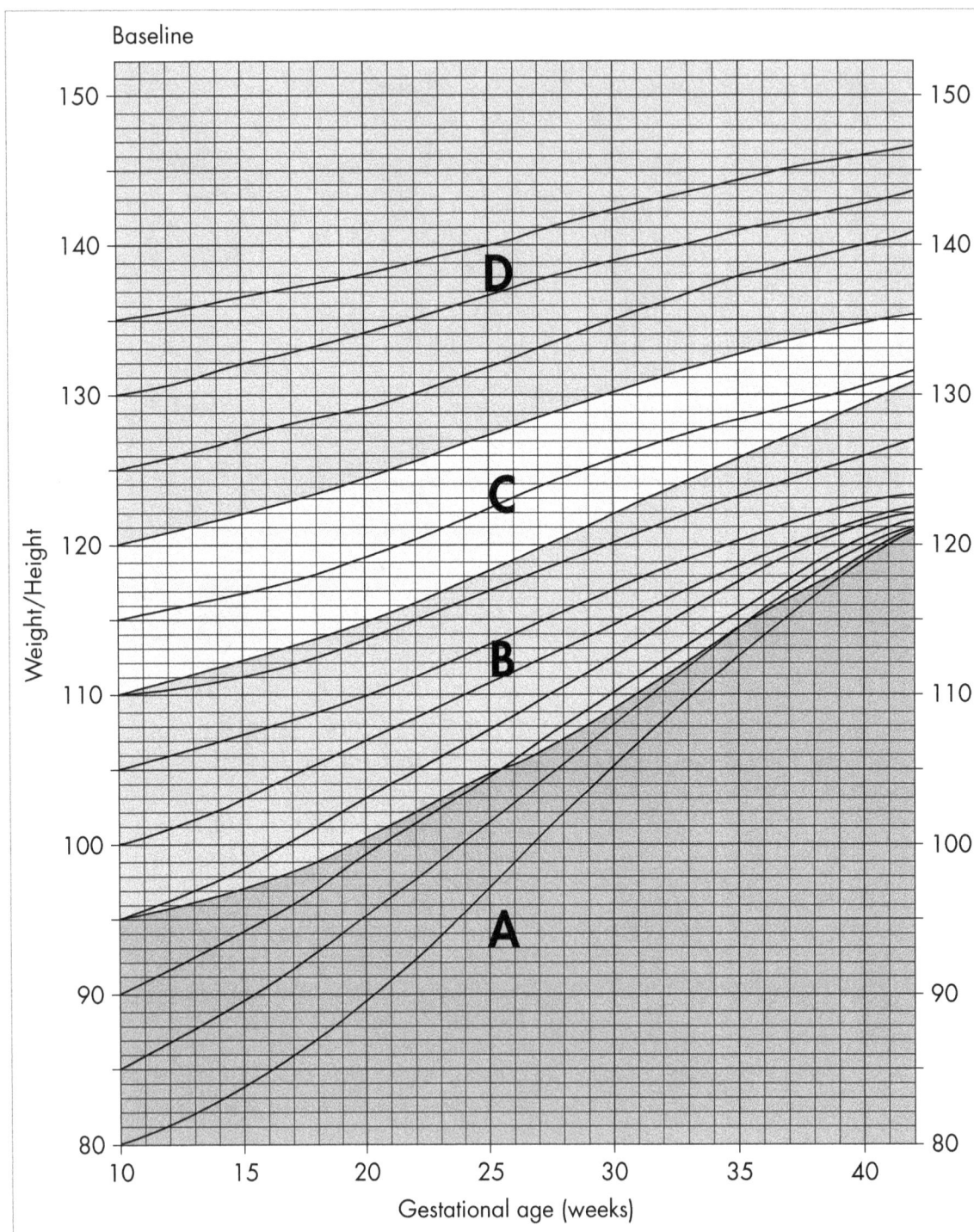

Figure 51.2 Chart of weight gain during pregnancy. A = underweight; B = normal weight; C = overweight; D = obese (adapted from Rasmussen & Yaktine, 2009)

Table 51.2

RDAs for non-pregnant, pregnant and lactating adolescents and women (National Academy of Sciences, 2017)

Age group	Non-pregnant 14–18	Non-pregnant 19–50	Pregnant 14–18	Pregnant 19–50	Lactating 14–18	Lactating 19–50
Energy (kcal)	2 368	2 403	+ 0 first trimester + 340 second trimester + 452 third trimester		+ 330 first six months + 400 second six months	
Energy (kJ)	9 950	10 100	+ 0 first trimester + 1 430 second trimester + 1 900 third trimester		+ 1 390 first six months + 1 680 second six months	
Protein (g)	46	46	71	71	71	71
Vitamin A (µg RE)	700	700	750	770	1 200	1 300
Vitamin D (µg)	15	15	15	15	15	15
Vitamin E (mgµ-TE)	15	15	15	15	19	19
Vitamin K (µg)	75	90	75	90	75	90
Vitamin C (mg)	65	75	80	85	115	120
Thiamine (mg)	1.0	1.1	1.4	1.4	1.4	1.4
Riboflavin (mg)	1.1	1.1	1.4	1.4	1.6	1.6
Niacin (mg NE)	14	14	18	18	17	17
Vitamin B6 (µg)	1.2	1.3	1.9	1.9	2	2
Folate (µg)	400	400	600	600	500	500
Vitamin B12 (µg)	2.4	2.4	2.6	2.6	2.8	2.8
Biotin (µg)	25	30	30	30	35	35
Pantothenic acid (mg)	5	5	6	6	7	7
Calcium (mg)	1 300	1 000	1300	1 000	1 300	1 000
Phosphorus (mg)	1 250	700	1250	700	700	700
Magnesium (mg)	360	310 (320 > 30 years)	400	350 (360 > 30 years)	360	310 (320 > 30 years)
Fluoride (mg)	3	3	3	3	3	3
Iron (mg)	15	18	27	27	10	9
Zinc (mg)	9	8	12	11	13	12
Iodine (µg)	150	150	220	220	290	290
Selenium (µg)	55	55	60	60	70	70

Energy

Energy requirements vary widely among women and are affected by factors such as age, pre-pregnancy weight, height and physical activity levels.

Energy requirements during the first trimester are the same as for the non-pregnant woman. This increases during the second trimester by 1 400 to 1 500 kJ/day (340 to 350 kcal/day) and by a further 470 kJ/day (110 kcal/day) during the third trimester. As a general rule, energy intakes of 11 500–12 000 kJ/day (2 730–2 850 kcal/day) during the second and third trimesters are adequate for most healthy pregnant women.

Since requirements vary widely, monitoring weight gain, adjusting individual energy intake and providing dietary counselling are essential to ensure that energy requirements are met.

Protein: Optimality and quality

An optimal protein intake is essential for the growth of the fetus and the maternal tissues. Proteins are essential components of the cell membranes, transport carriers, hormones, enzymes, the immune system and genetic material.

Approximately 42 per cent of protein is deposited in the fetus, with the remainder being taken up by the uterus (17 per cent), blood (14 per cent), placenta (10 per cent) and breasts (8 per cent) (Rasmussen & Yaktine, 2009). Most protein deposition occurs during the second half of pregnancy. Requirements therefore increase from the start of the second trimester and peak during the third trimester. The RDA for protein during the second and third trimesters of pregnancy is 25 g/day higher than for a non-pregnant woman. This is equivalent to an intake of 71 g of protein per day. Protein should supply 12–15 per cent of the total energy intake in the diet.

An optimal mix of protein and carbohydrates is needed. Protein intake cannot be separated from the total energy intake. If the energy obtained from carbohydrates and fats is inadequate to meet the energy requirements, proteins will be utilised as an energy source instead of being utilised for tissue growth and other vital functions. Thus, an adequate energy intake is essential for optimal protein utilisation.

The optimal quality of the protein in the diet must also be considered. The basic units of proteins are amino acids. Most amino acids can be synthesised by the body; these are known as the non-essential amino acids. There are, however, a number of amino acids that the human body cannot synthesise and which must be supplied by the diet. These are the essential amino acids. The quality of a dietary protein is determined by its amino acid composition. Foods that provide all the essential amino acids are said to be high-quality or complete proteins. These include meat, fish, poultry, eggs, milk and milk products. Proteins obtained from plant sources such as vegetables and whole grains do not contain all the essential amino acids and are therefore known as incomplete proteins. Some plant proteins, such as those in dried beans and soya, are known as complementary proteins since, when combined with other plant proteins, they provide a high-quality protein. It is very important that the diet during pregnancy not only provides an adequate amount of protein, but also an optimal mixture of proteins. Vegetarians and women whose animal food intake is limited need to be advised on how best to combine their food to obtain an optimal mix of essential and non-essential amino acids.

Carbohydrates

Carbohydrates are a major source of energy for the body. The fetus uses glucose as its major energy source. Furthermore, an adequate glucose supply is essential for fetal brain development. From 17 to 26 g of glucose are transferred from the mother to the fetus per day. Thus, it is essential that the carbohydrate intake is sufficient to meet the energy requirements of the mother and of the fetus.

The IOM (National Academy of Sciences, 2017) recommends carbohydrate intakes of 175 g/day during pregnancy to provide sufficient energy and to maintain appropriate glucose blood levels in mother and fetus. Carbohydrates should supply 55–65 per cent of the total daily energy intake. Preference should be given to unrefined carbohydrates such as wholewheat bread, wholegrain breakfast cereals, oats, rice and pasta, starchy vegetables such as potatoes and fresh fruit.

Fat

Dietary fats are an important and concentrated source of energy and in the body, fat is the major energy store. In addition, fats are essential for the absorption of the fat-soluble vitamins (vitamins A, D, E and K) and phytochemicals such as the carotenoids. Fats also provide the essential fatty acids (those the body cannot synthesise). Fats serve other vital functions in the body, including forming part of cell membranes, cushioning and holding internal organs in place and providing subcutaneous insulation to preserve body temperature. During pregnancy, maternal fat stores are built up to provide the mother with the energy needed during pregnancy and lactation.

There is no RDA for fat intake during pregnancy. The amount of fat in the diet depends on the energy requirements and adequate weight gain. As a rule, fat should not provide more than 30 per cent of the total energy intake. The IOM does, however, give recommendations for adequate intakes of the essential fatty acids linoleic acid and alpha-linolenic acid: 13 g and 1.4 g per day respectively (National Academy of Sciences, 2017). During lactation, adequate intakes of 13 and 1.3 g/day of linoleic and alpha-linolenic acid respectively are considered adequate to meet both the mother's and infant's needs.

Fibre

Adequate fibre intake helps prevent constipation, a common problem during pregnancy. The adequate intake (AI) for fibre during pregnancy is 28 g/day and during lactation, 29 g/day. These can be met by increasing intakes of wholewheat bread and cereals, wholegrain products, legumes, nuts, vegetables and fresh and dried fruit. A fluid intake of six to eight glasses per day is needed to form soft stools with the increased fibre intake.

Minerals

While requirements for all minerals increase during pregnancy and lactation, particular attention needs to be given to calcium, iron, zinc and iodine.

Calcium

Calcium is essential for the formation and maintenance of bones and teeth and plays a role in vascular and muscle contraction and nerve transmission. Approximately 30 g of calcium accumulates during pregnancy. Of this, 25 g is deposited in the fetal skeleton, mostly during the third trimester, and the remainder is stored in the maternal skeleton.

From Table 51.2 on page 811, it can be seen that the recommendations for calcium intake during pregnancy are the same as those for non-pregnant women of the same age (1 300 mg/day for adolescents and 1 000 mg/day for adults); this is because hormonal changes during pregnancy result in increased absorption and use of calcium. Calcium intakes lower than the recommendation may result in lowered bone density in the fetus and in loss of calcium from the mother's skeleton. Inadequate calcium intakes may also result in pre-eclampsia and hypertension. The best dietary sources of calcium are milk and milk products.

Since calcium intakes have been found to be low among South African women, the BANC programme requires that all women receive calcium supplements of 1 000 mg daily (two tablets orally, three times daily with food) to prevent pre-eclampsia (WHO, 2013). Women should be advised to take the tablets with meals, four hours before or after taking their iron supplement, to prevent the calcium interfering with iron absorption.

Iron

Iron plays an essential role in many body functions, including red blood cell (RBC) formation and function, myoglobin activity and enzyme activity. During pregnancy, RBC volume is increased by approximately 20 per cent, necessitating greatly increased iron intakes. In total, an additional 700 to 800 mg of iron is required during pregnancy. Of this, 500 mg is used for haematopoiesis (RBC formation) and 250–300 mg for fetal and placental tissues. Maternal and fetal demands are highest from week 20 of pregnancy.

Inadequate intakes of iron during pregnancy result in anaemia (serum Hb of below 10 g/dl). The risk of haemorrhage, maternal death, premature delivery, LBW and perinatal mortality are increased in the presence of anaemia.

The RDA for iron during pregnancy is 27 mg/day, 50 per cent higher than that of non-pregnant women and almost double that of a non-pregnant adolescent. Most women do not have sufficient iron stores at the beginning of pregnancy to meet their increased needs. Thus, an adequate intake of iron is vital. The best dietary sources of iron are liver, kidney, heart, lean meat, poultry and fish. Dried beans and some vegetables are also good sources of iron, but the availability of the iron to the body is lower than that of iron from animal sources. In South Africa, fortified bread and maize meal provide an important source of iron.

The high dietary requirement of iron during pregnancy is, however, difficult to meet through diet alone. It is recommended that, in addition to a well-balanced diet, all pregnant women receive preventive iron supplementation in the form of ferrous sulphate. The recommended iron supplementation protocol of the South African Department of Health (DoH) is shown in Table 51.3 on the next page. Milk, tea and coffee interfere with iron absorption and should not be consumed with the supplement. Beverages containing vitamin C, such as fresh orange juice, increase iron absorption.

Zinc

Zinc plays a role in a wide range of catalytic, structural and regulatory functions in the body. Zinc requirements are 40–50 per cent higher than normal during pregnancy. Zinc is accumulated in the fetal and maternal tissues throughout pregnancy, reaching a peak in the last months of pregnancy. Pregnant women whose diets lack adequate zinc are unable to mobilise zinc stored in the skeleton and are at high risk of developing zinc deficiency.

Table 51.3

Recommended iron supplementation protocol (DoH, 2015)

	Prevention	Treatment (mild anaemia)	Treatment (severe anaemia)
Serum Hb level	≥ 10 g/dl	7–9.9 g/dl	< 7 g/dl
Dosage: Ferrous sulphate (200 mg tablets containing 60 mg iron)	Single pregnancy: 200 mg daily (1 tablet) Multiple pregnancy: 200 mg twice daily (2 tablets)	200 mg 3 times daily (3 tablets)	Refer to hospital

The RDAs for zinc during pregnancy are 11 g and 12 g per day for adults and adolescents respectively. Good dietary sources of zinc are meat, fish, poultry, milk and milk products, wholegrain cereals, dried beans, and fortified maize meal and bread flour.

Iodine

Iodine is essential for brain development and for the production of thyroxin, a hormone secreted by the thyroid gland. Iodine plays a vital role in a number of functions, including the maintenance of body temperature, brain function, reproduction and growth.

The requirement for iodine during pregnancy is 47 per cent higher than for the non-pregnant woman, giving an RDA of 220 µg/day. Inadequate iodine intake during early fetal development can adversely affect neurological development, resulting in impaired cognitive function in infants. The most important sources of dietary iodine are iodated salt, fish, milk and milk products, meat and eggs.

Vitamins

As in the case of minerals, the requirements for all vitamins are increased during pregnancy and can be met by a well-balanced and varied diet. Some vitamins, however, are of particular concern during pregnancy.

Vitamin A

Vitamin A plays a role in gene differentiation and proliferation and thus in the development of the fetus. It is also essential for a healthy immune system.

The RDA for vitamin A is 750 µg/day and 770 µg/day for adolescents and adults respectively during pregnancy, slightly higher than the RDA of 700 µg/day for the non-pregnant woman. It is estimated that the fetal liver accumulates 50 µg/day of vitamin A during pregnancy. Excessive vitamin A intake during pregnancy may be harmful to the fetus.

The richest sources of vitamin A are liver and red meat. Dark green and orange vegetables and fruit are good sources of beta-carotene, which is converted to vitamin A in the body.

Folate (folic acid)

Folate is required by the enzymes that produce the DNA for normal cell division and growth. Folate requirements increase by 50 per cent during pregnancy to provide for the high rate of cellular division and for deposition in the fetus.

In the mother, folate deficiency results in megaloblastic anaemia and preterm delivery. For the fetus, an inadequate folate intake are associated with neural tube defect (NTD), a congenital defect that affects 11.7 to 22.6 babies per 10 000 births in South Africa annually (Zaganjor et al, 2016). Folate deficiency is also linked to other congenital defects, such as clubfoot and cleft palate. Folate deficiency develops over a period of 18 weeks of a low-folate diet or can develop due to a folate antagonist (medication that prevents the absorption of folate).

Dietary sources of folate include liver, green leafy vegetables and fortified bread flour and maize meal. Lean meat, wholewheat bread and dried beans are also good sources. It is, however, difficult to achieve the RDA of 600 µg/day through diet alone. The BANC programme recommends routine preventive supplementation for all pregnant women of 5 mg folic acid per day (Greenberg et al, 2011).

Vitamin B12

Vitamin B12 (cobalamin) functions as a co-enzyme in metabolic reactions. Adequate intakes are needed for normal blood formation and neurological functions.

The absorption of vitamin B12 from food takes place in the small intestines; this depends on the secretion of a glycoprotein that is a facilitating gastric intrinsic factor (GIF) in the stomach. A GIF is a glycoprotein produced by the parietal cells of the stomach. It is necessary for the absorption of vitamin B12 (cobalamin) later on in the small intestine. In humans, the GIF protein is encoded by the GIF gene. Thus, conditions which may decrease gastric secretion could lead to vitamin B12 deficiency.

The absorption of vitamin B12 appears to be reduced during pregnancy, as the drop in serum levels during the first trimester is greater than would be expected from haemodilution alone. Transfer of vitamin B12 by the placenta to the fetus is very efficient, resulting in fetal levels twice as high as those of the mother.

The RDA for vitamin B12 during pregnancy is 2.6 µg/day; 0.2 µg/day more than the non-pregnant recommendations. Vitamin B12 is found only in foods of animal origin, with the highest concentration in liver. Diets which provide sufficient protein from animal sources will therefore also provide adequate vitamin B12 and even a fairly small intake of these foods should be adequate to meet the requirements. Supplementation of vitamin B12 is needed for vegans (people who consume no animal products) or when intake of animal foods has been very limited over a long period.

Vitamin B6

Vitamin B6, also known as pyridoxine, helps the body metabolise protein, fats and carbohydrates. It also helps form new RBCs, antibodies and neurotransmitters, and is vital for the development of the fetal brain and nervous system.

Pregnant women need about 1.9 mg per day and breastfeeding women 2 mg daily. A woman need not take the recommended amount of vitamin B6 every day. Instead, she can aim for that amount as an average over the course of a few days or a week. Beans, nuts, lean meat and fish are good sources of vitamin B6. Fortified breads and cereals can also be good sources.

Research shows that very high doses of vitamin B6 may relieve nausea or vomiting for some women during pregnancy. However, since excessive doses of vitamin B6 may have harmful side effects, such as numbness and nerve damage, it should only be administered under the supervision of a medical practitioner. The tolerable upper intake level for the vitamin – the maximum amount considered safe by the Food and Nutrition Board of the IOM – is 100 mg for women (including pregnant and nursing women) 19 years and older, and 80 mg for women 18 years and younger (NIH, 2016).

Other B-complex vitamins

As can be seen in Table 51.2 on page 811, the RDAs for all other B-complex vitamins (thiamine, riboflavin, niacin, pantothenic acid and biotin) are increased during pregnancy. As a group, the B-complex vitamins play essential roles in all metabolic processes by acting as cofactors in the various enzyme systems that produce energy from food. It follows that higher intakes during pregnancy are needed to produce energy from the greater food intake and to provide for the high-energy needs of the mother and fetus.

The B-complex vitamins are present in a wide range of animal and plant foods, in addition to being added to fortified foods such as breakfast cereals. In South Africa, maize meal and bread flour are fortified with B-complex vitamins and therefore serve as an important dietary source. As already stated, mothers must be encouraged to consume a variety of foods to ensure that all their nutrient requirements are met.

Ascorbic acid (Vitamin C)

Ascorbic acid serves multiple functions in the body, including the formation of collagen, the repair of damaged tissues, the facilitation of iron absorption and a function in the immune system.

The RDA of 80–85 mg/day for ascorbic acid during pregnancy is 10–15 mg higher than the RDA for non-pregnant females. Rich sources of ascorbic acid include fruit such as oranges, guavas, paw-paw, mangoes and tomatoes.

In most healthcare systems, there are preparations of vitamins and minerals designed for pregnant women that have been tested for safety. Women are encouraged to use only prescribed substances that are declared safe.

51.4 Food guide during pregnancy

Food guides translate the recommended energy and nutrients into a simple, practical guide on the types and quantities of foods needed for optimum nutrition. Their main purpose is to assist individuals in choosing foods that will meet nutritional requirements. Usually food guides are based on food groups, specifying the amounts of foods from each group required to meet nutrient requirements. The pregnant woman's increased energy and other nutrient requirements can be met by following the daily food guide in Table 51.4 on the next page.

Maize, rice and bread

Maize, rice and bread are mostly starchy staple foods that are the basis of most diets, making up 55–60 per cent of what is eaten. Foods in this group include wholegrain cereals, for example maize, rice, millet, sorghum, oats, wheat and bread. They are rich in complex carbohydrates and good sources of fibre (if unrefined), some micronutrients and some protein. At times, they are fortified with some key micronutrients. The group also includes starchy roots and tubers, for example potato, sweet potato, cassava and starchy fruits such as bananas.

Table 51.4

Daily food guide and serving sizes during pregnancy and lactation

Food group	Number of servings per day			Serving size
	Non-pregnant	**Pregnant**	**Lactating**	
Bread, cereal, maize, rice	6–11	7–11	8–11	1 slice of bread (30–40 g) ½ cup cooked cereal 1 cup ready-to-eat cereal ½ large bun 3 crackers medium-sized muffin
Vegetables	3	3	3	150 ml vegetable juice ½ cup cooked vegetables 1 cup raw vegetables
Fruit	2	2	2	1 medium-sized fruit (apple, orange, banana) ½ large-sized fruit 1 cup chopped fruit
Milk	2	3	3–4	1 cup milk, amasi or yoghurt 60 g hard cheese (the size of a matchbox)
Meat, poultry, fish, eggs	2	2	2	70–80 g meat, fish, chicken or organ meat 2 eggs
Legumes, dry beans, lentils	1	1	1	½ cup cooked/canned beans or lentils 1 tablespoon peanut butter
Fats, oils, butter	Use sparingly	Use sparingly	Use sparingly	1 teaspoon or 5 g oil, margarine or mayonnaise
Sugar, jam, honey	Use sparingly	Use sparingly	Use sparingly	1 teaspoon (5 g)
Water	8 glasses	8 glasses	8 glasses	–

It is recommended that a pregnant woman consume 7–11 servings of these foods each day in pregnancy. One serving is approximately one slice of bread; half a cup of cooked cereal, rice or pasta; or one cup of ready-to-eat cereals.

Legumes, oily seeds and nuts

Legumes, oily seeds and nuts are good sources of proteins, carbohydrates, fibre and micronutrients. Some high-fat legumes, oily seeds and nuts are also rich in good fats and oils. Examples of foods in this group are dried beans, dried peas, lentils, nuts, groundnuts, mung beans, soya beans and pumpkin seeds.

Vegetables

Vegetables are a good source of a large number of micronutrients, such as vitamins (vitamin A and C, folic acid), minerals (including potassium and magnesium) and the best source of fibre, especially if eaten raw and with peels. Pregnant women must consume a large variety of vegetables, such as:

▶ dark green leafy vegetables, for example *imifino* or *morogo*, spinach, beetroot leaves, pumpkin leaves
▶ orange and deep yellow vegetables such as carrots, pumpkin, butternut, squash and orange-fleshed sweet potatoes

- starchy vegetables such as yellow corn and potatoes
- legumes, including a large variety of beans, such as green beans.

A pregnant woman should consume at least three servings of vegetables per day. Half a cup of cooked or chopped vegetables or one cup of raw vegetables is considered one serving.

Fruit

Fruit is the best source of vitamins A and C, potassium and fibre. Citrus fruits, for example oranges, lemons, grapefruit, naartjies, morula fruit and guava, are particularly high in vitamin C. The orange or deep yellow fruits, such as paw-paw, mango, apricots and yellow peaches, are rich in vitamin A. It is recommended that at least two servings per day be consumed, with one serving being half a large fruit, or one medium size or two small fruits, and half a cup of canned or cooked fruits. Seeing that some of the nutrients may be destroyed during preparation and cooking, fruit is best eaten whole and raw.

Meat, poultry, organ meat, fish and insects

These foods are good sources of complete proteins and a large number of minerals such as iron, zinc and vitamin A. Foods in this group include beef, mutton, animal organs (*mala, mogodu, dikilana le maotwana*, including liver), chicken, tinned fish and eggs. Most of the foods in this group are expensive and thus may be unaffordable. Furthermore, some religious practices forbid the consumption of animal foods, which complicates the situation. Caution should be exercised in selecting foods from this group, as they contain saturated fats and cholesterol, which is bad fat. Meat should be selected from a safe source and be well cooked if it is to be eaten by a pregnant woman, as it can transmit diseases.

Milk, yoghurt and cheese

These foods are rich sources of mineral calcium, but are also good sources of protein, carbohydrates, vitamin B, vitamin A and vitamin D. Full-cream milk products also contain saturated fats and cholesterol. In pregnancy it may at times be better to choose low-fat or fat-free (skimmed) milk, from which the fats have been removed. Two or three servings of these foods should be included in a pregnant woman's daily food intake. The serving size is one cup of milk, amasi, buttermilk or yoghurt, or 30 g cheddar or Gouda cheese (the size of a matchbox).

Fats and oils

Fats and oils, for example butter, margarine, vegetable oil and mayonnaise, are a major source of energy and contain a number of fat-soluble vitamins such as vitamin A and E. Generally, foods from animal sources such as meat and milk contain saturated fats, while most plant sources (maize, sunflower, peanuts, ground nuts, oily seeds and olives) contain unsaturated fats. There are no serving recommendations, but items in this group should be used sparingly because of their very high energy content and low nutrient content.

Sugar and sweet foods

Sugar and sweet foods, including sugar, honey, molasses, jam, carbonated ('fizzy') cold drinks, fruit squashes and many types of food with sugar added, such as biscuits, provide only energy and no nutritional value. There are no recommended servings for these types of food and it advisable to use them sparingly.

Water and other fluids

Currently, there are no scientifically based recommendations for water needs as with energy and other nutrients, as water requirements are regulated by thirst.

Fluids from beverages of various types, fruit and vegetables and other foods are sources of water, but if the woman is still thirsty, she should drink water. Pregnant women should be advised to limit their intake of caffeine-containing drinks, including coffee, black and green tea, energy drinks and cola drinks. Energy drinks have a very high energy content, with no or little nutritional value and are not advised. Although pure fruit juices contain some vitamins and minerals, the amounts are small and the energy content is high. Fruit juice should thus be used sparingly.

Breastfeeding mothers require more fluid than normal to replace water lost in the infant's milk.

Sample menu plan

With judicious selection of foods from each group, a balanced diet can be planned to ensure supply of the necessary nutrients. A sample menu plan demonstrates how the food guide can be translated to food on a plate. It is recommended that pregnant and lactating women eat five to six meals a day, starting with breakfast, followed by a midmorning snack, then lunch followed by an afternoon snack and then supper, if necessary followed by a late-night snack. Table 51.5 on the next page offers a sample menu for pregnant and lactating women.

Table 51.5

A sample menu

Main meals	Snacks
Breakfast 1 cup cereal 1 cup milk 2 teaspoons sugar	**Mid-morning** 1 medium fruit in season
Lunch 2 slices wholewheat bread 1 tablespoon peanut butter 1 cup fruit juice (100% juice)	**Afternoon** 6 crackers/2 cups *magewu* Jam/sugar to taste
Supper 1½ cup samp and beans (*umgqusho*) 90 g stewed chicken with vegetables 1 cup cooked spinach/any *morogo*	**Late evening** Boiled/braised corn on cob OR a sweet potato, preferably orange-fleshed 1 cup milk/amasi

The physiological changes during pregnancy may cause much of the discomfort experienced by the pregnant woman. The box below briefly describes how nausea, vomiting, constipation and heartburn can be relieved. The next section deals with the nutritional concerns of HIV-positive pregnant women.

Tips to alleviate common discomforts of pregnancy

Suggestions to alleviate nausea in pregnancy:
▶ On waking up, get up slowly.
▶ Eat dry toast, crackers or dry cereal.
▶ Chew gum or suck hard sweets.
▶ Eat small, frequent meals.
▶ Take ginger tea, ginger drinks or ginger-flavoured foods.
▶ Avoid foods with offensive smells.
▶ Avoid drinking liquids with meals.
▶ Avoid coffee, tea and spicy foods.
▶ Limit the intake of high-fat foods.

To prevent or alleviate constipation:
▶ Increase fibre intake by eating wholegrain breads and cereal.
▶ Drink at least eight glasses of liquid per day.
▶ Participate in regular exercise.
▶ Hot water with lemon or prune juice may be helpful, especially if taken first thing in the morning.
continued

To prevent or relieve heartburn:
▶ Relax and eat slowly.
▶ Eat small, frequent meals.
▶ Avoid liquid intake just before meals, with meals or immediately after meals.
▶ Drink liquid between meals, at least two hours before and after a meal.
▶ Avoid spicy, high-fat foods.
▶ Sit up while eating.
▶ Avoid lying down or bending over for an hour after meals.

51.5 Nutritional concerns for HIV-positive pregnant and lactating women

HIV-positive pregnant and lactating women are at high risk of mal- and undernutrition and thus require close monitoring. Improving nutrition prior to pregnancy should be the main goal to minimise the impact of HIV on the pregnancy outcome. This is unfortunately a huge challenge, because many women have unplanned pregnancies and only become aware of their HIV status once they are pregnant, while some women enter pregnancy with a poor nutritional status.

The effects of HIV on nutritional status

HIV affects nutrition by decreasing food consumption, reducing the absorption of nutrients and causing changes in metabolism. Poor nutritional status can speed up the progression of HIV-related diseases.

HIV-positive pregnant women, especially from developing communities, are vulnerable to nutrient deficiencies, mainly due to the increased nutrient requirements associated with HIV and the demands of pregnancy. Therefore, HIV increases the risk of maternal malnutrition, which in turn increases the risk of mother-to-child transmission (MTCT) and maternal and fetal morbidity and mortality. If HIV is associated with other infections, such as diarrhoea or tuberculosis, over a long period of time, it results in wasting.

Nutritional assessment

As with HIV-negative women, body weight measurements are the most commonly used method to assess gestational weight changes in HIV-positive pregnancies. However, some argue that weight alone may not be a good assessment indicator because of the increased total body water. In addition to weight, recommended measurements may include height, BMI and MUAC.

Nutritional requirements

During pregnancy and lactation, the requirements for energy, protein and various micronutrients increase to meet the demands for adequate weight gain during pregnancy and milk production during lactation.

▶ *Energy.* The recommended increases in energy intake in HIV-positive pregnant and lactating women – compared with non-pregnant and non-lactating women – are adapted as explained in the following recommendations. The recommended increase for HIV-positive women during the asymptomatic phase is 10 per cent, which increases to 20–30 per cent if signs of AIDS and other infections appear. For HIV-positive lactating women, 1 680 kJ (400 calories) should be added for lactation, in addition to 10 per cent in asymptomatic women and 20–30 per cent in symptomatic women.

▶ *Protein.* There are no current recommendations for HIV-positive pregnant and lactating women to increase protein intake as a result of HIV infection. Protein requirements are 12–15 per cent of energy intake, the same as for HIV-negative women.

▶ *Micronutrients.* There is inadequate evidence to estimate the micronutrient requirements of HIV-positive pregnant and lactating women. However, multi-micronutrient supplementation containing 100 per cent of the daily requirements of all micronutrients is associated with improved health outcomes for HIV-positive pregnant and lactating women (Siegfried et al, 2012).

Generally, the HIV-positive pregnant woman gains less weight and at a slower rate than the HIV-negative woman. The rate of weight gain decreases progressively during pregnancy. It is therefore very important that weight gain during pregnancy should be closely monitored. *Pregnancy weight gain of less than 1.5 kg per month in the second and early third trimester, or less than 10.5 kg during the entire pregnancy, is of serious concern.*

51.6 Drugs and other substances in pregnancy

The fetus is affected in some way by most of the substances administered to, ingested by or inhaled by the pregnant woman. The breastfed newborn baby will also be affected by the substances contained in the breast milk. In addition, if tobacco or any other drug is smoked in the vicinity of the baby, the baby may be affected by some of the chemical constituents. The baby is therefore greatly affected by the lifestyle of the parents, and the effects of many unhealthy parental habits are forced upon the fetus and the newborn baby.

In pregnancy, particularly in the first trimester, the developing fetus is vulnerable and can be affected by the harmful substances passed on through the mother when smoking, using drugs or alcohol. In late pregnancy, such habits may lead to fetal distress and demise.

Tobacco smoking and inhalation

Tobacco use and the subsequent inhalation or ingestion of nicotine can take the form of smoking cigarettes, cigars or pipes or using snuff. There is now clear evidence to show that cigarette smoking during pregnancy does have detrimental effects upon the fetus and the newborn infant.

There is a definite increase in the following conditions and therefore also in the subsequent complications of these conditions:

▶ Small-for-gestational age (SGA) babies
▶ A low average placental weight at birth (compared to non-smokers)
▶ Spontaneous abortion
▶ Preterm labour and therefore preterm babies
▶ The perinatal mortality rate.

There is a possible increase in congenital malformations (particularly NTDs), respiratory problems in the neonate and infant and neonatal and infant morbidity and mortality rates.

The detrimental effects of nicotine intake to the fetus can be prevented if pregnant women can be persuaded not to smoke. It would be even better to discourage all smoking. Women who smoke often also have affected taste and lower food intake.

The midwife should, at every opportunity, explain the dangers of smoking and encourage pregnant women to give up smoking. Heavy smokers should be encouraged to at least reduce the number of cigarettes to less than five a day.

Alcohol

It has been suspected for centuries that alcohol has potential teratogenic effects; however, it was only in 1973 that a specific pattern of malformations and neurological impairments was first described as fetal alcohol syndrome (FAS). Alcohol consumption during pregnancy is now known to result in a range of conditions collectively known as fetal alcohol spectrum disorders (FASD), with FAS as the most severe and complex.

The most debilitating effects of alcohol consumption are on the central nervous system (CNS) of the fetus, causing impaired mental function. Prenatal alcohol exposure may also result in physical abnormalities and defects of the heart, liver, kidneys, gastrointestinal (GI) tract and endocrine system. The clinical features of FAS are described on the next page.

Both chronic alcoholism and binge drinking are directly linked to FASD. However, moderate alcohol consumption (one drink per day) during pregnancy may also result in severe behavioural problems in children. The prevalence of FASD in South Africa is one of the highest in the world and alcohol consumption during pregnancy may be one of the leading causes of mental retardation in South Africa. Yet FASD is totally preventable by a complete avoidance of alcohol throughout pregnancy.

The dangers of alcohol consumption during pregnancy should be widely publicised and midwives should do their utmost to discourage this practice. In fact, women should be educated to understand that if they intend or are likely to become pregnant, they should abstain from alcohol, because the first month of pregnancy is the most critical.

Women suffering from chronic alcoholism should be encouraged to take effective birth control measures. Pregnant women suffering from alcoholism must be referred to appropriate healthcare professionals for counselling and support to reduce and stop their alcohol intake. It has also been suggested that chronic alcoholism could or should be an indication for termination of pregnancy.

In addition to the direct effects on the fetus, alcohol interferes with vitamin A absorption. Alcohol abusers tend to be malnourished and prone to unhealthy habits, including unhealthy sexual behaviour, smoking and drug abuse, increasing the risk of LBW and premature births.

Clinical features of fetal alcohol syndrome

▶ *Defects in growth.* Almost all children afflicted with FAS are small in height, weight and head size.
▶ *CNS dysfunction.* The IQ deviation of children with FAS, compared with the level of physical development delays, is particularly noted in verbal IQ and behaviour. It has also been noted that the most severely physically affected children have the greatest degree of mental retardation.
▶ *Abnormal facial characteristics.* Those with FAS have certain distinctive facial features, namely:
  • short palpebral fissures (the length of the eye opening or eye-slit is reduced and epicanthic folds are often present)
  • a flattened or absent philtrum (the furrow running from the base of the nose to the centre of the upper lip is shallow or absent)
  • a hypoplastic upper lip with a thin vermilion border (an under-developed upper lip).
▶ *Cardiac abnormalities.* Of children with FAS, 25–50 per cent have cardiac abnormalities. These include atrial and ventricular septal defects (ASD and VSD), patent ductus arteriosus (PDA) and Fallot's tetralogy.

▶ *Associated abnormalities.* Further abnormalities that have been associated with FAS include abnormalities of the neuroskeletal, urogenital and cutaneous systems. There also appears to be an association between chronic alcoholism of the mother and fetal liver damage.

Dependence-producing drugs

Narcotics and hallucinogenic drugs have detrimental effects upon the fetus and the newborn infant. However, it is difficult to estimate the actual harm done by these drugs alone, as pregnant women using these drugs are usually also subject to other problems, such as malnutrition, alcoholism, tobacco smoking and general neglect. To add to these problems, the newborn infant will often be reared in this same environment.

Drugs are excreted through breast milk in toxic levels. The effects of narcotics on the fetus are probably similar to those of smoking tobacco, but with an increased risk of fetal abnormalities. In addition, there is likely to be difficulty with the initiation and maintenance of respiration at birth and there are also the problems of neonatal drug withdrawal.

The effects of smoking dagga (marijuana, pot, hashish) are still being evaluated. It must be assumed, therefore, that the detrimental effects are at least the same as those of tobacco smoking.

In South Africa, the use of the drug *tik* (crystal meth) is very popular among young people and the poor. It is very dangerous, because it is often mixed with unknown substances that can be more harmful than the drug itself.

The midwife should be able to recognise a woman with a drug use problem during history taking and examination at the first antenatal visit, although the woman may go to great lengths to hide the problem. Dilation of the pupils, reddened eyes and an over-stimulated or excited state could be suggestive of hallucinogenic substances, while pinpoint pupils and a depressed and unresponsive state could be suggestive of narcotics. The withdrawal signs of any of these substances may be an over-excited state, with tremors, sweating and hallucinations.

Once the problem has been diagnosed, the woman should be referred to expert specialist care and the social welfare authorities should be notified.

Prescription drugs

All pregnant and breastfeeding women should be instructed not to take any unnecessary medication. Even medicines which can be bought without prescription and from supermarkets can have adverse effects upon the fetus and the breastfed baby.

If the woman has any minor ailments, such as a cold or cough, she should check with a qualified pharmacist before taking any medicine, to make sure that it is not harmful to the fetus. Any pregnant woman who has to be seen by a medical practitioner (or dentist) must inform that medical practitioner that she is pregnant and she should take any medication exactly as prescribed. Should any medication have an adverse effect, the woman should notify her medical practitioner immediately.

Every woman who has some disorder and is on medication should inform her medical practitioner or midwife if she intends to try to become pregnant and also as soon as she thinks she may be pregnant. If the medication she is taking could be detrimental to the fetus, the medical practitioner will substitute the medicine.

51.7   Conclusion

In South Africa, a midwife is often the only healthcare professional a woman will see during pregnancy and birth. Midwives therefore have an important role to play in assessing women's nutritional needs within the boundaries of their socioeconomic circumstances and cultures. Women need to be supported and provided with appropriate advice and information to maintain their health during pregnancy and lactation. If problems are identified, the woman needs to be referred for nutritional support from a registered nutritional specialist.

Section Eleven

Medication used in childbirth

Complementary and alternative medicines

LEARNING OBJECTIVES

On completion of this chapter, you must be able to:
▶ identify safe complementary and alternative medicines (CAMs) and traditional practices useful in obstetrics
▶ develop skills to advise and educate women on the safe use of CAMs in pregnancy and birth.

KNOWLEDGE ASSUMED TO BE IN PLACE

General knowledge of traditional substances and practices related to health that are used in communities

KEYWORDS

complementary • alternative • traditional medicine • Allied Health Professions Council of South Africa (AHPCSA)

52.1 Introduction

Complementary and alternative medicines (CAMs) and/or therapies are some of the many terms used to describe any approach to healing that is not traditional in Western medicine, though they may have a long history of use in many countries.

Traditional medicines refer to objects, substances and customs used in traditional health practice by traditional healers and traditional birth attendants (TBAs) for the diagnosis, treatment or prevention of a physical or mental illness.

It is important for midwives to understand the role of CAMs, traditional medicines and customs in pregnancy, labour and baby care.

52.2 Background: Complementary and alternative medicine in South Africa

People's increasing desire to self-medicate (a worldwide move to the use of alternative medicine) and the greater affordability of natural remedies are factors contributing to the growing popularity of CAMs.

In South Africa, traditional medicine still exerts a strong influence and the regulation thereof is a particularly sensitive subject. The Traditional Health Practitioners Act 22 of 2007 is used to regulate four groups of traditional healers: *sangomas*

(diviners), *izinyangas* (herbalists), TBAs and *iingcibi* (traditional surgeons). The trend seems to be not to overregulate but to encourage self-regulation, improve traditional practices with health knowledge and primary care, and promote a culture of tolerance and mutual respect.

There are 10 therapies or modalities that have statutory recognition in South Africa and which fall under the authority of the Allied Health Professions Council of South Africa (AHPCSA). CAM – the specific term for medicines and remedies used by 'natural' therapists or the public for self-treatment – is included under the authority of the AHPCSA. These include herbs, homeopathic remedies, flower essences, vitamins and minerals, sport and nutritional supplements, weight management products and even energy devices. Given the substantial increase in public support for CAMs, it is encouraging that government has taken steps towards appropriate regulations for the industry.

While the AHPCSA is empowered to monitor the treatment modalities that fall under its auspices and each modality also has its own professional regulatory body, over-the-counter (OTC) products and remedies are not controlled by any of these bodies. The Health Products Association of South Africa (HPASA) is a body that acts as a mouthpiece for the CAM market and has collaborated with the Department of Health (DoH) to formulate revised regulations. HPASA regularly communicates with member companies, practitioners and other interested parties to advise on regulatory changes, encourage ethical practices and promote manufacturing standards. In 2011, the Minister of Health published an amendment to the Regulations to the Medicine and Related Substances Act 101 of 1965 that calls for the regulation of CAMs. The roadmap to register CAMs in South Africa was published in December 2013 (DoH & MCC, 2013), and includes aspects of scope, control, registration, licensing of manufacturers, labelling and general advice to consumers, including contact details for information relating to the various products (see Thembo, nd). The roadmap set goals for licensing of all CAM substances with regard to withdrawal or banned and schedules substances, compliance of labelling, specific medication for use, for example antiviral cardiac and diabetic substances, slimming products and sexual stimulants, immune and muscle boosters, sport supplements and all pharmacological classification not included above.

The move to integrative medicine in recent years highlights the importance of the regulation of CAMs, as well as the need for Western health professionals to increase their knowledge of CAMs and the role that traditional healers and natural health practitioners can play in the health field.

52.3 Important perspectives for nurses and midwives

It is the author's standpoint that mothers are growing the next generation, shaping the future of humankind and nurturing the leaders of tomorrow. In short, they are doing the most important job on earth. Midwives and maternal and child health nurses are in the privileged and powerful position to help them, and natural therapies can be a powerful tool and catalyst in their hands. Furthermore, midwives and nurses are in a unique position to use their instinctive and trained skills to make a vast difference to women's lives. Recognising individuality, respecting preferences, working with nature, truly caring about the families in their care, promoting breastfeeding and being knowledgeable about natural therapies will make all the difference in providing superior care and service. The word midwife means 'with women' – probably the most important role possible, second only to mothering itself.

Midwives and nurses, as skilled birth attendants, can improve maternal and newborn health at grass-roots level. The role of midwives in caring for pregnant women and conducting deliveries is acknowledged and they should be encouraged to promote practices that help achieve the Sustainable Development Goals (SDGs) (which superseded the Millennium Development Goals, or MDGs) through sound primary healthcare (PHC) practices. In particular, the prevention, early recognition and emergency treatment of the major contributors to high maternal and child mortality are in the hands of midwives and nurses, who can influence TBAs and mothers to adopt healthier practices.

The use of complementary and alternative medicine

Alternative and supplementary therapies are often incorporated in nurses' repertoire of care. This may differ between regions. A study in the USA in 2009 (Hastings-Tolsma & Terada, 2009) indicated that 78 per cent of healthcare workers reported using CAMs in their practices. The respondents were middle-aged and qualified to Master's level. It is important that clinicians study the use of alternative and complimentary therapies if they want to incorporate these in their practice.

52.4 Terminology

The many terms used in complementary and traditional medicine need to be understood from the outset. The following explanation of the terminology particular to and descriptive of CAMs will assist you to develop an informed understanding of the practices and to distinguish approved practices from potentially harmful ones:

▶ *Complementary medicine.* The word 'complementary' literally means 'in addition to', but in this context it usually implies an active choice on the part of the consumer to use natural remedies or a measure resorted to when conventional medicine is not successful.

▶ *Natural medicines or remedies.* The word 'natural' is unfortunately misused, with most people assuming that it denotes something that possesses no potential for adverse reactions. Many naturally occurring substances have toxicity and in-depth knowledge is required in order to use these correctly. The use of natural substances without knowledge can cause damage and even lead to death.

▶ *Phytotherapy.* This literally means 'plant medicine', derived from the Greek word for 'plant' or 'that which grows'– *phyton.* Herbal and other plant remedies fall in this category. They are in all likelihood the most common category of medicinal substance known and their use is widespread. Phytotherapy encompasses many different approaches and systems, such as traditional Chinese medicine, Ayurvedic remedies, Western herbal medicine and traditional plant remedies used by rural cultures.

▶ *Homeopathy.* This is the term for a widely used complementary therapy, derived from the two Greek words *homoios* (similar) and *pathos* (suffering).

Homeopathy thus literally means 'similar suffering'. This gives a clue to its foundational diagnostic and therapeutic approach, which is based on the principle that every substance has the power to heal or to harm and that in-depth analysis of the symptoms with which a patient presents is essential in the selection of remedies. This selection must be based on the central Law of Similars (see the section on homeopathy on pages 828–829).

- *Allopathic medicine.* This is the term that many alternative health practitioners use to refer to conventional Western medicine. It is derived from the Greek word *allos*, meaning 'different' or 'other'. The term encapsulates the approach of using substances to treat conditions based on the principle of counteracting the perceived cause of pathology and its effects – an approach that is thus directly opposite to homeopathy's approach.
- *Neutraceuticals.* These medicines are also considered to be foods.
- *Vital force.* This is what many alternative health therapies call 'the inherent energy' that keeps a person in a state of dynamic well-being. It is not quantifiable, nor can it be seen with the naked eye, yet it is acknowledged by most disciplines as being present in all living beings. It is comparable with 'chi' in Chinese medicine.
- *Holism.* This is a theory of health based on the importance of taking a person's complete physical, mental and social conditions into account in the understanding and treatment of illness.
- *Teratogenic.* This term refers to a substance that can cause abnormalities of the fetus during its development. It is derived from the Greek words *teratoit*, meaning 'monster', and *genesis*, meaning 'generation' or 'producing'.
- *Abortifacient.* This is anything used to induce abortion of a fetus.
- *TBA.* A TBA is a person (usually a woman) who engages in traditional health practice and is registered under the Traditional Health Practitioners Act 22 of 2007. In remote and very small communities, there may be no TBAs and many women still deliver by themselves or with the help of a close female relative or friend. In cultures where there are TBAs, their work is often restricted to one extended family and they may do as few as 20 deliveries a year. Very few TBAs have a practice big enough to make it their main means of living. The *South African Demographic and Health Survey* (SADHS) (DoH, 2003: 125) indicated that in 2003 in South Africa, 6.6 per cent of women birthed at home and that in 4.7 per cent of births the carer was not known.

52.5 A brief overview of some complementary therapies

Complementary therapies (and in all likelihood traditional medicine too) operate on the principle that healing is performed by the human body and mind. Any therapy, such as a remedy taken, therapeutic massage done or procedure performed (that has positive effects on a person), is considered as merely a catalyst that triggers the restoration of balance or good health to the body and mind. This does not mean that illness is perceived to be all in the mind, as so many critics of complementary or natural therapies suppose. The basis for the success of some therapies is not always clear.

Women generally have less trouble accepting natural therapies, probably because they seek the gentlest and most effective way of restoring their families to health. As is true in conventional medicine, the therapy is only as good as the practitioner and the quality of the remedies; users need to ask relevant questions when choosing a practitioner or remedy.

An important cornerstone of complementary or alternative therapy is the emphasis laid on holism and the responsibility of the individual to get actively involved with his or her own health. Consider for a moment the word 'disease'. Separate it into syllables – dis / ease – and you will see disease translated into a condition of discomfort. CAMs and natural therapies have the intention of returning mind and body back to a state of ease. It does not claim to have all the answers or cure all conditions, but is of assistance in bringing balance physiologically and between body and mind. The concept 'psychosomatic' in Western medicine acknowledges the link between the mind and the body that cannot be replicated using medicine.

Complementary therapies

In this section, we will take a brief look at some therapies that actively use remedies or medicinal substances as the cornerstone of their treatment regimens. This will help you to understand the rationale behind the different CAMs available, within the context of the specific therapy. At the same time, it will become clear why it is important to distinguish between the mode of action, the benefits and the risks of individual therapies and the best way to select, use and monitor the use of CAMs.

Aromatherapy

Aromatherapists use essential oils, which are very potent oil extracts, from a great variety of plants; these have physical and psychological effects. In plants, these oils acts as pesticides, fungicides and bactericides and may also have hormone-like properties. The complex oils extracted are esters, alcohols, aldehydes, ketones and terpenes. Essential oils are diluted with an inactive base oil before treatment.

Essential oils affect the body in two ways:
1. As they are applied to the body, the person breathes in the vapours, which are then absorbed by the blood vessels in the lungs and rapidly transported throughout the body.
2. The skin also absorbs the oils at the point of application if the skin is clean and well prepared.

Each type of oil has specific properties that have a direct physiological effect on the body. Some stimulate activity, others relax the body processes and others have healing properties.

Once absorbed, the oils are dispersed to the extracellular fluid. They are excreted mainly through the lungs and the kidneys, and some are altered in the body, just as with drugs. Some are potentially toxic and the correct therapeutic dosage is important.

Not only are the inhaled vapours absorbed in the lungs, but the olfactory nerve in the nasal mucous membranes registers their presence and transmits their message to the centre in the brain responsible for emotional control and the memory process. Emotions are then affected by the treatment, depending on the properties of the oils. Aromatherapists believe that, to ensure maximum benefit, it is essential that the person instinctively likes the aroma of the oils used.

The concentration of essential oils holds the potential for side effects, which is of particular importance in pregnancy. Therapists must be chosen with care for their knowledge and experience. Some of the essential oils to be avoided in pregnancy are pennyroyal, basil, hyssop, marjoram, sage, cedarwood, rosemary, fennel, cinnamon and citronella. Despite the possibility of side effects, expectant women can profit from skilled aromatherapy treatment.

Guidelines for safety of use of aromatherapy in pregnancy

Alert: Not all essential oils are safe for use in pregnancy. The use of some aromatherapy in pregnancy is controversial. Guidelines for use by the National Association for Holistic Aromatherapy (NAHA) are available from www.naha.org/explore-aromatherapy/safety.

Most commercially available aromatherapeutic creams, lotions and oil products contain very diluted quantities of essential oils, if any at all, and pose no risk in pregnancy beyond topical allergy reactions to the base substances. Checking pack inserts and the manufacturer's instructions will provide added safeguards.

Herbal substances

Herbal remedies, also called phytotherapy, herbalism and plant medicine, have a history as old as humankind. All herbal remedies need to be used with caution, as these may have harmful as well as beneficial properties and the accumulation of active ingredients in the body is possible. Preparation methods may in some instances also pose risks and different people may react differently.

Some herbal medicines are strictly contraindicated in pregnancy and lactation and in small children; some may have teratogenic effects, some are abortifacients and some are highly toxic.

Herbal remedies have an action that is similar to conventional traditional drugs, which also have the potential for adverse effects. The quality of the raw material and agricultural methods used, the quality of manufacture and of the remedies themselves as well as the expertise and practices of the therapist all influence the outcomes achieved with herbal remedies.

Important general precautions include the following:
▶ Choose products that are manufactured from registered and approved sources.
▶ Keep strictly to the dosage instructions.
▶ Use for limited periods; thereafter take a break to avoid accumulation in the body.

Some herbal products can be used safely in pregnancy, but advice should be sought from an expert in the field. Topical cosmetic and treatment products containing well-known herbal ingredients are mostly less problematic in pregnancy, although some may cause allergy symptoms associated with base substances.

The culinary use of herbs, spices and teas will seldom pose a problem, unless significant quantities or extremely concentrated amounts are used quite frequently. When herbs are turned into medicines, the product is very concentrated and more likely to have adverse effects. A rule of thumb with herbal teas, to ensure safety, is to have no more than two or three cups a day and to ensure a weak infusion.

Homeopathy

Since the formalised inception of its principles in 1786, homeopathy has been accepted in the field of healing. Modern orthodox medicine is in fact a very new discipline by comparison, although it too developed in part from the age-old medicinal use of herbal remedies. There is a common misperception that homeopathy's roots are in the East, but as can be seen from history, its origins can be traced back to Europe.

Homeopathy is often mistakenly taken to be the same as herbal medicine. Although certain herbs and plants are sources of homeopathic remedies, there are significant differences, the main one being the absence of adverse effects in homeopathic remedy use.

Dr Samuel Hahnemann, a physician, chemist and visionary in Germany, is recognised as the initiator of modern homeopathic practice. After 10 years of meticulous experimentation and documentation of findings while using common medicinal substances, he formulated the Law of Similars. This stated that a substance that will relieve a set of symptoms in an ill person will cause those same symptoms in a healthy individual. Hahnemann coined the name 'homeopath', deriving it from the two Greek words *homoios* (similar) and *pathos* (suffering).

He realised that overdosage was an inherent risk with traditional substances used medicinally. He understood the concept of 'energy medicine' and proceeded to evolve the idea of potentising remedies, which involves diluting the original substance (called a mother tincture in homeopathy) and then succussing it (or shaking vigorously). This process transfers the molecular healing energy of the substance to the carrier base. In the process of dilution, any potential for adverse effects is removed. In short, one could say that homeopathy harnesses and transfers the healing essence of a substance through succussion to the base ingredient and discards potential toxicity by diluting to the stage of no material substance remaining (concentration is 10^{-6}).

The efficacy of this form of healing cannot merely be ascribed to a placebo effect, as is possibly most easily demonstrated by the regularity with which both animals and babies respond positively to treatment. One of the many myths about homeopathy is that it can only be used for minor complaints like 'the common cold'. The correctly chosen remedy can, however, relieve acute symptoms of illnesses such as tonsillitis, otitis media, conjunctivitis, bladder infection (cystitis) and premenstrual tension within a few hours. Chronic conditions such as rheumatism and emphysema will take longer to respond, due to long-term effects on the body. In pregnancy, during labour and for treatment of babies and children, homeopathy provides a safe and effective therapy.

It is important to be able to distinguish whether a remedy is homeopathic or herbal. As a very basic rule of thumb, if the ingredient units used are D6, 6x, 30 CH, etc, the remedies are homeopathic. If measured in micrograms, milligrams, grams, etc, or if one is advised to take a 'teaspoon' or medicine measure of the product, it is likely to be a herbal preparation. For instance, one of the common concerns in pregnancy is the use of the remedy arnica, which is known to promote bleeding when used in herbal form. Homeopathic arnica, however, would not pose any risk.

Homeopathy is not an esoteric system, nor is it linked to any religious belief. No mystical process is used to manufacture remedies. Scepticism usually comes in two forms – scientific criticism for supposed lack of research evidence and religious resistance from some sectors. It is generally believed that the discipline is linked to Eastern religions, which is simply not the case, and that the manufacturing process includes occult practices. Western health practitioners study and practise homeopathy and alternative healthcare, also its use in obstetrics.

The WHO (2008) raised concerns about the quality of homeopathic products being sold in some areas. Generally, the quality of homeopathic substances from Europe is good, but the same may not be true for the rest of the world.

In short, homeopathy is the medicinal therapy that can claim no adverse effects, has no cumulative drug effects, can be taken with other treatments and is totally safe in pregnancy, breastfeeding and for babies, if derived from an approved source and of an approved quality.

Tissue salt therapy

Tissue salts (also called 'cell salts') are basically homeopathically prepared mineral compounds. As a result, they possess or cause no adverse effects. Tissue salts, derived as they are from minerals, are related in some way to mineral therapy and are often more easily accepted by health practitioners and the public alike.

Some two or three hundred years ago, it was not known that the human body was made of water, inorganic and organic matter in perfect proportion. The concept of tissue cells was also foreign. That all changed when Dr Wilhelm Schuessler, a medical doctor, homeopath, physicist and biochemist, recognised the importance of twelve inorganic compounds in the body. Dr Schuessler lived and worked in Germany in the 19th century and although he was not the only scientist active in this field, the tribute for tissue salt therapy goes to him. He noted that these 'salts', or chemical compounds, were present in minute doses in the body and that they were essential to correct cell and body functioning.

Conventional mineral supplementation is vital in some cases. The 12 tissue salts have proven to be of immense benefit in preventive and healing therapy. Table 52.1 on page 834 gives details of their use in obstetrics.

Flower essences

Flower essences are made in a number of places in the world. English flower essences – originally introduced by Dr Edward Bach in the 1930s – are possibly the best known. In South

Africa, flower essences utilising the plants from the amazing floral kingdom of the Cape Peninsula have been commercially manufactured since 1995 and are distributed and used in 18 different countries.

Like homeopathy, flower essences are taken orally and work on the principle of vibrational healing, which is a form of energy medicine.

Flower essences are totally safe in pregnancy and lactation.

Selected non-remedy alternative therapies

Non-remedy alternative therapies are not substances, but physical therapies based on science. They include physical touch and are non-invasive and mostly non-harmful when performed by an experienced practitioner.

Reflexology

This therapy traces its roots to ancient Egypt, as shown in surviving artwork depicting foot-massage therapy taking place. Central to reflexology is the belief that every organ and every part of the body has invisible but corresponding reflexive endings on the feet and the hands. A specific massage technique has the dual benefits of greatly relaxing the person while stimulating the healing processes of the body at the same time. This therapy operates on the basis that humans all have energy fields that are intricately linked to both health and illness. The healing power of relaxation has been proven over and over by all disciplines and it is especially important in pregnancy.

Reflexology is safe for mother and baby, but certain parameters should be adhered to:

▶ Choose a therapist whose touch is not uncomfortably firm.

▶ The reflex area to the uterus should not be stimulated. It is unlikely that this would bring on premature labour, but the area would be very sensitive and no chances should be taken.

▶ The woman should not lie on her back during treatment from about the fifth month of pregnancy, to ensure good circulation to her baby.

Reflex areas to endocrine glands (such as the thyroid and ovaries) are usually more sensitive – this does not mean that something is wrong. Reflexology does not tickle, a concern many people have before they first try a treatment. Reflexology does not claim to treat specific complaints, although it certainly can aid the body in its own healing processes and is very relaxing and rejuvenating.

Many pregnant women report finding relief from bladder and vaginal infections and some experience substantial help with varicose veins and swelling linked to poor circulation in pregnancy. Most women report an increase in their overall sense of well-being.

Used for colic and restless infants after birth, gentle reflexology is a wonderful and soothing therapy. Constipation in babies also responds very well to treatment.

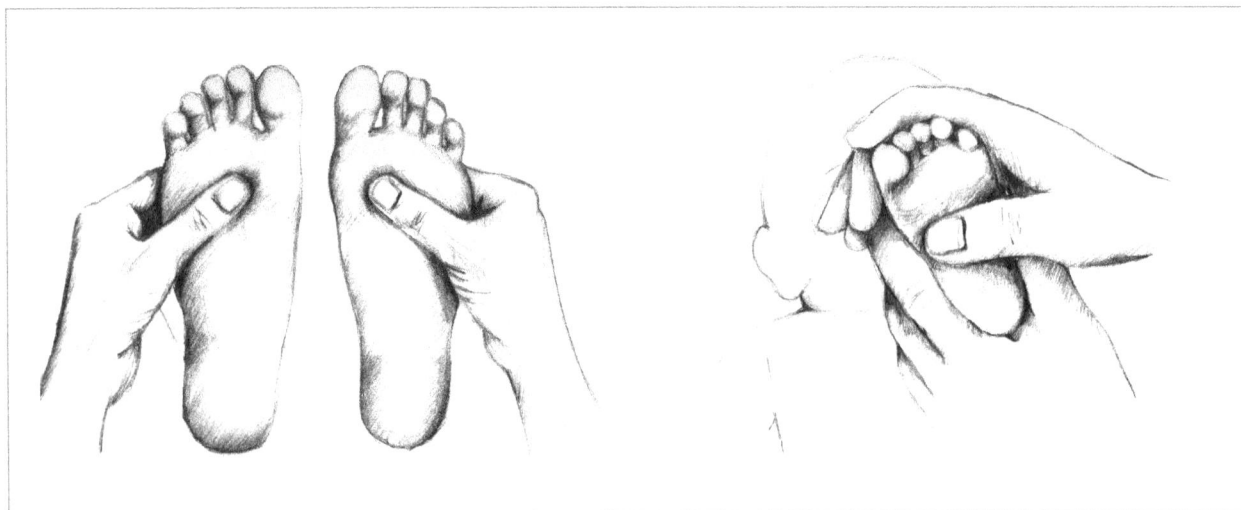

Figure 52.1 Reflexology for mother and baby

Acupuncture

Based on the concepts of traditional Chinese medicine, acupuncture has a history of more than 3 000 years. Acupuncture works on the basis of stimulating points on the body's surface to positively affect the physiological functioning of the whole body or specific parts. The ancient Chinese believed that we are born with inherent energy called 'qi' (or 'chi', as it is pronounced and mostly written) circulating in our bodies through 12 invisible channels or interconnected pathways called meridians.

Thin needles are inserted into different points along the meridians to redirect and regulate the flow of energy, creating balance and allowing organ systems to function properly. Between six and 20 needles are used during therapy and they are normally left in for at least 30 minutes.

As reported by Wang, Kain and White (2008), acupuncture is used in Western medicine mainly for pain relief and nausea and vomiting. There is still a lack of useful scientific information on the use of acupuncture and research is ongoing. Theoretically, the needles may change the blood flow, thus reducing nausea and vomiting, releasing neurotransmitters – endogenous opioid-like substances – and activating *c-fos* within the central nervous system (CNS), resulting in the relief of pain.

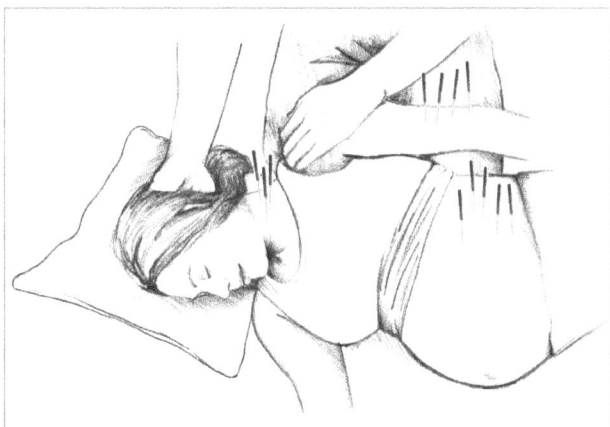

Figure 52.2 Acupunture in pregnancy

Acupuncture is ideally suited to obstetrics, particularly in cases where there are restrictions on the use of drugs. It is useful in the treatment of conditions such as morning sickness, migraine, backache and constipation, version of the fetus in breech presentation, non-medical stimulation of labour and pain relief in labour. After the birth, it may be used to treat haemorrhoids, mastitis, depression and other problems associated with this period.

Chiropractic

In South Africa, chiropractic practitioners graduate after six years of study and training from selected universities.

Chiropractors use pressure and manipulation of the spine to relieve irritation of the nerves that run through the centre of the spinal column. The spinal cord carries information throughout the body and is responsible for all bodily functions, so if the vertebrae are even slightly twisted or misaligned, this can affect the rest of the body. Spinal misalignment in babies usually occurs due to intrauterine position, difficult labour or delivery. Skeletal and muscle manipulation restores the alignment of the body to prevent blockages, much like in acupuncture.

Chiropractors must be informed of pregnancy and will then avoid certain techniques at different stages of pregnancy. The techniques used with babies differ somewhat from those used on adults, due to bone structure and strength. Women should be encouraged to choose experienced practitioners when pregnant.

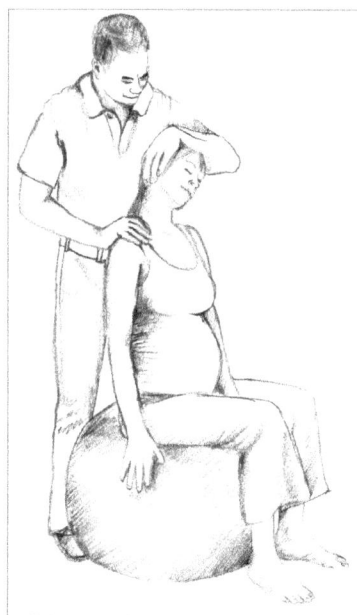

Figure 52.3 Chiropractic in pregnancy

52.6 Common remedies used in pregnancy, birth and childcare

In a study published in 2004 on the attitudes of midwives and obstetricians towards the use of CAMs during pregnancy in South Australia, Gaffney and Smith (2004) found that more than 90 per cent of midwives and obstetricians indicated that they need knowledge of CAMs. It is essential that midwives become knowledgeable about the remedies that women may use in pregnancy – including traditional substances, some of which may be harmful – so that they are able to give appropriate advice.

Phytotherapeutic or herbal remedies used in childbirth

Raspberry leaf

Raspberry leaf tea is one of the better-known herbal remedies for easing the process of labour. Raspberry plants (*Rubus idaeus*) are native to many parts of Europe and northern America and the leaves have been used in pregnancy and lactation since the 6th century. They are a rich source of iron, calcium, manganese and also magnesium; a mineral which helps to strengthen the uterine muscles and prevents uterine irritability. Raspberry leaf is also a valuable source of vitamins B1, B3 and E, which are important in pregnancy and lactation.

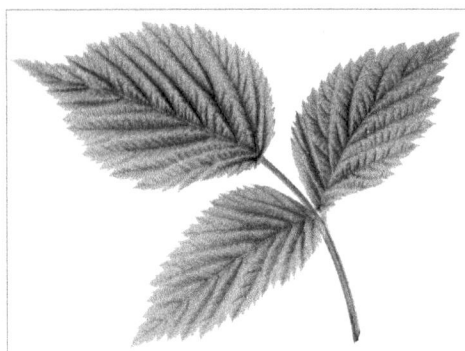

Figure 52.4 Raspberry leaves

Raspberry leaf tea has many uses in the female reproductive years. It is used to help regulate the menstrual cycle, aid fertility, ease the symptoms of morning sickness and lessen discomfort from Braxton-Hicks contractions.

Raspberry leaf tea has some clinical research to back up its use in labour, specifically from Australia (Simpson et al, 2001). Studies were initially observational, followed by a randomised controlled trial. The results showed clinically significant benefits, although statistically the research is not that compelling. The remedy was found to have a uterine stimulant and tonic action. Consensus is that raspberry leaf shortens the second stage of labour, helps avert the artificial rupture of membranes (AROM), reduces the need for assisted delivery by

forceps or vacuum and lowers the Caesarean rate. No adverse effects to usage throughout pregnancy were observed in the observational study, though in the clinical study the remedy was only used from 32 weeks, with no adverse effects being noted.

The stimulant action of raspberry leaf is why it should be avoided in the first trimester and not used in excess at any stage. Raspberry leaf tea can be taken in a tea bag, as loose leaves, as a tablet or as a tincture and is available from most herbalists and health food stores. The safest usage seems to be to use only in the last trimester and preferably from 34 weeks. Use one cup a day (or the tablet equivalent according to dosage instructions). From 36–37 weeks, the amount can be gradually stepped up to four cups over the course of a day. Once labour starts, raspberry leaf tea can be sipped throughout.

Black cohosh

Black cohosh, a perennial herb also known as black snakeroot (*Actaea racemosa* and *Cimicifuga racemosa*), is used in many parts of the world in female healthcare, with specific application in traditional labour assistance and menopause. Black cohosh is used for dysmenorrhoea and helps raise the pain threshold in labour. Recovery from birth is generally better.

It is also useful in the treatment of mild depression of both the postnatal period and menopause. It has oestrogen-like properties due to the isoflavonoids and triterpenoids and acts to relieve hot flushes and other common menopausal symptoms.

Alert: Black cohosh can potentially be overdosed or used inappropriately if not under the guidance of a trained or experienced herbalist. Excessive intake may cause nausea and vomiting, dizziness, diarrhoea, tremors, depressed heart rate and miscarriage. More than 5 g of the substance can be toxic.

Other herbs

Many herbs stimulate the uterus and are unsafe in concentrated usage in pregnancy. In concentrated essences, they could have adverse effects. These include aloe vera, rosemary, rue, sage, southernwood, thuja, parsley seed, pennyroyal, pokeweed, blue cohosh, celery seed, cinnamon and devil's claw. Parsley, celery and rocket in their natural form are useful for their vitamin and mineral properties, but the use of their seeds must be avoided in pregnancy.

The following can be useful in pregnancy:

▶ Chamomile tea is fairly safe in pregnancy in moderation, although babies will react sensitively, with restlessness and digestive discomfort, if too much is ingested. Used sparingly, it can safely assist with restful sleep and anxiety.

▶ Chewing a mint leaf for heartburn is an effective home remedy. A few drops of peppermint essence in a cup of hot water is another safe way of using this common garden herb.

▶ Fenugreek, fennel, caraway and milk thistle are all traditionally used to promote lactation.

▶ Rooibos remains a firm South African favourite and is proven to be totally safe and has wonderful antioxidant and other health benefits. Drinking vast quantities is sometimes thought to be linked to anaemia, especially in babies.

▶ Green tea is considered to be a very healthy drink for all ages and is safe to use in moderation in pregnancy too.

▶ Fennel and ginger tea can help with nausea and indigestion in pregnancy.

Homeopathic remedies in pregnancy and labour

Remedies used in pregnancy and birth need to be chosen carefully. The best possible results require a trained homeopathic practitioner to advise the most appropriate remedy. In labour, remedies are mainly used for their effect in supporting the natural birth process. Homeopathic remedies do not have a drug-type action, so their use will not remove pain altogether. They act to relax the cervix, stabilise uterine contractions, reduce the length and severity of the contractions (pain) and help to address specific tendencies, such as stress and anxiety, that will affect uterine contractions. The baby will suffer no negative side effects.

The following are homeopathic remedies that can be used in pregnancy and labour:

▶ *Caulophyllum* (blue cohosh) is one of the better-known labour remedies and a wide range of women can profit from its use. It relaxes the cervix and uterine muscle and consequently reduces the pain of labour. It may improve the co-ordination of uterine contractions. If labour seems to come and go (erratic and unco-ordinated), this is the indicated remedy. It is mostly taken as labour starts, in a dose every half to one hour. Nausea in labour also responds well to this substance. The potency range used is 30 CH to 200 CH.

▶ *Actaea racemosa* (black cohosh) in herbal form helps raise the pain threshold. Women who are pain-sensitive will probably need it. It is beneficial for restlessness and discomfort during labour, and for the tendency to feel hysterical or out of control.

▶ *Pulsatilla* is indicated for extreme anxiety, irritability and tearfulness in labour. It also gives direction to a slow-starting labour and strengthens a woman's resolve.

▶ *Nux vomica* is a widely used homeopathic remedy. It is helpful for a mother with an intense nature, who needs to relax to allow Mother Nature to do her job. It will also help for queasiness in labour.

Homeopathic remedies for the postnatal period

Some brief pointers only are given in this regard:

▶ *Arnica* promotes rapid healing, reduces swelling and helps prevent infection in the mother.

▶ *Hypericum* helps prevent infection, relieves nerve pain in the perineal area and heals cracked nipples.

▶ *Baryta carb* assists premature babies to catch up on milestones and thrive.

▶ *Calendula* is excellent for infection prevention, skin rashes and cracked nipples.

▶ *Chamomilla* is used for frequent crying, colic and teething in babies.

▶ *Ignatia* is used for mild depression and to help women cope with loss (for instance after miscarriage or stillbirth).

Tissue salts for the perinatal period

Tissue salt remedies provide a trusted and unique approach to health. They offer safe, natural treatment for the minor complaints of pregnancy, can support labour progress and relieve many postpartum and infant problems. Table 52.1 on the next page provides a summary of useful tissue salts and their use in obstetrics.

Traditional customs and herbal remedies used during pregnancy and labour

Many plants and herbs are used by rural women as traditional remedies in the reproductive years in most parts of the world. These have often become part of folklore and are handed down from one generation to another, mostly through the maternal line. TBAs and/or healers are also custodians of customs, practices and remedies used to:

▶ improve female health
▶ promote or delay conception
▶ induce abortion
▶ trigger the onset of delayed labour
▶ promote the labour process
▶ ensure effective uterine contraction after birth
▶ promote lactation.

Table 52.1

Tissue salts used in obstetrics

Pregnancy:	**Labour and birth:**	**For the baby:**
Calc fluor for stretchmarks, ligament pain, varicose veins, constipation, dental health of mother and baby	*Kali phos* to allay anxiety, raise pain threshold	*Calc fluor* for stronger teeth
Calc phos for growth of baby, immunity, anaemia, skeletal strength, dental health of mother and baby	*Mag phos* as an anti-spasmodic for pain relief, soothing cramping muscles	*Calc phos* for slow teething, a large anterior fontanelle that is slow to close, or for a baby who is often ill
Calc sulph for acne in pregnancy	*Ferrum phos* for burning pain, strength of spirit and body in labour and perineal protection during labour	*Calc sulph* for green, lumpy mucus and together with *ferrum phos* for sore throat
Ferr phos for strength of ligaments, as an anti-inflammatory in case of any infections, anaemia, oxygenation, acne	**Maternal use postnatally:**	*Ferrum phos* for fever, inflammation and infection
Kali mur (together with *calc sulph*) for vaginal thrush	*Ferrum phos* taken as an anti-inflammatory may reduce swelling and the chance of infection, prolapse of womb and vagina, anaemia, pain relief	*Kali mur* for thick, white-to-grey mucus, 'glue ear', oral thrush, cradle cap
Kali phos for baby's CNS development, emotions of pregnancy, aches and pains	*Kali phos* for nerve repair in the birth canal, healing, maternal anxiety	*Kali phos* for anxiety, very restless behaviour
Mag phos for uterine irritability, leg muscle cramping, baby hiccups in the womb, headaches	*Nat mur* for third-day blues or postnatal depression	*Kali sulph* for chronic skin rashes, yellow sticky mucus
Nat mur for dry, itchy skin, weepiness and depression, dry stools, mild swelling		*Mag phos* for colic, hiccups, cramps
Nat phos for nausea in pregnancy, heartburn, indigestion		*Nat mur* for watery mucus, excessive crying, constipation or diarrhoea to balance digestive system
Nat sulph for nausea, mild swelling		*Nat phos* for sour-smelling possetting, milia ('*babasuur*')
		Silicea to strengthen a scrawny body with a big head and weak neck, and back control

While some remedies are specific to a region, many are customary across various parts of the world.

Remedies are frequently used in combination with other practices, including incantations, visualisation, ancestral communication and culture-specific rituals. These customs and remedies often seem shrouded in secrecy, simply because they are more prevalent in remote areas and because Western medicine mostly censures their use; they are therefore often not talked about to outsiders.

Some traditional customs

Midwives, nurses and TBAs cannot control customs and rituals that have been in practice from time immemorial, but should be alert in order to assess if there is harm or risk for either mother or baby. Rituals often promote emotional support, relax the mother and relieve anxiety and are to be encouraged in the absence of risk. Midwives should respect these and other practices.

A few common customs are as follows:

▶ If there is a bundle of wood in the house or any other knotted items, TBAs or relatives accustomed to helping at deliveries will ask for these to be untied, believing that this will 'loosen up everything' in the woman and promote easy birth.

▶ The umbilical cord that eventually detaches from the baby is kept safe by the mother by tying it on the cloth that she has around her stomach. This she must then give to her mother-in-law and say 'Here is the child's mercy'. The cord is hung from the roof, which signifies that this is the baby's home and that he or she will 'know where home is when grown up and not give problems'.

▶ Every child born is greeted with the traditional praise cry '*Hala-la*' before being washed.

▶ The process of birth, greeting the baby and hanging up the umbilical cord is followed by *ukusoka*, the giving of presents, which also ensures that the baby will know where home is and have respect for the place.

◗ A man from the family will take some hair from a cow's tail in the kraal, go to the woman's home where she has given birth and roll it into a belt that will be tied around the baby's waist and neck. Various rituals then ensue and the mother and baby are both covered with a blanket so that people cannot see the mother's face. It is only once the belt is finished and worn by the baby that the mother can show her face again.

◗ In the Muslim culture, after birth, the baby will have a prayer said into its ear by a male. The baby is given a drop of holy water and a tiny piece of dates from Mecca, if available.

◗ *Efukweni* is a custom that causes some concern. Some women are told not to go to hospital to get antiretroviral (ARV) treatment for two weeks after birth until the umbilical cord falls off, to avoid exposing the child to evil spirits.

◗ Another concerning custom is the belief that a newborn baby should be given *isicakati* as a first feed for a few days. This increases the risk of transmission of HIV from mother to baby when breastfeeding commences thereafter.

◗ In some cultures, it is believed that a newborn baby should be taken to *ilawini*, a traditional healer, to get a remedy for the removal of evil spirits – *umoya uphumile*.

◗ Harmful practices such as putting cow dung on the umbilical cord are discouraged through health education.

Traditional herbal remedies

The use of herbs, traditional remedies and customs are often frowned upon and considered unscientific. This calls for an approach that respects practices and seeks to incorporate safe traditional customs into healthcare. The WHO (2008) has recognised traditional medicine as a positive integration of medical know-how and cultural (or ancestral) experience. Many countries are proactively studying these remedies to understand all their effects and make sure that they can be used safely, rather than simply being ignored or condemned.

Studies clearly demonstrate that there is a scientific basis to the innate knowledge of traditional healers and the plant remedies of their geographical areas. Surveys also show that many women who have moved to urban areas use a combination of traditional herbal remedies and Western medical care. Some of these are discussed below:

◗ *Imbelekisane* is a frequently encountered traditional remedy for female health. There is circumstantial and research evidence of its tonic effect and specific application in the perinatal period, as well as evidence suggesting potential toxicity and negative effects of ingestion on maternal and fetal health.

◗ *Isihlambezo* is a term commonly used in South Africa, especially among Zulu women, to describe a herbal compound used during pregnancy and labour. The primary benefits of *isihlambezo* are said to be ensuring adequate fetal growth, promotion of general maternal health and promoting an uncomplicated labour.

There is some concern about the toxicity of some of the plants used, which total about 60 species in various *isihlambezo* and *imbelekisane* mixtures. Pharmacological studies seem to confirm both therapeutic and harmful consequences of *isihlambezo* and *imbelekisane* use. It seems that the popularity of *isihlambezo* and *imbelekisane* among urban women is attributable to the high cost and inferior quality of public healthcare. It is believed that the use eases adaptation to urbanisation and it indicates how rural cultures integrate into new sociocultural situations and contribute to emerging cultural patterns.

TBAs prepare *imbelekisane* before touching a pregnant woman and then rub it in their hands when examining her. This is often combined with shaking the woman's belly to make the baby move and change position in case of breech, transverse or posterior lie – a procedure that is not without risk.

What follows is a brief overview of the effects of some well-known plants traditionally used in *isihlambezo* and *imbelekisane*:

◗ *Agapanthus africanus*, also known as *ubani*, *leta-la-phofu*, blue lily and *bloulelie*, is a common, attractive flowering plant found in many gardens. Preliminary studies show it to have direct smooth muscle activity, distinct uterotonic action and a mild laxative effect. The root is utilised to induce labour and water in which the plant is grown is used in pregnancy and labour. Both rectal and oral administration is known.

◗ *Gunnera perpensa*, also known as *ugobho*, river pumpkin, wild rhubarb and *rivierpampoen*, is often found in gardens. It has leaves similar to that of the pumpkin plant. The root is mostly used and it has a strong oxytocic effect. It is widely used for fertility, during pregnancy in small doses and postpartum to help expel the placenta. Incidences of severe contraction of the lower segment have been reported when used during labour, leading to fatalities.

◗ *Rhoicissus tridentata*, also known as *isinwazi*, wild grape and *bobbejaantou*, is commonly found in the eastern parts of southern Africa. The San used the tuberous roots medicinally and it can be seen on rock art. It is known to relieve various digestive symptoms of pregnancy, initiate labour and to help expel a retained placenta. **Alert:** Macerated leaves in water are used as an abortifacient.

A number of fatalities caused by CNS depression and respiratory failure have been linked to its use.

- *Combretum paniculatum*, also known as 'flame creeper', is used to expel a retained placenta. **Alert:** The fruits of the genus are regarded as toxic, avoided by wild animals and not used by healers. Fatalities have been reported from vaginal insertion of some species of combretum.

- *Clivia miniata*, also known as *umayime*, orange lily and *boslelie*, is a popular plant in shady gardens, with orange flowers being the most common. Only two varieties of clivia are used as traditional remedies. The action is reportedly to initiate overdue labour and facilitate the process of labour. Leaf extracts have been shown to have uterotonic effects. Alkaloids such as lycorine are contained in the rhizomes and are very toxic.

- *Adansonia digitata* is also known as the baobab tree. The fruit pulp is used as a porridge if lactation is deficient after birth.

- *Amaranthus caudatus*, also known as *marog*, is a common food in Africa. The leaves of *marog* are used as an abortifacient. In general, it is rich in protein (26–30 per cent), iron, calcium and vitamin A.

- *Aloe zebrine* is also known as *kgopalmabalamantsi*. The stems and leaves are used in a mixture to help expel the placenta and 'cleanse' the system. The species *aloe ferox* in concentrated doses can cause severe purging and promote abortion.

- *Chironia baccifera*, also known as *bitterbos*, is used extensively by the Khoi and others in a wide range of common ailments. An infusion of leaves, stems and fruits help expel a retained placenta but may cause non-severe diarrhoea. **Alert:** Toxicity in animals has been encountered, but seemingly not in humans.

- *Erythrina lysistemon* is also known as the common coral tree, *umsinsi*, *muvale* and *koraalboom*. Strips of the bark are cut from all four sides of the trunk, bound together and used to make an infusion to ease labour pains during birth. **Alert:** Alkaloids present in the substance are known to be highly toxic. Traditional usage supports the belief that the infusion has analgesic, antibacterial and anti-inflammatory properties.

52.7 Conclusion

A range of known and unknown substances are used by women in pregnancy. Midwives are tasked with providing advice on substances that may be harmful for the fetus. The rule is to only use substances that are tested and prescribed for the first trimester. All patients should be asked about the use of CAMs and self-medication, as there is the risk of interaction with prescription medication.

Any registered drug or unregistered substance (OTC medication), traditional medicine or illicit drug can cross the placenta and have serious consequences for the well-being of the fetus. Knowledge of the drugs, their contraindications, their effects and side (or adverse) effects is essential for safe practice and optimum outcomes for the mother and child.

Principles of pharmacology in obstetrics and the neonatal period

LEARNING OBJECTIVES
On completion of this chapter, you must be able to:
▸ apply the principles of drug therapy during pregnancy, birth and the puerperium, as well as in the neonatal period
▸ identify drugs to be avoided during pregnancy
▸ describe drugs commonly used in the newborn
▸ use the knowledge you have gained about drug therapy in pregnancy, birth, lactation and the neonatal period to assist with the facilitation of competent, safe and responsible practice.

KNOWLEDGE ASSUMED TO BE IN PLACE
Basic knowledge and understanding of the principles of pharmacology, with specific reference to the two major subdivisions, namely pharmacodynamics and pharmacokinetics
A sound knowledge of the principles, routes and methods of drug administration
The ability to access and interpret specific drug information, with particular reference to registered indications, warnings, contraindications, side effects and recommended dosing regimens

KEYWORDS
pharmacodynamics • pharmacokinetics • pharmacotherapy • teratogenesis

53.1 Introduction
One of the major medical challenges facing the practices of midwifery and neonatal nursing is that of drug therapy (also referred to as pharmacotherapy). A very important reason for this is the fact that drug therapy (ie the use of medication to attain certain clinical outcomes) may pose a significant risk during each of the vulnerable periods in the human reproductive cycle, as discussed in Section 53.2.

Pharmacology is a broad and complex subject. Therefore, this chapter will only focus on the principles of pharmacotherapy as they apply to pregnancy, childbirth, lactation and the neonatal period. The basic pharmacokinetic (PK) and pharmacodynamic (PD) terminology referred to in this chapter is summarised in Table 53.1 on page 839. Specific drug treatment aimed at particular conditions is discussed in the corresponding chapters and sections that deal with the various disorders and emergencies in question.

53.2 Risks of drug therapy in the human reproductive cycle

From fertilisation to complete implantation
During this period, the two greatest risks would be a spontaneous abortion or the reabsorption of the products of conception, both of which would probably go unnoticed. This period lasts for about two weeks (see Figure 53.1).

Intrauterine life
Drugs may cross the placental barrier and reach the systemic blood circulation of the unborn child, with potential adverse effects.

Embryonic development and organogenesis
The embryonic period lasts until the end of the eighth week after fertilisation, and the embryo is exceptionally vulnerable to structural abnormalities.

Fetal development and maturation

During the second and third trimesters, drugs usually only affect the growth and maturation of the fetus, since organogenesis is completed by the end of the embryonic period. However, the development of the external genitalia continues into the second trimester and the development of the central nervous system (CNS) is an ongoing process for the duration of the pregnancy (and beyond).

Mother and baby

The physiological processes of the mother are altered during pregnancy and birth due to the associated anatomical and hormonal changes. The baby's physiological systems are still immature and cannot necessarily metabolise and excrete foreign substances sufficiently.

The birthing process

Drugs used to manage the intrapartum period may have direct effects on the fetus during and directly after birth (for example,

administering pethidine to a mother during labour may cause respiratory depression in the newborn).

Breastfeeding

Drugs such as the ergot derivatives may be excreted in the mother's breast milk.

The development of the newborn child

All newborns are vulnerable, whether they are of normal gestational age (GA) and birth weight or not. Factors contributing to the challenges that pharmacotherapy pose for newborns include:

▶ their smaller body size
▶ the higher percentage of body water; premature babies have an even higher percentage of body water than neonates do (see Figure 53.3 on page 848)
▶ the fact that liver biotransformation, for example, is slower in the neonate
▶ the slower rate of renal elimination of certain drugs (due to the immaturity of the kidneys and the liver).

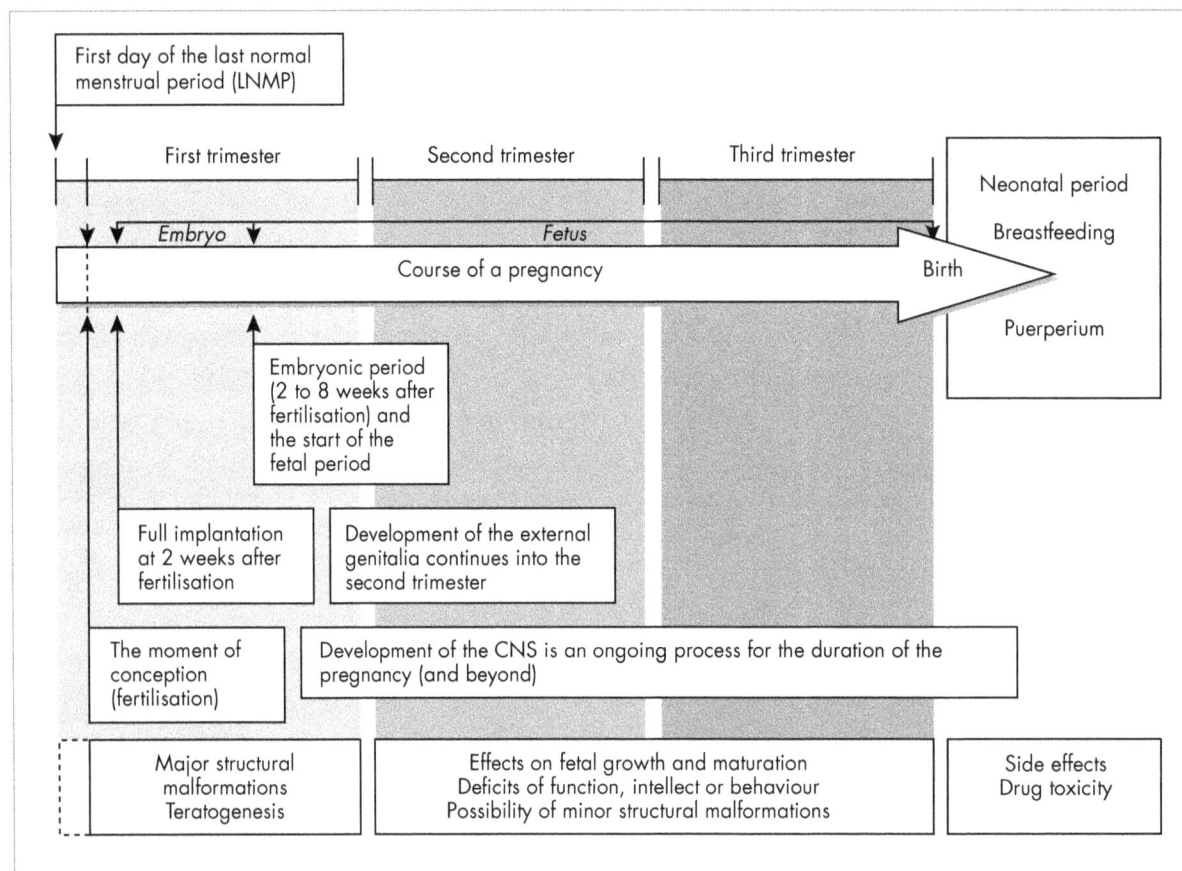

Figure 53.1 The vulnerability of the unborn child and neonate to drug therapy (also see colour illustration C2 on page 70)

Terminology

Table 53.1

Basic pharmacokinetic and pharmacodynamic terminology

Term	Definition
Pharmacokinetic terms	
Absorption	The process by which a drug proceeds from its site of administration to the central blood circulation (the site of measurement within the body). This process is not restricted to oral administration only, but is equally applicable to events that follow other routes of administration, ie IM and subcutaneous injection, rectal administration, etc. However, IV injected drugs enter the bloodstream directly and therefore do not require any absorption to take place
Apparent volume of distribution (V_d)	The apparent volume into which a drug distributes in the body's fluid compartments at equilibrium. This is the volume into which the specific drug dosage will need to be dissolved for it to reach the same concentration as it does in the plasma
Biopharmaceutical properties	The relationship between the physical and chemical properties of a drug, in a specific dosage form, and the pharmacological, toxicological or clinical effects that are observed following its administration. This information can be used to optimise drug availability at the site of action
Clearance (CL)	The volume of body fluid which is totally cleared of drug per unit of time
Elimination half-life ($t½$)	The time it takes for the drug's plasma concentration to be reduced by 50%
Pharmacokinetics	The study of the kinetics of drug absorption, distribution, metabolism and elimination/excretion in humans and animals. In other words, that which happens to the drug in the body
Plasma steady-state concentration	A stable plasma drug level (or plateau concentration) during which the drug's rate of absorption is equal to its rate of elimination (ie the drug's input equals its output). It takes approximately four to five half-lives to reach steady-state
Systemic bioavailability (F)	The fraction of an orally administered dosage which reaches the systemic blood circulation of the patient. It reflects the extent of absorption and pre-systemic elimination
Therapeutic drug monitoring (TDM)	• The mathematical relationship between a drug dosing regimen and its resulting serum concentrations (pharmacokinetics) • The relationship between drug concentrations at the site of action and the resultant pharmacological response (pharmacodynamics) • The use of serum drug concentrations to optimise drug therapy in individual patients, in conjunction with their clinical status and response to therapy
Pharmacodynamic terms	
Pharmacodynamics	The study of the biological effects resulting from the interaction between drugs and biological (body) systems. In other words, what the drug does to the body

53.3   Drug therapy during pregnancy, childbirth and lactation

Pharmacotherapy during pregnancy, childbirth and lactation may be required for a number of reasons, including:

▶ pregnancy-, labour- and lactation-related interventions (eg using drugs to induce labour or to strengthen uterine contractions), disorders and emergencies (eg the drug management of eclampsia)

▶ acute illness or trauma during the course of a pregnancy (eg a motor vehicle accident, perinatal infection, or an acute episode of upper respiratory tract infection)

▶ chronic illness or disability, including a few conditions that are of particular importance in this setting and that may impact upon maternal and perinatal mortality (even when treated), namely:

* HIV/AIDS
* diabetes mellitus
* hypertension
* asthma
* epilepsy
* migraine headaches
* mental health disorders (including depression and anxiety)
* conditions requiring long-term anticoagulant therapy (eg atrial fibrillation)
* cancer.

In a few instances, the fetus may actually be the target of the drug therapy given to the mother (as part of a so-called fetal therapy regimen).

In these settings, as in any other healthcare setting, it is of vital importance to carefully weigh up the possible benefits and risks of pharmacotherapy against the possible outcomes (for both mother and child) of not treating the condition at all. The decision to opt for drug therapy should always be a sound and rational one. The outcomes that the clinician is aiming to achieve should be realistic and he or she should take into consideration what the available drugs, under the specified conditions, may be reasonably expected to do when given to the patient in question.

Furthermore, it has to be mentioned that treatment cannot necessarily be interrupted, postponed or avoided altogether merely because a woman is pregnant or breastfeeding. This poses a complex clinical challenge that requires expert opinion and balanced, evidence-based decision making (see Figure 53.2 on page 846).

Aspects to consider when administering medication

Physiological changes during pregnancy that may affect drug action and kinetics

Certain physiological changes during pregnancy have implications for drug therapy and may affect any of the four basic kinetic processes, namely absorption, distribution, metabolism and elimination/excretion (ie the ADME processes). The following aspects could alter the way in which drug molecules are handled by the body (ie alter their pharmacokinetic profiles):

▶ Increased progesterone levels cause a decrease in gastrointestinal (GI) motility (with resultant constipation) as well as a decrease in oesophageal sphincter pressure (which causes heartburn). In addition, placenta-derived human chorionic gonadotropin (hCG) causes nausea and vomiting. The altered GI functioning caused by these changes could influence the rate and extent of drug absorption for orally administered drugs.

▶ Pregnancy also results in increased lung perfusion and pulmonary alveolar drug transfer (due to the improved cardiac output [CO]), meaning that absorption will be improved for drugs that are administered via the pulmonary route (ie via nebulisers and inhalers).

▶ The increased plasma volume that accompanies pregnancy may result in an increased volume of distribution of certain drugs. Furthermore, pregnancy brings about a decreased blood albumin level, which could result in an increased fraction of free drug molecules. This may be especially significant in the case of drugs that are highly protein-bound, also increasing their volumes of distribution and altering other kinetic properties. Note that only the free, unbound fraction will be able to cross the placental barrier. In these instances, the higher fraction of free drug molecules implies that there are higher levels of the active drug in circulation (for both mother and unborn child), which increases the likelihood of drug toxicity.

▶ Altered liver functioning may affect the plasma concentrations of drugs that follow the hepatic metabolism.

▶ The increased plasma volume increases CO, renal blood flow and glomerular filtration rate (GFR). This could increase the renal excretion of drugs that are significantly eliminated via this route.

▶ Drugs and their metabolites may also be excreted in breast milk. A nursing infant may therefore be exposed to the drug via the mother's milk. This could also apply to recreational drugs (such as dagga/cannabis) and environmental toxins.

Drug toxicity during pregnancy

Drugs may be toxic to the developing embryo and fetus. The first trimester of pregnancy (ie the stage of embryonic development and organogenesis) is of particular importance, since the teratogenic effects of certain drugs will influence normal development of the unborn child on a structural or functional level (see Figure 53.1 on page 838). A teratogen is a drug (or other chemical substance) that may affect normal embryonic development and cause recognisable congenital (birth) defects.

During the very early stages of pregnancy, the expectant mother may not even be aware of the fact that she is carrying a developing embryo (the excessive use of drinking alcohol, or ethanol, is of particular importance here). She may unknowingly harm her unborn child through the careless or indifferent use of drugs and other substances, including over-the-counter (OTC) medicines and other remedies. Therefore, this is an important topic to include in preconception care. Many pregnancies, however, are unplanned or unexpected, implying that preconception care would not have been rendered at all.

Also note that for drugs which have been shown to pose a significant risk to an unborn child, or in the case of drugs with insufficient evidence of relative safety during pregnancy, sufficient precautions in the form of patient education and the use of highly effective contraceptive methods need to be instituted when treating women of childbearing age or potential. Some drugs even need to be avoided in men who may father children while being treated with them.

Cross-placental transfer of drug molecules (and their metabolites)

Drug treatment during pregnancy implies that the unborn child will be exposed to either the effects of the drug on the mother, the direct effects of the drug on the embryo or fetus, or a combination of both.

The placenta acts as a barrier between the circulatory systems of mother and child throughout the duration of the pregnancy. However, in terms of drug molecules, this barrier is not very efficient, implying that when such molecules enter the maternal blood circulation, they have the potential of crossing this barrier and entering the fetal circulation as well. Lipid-soluble drugs are capable of crossing the placenta via simple diffusion. However, most water-soluble drugs can also cross the placenta because of the relative inefficiency of the barrier. Heparin is an exception. The box that follows highlights the four characteristics of drug molecules that are most likely to cross the placenta.

The characteristics that make drug molecules most likely to cross the placental barrier

- A high degree of fat-solubility (ie lipophilic molecules)
- A low degree of ionisation (ie molecules that do not carry charges)
- A low level of protein binding in the maternal bloodstream (drugs that are highly protein-bound have only small fractions of free molecules capable of crossing membranes)
- Low molecular mass (ie small molecules), especially in the case of water-soluble drugs. It is generally agreed that:
  - drug molecules with a molecular mass of less than 500 Da will readily cross the placenta
  - molecules of 500 to 1 000 Da will cross very slowly
  - molecules of more than 1 000 Da will not cross the placental barrier at all.

Excretion in breast milk

During lactation, drugs may pass from the bloodstream to the breast milk, especially if they are lipid-soluble or basic drugs (basic drugs will tend to ionise in the breast milk since it is more acidic than blood) or if they are water-soluble molecules with a relatively low molecular mass.

Drug safety during pregnancy and lactation

There is limited data available on the actual safety profiles of many drugs during pregnancy and lactation. (There are many reasons for this, similar to the ones that apply to drug therapy in the newborn). Drugs should therefore always be used with caution. However, many women will still take some medication during their pregnancy.

The prescriber must make pharmacotherapeutic decisions pertaining to each individual patient, with due consideration being given to the unique maternal, fetal and infant risk-benefit profiles. This highlights the importance of having a system that healthcare providers can use to make better and safer drug choices for their pregnant and lactating patients.

It is important to consult suitable drug references when prescribing and administering medicines to pregnant or lactating mothers. Known teratogens should obviously be avoided during pregnancy. However, situations may arise where the benefits of treating the mother with a certain drug may outweigh the possible harm that the drug may or may not do. For example, if aggressive cancer is endangering the life of an expectant mother, the decision to treat the mother's cancer may pose a considerable and unacceptable risk to the fetus, which could lead to the decision to abort the pregnancy to avoid the risk.

Pregnancy and lactation drug information and labelling safety rules

Towards the end of 2014, the Food and Drug Administration (FDA) in the USA announced its amendment of the content and format of its labelling requirements in the new Pregnancy and Lactation Labeling Rule. The FDA's goal with this amendment is to provide pregnant or breastfeeding mothers, as well as their healthcare providers, with the best possible information on the use of available agents during the various stages of pregnancy and lactation. These amendments came into effect on 30 June 2015.

Gaps in the previous FDA drug safety information

The previous FDA requirements for medication risks in pregnancy and breastfeeding consisted of the five-letter categories A, B, C, D and X. These categories attempted to broadly identify risk while using a specific medication. This simplified system did not provide sufficient information to allow healthcare providers to make the most informed decisions regarding drug choices for the pregnant or lactating mother. This system was misinterpreted as a grading system and the lack of information held a potential risk to both mother and fetus.

The new rule now consists of up-to-date and well-organised information to afford the healthcare provider with better information during the different stages of pregnancy. This labelling will also assist healthcare providers during the counselling of patients on the correct use of their medication during pregnancy and lactation.

New improved information labelling

The FDA also amended its requirements in terms of the relevant labelling subsections and their content. The subheadings 'Pregnancy', 'Labour and Delivery' and 'Nursing Mothers' have therefore been replaced or updated with 'Pregnancy' (to include labour and delivery), 'Lactation' (to include nursing mothers) and 'Females and Males of Reproductive Potential'. Both the pregnancy and lactation sections are further divided into a risk summary, clinical considerations and data section. The guideline also assists with the labelling of new products and reversing or amending existing labelling.

▶ *Pregnancy:* The pregnancy subsection provides information on the use of a specific drug during all three trimesters of pregnancy. This subsection also includes registers that collect and maintain data on how the said drug can affect pregnancy during certain trimesters, or after birth and into childhood.

continued

The new label will also include information on physiological changes during pregnancy and how these will affect dosage and risk during the stages of pregnancy, as well as the postpartum period. Information will be provided on maternal adverse reactions, fetal or neonatal adverse reactions and drug effects on delivery or labour. Disease-associated risks to mothers, embryos and fetuses are also included.

▶ *Lactation:* The lactation subsection provides more information on whether the active ingredient will have an effect on the infant during breastfeeding.

▶ *Females and males of reproductive potential:* This new subsection has information on how certain medications can affect fertility, pregnancy testing and contraception.

The package inserts and patient information leaflets of registered medicines should also be consulted for specific information on the use of such agents in the treatment of pregnant and lactating women, or even in women who are of childbearing potential but not yet pregnant (see the next section for more information on accessing and interpreting drug information via approved package inserts and patient information leaflets).

Well-known examples of teratogenic drugs include isotretinoin (used in the treatment of severe forms of acne), methotrexate (an antineoplastic and immunosuppressant agent), the anti-epileptic agents phenytoin and valproate, the antiretroviral (ARV) agent efavirenz (EFV), and warfarin (an oral anticoagulant). Using ethanol (drinking alcohol) during pregnancy may cause fetal alcohol syndrome (FAS). There are many more examples. Table 53.2 gives various examples of known teratogenic drugs to avoid during pregnancy. Note that drugs that are not listed here are not necessarily safe to use.

HIV, drugs and pregnancy (see Chapter 50)

Did you know?

Although EFV appears in the list of known teratogenic drugs and used to be contraindicated during pregnancy, this drug is currently included as part of the first-line treatment regimen, regardless of the GA of the unborn fetus. According to the WHO (2012), 'the available data and programmatic experience provides reassurance that exposure to EFV in early pregnancy has not resulted in increased birth defects or other significant toxicities'. Manufacturers are, however, still warning about the potential dangers of using EFV during the first trimester of pregnancy.

Table 53.2

Teratogenic agents

Teratogen	Effect
Alcohol	FAS Abnormal functioning of the CNS Disturbances of behaviour
Anticonvulsants	Valproate is associated with neural tube defects (NTDs), as is carbamazepine. Phenytoin may cause malformations in the CNS and adversely affect fetal growth.
Anticoagulants	Warfarin is associated with: ▶ haemorrhage in the fetus ▶ malformations in the CNS ▶ malformations in the skeletal system.
Antihypertensive agents	Angiotensin-converting enzyme (ACE) inhibitors cause renal damage and may restrict normal growth patterns in the unborn child.
Antineoplastic (anticancer or chemotherapeutic) drugs	High risk of multiple congenital malformations
ARV agents	EFV may be associated with NTD.
Isotretinoin (acne)	High risk of multiple congenital malformations
Misoprostol	Malformations of the CNS and limbs
Neuroleptic drugs	Lithium is associated with congenital defects of the cardiovascular system.
Non-steroidal anti-inflammatory drugs (NSAIDs)	Premature closing of the ductus arteriosus
Tetracyclines	Malformations of teeth (as well as permanent discolouration) and bone
Thalidomide	Malformations of the internal organs and limbs

In addition, the following drugs are associated with withdrawal symptoms in the newborn infant:

▶ Barbiturates
▶ Benzodiazepines
▶ Opioid analgesics
▶ Tricyclic antidepressants.

Interpreting drug information from package inserts and patient information leaflets

Package inserts and patient information leaflets have to contain all of the information regarded as essential and applicable to the registration status of a specific drug or medicinal product by the relevant regulatory authority. Information that may be found in an approved package insert and its accompanying patient information leaflet can be used to answer the following questions relating to the medicine's use in clinical practice (Schellack, 2010).

What type of product is it and how does it work?

Consider the pharmacological classification and description of the drug's mechanism of action and relevant pharmacodynamic properties.

Information on the composition of the product or medicine will include all of the active pharmaceutical ingredients (the drug, or, in the case of a fixed-dose combination [FDC], the drugs that make up the product) as well as all of the

843

excipients (the inactive ingredients used in the pharmaceutical formulation) required by the regulatory authority. The active ingredients (the actual drugs) are identified by their generic or non-proprietary names, for ease of reference.

What is or can this product be used for?

It is of vital importance that the approved indications are carefully considered. For each of the listed indications, scientific evidence of the drug's, medicine's or product's efficacy and safety would have been provided to the regulatory authority. Products may only be marketed and sold in accordance with their approved label, ie those indications that emerged from a comprehensive development plan and subsequently passed the scrutiny of the regulatory authorities.

It does, however, happen that drugs are sometimes used for other reasons or indications than those that have already been approved. In these situations, the drug or product concerned is being used off-label, which needs to be in the patient's best interest at all times, and should preferably be evidence-based (backed by scientific evidence or proof).

What will the body do with the drug(s)?

Consider all of the relevant biopharmaceutical and pharmacokinetic properties of the drug or drug combination that are described in relation to the kinetic processes, as well as important pharmacokinetic parameters, where applicable. These may include aspects such as the bioavailability, elimination half-life, hepatic or renal clearance, information on active drug metabolites, etc.

How safe and effective is the product?

At the recommended dosage, a drug's efficacy or therapeutic benefit should outweigh its possible risks or detrimental effects. Certain adverse drug reactions (or side effects) may be life-threatening and even fatal, although this is rare.

Many factors contribute towards a drug's risk-to-benefit ratio, including aspects such as age, gender, pregnancy and lactation, concomitant medication and other treatments, as well as co-morbid (coexisting) and intercurrent illnesses (occurring during the course of the illness already being treated).

In light of the above, careful consideration must be given to the following important aspects of the package insert:
- Boxed warnings are of significant importance and will be found as bold-type text enclosed in a text box, if and when required by the regulatory authorities. Read these warnings very carefully, since they could have a significant impact on the risk-to-benefit ratio for specific patients in given situations.
- Contraindications may be absolute or relative and need to be considered against the background of

the patient's health status and risk assessment, since relative contraindications only apply in certain patient populations or in the presence of specific risk factors. Relative contraindications are listed or described under warnings. Absolute contraindications, however, will prohibit the use of a specific drug, medicine or product, if and when they are present. This includes known hypersensitivity to any of the ingredients contained in the product. Certain drugs may also be contraindicated for use together with the specific product due to the likelihood of serious, dangerous or life-threatening drug interactions. Furthermore, the product or medicine may be contraindicated during pregnancy and lactation, if appropriate.
- Pay careful attention to warnings (including relative contraindications), adverse reactions (side effects), special precautions, drug interactions and the use of the specific product in special patient populations. These populations could include pregnant or breastfeeding mothers, infants and children, the elderly, patients with hepatic or renal impairment, gender and race (if applicable), smokers, implications for fertility and women of childbearing potential, and porphyria.
- Clinically significant interactions may also be listed for certain foodstuffs and beverages (eg grapefruit juice) as well as certain herbal remedies (eg St John's wort). A description of the effects of the product or medicine on the patient's ability to drive a motor vehicle or to operate machinery may be required by the regulatory authority. Also consider any statements on specific circumstances or instances for which safety and efficacy of the product have not been established.

How should the drug be administered to the patient? What dosage should the patient receive and how often?

The package insert will provide clear instructions on any special preparations, such as reconstitution, that need to be made before administering the product to a patient, as well as the route of administration for each individual dosage form, the recommended dosage for each of the approved indications, dosing intervals and the recommended duration of treatment.

Aspects such as dosing adjustments for specific patients or clinical conditions, as well as dosing adjustments for specific age groups, may be included. Information on maximum recommended dosages, correct usage, taking of the product or medicine in relation to meals, dose titration, dose tapering and monitoring of the patient's reaction to the treatment may be included as needed, or as required by the regulatory authority.

Other useful information

Regulatory authorities have different ways of limiting consumer access to medicinal products, which may be based on their potential to be abused or the perceived dangers involved in using them without the guidance and supervision of a qualified healthcare provider who is authorised to prescribe such medication. A clear distinction is made between OTC medicines and prescription-only medicines. The package insert will therefore reflect the status of the product in relation to the abovementioned explanation. In South Africa, for example, the package insert will reflect the product's scheduling status in accordance with the applicable legislation.

The information on a drug overdose, whether accidental or intentional, contained in the package insert is aimed at describing the clinical manifestations and possible complications of an overdose, as well as recommendations on how such an overdose should be managed. Management may include the administration of a known antidote, if applicable, interventions aimed at limiting the patient's exposure to the active ingredient(s), careful monitoring of the patient's condition and the use of standard symptomatic and supportive treatment.

The package insert will also contain information on how the product may be identified, its packaging and presentation, the relevant storage instructions and guidance on how the product should be handled.

Information aimed directly at the consumer is contained in the patient information leaflet.

Choices in drug therapy

Many different factors determine the choice and possible outcomes of drug therapy during pregnancy, childbirth and lactation. These factors include:

- age, obstetric history and gestation
- physical characteristics (eg size and body mass index [BMI])
- diet and nutritional status
- gene pool and genetic factors
- previous responses and reactions to drug treatment (including allergic reactions and anaphylaxis)
- other drugs already in use which may give rise to drug interactions, including OTC medicines and herbal remedies
- the influence of current and pre-existing illnesses
- the person's health status and general standard of living
- unwanted and toxic effects of the drugs in question
- patient compliance
- the pharmacological profile of the drug in question, since the altered physiology during pregnancy may alter the

way in which the body responds to the drug, as well as how the body deals with the drug molecules and their metabolites.

Treatment principles pertaining to drug therapy

The following treatment principles may be applied when considering or continuing drug therapy during pregnancy and lactation:

- Preferably choose drugs that are well known to be safe and effective during pregnancy and lactation.
- Use the lowest possible dosage of the drug with the shortest plasma half-life, for the shortest possible duration of treatment.
- Avoid new drugs due to the lack of data and clinical experience.
- All known teratogens (eg excessive dosages of vitamin A) should be avoided in women of childbearing potential, even if they are not pregnant, and sometimes even in fertile males.
- Discourage self-medicating practices and the indiscriminate use of OTC drugs, herbal and traditional remedies and nutritional supplements.
- Carefully consider possible drug interactions. Commonly used concomitant medications in pregnancy include the use of antacids, for example, which may interfere with drug absorption from the GI tract.
- Always refer to the most up-to-date information available on each drug in question.
- Drugs should never be administered to a pregnant woman, or any other patient, without performing a proper assessment, including history taking, current medication use, drug and food allergies, and other relevant information.

53.4   Drug therapy in the newborn

A newborn infant is exceptionally vulnerable to the effects of drugs and cannot communicate the adverse effects being experienced in the way that older children and adults would. Great care needs to be exercised when administering medication to a newborn.

Several drugs are prescribed and administered to newborns in spite of a lack of clinical evidence in this patient population. Infants treated in ICUs may often receive at least one drug that is unlicensed (not yet registered by the regulatory authority in question, possibly because it is still under clinical investigation) or off-label (used for an indication or a reason other than what has already been approved). There are several reasons for this, many of which pertain to the relative scarcity of clinical trial data in this patient population. This is due to factors such as:

▶ the nature of the patient population in question, which is very limited, high-risk and extremely vulnerable

▶ difficulties in conducting suitable clinical trials, both on ethical and technical grounds.

Clinicians therefore have to rely on preclinical trial data (derived from animal testing), case reports and surveillance data, which makes it difficult to predict the effects and possible outcomes of drug therapy in certain circumstances.

Newborn infants form part of the broader paediatric patient population and many of the general principles of paediatric pharmacotherapy apply to neonates, in addition to principles that aim to address their unique needs. The broader paediatric patient population comprises a diverse group of patients with a variety of characteristics, ranging from the preterm newborn to the adolescent on the brink of adulthood (see Table 53.3).

Table 53.3

Paediatric age groups according to the Eunice Kennedy Shriver National Institute of Child Health and Human Development (NICHD) classification system (NICHD, nd)

Neonatal	Full-term birth to 27 days old
Infancy	Full-term birth to 12 months
Toddlerhood	13 months to two years
Early childhood	2–5 years
Middle childhood	6–11 years
Early adolescence	12–18 years
Late adolescence	19–21 years

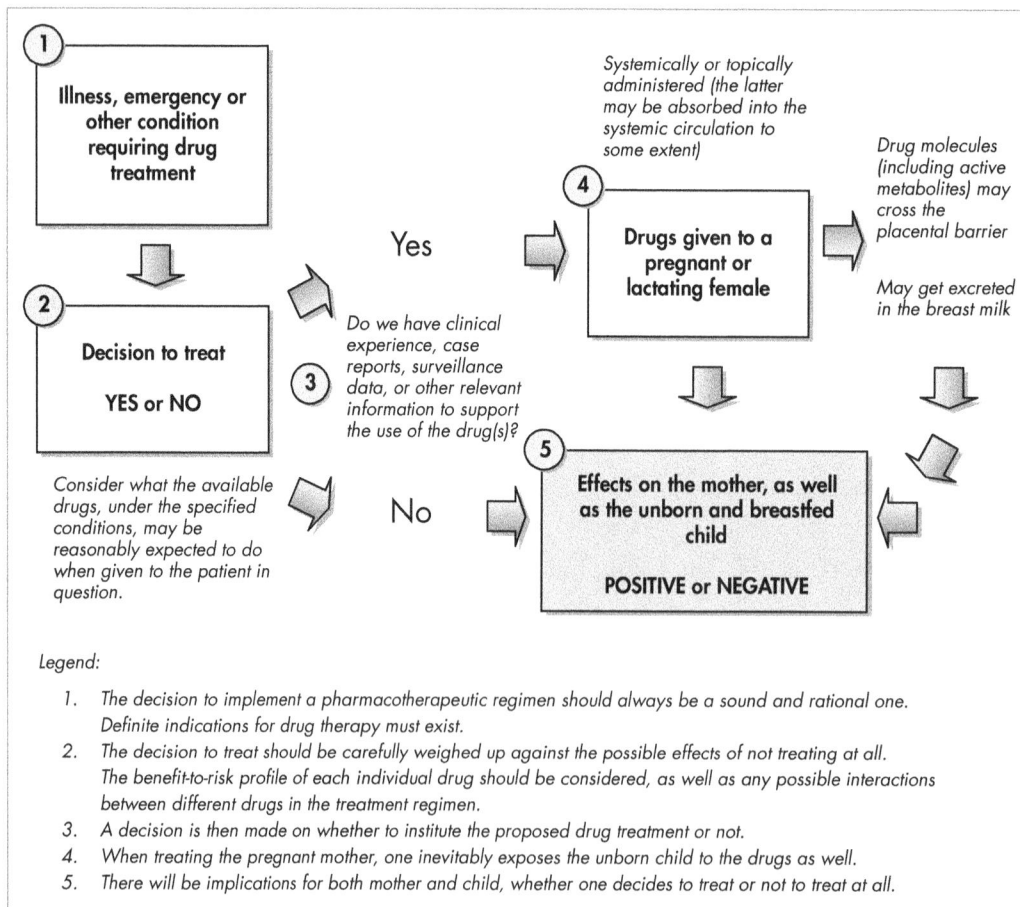

Legend:

1. The decision to implement a pharmacotherapeutic regimen should always be a sound and rational one. Definite indications for drug therapy must exist.
2. The decision to treat should be carefully weighed up against the possible effects of not treating at all. The benefit-to-risk profile of each individual drug should be considered, as well as any possible interactions between different drugs in the treatment regimen.
3. A decision is then made on whether to institute the proposed drug treatment or not.
4. When treating the pregnant mother, one inevitably exposes the unborn child to the drugs as well.
5. There will be implications for both mother and child, whether one decides to treat or not to treat at all.

Figure 53.2 A simplified diagram of pharmacotherapeutic decision making during pregnancy, childbirth, lactation and the neonatal period

Neonatal prescribing and dosing

Drug prescribing in this population has to follow the general principles of rational drug use, as prescribed by the 1996 National Drug Policy (NDP) for South Africa. These include (DoH, 1996):

- the correct drug (for the illness or infection being treated)
- the appropriate indication
- the appropriate drug (for the patient and condition being treated)
- the appropriate dosage, administration and duration of treatment
- the appropriate patient.

A practitioner should also consider giving drugs at the lowest possible cost to the patient and the community of concern. Figure 53.2 is a simplified diagram to illustrate the intricacies of clinical decision making when considering drug therapy in any of these vulnerable patient populations.

Paediatric dosing handbooks use various methods to calculate the correct drug dosage for paediatric patients. The patient's age, weight, height and body surface area (BSA), as well as relevant pharmacokinetic principles, may be taken into consideration. The BSA may be calculated by using Mosteller's formula (see the box below).

Mosteller's formula for calculating body surface area

$$\sqrt{\text{BSA (m}^2) = [\text{weight (kg)} \times \text{height (cm)}] \div 3\ 600}$$

The BSA refers to the total skin surface area covering the human body. Clinically, the BSA has huge application value, from calculating accurate drug dosages in neonates to determining ideal fluid intake, renal clearance and other parameters. Mosteller's formula uses body weight (in kg) and height (in cm) – or length, in the case of infants – in a simplified method of calculating the BSA. The average BSA value for a neonate is 0.25 m²; for an adult woman it is 1.6 m².

The BSA is of particular importance when calculating the dosages of certain ARV agents in paediatrics, such as didanosine (ddI) and the lopinavir/ritonavir (LPV/r) combination.

Additionally, in the neonatal population, specific factors such as GA and birth weight need to be taken into consideration. The specific terminology relating to the calculation of neonatal dosages is presented in Table 53.4.

Table 53.4

Neonatal dosing terminology

Term	Definition
GA	*By dates.* The number of weeks from the onset of the mother's last normal menstrual period until birth *By examination.* Assessment of gestation (time from conception until birth) using a physical and neuromuscular examination
Low birth weight (LBW)	< 2 500 g
Very low birth weight (VLBW)	< 1 500 g
Appropriate for gestational age (AGA)	Birth weight between the 10th and 90th percentile for GA
Large for gestational age (LGA)	Birth weight > 90th percentile for GA
Preterm neonate/infant	< 37 completed weeks GA at birth
Full-term neonate/infant	38 to 42 weeks GA at birth

Pharmacokinetics and pharmacodynamics in the neonate

Drug therapy, prescribing and dosing should consider the differences between the preterm neonate, full-term neonate and young infant in terms of drug disposition (absorption, distribution, metabolism and elimination/excretion).

Absorption

The neonatal period is characterised by problems related to drug disposition, as the digestive system is undergoing major adjustments, and the absorption of any orally administered substance is variable. Relative achlorhydria (the absence of hydrochloric acid from the gastric secretions) is present for the first 10–15 days after birth. Compared to that of an adult, gastric emptying is also delayed. The reduced gastric acid secretion increases the bioavailability of acid-labile drugs (eg penicillin) and decreases the bioavailability of weak acidic drugs (eg phenobarbitone).

IM administration of drugs in the neonate is generally not used, because it is considered to be too painful. In addition,

IM absorption is erratic in neonates due to scarce muscle and adipose tissue. Transdermal absorption may be a preferred method of delivering drugs to the systemic circulation, as it bypasses the immature GI system. However, physiological factors such as the presence of brown fat under the skin surface, the presence of pigmented lesions on the skin, and conditions such as hyperbilirubinaemia, hyperviscosity or vasculitis may lead to inter-individual variation in drug absorption from one infant to the next. The ratio of skin surface to body weight is approximately three times greater in infants than in adults. Premature neonates have an incompletely formed stratum corneum (the outermost layer of the skin, which acts as a protective barrier when developed). This can lead to systemic toxicity due to the absorption of toxic compounds such as aniline dyes, hexachlorophene and alcohol through the skin (Choonara & Tieder, 2002; Pelletier, Perez & Jacob, 2016).

Distribution

The volume of distribution (V_d) also differs with age (see Figure 53.3 for an illustration of these differences from the neonatal period to old age). Even the water content differs between a preterm infant (80 per cent) and a full-term infant (70 per cent). These differences are important when determining suitable dosages for drugs such as the aminoglycosides. The V_d of the aminoglycosides is approximately 0.6 ℓ/kg in the neonate, whereas in adults the V_d is 0.2 to 0.3 ℓ/kg.

Figure 53.3 also shows that the premature neonate has lower total protein contents than the other paediatric age groups. Neonates have decreased levels of protein binding when compared to adults. This influences drug availability. The comparative protein binding for the newborn versus the adult in the case of ampicillin, for example, is 10 per cent versus 18 per cent and for theophylline it is 36 per cent in neonates versus 56 per cent in adults.

The risk of the neonate developing kernicterus (bilirubin encephalopathy) is also increased, since the neonate has decreased blood albumin levels. There are several drugs that are thought to compete with or displace bilirubin from its binding site on the albumin molecule, which increases the risk of developing kernicterus.

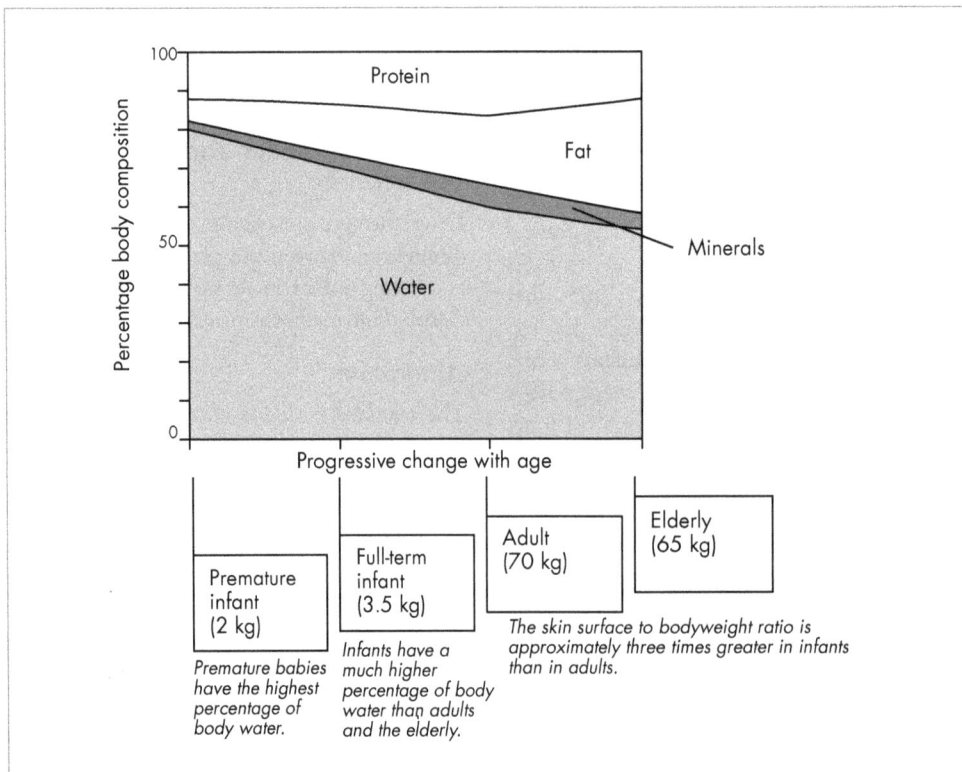

Figure 53.3 Proportionate changes in body composition with age (adapted from Puig, 1996)

The antibacterial agent ceftriaxone is an example of a drug that displays one of the highest levels of bilirubin displacement. In addition, it is believed that cotrimoxazole, based on its pharmacological properties, displaces bilirubin from its albumin binding sites, thereby increasing bilirubin levels. This, in turn, could also result in kernicterus.

Metabolism

Some drugs may pass through the body entirely unchanged, or they may be biotransformed (metabolised) into some other substance (a metabolite). The metabolite can be either pharmacologically active or inactive, and will be more water-soluble than the administered drug (or parent compound), causing it to be excreted more rapidly. The conversion of theophylline to caffeine is an example of the formation of an active metabolite, and is of significant importance in the neonatal population, since caffeine has an elimination half-life of 100 hours; this can result in a noteworthy accumulation of the active metabolite.

The cytochrome P450 (CYP) enzyme system is an extremely important system for drug metabolism. Furthermore, the CYP system can be induced or inhibited by certain drugs such as phenobarbitone, which induces enzyme activity, not only increasing its own hepatic elimination (an example of auto-induction), but also that of other substances such as bilirubin.

Elimination/excretion

The renal system is not the only system responsible for excretion. Other systems involved in drug excretion include the biliary system and the pulmonary system. The exocrine glands can also participate in this process. Excretion is the last of the four kinetic processes.

Renal plasma flow is low at birth (12 ml/min) and gradually reaches the adult level of 140 ml/min by the age of one year. Renal excretion includes three processes, namely glomerular filtration, active tubular secretion and passive tubular reabsorption. The first two processes reach adult values at about 6 months of age. The changes in the half-life of theophylline clearly illustrate the changes in these processes. Its half-life is 30 hours in the preterm infant, 14 hours in the full-term infant less than 6 months of age, 4.6 hours in infants between 6 and 11 months of age, and 3.4 hours in children between 1 and 4 years old. These differences are due to the maturation of kidney and liver function. A better understanding of these processes could prevent inadvertent overdose in infants younger than 1 year of age and the risk of suboptimal dosing in children of 1 to 4 years of age.

Drugs used in the neonatal period

Table 53.5 summarises the classes of drugs most widely used in the neonatal setting. These are described with reference to their generic names, mechanisms of action, clinical uses and special nursing implications (which incorporate adverse effects that are of particular interest, as well as special precautions, warnings and contraindications). The Anatomical Therapeutic Chemical (ATC) classification system of the WHO has been used to organise the content. The ATC classification system divides drugs into different groups according to the organ and system on which they act and their pharmacological, therapeutic and chemical characteristics. (Visit http://www.who.int/classifications/atcddd/en/ and http://www.whocc.no/atc_ddd_index/ for more information on this classification system.)

Table 53.5

Commonly encountered pharmacotherapeutic agents used in the neonate, grouped according to the WHO's ATC classification system

Generic name	Mechanism of action or uses	Nursing implications
A → Alimentary tract and metabolism		
Metoclopramide (nausea/vomiting)	GI dysmotility or gastro-oesophageal reflux disease (GERD): used as a prokinetic agent to promote enteral feeding, to treat and manage gastric stasis.	The adverse effects seem to be related to the dosage given. Higher dosages may lead to a higher likelihood of side effects. High dosages may precipitate extrapyramidal effects (eg oculogyric crisis with torticollis and neck pain). It should be administered 6-hourly, 30 minutes prior to a feeding (for optimum effectiveness).

continued

Generic name	Mechanism of action or uses	Nursing implications
	The prokinetic effects may be due to dopamine receptor (D2) antagonism, but also due to its effect on acetylcholine release from the postganglionic nerve terminal, peripherally related to the drug's effect on the smooth muscle of the GI tract. In higher dosages it may be used for its anti-emetic properties in older children and adults.	
Ranitidine (acid-reflux control)	To increase gastric pH in patients at risk of GI haemorrhage, eg GERD, etc. It is a competitive antagonist of histamine at the H2-receptors, including receptors on the gastric cells.	Careful consideration should be given before administration of ranitidine in the neonate, as the H2-receptor antagonism may increase the risk of developing necrotising enterocolitis (NEC), especially in VLBW neonates. There are fewer drug interactions with ranitidine than with cimetidine. Do not co-administer with antacids. Delay administration of ranitidine after administration of an antacid. Dosages should be adjusted in patients with renal or hepatic impairment, since ranitidine is excreted primarily by the kidneys and metabolised by the liver.

B → Blood and blood-forming organs

Generic name	Mechanism of action or uses	Nursing implications
Vitamin K1 (phytonadione)	This is used as prophylaxis and treatment of haemolytic disease of the newborn (HDN). It is important in the synthesis of coagulation factors II, VII, IX and X.	IM administration (an exception to the general guideline) of vitamin K seems to prevent both early and late presentation of HDN, and IM administration seems to be more effective than oral administration. Administer within 1 hour after birth.

C → Cardiovascular system

Generic name	Mechanism of action or uses	Nursing implications
Furosemide	This is a high-ceiling (loop) diuretic. It is used to treat oedema in renal, hepatic, pulmonary and heart disease. It may be used to treat neonatal hypertension and hypercalcaemia. This is used when a greater diuretic effect is needed than that provided by thiazide diuretics.	It may cause dehydration and electrolyte imbalances (especially potassium and sodium depletion). Supplement these when needed. When used with an aminoglycoside, furosemide may potentiate the risk of developing ototoxicity. Monitor glucose levels, as it may cause hyperglycaemia and glycosuria. In preterm infants, use the minimum effective dosage. During long-term therapy, alternate day therapy may be considered. When administered orally, a higher dosage may be required because of a reduction in its bioavailability.

continued

Generic name	Mechanism of action or uses	Nursing implications
Hydrochlorothiazide	This is a low-ceiling thiazide diuretic. It is used for neonatal hypertension. It is often used in combination with spironolactone to treat pulmonary fluid accumulation in chronic lung diseases, eg bronchopulmonary dysplasia (BPD).	This may cause dehydration. Electrolyte disturbances (eg hyponatraemia and hypokalaemia) may occur when it is administered on its own. Caution should be taken when administering with spironolactone, since it may cause hyperkalaemia.
Dopamine	Administer via continuous IV infusion. Do not administer via the umbilical arterial catheter or any other artery. Use a large vein for IV administration. *Low dosages:* 1–5 mcg/kg/minute provides a diuretic effect via increased renal blood flow (dopamine-receptor effects). *Intermediate dosages:* 5–15 mcg/kg/minute increases both renal blood flow and cardiac output (b-receptor effects); both heart rate and cardiac contractility are increased, which also increases the arterial BP. *High dosages:* At > 15 mcg/kg/minute, α-receptor effects begin to predominate, with subsequent vasoconstriction that leads to increased peripheral vascular resistance.	Correct any fluid deficit prior to administration. Side effects are dosage-related. Adverse effects are usually seen at dosages above 20 mcg/kg/minute. Blanching along the vein into which it is being administered may result; this is usually not harmful. Avoid extravasation (infusing the drug into the tissue), as this may cause gangrene.

H → Systemic hormonal preparations (excluding sex hormones and insulins)

Generic name	Mechanism of action or uses	Nursing implications
Dexamethasone	This is a long-acting corticosteroid with minimal sodium-retaining potential. It is used: • as an anti-inflammatory agent to prevent chronic lung disease • as an immunosuppressant • for the treatment of airway oedema prior to endotracheal extubation • for BPD, to shorten the length of time required for mechanical ventilation.	Monitor for hypertension and hyperglycaemia immediately after administration of the dosage. If used for a prolonged period of time, monitor for signs of infection, especially fungal infections. If used for prolonged periods of time, monitor growth parameters and neurodevelopmental markers. Use the lowest possible dosage for the shortest period of time.

J → Anti-infectives for systemic use

J01 → Antibacterials for systemic use

J01C → Beta-lactam antibacterials, penicillins

Generic name	Mechanism of action or uses	Nursing implications
Benzylpenicillin	This is a beta-lactam antibiotic. It is used in combination with an aminoglycoside as empirical treatment to prevent early sepsis.	Observe the IV site to prevent extravasation. Observe for hypersensitivity reactions. The IV infusion should be diluted with dextrose 5% or normal saline. Do not mix with other drugs, especially the aminoglycosides. Aminoglycosides are inactivated by high dosages of IV benzylpenicillin.

continued

Generic name	Mechanism of action or uses	Nursing implications
Amoxicillin	This beta-lactam antibiotic is an extended-spectrum penicillin with more or less the same spectrum as ampicillin. It is preferred over ampicillin for oral therapy, as it causes less GI side effects, requires smaller daily dosages and is better absorbed orally. It is often used in combination with either an aminoglycoside or a cephalosporin for the management of meningitis in the neonate due to *Listeria monocytogenes*. It is used for urinary tract infection (UTI) prophylaxis in infants younger than 1–2 months of age. It is also used for the prevention of bacterial endocarditis and the treatment of acute otitis media.	Observe for hypersensitivity reactions. Monitor for diarrhoea. Do not mix in the same syringe as the aminoglycosides, or administer in the same IV line, as the risk of inactivation of the aminoglycosides exists.
Piperacillin and tazobactam combination	Piperacillin is an antipseudomonal penicillin. The combination with tazobactam extends the spectrum to include beta-lactamase-producing bacteria. When used in combination with an aminoglycoside, synergism is achieved.	Do not mix in the same syringe as the aminoglycosides, or administer in the same IV line, as the risk of inactivation of the aminoglycosides exists. Monitor for signs of oedema or hypernatraemia and hypokalaemia.

J01D → Other beta-lactam antibacterials

Generic name	Mechanism of action or uses	Nursing implications
Meropenem	This broad-spectrum antibiotic has excellent Gram-negative activity. It is only registered for use in infants over 3 months of age, although kinetic studies have been done in infants younger than 3 months. In children over 3 months, it is used for serious infections (eg meningitis).	Do not use routinely, to prevent possible resistance. Monitor for the occurrence of rash and diarrhoea.
Cephalosporins (cefotaxime and ceftazidime)	These are third-generation cephalosporins. They are semi-synthetic beta-lactam antibiotics. They are used as empiric antibiotic therapy for suspected meningitis. They should preferably be used in combination with an aminoglycoside, to prevent resistance.	Resistance is a major problem with the cephalosporins and they should be used judiciously. Monitor for rash and/or diarrhoea.

J01E → Sulphonamides and trimethoprim

Generic name	Mechanism of action or uses	Nursing implications
Cotrimoxazole	This is a broad-spectrum antibiotic. It is used as prophylaxis and treatment of *Pneumocystis jirovecii* (formerly *P carinii*).	It should preferably only be used from 6 weeks of age, due to an increased risk of kernicterus developing in the jaundiced infant. Prevent dehydration in the infant receiving cotrimoxazole. Monitor for rash and/or diarrhoea.

continued

Generic name	Mechanism of action or uses	Nursing implications
		Some preparations may contain either benzyl alcohol or propylene glycol. Either of these ingredients in large quantities may have toxic side effects. The former may cause the so-called gasping syndrome in neonates, and the latter may result in hyperosmolality, lactic acidosis, depressed breathing and seizure activity.

J01F → Macrolides, ketolides and lincosamides

Generic name	Mechanism of action or uses	Nursing implications
Erythromycin	This is used for atypical infections in the neonate caused by *Chlamydia trachomatis* pneumonitis, *Ureaplasma urealyticum* and other atypical organisms. It is also used for its prokinetic effects in the GI tract (where it stimulates the motilin receptors).	Monitor for signs and symptoms of gastric intolerance, as it can cause infantile hypertrophic pyloric stenosis. It can cause pain at the site of infusion and vein irritation; monitor the IV site. Monitor for signs of diarrhoea.

J01G → Aminoglycoside antibacterials

Generic name	Mechanism of action or uses	Nursing implications
Amikacin Gentamicin	These are broad-spectrum protein synthesis inhibitors. They are most often used in synergistic relationship with a penicillin. They have excellent Gram-negative coverage. They are used for the treatment of serious infections caused by sensitive Gram-negative organisms.	Therapeutic drug monitoring should be requested to establish safety (it can cause oto- and nephrotoxicity). It should not be administered in the same syringe or IV line as the penicillins. Monitor renal function. In patients with impaired renal function, therapeutic drug monitoring should be done to preserve renal function. It should be infused over 30 minutes. Administration is once daily.
Tobramycin	As for gentamicin. However, a comparison between tobramycin and gentamicin has suggested less nephrotoxicity with tobramycin and a greater activity against *Pseudomonas* spp with tobramycin. These comparisons were done in adults.	As for gentamicin

J01M → Quinolone antibacterials

Generic name	Mechanism of action or uses	Nursing implications
Ciprofloxacin	This broad-spectrum antibiotic (may be reserved for *Pseudomonas aeruginosa* and *Klebsiella pneumoniae*) acts by inhibiting DNA gyrase. It is used in paediatrics where the benefits outweigh the risk. Its use is restricted in neonates and children due to the potential side effects on joint cartilage.	Subsequent studies have suggested that it may be used with caution in neonates with septicaemia due to multi-drug-resistant organisms.

continued

Generic name	Mechanism of action or uses	Nursing implications
J01X → Other antibacterials		
Vancomycin	This is a bacterial cell wall synthesis inhibitor. It should be reserved for serious Staphylococcal infections, especially methicillin-resistant *Staphylococcus aureus* (MRSA) and *S epidermidis* (MRSE). In neonates it is also effective against *Listeria monocytogenes*.	Routine therapeutic drug monitoring in the neonate is not indicated. It causes ototoxicity. Refer for regular audiological examination. This is not as frequent if vancomycin levels are kept within the therapeutic range. Nephrotoxicity is not as common anymore; however, it is important to monitor urinary output and renal markers. 'Red man' (or 'red baby') syndrome may develop due to rapid infusion of vancomycin. A rapid infusion causes massive histamine release from mast cells. Therefore, always dilute well and infuse slowly.
J02 → Antimycotics for systemic use		
Fluconazole	This fungistatic is a member of the azole class of antifungal agents. It is an inhibitor of ergosterol in the fungal cell membrane. It is used as the main alternative to amphotericin B when treating neonatal candidiasis. It is used in the prevention of cryptococcal meningitis.	Resistance is developing from overuse. Monitor for GI symptoms such as diarrhoea and feeding intolerance. Monitor liver functions, especially in patients with jaundice.
Voriconazole	This belongs to the same class of antifungal agents as fluconazole. It may be used for severe fungal infections in the neonate.	There is limited pharmacokinetic data available for the neonatal patient population.
Amphotericin B	This is a polyene macrolide antibiotic. It has fungicidal effects through binding to the sterol moiety (ergosterol) in sensitive fungi, leading to leakage of the intracellular ions, which eventually results in cell death. Most species of *Candida* are considered susceptible; however, resistance has emerged in *C krusei* and *C glabrata*, for example. It is the drug of choice for all life-threatening mycotic infections.	Infusion-related toxicity is a reaction that consists of fever, chills, muscle spasms, vomiting, headache and hypotension. Pre-medicating with antipyretics, antihistamines and corticosteroids could be helpful. Do not administer rapidly. Administer over 4 hours. Renal toxicity has been described as dosage-dependent. Ensure good hydration and monitor renal markers. Monitor potassium and magnesium levels (it may cause hypokalaemia and hypomagnesaemia). Monitor liver functions weekly, as it may cause liver damage. Administration of a test dose is a contentious issue and should be gauged by the clinical condition of the patient. Do not mix with saline solution. Dextrose is recommended.

continued

Generic name	Mechanism of action or uses	Nursing implications
J05 → Antivirals for systemic use (see Chapter 50)		
M → Musculoskeletal system		
Indomethacin	This is an NSAID. It is used in the pharmacological closure of patent ductus arteriosus (PDA) in preterm infants. It is also used in the prevention of intraventricular haemorrhage (IVH).	Ibuprofen (see below) has been proven to be equally effective with fewer side effects (eg oliguria). Monitor renal function, as renal impairment has been noted, and can be clinically monitored by monitoring urinary output. It may have GI effects, eg abdominal distention, bleeding and even perforation. If abdominal distension is noted, discontinue the drug. Inhibition of platelet aggregation has been noted. Monitor platelet counts. A regimen of indomethacin normally constitutes three IV dosages, staggered at intervals of 12–24 hours. If unsuccessful and if urine output is normal, a second course (one to two doses) may be administered.
Ibuprofen	This is an NSAID.	Calculate dosages based on birth weight. Monitor urine output for signs of renal impairment.
Pancuronium	This is a non-depolarising, neuromuscular blocking agent. It is used for skeletal muscle relaxation during surgery (general anaesthesia) and for mechanical ventilation.	The drug should only be administered by an experienced medical practitioner, and only if facilities for endotracheal intubation, artificial ventilation and oxygen supplementation are available. The medical practitioner should be prepared to assist and support ventilation. Neonates are very sensitive to the effects of the non-depolarising skeletal muscle relaxing agents, and should be tested (with a test dosage) for responsiveness. The long-term use of pancuronium has been associated with methaemoglobinaemia and prolonged, severe skeletal muscle weakness. Antagonists such as pyridostigmine and neostigmine in combination with atropine should be readily available.
N → Nervous system		
Midazolam	This is a short-acting benzodiazepine. It is used as a sedative in infants undergoing procedures in the ICU, eg mechanical ventilation. It does not provide any pain relief.	Continued use in the NICU is not justified and may lead to unpleasant withdrawal symptoms. GA has a marked effect on the drug's half-life and clearance changes rapidly within the first few weeks of life. High dosages, rapid administration or concurrent use with an opioid lead to an increased chance of respiratory depression.

continued

Generic name	Mechanism of action or uses	Nursing implications
		If used continuously for more than one week, the risk of physiological dependency is increased. The dosage must be tapered to minimise withdrawal symptoms. Withdrawal can be achieved by tapering the dosage every second day, decreasing the dosage by about 10%, as tolerated. Use the lowest effective dosage for the shortest period of time. The antidote for midazolam is flumazenil.
Pethidine (syn meperidine)	This is an opioid analgesic. It is used for the management of severe pain in the neonate, eg post-operative pain. This is best used in conjunction with a neonatal pain scale to assess the severity of pain. Morphine is an alternative to pethidine for the management of severe pain. **The routine use of pethidine in neonates is not recommended (if used, it should be discontinued in ≤ 48 hours).**	Increasing the dosage or concurrent use with a benzodiazepine may increase the risk of respiratory depression. The antidote for pethidine is naloxone. It can cause addiction. Do not discontinue abruptly. Tolerance develops to the drug. The toxic metabolite is norpethidine (syn normeperidine), which may cause seizures in neonates. However, the rate of accumulation is slow. Accumulation is more likely in neonates with renal failure, or when extremely high dosages of pethidine are administered. After administration, observe BP and heart rate. Observe the level of sedation and pain relief. After long-term administration, observe and monitor for withdrawal symptoms.
Morphine	This is an opioid analgesic. It is used for pain relief, endotracheal intubation and neonatal abstinence syndrome. Its analgesic effects – through its actions on the opioid receptors in the CNS, and by inhibiting the ascending pain pathways – produces a generalised CNS depression. It is best used in conjunction with a neonatal pain scale to assess the severity of pain.	See the guidelines for pethidine. Monitor breathing rate, oxygen saturation, mental status, arterial BP, heart rate, the level of pain relief and sedation, as well as for signs of misuse, abuse and addiction. Titrate dosages according to the desired effect.
Phenobarbitone (syn phenobarbital)	This is a barbiturate anticonvulsant, with sedative-hypnotic properties. It is used in the management of neonatal seizures. Therapeutic drug monitoring (TDM) is recommended, especially in infants with hepatic disorders. It is a hepatic enzyme inducer; it may increase the elimination of not only certain other drugs and bilirubin, but also of phenobarbitone itself (auto-induction).	There is a lack of evidence for the prophylactic use of oral phenobarbitone in preventing phototherapy in jaundiced patients; this has not been proven by evidence-based medicine. Monitor the patient for respiratory depression, especially if used with other opioids or benzodiazepines. Taper the drug carefully, as abrupt withdrawal may cause seizures.

continued

Generic name	Mechanism of action or uses	Nursing implications
P → Antiparasitic products, insecticides and repellents		
Metronidazole	This is used for anaerobic sepsis in the neonate (anaerobic Gram-positive and anaerobic Gram-negative bacteria, eg *Bacteroides fragilis*, and protozoa).	This is best used in combination with other antimicrobials, as it does not include aerobic organisms in its spectrum of activity. Monitor for clinical improvement. It is used in prophylaxis of high-risk abdominal surgery. Monitor full blood count (FBC) for neutropaenia.
R → Respiratory system		
Aminophylline	This is classified as a methylxanthine. It is used in the prevention of apnoea of prematurity (AOP) in the neonatal population (caffeine may be preferred for this indication). It may also be used to reduce the risk of BPD. The proposed mechanism of action for this indication is via adenosine antagonism, which increases the sensitivity of the respiratory centres to carbon dioxide, thus acting as a driver for inspiration.	The therapeutic range is narrow and serum levels should be monitored. The lowest possible therapeutically active dosage should be given to avoid adverse effects. Adverse effects include tachycardia, tachypnoea, hyperactivity, nausea, vomiting and headache. CNS side effects may be more frequent with increased dosages. Monitor the heart rate. If it is above 180 bpm, it may be due to aminophylline toxicity and should be investigated, and the next dosage skipped. Re-evaluate. In patients with NEC, oral theophylline should be discontinued.
Caffeine	This is classified as a methylxanthine. It is used in the prevention of AOP in the neonatal population. It stimulates the respiratory centres via adenosine antagonism, increasing the sensitivity to carbon dioxide, thus acting as a driver for inspiration.	Therapeutic drug monitoring of caffeine remains controversial, as the drug is usually well tolerated. Monitor for clinical signs of toxicity, eg tachycardia (> 180 bpm), jitteriness, irritability and feeding intolerance.
Poractant alfa (Curosurf®)	This is a porcine surfactant consisting of 99% polar lipids (mainly phospholipids) and 1% hydrophobic proteins of low molecular weight. It is used to reduce the morbidity and mortality associated with respiratory distress syndrome (RDS, or hyaline membrane disease [HMD]). (Physiologically, surfactant plays a vital role in reducing the surface tension at the air–liquid interface of the alveoli during lung ventilation, effectively preventing alveolar collapse at resting trans-pulmonary pressures).	**This is for endotracheal administration only.** Monitor saturation while administering the drug, as desaturation may occur during administration. Transient episodes of bradycardia and hypotension may occur upon administration. Follow the manufacturer's guidelines. Store the drug in a medicine fridge (2–8 °C). Warm to room temperature prior to use. (Vials are for single use only; do not warm and then refrigerate again.) **Protect from light and do not shake.** If dispersion of particles occur, swirl vial.

continued

Generic name	Mechanism of action or uses	Nursing implications
Beractant (Survanta®)	This is a natural bovine lung extract. It contains phospholipids, neutral lipids, fatty acids and surfactant-associated proteins, to which colfosceril palmitate, palmitic acid and tripalmitin have been added. These are added to mimic naturally occurring human surfactant with surface-lowering properties. It is used in RDS (or HMD). (Physiologically, surfactant plays a vital role in reducing the surface tension at the air–liquid interface of the alveoli during lung ventilation, effectively preventing alveolar collapse at resting trans-pulmonary pressures.)	**This is for endotracheal use only.** Frequent monitoring of saturation is necessary, as rapid improvements in oxygenation may occur. Frequent monitoring prevents hyperoxia. Follow the manufacturer's guidelines for administration. **Do not shake vial. If dispersion of particles occur, swirl vial.** Artificial warming techniques should not be followed. The drug should be warmed to room temperature 20 minutes prior to administration or warmed in the hand for at least eight minutes. Store in the refrigerator between 2–8 °C. Do not remove from the fridge for more than 24 hours. Bradycardia and desaturation may occur while administering the drug; ensure proper monitoring. Protect from light. Hypo- or hypertension may occur.

53.5   Conclusion

The use of drug therapy in pregnancy, childbirth, lactation and the newborn infant requires careful consideration by all healthcare providers involved. Altered physiology changes the pregnant woman's and neonate's ability to absorb, transport, metabolise and excrete drugs. There are several drugs for which the optimal therapeutic dosages and safety parameters have not been established in this population, leaving practitioners, pregnant women and neonates at potential risk. For this reason, midwives need a thorough understanding of the use of medication in obstetrics and neonatology, and the potential dangers to both mother and baby. A number of drugs have been used very successfully and, as more experienced is gained, with a wider variety of therapeutic agents, more options – as well as additional challenges – will arise.

Annexure A : ICD-10 codes

The International Statistical Classification of Diseases and Related Health Problems 10th Revised Version for 2007 is a system to classify the health status of a person for statistical purposes and to determine health profiles and healthcare costs for healthcare planning. It assists in standardising diagnosis and care.

The ICD-10 codes have been accepted and used in the public sector in South Africa since 2004. The private healthcare sector also uses the system.

All medical practitioners are required by medical insurance companies to indicate the correct codes of the conditions that a person presents with or is diagnosed with. The ICD codes indicate:

▶ primary diagnosis
▶ secondary diagnosis
▶ comorbidities
▶ events.

CPT4 codes are related to the ICD-10 codes and are the interventions (medical and nursing) to treat the condition.

The complete diagnostic possibility is arranged in systems and linked to the alphabet.

Gynaecology and obstetrics are represented from N to Q as indicated in the table that follows.

The conditions are listed from 0–99 for each alphabetical category. The specific description is further indicated, for example 0.0; 0.1; 0.2.

The following tables give the main categories of conditions for gynaecological and obstetric conditions only.

Comorbidities from any other system can be added.

Each ICD-10 code consists of seven alphanumeric characters. The second through seventh characters mean the same thing within each section, but may mean different things in other sections. Each character can be any of 34 possible values, the ten digits 0-9 and the 24 letters A–H, J–N and P–Z may be used, in each character. There are no decimals in ICD-10-PCS. For more information, visit https://www.practicefusion.com/icd-10/clinical-concepts-for-obgyn/icd-10-codes/.

Key for obstetrics

▶ Character 1 = Section
▶ Character 2 = Body system
▶ Character 3 = Root operation
▶ Character 4 = Body part
▶ Character 5 = Approach
▶ Character 6 = Device
▶ Character 7 = Qualifier

Chapter XIV	N00-N99	**Diseases of the genitourinary system**
Chapter XV	O00-O99	**Pregnancy, childbirth and the puerperium**
	O00-O08	Pregnancy with abortive outcome
	O10-O16	Oedema, proteinuria and hypertensive disorders in pregnancy, childbirth and the puerperium
	O20-O29	Other maternal disorders predominantly related to pregnancy

continued

	O30-O48	Maternal care related to the fetus and amniotic cavity and possible delivery problems
	O60-O75	Complications of labour and delivery
	O80-O84	Delivery
	O85-O92	Complications predominantly related to the puerperium
	O94-O99	Other obstetric conditions, not elsewhere classified
Chapter XVI	P00-P96	**Certain conditions originating in the perinatal period**
	P00-P04	Fetus and newborn affected by maternal factors and by complications of pregnancy, labour and delivery
	P05-P08	Disorders related to length of gestation and fetal growth
	P10-P15	Birth trauma
	P20-P29	Respiratory and cardiovascular disorders specific to the perinatal period
	P35-P39	Infections specific to the perinatal period
	P50-P61	Haemorrhagic and haematological disorders of the fetus and newborn
	P70-P74	Transitory endocrine and metabolic disorders specific to the fetus and newborn
	P75-P78	Digestive system disorders of fetus and newborn
	P80-P83	Conditions involving the integument and temperature regulation of fetus and newborn
	P90-P96	Other disorders originating in the perinatal period
Chapter XVII	Q00-Q99	**Congenital malformations, deformations and chromosomal abnormalities**
	Q00-Q07	Congenital malformations of the nervous system
	Q10-Q18	Congenital malformations of eye, ear, face and neck
	Q20-Q28	Congenital malformations of the circulatory system
	Q30-Q34	Congenital malformations of the respiratory system
	Q35-Q37	Cleft lip and cleft palate
	Q38-Q45	Other congenital malformations of the digestive system
	Q50-Q56	Congenital malformations of genital organs
	Q60-Q64	Congenital malformations of the urinary system
	Q65-Q79	Congenital malformations and deformations of the musculoskeletal system
	Q80-Q89	Other congenital malformations
	Q90-Q99	Chromosomal abnormalities, not elsewhere classified

Annexure B: Competencies, interventions and procedures in obstetrics

Essential (life-saving) obstetric interventions and competencies for skilled attendants	Interventions by independent midwives	Medical procedures	Procedures that midwives perform under supervision/ collaboration
Breech delivery	Artificial rupture of membranes (AROM)	Infertility investigations	IOL
Premature delivery	Episiotomy (cut and suture)	Induction of labour (IOL)	Augmentation of labour
Ventouse delivery	Suture of first- and second-degree tears and episiotomy	Anaesthesia/general/epidural and spinal	
Prolapsed cord	Termination of pregnancy (TOP) before 12 weeks	Augmentation of labour	Vaginal birth after caesarian section (VBAC)
Fetal distress/neonatal asphyxia	Insertion of intrauterine contraceptive device (IUCD)	Forceps delivery	Emergency care in pregnancy-induced hypertension (PIH)
Uterine rupture	Limited obstetric ultrasound	Suture of cervical tear	Sepsis management
Shoulder dystocia	Administration of pethidine and oxytocin (third stage) (independent)	Suture of third-degree tear	Administration of Entonox®
Ante- and postpartum haemorrhage/hypovolaemia	Transcutaneous electrical nerve stimulation (TENS)	TOP after 12 weeks	Pain management
Inversion of the uterus (emergency care)	External version	Obstructed labour	
Intubation (mother and newborn)	Administer local anaesthetic	Caesarean section	
Eclampsia	External version (second twin)	Manual removal of a placenta	
	Hydrotherapy	Surgical evacuation of the products of conception	
	Ventouse delivery	Prescription and administration of medication	
	Resusitation	Suppression of labour	
		Inversion of uterus (curative)	
		Amniocentesis	
		External and internal version	

Glossary

A

abdominal pregnancy: an extrauterine, intra-abdominal pregnancy

abortion: the termination of a pregnancy before the fetus is 'viable'

afterpains: cramp-like pains of the uterus, which may occur after the birth of the child

AIDS: Acquired Immune Deficiency Syndrome

alpha-fetoprotein (AFP): the major circulating protein of the early human fetus

amelia: the absence of a limb

amniocentesis: the insertion of a needle abdominally into the amniotic sac for the removal of amniotic fluid

amnion: the inner of the two membranes forming the sac that contains the amniotic fluid and the fetus

amniotic fluid: the fluid contained within the amniotic sac and surrounding the fetus

amniotic fluid embolism: maternal embolism caused by amniotic fluid being forced into the maternal circulation at birth

amniotomy: artificial rupture of membranes (AROM) or surgical induction

anaphylaxis: a life-threatening physiological immunological reaction (including drug hypersensitivity) to a known or unknown agent

android pelvis: a 'male-type' or male-shaped pelvis

anencephaly: a congenital abnormality resulting in the absence of the cranial vault and the brain

anoxia: the absence of oxygen in the body tissues

antenatal: prenatal or preceding birth

antepartum: preceding labour

anterior fontanelle: the larger diamond-shaped fontanelle situated anteriorly, also known as the bregma

anthropoid pelvis: a pelvis in which the anteroposterior diameters are enlarged and the transverse diameters are reduced

anti-D: a specific gamma globulin (IgG) containing anti-Rh V antibodies. This is obtained by a cold alcohol method of fractionation of carefully screened human plasma (RHOGAM) and is used in the prevention of Rh isoimmunisation

Apgar score: a numeric description of the condition of the newborn, designed for rapid assessment at birth, developed by Dr Virginia Apgar

apnoea: a temporary cessation of breathing

apnoea neonatorum: the disturbance of the respiratory mechanism in an infant at birth or shortly after

appropriate for gestational age (AGA): newborn babies with a birth weight between the 10th and 90th percentiles

asphyxia neonatorum: a condition in which a viable newborn infant fails to initiate and/or sustain respiration after delivery

asynclitism: the lateral tilting of the fetal head in order to channel the head through the pelvic brim

atelectasis: the partial or complete non-expansion of the lungs of a newborn baby

atresia: congenital closure of a usual opening or canal, such as oesophageal atresia

attitude of the fetus: the relation of the fetal parts to one another *in utero*

auscultation: assessment by listening to sound within the body, for example the fetal heart

B

baby-friendly: conditions that consider the needs of a baby

ballottement: a technique of palpation to detect or examine a floating object in the body, for example the fetal head in the amniotic fluid

Bandl's ring: a pathological uterine retraction ring, seen abdominally in obstructed labour

Bartholin's glands: two small mucus-secreting glands situated one on either side of the vaginal opening, to which they are connected by small ducts

battering: repeated and steady beating, which is usually physical but could also be psychological; the effects of battering remain in the memory for a long time

betamimetics: any drug that mimics the stimulation of the beta-adrenergic receptors of the sympathetic nervous system (in childbirth, mainly used for suppression of contractions and fetal lung maturity)

Better Birth Initiative: principles of evidence-based care related to childbirth

bicornuate uterus: a congenital uterine abnormality where the uterine fundus is divided into two parts

biophysical profile: a sophisticated means of assessing fetal well-being

bonding: the relationship process that links two individuals

brachial palsy: partial or complete paralysis of a portion of a baby's arm resulting from a difficult delivery, for example Erb-Duchenne and Klumpke's paralyses

Brandt-Andrews' manoeuvre: modified controlled cord traction used to remove the placenta after the delivery of the baby

Braxton-Hicks contractions: painless uterine contractions during pregnancy

breast engorgement: excessive fluid and swelling in the breasts in the puerperium

breech presentation: where the buttocks and possibly the feet of the fetus, instead of the head, lie in the lower pole of the uterus

bregma: the large, diamond-shaped anterior fontanelle

brown fat: a source of energy for heat production unique to the neonate but reduced or absent in the preterm baby

C

Caesarean section: the surgical removal, by abdominal incision, of the products of conception as a viable fetus

caput succedaneum: an oedematous subcutaneous swelling on the presenting part of the fetal head, caused by pressure during labour

cardiomyopathy: pathological enlargement of the cardiac muscle

cardiotocography: monitoring of the fetal heart and the maternal uterine contractions using an electronic monitoring machine; used in high-risk pregnancies

caul: the portion of the amnion which covers the baby's face if the baby is born with the membranes intact

cephalohaematoma: a swelling on the head of the newborn caused by bleeding under the periosteum of the skull, usually the parietal bone/s

cephalopelvic disproportion (CPD): disproportion between the size of the fetal head and the size of the mother's pelvis

cervical dystocia: non-dilatation of the cervix in the presence of efficient uterine contractions, resulting in difficult labour

cervical os: the internal and/or external opening of the cervical canal

chloasma: brown pigmentation on the skin of the face during pregnancy and in some women who are taking oral contraceptives; also called 'the mask of pregnancy'

choanal: pertaining to the nose

chorioamnionitis: inflammation of the fetal membranes due to infection in the liquor amnii

chorioepitheliorna: a rapidly developing malignant condition of the epithelium of the chorionic villi, which may be found after hydatidiform mole

chorion: the outer fetal membrane

coitus: sexual intercourse, copulation

colloids: particles that do not break down in water, larger than 30 kilodaltons (kDa) (used in hypovolaemia). Dalton (Da) is an alternate name for the atomic mass unit, and kilodalton (kDa) is 1 000 daltons. Albumin is the principal natural colloid, comprising 50 to 60 per cent of all plasma proteins. Albumin consists of a single polypeptide chain of 585 amino acids, with a molecular weight of 69 000 Dalton

colostrum: a yellow secretion from the breasts during pregnancy and prior to true lactation

competency: knowledge, skill or attitude that enables one to effectively perform the activities of a given occupation or function to the standards expected in employment

conceptus: the products of conception

confinement: the period of labour, the delivery and the early puerperium

congenital: present or existing in the baby, before and at birth

conjoined twins: twins who are physically joined; Siamese twins

constriction ring: an internal localised spasm of the uterine muscle, for example an 'hour-glass' constriction ring

continuous positive airway pressure (CPAP): a method of artificial respiration

contraction and retraction: the tightening and shortening of the uterine muscle fibres during labour

Coomb's test: a test to determine the presence of Rh-positive antibodies

Couvelaire uterus: bleeding into the uterine muscle due to placental abruption

craniostenosis (craniosynostosis): premature closure of the sutures of the skull bones in the newborn

crowning of the head: the distending of the vaginal orifice by the widest diameter, the biparietal diameter, of the fetal head during birth

crystalloids: substances from crystals (sodium and chloride) that break down in water with a weight of 30 kDa (used as an intravenous volume expander)

curve of Carus: the pathway which the fetus takes as it passes through the pelvis (the 90 degree curve of the birth canal)

D

decidua: the lining of the uterus (the endometrium) during pregnancy

delivery: the birth of the baby, the placenta and membranes

denominator: that part of the presentation which gives the position its name

deprivation: to suffer due to absence of something essential

desquamation: shedding of the epithelial cells of the skin and mucous membranes

dextrocardia: a congenital abnormality where the heart is situated on the right-hand side of the thorax

dextrorotation of the uterus: the pregnant uterus is usually rotated slightly towards the right-hand side by 20 weeks, because it is displaced by the rectum and sigmoid colon on the left-hand side of the body

diagonal conjugate: an important measurement, gauged digitally, and used to assess the size of the pelvis. The measurement is taken from the lower border of the symphysis pubis to the promontory of the sacrum

diaphragmatic hernia: a congenital abnormality of the diaphragm, allowing the abdominal organs to protrude into the thoracic cavity

diastasis of the rectus abdominis muscles: a parting along the centre of the rectus abdominis muscles, often found after repeated pregnancies

dilatation of the cervix: the dilating of the cervix during labour, brought about by uterine contraction and retraction

disparate twins: twins who are noticeably different in weight and colour, as found in twin transfusion syndrome

disseminated intravascular coagulation (DIC): fibrin degradation products in the blood circulation, resulting in severe haemorrhage

dizygotic twins: binovular or non-identical twins

Doderlein bacillus: the Gram-positive bacterium found in normal vaginal secretions

doula: an assistant who provides non-medical and non-midwifery support (physical and emotional) in childbirth

Down's syndrome (or trisomy 21): a chromosomal defect resulting from the presence of an extra chromosome on the twenty-first pair

Dubowitz assessment: a set of criteria used to assess the gestational age of a newborn baby

ductus arteriosus: a temporary duct between the aorta and the pulmonary artery in the fetal circulation

ductus venosus: a temporary connection between the umbilical vein and the inferior vena cava in the fetal circulation

dyspareunia: painful and/or difficult sexual intercourse

dystocia: very painful, difficult and/or prolonged labour

E

eclampsia: a severe complication of pregnancy arising from a pre-eclamptic condition of unknown cause, characterised by hypertension, proteinuria and often generalised oedema, culminating in convulsions

ectoderm: the outer layer of cells in the developing embryo, which gives rise to the nervous system, skin, nails and hair

ectopic pregnancy: an extrauterine pregnancy

effacement of the cervical canal: shortening and thinning (taking up) of the cervical canal

embryo: the developing conceptus from the beginning of the fourth week to the end of the eighth week

endoderm: the inner layer of cells of the embryo, which gives rise to the internal organs

endometrium: the mucous membrane lining the inner surface of the uterus in the non-pregnant state

engagement of the fetal head: when the largest diameters of the presenting part of the fetal head, including the biparietal diameter, have passed through the pelvic brim or inlet

epidural analgesia: analgesia now used extensively during labour, and given by administering a local anaesthetic into the epidural space

episiotomy: an incision into the perineum in order to increase the size of the vaginal orifice to facilitate delivery and to avoid severe laceration

ergometrine: an oxytocic substance resulting in a long, sustained contraction of the uterine muscle, and which may only be used after delivery for contracting the uterus

erythroblastosis fetalis: an abnormal condition affecting the newborn baby as a result of Rh isoimmunisation, and characterised by a raised serum bilirubin level (haemolytic disease of the newborn, or HDN)

eutocia: normal labour

exchange transfusion of the newborn: 70–80 per cent of circulating blood in the newborn baby suffering from erythroblastosis fetalis will be replaced with group O Rh-negative donor blood

exomphalos: a congenital anomaly characterised by the absence of the anterior abdominal wall and resulting in protrusion of abdominal viscera

exsanguination: loss of a large quantity of blood

F

face presentation: where the face of the fetus, instead of the vertex, lies in the lower pole of the uterus

false labour: unequal, arythmical, early uterine contractions which do not result in cervical dilatation

false pelvis: that portion of the pelvis situated above the pelvic brim or inlet

female genital mutilation (FGM): female circumcision

Ferguson reflex: reflex contractions of the uterus after stimulation of the cervix by a well-fitting presenting part

ferning: the appearance of a branching pattern in dried smears of uterine cervical mucus in the presence of oestrogen

fetal acidosis: the disturbance of the acid balance due to lack of oxygen. Also see 'asphyxia neonatorum'

fetal alcohol syndrome (FAS): a syndrome caused by maternal alcohol ingestion and resulting in typical neonatal facial anomalies, possible mental retardation and personality disorders later on in life

fetal growth restriction: see 'intrauterine growth restriction'

fetus: the conceptus, from the beginning of the ninth week after conception to term

fetus papyraceous: a twin that has died *in utero* and been retained to term, when it is expelled with the placenta. The body fluids will have been reabsorbed and the fetus will have a flattened and 'paper-like' appearance

fistula: an abnormal passage, for example a tracheo-oesophageal fistula

flexion: bending or being bent; the opposite of extension

fontanelle: a space at the intersection of the sutures in the fetal skull

footling presentation: the extension of a leg in a breech presentation

foramen ovale: a temporary opening in the interatrial septum of the heart, in the fetal circulation

frank breech presentation: the fetus lies as a breech presentation, with both legs flexed at the hips but extended at the knee

fundus: the upper portion of the uterus, between the Fallopian tubes

funic: pertaining to a cord, such as the umbilical cord

G

galactagogue: an agent causing an increase in the flow of milk

galactorrhoea: the excessive secretion of milk

galactosaemia: an inability in infants to metabolise lactose and galactose

gender violence: the social pathology of violence between genders

genetics: a branch of biology concerned with the study of heredity (the transmission of characteristics from parents to their offspring) and the variation (the differences observed between living things)

gestation: pregnancy

gestational age (GA): the age of the embryo or fetus, estimated from the first day of the last normal menstrual period

gestational diabetes: diabetes mellitus that becomes apparent during pregnancy

glabella: that part of the sinciput situated above the root of the nose and between the eyebrows

golden minute: the time period and the steps that a birth attendant must take immediately after birth to evaluate the baby and stimulate breathing

good-enough mothering: mothering that provides a holding environment in which the child can develop, including micro-interactions between the mother and child as central to the development of the child's internal world

grand multipara: a woman who has had five or more viable babies

gravid: pregnant

gravida: a pregnant woman

gynaecoid pelvis: a typical female pelvis

H

haemorrhagic disease of the newborn: a bleeding disorder in the newborn due to a lack of vitamin K

Hegar's sign of pregnancy: a method to detect early pregnancy and to determine an approximate gestational age of the fetus

HELLP syndrome: a complication of pre-eclampsia and eclampsia, characterised by haemolysis, elavated liver enzymes and low platelets

HIV: human immunodeficiency virus

human chorionic gonadotrophin (hCG): a hormone of pregnancy produced by the chorionic villi

human placental lactogen (HPL): a hormone that is only found in pregnant women and that has growth hormone properties

hyaline membrane disease (HMD): a hyaline membrane forms in respiratory distress syndrome and on autopsy is found lining the lungs

hydatidiform mole: proliferation of the trophoblast, resulting in grape-like vesicles and vaginal bleeding. There is usually no development of the embryo

hydrocephaly: a condition in which excessive cerebrospinal fluid in the brain leads to rapid head growth

hydrops fetalis: the most severe form of erythroblastosis fetalis, causing severe oedema and cardiac failure which is usually fatal

hyperbilirubinaemia: excessive amounts of serum bilirubin

hypercapnia: an increased amount of carbon dioxide in the arterial blood

hyperemesis gravidarum: excessive vomiting during pregnancy after the first trimester

hypofibrinogenaernia: low levels of fibrinogen in the blood

hypogastric arteries: temporary structures carrying deoxygenated blood from the fetus to the placental tissues; also known as the umbilical arteries

hypoxia: an inadequate level of oxygen in the blood

hysterectomy: surgical removal of the uterus

hysterotomy: surgical incision into the uterus, performed to remove the products of conception before viability

I

iatrogenic: an abnormality caused by medical treatment, for example retrolental fibroplasia

ichthyosis: a congenital skin disease characterised by the desquamation of plaques or scales of smooth, dry, horny skin

imperforated anus: a condition in which there is no anal opening to the rectum at birth. This condition may be associated with a fistula

implantation: the attachment of the products of conception to the uterine wall in a normal pregnancy

incidental antepartum haemorrhage: antepartum haemorrhage other than placenta praevia or placental abruption

incompetent cervix: a cause of habitual abortion or preterm labour, where the cervix is unable to retain the products of conception

inco-ordinate uterine action: a type of disordered, arhythmical uterine action, where the fundal dominance is lost, for example in a 'colicky' uterus

induction: the artifical initiation of labour

infant mortality: death of a child in the first year of life

intermittent positive pressure ventilation: a type of artificial respiration

intertuberous diameter: the distance between the ischial tuberosities, used in the assessment of the pelvic outlet

intervillous spaces: open maternal blood spaces within the placenta, allowing materno-fetal exchange to occur

intrauterine anoxia: an absence of oxygen to the fetus

intrauterine growth restriction (IUGR): usually caused by placental insufficiency and resulting in a small-for-gestational-age (SGA) baby

introitus: an opening, particularly the entrance to the vagina

inversion of the uterus: where the uterus is turned inside out after the delivery of the baby; this is usually acute

inverted nipple: an abnormal condition where the nipple does not protrude from the breast

involution (of the uterus): the gradual process whereby the uterus and other reproductive organs resume their normal size and function after delivery

ischial spines: spines situated on the ischial bones and protruding into the birth canal on either side

isoimmunisation: the development of antibodies in the mother against an antigen from the fetus, for example the Rh factor

J

Jacquemier's/Chadwick's sign: a method to detect early pregnancy; a dark purplish discolouration of the mucous membranes of the cervix, vagina and vulva

K

kangaroo-mother-care (KMC): care of a small infant needing incubation by placing the infant skin-to-skin on the mother's chest 24 hours a day

karyotype: the arrangement of the chromosomes in a set pattern or order

kernicterus: high levels of circulating unconjugated bilirubin in the bloodstream, causing staining of the basal ganglia of the brain and resulting in athetoid paralysis or death

ketosis: the presence of ketone bodies in the blood, detected by urinalysis

kick count: an evidence-based low-cost method to monitor fetal well-being *in utero*

Klinefelter's syndrome: a sex chromosomal defect resulting in karyotype XXY, with three sex chromosomes being present, ie 47 instead of 46 chromosomes. The individual is a male with some female characteristics and the condition is compatible with life

L

labour: the process whereby the conceptus is expelled from the uterus and delivered; also known as parturition or confinement

lactation: the process of milk secretion and excretion

lactiferous sinus: the distended area of the lactiferous ducts, located just beneath the areola of the breast

lactosuria: the presence of lactose in the urine during late pregnancy and lactation; it may be confused with glycosuria during lactation

lanugo: fine, soft hair which often covers the fetus from about 20 weeks until birth

large for gestational age (LGA): where the fetus is unusually large in relation to gestational age (above the 90th percentile); also known as macrosomia and often found in mothers with diabetes mellitus

lecithin: a phospholipid that lowers the surface tension of the alveoli of the lungs and which is important in respiratory distress syndrome (RDS). The lecithin-sphingomyelin test is used to determine fetal lung maturity and the presence of surfactant

left lateral position: when the mother lies in this position during pregnancy and early labour, the oxygen supply to the fetus is increased, preventing supine hypotensive syndrome. During labour this position facilitates more controlled labour and easier access by attendants, and is also known as the Queen Charlotte or the Rotunda position for delivery

let-down: the milk ejection reflex, also known as the 'draught'

leucorrhoea: normal vaginal discharge

levator ani muscles: large specialised muscles of the pelvic floor which direct the fetus in the mechanism of labour

lie of the fetus: the relationship of the long axis of the fetus to the long axis of the uterus; may be longitudinal, transverse or oblique

lightening: the descent of the uterus within the abdominal cavity around 36 weeks, which results in a lowering of the fundal height and therefore a reduction of pressure on the diaphragm

linea nigra: a brown pigmented line on the skin of the anterior abdominal wall, which runs from the umbilicus to the symphysis pubis and which occurs during pregnancy

liquor amnii: the fluid contained within the amniotic sac and surrounding the fetus

lithotomy position: the woman lies on her back with her knees drawn up and her feet in stirrups which are attached to lithotomy poles

litigation: legal action against a person

living ligatures: the middle, criss-cross layer of uterine muscle fibres which are arranged in such a way that they ligate the maternal blood vessels in the third stage of labour and prevent postpartum haemorrhage (PPH)

lochia: the vaginal discharge during the puerperium

Lovset's manoeuvre: the remedial manoeuvre used when there are extended arms in the nuchal position, in a breech delivery

low forceps delivery: the application of forceps to lift the fetal head out once it has passed the midpelvis and has reached the perineum

M

macerated fetus: the process of degeneration of a fetus that has died *in utero*

macrosomia: a condition where the baby is large for gestational age (LGA)

malposition: a posterior position in a vertex presentation

malpresentation: when the presentation is other than a normal vertex presentation

mammary gland: compound milk-secreting gland of the female breast

mastitis: inflammation of breast tissue

maternal containment: the psychological component of the mother–infant relationship. The mother is able to understand what the infant wants and responds appropriately. The infant's inner life is then in order, which creates comfort and alleviates anxieties in the neworn

Maurice Smellie-Veit manoeuvre: the remedial manoeuvre used for an extended head in a breech delivery, and which may be used for delivery of the head in any breech presentation

meatus: an external opening to an internal passage leading to an organ, for example the urinary meatus of the urethra

mechanism of labour: a series of passive movements by which the fetus is moved through the birth canal

meconium: the greenish-black contents of the fetal bowel and the first stools of the neonate

meconium aspiration syndrome (MAS): an obstruction of the airways in the baby at birth due to the aspiration of meconium into the lungs

meconium flown: an obstruction of the bowel of the newborn caused by the compaction of viscid meconium in babies suffering from cystic fibrosis

meconium-stained fluid: the presence of meconium in the liquor amnii as a result of hypoxia in the fetus

meiosis: cell division occurring in germ (sex) cells

Mendelson's syndrome: a potentially fatal complication in pregnancy and birth where stomach contents are aspirated

meningomyelocele: a congenital neural tube defect (NTD) where both the meninges and the spinal cord protrude through the non-union of the spinous processes of one or more vertebrae (spina bifida)

mentum: the denominator in a face presentation, for example right mentoanterior (RMA)

mesoderm: the middle layer of cells in the developing embryo, which gives rise, for example, to muscles, the circulatory system and epithelial tissue

metritis: inflammation of the uterine wall

microcephaly: an abnormally small head

micrognathia: an abnormally small lower jaw

micturition: passing of urine

mid-cavity forceps delivery: the use of forceps when the head is held up in the mid-cavity of the pelvis, especially in posterior positions of the vertex when the ischial spines are prominent

millia: tiny white spots seen on the face of the neonate, particularly around the nose. They are of no significance and soon disappear

missed abortion: when the fetus dies *in utero* but the products of conception are not aborted

mitosis: cell division occurring in somatic cells

Mongolian spot: a pigmented area found on the lower back and buttocks of some newborn babies and which is of no significance

moniliasis: infection of the mucous membrane by *Candida albicans* (thrush)

monozygotic twins: uniovular or identical twins

Montgomery's follicles: sebaceous glands in the areola surrounding the nipple which hypertrophy during pregnancy and appear as small lumps

morbidity: sequelae of abnormal conditions

morning sickness: nausea, sometimes vomiting, occurring in early pregnancy. It is a normal condition and can occur at any time of day. If it should become abnormal, it results in hyperemesis gravidarum

Moro reflex: the 'startle' reflex found in the normal neonate

mortality: death

morula: the ball of cells, looking rather like a tiny mulberry, which normally develops in the uterine tubes as a result of cell division after fertilisation

moulding: the shaping of the fetal head as it passes through the birth canal. The presenting diameters are decreased by the overlapping of the skull bones at the sutures and fontanelles

Müllerian ducts: two tubular embryonic structures from which the female genital organs evolve

multigravida: a woman who is pregnant for the second or any subsequent time

multipara: a woman who has had more than one viable baby

mutation: a change in a chromosome or gene

myoepithelial cells: contractile cells around the alveoli in the breast, facilitating the expression of milk into the mammary ducts

myometrium: the muscle layers of the uterus

N

Naegele's rule: to establish the approximate estimated date of delivery (EDD), seven days and then nine months (or one year less three months, plus seven days) are added to the first day of the last normal menstrual period

naevus: a birthmark

necrotising enterocolitis (NEC): a rare condition resulting in necrosis of the bowel in the newborn; it may occur in artificially fed babies and following umbilical catheterisation

neonatal mortality: death of the infant in the first four weeks of life

neonate: an infant from birth until four weeks of age

non-shivering thermogenesis: the process by which the newborn produces heat by increasing the metabolic rate

non-stress test (NST): a test for fetal well-being using the cardiotocograph machine

nosocomial: pertaining to a hospital

nulligravida: a woman who has never been pregnant

nullipara: a woman who has never delivered a viable baby

nurse midwife: a midwife who is also trained as a general professional nurse

O

obstructed labour: no descent of the presenting part in the presence of efficient uterine contractions, usually due to cephalopelvic disproportion (see 'Bandl's ring')

occipitoposterior position: the malposition of the occiput, with the occiput lying in a posterior segment of the mother's pelvis

occiput: the most posterior skull bone, which is also the denominator in a vertex presentation

oligohydramnios: an insufficiency of amniotic fluid

oliguria: diminished secretion of urine

omphalitis: inflammation of the umbilicus

oogenesis: maturation of the ova

operculum: a mucus plug sealing off the cervical canal during pregnancy

ophthalmia neonatorum: a gonococcal infection of the eye in the newborn, which can result in blindness

orifice: an opening, for example the anus

Ortolani's manoeuvre: a procedure to detect congenital dislocation of the hip in the newborn

os: an opening or mouth, for example the external cervical os

Osiander's sign: a method to detect early pregnancy. Increased pulsation is felt in the lateral fornices of the vagina

osteogenesis imperfecta: a congenital abnormality characterised by brittle bones

outlet dystocia: the fetus has difficulty in negotiating an inadequate pelvic outlet

oxytocin: a substance which stimulates uterine contractions

P

PaCO$_2$: arterial carbon dioxide tension – the percentage of carbon dioxide in arterial blood indicating the pH (acidity) of an arterial blood sample, oxygen content (O$_2$CT) and oxygen saturation (SaO$_2$)

palpation: physical examination using the hands

PaO$_2$: arterial oxygen tension – the partial pressure of arterial oxygen, giving a comparison between the oxygen level in the blood and the oxygen concentration that is breathed in

Papanicolaou's test (Pap smear): a test for cervical cancer

para: a woman who has delivered one or more viable infants

parent: a person who takes care of a child; either the biological parent or an unrelated person

parity: the number of viable infants that a woman has delivered

parous: a woman who has delivered one or more viable infants

partogram (cervicograph): a graphic representation of the progress of labour used in the active management of labour for the early detection of abnormalities

parturition: the process of giving birth

patent: open

Pawlik's grip: a grip used in abdominal palpation to determine the presenting part of the fetus

PCO$_2$: carbon dioxide partial pressure. CO2 levels will directly affect the levels of acid in the blood

PCV: packed cell volume or haematocrit

pelvic axis: an imaginary line which bisects all the anteroposterior diameters of the pelvis and is the pathway which the fetus takes as it passes through the pelvis (see 'curve of Carus')

pelvic brim or inlet: the plane of division between the true and the false pelvis

pelvic outlet: the diamond-shaped outlet of the pelvis

pelvimetry: assessment of pelvic size

pendulous abdomen: when the uterus falls forward due to lack of muscle tone of the rectus abdominis muscles. The condition is also known as anterior obliquity of the uterus

perimetrium: a layer of peritoneum covering the uterus

perinatal mortality: death of the infant during the first week of life, including stillbirth

perineal body: a triangular-shaped wedge of muscle situated behind the perineum and between the vagina and rectum

perineorrhaphy: suturing of the perineum

perineum: the surface area between the vagina and the anus

period of gestation: the length of a particular pregnancy, calculated in days, weeks or months

persistent occipitoposterior position (POP): when the occiput fails to rotate forward in an occipitoposterior position; commonly known as a 'face-to-pubes' delivery

pharmacodynamics: the study of the physiological effects of drugs on the body

pharmacokinetics: the study of what the body does to a drug

pharmacotherapy: the treatment of disease through the administration of drugs

phenylketonuria: an inherited autosomal recessive trait, resulting in a defect in the metabolism of the amino acid phenylalanine. If untreated, this will result in mental retardation

phimosis: excessive tightness of the penile foreskin

phocomelia: a genetic anomaly resulting in the shortening or absence of the long bones of the limbs

phototherapy: the use of light energy to dispel the bilirubin present under the skin of a jaundiced infant

pica: the craving to eat unusual substances, such as mud

Pierre-Robin syndrome: a congenital abnormality characterised by micrognathia, a small tongue, a cleft palate and possibly a cleft lip

pinna: the cartilaginous portion of the ear

placenta: a temporary organ which links the mother and the fetus during pregnancy and, among other functions, facilitates the exchange of substances

placenta accreta: a morbidly adherent placenta. The use of the terms 'increta' and 'percreta' indicate the depth of adherence

placental abruption: partial or total premature separation of a normally situated placenta

placental infarcts: various abnormal areas sometimes found on the placenta

placental insufficiency: placental dysfunction

placenta praevia: a placenta implanted in the lower, instead of the upper, uterine segment and which almost always results in antepartum haemorrhage (APH)

platypelloid pelvis: a pelvis in which the anteroposterior diameter is reduced

plethoric: congested and dark red in colour

polycythaemia: an increase in the number of red blood cells

polydactyly: a congenital anomaly characterised by extra digits on the hands and/or feet

polyhydramnios: an excess of amniotic fluid

porphyria: a group of disorders that involve the biosynthesis of haem and cause an excessive renal excretion of porphyrins or their precursors

position (of the fetus): the relationship of the denominator to the brim of the mother's pelvis

posterior fontanelle: the small triangular fontanelle situated posteriorly, also known as the lambda

postpartum (postnatal): after childbirth

postpartum haemorrhage (PPH): excessive bleeding after the birth of the baby and/or in the puerperium

post-term: a pregnancy lasting longer than 42 full weeks. ('Post-mature infant' is suggestive of an abnormal condition.)

precipitate labour: an unusually short labour

pre-eclampsia: a complication of pregnancy characterised by hypertension, proteinuria and possibly oedema, which may culminate in eclampsia. The cause of this condition is not known

premature rupture of the membranes (PROM): rupture of membranes before the onset of labour

premonitory (prodromal) signs: signs or symptoms serving as a warning

prepuce: foreskin

presentation: that part of the fetus which lies over the brim of the pelvis

presenting part: that part of the presentation lying over the internal cervical os

preterm infant: a viable infant born before 37 full weeks' gestation

primigravida: a woman pregnant for the first time

primipara: a woman who has delivered one viable baby

progesterone: a female hormone

prolactin: a hormone produced by the anterior pituitary gland responsible for the manufacture of milk. It is inhibited by the presence of high levels of oestrogen in the blood

prolonged pregnancy: a pregnancy lasting more than 42 completed weeks' gestation

promontory of the sacrum: that part of the sacrum which juts into the pelvic brim at the junction of the superior surface of the sacrum and the inferior surface of the fifth lumbar vertebra

prone: lying flat, face downwards

prostaglandins: compounds that stimulate contractions of smooth muscles, particularly the uterine muscles

proteinuria: the presence of protein in the urine

pruritis: itching

pseudocyesis: false pregnancy

psychoprophylaxis: one of the methods of preparation for labour

ptyalism: an excessive amount of saliva, which may occur during early pregnancy

pudendal nerve block: the injection of local anaesthetic around the pudendal nerve on either side of the pelvis

puerperal infection (sepsis): infection of the genital tract following childbirth

puerperium: a period of time extending from the end of the third stage of labour to the end of the sixth week following delivery

Q

quickening: the movements of the fetus *in utero* which are felt by the mother. Fetal movements only become apparent to the mother between the 16th and 20th weeks, when the uterus becomes an abdominal organ, although slight movements have been taking place since early fetal development

R

recommended dietary allowances (RDAs): the evidence-based level of intake of food substances that is required and safe

rectovaginal fistula: see 'vesicovaginal fistula'

regulatory authority: the Medicines Control Council (MCC) is the South African drug regulatory authority, which registers new medicines and approves their package inserts and patient information leaflets

relaxin: a hormone of pregnancy causing a relaxation of smooth muscle and cartilage

respiratory distress syndrome (RDS): in the newborn, this condition is due to a lack of surfactant in the lungs (see also 'hyaline membrane disease' and 'lecithin')

restitution: resumption of the original position, for example external restitution after internal rotation of the fetal head during birth

retraction of uterine muscle: a property unique to the uterine muscle. Retraction is a progressive shortening of each longitudinal muscle fibre with every successive contraction

retraction ring: an imaginary physiological ring being the demarcation between the upper and lower uterine segments (for pathological retraction ring see 'Bandl's ring')

retrolental fibroplasia: an iatrogenic condition in the newborn causing blindness, which is due to a high arterial oxygen tension; the preterm baby is more susceptible

Rh factor: a group of antigens that may be present on the envelope of the red blood cells

rhonchi: coarse, snoring, auscultatory sounds made when mucous plugs obstruct the passage of air in the lungs

Ringer's lactate: sodium chloride, sodium lactate, potassium

ripening of the cervix: softening of the cervix as the pregnancy approaches term and labour

rooting reflex: the instinctive turning of a normal newborn's mouth towards any facial sensory stimulant, such as the nipple

rotation of the head, internal and external: some of the passive movements of the fetal head made during the mechanism of labour

S

Safe Motherhood Initiative (SMI): the movement to make birth a safer process

sagittal suture: the suture situated between the parietal bones and running into the anterior and posterior fontanelles

shoulder girdle dystocia (impacted shoulders): obstruction of the shoulders by the bony pelvis after the head is born in a cephalic lie

show: the appearance of the displaced operculum at the vaginal introitus. This is sometimes accompanied by a small amount of blood

simian crease: a single palmar crease usually found in infants with Down's syndrome

Sims' position: the lateral positioning of the body; the exaggerated Sim's position is used in umbilical cord prolapse

sinciput: the forehead or brow in the fetus (the two frontal bones)

small for gestational age (SGA): where the fetus is unusually small in relation to gestational age (below the 10th percentile)

souffle: the swishing sound, detected on abdominal auscultation, of blood passing through the arteries. Funic (umbilical), placental and uterine souffles may be detected

Spalding's sign: the overlapping of the skull bones detected in a macerated fetus on X-ray

spina bifida: the lack of fusion of the spinous processes of a vertebra

station of the presenting part: the level of the descending presenting part in relation to the ischial spines

stem cells: cells found in all multicellular organisms, characterised by the ability to renew themselves through mitotic cell division

stress urinary incontinence (SUI): when the bladder leaks when coughing or laughing

striae gravidarum: the stretch marks occurring on the mother's skin in pregnancy

stripping of the membranes: a means of inducing uterine contractions by digitally stripping the membranes from around the cervical os

sub-involution of the uterus: an abnormal reduction in the rate of involution of the uterus

supernumerary nipples (auxiliary breasts): additional nipples, with or without breast tissue, found in some people

supine: lying flat, face upwards

supine hypotensive syndrome: a restriction of venous blood flow from the uterus and lower limbs due to pressure exerted on the inferior vena cava when the woman adopts a supine position. This results in maternal hypotension and a reduced oxygen supply to the fetus

surfactant: a combination of enzymes which lowers the surface tension of the alveoli of the lungs

sutures of the fetal skull: the membranous spaces situated between the skull bones of the fetus or newborn, where ossification has not yet taken place

symphysiotomy: artificial or spontaneous division of the ligaments of the symphysis pubis, resulting in enlargement of the diameters of the bony pelvis

syndactyly: webbing or fusion of the fingers or toes

T

tachypnoea: an excessively rapid respiration rate

talipes: a congenital abnormality of the feet, such as clubfoot

teratogen: any environmental agent causing a malformation of the developing embryo or fetus

term: the full gestational period of 40 weeks in the human. The period from the beginning of 38 weeks to 42 completed weeks' gestation is also considered to be normal

termination of pregnancy (TOP): by medical indication or by a woman's choice for social reasons

tetanic contraction of the uterus: a uterine contraction that is longer and stronger than normal, usually resulting from the misuse of oxytocics

third-degree tear: a laceration of the perineum extending through the muscles of the anal sphincter

thrush in the newborn: a fungal infection of the oral mucous membranes of the newborn caused by *Candida albicans*

titration: sequentially administering carefully measured amounts or dosages of a drug until the desired effect is achieved

tocolytic drug: a drug used to suppress uterine contractions in preterm labour

tonic contractions: see 'tetanic contraction of the uterus'

tonic neck reflex: a normal reflex of the newborn, resulting in the so-called fencing position

TORCH organisms: a group of organisms causing intrauterine and neonatal infections that may cause fetal abnormality or death (toxoplamosis, other, rubella, cytomegalovirus and herpes)

trial of labour: continuous careful assessment of the progress of labour in possible cephalopelvic disproportion. Any labour, particularly primigravid labour, may also be regarded as a trial of labour

trimester: the nine-month gestational period is divided into three trimesters of three months each

trisomy 21: see 'Down's syndrome'

trophoblast: by the seventh day after fertilisation, the morula has developed two specialised outer layers of cells and is known as the trophoblast

true pelvis: that portion of the pelvis forming the bony passage of the birth canal

Turner's syndrome: a sex chromosomal defect resulting in karyotype X0, with only one sex chromosome being present, meaning that there are only 45 instead of 46 chromosomes. The individual has a female appearance and the condition is compatible with life, but serious physical defects may be present

twin transfusion syndrome (parabiotic syndrome): an abnormal condition which occasionally occurs in identical twins when there is anastomosis of the fetal blood vessels causing feto-fetal blood transfer. One twin receives most of the blood and becomes polycythaemic while the other twin suffers from anaemia. Occasionally, the anaemic twin may die, be retained and give rise to a fetus papyraceous

U

ultrasonography: the use of ultrasound waves to visualise soft tissue by means of sound waves, and to record these photographically

umbilical catheterisation: the insertion of a catheter into the umbilical vein in order to feed the critically ill newborn baby and to enable blood tests, such as the Astrup test, to be performed (an umbilical artery may also sometimes be used) and also to administer medication

umbilical cord (funis): the cord which connects the fetus to the placenta

umbilical cord presentation: the cord lies in front of the presenting part, with the membranes intact

umbilical cord prolapse: the cord lies in front of the presenting part, with the membranes ruptured

uterine inertia: disordered, hypotonic uterine action, most commonly occurring in the nullipara. In primary uterine inertia there is ineffective uterine action resulting in little or no dilatation of the cervix, while in secondary uterine inertia, the uterus has become exhausted due to obstructed labour and the contractions have ceased temporarily

uterine tetany: tonic contraction of the uterus brought about by the misuse of oxytocic medications

V

vacuum extraction: the extraction of the fetal head from the birth canal by means of a vacuum cup or ventouse extractor

Valsalva manoeuvre (bearing down): forcible exhalation effort against a closed glottis: the resultant increase in intra-thoracic pressure interferes with the venous return to the heart

vasa praevia: this condition occurs in a velamentous insertion of the cord where the fetal blood vessels, which run through the membranes, lie in front of the presenting part. The danger is rupture of the fetal vessels and possible fetal exsanguination

velamentous insertion of the cord: the cord is abnormally inserted into the membranes instead of into the substance of the placenta

vernix caseosa: a cheeselike, greasy, white substance which is secreted by the fetal sebaceous glands from the second trimester of pregnancy and which protects the fetal skin *in utero*. It is present at term and acts as a lubricant during the birth

version: the turning of the fetus so that there is a different presenting part. Version can be either spontaneous or by manipulation

vertex: the highest portion of the fetal skull, which is bounded by the anterior fontanelle in front, the posterior fontanelle at the back and the parietal eminences at the sides. It is this portion of the fetal skull which presents in a normal well-flexed vertex presentation

vesicovaginal fistula: a fistula occurring between the bladder or urethra and the vagina as a result of obstructed labour (a rectovaginal fistula can also occur between the rectum and the vagina)

viability: the ability of a fetus to sustain life outside the uterus. This is six months or 26 weeks after conception, according to South African law

W

Wharton's jelly: the jelly-like substance contained within the umbilical cord and surrounding the umbilical blood vessels

Bibliography

General: Acts, bills, policies, protocols and guidelines

Cadegan, M. 2012. *A Brief Summary of the Strategic Plan for Maternal, Newborn, Child and Women's Health (MNCWH) and Nutrition in South Africa 2012–2016.* http://www.hst.org.za/publications/Kwik%20Skwiz/KS_V2Issue2MaternalHealth_31Oct2012_0.pdf (HST.KS_V2Issue) (Accessed 5 October 2017).

DoH (Department of Health). nd(a). *Strategic Priorities for the National Health System 2004–2009.* https://www.gov.za/sites/default/files/stratpriorities_0.pdf (Accessed 5 October 2017).

DoH. nd(b). *National Guideline for Cervical Cancer Screening Programme.* http://www.kznhealth.gov.za/cervicalcancer.pdf (Accessed 5 October 2017).

DoH. nd(c). *Negotiated Service Delivery Agreement (NDSA 2010–14) Programme of action.* http://www.poa.gov.za/POA%20Overview%20Files/Outcome%2002%20Health.pdf (Accessed 5 October 2017).

DoH. nd(d). *Human Genetics Policy Guidelines for the Management and Prevention of Genetic Disorders, Birth Defects and Disabilities.* https://www.gov.za/sites/default/files/humangenetics_0.pdf (Accessed 5 October 2017).

DoH. 1965. Medicines and Related Substances Act & Regulations 101 of 1965. Reg 777, 10 April 1981 (as amended). *Government Gazette* No 24747, 10 April 2003. http://www.hpcsa.co.za/Uploads/editor/UserFiles/downloads/legislations/acts/medicines_and_related_sub_act_101_of_1965.pdf (Accessed 5 October 2017).

DoH. 1980. Regulation Governing Private Hospitals and Unattached Operating Theatre Units. No R 158. *Government Gazette* No 6832, 1 February 1980. pp. 32–63. http://www.kznhealth.gov.za/regulations/pvthosp.pdf (Accessed 5 October 2017).

DoH. 1996. Choice on Termination of Pregnancy Act 92 of 1996. *Government Gazette* No 17602, 22 November 1996. https://www.gov.za/sites/default/files/Act92of1996.pdf (Accessed 5 October 2017).

DoH. 1997. White Paper for the Transformation of the Health System in South Africa. Notice 667, *Government Gazette* No 17910, vol 382, 16 April 1997. https://www.gov.za/sites/www.gov.za/files/17910_gen667_0.pdf (Accessed 5 October 2017).

DoH. 1998. Sterilisation Act 44 of 1998. Pretoria: Government Printer.

DoH. 1999. *Draft Policy Guidelines for Adolescent and Youth Health.* http://www.youth-policy.com/Policies/South%20Africa%20Policy%20Guidelines%20for%20Adolescent%20&%20Youth%20Health.pdf (Accessed 5 October 2017).

DoH. 2003. National Health Act 61 of 2003. *Government Gazette* No 26595, Vol 469, 23 July 2004. https://www.gov.za/sites/default/files/a61-03.pdf (Accessed 5 October 2017).

DoH. 2005a. Nursing Act 33 of 2005. http://www.sanc.co.za/pdf/Nursing%20Act%202005.PDF (Accessed 5 October 2017).

DoH. 2005b. *National Sexual Assault Policy.* http://www.svri.org/sites/default/files/attachments/2016-07-05/South%20Africa%20National%20Sexual%20Assault%20Policy%20-%202005%20scanned.pdf (Accessed 5 October 2017).

DoH. 2005c. Sterilisation Amendment Act 3 of 2005. Pretoria: Government Printer.

DoH. 2007. The Traditional Health Practitioners Act 22 of 2007. *Government Gazette* No 30660, Vol 511, 10 January 2008. https://www.gov.za/sites/www.gov.za/files/a22-07.pdf (Accessed 5 October 2017).

DoH. 2011. *Human Resources for Health South Africa: HRH Strategy for the Health Sector. 2012/13–2016/17.* https://www.gov.za/sites/default/files/hrh_strategy_0.pdf (Accessed 5 October 2017).

DoH. 2012a. *Adolescent and Youth Health Policy.* http://www.youthmetro.org/uploads/4/7/6/5/47654969/adolescent_

youth_health_policy_draft.pdf
(Accessed 5 October 2017).

DoH. 2012b. *Standard Treatment Guidelines and Essential Medicines List for South Africa Primary Health Care Level.* http://www.kznhealth.gov.za/pharmacy/edlphc2014a.pdf (Accessed 5 October 2017).

DoH. 2012c. *National Vitamin A Supplementation Policy Guidelines for South Africa.* http://www.adsa.org.za/Portals/14/Documents/DOH/Vit%20A%20policy%20guidelines%20OF%20S%20A%20-%20recent_1.pdf (Accessed 5 October 2017).

DoH. 2012d. *Integrated School Health Policy.* https://www.health-e.org.za/wp-content/uploads/2013/10/Integrated_School_Health_Policy.pdf (Accessed 5 October 2017).

DoH. 2013a. *Essential Newborn Care Quality Improvement Toolkit.* http://www.lincare.co.za/wp-content/uploads/2016/06/Essential-Newborn-Care-Quality-Improvement-Toolkit-2013-1.pdf (Accessed 5 October 2017).

DoH. 2013b. *Infant and Young Child Feeding Policy.* https://www.health-e.org.za/wp-content/uploads/2013/09/IYCF_Policy_2013.pdf (Accessed 5 October 2017).

DoH. 2013c. *The National Strategic Plan for Nurse Education, Training and Practice 2012/13–2016/17.* http://www.sanc.co.za/archive/archive2013/linked_files/Strategic_Plan_for_Nurse_Education_Training_and_Practice.pdf (Accessed 5 October 2017).

DoH. 2014a. *Saving Mothers 2011–2013. Sixth Report on the Confidential Enquiries into Maternal Deaths in South Africa.* https://www.health-e.org.za/wp-content/uploads/2016/05/Saving-Mothers-2011-2013-short-report.pdf (Accessed 6 October 2017).

DoH. 2014b. *Newborn Care Charts. Routine Care at Birth and Management of the Sick and Small Newborn in Hospital.* http://www.kznhealth.gov.za/kinc/Newborn_care_charts_March_2014.pdf (Accessed 6 October 2017).

DoH. 2015a. *Guidelines for Maternity Care in South Africa. A Manual for Clinic, Community Health Centres and District Hospitals.* https://www.health-e.org.za/wp-content/uploads/2015/11/Maternal-Care-Guidelines-2015_FINAL-21.7.15.pdf (Accessed 6 October 2017).

DoH. 2015b. *National Consolidated Guidelines for the Prevention of Mother-to-Child Transmission of HIV (PMTCT) and the Management of HIV in Children, Adolescents and Adults.* http://www.sahivsoc.org/Files/ART%20Guidelines%2015052015.pdf (Accessed 6 October 2017).

DoH. 2015c. National Perinatal Morbidity and Mortality Committee (NaPeMMCo). http://www.health.gov.za/index.php/shortcodes/2015-03-29-10-42-47/2015-04-30-08-18-10/2015-04-30-08-24-27?download=889:national-perinatal-morbidity-and-mortality-committee-napemmco (Accessed 6 October 2017).

DoH. 2016. *Ideal Clinic Manual. Version 16.* http://www.kznhealth.gov.za/family/Ideal-Clinic-Manual-Oct2015.pdf (Accessed 6 October 2017).

DoJ (Department of Justice). 2005. Children's Act 38 of 2005. *Government Gazette* No 28944, Vol 492, 19 June 2006. https://www.gov.za/sites/www.gov.za/files/a38-05_3.pdf (Accessed 6 October 2017).

DPSA (Department of Public Service and Administration). 1997. *Batho Pele White Paper on Transforming Public Service Delivery.* Notice 1459 of 1997. *Government Gazette* No 18340, Vol 388, 1 October 2001. http://www.justice.gov.za/paja/docs/1997_batho.pdf (Accessed 6 October 2017).

Futures Group. 2013. A seven step implementation plan for maternal and neonatal health at the facility level in South Africa. Unpublished document.

HST (Health Systems Trust). nd. *Reducing Maternal and Child Mortality through Strengthening Primary Healthcare (RMCH) 2012–2015.* https://www.blacksash.org.za/index.php/sash-in-action/2017-07-09-15-09-47/reproductive-mother-and-child-health (Accessed 6 October 2017).

Moodley, J. 2008. *Saving Mothers 1999–2001. Executive Summary. Reports on Confidential Enquiry into Maternal Deaths in South Africa.* http://www.samj.org.za/index.php/samj/article/view/2163/1441 (Accessed 6 October 2017).

MRC Unit for Maternal and Infant Healthcare Strategies. 2003. *Saving Babies 2003. Fourth Perinatal Care Survey of South Africa.* https://www.ppip.co.za/wp-content/uploads/Saving-babies-2003.pdf (Accessed 6 October 2017).

MRC Unit for Maternal and Infant Healthcare Strategies. 2007. *Saving Babies 2006–2007. Sixth Report on Perinatal Care in South Africa.* https://www.ppip.co.za/wp-content/uploads/Saving-babies-2006-7.pdf (Accessed 6 October 2017).

NICE (National Institute for Health and Care Excellence). 2009. Guidelines. https://www.nice.org.uk/guidance (Accessed 6 October 2017).

Packhard Foundation. 2006. *Save the Children. State of the World's Mothers. Saving the Lives of Mothers and Newborns.* Packhard Foundation: Westport, Connecticut.

Pattinson, RC. 2007. *Saving Mothers. Fourth Report on Confidential Enquiries into Maternal Deaths in South Africa. 2005–2007.* NCCEMD.

Ramsey, EM. 1965. 'The placenta and fetal membranes', in *Obstetrics,* edited by JP Greenhill, 13th ed. Philadelphia: WB Saunders.

Robertson-Sutton, A. 2011. *Improving newborn care in South Africa: Lessons learned from Limpopo Initiative for Newborn Care (LINC)*. UNICEF, DoH, Save the Children. http://www.lincare.co.za/wp-content/uploads/2016/06/Improving_Newborn_Care_LINC_2011.pdf (Accessed 6 October 2017).

SANAC (South African National AIDS Council). 2017. *Summary Brochure: National Strategic Plan on HIV, TB and STIs 2017–2022*. http://sanac.org.za/2017/04/03/summary-brochure-national-strategic-plan-on-hiv-tb-and-stis-2017-2022/ (Accessed 6 October 2017).

Tshwane Declaration of Support for Breastfeeding in South Africa. 2011. *S Afr J Clin Nutr* 24(4). http://www.sajcn.co.za/index.php/SAJCN/article/viewFile/586/820 (Accessed 6 October 2017).

UN (United Nations). nd. International day for the elimination of violence against women. http://www.un.org/en/events/endviolenceday/ (Accessed 6 October 2017).

UN. 1979. Convention on the elimination of all forms of discrimination against women (Art 5(a), adopted by the General Assembly resolution 34/180 of 18 December 1979). http://www.un-documents.net/a34r180.htm (Accessed 6 October 2017).

UNICEF (United Nations Children's Fund). 2009. *Newborn Care Charts. Management of Sick and Small Newborns in Hospital*. Save the children/Limpopo Provincial Government. https://www.healthynewbornnetwork.org/resource/newborn-care-charts-management-of-sick-and-small-newborns-in-hospital/ (Accessed 6 October 2017).

WHO. 2001 & 2008. Female Genital Mutilation Policy No 5. The prevention and management of health complications. Policy guidelines for nurses and midwives. http://www.who.int/reproductivehealth/publications/fgm/RHR_01_18/en/ (Accessed 6 October 2017).

WHO. 2009. WHO Guidelines on Nutrition. http://www.who.int/publications/guidelines/nutrition/en/ (Accessed 6 October 2017).

WHO. 2011. *Vitamin A Supplementation for Infants and Children 6–59 Months of Age*. http://www.who.int/nutrition/publications/micronutrients/guidelines/vas_6to59_months/en/ (Accessed 6 October 2017).

Section 1: Maternal and child healthcare

AHO (African Health Observatory). 2010. The Ouagadougou Declaration on primary health care and health systems in Africa: Achieving better health for Africa in the new millennium. *African Health Monitor*, 12. https://www.aho.afro.who.int/en/ahm/issue/12/reports/ouagadougou-declaration-primary-health-care-and-health-systems-africa-achieving (Accessed 6 October 2017).

Alberts, LL, Selder, KD & Guelich, B. 1999. 'Midwifery care: the "Golden Standard" for normal childbirth'. *Birth*, 21: 53–54.

ANC. 2004. Report on Delivery to Women. http://www.anc.org.za/content/report-delivery-women (Accessed 6 October 2017).

Ancestors South Africa: Genealogical Research Services. nd. Mothers, midwifery, births and babies. http://www.ancestors.co.za/mothers-midwifery-births-babies/ (Accessed 6 October 2017).

Angelini, DJ. 1999. 'Obstetric triage: The realm of the midwife. Part 2'. *Journal of Nurse-Midwifery*, 44: 536.

Avery, MD. 2005. 'The history and evolution of the core competencies for basic midwifery practice'. *American College of Nurse-Midwives*, 50: 102–106.

Avery, MD. 2007. 'The DNP entry into midwifery practice: An analysis'. *Journal of Midwifery and Women's Health*, 52: 14–20.

Banda, J. 2012. Why CARMMA? www.carmma.org/page/why-carmma (Accessed 11 October 2017).

BAPCA (British Association for the Person-centred Approach). 2015. What is the person-centred approach? http://www.bapca.org.uk/about/what-is-it.html (Accessed 6 October 2017).

Bergstrom, L. 1997. 'Midwifery as a discipline'. *Journal of Nurse-Midwifery*, 42: 417–420.

Better Birth Initiative. 2006. Implementation aids: An introduction to the better birth initiative. A global initiative to promote humane, evidence-based childbirth care. *The WHO Reproductive Health Library*, no 9.

Bettercare. 2000. The primary health care package for SA: A set of norms and standards. http://bettercare.co.za/wp-content/uploads/2013/01/The-Primary-Health-Care-Package-for-South-Africa-a-set-of-norms-and-standards.htm (Accessed 6 October 2017).

Biblesoft. 2006. New Exhaustive Strong's Numbers and Concordance with Expanded Greek-Hebrew Dictionary. Biblesoft, Inc. & International Bible Translators, Inc.

Black Sash. 2017. Strengthening community accountability mechanisms to improve maternal and child health services. https://www.blacksash.org.za/index.php/sash-in-action/2017-07-09-15-09-47/reproductive-mother-and-child-health (Accessed 17 November 2017).

Blais, R, Maxeux, B, Lambert, J, Loisette, J, Gauthier, N & Framarin, A. 1994. 'Midwifery defined by physicians, nurses and midwives: The birth of consensus'. *Canadian Medical Association Journal*, 150: 691–697.

Blix, E, Sviggum, O, Koss, KS & Qian, L. 2003. 'Inter-observer variation in assessment of 845 labour admission tests: Comparison between midwives and obstetricians in the clinical setting and two experts'. *Drcog Bjog: An International Journal of Obstetrics and Gynaecology*, 110: 1–5.

Bobadilla, JL. 1992. 'Evaluation of maternal health programs: Approaches, methods and indicators'. *International Journal of Gynaecology and Obstetrics*, 38: 67–73.

Brennan, TA, Leape, LL, Laird, NM, Hebert, L, Localio, R, Lawthers, AG, Newhouse, JP, Weiler, PC & Hiatt, HH. 1991. 'Incidence of adverse events and negligence in hospitalized patients — Results of the Harvard Medical Practice Study'. *Engl J Med*, 324: 370–376. DOI: 10.1056/NEJM199102073240604 (Accessed 11 October 2017).

Broad, E. 1991. *Strengthening Nursing and Midwifery in Support of Strategies for Health for All*. apps.who.int/iris/bitstream/10665/170431/1/EB89_13_eng.pdf (Accessed 6 October 2017).

Bruce J, Dippenaar, J, Mphuti, D, Schmollgruber, S & Huiskamp, A. 2017. Advancing nursing scholarship: the Mozambique model. (Accepted for publication). Global Health Action. Ref: ZGHA-2016-0049R2.

Cadegan, M. 2012. *A Brief Summary of the Strategic Plan for Maternal, Newborn, Child and Women's Health (MNCWH) and Nutrition in South Africa 2012–2016*. http://www.hst.org.za/publications/Kwik%20Skwiz/KS_V2Issue2 MaternalHealth_31Oct2012_0.pdf (HST.KS_V2Issue) (Accessed 6 October 2017).

CAM ACSF (Canadian Association of Midwives). 2017. Midwifery across Canada. https://canadianmidwives.org/midwifery-across-canada/ (Accessed 6 October 2017).

Cara, C. 2003. A pragmatic view of Jean Watson's Caring Theory. https://pdfs.semanticscholar.org/1eac/3d84e2725 b5d5aa113589f1d209d0a8ca7b3.pdf (Accessed 9 October 2017).

Carlough, M & McCall, M. 2005. 'Skilled birth attendance: What does it mean and how can it be measured? A clinical skill assessment of maternal and child health workers in Nepal'. *International Journal of Gyneacology and Obstetrics*, 89: 200–208.

Carr, KC. 1994. 'Characteristics of the supportive and non-supportive childbirth environment'. *International Journal of Childbirth Education*, 9: 10–13.

Chalmers, B. 1990. *African birth: Childbirth in cultural transition*. Johannesburg: Berev Publications.

Chaponda, A, Brokenshire-Scott, C, Strydom, T, Nyathikazi, M, Mabela, P, Maphanga, T, Shaver, T & Livinski, A. 2004. Concept Paper for the Establishment of a White Ribbon Alliance for Safe Motherhood and Secretariat in South Africa. South Africa. *The Cochrane Collaboration*. 2006. Cochrane Library.

Childbirth Connection. nd. The rights of childbearing women. http://www.nationalpartnership.org/research-library/maternal-health/the-rights-of-childbearing-women.pdf (Accessed 17 November 2017).

Citizens for Midwifery. 2007. Mother-friendly childbirth: Highlights of the evidence. http://www.motherfriendly.org/Resources/Documents/Mother-Friendly%20 Childbirth-Highlights%20of%20the%20Evidence.pdf (Accessed 9 October 2017).

CMS (Council for Medical Schemes). 2015. *Annual Report 2014–2015*. https://www.medicalschemes.com/files/Annual%20Reports/AR2014_2015.pdf (Accessed 9 October 2017).

CMS. 2016. *Annual report 2015/2016*. Annexures. https://www.medicalschemes.com/files/Annual%20Reports/CMS%20Annual%20Report%202015-2016%20 Annexures.pdf (Accessed 9 October 2017).

Comino, EJ & Harris, E. 2003. 'Maternal and infant services: Examination of access in a culturally diverse community'. *Journal of Pediatric and Child Health*, 39: 95–99.

Copcutt, DI. 1975. 'Midwifery in the 18th century'. *SA Nursing Journal*, 18–20.

Copcutt, DI. 1976a. 'Midwifery in the 19th century. Part I'. *SA Nursing Journal*, 22–24.

Copcutt, DI. 1976b. 'Midwifery in the 19th century. Part 11'. *SA Nursing Journal*, 15–17.

Core Competencies for Midwives. 2002. 'The core competencies for basic midwifery practice'. (Adopted by the American College of Nurse Midwives) *Journal of Midwifery and Woman's Health*, 47: 402–406.

Cullinan, K. 2006. Health services in SA: A basic introduction. https://www.health-e.org.za/2006/01/29/health-services-in-south-africa-a-basic-introduction/ (Accessed 9 October 2017).

Cullinan, K. 2015. Antidote to poor health services? https://www.health-e.org.za/2015/04/29/antidote-to-poor-health-services/ (Accessed 9 October 2017).

Currentnursing.com. 2012. Theory of interpersonal relations. http://currentnursing.com/nursing_theory/interpersonal_theory.html (Accessed 9 October 2017).

Daviaud, E & Chopra, M. 2008. 'How much is not enough? Human resource requirements for primary health care: A case study from South Africa'. *Bulletin of the World Health Organization*, 86: 46–50.

Davies, R. 1998. 'Midwives role still undervalued'. *Australian Nursing Journal*, 5(11): 32.

Davis-Floyd, R. 2000. 'Anthropological perspectives on global issues in midwifery'. *Midwifery Today*, 53.

De Divitiis, E, Cappabianca, P & De Divitiis, O. 2004. 'The "schola medica salernitana": The forerunner of the modern university medical schools'. *Neurosurgery*, 5(4): 722–744.

De Kock, J & Van Der Walt, C. 2004. *Maternal and newborn care*. Cape Town: Juta.

De la Santé, OM. 1995. Strengthening nursing and midwifery. WHO. apps.who.int/iris/bitstream/10665/172797/1/EB97_Inf.Doc-2_eng.pdf (Accessed 9 October 2017).

De Maayer, IL. 2000. The reason for choosing a private practising midwife as birth attendant. Master's thesis. Johannesburg: Rand Afrikaans University.

De Veer, AJ & Meijer, WJ. 1996. 'Obstetric care: Competition or co-operation'. *Midwifery*, 12: 4–10.

DoH (Department of Health). nd(a). *National Guideline for Cervical Cancer Screening Programme*. http://www.kznhealth.gov.za/cervicalcancer.pdf (Accessed 6 April 2017).

DoH. nd(b). *Human Genetics Policy Guidelines for the Management and Prevention of Genetic Disorders, Birth Defects and Disabilities*. https://www.gov.za/sites/default/files/humangenetics_0.pdf (Accessed 6 October 2017)

DoH. nd(c). *NSDA: A long and healthy life for all South Africans*. http://nhrec.org.za/index.php/2014-08-15-12-54-26/category/94-2013s? (Accessed 9 October 2017).

DoH. 1998. *South African Demographic and Health Survey 1998: Preliminary Report*. http://www.mrc.ac.za/bod/dhsfin1.pdf (Accessed 9 October 2017).

DoH. 1999. *Draft Policy Guidelines for Adolescent and Youth Health*. Available: http://www.youth-policy.com/Policies/South%20Africa%20Policy%20Guidelines%20for%20Adolescent%20&%20Youth%20Health.pdf (Accessed 9 October 2017).

DoH. 2002. *A District Hospital Service Package for South Africa: A set of norms and standards*. http://www.kznhealth.gov.za/norms.pdf (Accessed 9 October 2017).

DoH. 2005. *National Sexual Assault Policy*. http://www.svri.org/sites/default/files/attachments/2016-07-05/South%20Africa%20National%20Sexual%20Assault%20Policy%20-%202005%20scanned.pdf (Accessed 9 October 2017).

DoH. 2011a. R655 National Health Act (61/2003): Regulations Relating to Categories of Hospitals. *Government Gazette* No 9570; Government Printer, Pretoria: National DoH.

DoH. 2011b. *National Core Standards for Health Establishments in South Africa*. http://www.phango.org.za/home/144-national-core-standards-ndoh (Accessed 9 October 2017).

DoH. 2012. *Integrated School Health Policy*. https://www.health-e.org.za/wp-content/uploads/2013/10/Integrated_School_Health_Policy.pdf (Accessed 09 October 2017)

DoH. 2013a. *The National Strategic Plan for Nurse Education, Training and Practice 2012/13–2016/17*. http://www.sanc.co.za/archive/archive2013/linked_files/Strategic_Plan_for_Nurse_Education_Training_and_Practice.pdf (Accessed 9 October 2017).

DoH. 2013b. *The HHAPI-Ness Road Map for Healthy Babies in South Africa*. http://studylib.net/doc/6759735/1.-what-is-hhapi---ness (Accessed 11 October 2017).

DoH. 2013c. *Infant and Young Child Feeding Policy*. https://www.health-e.org.za/wp-content/uploads/2013/09/IYCF_Policy_2013.pdf (Accessed 9 October 2017).

DoH. 2013d. *Essential Newborn Care Quality Improvement Toolkit*. http://www.lincare.co.za/wp-content/uploads/2016/06/Essential-Newborn-Care-Quality-Improvement-Toolkit-2013-1.pdf (Accessed 9 October 2017)

DoH. 2014. *Saving Mothers 2011–2013. Sixth Report on the Confidential Enquiries into Maternal Deaths in South Africa*. https://www.health-e.org.za/wp-content/uploads/2016/05/Saving-Mothers-2011-2013-short-report.pdf (Accessed 9 October 2017).

DoH. 2015a. *Guidelines for Maternity Care in South Africa. A Manual for Clinic, Community Health Centres and District Hospitals*. https://www.health-e.org.za/wp-content/uploads/2015/11/Maternal-Care-Guidelines-2015_FINAL-21.7.15.pdf (Accessed 9 October 2017).

DoH. 2015b. *National Health Insurance for South Africa. Towards Universal Health Coverage*. https://www.health-e.org.za/wp-content/uploads/2015/12/National-Health-Insurance-for-South-Africa-White-Paper.pdf (Accessed 9 October 2017).

DoH. 2015c. *The Comprehensive Primary Health Care Services Package*. www.kznhealth.gov.za/PHC%20Services%20Package.PDF (Accessed 9 October 2017).

DoH. 2016. *Ideal Clinic Manual. Version 16*. http://www.kznhealth.gov.za/family/Ideal-Clinic-Manual-Oct2015.pdf (Accessed 9 October 2017).

Dörfling, CS. 1993. Wetgewing wat die Praktyk van die Vroedvrou Beheer. Doctoral thesis. Johannesburg: Rand Afrikaans University.

Dower, CM, Miller, JE, O'Neil, EH & The Taskforce of Midwifery. 1999. 'Charting a course for the 21st century'.

Pew Health Professions Commission and The UCSF Center for the Health Professions, 44(4): 337–424.

Editorial. 1991. 'Midwives and the empowerment of women. An international perspective'. *Journal of Nurse-Midwifery*, 36(2): 85.

Edwards, N. 2004. 'Protection – regulations and standards: Enabling or disabling?' *Midwives. The Official Journal of the Royal College of Midwives*, 7: 116–119.

Erasmus, DGJ. 1996. Die Kennis en Vaardighede van Vroedvroue in Suid Afrika. Doctoral thesis. Johannesburg: Rand Afrikaans University.

Farley, C & Carr, KC. 2003. 'New directions in midwifery education: The masters of science in midwifery degree'. *Journal of Midwifery and Women's Health*, 48: 134–137.

Farquhar, M, Camilleri-Ferrante, C & Todd, C. 2000. 'Continuity of care in maternity services: Women's views of one team midwifery scheme'. *Midwifery*, 16: 35–47.

Ford, K, Byrt, R & Dooher, J. 2010. 'Preventing and reducing aggression and violence in health and social care'. *Nurs Manag*, 17(7). https://www.ncbi.nlm.nih.gov/pubmed/27653535 (Accessed 9 October 2017).

Foster, J, Requeira, Y, Burgos, RI & Sanchez, SH. 2005. 'Midwifery curriculum for auxiliary maternity nurses. A study in the Dominican Republic'. *Journal of Midwifery and Women's Health*, 50: 45–49.

Friedman, I. 1999. 'Poverty, human rights and health. Chapter 1'. *South African Health Review*. http://www.hst.org.za/publications/South%20African%20Health%20Reviews/SAHR2010.pdf (Accessed 9 October 2017).

Frith, L (ed). 1999. *Ethics and midwifery*. Oxford: Butterworth Heinemann.

Fullerton, JT & Thompson, JB. 2005. 'Examining the evidence for the International Confederation of Midwives' essential competencies for midwifery practice'. *Midwifery*, 21: 2–13.

Fullerton, J, Severino, R, Brogan, K & Thompson, J. 2003. 'The International Confederation of Midwives' study of essential competencies of midwifery practice'. *Midwifery*, 19: 174–190.

Geyer, N. 1995. 'Professional indemnity'. *Nursing News*, 37–38.

Geyer, N. 2005. *Record keeping*. Cape Town: Juta.

Girot, EA, Enderz, BC & Wright, J. 2005. 'Transforming the obstetric nursing workforce in NE Brazil through international collaboration'. *Journal of Advanced Nursing*, 50: 651–660.

Green, A. 2006. 'Nursing and midwifery: Millennium Development Goals and the global human resource crisis'. *International Nursing Review*, 53(1): 13–15.

http://onlinelibrary.wiley.com/doi/10.1111/j.1466-7657.2006.00482.x/full (Accessed 9 October 2017).

Hatem, M, Sandall, J, Devane, D, Soltani, H & Gates, S. 2008. 'Midwife-led versus other models of care for childbearing women'. *Cochrane Database Syst Rev* (4): CD004667. DOI: 10.1002/14651858.CD004667.pub2 (Accessed 11 October 2017).

Henney, NM. 2013. Successes and Challenges of MBFI Implementation. https://www.westerncape.gov.za/assets/departments/health/breastfeeding_restoration_conferance_2013_nmh_final_2.pdf (Accessed 9 October 2017).

Honikman, S, Fawcus, S & Meintjes, I. 2015. 'Abuse in South African maternity settings is a disgrace: Potential solutions to the problem'. *SAMJ*, 105(4): 284–286. http://www.samj.org.za/index.php/samj/article/view/9582/6685 (Accessed 9 October 2017).

Hotelling, BA. 2004. 'Is your perinatal practice mother-friendly? A strategy for improving maternity care'. *Birth*, 31: 143–147.

HST (Health Systems Trust). 2016. *District Health Barometer 2015/16*. http://www.hst.org.za/publications/District%20Health%20Barometers/Complete_DHB_2015_16_linked.pdf (Accessed 9 October 2017).

Hundley, VA, Milne, JM, Glazener, CM & Mollison, J. 1997. 'Satisfaction and the three Cs: Continuity, choice and control. Women's views from a randomised controlled trial of midwifery-led care'. *British Journal of Obstetrics and Gynaecology*, 11: 1273–1280.

Hunter, B. 2010. 'Mapping the emotional terrain of midwifery: What can we see and what lies ahead'. *Int J Work Organisation and Emotion*, 3(3): 253–269.

Hussein, J, Bell, J, Nazzar, A, Abbey, M, Adjei, S & Graham, W. 2004. 'The skilled attendance index. Proposal for a new measure of skilled attendance at delivery'. *Reproductive Health Matters*, 12(24): 160–170.

ICM (International Confederation of Midwives). 2013. Essential competencies for basic midwifery practice. http://internationalmidwives.org/what-we-do/education-coredocuments/essential-competencies-basic-midwifery-practice/ (Accessed 9 October 2017).

ICM. 2014a. *Philosophy and Model of Midwifery Care*. http://internationalmidwives.org/assets/uploads/documents/CoreDocuments/CD2005_001%20V2014%20ENG%20Philosophy%20and%20model%20of%20midwifery%20care.pdf (Accessed 9 October 2017).

ICM. 2014b. *International Code of Ethics for Midwives*. http://internationalmidwives.org/assets/uploads/documents/CoreDocuments/CD2008_001%20V2014%20ENG%20

International%20Code%20of%20Ethics%20for%20 Midwives.pdf (Accessed 9 October 2017).

ICM. 2014c. *Midwives' Provision of Abortion-related Services*. http://internationalmidwives.org/assets/uploads/ documents/Position%20Statements%20-%20English/ Reviewed%20PS%20in%202014/PS2008_011%20 V2014%20Midwives'%20provision%20of%20 abortion%20related%20services%20ENG.pdf (Accessed 9 October 2017).

ICM. 2017. ICM international definition of the midwife. internationalmidwives.org/who-we-are/policy-and-practice/icm-international-definition-of-the-midwife/ (Accessed 9 October 2017).

ICN (International Council of Nurses), International Hospital Federation, International Pharmaceutical Federation, World Confederation for Physical Therapy, World Dental Federation & World Medical Association. 2008. Positive practice environments for health care professionals. http://www.whpa.org/ppe_fact_health_pro. pdf (Accessed 9 October 2017).

Index Mundi. 2017. South Africa demographics profile 2017. http://www.indexmundi.com/south_africa/demographics_ profile.html (Accessed 9 October 2017).

Islam, M. 2007. 'The Safe Motherhood Initiative and beyond'. *Bulletin of the World Health Organization*, 85(10): 733–820. http://www.who.int/bulletin/ volumes/85/10/07-045963/en/ (Accessed 9 October 2017).

Jacobs, M, Wighton, A, Makhanya, N & Ngcobo, B. 1997. 'Maternal, child and women's health'. *South African Health Review*, Chapter 16. http://www.hst.org.za/publications/ South%20African%20Health%20Reviews/sahr97.pdf (Accessed 17 October 2017).

Janssen, B & Wiegers, TA. 2006. 'Strengths and weaknesses of midwifery care from the perspective of women'. *The Royal College of Midwives. Evidence-based Midwifery*, 4(2): 53–59.

Jewkes, R, Abraham, N & Mvo, Z. 1998. 'Why do nurses abuse patients? Reflections from South African obstetric services'. *Social Science and Medicine*, 47: 1781–1795.

Jobson, M. 2015. Structure of the health system in South Africa. https://www.khulumani.net/active-citizens/item/ download/225_30267364dfc1416597dcad919c37ac71. html (Accessed 6 October 2017).

Kanter, RM. 1993. *Men and women of the corporation*. 2nd ed. [1977]. New York: Basic Books.

Kendall, T. 2015. *Critical Maternal Health Knowledge Gaps in Low- and Middle-Income Countries for Post-2015: Researchers' Perspectives*. Women and health initiative

working Paper 2. Women and health initiative, Harvard TH Chan School of Public Health: Boston, MA. https://cdn2.sph.harvard.edu/wp-content/uploads/ sites/32/2015/02/Knowledge_gaps_MH_post2015.pdf (Accessed 9 October 2017).

Kennedy, HP, Rousseau, AL & Low, LK. 2003a. 'Essential elements of midwifery care'. *Journal of Midwifery and Women's Health*. http://onlinelibrary.wiley.com/ doi/10.1111/j.1542-2011.2004.tb04413.x/full (Accessed 13 October 2017).

Kennedy, HP, Rousseau, AL & Low, LK. 2003b. 'An exploratory metasynthesis of midwifery practice in the United States'. *Midwifery*, 19(3): 203–214.

Kerber, KJ, De Graft-Johnson, E, Bhutta, ZA, Starrs, A & Lawn, JE. 2007. Continuum of care for maternal, new-born and child health. From slogan to service delivery. http://www.who.int/pmnch/topics/20071003lancet.pdf (Accessed 9 October 2017).

Khan, KS, Wojdyla, D, Say L, lmezoglu, AM & Van Look, PF. 2006. 'WHO analysis of causes of maternal death: A systematic review'. *Lancet*, 36: 1066–1074.

King, SS, Mhlanga, RE & De Phino, H. 2006. 'The context of maternal and child health. Chapter 7'. *SA Health Review*. https://www.popline.org/node/196335 (Accessed 13 October 2017).

Knol, J & Van Linge, R. 2009. 'Innovative behaviour: The effect of structural and psychological empowerment on nurses'. *Journal of Advanced Nursing*, 65(2): 359–370. http://onlinelibrary.wiley.com/doi/10.1111/j.1365-2648.2008.04876.x/abstract (Accessed 9 October 2017).

Koff, ZS. 2016. *Nursing in the European Union: Anatomy of a profession*. Vol 1. New York: Transaction Publishers.

Kortenbout, E. 1998. 'Production of nurses in South Africa'. Chapter 6. *South African Health Review*. http://www.hst. org.za/publications/South%20African%20Health%20 Reviews/SAHR98.pdf#search=Sa%20health%20 review%201998 (Accessed 17 November 2017).

Kotzé, W. 1995. The South African Nursing Council: 50 years of self-regulation. http://www.curationis.org.za/ index.php/curationis/article/view/1358 (Accessed 9 October 2017).

Kritzinger, S. 2005. *The politics of birth*. London: Elsevier.

KWT Dominican Sisters. 2014. Chapter 37. http:// www.kwtdominicans.org/wp-content/uploads/ Allforgodspeople/afgp-chapter-37.pdf (Accessed 17 November 2017).

Langer, A. 2006. 'Continuous support for women during childbirth'. *WHO Reproductive Health Library*, no 9. Oxford: Update Software Ltd.

Laschinger, HK. 1996. 'A theoretical approach to studying work empowerment in nursing: A review of studies testing Kanter's theory of structural power in organizations'. *Nursing Administration Quarterly*, 20(2): 25–41.

Laschinger, HKS, Finegan, J & Shamian, J. 2001. 'The impact of workplace empowerment and organizational trust on staff nurses' work satisfaction and organizational commitment.' *Health Care Management Review*, 26(3): 7–23.

Lavender, T & Baker, L. 2002. 'The Dutch maternity care: Best practice mission 2002'. *British Journal of Midwifery*, 11(3): 150–151.

Leach, J, Dowswell, T, Hewison, J, Baslington, H & Warrilow, J. 1998. 'Women's perceptions of maternity carers'. *Midwifery*, 14(1): 48–53.

Littlejohn, M. 2014. Midwifery and apartheid in South Africa. http://www.spiritualbirth.net/midwifery-and-apartheid-in-south-africa (Accessed 9 October 2017).

Lyon, DS, Mokhtarian, PL & Reever, MM. 1999. 'Predicting style-of-care preferences of obstetric patients. Medical vs. midwifery model'. *Journal of Reproductive Medicine*, 44(2): 101–106.

Malherbe, J. 2013. 'Counting the cost: The consequences of increased medical malpractice litigation in South Africa'. *S Afr Med J*, 103(2): 83–84. http://www.samj.org.za/index.php/samj/article/view/6457/4857 (Accessed 9 October 2017).

Markowitz, L & Tice, KW. 2002. 'Paradoxes of professionalisation'. *Gender and Society*, 16: 941.

Maropeng. 2009. New 'home' for Taung child. http://www.maropeng.co.za/news/entry/new_home_for_taung_child (Accessed 9 October 2017).

Maropeng. 2017. The age of Australopithecus. http://www.maropeng.co.za/content/page/the_age_of_emaustralopithecus (Accessed 9 October 2017).

Mashaba, TG. 1995. *Rising to the challenge of change. A history of black nursing in South Africa*. Cape Town: Juta.

Matthews, A, Scott, AP, Gallagher, P. 2009. 'The development and psychometric evaluation of the Perceptions of Empowerment in Midwifery Scale'. *Midwifery*, 25(3): 327–335. http://www.midwiferyjournal.com/article/S0266-6138(07)00043-5/fulltext (Accessed 9 October 2017).

Matthews, A, Scott, PA, Gallagher, P & Corbally, MA. 2005. 'An exploratory study of the conditions important in facilitating the empowerment of midwives'. *Midwifery*, 22(2): 181–191. https://www.ncbi.nlm.nih.gov/pubmed/16359761 (Accessed 11 October 2017).

McCool, WF, Guidera, M, Hakala, S & Delaney, EJ. 2007. 'The role of litigation in midwifery practice in the United States: Results from a nationwide survey of certified nurse-midwives/certified midwives'. *J Midwifery Women's Health*, 52(5): 458–464.

McKenna, H & Hasson, F. 2002. 'A study of skill-mix issues in midwifery: A multi-method approach. Nursing and healthcare management issues'. *Journal of Advanced Nursing*, 37: 52–56.

McKenna, H, Hasson, F & Smith, M. 2002. 'A delphi survey of midwives and midwifery to identify non-midwifery duties'. *Midwifery*, 18: 314–322.

McKenzie A, Schneider H, Schaay, N, Scott, V & Sanders, D. 2016. Primary Care Systems Profiles & Performance (PRIMASYS): South Africa Case Study. Technical report for the Alliance for Health Policy and Systems Research, Geneva.

Moore, W & Slabbert, MN. 2013. 'Medical information therapy and medical malpractice litigation in South Africa'. *South African Journal of Bioethics and Law*. http://www.sajbl.org.za/index.php/sajbl/article/view/277/316 (Accessed 9 October 2017).

Motsoaledi. A. 2012. District clinical specialist teams in South Africa. http://www.health.gov.za/index.php/2014-08-15-12-55-04/category/100-2012rp?download=186:district-clinical-specialist-teams-in-south-africa-ministerial-task-team-report (Accessed 9 October 2017).

Muller, M. 2002. *Nursing dynamics*. 3rd ed. Cape Town: Heinemann.

Munjanja, OK, Kibuka, S & Dovlo, D. 2005. *The nursing workforce in sub-Sahara Africa*. Issue 7. ICN Switzerland. https://www.ghdonline.org/uploads/The_nursing_workforce_in_sub-Saharan_Africa.pdf (Accessed 11 October 2017).

Naledi, T, Barron, P & Schneider, S. 2011. 'Primary health care in SA since 1994 and implications of the new vision for PHC re-engineering'. *Health Review*. http://www.hst.org.za/publications/South%20African%20Health%20Reviews/sahr_2011.pdf (Accessed 11 October 2017).

Nghiem, C. 2008. Resurrection in the present moment. http://www.mindfulnessbell.org/archive/2015/02/resurrection-in-the-present-moment (Accessed 9 October 2017).

Nicholls, L & Webb, C. 2006. 'What makes a good midwife? Implications for midwifery practice'. *Royal College of Midwives. Evidence-based midwifery*, 4: 65–70.

Nursing Council of New Zealand. 2012. *Guidelines: Professional boundaries*. http://www.nursingcouncil.

org.nz/index.php/content/download/707/2829/ file/Guidelines%20Professional%20Boundaries%20 printer%20friendly.pdf (Accessed 9 October 2017).

OHCHR (Office of the United Nations High Commissioner for Human Rights). 2014. Birth registration and the right of everyone to recognition everywhere as a person before the law. Report of the Office of the United Nations High Commissioner for Human Rights. http://www.ohchr. org/EN/HRBodies/HRC/RegularSessions/Session27/ Documents/A_HRC_27_22_ENG.doc (Accessed 9 October 2017).

Olsen, O & Jewell, MD. 2002. 'Home versus hospital birth'. *Cochrane Database Syst Rev,* 2: CD000352.

Page, L. 2001. 'Human resources for maternity care: The present system in Brazil, Japan, North America, Western Europe and New Zealand'. *International Journal of Gynaecology & Obstetrics,* 75(1): S81–S88.

Page, L. 2003. 'One-to-one midwifery: Restoring the "with woman" relationship in midwifery'. *Journal of Midwifery and Women's Health,* 48(2): 119–125.

Paine, LL, Dower, CM & O'Neil, EH. 1999. 'Midwifery in the 21st century. Recommendations from The Pew Health Professions Commission/UCSF centre for the health professions 1998 taskforce on midwifery'. *Journal of Nurse Midwifery,* 44(4): 341–348.

Parkhurst, J, Penn-Kekana, L, Blaauw, D, Balabanova, D, Danishevski, K, Rahman, SA, Onama, V & Sengooba, F. 2005. 'Health system factors influencing maternal health services: A four-country comparison'. *Health Policy,* 73: 127–138. http://ehrn.co.za/publications/download/62.pdf (Accessed on 9 October 2017).

Parratt, J & Johnston, J. 2002. 'Planned homebirths in Victoria. 1995–1998'. *Australian Journal of Midwifery,* 15(2): 16–25.

Pattinson RC & Rhoda, N (for the PPIP group). 2014. *Saving Babies 2012–2013: Ninth Report on Perinatal Care in South Africa.* Pretoria: Tshepesa Press. http://www.ppip. co.za/wp-content/uploads/Saving-Babies-2012-2013.pdf (Accessed 11 October 2017).

Pattinson, RC, Makin, JD, Pillay, Y, Van den Broek, N & Moodley, J. 2015. 'Basic and comprehensive emergency obstetric and neonatal care in 12 South African health districts'. *SAMJ,* 105(4): 256–260. http://dx.doi. org/10.7196/SAMJ.9181 (Accessed 9 October 2017).

Penn-Kekana, L & Blaauw, D. 2004. A rapid appraisal of maternal health services in South Africa. A health system approach. HSD/W/01/02. HSD. Centre of Health System Development Programme. https://assets.

publishing.service.gov.uk/media/57a08d49ed915d622c00 18d1/01-02_south_africa.pdf (Accessed 9 October 2017).

PMNCH. 2011. *Knowledge Summaries: #14 – Save lives: Invest in midwives.* PMNCH. http://www.who.int/ pmnch/knowledge/publications/summaries/ks14. pdf?ua=1 (Accessed 13 October 2017).

PoA (Programme of action). nd. *Negotiated Service Delivery Agreement (NDSA) 2010–2014.* http://www.poa.gov.za/ POA%20Overview%20Files/Outcome%2002%20Health. pdf (Accessed 9 October 2017).

Pretorius, C. 1976. 'Pionier vroedvroue in Suid Afrika'. *Geneeskunde,* 18: 45–47.

Price, CH. 1962. Cape of Good Hope 1652–1807. https:// www.ncbi.nlm.nih.gov/pmc/articles/PMC1034703/ (Accessed 9 October 2017).

Quilliam, S. 1999. 'Clinical risk management in midwifery. What are midwives for?' *MIDIRS (Midwives information resource service) Midwifery Digest,* 11(3), Supplement 2: S22–S26.

Republic of South Africa. 2013. Municipal Health Services. *Government gazette* 36849, vol 579, 20 September 2013, page 6. https://www.greengazette.co.za/documents/ national-gazette-36849-of-20-september-2013-vol-579_20130920-GGN-36849 (Accessed 9 October 2017).

Rhodes, P. 1990. 'Obstetrics in 17th century England'. *Nursing RSA,* 5: 29–31.

Robertson-Sutton, A. 2011. *Improving newborn care in South Africa: Lessons learned from Limpopo Initiative for Newborn Care (LINC).* UNICEF, DoH, Save the Children. http://www.lincare.co.za/wp-content/uploads/2016/06/ Improving_Newborn_Care_LINC_2011.pdf (Accessed 9 October 2017).

Rogers. C. 1967. The therapeutic conditions antecedent to change: A theoretical view. http://www. centerfortheperson.org/pdf/therapeutic-conditions-antecedent-to-change.pdf (Accessed 9 October 2017).

Rooks, JP. 1999. 'The midwifery model of care'. *Journal of Nurse Midwifery,* 44(4): 370–374.

Rooks, JP & Ernst, EKM. 1999. 'The future of midwifery'. *International Journal of Childbirth Education,* 14: 16.

Rosenfield, A. 1997. 'The history of the Safe Motherhood Initiative'. *International Journal of Gynecology and Obstetrics,* 59(2):S7–9. https://www.popline.org/ node/271539 (Accessed 9 October 2017).

Sadan, E. 2004. Empowerment: Definitions and meanings. http://www.mpow.org/elisheva_sadan_empowerment_ chapter2.pdf (Accessed 9 October 2017).

Samson, JP. 1978. 'Education and the black nurse'. *Curationis*, 1(1). http://www.curationis.org.za/index.php/curationis/article/view/206 (Accessed 9 October 2017).

SANAC (South African National AIDS Council). 2017. *Summary Brochure: National Strategic Plan on HIV, TB and STIs 2017–2022.* http://sanac.org.za/2017/04/03/summary-brochure-national-strategic-plan-on-hiv-tb-and-stis-2017-2022/ (Accessed 9 October 2017).

SANC (South African Nursing Council). 1990. Regulations relating to the conditions under which registered midwives may carry on their profession. No R 2488. *Government Gazette* No 12805. 26 October 1990. 30–46.

SANC. 2004. *Draft Charter of Nursing Practice.* Pretoria: SANC.

SANC. 2006. 'Where are the Nurses? March workshop Durban'. *Nursing Update*, 30(4): 42–45.

Sandall, J, Soltani, H, Gates, S, Shennan, A & Devane, D. 2016. 'Midwife-led continuity models versus other models of care for childbearing women'. *Cochrane Review.* http://onlinelibrary.wiley.com/doi/10.1002/14651858. CD004667.pub5/abstract (Accessed 9 October 2017).

SA Private Hospitals. 2017. www.saprivatehospitals.com (Accessed 9 October 2017).

Searle, C. 1964. A socio-historical survey of the development of nursing in South Africa between 1652 and 1960. Doctoral thesis. Pretoria: University of Pretoria.

Seedat, BA & Blaauw, D. 2008. 'Comparison of a midwifery private obstetric unit and a private consultant obstetric unit'. *Baby Talk. Professional Forum for Childbirth Educators*: 18.

Segovia, I. 1998. 'The midwife and her functions by level of care'. *International Journal of Gynecology and Obstetrics*, 63: 61–66.

Seyer, J & Duncan, N. 2008. 'Health professions demand strong principles for task shifting'. *Press Information Uganda*, 11. http://www.whpa.org/pr03_08.htm (Accessed 9 October 2017).

Shaver, T. 2000. *Awareness, mobilisation and action for safe motherhood. A field guide.* The White Ribbon Alliance. Washington DC: NGO Network for Health USA.

Spreitzer, GM. 1996. 'Social structural characteristics of psychological empowerment'. *Academy of Management Journal*, 39(2): 483–504.

Stats SA. 2015. *Millennium Development Goals: Improve Maternal Health.* http://www.statssa.gov.za/MDG/MDG_Goal5_report_2015_.pdf (Accessed 13 October 2017).

Stats SA. 2016a. *Recorded Live Births 2013–2015.* http://www.statssa.gov.za/publications/P0305/P03052015.pdf (Accessed 9 October 2017).

Stats SA. 2016b. *South African Demographic and Health Survey 2016: Key Indicators Report.* http://www.mrc.ac.za/bod/SADHS2016.pdf (Accessed 9 October 2017).

Strauss, SA. 1984a. *Legal handbook for nurses and health personnel.* 5th ed. Cape Town: King Edward VII Trust.

Strauss, SA. 1984b. *Doctor, patient and the law.* 2nd ed. Pretoria: JL van Schaik.

Tshwane Declaration of Support for Breastfeeding in South Africa. 2011. *S Afr J Clin Nutr*, 24(4). http://www.sajcn.co.za/index.php/SAJCN/article/viewFile/586/820 (Accessed 9 October 2017).

UN (United Nations). nd. Every Woman Every Child. https://sustainabledevelopment.un.org/sdinaction/everywomaneverychild (Accessed 9 October 2017).

UN. 2015. Sustainable Development Goals. https://sustainabledevelopment.un.org (Accessed 9 October 2017).

UNICEF (United Nations Children's Fund). nd. The reality of malaria. https://www.unicef.org/health/files/health_africamalaria.pdf (Accessed 9 October 2017).

UNICEF. 2013a. One in 3 children under five does not officially exist. https://www.unicef.org/media/media_71508.html (Accessed 11 October 2017).

UNICEF. 2013b. Keeping mothers and children alive and healthy: Tracking South Africa's progress. https://www.unicef.org/southafrica/survival_devlop_13314.html (Accessed 9 October 2017).

UNICEF. 2016a. Undernourishment in the womb can lead to diminished potential and predispose infants to early death. https://data.unicef.org/topic/nutrition/low-birthweight/ (Accessed 9 October 2017).

UNICEF. 2016b. Girl's education and child protection. http://carmma.org/event/girls%E2%80%99-education-child-protection-unicef-carves-niche-africa%E2%80%99s-agenda-2063 (Accessed 9 October 2017).

Van Rensburg, HCJ, Benator, SR, Doherty, JE, Heunis, JC, Mcintyre, DE, Ngwena, CG, Pelser, AJ, Pretorius, E, Redelinghuys, N & Summerton, JV. 2004. *Health and healthcare in South Africa.* Pretoria: Van Schaik.

Wagner, M. 1995. 'A global witch-hunt'. *Lancet*, 346: 1050.

Wallace, M. 2001. The European Union standards for nursing and midwifery. Information for accession countries. The midwifery directives (80/154/EEC and 80/155/EEC). Copenhagen: WHO regional office for Europe.

Watson, J. 2008. *Nursing: The philosophy and science of caring.* Boulder: Boulder University Press.

Wells, D. 2003. 'Midwives taking on more roles: The 1st on call project: Extending the role of the midwife does not always mean an end to one-on-one care'. *RCM Midwives Journal.* http://europepmc.org/abstract/med/12630287 (Accessed 11 October 2017).

The White Ribbon Alliance. 2008. Our history. http://whiteribbonalliance.org/about-us/history/ (Accessed 9 October 2017).

WHO. 1985. *Having a baby in Europe.* Copenhagen: Regional Office of Europe.

WHO. 1996. *Nursing Practice. Report of a WHO Expert Committee.* Geneva: WHO.

WHO. 2000a. *Strengthening Nursing and Midwifery.* 54th World Health Assembly. Agenda 13.4. http://www.who.int/hrh/resources/WHA54-12.pdf (Accessed 9 October 2017).

WHO. 2000b. *Global Advisory Group on Nursing and Midwifery: Report of the Sixth Meeting, Geneva, 19–22 November 2000.* http://apps.who.int/iris/handle/10665/68763 (Accessed 17 November 2017).

WHO. 2001a. WHO consultation on integrated management of pregnancy and childbirth. http://www.who.int/maternal_child_adolescent/topics/maternal/impac/en/ (Accessed 9 October 2017).

WHO. 2001b. 'Management of pregnancy, childbirth and the postpartum period in the presence of female genital mutilation'. *WHO Technical Report Series.* Geneva: WHO/. http://apps.who.int/iris/bitstream/10665/66805/1/WHO_FCH_GWH_01.2.pdf (Accessed 9 October 2017).

WHO. 2002a. *Making Pregnancy Safer.* http://apps.who.int/iris/bitstream/10665/107588/1/E84613.pdf (Accessed 12 October 2017).

WHO. 2002b. Advisory group on management of nursing and midwifery workforce. Report of the first meeting: New Delhi, December 2001. http://apps.searo.who.int/PDS_DOCS/B3578.pdf (Accessed 9 October 2017).

WHO. 2003a. *Managing Complications in Pregnancy and Childbirth: A Guide for Midwives and Doctors.* SHR Department of Reproductive Health and Research Family and Community Health. Geneva: WHO.

WHO. 2003b. Nursing and midwifery workforce management. Conceptual framework. *Searo Technical Publication 25.* http://www.who.int/management/resources/staff/NursingMidwiferyWorkforceManagement.pdf (Accessed 13 October 2017).

WHO. 2003c. Strengthening Nursing and Midwifery. 56th World Health Assembly. A56/19.

WHO. 2003d. Strategic directions for strengthening nursing and midwifery services 2002–2008. A brief produced by The Global Network of WHO Collaborating Centres for Nursing and Midwifery Development. http://www.wpro.who.int/hrh/about/nursing_midwifery/strategic_directions_for_strengthening_nursing_and_midwifery_services.pdf (Accessed 9 October 2017).

WHO. 2004. Primary health care. http://www.euro.who.int/en/health-topics/Health-systems/primary-health-care (Accessed 9 October 2017).

WHO. 2006. *Reproductive Health Indicators. Guidelines for their Generation, Interpretation and Analysis for Global Monitoring.* Geneva: WHO Reproductive Health and Research.

WHO. 2007a. International statistical classification of diseases and related health problems. 10th revision version for 2007. http://apps.who.int/classifications/icd10/browse/2016/en (Accessed 17 October 2017).

WHO. 2007b. *Health System Development. Nursing and Midwifery Regional Initiatives.* Geneva: WHO Regional Office of South East Asia.

WHO. 2007c. Proportion of births attended by a skilled attendant: 2007 updates. Department of Reproductive Health and Research. http://apps.who.int/iris/bitstream/10665/69949/1/WHO_RHR_07.16_eng.pdf (Accessed 9 October 2017).

WHO. 2007d. Continuum of care for maternal, newborn, and child health: From slogan to service delivery. www.who.int/pmnch/knowledge/topics/coc_slogantodelivery/en/ (Accessed 9 October 2017).

WHO. 2008a. Nursing midwifery progress report 2008–2012. http://www.who.int/hrh/nursing_midwifery/progress_report/en/ (Accessed 9 October 2017).

WHO. 2008b. ICN global standards for initial education of professional nurses and midwives. http://www.who.int/hrh/resources/standards/en/ (Accessed 9 October 2017).

WHO. 2009a. WHO Guidelines on Nutrition. http://www.who.int/nutrition/publications/nutrient/en/ (Accessed 9 October 2017).

WHO. 2009b. *Women and Health. Today's evidence, tomorrow's agenda.* Geneva: WHO.

WHO. 2009c. *Global Standards for the Initial Education of Professional Nurses and Midwives.* http://www.who.int/hrh/nursing_midwifery/hrh_global_standards_education.pdf (Accessed 17 November 2017).

WHO. 2011a. Country stillbirth rates per 1000 total births for 2009. http://www.who.int/pmnch/media/news/2011/stillbirths_countryrates.pdf (Accessed 9 October 2017).

WHO. 2011b. PMNCH Fact Sheet: RMNCH continuum of care. http://www.who.int/pmnch/about/continuum_of_care/en/ (Accessed 9 October 2017).

WHO. 2012. *Nursing Midwifery Progress Report 2008–2012.* www.who.int.hrh (Accessed 3 March 2017).

WHO. 2014a. WHA *Global Nutritional Targets 2025. Low Birth Weight Policy Brief.* http://www.who.int/nutrition/topics/globaltargets_lowbirthweight_policybrief.pdf (Accessed 9 October 2017).

WHO. 2014b. Primary health care. http://www.euro.who.int/en/health-topics/Health-systems/primary-health-care (Accessed 13 October 2017).

WHO. 2015a. Health equity monitoring. http://www.who.int/gho/health_equity/about/en/ (Accessed 9 October 2017).

WHO. 2015b. MDG 6: Combat HIV/AIDS, malaria and other diseases. http://www.who.int/topics/millennium_development_goals/diseases/en/ (Accessed 9 October 2017).

WHO. 2017a. Stillbirths. http://www.who.int/maternal_child_adolescent/epidemiology/stillbirth/en/ (Accessed 9 October 2017).

WHO. 2017b. The Partnership for Maternal, Newborn and Child Health. http://www.who.int/life-course/partners/pmnch/en/ (Accessed 9 October 2017).

World Bank. 2017. Birth rate, crude (per 1 000 people). data.worldbank.org/indicator/SP.DYN.CBRT.IN (Accessed 9 October 2017).

The World Factbook. 2016. https://www.cia.gov/library/publications/resources/the-world-factbook/index.html (Accessed 9 October 2017).

Zhar, C & Royston, E. 1991. Maternal mortality – a global factbook. apps.who.int/iris/bitstream/10665/38317/1/WHO_MCH_MSM_91.3.pdf (Accessed 9 October 2017).

Section 2: The female reproductive system

Ballard, OJD & Morrow, AL. 2013. 'Human milk composition: Nutrients and bioactive factors'. *Pediat Clin Nort Am*, 60(1): 49–74. https://www.ncbi.nlm.nih.gov/pmc/articles/PMC3586783/ (Accessed 10 October 2017).

Baskett, TF & Nagele, F. 2000. 'Naegele's rule: A reappraisal'. *British Journal of Obstetrics and Gynaecology*, 107: 1433–1435. http://onlinelibrary.wiley.com/doi/10.1111/j.1471-0528.2000.tb11661.x/pdf (Accessed 10 October 2017).

Blackburn, ST. 2003. *Maternal, fetal and neonatal physiology: A clinical perspective.* 2nd ed. St Louis: Saunders.

Brooks, M. 1999. *Get a grip on genetics.* Hong Kong: Ivy Press.

Burnett, CWF. 1979. *The anatomy and physiology of obstetrics.* 6th ed. (rev MM Anderson). London: Faber and Faber.

CDC (Centres for Disease Control and Prevention). 2011. Office on Women's Health (US). The Surgeon General's call to action to support breastfeeding. (Rockville MD). The importance of breastfeeding. NCBI. https://www.ncbi.nlm.nih.gov/books/NBK52682/ (Accessed 10 October 2017).

Chard, T & Klopper, A. 1982. 'Placental enzymes', in *Placental function tests*, by T Chard & A Klopper. London: Springer: 34–38. link.springer.com/chapter/10.1007%2F978-1-4471-3508-1_4 (Accessed 10 October 2017).

Chudleigh, P & Pearce, JM. 1995. *Obstetric ultrasound: How, why and when.* 2nd ed. London: Churchill Livingstone.

DoH (Department of Health). nd(a). Birth defects. Fact sheet. https://www.westerncape.gov.za/text/2003/birthdefects.pdf (Accessed 13 October 2017).

DoH. nd(b). *Human Genetic Policy Guidelines for the Management and Prevention of Genetic Disorders, Birth Defects and Disabilities.* https://www.gov.za/sites/default/files/humangenetics_0.pdf (Accessed 10 October 2017).

DoH. 2013. *Infant and Young Child Feeding Policy.* https://www.health-e.org.za/wp-content/uploads/2013/09/IYCF_Policy_2013.pdf (Accessed 10 October 2017).

Emery, AEH. 1983. *Elements of medical genetics.* 6th ed. Edinburgh: Churchill Livingstone.

Fox, H. 1966. 'Haemangiomata of the placenta'. *J Clin Path*, 19(2): 133–137. https://www.ncbi.nlm.nih.gov/pmc/articles/PMC473204/ (Accessed 11 October 2017).

Freeman, WH & Bracegirdle, B. 1967. *An atlas of histology.* 2nd ed. London: Heinemann Educational Books.

Garfield, RE & Maner, WLJ. 2007. 'Physiology and electrical activity of uterine contractions'. *Seminars in Cell and Developmental Biology*, 18: 289–295.

Garrey, MM, Govan, ADT, Hodge, CH & Callander, R. 1974. *Obstetrics illustrated.* 2nd ed. Edinburgh and London: E and S Livingstone.

Godhia, ML & Patel, N. 2013. 'Colostrum, its composition, benefits as a neutraceutical: A review'. *Curr Res Nutr Food Sci*, 1(1): 37–47. http://www.foodandnutritionjournal.org/volume1number1/colostrum-its-composition-benefits-as-a-nutraceutical-a-review/ (Accessed 9 October 2017).

Grimbizis, GF, Gordts, S, Di Spiezio Sardo, A, Brucker, S, De Angelis, C, Gergolet, M, Li, T, Tanos, V, Brölmann, H, Gianaroli, L & Campo, R. 2013. 'The ESHRE/ESGE consensus on the classification of female genital tract congenital anomalies'. *Hum Reprod*, 28(8): 2032–2044. https://www.eshre.eu/conuta (Accessed 9 October 2017).

Harrison, V. 2008. *The newborn baby*. 5th ed. Cape Town: Juta.

Harvey, MA. 2003. 'Pelvic floor exercises during and after pregnancy: A systematic review of their role in preventing pelvic floor dysfunction'. *J Obstet Gynaecol Can*, 25(6): 487–498. https://www.ncbi.nlm.nih.gov/pubmed/12806450 (Accessed 17 November 2017).

ICN (International Council of Nurses). 2008. *Nursing Matters. Female genital mutilation*. http://www.icn.ch/images/stories/documents/publications/fact_sheets/10e_FS-Female_Genital_Mutilation.pdf (Accessed 10 October 2017).

Innis, SM, Gilley, J & Werker, J. 2001. 'Are human milk long-chain poly-unsaturated fatty acids related to visual and neural development in breastfed term infants?' *Journal of Pediatrics*, 139(4): 532–538. https://www.ncbi.nlm.nih.gov/pubmed/11598600 (Accessed 10 October 2017).

Johnston-Robledo, I & Chrisler, JC. 2011. *The menstrual mark: Menstruation as social stigma*. Springer Science+Business Media, LLC. https://www.researchgate.net/profile/Joan_Chrisler/publication/225143159_The_Menstrual_Mark_Menstruation_as_Social_Stigma/links/55d5f08a08aec156b9a6da8f.pdf (Accessed 10 October 2017).

La Cerva, V. 1981. *Breastfeeding: A manual for healthcare professionals*. New York: Medical Examination Publishing.

Lain, KY & Roberts, JM. 2002. 'Contemporary concepts of pathogenesis and management of preeclampsia'. *JAMA*, 287(24): 3183–3186. https://www.ncbi.nlm.nih.gov/pubmed/12076198 (Accessed 10 October 2017).

La Leche League International. 1981. *The womanly art of breastfeeding*. Illinois: Franklin Park.

Lawrence, EA & Lawrence, EM. 2015. *Breastfeeding: A guide for the medical profession*. 8th ed. Elsevier. https://books.google.co.za/books?isbn=0323394205 (Accessed 10 October 2017).

Lebese, V, Aldous, C & Malherbe, HL. 2016. 'South African congenital disorders data, 2006–2014'. *S Afr Med J*, 106(10): 992–995. http://www.samj.org.za/index.php/samj/article/view/11314 (Accessed 17 October 2017).

Lim, CT, Grossman, A & Khoo, B. 2014. 'Normal physiology of ACTH and GH release in the hypothalamus and anterior pituitary in man'. https://www.ncbi.nlm.nih.gov/books/NBK279116/ (Accessed 10 October 2017).

Llewellyn-Jones, D. 1992. *Fundamentals of obstetrics and gynaecology*. London: Faber and Faber.

Marshall, J, Raynor, M & Nolte, A. 2014. *Myles textbook for midwives*. 3rd African ed. Johannesburg: Elsevier.

Marshall, WM & Tanner, JM. 1970. 'Variations in the pattern of pubertal changes in boys'. *Archives of Disease in Childhood*, 45, 13. http://adc.bmj.com/content/archdischild/45/239/13.full.pdf (Accessed 10 October 2017).

Merten, S, Dratva, J & Ackermann-Liebrich, U. 2005. 'Do baby-friendly hospitals influence breastfeeding duration on a national level?' *Pediatrics*, 116: E702–708.

Meyer, GP, Labidi, S, Podewski, E, Sliwa, K, Drexler, H & Hilfiker-Kleiner, D. 2010. 'Bromocriptine treatment associated with recovery from peripartum cardiomyopathy in siblings: Two case reports'. *Journal of Medical Case Reports*, 4(80). DOI: 10.1186/1752-1947-4-80. https://jmedicalcasereports.biomedcentral.com/articles/10.1186/1752-1947-4-80/open-peer-review (Accessed 10 October 2017).

Moore, KL. 1983. *Before we are born*. 2nd ed. Toronto/Philadelphia: WB Saunders.

MRC (Medical Research Council). 2005. *Intra partum care in South Africa*. South Africa: MRC.

Muir, BL. 1983. *Essentials of genetics for nurses*. New York/Toronto: John Wiley.

Naeye, RL. 1987. 'Functionally important disorders of the placenta, umbilical cord and fetal membranes'. *Human Pathology*, 18: 680–690.

NHGRI (National Human Genome Research Insitute). 2015. All about the Human Genome Project. https://www.genome.gov/10001772/all-about-the--human-genome-project-hgp/ (Accessed 10 October 2017).

Nilson, L, Ingelman-Sundberg, A & Wirsen, C. 1967. *The everyday miracle*. London: Penguin Press.

O'Brien, M, Buikstra, E & Hegney, D. 2008. 'The influence of psychological factors on breastfeeding duration'. *Journal of Advanced Nursing*, 63: 397–408.

Patel, RR, Steer, P, Doyle, P, Little, MP & Elliott, P. 2004. 'Does gestation vary by ethnic group? A London-based study of over 122,000 pregnancies with spontaneous onset of labour'. *Int J Epidemiol*, 33(1): 107–113. https://www.ncbi.nlm.nih.gov/pubmed/15075154 (Accessed 10 October 2017).

Picciano, MF. 1984. 'What constitutes a representative human milk sample?' *Journal of Pediatric Gastroenterology and Nutrition*, 3: 280–283.

Pronczuk, J, Akre, J, Moy, J & Vallenas, C. 2002. 'Global perspectives in breast milk contamination: infectious and toxic hazards'. The National Institute of Environmental Health Sciences (NIEHS). *Environmental Health Perspectives*, 110: 349.

Richter L. 2016. Why breastfeeding in South Africa still needs champion. https://www.wits.ac.za/news/latest-news/in-their-own-words/2016/2016-08/why-breastfeeding-in-south-africa-still-needs-champion.html (Accessed 10 October 2017).

Rojas-Burke, J. 2010. Starting in the womb, females have an advantage over males. *The Oregonian.* http://www.oregonlive.com/health/index.ssf/2010/06/starting_in_the_womb_females_h.html (Accessed 11 October 2017).

Siziba, LP, Jerling, J, Hanekom, SM & Wentzel-Viljoen, E. 2015. 'Low rates of exclusive breastfeeding are still evident in four South African provinces'. *SAJCN*, 28(4): 170–179. www.sajcn.co.za/index.php/SAJCN/article/view/996 (Accessed 10 October 2017).

Smith, LJ. 1997. How mother's milk is made. BFLRC. https://www.bflrc.com/ljs/breastfeeding/MakeMilk.html (Accessed 30 November 2017).

Smith, H, Brown, H, Hofmeyr, GJ & Garner, P. 2004. 'Evidence-based obstetric care in South Africa – influencing practice through the "Better Births Initiative"'. *S Afr Med J*, 94(2): 117–120. https://www.ncbi.nlm.nih.gov/pubmed/15034990 (Accessed 10 October 2017).

Solomon, EP & Davis, PW. 1983. *Human anatomy and physiology.* Philadelphia: Saunders College Publishing.

Stuebe, A. 2009. 'The risks of not breastfeeding for mothers and infants'. *Rev Obstet Gynecol*, 2(4): 222–231. https://www.ncbi.nlm.nih.gov/pmc/articles/PMC2812877/ (Accessed 10 October 2017).

Tanner, JM. 1948. Puberty and the Tanner stages. Child growth foundation. http://www.childgrowthfoundation.org/CMS/FILES/Puberty_and_the_Tanner_Stages.pdf (Accessed 10 October 2017).

Tshwane declaration of support for breastfeeding in South Africa. 2011. *S Afr J Clin Nutr*, 24(4). http://www.sajcn.co.za/index.php/SAJCN/article/view/586/820 (Accessed 10 October 2017).

Uechi, M, Ikezawa, Y & Kosuge, K. 2007. 'Anti-infective substances in human colostrum and milk'. *Pediatrics International*, 24: 245–251.

UNICEF (United Nations Children's Fund). 2015. Breastfeeding and nutrition. https://www.unicef.org/nutrition/index_24824.html (Accessed 10 October 2017).

USAID (United States Agency for International Development). 2010. Fistula care projects. https://fistulacare.org/ (Accessed 17 October 2017).

Whirledge, S & Cidlowski, JA. 2010. 'Glucocorticoids, stress, and fertility'. *Minerva Endocrinol*, 35(2): 109–125. https://www.ncbi.nlm.nih.gov/pmc/articles/PMC3547681/ (Accessed 10 October 2017).

WHO. nd. World breastfeeding week. http://www.who.int/life-course/news/events/2017-breastfeeding-week/en/ (Accessed 10 October 2017).

WHO. 2001. Female genital mutilation. The prevention and management of health complications. Policy guidelines for nurses and midwives. WHO/Fch/Gwh/015./Who/Rhr/01/18. Geneva: WHO.

WHO. 2003. *Global Strategy for Infant and Young Child Feeding.* http://www.who.int/nutrition/publications/gs_infant_feeding_text_eng.pdf (Accessed 10 October 2017).

WHO 2017. Infant and young child feeding. http://www.who.int/mediacentre/factsheets/fs342/en/ (Accessed 4 October 2017).

Williams, PL & Warwick, R. 1980. *Gray's anatomy.* 36th ed. London: Churchill Livingstone.

World Bank. nd. World development indicators. Exclusive breastfeeding rates. https://data.worldbank.org/indicator/SH.STA.BFED.ZS (Accessed 10 October 2017).

Section 3: Psychosocial and cultural aspects of childbirth

AACN (American Association of Colleges of Nursing). 2008. Cultural competency toolkit for Baccalaureate Nurses. http://www.aacnnursing.org/Portals/42/AcademicNursing/CurriculumGuidelines/Cultural-Competency-Bacc-Tool-Kit.pdf?ver=2017-05-18-143552-023 (Accessed 10 October 2017).

Abdollahi, F, Lye, M-S, Zain, A, Ghazali, SS & Zarghami, M. 2011. 'Postnatal depression and its associated factors in women from different cultures'. *Iran J Psychiatry Behav Sci*, Autumn-Winter; 5(2): 5–11. https://www.ncbi.nlm.nih.gov/pmc/articles/PMC3939973/ (Accessed 10 October 2017).

Ahmed, BZS. 2005. Poverty, family stress and parenting. http://www.humiliationstudies.org/documents/AhmedPovertyFamilyStressParenting.pdf (Accessed 10 October 2017).

Ainsworth, MD. 1985. 'Patterns of infant mother attachment'. *Bulletin of the New York Academy of Medicine*, 61: 792–812.

AIS (The American Institute of Stress). 2017. The Holmes-Rahe stress inventory. https://www.stress.org/holmes-rahe-stress-inventory/ (Accessed 10 October 2017).

Atif, N, Lovell, K & Rahman, A. 2015. 'Maternal mental health: The missing M in the global maternal and child agenda'. *Seminars in Perinatology,* 39(5): 345–352. http://

www.seminperinat.com/article/S0146-0005(15)00054-3/ abstract (Accessed 10 October 2017).

Baird, SF. 1976. 'Crisis intervention theory in maternal-infant nursing'. *JOGNN*, 5(1): 30–39. http://onlinelibrary.wiley.com/doi/10.1111/jogn.1976.5.issue-1/issuetoc (Accessed 17 November 2017).

Blackie, D. 2014. Fact sheet on child abandonment research in South Africa, 20 May 2014. http://www.adoptioncoalitionsa.org/wp-content/uploads/2014/05/Fact-Sheet-Research-on-Child-Abandonment-in-South-Africa_Final2.pdf (Accessed 10 October 2017).

Bolby, J. 1969. *Attachment and loss. Vol. 1: Attachment*. New York: Basic Books.

Bowen, SM & Miller, BC. 1980. 'Paternal attachment behavior as related to presence at delivery and preparenthood classes: A pilot study'. *Nursing Research*, 29(5): 269. http://journals.lww.com/nursingresearchonline/Abstract/1980/09000/Paternal_Attachment_Behavior_as_Related_to.10.aspx (Accessed 10 October 2017).

Brazelton, TB. 1983. *Infants and mothers: Differences in development*. Revised edition. New York: Dell.

Campinha-Bacote, J. 2009. 'A culturally competent model of care for African Americans'. *Urologic Nursing*, 29(1): 49–54. https://www.suna.org/download/members/unjarticles/2009/09feb/49.pdf (Accessed 10 October 2017).

Cartwright, JE, Fraser, R, Leslie, K, Wallace, AE & James, JL 2010. 'Remodelling at the maternal-fetal interface: relevance to human pregnancy disorders'. *Reproduction*, Dec 140(6): 803–813. DOI: 10.1530/REP-10-0294. https://www.ncbi.nlm.nih.gov/pubmed/20837731 (Accessed 10 October 2017).

Chalmers, B. 1983. 'Psycho-social factors and obstetric complications'. *Psychological Medicine*, 13: 333–339.

Chalmers, B. 1984a. *Early parenthood: Heaven or hell*. Cape Town: Juta.

Chalmers, B. 1984b. 'Behavioural associations of pregnancy complications'. *Journal of Psychosomatic Obstetrics and Gynaecology*, 3: 27–35.

Chalmers, B. 1987a. 'Pregnancy: the Pedi woman's veil of secrecy'. *South African Journal of Psychology*, 17: 30–31.

Chalmers, B. 1987b. 'Urban–rural differences regarding Pedi childbirth experiences'. *Journal of Psychosomatic Obstetrics and Gynaecology*, 7: 131–139.

Chalmers, B. 1987c. 'Black women's birth experiences: changing traditions'. *Journal of Psychosomatic Obstetrics and Gynaecology*, 6: 211–224.

Chalmers, B. 1987d. 'Social support in pregnancy and the puerperium amongst Pedi women'. *Journal of Psychosomatic Obstetrics and Gynaecology*, 7: 63–70.

Chalmers, B. 1987e. 'Knowledge about pregnancy, birth and the postpartum period amongst Pedi women'. *Journal of Psychosomatic Obstetrics and Gynaecology*, 7: 51–61.

Chalmers, B. 1990. *African birth*. South Africa: Berev Publications.

Chapman, RR. 2003. 'Endangering safe motherhood in Mozambique: Prenatal care as pregnancy risk'. *Social Science and Medicine*, 57: 355–374.

Charles, VE, Polis, CB, Sridhara, SK & Blum, RW. 2008. 'Abortion and long-term mental health outcomes: A systematic review of the evidence'. *Contraception*, 78(6): 436–450. DOI: 10.1016/j.contraception.2008.07.005. https://www.ncbi.nlm.nih.gov/pubmed/19014789 (Accessed 20 October 2017).

Cobb, J. 1980. *Babyshock: A mother's first five years*. London: Hutchinson.

Collier, P. 1982. 'Understanding Couvades'. *Maternal Child Nursing*, 7: 114–115.

Condon, JT, Boyce, P & Corkindale, CJ. 2004. 'The First-Time Fathers Study: A prospective study of the mental health and wellbeing of men during the transition to parenthood'. *Australian and New Zealand Journal of Psychiatry*, 38: 56–64. https://www.researchgate.net/profile/Philip_Boyce2/publication/8913480_The_First-Time_Fathers_Study_A_prospective_study_of_the_mental_health_and_wellbeing_of_men_during_the_transition_to_parenthood/links/0fcfd51141ed95c6f8000000.pdf (Accessed 10 October 2017).

Cronenwett, L & Kunst-Wilson, W. 1981. 'Stress, social support and transition to fatherhood'. *Nursing Research*, 30(4): 196–201.

Davis, T. 2011. Rites of passage in Africa. Birth of adulthood. African holocaust. http://africanholocaust.net/ritesofpassage/ (Accessed 10 October 2017).

Davis, M & Walbridge, D. 1981. *Boundary and space: An introduction to the work of DW Winnicott*. London: Karnac Books.

Dawson, E, Gauld, R & Ridler, J. 1993. 'Empowering mothers'. *Nursing RSA*, 84: 10.

Dick-Read, G. 2005. *Childbirth without fear*. London: Pinter and Martin Publishers.

DoH (Department of Health). 2003. *South African Demographic and Health Survey*. Full report. https://dhsprogram.com/pubs/pdf/FR206/FR206.pdf (Accessed 17 October 2017).

DoH. 2016. *Ideal Clinic Manual. Version 16.* http://www.kznhealth.gov.za/family/Ideal-Clinic-Manual-Oct2015.pdf and https://www.idealclinic.org.za/docs/2016/Ideal%20Clinic%20Manual%20v16%20-%2023Jun16.pdf (Accessed 10 October 2017).

DoH & MRC (Medical Research Council). 1998. *Demographic and Health Survey 1998, South Africa.* https://www.datafirst.uct.ac.za/dataportal/index.php/catalog/364 (Accessed 11 October 2017).

DoJ & CD (Department of Justice and Constitutional Development). 2017. What is ukuthwala? http://www.justice.gov.za/brochure/ukuthwala/ukuthwala.html (Accessed 10 October 2017).

DPSA (Department of Public Service and Administration). nd. *The Batho Pele Vision: A better life for all South Africans by putting people first.* www.dpsa.gov.za/documents/Abridged%20BP%20programme%20July2014.pdf (Accessed 10 October 2017).

Drugs.com. 2017. Valproic acid: Pregnancy and breastfeeding warnings. https://www.drugs.com/pregnancy/valproic-acid.html (Accessed 10 October 2017).

Eberstat, N. 2015. China's demographics in the one-child policy era. http://www.aei.org/publication/chinas-demographics-in-the-one-child-policy-era-answered-and-unanswered-questions/ (Accessed 10 October 2017).

Edinburgh Postnatal Depression Scale (EPDS). www.fresno.ucsf.edu/pediatrics/downloads/edinburghscale.pdf (Accessed 10 October 2017).

Erikson, E. 1983. *Identity: Youth and crisis.* London: Faber and Faber.

Ewing, J. 1984: 'Detecting alcoholism. The CAGE questionnaire'. *JAMA,* 252(14): 1905–1907.

Farquhar, M, Camilleri-Ferrante, C & Todd, C. 2000. 'Continuity of care in maternity services: Women's views of one team midwifery scheme'. *Midwifery,* 16(1): 35–47.

Fildes, V. 1988. 'The English wet nurse and her role in infant care 1538–1800'. *Medical History,* 32: 142–173.

Finlay, L. 2015. *Relational integrative psychotherapy: Process and theory in practice.* Chichester, Sussex: Wiley. http://eu.wiley.com/WileyCDA/WileyTitle/productCd-1119087309.html (Accessed 10 October 2017).

Fishbein, EG. 1981. 'Fatherhood and disturbances of health. A review'. *Journal of Psychiatric Nursing,* 19(7): 24–27. https://www.ncbi.nlm.nih.gov/pubmed/6267272 (Accessed 10 October 2017).

Fisher, E. 1987. *Psychology for nurses.* 6th ed. Cape Town: Juta.

Flenady, V, Boyle, F, Koopmans, L, Wilson, T, Stones, W & Cacciatore, J. 2014. 'Meeting the needs of parents after a stillbirth or neonatal death'. *BJOG: An International Journal of Obstetrics and Gynaecology* 121(4): 137–140. http://onlinelibrary.wiley.com/doi/10.1111/1471-0528.13009/pdf (Accessed 10 October 2017).

Forray, A. 2016. 'Substance use during pregnancy'. US National Library of Medicine National Institutes of Health Version 1. F1000Res. 2016; 5: F1000 Faculty Rev-887. https://www.ncbi.nlm.nih.gov/pmc/articles/PMC4870985/ (Accessed 10 October 2017).

Foster, EM. 2001. 'Expenditures and sustainability in systems of care'. *Journal of Emotional and Behaviour Disorders,* 9: 53–62.

Freud, A. 1989. *Normality and pathology in childhood.* London: Karnac Books.

FSU (Florida State University). 2016. *Promoting attachment security in pediatric practice: Using the circle of security.* Paediatric Brief 1, Center for Prevention and Early Intervention Policy. http://cpeip.fsu.edu/mma/documents/ECHO%20Pediatrician%20Brief%201%20-%20Promoting%20Attachment%20Security%20-%20Using%20the%20Circle%20of%20Security.pdf (Accessed 4 October 2017).

Gay, J. 1981. 'A conceptual framework of bonding'. *JOGNN,* 10(6): 440–444. http://www.jognn.org/article/S0090-0311(15)30715-8/fulltext (Accessed 10 October 2017).

Gelaye, B, Rondon, M, Araya, R & Williams, MA. 2016. 'Epidemiology of maternal depression, risk factors, and child outcomes in low-income and middle-income countries'. *Lancet Psychiatry,* 3(10): 973–982. DOI: 10.1016/S2215-0366(16)30284-X. https://www.ncbi.nlm.nih.gov/pubmed/27650773 (Accessed 10 October 2017).

Giger, JN & Davidhizar, R. 2002. 'The Giger and Davidhizar Transcultural Assessment Model'. *J Transcult Nurs,* Jul 13(3): 185–188. https://www.ncbi.nlm.nih.gov/pubmed/12113147 (Accessed 10 October 2017).

Givengain.com. 2017. Tears Foundation. https://www.givengain.com/c/tears/about/ (Accessed 10 October 2017).

Hangsleben, KL. 1983. 'Transition to fatherhood: An exploratory study'. *JOGNN,* 12(4): 265–270. http://www.jognn.org/article/S0090-0311(15)30806-1/fulltext (Accessed 10 October 2017).

Harlow, BL, Vitonis, AF, Sparen, P, Cnattingius, S, Joffe, H & Hultman, CM. 2007. 'Incidence of hospitalization for postpartum psychotic and bipolar episodes in women with and without prior prepregnancy or prenatal psychiatric hospitalizations'. *Arch Gen Psychiatry,* Jan, 64(1): 42–48.

https://www.ncbi.nlm.nih.gov/pubmed/17199053 (Accessed 10 October 2017).

Haub, C. 2012. World population data sheet. Population Reference Bureau. http://www.prb.org/Publications/Datasheets/2012/2012-world-population-data-sheet.aspx (Accessed 10 October 2017).

ICM (International Confederation of Midwives). 2005. *Female genital mutilation.* http://internationalmidwives.org/assets/uploads/documents/Position%20Statements%20-%20English/PS2011_007%20ENG%20Female%20Genital%20Mutilation%20(FGM).pdf (Accessed 10 October 2017).

Javadifar, N, Majilesi, F, Nasrabadi, AN, Nedjat, S & Montazeni, A. 2013. 'Internal conflicts of Iranian first-time mothers in adaptation to maternal role'. *Iran J Nurse Midwifery Res,* 18(3): 222–227. https://www.ncbi.nlm.nih.gov/pmc/articles/PMC3748542/ (Accessed 10 October 2017).

Jewkes, R, Abraham, N & Mvo, Z. 1998. 'Why do nurses abuse patients? Reflections from South African obstetric services'. *Social Science and Medicine,* 47: 1781–1795.

Jewkes, R, Levin, J & Penn-Kekana, L. 2002. 'Risk factors for domestic violence: Findings from a South African cross-sectional study'. *Social Science and Medicine,* 55: 1603–1617.

Jomeen, J. 2004. 'The importance of assessing psychological status during pregnancy, childbirth and the postnatal period as a multidimensional construct: A literature review'. *Clinical Effectiveness in Nursing,* 8: 144–155.

Jordan, RG, Engstrom, J, Marfell, J & Farley, CL. 2013. *Prenatal and postnatal care.* Wiley Blackwell.

Keller, KT. 2001. *Parenting an infant. Skills for teens who parent.* Minnesota: Capstone Press.

Kendell, RE, Chalmers, JC & Platz, C. 1987. 'Epidemiology of puerperal psychoses'. *The British Journal of Psychiatry,* May 150(5): 662–673. DOI: 10.1192/bjp.150.5.662. http://bjp.rcpsych.org/content/150/5/662 (Accessed 10 October 2017).

Kersting, A & Wagner, B. 2012. 'Complicated grief after perinatal loss'. *Dialogues Clin Neurosci,* 14(2): 187–194. https://www.ncbi.nlm.nih.gov/pmc/articles/PMC3384447/ (Accessed 10 October 2017).

Kiehl, EM & White, MA. 2003. 'Maternal adaptation during childbearing in Norway, Sweden and the United States'. *Caring Science,* 17(2): 96–103. https://www.ncbi.nlm.nih.gov/pubmed/12753509 (Accessed 10 October 2017).

Kitzinger, S. 1978. *The experience of childbirth.* London: Penguin.

Klaus, MH & Kennell, JH. 1982. *Parent–infant bonding.* 2nd ed. St. Louis: The CV Mosby Company.

Kleinschmidt, I, Adamchak, S, Janowitz, B & Cuthbertson, C. 2004. *Involving men in maternity care in South Africa.* US Aid. http://pdf.usaid.gov/pdf_docs/Pnada931.pdf (Accessed 10 October 2017).

Kübler-Ross, E. 1969. *On death and dying.* Scribner.

Kübler-Ross, E & Kessler, D. 2005. *On grief and grieving.* Simon and Schuster.

Lamb, GS & Lipkin, M. 1982. 'Somatic symptoms of expectant fathers'. *Maternal and Child Nursing,* 7:110–113.

Leininger, MM. 1991. *Culture care diversity and universality: A theory of nursing.* National League for Nursing Press.

Leininger, M. 2006. 'Madeleine Leininger's cultural care: Diversity and universality'. Chapter 15. http://nursing.jbpub.com/sitzman/ch15pdf.pdf (Accessed 10 October 2017).

Li, J & Karakowsky, L. 2001. 'Do we see eye-to-eye? Implications of cultural differences for cross-cultural management research and practice'. *The Journal of Psychology,* 135(5): 501–517. https://www.ncbi.nlm.nih.gov/pubmed/11804004 (Accessed 10 October 2017).

Lipka, M. 2014. Africans among the most morally opposed to contraception. http://www.pewresearch.org/fact-tank/2014/04/16/africans-among-the-most-morally-opposed-to-contraception/ (Accessed 10 October 2017).

Lothian, JA. 2008. The journey of becoming a mother. https://www.ncbi.nlm.nih.gov/pubmed/19436533 (Accessed 10 October 2017).

Lundqvist, C & Sabel, KS. 1999. The Brazelton neonatal behaviour assessment scale detects differences among newborn infants of optimal health. https://academic.oup.com/jpepsy/article/25/8/577/914725/The-Brazelton-Neonatal-Behavioral-Assessment-Scale (Accessed 10 October 2017).

Mahery, P & Proudlock, P. 2011. *Legal guide to age thresholds for children and young people.* Children's Institute, University of Cape Town. http://www.ci.uct.ac.za/sites/default/files/image_tool/images/367/Law_reform/Children_Act_guides/Ages%20Guide%20April%202011%20print%20version.pdf (Accessed 10 October 2017).

Maimbolwa, MC, Yamba Yiwan, Y & Yansjo-Yrvidson, Y. 2003. 'Issues and innovations in nursing practice. Cultural childbirth practices and beliefs in Zambia'. *Journal of Advanced Nursing,* 43: 263–274.

Mashita, RJ, Themane, MJ, Monyeki, KD & Kemper, HCG. 2011. 'Current smoking behaviour among rural

South African children: Ellisras longitudinal study'. *MC Pediatrics*, 11: 58. DOI: 10.1186/1471-2431-11-58. https://bmcpediatr.biomedcentral.com/articles/10.1186/1471-2431-11-58 (Accessed 10 October 2017).

Matria, B. 1995. 'Giving due consideration to the family's race and criteria background', in *Assessment of parenting: Psychiatric and psychological contributions*, by P Reder & C Lucey. London: Routledge.

May, AK. 2006. 'Active involvement of expectant fathers in pregnancy'. *Journal of Obstetrics, Gynegologic and Neonatal Nursing*, 7: 7–12.

McCool, W, Guidera, M, Stenson, M & Dauphinee, L. 2009. 'The pain that binds us: Midwives' experiences of loss and adverse outcomes around the world'. *Health Care for Women International*, 30: 1003–1013.

McLeod, P. 2007. Bowlby's attachment theory. https://www.simplypsychology.org/bowlby.html (Accessed 11 October 2017).

Meny-Gilbert, S & Chiumia, S. 2016. Where do South African international migrants come from? https://africacheck.org/factsheets/geography-migration/ (Accessed 11 October 2017).

Mercer, R. 2004. 'Becoming a mother versus maternal role attainment'. *J Nurs Scholarship*, 36(3): 226–232. https://www.ncbi.nlm.nih.gov/pubmed/15495491 (Accessed 11 October 2017).

Mercer, R. 2016. Maternal role attainment theory. http://www.nursing-theory.org/theories-and-models/mercer-maternal-role-attainment-theory.php (Accessed 11 October 2017).

MHRA (Medicines and Healthcare Products Regulatory Agency). 2016. Toolkit on the risks of valproate medicines in female patients. https://www.gov.uk/government/publications/toolkit-on-the-risks-of-valproate-medicines-in-female-patients (Accessed 11 October 2017).

Murphy, SC. 2006. Mapping the literature of transcultural nursing. *J Med Lib Ass*, 9(2Suppl) E143–151. https://www.ncbi.nlm.nih.gov/pmc/articles/PMC1463039/ (Accessed 11 October 2017).

National Adoption Coalition SA. nd. Fact sheet on child abandonment research in South Africa. http://www.adoptioncoalitionsa.org/wp-content/uploads/2014/05/Fact-Sheet-Research-on-Child-Abandonment-in-South-Africa_Final2.pdf (Accessed 11 October 2017).

Ngunyulu, RN & Malaudzi, FM. 2009. 'Indigenous practices regarding postnatal care at Sikhunyani village in the Limpopo province of South Africa'. *African Journal of Nursing and Midwifery*, 2(1): 48–64. https://repository.

up.ac.za/bitstream/handle/2263/10507/Ngunyulu_Indigenous(2009).pdf?sequence=1 (Accessed 11 October 2017).

NICE (National Institute for Health and Care Excellence). 2003. *National Institute for Health and Care Excellence: Clinical Guidelines*. London: NICE. https://www.ncbi.nlm.nih.gov/books/NBK11822/ (Accessed 11 October 2017).

NICE. 2009. Child maltreatment: When to suspect maltreatment under 18: Clinical guidelines. https://www.nice.org.uk/guidance/cg89 (Accessed 11 October 2017).

NICE. 2011. Common mental health problems: Identification and pathways to care. Clinical guideline [CG123]. https://www.nice.org.uk/guidance/cg123 (Accessed 11 October 2017).

NICE. 2016. Antenatal and postnatal mental health. QS115. https://www.nice.org.uk/guidance/qs115 (Accessed 11 October 2017).

Oakley, A. 1980. *Women confined: Towards a sociology of childbirth*. London: Penguin.

O'Brien, CP. 2008. Detecting alcoholism: The CAGE questionnaire. *JAMA*, 300(17): 2054–2056. DOI: 10.1001/jama.2008.570. http://jamanetwork.com/journals/jama/fullarticle/182810 (Accessed 11 October 2017).

O'Connor, TG, Heron, J, Golding, J & Beveridge, VG. 2002. 'Maternal anxiety and children's behaviour/emotional problems at 4 years'. *The British Journal of Psychiatry*, 180(6): 502–508. http://bjp.rcpsych.org/content/bjprcpsych/180/6/502.full.pdf (Accessed 11 October 2017).

Office of the Status of Women. South African Office of the Presidency. 2000. *South Africa's National Policy Framework for Women's Empowerment and Gender Equality*. https://www.parliament.gov.za/storage/app/media/ProjectsAndEvents/2015_womens_roundtable_discussion/docs/National_Gender_Framework.pdf (Accessed 11 October 2017).

OHCHR (Office of the High Commissioner of Human Rights). 1979. Fact Sheet no 23. http://www.ohchr.org/Documents/Publications/FactSheet23en.pdf (Accessed 11 October 2017).

Olsen, O & Jewell, MD. 2002. 'Home versus hospital birth'. *Cochrane Database Syst Rev*, 2: CD 000352.

OSG (Office of the Surgeon General). 2004. 'Respiratory diseases'. In *The health consequences of smoking: A report of the surgeon general*. Atlanta (GA): CDC. https://www.ncbi.nlm.nih.gov/books/NBK44694/?report=reader (Accessed 11 October 2017).

Parke, RD. 1978. 'The father's role in infancy'. *Birth and Family Journal,* 5: 211.

Parke, RD. 1981. *Fathering.* Glasgow: William Collins.

Penn-Kekana, L & Blaauw, D. 2004. *A Rapid Appraisal of Maternal Health Services in South Africa. A Health System Approach.* HSD/W/01/02. HSD. Centre of Health Systems Development Programme. https://assets. publishing.service.gov.uk/media/57a08d49ed915d622c00 18d1/01-02_south_africa.pdf (Accessed 11 October 2017).

Prince, J & Adams, ME. 1978. *Minds, mothers and midwives: The psychology of childbirth.* Edinburgh: Churchill Livingstone.

Pratt, D. 1990. 'The partner's role in pregnancy'. *Midwifery,* 4: 23–25.

Pruett, KD. 1997. How men and children affect each other's development. https://www.zerotothree.org/ resources/1075-how-men-and-children-affect-each-other-s-development (Accessed 11 October 2017).

Purnell, L. 2002. 'The Purnell model for cultural competence'. *J Transcult Nurs,* Jul 13(3): 193–196. https:// www.ncbi.nlm.nih.gov/pubmed/12113149 (Accessed 11 October 2017).

Rahman, A, Fisher, J, Bower, P, Luchters, S, Tran, T, Yasamy, MT, Saxena, S & Waheed, W. 2013. 'Interventions for common perinatal mental disorders in women in low- and middle-income countries: A systematic review and meta-analysis'. *Bull World Health Organization,* Aug 1, 91(8): 593–601. DOI: 10.2471/BLT.12.109819. https:// www.ncbi.nlm.nih.gov/pubmed/23940407 (Accessed 11 October 2017).

Rao, DB, Lakshmi, VV, Rao, VV & Krishna, VV. 2000. *Status and advancement of women.* New Delhi: APH.

RCOG (Royal College of Obstetricians and Gynaecologists). 2011. 'Management of women with mental health illness during pregnancy'. *Good practice,* 14. https:// www.rcog.org.uk/globalassets/documents/guidelines/ managementwomenmentalhealthgoodpractice14.pdf (Accessed 11 October 2017).

Richter, L. 2006. *BABA. Men and fatherhood in South Africa.* Cape Town: HSRC Press.

Salomonsson, B. 2014. *Psychoanalytic therapy with infants and their parents. Practice theory and results.* New York: McGraw-Hill.

SANC (South African Nursing Council). 2016. Nurses' Pledge. www.sanc.co.za/aboutpledge.htm (Accessed 11 October 2017).

Schwartz, J. 2002. 'Enhancing the birth experience. The doula as part of the hospital maternity program'. *International Journal of Childbirth Education,* 17(1): 18–19.

Sewpaul, V. 1999. 'Culture, religion and infertility: A South African perspective'. *The British Journal of Social Work,* 29(5): 741. https://www.popline.org/node/528371 (Accessed 11 October 2017).

Silva, EB (ed). 1996. *Good enough mothering.* London: Routledge.

Spector, R. 2009. *Cultural diversity in health and illness.* 7th ed. Upper Saddle River, NJ: Prentice Hall.

Stone, PW, Swanziger, J, Walker, PH & Bueting, J. 2000. 'Analysis of two models of low-risk maternity care: Freestanding birth centres compared to traditional settings'. *Research in Nursing & Health,* 23(4): 279–289.

The Tembisan. 2015. One in six women killed by intimate partner – POWA. 11 August. http://tembisan. co.za/20652/one-six-women-killed-intimate-partner-powa/ (Accessed 11 October 2017).

Thurow, R & Hansen, KE. 2016. The first 1 000 days: A crucial time for mothers and children – and the world. live.worldbank.org/the-first-one-thousand-days (Accessed 11 October 2017).

UN. nd. Fourth World Conference on Women: Beijing Declaration. http://www.un.org/womenwatch/daw/ beijing/platform/ (Accessed 11 October 2017).

UN. 1994. Further promotion and encouragement of human rights and fundamental freedoms, including the question of the programme and methods of work of the commission alternative approaches and ways and means within the United Nations system for improving the effective enjoyment of human rights and fundamental freedoms. Fiftieth session. hrlibrary.umn.edu/commission/ thematic51/42.htm (Accessed 11 October 2017).

UN. 2006. United Nations Millennium Project. Millennium Development Goals: Commissioned by the UN Secretary and Supported by the UN Development group 2002–2006. http://www.un.org/millenniumgoals/reports.shtml (Accessed 17 October 2017).

UN. 2015. Sustainable Development Goals. http://www. un.org/sustainabledevelopment/sustainable-development-goals/ (Accessed 11 October 2017).

UNFPA (United Nations Population Fund). 2014. Population and poverty. http://www.unfpa.org/resources/ population-and-poverty (Accessed 22 January 2017).

UNFPA. 2015. World population trends. www.unfpa.org (Accessed 11 October 2017).

UNICEF (United Nations Children's Fund). 2005. Early marriage. A harmful traditional practice. A statistical exploration. https://www.unicef.org/publications/files/ Early_Marriage_12.lo.pdf (Accessed 11 October 2017).

UNICEF. 2013a. *Ending Child Marriage: Progress and Prospects.* https://www.unicef.org/media/files/Child_ Marriage_Report_7_17_LR..pdf (Accessed 11 October 2017).

UNICEF. 2013b. Joint press release. Child marriages: 39 000 every day. https://www.unicef.org/media/media_68114. html (Accessed 11 October 2017).

UNICEF. 2015. *A Post 2015 World Fit for Children: A Review of the OWG Report on SDGs from a Child Rights Perspective.* https://www.unicef.org/agenda2030/files/Post_2015_ OWG_review_CR_FINAL.pdf (Accessed 11 October 2017).

UNICEF. 2016. *Female genital mutilation/cutting: A global concern.* https://www.unicef.org/media/files/ FGMC_2016_brochure_final_UNICEF_SPREAD.pdf (Accessed 11 October 2017).

UNICEF. 2017. Child marriage is a violation of human rights, but is all too common. https://data.unicef.org/ topic/child-protection/child-marriage/ (Accessed 11 October 2017).

UNICEF, HSRC (Human Sciences Research Council) & DoE (Department of Education). 2009. *Teenage pregnancy in SA.* https://www.education.gov.za/LinkClick.aspx?fileti cket=uIqj%2BsyyccM%3D (Accessed 11 October 2017).

Uys, L & Middleton, L. 2013. *Mental health nursing.* 6th ed. Cape Town: Juta.

Vaughan, VC & Brazelton, TB. 1976. *The family: Can it be saved?* Yearbook of Medical Publishers.

Waddell, M. 1998. *Inside lives: Psychoanalysis and the growth of the personality.* London: Gerald Duckworth.

Walker-Smith, J & Murch, S. 1999. *Diseases of the small intestines in childhood.* 4th ed. UK: Isis Medical Media.

WHO. 2001. *Female genital mutilation.* http:// internationalmidwives.org/assets/uploads/documents/ Position%20Statements%20-%20English/ PS2011_007%20ENG%20Female%20Genital%20 Mutilation%20(FGM).pdf (Accessed 11 October 2017).

WHO. 2002. *World report on violence and health.* Released 3 October. http://apps.who.int/iris/ bitstream/10665/42495/1/9241545615_eng.pdf (Accessed 11 October 2017).

WHO. 2003. Maternal mental health. http://www.who.int/ mental_health/prevention/suicide/mmh&chd_chapter_3. pdf (Accessed 11 October 2017).

WHO. 2008. *Maternal Mental Health and Child Development in Low and Middle Income Countries.* http://www.who.int/ mental_health/prevention/suicide/mmh_jan08_meeting_ report.pdf (Accessed 11 October 2017).

WHO. 2013. *Mental Health Action Plan 2013–2020.* http:// www.who.int/mental_health/publications/action_plan/en/ (Accessed 11 October 2017).

WHO. 2016. Violence against women: Intimate partner and sexual violence against women. http://www.who.int/ mediacentre/factsheets/fs239/en/ (Accessed 11 October 2017).

WHO. 2017. Violence and injury prevention. http://www. who.int/violence_injury_prevention/en/ (Accessed 11 October 2017).

Willen, S. 2013. *A Review of Teenage Pregnancy in South Africa – Experience of Schooling and Knowledge and Access to Sexual and Reproductive Health Services.* http://www. hst.org.za/publications/NonHST%20Publications/ Teenage%20Pregnancy%20in%20South%20Africa%20 Final%2010%20May%202013.pdf (Accessed 11 October 2017).

Xu, F, Sullivan, E & Homer, CSE. 2016. 'Mental disorders in new parents before and after birth: A population-based cohort study'. *BJ PSych,* 2(3): 233–243. https://www.ncbi. nlm.nih.gov/pubmed/27703780/ (Accessed 11 October 2017).

Zitzow, D & Estes, G. 1981. 'Heritage consistency as a consideration in counseling Native Americans'. https:// eric.ed.gov/?id=ED209035 (Accessed 11 October 2017).

Section 4: Pregnancy

AAFP (American Academy of Family Physicians). 2010. Should pregnant women wear seatbelts? National Highway Transportation Safety Administration. https:// www.nhtsa.gov/risky-driving/seat-belts (Accessed 12 October 2017).

Ablove, RH & Ablove, TS. 2009. 'Prevalence of carpel tunnel syndrome in pregnant women'. *Wisconsin Medical Journal,* 108(4): 194–196.

ACS (American Cancer Society). 2016. Chemotherapy for breast cancer. Revised August 18, 2016. http:// www.cancer.org/cancer/breastcancer/moreinformation/ pregnancy-and-breast-cancer (Accessed 12 October 2017).

Adewole, IF. 2002. 'Prophylactic antibiotics for inhibiting preterm labour with intact membranes'. *The WHO Reproductive Health Library.* Geneva: WHO.

Agampodi, SB, Wickramasinghe, ND, Horton, J & Agampodi, TC. 2013. 'Minor ailments in pregnancy are not a minor concern for pregnant women: A morbidity assessment survey in rural Sri Lanka'. *PLOS ONE.* DOI: 10.1371/

journal.pone.0064214. http://www.ncbi.nlm.nih.gov/pmc/articles/PMC3651131/ (Accessed 12 October 2017).

Ajayi, IO, Osakinle, DC & Osakinle, EO. 2013. 'Quality assessment of the practice of focused antenatal care (FANC) in rural and urban primary health centres in Ekiti State'. *Open Journal of Obstetrics and Gynecology*, 3(3): 319–326. http://www.scirp.org/journal/ojog/ (Accessed 12 October 2017).

Alfirevic, Z, Sundberg, K & Brigham, S. 2006. 'Amniocentesis and chorionic villus sampling for prenatal diagnosis (Cochrane Review)'. *The Reproductive Health Library* 9. https://www.ncbi.nlm.nih.gov/pubmed/12917956 (Accessed 12 October 2017). Reprinted from *The Cochrane Library*, Issue 1, 2006. Chichester, UK: John Wiley.

Al-Jaafry, A. 2015. *Polyhydramnios and oligohydramnios*. Qassim University, Faculty of Medicine, Obstetrics and Gynaecology.

American Pregnancy Association. nd. Pregnancy Complications/Hyperemesis Gravidarum. http://americanpregnancy.org/pregnancy-complications/hyperemesis-gravidarum/ (Accessed 12 October 2017).

American Pregnancy Association. 2015. Hyperemesis gravidarum. http://americanpregnancy.org/pregnancy-complications/hyperemesis-gravidarum/ (Accessed 12 October 2017).

American Thyroid Association. 2017. Pregnancy and thyroid disease. http://www.thyroid.org/thyroid-disease-pregnancy/ (Accessed 17 November 2017).

ANZCA (Australian and New Zealand College of Anaesthetists). 2008. Management of pre-eclampsia and eclampsia. http://www.anzca.edu.au/documents/mark-brown-medical-management-of-pre-eclampsia (Accessed 12 October 2017).

Australian government. Department of Health. nd. National antenatal care guidelines. http://www.health.gov.au/antenatal (Accessed 12 October 2017).

Baby2see.com. nd. Pregnancy Information. Fundal symphysis height measurement. http://www.baby2see.com/medical/fundal_height.html 2015/09/29 (Accessed 12 October 2017).

Babycenter.com. 2017. Lower back pain during pregnancy. https://www.babycenter.com/0_lower-back-pain-during-pregnancy_9402.bc (Accessed 13 October 2017).

Badr, S, Ghareep, A-N, Abdulla, LM & Hassanein, R. 2013. 'Ectopic pregnancy in uncommon implantation sites'. *The Egyptian Journal of Radiology and Nuclear Medicine*, 44(1): 121–130. http://www.sciencedirect.com/science/article/pii/S0378603X1200099X#! (Accessed 16 October 2017).

Baha, M & Sibia, MD. 2005. 'Magnesium sulphate prophylaxis in pre-eclampsia. Evidence from randomised control trials'. *Clinical Obstetrics and Gynaecology*, 48(2): 478–487.

Bakker, R & Smith, CV. 2016. Placenta previa. Medscape. http://emedicine.medscape.com/article/262063-overview#a5 (Accessed 16 October 2017).

Baston, H & Hall, J. 2009. *Midwifery essentials, Antenatal*, 2. New York: Elsevier.

Batra, P, Kuhn, L & Denny, L. 2010. 'Utilisation and outcomes of cervical cancer prevention services among HIV-infected women in Cape Town'. *South African Medical Journal*, 100(1): 39–44. http://www.samj.org.za/index.php/samj/article/view/3492 (Accessed 16 October 2017).

Beckman, CRB, Ling, FW, Barzansky, BM, Herbert, WNP, Laube, DW & Smith, RP. [in collaboration with ACOG]. 2009. *Obstetrics and Gynecology*. 6th ed. New York: Lippincott, Williams and Wilkins.

Berkow, R, Fletcher, AJ & Beers, MH. 1992. *Merck manual*. 16th ed. New York: Merck Research Laboratories.

Bettercare. nd. The Better Births Initiative (BBI). http://ls.bettercare.co.za/maternal-mental-health/4.html#the-better-births-initiative-bbi (Accessed 17 November 2017).

Bharj, KK & Henshaw, AM. 2011. 'Confirming pregnancy and care of the pregnant woman', in *Mayes' midwifery*, edited by S Macdonald & J Maggill-Cuerden. 14th ed. Sydney: Bailliere Tindall: 411–414.

Blencowe, H, Cousens, S, Oestergaard, M, Chou, D, Moller, AB, Narwal, R, Adler, A, Garcia, CV, Rohde, S, Say, L & Lawn, JE. 2012. 'National, regional and worldwide estimates of preterm birth'. *The Lancet*, 9: 379(9832): 2162–2172. http://www.who.int/mediacentre/factsheets/fs363/en/; http://www.cdc.gov/features/prematurebirth/ (Accessed 16 October 2017).

Bloom, ML & Van Dongen, L. 1972. *Clinical gynaecology — Integration of structure and function*. London: William Heinemann Medical Books.

Bojö, AFS, Hall-Lord, ML, Axelsson, O, Udé, G & Larsson, BW. 2004. 'Midwifery care: Development of an instrument to measure quality based on the World Health Organization's classification of care in normal birth'. *Journal of Clinical Nursing*, 13: 75–83.

Boulvain, M. 2006. 'Amnioinfusion for meconium-stained amniotic fluid: RHL commentary'. *The WHO Reproductive Health Library* 9. Geneva: WHO.

Bradshaw, E. 2003. *Exercises for pregnancy and childbirth*. London: BFM.

Brummer, WE, Cronje, HS, Grobler, CJF & Visser, AJ. 1990. *Verloskunde*. 3rd ed. Pretoria: Academica.

Buchmann, E. 2003. 'Routine symphysis-fundal height measurement during pregnancy: RHL commentary'. *The WHO Reproductive Health Library*. Geneva: WHO.

Burd, I & Fink, A. 2016. Common tests during pregnancy. https://www.urmc.rochester.edu/encyclopedia/content.aspx?ContentTypeID=85&ContentID=P01241 (Accessed 16 October 2017).

Carter, BS, 2015: 'Polyhydramnios and oligohydramnios clinical presentation'. Medscape. http://reference.medscape.com/article/975821-clinical#b5 (Accessed 16 October 2017).

Caughey, AB. 2016. 'Postterm pregnancy'. Medscape. http://emedicine.medscape.com/article/261369-overview (Accessed 16 October 2017).

CDC (Centers for Disease Control and Prevention). nd. What is premature birth? http://www.cdc.gov/Features/PrematureBirth/ (Accessed 16 October 2017).

CDC. 2014. National premature awareness month. https://www.cdc.gov/media/releases/2016/s1103-prematurity-awareness.html (Accessed 16 October 2017).

Chapman, RR. 2003. 'Endangering safe motherhood in Mozambique: Prenatal care as pregnancy risk'. *Social Science and Medicine*, 57: 355–374.

Cobo, E. 2006. 'Continuous electronic heart rate monitoring for fetal assessment during labour: RHL commentary'. *The WHO Reproductive Health Library* 9. Geneva: WHO.

Corry, M & Rooks, J. 1999. 'Public education. Promoting the midwifery model of care in partnership with the Maternity Centre Association'. *Journal of Nurse-Midwifery*, 44: 47.

Crews, C. nd. Fetal movement counting. http://www.midwiferyservices.org/FetalMovementCt.pdf (Accessed 16 October 2017).

Cronje, HS & Grobler, CJF. 2003. *Obstetrics in southern Africa*. Pretoria: Van Schaik.

Cronk, M & Flint, C. 1998. *Community midwifery. A practical guide*. London: Heinemann Medical Books.

Dale, B & Roeber, J. 1982. *Exercises for childbirth*. London: Century Publishing.

Deering, SH & Smith, CV. 2016. Abruptio placentae. Medscape. emedicine.medscape.com/article/252810-overview (Accessed 16 October 2017).

De Kock, J & Van Der Walt, C. 2004. *Maternal and newborn care*. Cape Town: Juta.

Dick-Read, G. 1959. *Childbirth without fear. The principles and practice of natural birth*. UK: Pinter & Martin.

DoH (Department of Health). 1998. *South African Demographic Health Survey*. http://www.mrc.ac.za/bod/dhsfin1.pdf (Accessed 16 October 2017).

DoH. 2002. *National Guideline on the Management of Asthma for Adults at Primary Care Level*. https://www.westerncape.gov.za/text/2003/national_guideline_management_asthma_adults_primary_level.pdf (Accessed 16 October 2017).

DoH. 2003. *South African Demographic Health Survey*. https://dhsprogram.com/pubs/pdf/FR206/FR206.pdf (Accessed 16 October 2017).

DoH. 2011. *National Core Standards for Health Establishments in South Africa*. http://www.phango.org.za/home/144-national-core-standards-ndoh (Accessed 16 October 2017).

DoH. 2014. *Saving Mothers 2011–2013. Sixth Report on the Confidential Enquiries into Maternal Deaths in South Africa*. https://www.health-e.org.za/wp-content/uploads/2016/05/Saving-Mothers-2011-2013-short-report.pdf (Accessed 16 October 2017).

DoH. 2015a. *Guidelines for Maternity Care in South Africa. A Manual for Clinic, Community Health Centres and District Hospitals*. https://www.health-e.org.za/wp-content/uploads/2015/11/Maternal-Care-Guidelines-2015_FINAL-21.7.15.pdf (Accessed 16 October 2017).

DoH. 2015b. *Saving Mothers 2014. Annual Report and Detailed Analysis of Maternal Deaths due to Non-pregnancy Related Infections*. Pretoria: DoH.

DoH. 2016. *Ideal Clinic Manual. Version 16*. https://www.idealclinic.org.za/docs/2016/Ideal%20Clinic%20Manual%20v16%20-%2023Jun16.pdf (Accessed 16 October 2017).

Donnet, ML, Howie, PW, Marnie, M, Cooper, W & Lewis, M. 1990. 'Return of ovarian function following spontaneous abortion.' *Clin Endocrinol* (Oxf), 33(1): 13–20. https://www.ncbi.nlm.nih.gov/pubmed/2401092/ (Accessed 16 October 2017).

Douglas, G, Nicol, F & Robertson, C (eds). 2009. *Macleod's clinical examination*. 11th ed. London: Churchill Livingstone.

Duggan, PM. 1998. 'Which Korotkoff sound should be used for the diastolic blood pressure in pregnancy?' *Aust N Z J Obstet Gynaecol*, 38(2): 194–197. https://www.ncbi.nlm.nih.gov/pubmed/9653859 (Accessed 13 October 2017).

Duly, L & Henderson-Smart, D. 2002. 'Magnesium sulphate versus phenytoin for eclampsia'. *Cochrane Database Syst Rev*, 4: CD000128.

Duly, L, Matar, HE, Almeric, MQ & Hall, DR. 2010. 'Alternative magnesium sulphate regimes for women with pre-eclampsia and eclampsia'. *The Cochrane Collaboration* 8. http://onlinelibrary.wiley.com/doi/10.1002/14651858. CD007388.pub2/full (Accessed 16 October 2017).

Du Plessis, DW. 2008. *Juta's clinical guide for midwives.* Cape Town: Juta.

Duque, S, Reche, M & López-Serrano, MC. 2002. 'Asthma and pregnancy'. *Alergologia e Inmunologia Clinica,* 17: 285–290. https://www.researchgate.net/publication/287707528_Asthma_and_pregnancy (Accessed 13 October 2017).

Ekabua, J, Ekabua, K & Njoku, C. 2011. 'Proposed framework for making focused antenatal care services accessible: A review of the Nigerian setting'. *Obsterics and Gynaecology,* 253964. Hindawi Publishing Corporation. https://www.hindawi.com/journals/isrn/2011/253964/ (Accessed 16 October 2017).

Enkin, M & Chalmers, I (eds). 1980. *Effectiveness and satisfaction in ante-natal care.* London: Spastics International Medical Publications.

Fletcher, GE. 2015. Multiple births. Medscape. http://emedicine.medscape.com/article/977234-overview#a6 (Accessed 13 October 2017).

Franck, LS & Callery, P. 2004. 'Re-thinking family-centered care across the continuum of children's healthcare'. *Child Care, Health and Development,* 30: 265–277.

Frank, K, Lombard, H & Pattinson, RC. 2009. 'Does completion of the Essential Steps in Managing Obstetric Emergencies (ESMOE) training package result in improved knowledge and skills in managing obstetric emergencies?' *South African Journal of Obstetrics and Gynaecology,* 15(3): 94–99. https://www.researchgate.net/publication/279581358_Does_completion_of_the_Essential_Steps_in_Managing_Obstetric_Emergencies_ESMOE_training_package_result_in_improved_knowledge_and_skills_in_managing_obstetric_emergencies (Accessed 30 November 2017).

Frier, EM, McKay, G & Carty, DM. 2017. 'Metformin in pregnancy. Drug notes'. *Practical Diabetes,* 34(5). http://www.practicaldiabetes.com/wp-content/uploads/sites/29/2017/06/DN-Metformin-in-pregnancy_P.pdf (Accessed 13 October 2017).

Galal, M, Symonds, I, Murray, H, Petraglia, F & Smith, R.. 2012. 'Postterm pregnancy'. *Facts Views Vis Obgyn,* 4(3): 175–187. https://www.ncbi.nlm.nih.gov/pmc/articles/PMC3991404/ (Accessed 29 November 2017).

Gandhi, A. 2016. 'Haemolytic disease of the fetus and newborn'. https://patient.info/doctor/haemolytic-disease-of-the-fetus-and-newborn (Accessed 19 August 2017).

Garrey, MM, Govan, ADT, Hodge, CH & Callander, R. 1978. *Obstetrics illustrated.* 2nd ed. Edinburgh and London: E and S Livingstone.

Glover, P. 1999. 'Acmi competency standards for midwives – what it means for your practice'. *Australian College of Midwives Incorporate Journal,* 12: 12–17.

Granados, JL. 1984. 'Survey of the management of post-term pregnancy'. *Journal of Obstetrics and Gynecology,* 63(5): 651–653.

Greenhill, JP & Friedman, EA. 1974. *Biological principles of modern obstetrics.* Toronto: WB Saunders.

Grosse, SD, Odame, I, Atrash, HK, Amendah, DD, Piel, FP & Williams, TN. 2011. 'Sickle cell disease in Africa: A neglected cause of early childhood mortality'. *Am J Prev Med,* 41(6): S398–S405. DOI: 10.1016/j.amepre.2011.09.013. https://www.ncbi.nlm.nih.gov/pmc/articles/PMC3708126/ (Accessed 29 November 2017).

Gulmezoglu, AM & Hofmyer, GJ. 2002. 'Bed rest in hospital for suspected impaired fetal growth'. *Cochrane Database Syst Rev,* 2: CD000034.

Healthline. nd. What is an HCG urine test? http://www.healthline.com/health/hcg-in-urine. 2015/10/12 (Accessed 16 October 2017).

Heslehurst, N, Rankin, Wilkinson, JR & Summerbell, CB. 2010. 'A nationally representative study of maternal obesity in England: UK: trends in incidence and demographic inequalities in 619 3323 births 1989–2007'. *International Journal of Obesity,* 34(3): 420-428. https://www.ncbi.nlm.nih.gov/pubmed/20029373 (Accessed 16 October 2017).

Hobbs, L. 1997. *The independent midwife.* 2nd ed. England: Books for Midwives Press. Hochland and Hochland Ltd.

Impey, L & Child, T. 2008. *Obstetrics and gynaecology.* 3rd ed. Wiley Blackwell: London.

INCIP (International Network on Cancer, Infertility and Pregnancy). nd. Ovarian cancer. https://www.cancerinpregnancy.org/ovarian-cancer (Accessed 16 October 2017).

Jazayeri, A. 2016. Premature rupture of membranes. Medscape. http://emedicine.medscape.com/article/261137-overview (Accessed 16 October 2017).

Jowett, M. 2000. 'Safe motherhood interventions in low-income countries: An economic justification and evidence of cost-effectiveness'. *Health Policy,* 53: 201–288.

Kane, A. 2002. 'Ethical and legal issues in reproductive health: Considerations for the childbirth educator'. *International Journal of Childbirth Education,* 17: 15–17.

Karam, A. 2017. Cervical cancer in pregnancy. UpToDate. https://www.uptodate.com/contents/cervical-cancer-in-

pregnancy?source=search_result&search=cervical+cancer+i
npregnancy&selectedTitle=2~150
(Accessed 16 October 2017).

Kavitha, N, De, S & Kanagasabai, S. 2013. 'Oral
hypoglycaemic agents in pregnancy: An update'. *Journal of
Obstetrics & Gynecology of India*, 62(2): 82–87. http://www.
ncbi.nlm.nih.gov/pmc/articles/PMC3664692/
(Accessed 16 October 2017).

Keller, TM, Rake, A, Michel, SCA, Seifert, B, Efe, G,
Treiber, K, Huch, R, Marincek, B & Kubik-Huch,
R. 2003. 'Obstetric MR pelvimetry: Reference values
and evaluation of inter- and intraobserver error and
intraindividual variability.' *Radiology*, 227(1). http://pubs.
rsna.org/doi/abs/10.1148/radiol.2271011658?journalCode
=radiology& (Accessed 5 October 2017).

Keyser, EA, Staat, BC, Fausett, MB & Shields, AD. 2012.
'Pregnancy-associated breast cancer.' *Obstetrics &
Gynecology*, 5(2): 94–99. https://www.ncbi.nlm.nih.gov/
pmc/articles/PMC3410508/ (Accessed 16 October 2017).

Knowles, M. 1990. *The adult learner: A neglected species*. 4th ed.
Houston: Gulf Publications.

Komal, PS & Mestman, JH. 2010. 'Graves hyperthyroidism
and pregnancy: A clinical update'. *Endocrine Practice*,
16(1): 118–129.

Leunen, K, Hall, D, Odendaal, HJ & Grové, D. 2003. 'The
profile and complications of women with placental
abruption and intrauterine death'. *Journal of Tropical
Pediatrics*, 49(4): 231–234. DOI: 0.1093/tropej/49.4.231.
https://www.researchgate.net/publication/10604365_
The_profile_and_complications_of_women_with_
placental_abruption_and_intrauterine_death
(Accessed 16 October 2017).

Lincetto, O, Mothebesoane-Anoh, S, Gomez, P & Munjanja,
S. nd. *Antenatal care*. World Health Organisations
Publications. http://www.who.int/pmnch/media/
publications/aonsectionIII_2.pdf
(Accessed 16 October 2017).

Llewellyn-Jones, D. 1982. *Fundamentals of obstetrics and
gynaecology*. 3rd ed. London: Faber & Faber.

Llewellyn-Jones, D. 1992. *Fundamentals of obstetrics and
gynaecology*. London: Faber and Faber.

Luesley, DM & Kilby, MD. 2016. *Obstetrics and gynecology:
An evidence-based text for the MRCOG*. 3rd ed. Boca
Raton: CRC Press.

MacDonagh, S. 2005. *Achieving skilled attendance for all, a
synthesis of current knowledge and recommended actions for
scaling up*. London: DFID Health Resource Centre.

Macdonald, S & Magill-Cuerden, J (eds). 2011. *Mayes'
midwifery*. 14th ed. Elsevier.

Major, CA. 2010. 'Using oral hypoglycemics in pregnancy to
manage type 2 and gestational diabetes'. *Contemporary OB/
GYN*, 34–38. https://www.smfm.org/publications/106-
using-oral-hypoglycemics-in-pregnancy-to-manage-type-
2-gestational-diabetes (Accessed 16 October 2017).

Mantle, J & Haslam, J. 2001. 'Raising pelvic floor awareness'.
Physiotherapy, 87: 618–619.

Marshall, S & Gilbert, W. 2015. External cephalic version for
breech delivery. http://www.webmd.com/baby/external-
cephalic-version-version-for-breech-position
(Accessed 16 October 2017).

Mason, L, Glenn, S, Walton, I & Hughes, C. 2001. 'Do
women practise pelvic floor exercises during pregnancy or
following delivery?' *Physiotherapy*, 87(12): 662–670.

Matthews, JE, George, S, Mathews, P, Mathai, E,
Brahmadathan, KN & Seshadri, L. 1998. 'The Griess
test: An inexpensive screening test for asymptomatic
bacteriuria in pregnancy'. *Aust N Z J Obstet Gynaecol*,
38(4): 407–410.

Matthews, A, Haas, D, O'Mathúna, DP & Dowswell,
T. 2015. 'Interventions for nausea and vomiting in
early pregnancy'. *Cochrane Database Syst Rev*, 9. DOI:
10.1002/14651858.CD007575.pub4
(Accessed 17 November 2017).

McCauley, ME, Van den Broek, N, Dou, L & Othman, M.
2015. 'Vitamin A supplementation during pregnancy
for maternal and newborn outcomes'. *Cochrane Database
Syst Rev*, 10: CD008666. DOI: 10.1002/14651858.
CD008666.pub3.

McWhirter, N & Russell, A. 1988. *Guinness book of world's
records*. New York: Bantam Books.

Measure Evaluation. Safe Motherhood. nd. https://www.
measureevaluation.org/prh/rh_indicators/specific/sm
(Accessed 16 October 2017).

MedicineNet. nd. Childbirth complications. https://www.
webmd.com/baby/features/childbirth-complications#1
(Accessed 16 October 2017).

Medscape. 2017. Effect of maternal heart disease on
pregnancy outcomes: Effect of heart disease on
pregnancy outcomes. http://www.medscape.org/
viewarticle/728031_6 (Accessed 13 October 2017).

Meniham, CA. 2000. 'Limited sonography in collaborative
midwifery practice'. *Journal of Midwifery and Women's
Health*, 45: 508–516.

Mills, L & Napier, JAF. 1988. 'Massive feto-maternal
haemorrhage: Effect of passively administered Anti D in
prevention of Rh sensitization and haemolytic disease of
the newborn'. *British Journal of Obstetrics and Gynaecology*,
95: 1007–1012.

Moore, L. 2016. Hydatidiform mole. Medscape. http://emedicine.medscape.com/article/254657-overview#a6 (Accessed 16 October 2017).

MRC Research Unit for Maternal and Infant Healthcare Strategies, PPIP users & the Saving Babies Technical Task Team. 2011. *Saving Babies 2008–2009. Seventh Report on Perinatal Care in South Africa*. https://www.ppip.co.za/wp-content/uploads/Saving-Babies-2008-9.pdf (Accessed 7 December 2017).

Murphy, PA & Fullerton, JT. 2001. 'Measuring outcomes of midwifery care: Development of an instrument to assess optimality'. *Journal of Midwifery and Women's Health*, 46: 5.

Murray, I & Hassall, J. 2009. 'Change and adaptation in pregnancy', in *Myles textbook for midwives*, edited by DM Fraser & MA Cooper. Nottingham: Churchill Livingstone.

Nahum, GG. 2016. Uterine rupture in pregnancy. Medscape. http://reference.medscape.com/article/275854-overview (Accessed 16 October 2017).

NCBI (National Center for Biotechnology Information). nd. What is thyroid disease? http://www.ncbi.nlm.nih.gov/pmc/articles/PMC3664692/ (Accessed 16 October 2017).

NCC-WCH (National Collaborating Centre for Women's and Children's Health). 2008. *Antenatal care: Routine care for the healthy pregnant woman*. London: RCOG Press.

Neilson, JP. 2003. 'Interventions for suspected placenta previa'. *Cochrane Database Syst Rev*, 2: CD 001998.

Neilson, JP & Alfirevic, Z. 2000. 'Doppler ultrasound for fetal assessment in high risk pregnancies'. *Cochrane Database Syst Rev*, 2: CD000073.

Ngxongo, SM & Sibiya, MN. 2013. 'Factors influencing successful implementation of the basic antenatal care approach in primary health care facilities in eThekwini district, KwaZulu-Natal'. *Curationis*, 7 May 2013.

NICE. 2014. Antenatal care clinical guideline 62. https://www.nice.org.uk/guidance/qs22/resources/antenatal-care-pdf-2098542418117 (Accessed 16 October 2017).

Nickens, MA, Craig, R & Geraci, SA. 2013. 'Cardiovascular disease in pregnancy'. *Southern Medical*, 106(11): 624–630.

NIDDK (National Institute of Diabetes and Digestive and Kidney Diseases). nd. How does hyperthyroidism affect the mother and baby? http://www.niddk.nih.gov/health-information/health-topics/endocrine/pregnancy-and-thyroid-disease/Pages/fact-sheet.aspx (Accessed 16 October 2017).

NMC (Nursing and Midwifery Council). 2009. *Record-keeping: guidance for nurses and midwives*. http://www.nipec.n-i.nhs.uk/Image/SitePDFS/ nmcGuidanceRecordKeepingGuidancefor NursesandMidwives.pdf (Accessed 16 October 2017).

Nolte, AGW, Slabber, CF, Visser, AA & Brummer, WE. 1987. *Verloskunde vir verpleegkundiges*. Pretoria: Academia.

O'Donnell, MJ, Elio, R & Day, D. 2010. *Carpal tunnel syndrome*. In practice. http://nwhjournal.org/article/S1751-4851(15)30511-0/pdf (Accessed 13 October 2017).

Ogunyemi, DA. 2010. 'Autoimmune thyroid disease and pregnancy. Medscape.www.emedicine.medscape.com/article/261913-overview (Accessed 16 October 2017).

Ogunyemi, DA & Isaacs, C. 2017. Hyperemesis gravidarum. Medscape.http://emedicine.medscape.com/article/254751-overview (Accessed 16 October 2017).

O'Hara Padden, M. 1999. 'HELLP syndrome: Recognition and perinatal treatment'. *American Family Physician*, 60(3): 829–836. http://www.aafp.org/afp/1999/0901/p829.html (Accessed 5 October 2017).

O'Meara, C. 1993. 'An evaluation of consumer perspective of childbirth and parenting education'. *Midwifery*, 9: 210–219.

Osman, NB. 2007. 'Interventions for suspected placenta praevia: RHL Commentary'. *The WHO Reproductive Health Library*. Geneva: WHO.

Padden, MO. 1999. 'HELLP syndrome. Recognition and perinatal management'. *Am J Obstet Gynecol*, 195: 723–728.

Parnas, M, Sheiner, E, Shoham-Vardi, I, Burstein, E, Yermiahu, T, Levi, I, Holcberg, G & Yerushalmi, R. 2006. 'Moderate to severe thrombocytopenia during pregnancy'. *European Journal of Obstetrics and Gynecology and Reproductive Biology*. http://williams.medicine.wisc.edu/pregnancythrombocytopenia.pdf (Accessed 13 October 2017).

Patience, NTS, Sibiya, MN & Gwele, NS. 2016. 'Evidence of application of the Basic Antenatal Care principles of good care and guidelines in pregnant women's antenatal care records'. *African Journal of PHC and FM*, 8(2): 1016. https://www.ncbi.nlm.nih.gov/pmc/articles/PMC4913450/ (Accessed 16 October 2017).

Pattinson, RC. 2007. *Basic Antenatal Care Handbook*. MRC. Pretoria: University of Pretoria.

Pattinson, R, Fawcus, S & Moodley, J. 2013. *Tenth Interim Report on Confidential Enquiries into Maternal Deaths in South Africa 2011 and 2012*. http://www.sexrightsafrica.net/wp-content/uploads/2016/11/Tenth-Interim-Report-Maternal-Deaths-2011-and-2012-copy.pdf (Accessed 16 October 2017).

Pattinson, RC & Rhoda, N (for the PPIP group). 2014. *Saving Babies 2012–2013: Ninth Report on Perinatal Care in South Africa*. Pretoria: Tshepesa Press. http://www.ppip.

co.za/wp-content/uploads/Saving-Babies-2012-2013.pdf
(Accessed 16 October 2017).

Pattinson, RC & Theron, GB. 1989. 'Inter-observer variation in symphysis-fundus measurements. A plea for individualised antenatal care'. *South African Medical Journal*, 76: 621–622.

Permaul-Woods, JA, Carroll, JC, Reid, AJ, Woodward, CA, Ryan, G, Domb, S, Arbitman, S, Fallis, B & Kilthei, J. 1999. 'Going the distance: the influence of practice location on the Ontario Maternal Serum Screening Program'. *Canadian Medical Association Journal*, 61: 381–385.

Pettker, CM & Lockwood, CJ. 2015. 'Thromboembolic disease: Diagnosis and treatment during pregnancy'. *Gynecology and Reproductive Sciences*. New Haven, Connecticut: Yale University of Medicine.

Phelan, JP. 2005. What constitutes fetal distress. http://www.obgyn.net/print.asp (Accessed 16 October 2017).

Phillips, C. 1999. 'Family-centred maternity care. Past, present and future'. *International Journal of Childbirth Education*, 14: 33.

Pollack, A. 2012. Before birth, Dad's ID. *The New York Times*, June 19, 2012. http://www.nytimes.com/2012/06/20/health/paternity-blood-tests-that-work-early-in-a-pregnancy.html (Accessed 16 October 2017).

Preboth, M. 2000. 'ACOG guidelines on antepartum fetal surveillance'. *Am Fam Physician*, 62(5): 1184–1188.

Preeclampsia Foundation. 2013. Preeclampsia and maternal mortality: A global burden. https://www.preeclampsia.org/health-information/149-advocacy-awareness/332-preeclampsia-and-maternal-mortality-a-global-burden (Accessed 16 October 2017).

Psychology Wiki. nd. Down's syndrome. http://psychology.wikia.com/wiki/Downs_syndrome (Accessed 22 August 2017).

Rana, TG, Rajopadhyaya, R, Bajracharya, B, Karmacharya, M & Osrin, D. 2003. 'Comparison of midwifery-led and consultant-led maternity care for low-risk deliveries in Nepal'. *Health Policy Planning*, 18: 330–337.

RANZCOG (The Royal Australian and New Zealand College of Obstetricians and Gynaecologists). 2013. C-Gyn 30: Guidelines for gynaecological examinations and procedures. https://www.ranzcog.edu.au/RANZCOG_SITE/media/RANZCOG-MEDIA/Women's%20Health/Statement%20and%20guidelines/Clinical%20-%20Gynaecology/Guidelines-for-gynaecological-examinations-and-procedures-(C-Gyn-30)-Review-March-2016.pdf?ext=.pdf (Accessed 16 October 2017).

RCOG (Royal College of Obstetricians and Gynaecologists). 2001. *The use of electronic fetal monitoring. Evidence-based clinical guideline 8*. Clinical Effectiveness Support Unit. http://ctgutbildning.se/images/Referenser/RCOG-2001.pdf (Accessed 17 November 2017).

RCOG. 2002a. *Green top guideline 1(B). Tocolytic drugs for women in preterm labour*. https://www.rcog.org.uk/en/guidelines-research-services/guidelines/gtg1b/ (Accessed 16 October 2017).

RCOG. 2002b. *Green top guideline 31. The investigations and management of the small-for-gestational-age fetus*. https://www.rcog.org.uk/en/guidelines-research-services/guidelines/gtg31/ (Accessed 16 October 2017).

RCOG. 2006. *Green top guideline 10A. The management of severe preeclampsia/eclampsia*. https://www.rcog.org.uk/en/guidelines-research-services/guidelines/gtg10a/ (Accessed 16 October 2017).

RCOG. 2008. *Green top guideline 47. Blood transfusion in obstetrics*. https://www.rcog.org.uk/en/guidelines-research-services/guidelines/gtg47/ (Accessed 16 October 2017).

RCOG. 2011. *Placenta praevia, placenta praevia accreta and vasa praevia: Diagnosis and management. Green-top Guideline no 27*. https://www.rcog.org.uk/globalassets/documents/guidelines/gtg_27.pdf (Accessed 16 October 2017).

Roberts, D & Dalziel, SR. 2006. 'Antenatal corticosteroids for accelerating fetal lung maturation for women at risk of preterm birth'. *Cochrane Database of Systematic Reviews* 3: CD004454. DOI: 10.1002/14651858.CD004454.pub2 (Accessed 16 October 2017).

Rubio, C, Simon, C, Vidal, F & Pellicer, A. 2003. 'Chromosomal abnormalities and embryo development in recurrent miscarriage couples'. *Human Reproduction*, 18(1): 182–188. DOI: 10.1093/humrep/deg015. https://www.researchgate.net/publication/5449676_Chromosomal_abnormalities_and_embryo_development_in_recurrent_miscarriage_couples (Accessed 16 October 2017).

Sackett, D. 2000. What is evidence-based practice? http://guides.mclibrary.duke.edu/c.php?g=158201&p=1036021 (Accessed 16 October 2017).

Safe Motherhood. nd(a). Current priorities. http://www.safemotherhood.org/priorities/index.html (Accessed 16 October 2017).

Safe Motherhood. nd(b). Welcome to safe motherhood. http://Safemotherhood.Org/Facts_And_Figures? Maternal_Health.Htm (Accessed 22 November 2004).

SANBS (South African National Blood Service). 2014. *Clinical Guideline for the Use of Blood Products in South Africa*. 5th ed. http://www.wpblood.org.za/village/

wpbnew/sites/default/files/clinical_guidelines_5th%20 Edition_2014.pdf (Accessed 16 October 2017).

Sandenbergh, H. 2015. Ectopic pregnancy. Department of Obstetrics & Gynaecology. University of Stellenbosch. http://www.health24.com/Medical/Diseases/Ectopic-pregnancy-Client-20120721 (Accessed 16 October 2017).

Sanders, LB. 2003. 'Advanced directives and midwifery care'. *Journal of Midwifery and Women's Health*, 48(4): 278–281.

Sanders, J, Somerset, M, Jewell, D & Sharp, D. 1999. 'To see or not to see? Midwives' perceptions of reduced antenatal attendances for "low-risk" women'. *Midwifery*, 15: 257–263.

SANGO Pulse. 2012. Preterm birth. http://www.ngopulse. org/press-release/time-focus-84-ooo-preterm-births-south-africa (Accessed 16 October 2017).

Say, L. 2004. *Treatment of Hypertension in Pregnancy. Postgraduate training course in reproductive health*. Geneva: WHO. https://www.gfmer.ch/Medical_education_En/ PGC_RH_2004/Pdf/Hypertension_pregnancy.pdf (Accessed 16 October 2017).

Seftel, H. nd. Diagnosis, treatment and complications of diabetes. Unpublished.

Shield, AD. 2014. Pregnancy diagnosis. Medscape. http:// emedicine.medscape.com/article/262591.overview (Accessed 16 October 2017).

Shields, L, Lee, R, Druzin, M, McNulty, J & Mason, H. 2003. Blood product replacement. Obstetric haemorrhage. *CMQCC:1–7*. https://www.cmqcc.org/resource/916/ download (Accessed 16 October 2017).

Shomon, M. 2016. Hyperthyroidism and Graves' disease during pregnancy. https://www.verywell. com/hyperthyroidism-and-graves-disease-during-pregnancy-3232953 (Accessed 16 October 2017).

Shrivastava, V, Kotur, P & Jauhari, A. 2014. 'Maternal and fetal outcome among abruptio placentae cases at a rural tertiary hospital in Karnataka, India: A retrospective analysis.' *Int J Res Med Sci*, 2(4): 1655–1658. http:// www.ejmanager.com/mnstemps/93/93-1412163088.pdf (Accessed 16 October 2017).

Sibia, BM. 2005. 'Magnesium sulphate prophylaxis in pre-eclampsia. Evidence from randomised trials'. *Clinical Obstetrics and Gynecology*, 48(2): 478–488.

Sliwa, K, Blauwet, L, Tibazarwa, K, Libhaber, E, Smedema, JP, Becker, A, McMurray, J, Yamac, H, Labidi, S, Struman, I & Hilfiker-Kleiner, D. 2015. 'Evaluation of bromocriptine in the treatment of acute severe peripartum cardiomyopathy'. *Circulation*, 121: 1465–1473. http://circ. ahajournals.org/content/121/13/1465 (Accessed 17 October 2017).

Sliwa, K, Förster, O, Libhaber, E, Fett, JD, Sunstrom, JB, Hilfiker-Kleiner, D & Ansari, AA. 2005. 'Peripartum cardiomyopathy, inflammatory markers as predictors of outcomes in 100 prospective patients'. *European Heart Journal*, 27(4): 441–446. https://doi.org/10.1093/ eurheartj/ehi481 (Accessed 16 October 2017).

Sliwa, K, Hilfiker-Kleiner, D, Petrie, MC, Mebazaa, A, Pieske, B, Buchmann, E, Regitz-Zagrosek, V, Schaufelberger, M, Tavazzi, L, Van Veldhuisen, DJ, Watkins, H, Shah, AJ, Seferovic, PM, Elkayam, U, Pankuweit, S, Papp, Z, Mouquet, F & McMurray, JJV. 2010. 'Current state of knowledge on aetiology, diagnosis, management, and therapy of peripartum cardiomyopathy: A position statement from the Heart Failure Association of the European Society of Cardiology Working Group on Peripartum Cardiomyopathy.' *European Journal of Heart Failure*, 12: 767–778. DOI: 10.1093/eurojhf/hfg120. http://www.hefssa.org/images/uploads/ppcm_position_ statement_2010.pdf (Accessed 17 October 2017).

Smaiil, FM & Vazquez, JC. 2015. 'Antibiotics for asymptomatic bacteriuria in pregnancy'. *Cochrane Database Syst Rev*, 8: CD000490.

Smith, H, Brown, H, Hofmeyr, GJ & Garner, P. 2004. 'Evidence-based obstetric care in South Africa: Influencing practice through the "Better Births Initiative"'. *S Afr Med J*, Feb 94(2): 117–120. https://www.ncbi.nlm. nih.gov/pubmed/15034990 (Accessed 17 November 2017).

Snyman, LC. 2009. 'Gestational trophoblastic disease: An overview'. *SA Journal of Gynaecological Oncology*, 1(1): 32–37.

Society for Maternal–Fetal Medicine. nd. Using oral hypoglycemics in pregnancy to manage type 2 gestational diabetes. https://www.smfm.org/publications/106-using-oral-hypoglycemics-in-pregnancy-to-manage-type-2-gestational-diabetes (Accessed 17 October 2017).

Soma-Pillay, P, MacDonald, AP, Mathivha, TM, Bakker, JL & MacKintosh, MO. 2008. 'Cardiac disease in pregnancy. A 4-year audit at Pretoria Academic hospital'. *South African Medical Journal*, 98: 553–556.

Stahl, K & Hundley, V. 2003. 'Risk and risk management in pregnancy – do we scare because we care?' *Midwifery*, 19(4): 238–309.

Stapleton, H, Kirkham, M & Thomas, G. 2002. 'Evidence-based patient information leaflets in maternity care had limited visibility and did not promote informed choice of childbearing women'. *British Medical Journal*, 324: 639–643.

Stöppler, MC & Davis, CP. 2015. Pregnancy: Pre-eclampsia and eclampsia. MedicineNet. http://www.medicinenet.com/pregnancy_preeclampsia_and_eclampsia/article.htm (Accessed 17 October 2017).

Taylor, S, Tudur Smith, C, Williamson, PR & Marson, AG. 2002. 'Phenobarbitone versus phenytoin monotherapy for partial onset seizures and generalized onset tonic-clonic seizures'. *Cochrane Database Syst Rev*, 4: CD002217.

Thomas, LH, McColl, E, Cullum, N, Rousseau, N & Soutter, J. 1999. 'Clinical guidelines in nursing, midwifery and the therapies: A systematic review'. *Journal of Advanced Nursing*, 30: 40–50.

Traynor, JD & Peaceman, AM. 1998. 'Maternal hospital charges associated with trial of labour versus elective repeat caesarean section'. *Birth Issues in Perinatal Care*, 25(2): 81–84.

Tucker, SM. 1988. *Fetal monitoring. Pocket nurse guide*. Toronto: Mosby.

Tucker, JS, Hall, MH, Howie, PW, Reid, ME, Barbour, RS, Florey, CD & McIlwaine, GM. 1996. 'Should obstetricians see women with normal pregnancies? A multi-centre randomised controlled trial of routine antenatal care by general practitioners and midwives compared with shared-care led by obstetricians'. *British Medical Journal*, 312: 554–559.

Tulandi, T & Al-Fozan, HM. 2017. 'Spontaneous abortion: Risk factors, etiology, clinical manifestations, and diagnostic evaluation'. UpToDate. https://www.uptodate.com/contents/spontaneous-abortion-risk-factors-etiology-clinical-manifestations-and-diagnostic-evaluation (Accessed 17 October 2017).

Vazquez, JC & Villar, J. 2003. 'Treatment for symptomatic urinary tract infections during pregnancy'. *Cochrane Database Syst Rev*, 4: CD002256.

VBAC.com. nd. What is a uterine rupture and how often does it occur? http://www.vbac.com/what-is-a-uterine-rupture-and-how-often-does-it-occur/ (Accessed 17 October 2017).

Villar, J, Carroli, G, Khan-Neeloufer, D, Piaggio, G & Gülmezoglu, M. 2001. 'Patterns of routine antenatal care for low-risk pregnancy'. *Cochrane Database Syst Rev*, 4: CD000934.

Villar, J & Gülmezoglu, AM. 1998. Maternal health. *Annual Technical WHO Report*: 172–181.

Walker, J. 2005. 'Informed choice and the concept of risk'. *Midwives*, 8: 40–41.

WHO. nd. Maternal, newborn, child and adolescent health. Stillbirths. http://www.who.int/maternal_child_adolescent/epidemiology/stillbirth/en/ (Accessed 17 October 2017).

WHO. 1999. Every pregnancy is at risk. Current approaches to reduction of maternal mortality. http://onlinelibrary.wiley.com/doi/10.1111/j.1471-0528.2005.00718.x/full (Accessed 17 October 2017).

WHO. 2003a. *Integrated Management of Pregnancy and Childbirth. Managing Complications in Pregnancy and Childbirth: A Guide for Midwives and Doctors.* Department of Reproductive Health and Research Family and Community Health. Geneva: WHO.

WHO. 2003b. WHO/ISH hypertension guidelines. http://www.who.int/cardiovascular_diseases/guidelines/hypertension/en/ (Accessed 17 October 2017).

WHO. 2006a. *Provision of Effective Antenatal Care. Integrated Management of Pregnancy and Childbirth (IMPAC).* http://www.who.int/reproductivehealth/publications/maternal_perinatal_health/effective_antenatal_care.pdf (Accessed 17 October 2017).

WHO. 2006b. *Neonatal and Perinatal Mortality: Country, Regional and Global Estimates.* http://apps.who.int/iris/bitstream/10665/43444/1/9241563206_eng.pdf (Accessed 19 August 2017).

WHO. 2007. *Recommendations for the Prevention of Postpartum Haemorrhage.* Geneva: WHO. hhttp://apps.who.int/iris/bitstream/10665/75411/1/9789241548502_eng.pdf (Accessed 17 October 2017).

WHO. 2014a. Preterm birth. http://www.who.int/mediacentre/factsheets/fs363/en/ (Accessed 17 October 2017).

WHO. 2014b. *Report of the Sixth Global Forum for Government Chief Nurses and Midwives. Nursing and Midwifery Workforce and Universal Health Coverage (UHC).* http://www.who.int/hrh/documents/report_forGCNMO.pdf (Accessed 17 October 2017).

WHO. 2016. *WHO Recommendations on Antenatal Care for a Positive Pregnancy Experience.* http://apps.who.int/iris/bitstream/10665/250796/1/9789241549912-eng.pdf?ua=1 (Accessed 17 October 2017).

WHO. 2017a. About WHO. Constitution of WHO: Principles. www.who.int/about/mission/en/ (Accessed 17 October 2017).

WHO. 2017b. Baby-friendly hospital initiative. http://www.who.int/nutrition/topics/bfhi/en/ (Accessed 30 November 2017).

Wikipedia. nd(a). External cephalic version. https://en.wikipedia.org/wiki/External_cephalic_version (Accessed 17 October 2017).

Wikipedia. nd(b). Evidence-based medicine. https://en.wikipedia.org/wiki/Evidence-based_medicine 2015/10/13 (Accessed 17 October 2017).

Wikipedia. nd(c). Glucose tolerance test. https://en.wikipedia.org/wiki/Glucose_tolerance_test (Accessed 17 October 2017).

Wikipedia. nd(d). Polyhydramnios. https://en.wikipedia.org/wiki/Polyhydramnios (Accessed 17 October 2017).

Wikipedia. nd(e). Preterm birth. https://en.wikipedia.org/wiki/Preterm_birth (Accessed 17 October 2017).

Wikipedia. nd(f). Oligohydramnios. https://en.wikipedia.org/wiki/Oligohydramnios (Accessed 17 October 2017).

Wikipedia. 2015. Cardiotocography. https://en.wikipedia.org/wiki/Cardiotocography (Accessed 17 October 2017).

Wikipedia. 2016a. Hyperemesis gravidarum. https://en.wikipedia.org/w/index.php?title=Hyperemesis_gravidarum&oldid=706274737 (Accessed 19 August 2017).

Wikipedia. 2016b. Teenage pregnancy. https://en.wikipedia.org/wiki/Teenage_Pregnancy (Accessed 19 August 2017).

Wikipedia. 2017a. Symphysis pubis dysfunction. https://en.wikipedia.org/wiki/Symphysis_pubis_dysfunction (Accessed 17 October 2017).

Wikipedia. 2017b. Pre-eclampsia. https://en.wikipedia.org/wiki/Pre-eclampsia (Accessed 17 October 2017).

Wikipedia. 2017c. Hashimoto's thyroiditis. https://en.wikipedia.org/wiki/Hashimoto%27s_thyroiditis (Accessed 13 October 2017).

Wikipedia. 2017d. Postpartum bleeding. https://en.wikipedia.org/wiki/Postpartum_bleeding (Accessed 13 October 2017).

Wikipedia. 2017e. Rh disease. https://en.wikipedia.org/wiki/Rh_disease (Accessed 19 August 2017).

Wikipedia. 2017f. Polyhydramnios. https://en.wikipedia.org/wiki/Polyhydramnios (Accessed 19 August 2017).

Wikipedia. 2017g. Twin. https://en.wikipedia.org/wiki/Twin (Accessed 22 August 2017).

Wilkins, C. 2006. 'A qualitative study exploring the support needs of first time mothers on their journey towards intuitive parenting'. *Midwifery*, 22(2): 169–180.

Wylie, L & Bryce, H. 2008. *The midwives' guide to key medical conditions. Pregnancy and childbirth.* Edinburgh: Churchill Livingstone Elsevier.

Yeast, JD. 2006. 'Polihydramnios and oligohydramnios in twin pregnancy'. *Neo Reviews*, 7: e305–e309. http://neoreviews.aappublications.org/content/7/6/e305?sso=1&sso_redirect_count=1&nfstatus=401&nftoken=00000000-0000-0000-0000-000000000000&nfstatusdescription=ERROR%3a+No+local+token (Accessed 17 October 2017).

Young, D, Shield, N, Holmes, A, Turnbill, D & Twaddle, S. 1997. 'Aspects of antenatal care, a new style of midwife-managed antenatal care: Costs and satisfaction'. *British Journal of Midwifery*, 5: 540–545.

Section 5: Birth

AAP (American Academy of Pediatrics) & AHA (American Heart Association). 2011. *Textbook of neonatal resuscitation.* 6th ed. Elk Grove Village, IL: American Academy of Pediatrics and American Heart Association.

Abalos, E. 2009. 'Effect of timing of umbilical cord clamping of term infants on maternal and neonatal outcomes: RHL Commentary'. *The WHO Reproductive Health Library.* Geneva: WHO.

Abdel-Aleem, H. 2006. 'Misoprostol for induction of labour'. *The WHO Reproductive Health Library* 9. Geneva: WHO.

ACOG (American College of Obstetricians and Gynecologists). 1995. *Fetal heart rate patterns: monitoring, interpretation, and management.* ACOG technical bulletin 207. Washington, DC: ACOG.

ACOG. 2000a. *Fetal macrosomia.* Practice Bulletin 22. Washington DC: ACOG.

ACOG. 2000b. *Assisted vaginal delivery.* Practice Bulletin 17. Washington DC: ACOG.

ACOG. 2002. *Shoulder dystocia.* Practice Bulletin 40. Washington, DC: ACOG.

ACOG. 2005. Committee on Obstetric Practice. 'Inappropriate use of the terms fetal distress and birth asphyxia'. Committee Opinion, 326. https://www.ncbi.nlm.nih.gov/pubmed/16319282 (Accessed 6 October 2017).

ACOG. 2013. Ob-gyns redefine meaning of term pregnancy. http://www.acog.org/About-ACOG/News-Room/News-Releases/2013/Ob-Gyns-Redefine-Meaning-of-Term-Pregnancy (Accessed 6 October 2017).

ACOG. 2014. Task Force on Neonatal Encephalopathy; American Academy of Pediatrics. *Neonatal encephalopathy and neurologic outcome.* 2nd ed. Washington, DC: ACOG.

ACS (American College of Surgeons). 2017. ALTS. https://www.facs.org/quality-programs/trauma/atls (Accessed 6 October 2017).

AHA. 2002. *Pals provider manual.* South Deerfield: Channing Bete Company.

Alfirevic, Z, Kelly, AJ & Dowswell, T. 2009. 'Intravenous oxytocin alone for cervical ripening and induction of labour'. *Cochrane Database of Systemic Reviews.* http://onlinelibrary.wiley.com/doi/10.1002/14651858.CD003246/otherversions (Accessed 11 October 2017).

Amriom, M. 2009. 'Early amniotomy and early oxytocin for prevention of, or therapy for, delay in first stage spontaneous labour compared with routine care: RHL Commentary'. *The WHO Reproductive Health Library* 10. Geneva: WHO.

Anderson, G. 2003. 'A concept analysis of "normal birth"'. *The Royal College of Midwives Evidence-based Midwifery,* 1(2): 48–54.

APA (American Pregnancy Association). 2015. Cephalopelvic disproportion (CPD). http://americanpregnancy.org/labor-and-birth/cephalopelvic-disproportion/ (Accessed 6 October 2017).

Apgar, V. 1953. 'A proposal for a new method of evaluation of the newborn infant'. *Curr Res Anesth Analg,* 32: 260–267.

Apgar, V, Holiday, DA, James, LS, Weisbrot, IM & Berrien, C. 1958. Evaluation of the newborn infant: second report. *JAMA,* 168: 1985–1988.

Athukorala, C, Middleton, P & Crowther, CA. 2006. 'Intrapartum interventions for preventing shoulder dystocia'. *Cochrane Database of Systematic Reviews.* http://www.cochrane.org/CD005543/PREG_intrapartum-interventions-for-preventing-shoulder-dystocia (Accessed 11 October 2017).

Attilakos, G, Sibanda, T, Winter, C, Johnson, N & Draycott, T. 2005. 'A randomised controlled trial of a new handheld vacuum extraction device'. *BJOG,* 112: 1510–1515.

Bain, C, Burton, K & McGavigan, C. 2011. *Gynaecology illustrated.* 6th ed. Edinburgh: Churchill Livingstone.

Baker A, Ferguson, SA, Roach, GD & Dawson, D. 2001. 'Perceptions of labour pain by mothers and their attending midwives'. *Journal of Advanced Nursing,* 35(2): 171–179.

Balaskas, J. 1983. *Active birth.* London: Unwin Paperbacks.

Balaskas, J. & Yehudi, G. 1992. *Water birth.* London: Thorsons Harper Collins.

Baldisseri, MR. 2009. Shock and pregnancy. Medscape. http://emedicine.medscape.com/article/169450-print (Accessed 6 October 2017).

Banyana, CM & Crow, R. 2003. 'A qualitative study of information about available options for childbirth venues and pregnant women's preference for a place of birth'. *Midwifery,* 19: 328–336.

Barrett, JM. 1991. 'Funic reduction for the management of umbilical cord prolapse'. *Am J Obstet Gynecol,* 165: 654–657.

Basevi, V & Lavender, T. 2000. 'Routine perineal shaving on admission in labor'. *Cochrane Database of Systematic Review* 4: CD001236. DOI:10.1002/ 1465858. cd001236. http://onlinelibrary.wiley.com/doi/10.1002/14651858. CD001236.pub2/full (Accessed 5 October 2017).

Beall, MH, Spong, CY & Ross, MG. 2003. 'A randomized controlled trial of prophylactic maneuvers to reduce head-to-body delivery time in patients at risk for shoulder dystocia'. *Obstet Gynecol,* 102(1): 31–35. https://www.ncbi.nlm.nih.gov/pubmed/12850603 (Accessed 30 November 2017).

Beaton, M. 1983. *Childbirth by Caesarean.* Cape Town: Juta.

Beckmann, CRB, Ling, FW, Barzansky, BM, Herbert, WNP, Laube, DW & Smith, RP. 2010. *Obstetrics and gynecology.* 6th ed. Philadelphia, PA: Lippincott Williams & Wilkins.

Beischer, NA & Mackay, EV. 1981. *Obstetrics and the newborn.* 2nd ed. London: Bailliere Tindall.

Benioff Children's Hospital. nd. Birth asphyxia. http://www.ucsfbenioffchildrens.org/conditions/birth_asphyxia/ (Accessed 6 October 2017).

Bennett, VR & Brown, LK. 1989. *Myles textbook for midwives.* 11th ed. Edinburgh: Churchill Livingstone.

Benson, R. 1983. *Handbook of obstetrics and gynaecology.* 8th ed. Los Altos. California: Langa Medical Publications.

Bettercare.co.za. nd. *Maternal care.* Chapter 10. http://ls.bettercare.co.za/maternal-care/10.html#pain-relief-in-labour (Accessed 6 October 2017).

Bharathi, BJ. 2010. 'Effective nursing interventions on pain during labour among primi mothers'. *The Nursing Journal of India.* CI 6. https://www.unboundmedicine.com/medline/citation/23520818/Effective_nursing_interventions_on_pain_during_labour_among_primi_mothers_ (Accessed 12 October 2017).

Blackburn, S. 2008. 'Physiological third stage of labour and birth at home', in *Community midwifery practice,* edited by J Edwins. Oxford: Blackwell.

Bord, I, Gemer, O, Anteby, EY & Shenhav, S. 2011. 'The value of bladder filling in addition to manual elevation of presenting fetal part in cases of cord prolapse'. *Arch Gynecol Obstet,* 283: 989–991.

Boulvain, M, Kelly, AJ & Irion, O. 2008. 'Intracervical prostaglandins for induction of labour'. *Cochrane Database of Systematic Reviews* 1. http://onlinelibrary.wiley.com/doi/10.1002/14651858.CD006971/full (Accessed 11 October 2017).

Boulvain, M, Ceysens, G, Haelterman, E & Zhang, W-H. 2010. 'Repeat digital cervical assessment in pregnancy for identifying women at risk of preterm labour'. (Review). *Cochrane Database of Systematic Reviews.* https://www.ncbi.nlm.nih.gov/pubmed/20556763 (Accessed 6 October 2017).

Bowes, WA. 2010. "Management of the fetus in transverse lie". UpToDate. http://cursoenarm.net/UPTODATE/contents/mobipreview.

htm?17/61/18398?source=HISTORY (Accessed 7 December 2017).

Boyle, JJ & Katz, VL. 2005. 'Umbilical cord prolapse in current obstetric practice'. *J Reprod Med*, 50: 303–306.

Breeze, AC & Lees, CC. 2004. 'Managing shoulder dystocia'. *Lancet*, 364(9452): 2160–2161. http://middleeast.thelancet.com/journals/lancet/article/PIIS0140-6736(04)17607-1/abstract (Accessed 12 October 2017).

Bricker, L & Luckas, M. 2000. 'Amniotomy alone for induction of labour'. *Cochrane Database of Systematic Reviews* 4. http://www.cochrane.org/CD002862/PREG_amniotomy-alone-for-induction-of-labour (Accessed 12 October 2017).

Bromage, PR. 1978. *Epidural analgesia*. Philadelphia: WB Saunders Company.

Brown, H, Nikodem, C, Garener, P & Hofmyer, J. 2000. 'Evidence-based maternity care and labour support'. *International Journal of Childbirth Education*, 15: 26–31.

Buhimschi, CS, Buhimschi, IA, Malinow, IA & Weiner, CP. 2001. 'Use of McRoberts' position during delivery and increase in pushing efficiency'. *Lancet*, 358: 470–471.

Casey, BM, McIntire, DD, & Leveno, KJ. 2001. 'The continuing value of the Apgar score for the assessment of the newborn infants'. *N Engl J Med*, 344: 467–471.

Caspi, E, Lotan, Y & Schrever, P. 1983. 'Prolapse of the cord: Reduction of perinatal mortality by bladder instillation and Caesarean section'. *Isr J Med Sci*, 19: 541–545.

Catlin, EA, Carpenter, MW, Brann, BS IV, Mayfield, SR, Shaul, PW & Goldstein, M. 1986. 'The Apgar score revisited: influence of gestational age'. *J Pediatr*, 109: 865–868.

Cecatti, JG. 2005. 'Antibiotic prophylaxis for caesarean section: RHL Commentary'. *The WHO Reproductive Health Library*. Geneva: WHO.

Clark, SL, Belfort, MA, Hankins, GD, Meyers, JA & Houser, FM. 2007. 'Variation in the rates of assisted delivery in the United States'. *Am J Obstet Gynecol*, 196: 526 (e1–526.e5).

Cluett, ER, Nikodem, RE, McCandish, ER & Burnes, EE. 2004. 'Emersion in water in pregnancy, labour and birth'. *Birth*, 31. *Cochrane Review* 3.

Cohen, WR. 1977. 'Influence of the duration of second stage labor on perinatal outcome and puerperal morbidity'. *Obstet Gynecol*, 49: 266–269.

Conley, O. 2010. 'Birth without Violence (1975), by Frederick Leboyer'. Embryo Project Encyclopedia. https://embryo.asu.edu/pages/birth-without-violence-1975-frederick-leboyer (Accessed 6 October 2017).

Cooley, SM, Geary, MP, O'Connell, MP, McQuillan, K, McParland, P & Keane, D. 2010. 'How effective is amniotomy as a means of induction of labour?' *Ir J Med Sci*, 179(3): 381–383.

Cottingham, CA. 2006. 'Resuscitation of traumatic shock: A hemodynamic review'. *Advanced Critical Care Nursing*, 17: 317–326.

Craig, T, Hatrick, MDJ, Kovan, JP & Shapiro, S. 2003. 'The numeric rating scale for clinical pain measurement: A ratio measure?' *Pain Practice*, 3: 9310–9316.

Critchlow, CW, Leet, TL, Benedetti, TJ & Daling, JR. 1994. 'Risk factors and infant outcomes associated with umbilical cord prolapse: A population-based case-control study among births in Washington State'. *Am J Obstet Gynecol*, 170: 613–618.

Cronje, HS & Grobler, CJF. 2003. *Obstetrics in southern Africa*. Pretoria: Van Schaik.

Cuervo, LG. 2006. 'Interventions for preventing or improving the outcome of delivery at or beyond term: RHL Commentary'. *The WHO Reproductive Health Library* 9.

Cunningham, T, Levano, K, Bloom, S, Hauth, Rouse, P & Spong, Y. 2010. 'Abnormalities of the placenta, umbilical cord and membranes', in *Williams obstetrics*. 23rd ed. United States: McGraw-Hill.

David, K. 2007. IV Fluids: Do you know what's hanging and why? http://www.modernmedicine.com/content/iv-fluids-do-you-know-whats-hanging-and-why (Accessed 12 October 2017).

De Kock, J & Heyns, T. 2008. The ABC of haemorrhagic shock in the pregnant woman'. *Professional Nurse Today*, 12: 54–57.

De Kock, J, Heyns, T & Van Rensburg, GH. 2008. 'The ABC of haemorrhagic shock in the pregnant woman'. *PNT* Sep/Oct, 12(5): 55–57. https://repository.up.ac.za/bitstream/handle/2263/9644/DeKock_ABC(2008).pdf?sequence=1 (Accessed 17 November 2017).

Dellinger, RP, Carlet, JM, Masur, H, Gerlach, H, Calandra, T, Cohen, J, Gea-Banacloche, J, Keh, D, Marshall, JC, Parker, MM, Ramsay, G, Zimmerman, JL, Vincent, JL and Levy, MM. 2004. 'Surviving sepsis campaign guidelines for management of severe sepsis and septic shock'. *Crit Care Med*, 32(3): 858–873.

Dick-Read, G. 1959. *Childbirth without fear. The principles and practice of natural birth*. UK: Pinter & Martin.

Dodd, JM & Crowther, CA. 2010. 'Misoprostol for induction of labour to terminate pregnancy in the second or third trimester for women with a fetal anomaly or after intrauterine fetal death'. *Cochrane Database of Systematic Reviews* 4. http://onlinelibrary.wiley.com/doi/10.1002/14651858.CD004901.pub2/full (Accessed 12 October 2017).

DoH (Department of Health). 2015. *Guidelines for Maternity Care in South Africa. A Manual for Clinic, Community Health Centres and District Hospitals.* https://www.health-e.org.za/wp-content/uploads/2015/11/Maternal-Care-Guidelines-2015_FINAL-21.7.15.pdf (Accessed 12 October 2017).

Downe, S, Gyte, GM, Dahlen, HG & Singata, M. 2013. 'Routine vaginal examinations for assessing progress of labour to improve outcomes for women and babies at term'. (Review). *Cochrane Database of Systematic Reviews*, 7. http://onlinelibrary.wiley.com/doi/10.1002/14651858.CD010088.pub2/pdf (Accessed 6 October 2017).

Drobin, D & Hahn, RG. 1999. 'Volume kinetics of Ringer's solution in hypovolemic volunteers'. *Anaesthesiology*, 90: 81–91.

Dubin, AE & Patapoutian, A. 2010. 'Nociceptors: The sensors of the pain pathway'. *J Clin Invest*, 120(11): 3760–3772. DOI: 10.1172/JCI42843. https://www.jci.org/articles/view/42843 (Accessed 6 October 2017).

Du Plessis, DW. 2008: *Juta's clinical guide for midwives.* Cape Town: Juta.

Edwards, B. 2007. 'Walking in: Initial visualisation and assessment'. *Accident and Emergency Nursing*, 15: 73–78.

Ehrenstein, V. 2009. 'Association of Apgar scores with death and neurologic disability'. *Clin Epidemiol*, 1: 45–53.

England, P & Horowitz, R. 2000. '"The Birthing From Within Holistic Sphere": A Conceptual Model for Childbirth Education'. *J Perinat Educ*, 9(2): 1–7. DOI: 10.1624/105812400X87590 https://www.ncbi.nlm.nih.gov/pmc/articles/PMC1595018/ (Accessed 17 November 2017).

Ezebialu, IU, Eke, AC, Eleje, GU & Nwachukwu, CE. 2015. 'Methods for assessing pre-induction cervical ripening'. (Review). *Cochrane Database of Systematic Reviews.* http://www.cochrane.org/CD010762/PREG_methods-for-assessing-pre-induction-cervical-ripening-the-ability-of-the-cervix-to-open-in-response-to-spontaneous-uterine-contractions (Accessed 6 October 2017).

Fantu, S, Segni, H & Alemseged, F. 2010. 'Incidence, causes and outcome of obstructed labor in Jimma University specialized hospital'. *Ethiop J Health Sci*, 20(3):145–151. https://www.ncbi.nlm.nih.gov/pmc/articles/PMC3275845/ (Accessed 6 October 2017).

Farrell, EM & Pattinson, R. 2005. *Intrapartum care in South Africa.* Medical Research Council.

Fischer, R. 2016. Breech presentation. Medscape. http://emedicine.medscape.com/article/262159-overview (Accessed 6 October 2017).

Freeman, JM & Nelson, KB. 1988. 'Intrapartum asphyxia and cerebral palsy'. *Pediatrics*, 82: 240–249.

French, L. 2001. 'Oral prostaglandin E2 for induction of labour'. *Cochrane Database of Systematic Reviews.* https://www.ncbi.nlm.nih.gov/pubmedhealth/PMH0011814/ (Accessed 16 October 2017).

Galvagno, SM & Camann, W. 2009. 'Sepsis and acute renal failure in pregnancy'. *Obstetric Anesthesiology*, 108: 572–575.

Garrey, MM, Govan, ADT, Hodge, C & Callander, R. 1974. *Obstetrics illustrated.* 2nd ed. Edinburgh: Churchill Livingstone.

Gebbie, D. 1966. 'Vacuum extraction and symphysiotomy in difficult vaginal delivery in a developing community'. *British Medical Journal*, 2: 1490–1493.

Gerber, S, Vial, Y & Hohlfield, P. 1999. 'Maternal and neonatal prognosis after a prolonged second stage of labor'. [in French] *J Gynecol Obstet Biol Reprod*, 28: 145–150.

Gherman, RB. 2001. 'Fetal abdominal circumference and macrosomia'. *J Reprod Med*, 46: 699–700.

Gherman, RB. 2002. 'Shoulder dystocia: An evidence-based evaluation of the obstetrical nightmare'. *Clinical Obstet and Gynecol*, 45: 345–361.

Gherman, RB, Tramont, J, Muffley, P & Goodwin, TM. 2000. 'Analysis of McRoberts' Maneuver by X-ray pelvimetry'. *Obstet Gynecol*, 95: 43–47.

Gilby, JR, Williams, MC & Spellacy, WN. 2000. 'Fetal abdominal circumference measurements of 35 and 38 cms as predictors of macrosomia: A risk factor for shoulder dystocia'. *J Reprod Med*, 45: 936–938.

Ginsberg, NA & Moisidis, C. 2001. 'How to predict recurrent shoulder dystocia'. *Am J Obstet Gynecol*, 184: 1427–1430.

Gonen, R, Bader, D & Ajami, M. 2000. 'Effects of a policy of elective caesarean delivery in cases of suspected fetal macrosomia on the incidence of brachial plexus injury and the rate of cesarean delivery'. *Am J Obstet Gynecol*, 183: 1296-1300.

Gonik, B, Walker, A & Grimm, M. 2000. 'Mathematic modeling of forces associated with shoulder dystocia: A comparison of endogenous and exogenous sources'. *Am J Obstet Gynecol*, 182: 689-691.

Government of Western Australia, Department of Health. nd. Fetal heart monitoring: Intrapartum. Women and newborn health service. King Edward Memorial hospital. http://www.kemh.health.wa.gov.au/development/manuals/O&G_guidelines/sectionb/index.htm (Accessed 6 October 2017).

Graham, ID, Logan, J, Davies, B & Nimrod, C. 2004. 'Changing the use of electronic fetal monitoring and labor support: A case study of barriers and facilitators'. *Birth*, 31: 293–301.

Greenhill, JP & Friedman, EA. 1974. *Biological principles and modern practice of obstetrics*. Philadelphia: Saunders.

Gudmundsson, S, Henningsson, AC & Lindqvist, P. 2005. 'Correlation of birth injury with maternal height and birthweight'. *BJOG*, 112(6): 764–767.

Gülmezoglu, M. 2006. 'Antibiotics for prelabour rupture of membranes at or near term: RHL Commentary'. *The WHO Reproductive Health Library*, 9. Geneva: WHO.

Gülmezoglu, AM, Crowther, CA & Middleton, P. 2009. 'Induction of labour for improving birth outcomes for women at or beyond term'. *Cochrane Database Of Systematic Reviews*, 4. http://onlinelibrary.wiley.com/doi/10.1002/14651858.CD004945.pub3/full (Accessed 16 October 2017).

Gupta, JK & Hofmeyr, GJ. 2006. 'Position in the second stage of labour for women without epidural anaesthesia'. *The WHO Reproductive Health Library*. https://www.researchgate.net/publication/317188234_Position_in_the_second_stage_of_labour_for_women_without_epidural_anaesthesia (Accessed 16 October 2017).

Gurewitsch, ED, Johnson, TL & Allen, RH. 2007. 'After shoulder dystocia: Managing the subsequent pregnancy and delivery'. *Semin. Perinatol*, 31(3): 185–195. https://www.ncbi.nlm.nih.gov/pubmed/17531900 (Accessed 16 October 2017).

Gutierrez, G, Reines, HD & Wulf-Gutierrez, E. 2004. *Clinical review: Hemorrhagic shock*. https://www.ncbi.nlm.nih.gov/pmc/articles/PMC1065003/ (Accessed 16 October 2017).

Hartfield, VJ. 1973. 'Comparison of early and late effects of subcutaneous symphysiotomy and of lower segment caesarean section'. *Journal of Obstetrics and Gynaecology of the British Commonwealth*, 80: 508–514. http://onlinelibrary.wiley.com/doi/10.1111/j.1471-0528.1973.tb15971.x/full (Accessed 16 October 2017).

Hartrick, CT, Kovan, JP & Shapiro, S. 2003. 'The numeric rating scale for clinical pain measurement: A ratio measure'. *Pain Practice*, 3: 9310–9316.

Hassan, SJ, Sundby, J, Hussein, A & Bjertness, E. 2012. 'The paradox of vaginal examination practice during normal childbirth: Palestinian women's feelings, opinions, knowledge and experiences'. *Reproductive Health*, 9:16. https://reproductive-health-journal.biomedcentral.com/articles/10.1186/1742-4755-9-16 (Accessed 16 October 2017).

Hegyi T, Carbone, T, Anwar, M, Ostfeld, B, Hiatt, M, Koons, A, Pinto-Martin, J & Paneth, N. 1998. 'The Apgar score and its components in the preterm infant'. *Pediatrics*, 101: 77–81.

Hodnett, E, Kennell, JH & Klaus, MH. 2003. 'Continuous nursing support during labor'. *Journal of the American Medical Association*, 289: 175–176.

Hofmyer, GJ. 2005. 'Evidence-based intra partum care. Best practice and research'. *Clinical Obstetrics and Gynecology*, 19: 103–115.

Holbrook, BD & Phelan, ST. 2013. 'Umbilical cord prolapse'. *Obstet Gynecol Clin North Am*, 40: 1–14.

Holcroft Argani, C & Satin, AJ. 2017. 'Occiput posterior position'. UpToDate. http://www.uptodate.com/contents/occiput-posterior-position (Accessed 14 October 2017).

Howarth, G & Botha, DJ. 2001. 'Amniotomy plus intravenous oxytocin for induction of labour'. *Cochrane Database of Systematic Reviews*, 3. CD003250. http://onlinelibrary.wiley.com/doi/10.1002/14651858.CD003250/pdf (Accessed 16 October 2017).

Hulton, EK & Mozurkewich, EL. 2001. 'Extra-amniotic prostaglandin for induction of labour'. *Cochrane Database Systematic Reviews*, 2: CD003092. http://onlinelibrary.wiley.com/doi/10.1002/14651858.CD003092/pdf (Accessed 16 October 2017).

Inturrisi, M & Lambert, L. 1998. 'LOS for uncomplicated vaginal birth. A perinatal continuous quality improvement project'. *Journal of Perinatal and Neonatal Nursing*, 12: 11–22.

Jain, L, Ferre, C, Vidyasagar, D, Nath, S & Sheftel, D. 1991. 'Cardiopulmonary resuscitation of apparently stillborn infants: Survival and long-term outcome'. *J Pediatr*, 118: 778–782.

Javed, I, Bhutta, S & Shoaib, T. 2007. 'Role of the partogram in preventing prolonged labor'. *Journal of the Pakistan Medical Association*, 57: 408–411.

Jensen, MD, Benson, RC & Bobak, IM. 1981. *Maternity care*. 2nd ed. St. Louis: The CV Mosby Company.

Jhalta, D. 2013. 'Abnormal uterine actions'. *Health & Medicine*, Jun 13. https://www.slideshare.net/drpawanj/abnormal-uterine-action-22808834 (Accessed 6 October 2017).

Johnson, R & Taylor, W. 2010. *Skills for midwifery practice*. 3rd ed. Edinburgh: Churchill Livingstone Elsevier.

Joint policy statement on normal childbirth. 2008. *Journal of Obstetrics and Gynaecology Canada*, 12: 1163–1165.

Kahana, B, Sheiner, E, Levy A, Lazer, S & Mazor, M. 2004. 'Umbilical cord prolapse and perinatal outcomes'. *Int J Gynaecol Obstet*, 84: 127–132.

Kalur, JS, Martin, JN, Kirchner, KA & Morrison, JC. 1991. 'Postpartum preeclampsia-induced shock and death: A report of three cases'. *American Journal of Obstetrics and Gynecology*, 165(1): 1362–1368.

Kaplow, R & Hardin, SR. 2007. *Critical care nursing: Synergy for optimal outcomes*. London: Jones and Bartlett.

Karri, K, Raghavan, R & Shahid, J. 2009. 'Severe anaphylaxis to Volplex, a colloid solution during cesarean section: A case report and review'. *Obstetrics and Gynecology International*. https://www.researchgate. net/publication/40039783_Severe_Anaphylaxis_ to_Volplex_a_Colloid_Solution_during_Cesarean_ Section_A_Case_Report_and_Review (Accessed 16 October 2017).

Kasdorf, E, Laptook, A, Azzopardi, D, Jacobs, S & Perlman, JM. 2015. 'Improving infant outcome with a 10 min Apgar of 0'. *Arch Dis. Child Fetal Neonatal Ed*, 100(2): F102–105.

Katz, Z, Lancet, M & Borenstein, R. 1982. 'Management of labor with umbilical cord prolapse'. *Am J Obstet Gynecol*, 142: 239–241.

Khan, KS, Wojdyla, D, Say, L, Gülmezoglu, AM & Van Look, PF. 2006. 'WHO analysis of causes of maternal death: a systematic review'. *Lancet*, 367: 1066–1074.

Kish, K & Collea, JV. 2003. 'Malpresentation and cord prolapse', in *Current obstetric and gynecologic diagnosis and treatment*, edited by AH DeCherney. London: Lange/ McGraw-Hill.

Kitzinger, S. 2000. *Rediscovering birth*. London: Simon & Schuster.

Kleinpell, RM. 2006. 'Stop severe sepsis in its tracks'. *Critical Care Nursing*, 1: 20–26.

Knight, M, Berg, C, Brocklehurst, P, Kramer, M, Lewis, G, Oats, J, Roberts, CL, Spong, C, Sullivan, E, Van Roosmalen, J & Zwart, J. 2012. 'Amniotic fluid embolism incidence, risk factors and outcomes: A review and recommendations.' *BMC Pregnancy and Childbirth*, 12(7). DOI: 10.1186/1471-2393-12-7. https://bmcpregnancychildbirth.biomedcentral.com/ articles/10.1186/1471-2393-12-7 (Accessed 6 October 2017).

Koonings, PP, Paul, RH & Campbell, K. 1990. 'Umbilical cord prolapse. A contemporary look'. *J Reprod Med*, 35: 690–692.

Kozak, LJ & Weeks, JD. 2002. 'Trends in obstetric procedures, 1990–2000'. *Birth*, 29: 157–161.

Krausz, MM. 2006. 'Initial resuscitation of hemorrhagic shock'. *World Journal of Emergency Surgery*, 1: 14.

Langer, A. 2006. 'Continuous support for women during childbirth'. *The WHO Reproductive Health Library*, 9. Geneva: WHO.

Lasbrey, AH. 1963. 'The symptomatic sequelae of symphysiotomy'. *South African Medical Journal*, 37: 231–234.

Latto, C. 2008. 'An overview of sepsis'. *Dimensions of Critical Care Nursing*, 27: 195–199.

Lauzon, L & Hodnett, E. 2002. 'Labour assessment programs to delay admission to labour wards'. *Cochrane Database Syst Rev*, 3: CD000936.

Lawrence, A, Lewis, L, Hofmeyr, GJ, Dowswell, T & Styles, C. 2009. 'Maternal positions and mobility during first stage labor'. *Cochrane Database of Systematic Reviews*, 2. http://onlinelibrary.wiley.com/doi/10.1002/14651858. CD003934.pub4/full (Accessed 13 October 2017).

Leduc, D, Biringer, A, Lee, L & Dy, J. 2013. 'Induction of labour'. *Journal of Obstetrics and Gynecology Canada*, 35(9).

Leong, A, Rao, J, Opie, G & Dobson, P. 2004. 'Fetal survival after conservative management of cord prolapse for three weeks'. *BJOG*, 111: 1476–1477.

Lerner, H. 2017. Incidence. http://www.shoulderdystociainfo. com/incidence.htm (Accessed 6 October 2017).

Levy, V & Moore, J. 1985. 'The midwife's management of the third stage'. Occasional Paper. *Nursing Times*, 81(5).

Lewis, TLT & Chamberlain, GVP. 1990. *Obstetrics by ten teachers*. 15th ed. London: Edward Arnold.

Li, F, Wu, T, Lei, X, Zhang, H, Mao, M & Zhang, J. 2013. 'The Apgar score and infant mortality'. *PLoS One*, 8: e69072.

Lie, KK, Grøholt, EK & Eskild, A. 2010. 'Association of cerebral palsy with Apgar score in low and normal birth weight infants: Population based cohort study'. *BMJ*, 341: c4990.

Liljestrand, J. 2003. 'Episiotomy for vaginal birth: RHL Commentary'. *The WHO Reproductive Health Library*. Geneva: WHO.

Lin, MG. 2006. 'Umbilical cord prolapse'. *Obstet Gynecol Surv*, 61: 269–277.

Littlefield, VM. 1986. *Health education for women, a guide for nurses*. Norwalk, CT: Appleton-Century-Crofts.

Llewellyn-Jones, D. 1982. *Fundamentals of obstetrics & gynaecology. Vol I: Obstetrics*. London: Faber & Faber.

Longo, LD. 1978. 'Classic Pages', in *Obstetrics and gynaecology*. St. Louis: The CV Mosby Company.

Lopriore, E, Van Burk F, Walther, F & Arnout, J. 2004. 'Correct use of the Apgar score for resuscitated and intubated newborn babies: Questionnaire study'. *BMJ*, 329: 143–144.

Luckas, M & Bricker, L. 2000. 'Intravenous prostaglandin for induction of labour'. *Cochrane Database of Systematic Reviews,* 4. http://onlinelibrary.wiley.com/doi/10.1002/14651858.CD002864/pdf (Accessed 13 October 2017).

Macones, GA, Hankins, GD, Spong, CY, Hauth, J & Moore, T. 2008. 'The 2008 National Institute of Child Health and Human Development workshop report on electronic fetal monitoring: Update on definitions, interpretation, and research guidelines'. *Obstet Gynecol,* 112: 661–666.

Malin, GL, Morris, RK & Khan, KS. 2010. 'Strength of association between umbilical cord pH and perinatal and long term outcomes: Systematic review and meta-analysis'. *BMJ,* 340: c1471.

Malmström, T. 1957. 'The vacuum extractor: An obstetrical instrument'. *Acta Obstet Gynecol Scand,* 36: 5–50.

Marino, TM. 2016. Face and brow presentation. Medscape. https://emedicine.medscape.com/article/262341-overview (Accessed 14 October 2017).

Marshall, J, Raynor, M & Nolte, A. 2016. *Myles textbook for midwives.* African edition. London: Elsevier.

Martel, M. 2002. 'Hemorrhagic shock. SOCG clinical guidelines'. *Journal of Obstetrics and Gynaecology Canada,* 24: 1–8. https://sogc.org/wp-content/uploads/2013/01/115E-CPG-June2002.pdf (Accessed 6 October 2017).

Martin, JA, Hamilton, BE, Sutton, PD, Ventura, SJ, Menacker, F, Kirmeyer, S, Munson, ML, Center for Disease Control and Prevention, National Center for Health Statistics & National Vital Statistics System. 2007. 'Births: Final data for 2005'. *Natl Vital Stat Rep,* 56: 1–103.

Martin, JA, Hamilton, BE, Ventura, SJ, Menacker, F, Park, M & Sutton, PD. 2002. 'Births: Final data for 2001'. *National Vital Statistics Reports,* 51: 1–102.

Martis, R. 2007. 'Continuous support for women during childbirth. RHL Commentary'. *The WHO Reproductive Health Library.* Geneva: WHO.

Massyn, H, Peer, N, Padarath, A, Barron, P & Day, C. 2015. *District health barometer 2014/2015.* Westville: HST. http://www.hst.org.za/publications/District%20Health%20Barometers/Complete_DHB_2014_15_linked.pdf#search=district%20health%20barometer%202014 (Accessed 9 October 2017).

Mayer, BH (ed). 2007. *Emergency nursing made incredibly easy.* Philadelphia: Lippincott Williams & Wilkins.

Mazouni, C, Porcu, G, Cohen-Solai, E, Heckenroth, H, Guidicelli, B, Bonnier, P & Gamerre, M. 2006. 'Maternal and anthropomorphic risk factors for shoulder dystocia'. *Acta Obstet Gynecol Scand,* 85(5): 567–570.

McCormick, C. 2009. 'The first stage of labour: physiology and early care', in *Myles textbook for midwives,* edited by D Fraser & MA Cooper. 15th ed. Edinburgh: Churchill Livingstone Elsevier.

McDonald, S. 2009. 'Physiology and management of the third stage of labour', in *Myles textbook for midwives,* edited by D Fraser D & MA Cooper. 15th ed. Edinburgh: Churchill Livingstone Elsevier.

McDonald, SJ & Middleton, P. 2008. 'Effect of timing of umbilical cord clamping of term infants on maternal and neonatal outcomes'. *Cochrane Database of Systematic Reviews,* 2. http://onlinelibrary.wiley.com/doi/10.1002/14651858.CD004074.pub2/abstract (Accessed 13 October 2017).

McQuillan, KA, Makic, MBF & Whalen, E. 2009. *Trauma nursing: From resuscitation through rehabilitation.* 4th ed. Philadelphia: Saunders Elsevier.

Mead, MMP & Kornbrot, D. 2002. 'An intrapartum intervention scoring system for the comparison of maternity units' intrapartum care of nulliparous women suitable for midwifery-led care'. *Midwifery,* 2: 15–26.

Melzack, R & Wall, PD. 1965. 'Pain mechanisms: A new theory'. *Science,* 150(3699): 971–979. https://www.ncbi.nlm.nih.gov/pubmed/5320816 (Accessed 9 October 2017).

Michaels, PA. 2010. 'A chapter from Lamaze history: Birth narratives and authoritative knowledge in France, 1952–1957'. *J Perinat Educ,* 19(2): 35–43. DOI: 10.1624/105812410X495532. https://www.ncbi.nlm.nih.gov/pmc/articles/PMC2866433/ (Accessed 9 October 2017).

Mitchell, MD, Flint, AP, Bibby, J, Brunt, J, Arnold, JM & Anderson, AB. 1977. 'Rapid increases in plasma prostaglandin concentrations after vaginal examination and amniotomy'. *Br Med J,* 2(6096): 1183–1185.

Moir, DD. 1986. *Pain relief in labour: A handbook for midwives.* 5th ed. Edinburgh: Churchill Livingstone.

Moka, E. 2011. Safety of epidural anaesthesia. 30th annual ESRA congress. Dresden, Germany. 7 to 10 September. http://www.esrahellas.gr/uploads/files/slides%20dresden%20last%20esra%20hellas%201%20locked.pdf (Accessed 14 October 2017).

Moore, KL. 1983. *Before we are born.* 2nd ed. Toronto/Philadelphia: WB. Saunders Company.

Moore, ML. 1983. *Realities in childbearing.* 2nd ed. Philadelphia: WB Saunders Company.

Morton, PG, Fontaine, DK, Hudak, CM & Gallo, BM. 2005. *Critical care nursing: A holistic approach.* 8th ed. Philadelphia: Lippincott Williams Wilkins.

Moster, D, Lie, RT, Irgens, LM, Bjerkedal, T & Markestad, T. 2001. 'The association of Apgar score with subsequent death and cerebral palsy: A population-based study in term infants'. *J Pediatr,* 138: 798–803.

Mowafi, DM. 2016. Obstetrics simplified. http://www.gfmer. ch/Obstetrics_simplified/abnormal_uterine_action.htm (Accessed 9 October 2017).

MRC Research Unit for Maternal and Infant Healthcare Strategies, PPIP users, DoH & Saving Babies Technical Task Team. 2003. *Saving Babies 2003. Fourth Perinatal Care Survey of South Africa.* https://www.ppip.co.za/ wp-content/uploads/Saving-babies-2003.pdf (Accessed 9 October 2017).

Murphy, DJ & MacKenzie, IZ. 1995. 'The mortality and morbidity associated with umbilical cord prolapse'. *Br J Obstet Gynaecol,* 102: 826–830.

Murray, A & McKinney, A. 2006. *Intrapartum complications. Foundations of maternal-newborn and women's health nursing,* 5th ed. Saunders Elsevier.

Mustafa, SS. 2017. Anaphylaxis. Medscape. https:// emedicine.medscape.com/article/135065-overview#a3 (Accessed 30 November 2017).

Myles, TD & Santolaya, J. 2003. 'Maternal and neonatal outcomes in patients with a prolonged second stage of labor'. *Obstet Gynecol,* 102: 52–58.

Nachum, Z, Garmi, G, Kadan, Y, Zafran, N, Shalev, E & Salim, R. 2010. 'Comparison between amniotomy, oxytocin or both for augmentation of labor in prolonged latent phase: A randomized controlled trial'. *Reprod Biol Endocrinol,* 8: 136.

Nelson, KB & Ellenberg, JH. 1981. 'Apgar scores as predictors of chronic neurologic disability'. *Pediatrics,* 68: 36–44.

NICE (National Institute for Health and Care Excellence). 2007. *Intrapartum care: Care of healthy women and their babies during childbirth.* Clinical guideline 55. https://www. nice.org.uk/guidance/cg55 (Accessed 13 October 2017).

NICE. 2008. *CG 70: Induction of labour.* http://www.nhs. uk/planners/pregnancycareplanner/documents/nice_ induction_of_labour.pdf (Accessed 9 October 2017).

NICE. 2013. Performing induction. https://pathways. nice.org.uk/pathways/induction-of-labour/performing- induction-of-labour (Accessed 9 October 2017).

NICHD (National Institute of Child Health and Human Development) Research Planning Workshop. 1997. 'Electronic fetal heart rate monitoring: Research

guidelines for interpretation'. *Am J Obstet Gynecol,* 177: 1385–1390.

NMC (Nursing and Midwifery Council). 2004. Midwives rules and standards. https://www.nmc.org.uk/news/ news-and-updates/revised-midwives-rules-and-standards- come-into-force/ (Accessed 13 October 2017).

NMC. 2008. *The Code: Standards of Conduct, Performance and Ethics for Nurses and Midwives.* http://www.rayson-homes. com/staff/wp-content/uploads/nmc.pdf (Accessed 9 October 2017).

NMC. 2009. *Record-keeping: Guidance for Nurses and Midwives.* http://www.nipec.n-i.nhs.uk/Image/ SitePDFS/nmcGuidance RecordKeepingGuidance forNursesandMidwives.pdf (Accessed 9 October 2017).

Nolte, A. 2008. *The partograph and how to assess labour.* Cape Town: Juta.

Notzon, FC. 1990. 'International differences in the use of obstetric interventions'. *Journal of the American Medical Association,* 263: 3286–3291.

Odent, M. 1985. *Entering the world.* Liarmondsworth, Middlesex: Penguin Books.

O'Driscoll, K & Meagher, D. 1986. *Active management of labour.* 2nd ed. London: Ballierre Tindall.

Olds, SB, London, ML, Ladewig, PA & Davidson, SV. 1980. *Obstetric nursing.* Menlo Park, California: Addison-Wesley.

O'Shea, RA. 2005. *Principles and practice of trauma nursing.* Oxford: Elsevier.

Othman, M, Neilson, JP & Alfirevic, Z. 2007. 'Probiotics for preventing preterm labour'. *Cochrane Database of Systematic Reviews,* 1: CD005941.

Pairman, S, Pincombe, J, Thorogood, C & Tracy, S (eds). 2015. *Midwifery: Preparation for practice.* 3rd ed. Sydney: Elsevier Australia.

Pairman, S, Tracy, S, Thorogood, C & Pincombe, J. 2010. *Midwifery: Preparation for practice.* 2nd ed. Chatswood, NSW: Elsevier Australia.

Papile, LA. 2001. 'The Apgar score in the 21st century'. *N Engl J Med,* 344: 519–520.

Parratt, JA & Fahy, KM. 2004. 'Creating a safe place for birth: An empirically grounded theory'. *New Zealand College of Midwives Journal,* 30: 11–14.

Pattinson, RC & Rhoda, N (for the PPIP group). 2014. *Saving Babies 2012–2013: Ninth Report on Perinatal Care in South Africa.* Pretoria: Tshepesa Press. http://www.ppip. co.za/wp-content/uploads/Saving-Babies-2012-2013.pdf (Accessed 9 October 2017).

Paul, M. 2015. Eating the placenta: Trendy but no proven health benefits and unknown risks. https://news. northwestern.edu/stories/2015/06/eating-the-placenta-trendy-but-no-proven-health-benefits-and-unknown-risks-- (Accessed 9 October 2017).

Philpott, RH. 1982. *Obstetric problems in the developing world — Clinics in obstetrics and gynaecology.* London: WB Saunders Company Ltd.

Philpott, RH, Ross, SM & Axton, JHM. 1986. *Obstetrics, family planning and paediatrics.* 3rd ed. Pietermaritzburg: University of Natal Press.

Pollak, AN. 2008. *Nancy Caroline's emergency care in the streets.* 6th ed. London: Jones and Bartlett Publishers International.

Prendiville, WJ, Elbourne, D & McDonald, S. 2006. 'Active versus expectant management in the third stage of labour'. (Cochrane Review). *The Reproductive Health Library,* 9. https://www.ncbi.nlm.nih.gov/pubmed/19588315 (Accessed 9 October 2017).

Pritchard, JA, Macdonald, PC & Gant, NF. 1985. *Williams obstetrics.* 17th ed. Connecticut: Appleton-Century-Crofts.

Proehl, JA. 2009. *Emergency nursing procedures.* 4th ed. Missouri: Saunders.

Quijano, C. 2007. 'Methods of repair for obstetric anal sphincter injury: RHL commentary'. *The WHO Reproductive Health Library.* Geneva: WHO.

RANZCOG (The Royal Australian and New Zealand College of Obstetricians and Gynaecologists). 2013. C-Gyn 30: Guidelines for gynaecological examinations and procedures. https://www.ranzcog.edu.au/RANZCOG_SITE/media/RANZCOG-MEDIA/Women's%20Health/Statement%20and%20guidelines/Clinical%20-%20Gynaecology/Guidelines-for-gynaecological-examinations-and-procedures-(C-Gyn-30)-Review-March-2016.pdf?ext=.pdf (Accessed 9 October 2017).

RCM (The Royal College of Midwives). 1997. *Campaign for normal birth.* https://www.rcm.org.uk/tags/campaign-for-normal-birth (Accessed 9 October 2017).

RCOG (Royal College of Obstetricians and Gynaecologists). 2005. *Green Top Guideline 42. Shoulder dystocia.* https://www.rcog.org.uk/en/guidelines-research-services/guidelines/gtg42/ (Accessed 9 October 2017).

RCOG. 2008. RCOG statement on umbilical non-severance or 'lotus birth'. https://www.rcog.org.uk/en/news/rcog-statement-on-umbilical-non-severance-or-lotus-birth (Accessed 17 November 2017).

Reid, PC & Osuagwu, FI. 1999. 'Symphysiotomy in shoulder dystocia'. *Journal of Obstetrics and Gynaecology,* 19(6): 664–666.

Resuscitation Council UK. 2008. *Emergency treatment of anaphylactic reaction.* London: Resuscitation Council UK. https://www.resus.org.uk/search/?q=emergency+treatment (Accessed 9 October 2017).

Reveiz, L, Gaitan, HG & Cuervo, LG. 2007. 'Enemas during labor'. *Cochrane Database of Systematic Reviews,* 4: CD000330. DOI:10.1002/146551858.CD000330.pub2. http://www.cochrane.org/reviews/en/ab000330.html (Accessed 9 October 2017).

Roberts, L, Gulliver, B, Fisher, J & Cloyes, KG. 2010. 'The coping with algorithm: An alternative pain assessment tool for the laboring woman'. *Journal of Midwifery and Women's Health,* 55: 107–116.

The Royal Women's Hospital. 2017. *Cardiotocograph (CTG) interpretation and response.* https://thewomens.r.worldssl.net/images/uploads/downloadable-records/clinical-guidelines/ctg-interpretation-and-response_160517.pdf (Accessed 17 November 2017).

Rudra, A, Chatterjee, S, Sengupta, R, Wankhade, S, Sirohia, S & Das, T. 2006. 'Fluid resuscitation in trauma'. *Indian Journal of Critical Care Medicine,* 10: 241–249.

SANC (South African Council of Midwives). 1990. Regulations relating to the conditions under which registered midwives and enrolled midwives may carry on their profession. Government notice R2488. http://www.sanc.co.za/regulat/Reg-cmi.htm (Accessed 9 October 2017).

Sandmire, HF. 1996. 'A guest editorial: Every obstetric department should have a caesarean section birth monitor'. *Obstetrical and Gynaecological Survey,* 51: 703–704.

Sarsam, S. 2014. 'Abnormal labor and abnormal uterine contractions (dystocia)'. Scribd. https://www.scribd.com/document/239157996/Abnormal-Labor-and-Abnormal-Uterine-Contractions-Dystocia-2 (Accessed 14 October 2017).

Satpathy, HK: Labor and delivery, analgesia, regional and local. Medscape. http://emedicine.medscape.com/article/149337-overview (Accessed 9 October 2017).

Schreiber, LA & Vlok, ME. 1987. *Manual of advanced nursing.* 5th ed. Cape Town: Juta.

Schwartz, ML. 1975. 'Zatuchni-Andros prognostic scoring index'. *American Journal of Obstetrics and Gynecology,* 123(1): 108. http://www.ajog.org/article/0002-9378(75)90959-X/abstract (Accessed 9 October 2017).

Seaward, PG, Hannah, ME, Myhr, TL, Farine, D, Ohlsson, A, Wang, EE, Hague, K, Weston, JA, Hewson, SA, Ohel, G & Hodnett, ED. 1997. 'International multicentre term prelabor rupture of membranes study: Evaluation of predictors of clinical chorioamnionitis and postpartum fever in patients with prelabor rupture of membranes at term'. *Am J Obstet Gynecol*, 177(5): 1024–1029.

Selo-Ojeme, DO, Pisal, P, Lawal, O, Rogers, C, Shah, A & Sinha, S. 2009. 'A randomised controlled trial of amniotomy and immediate oxytocin infusion versus amniotomy and delayed oxytocin infusion for induction of labour at term'. *Arch Gynecol Obstet*, 279(6): 813–820.

Siassakos, D, Hasafa, Z, Sibanda, T, Fox, R, Donald, F, Winter, C & Draycott, T. 2009. 'Retrospective cohort study of diagnosis-delivery interval with umbilical cord prolapse: the effect of team training'. *BJOG*, 116: 1089–10

Silva, M & Halpern, SH. 2010. 'Epidural analgesia for labor: Current techniques'. *Anesthesiology*, Mar; 112(3): 530–545. http://www.ncbi.nlm.nih.gov/pmc/articles/PMC3417963/ (Accessed 9 October 2017).

Smith, JR & Brennan, BG. 2009. Management of the third stage of labour. Medscape. http://emedicine.medscape.com/article/275304-overview (Accessed 9 October 2017).

Smith, JR & Brennan, BG. 2010. Postpartum hemorrhage. Medscape. http://emedicine.medscape.com/article/275038-overview (Accessed 9 October 2017).

Smyth, RM, Alldred, SK & Markham, C. 2007. 'Amniotomy for shortening spontaneous labour'. *Cochrane Database Systematic Review*, 4: CD006167.

Soni, BL. 2009. 'Effect of partogram use on outcomes for women in spontaneous labor at term: RHL Commentary'. *The WHO Reproductive Health Library*. Geneva: WHO.

Spaniol, JR, Knight, AR, Zembley, JL, Anderson, D & Pierce, JD. 2007. 'Fluid resuscitation therapy for hemorrhagic shock'. *Journal of Trauma Nursing*, 14: 152–160.

SPNP (Society of Private Nursing Practitioners). 2008. Guidelines for midwife home births. *PNT Online*, 12(3): 19–20. http://ww.pntonline.co.za/index.php/PNT/article/view/255/247 (Accessed 17 November 2017).

Stables, D & Rankin, J. 2010. *Physiology in childbearing with anatomy and related biosciences.* 3rd ed. Edinburgh: Elsevier.

Sweet, BR. 1988. *Mayes' midwifery.* 11th ed. London: Bailliere Tindall.

Thacker, SB & Banta, HD. 2009. 'Benefits and risks of episiotomy: An interpretative review of English language literature 1860-1980'. *Obstetrical And Gynaecological Survey,* 38: 324.

Thurlow, JA & Kinsella, SM. 2002. 'Intrauterine resuscitation: active management of fetal distress'. *International Journal of Obstetric Anesthesia,* 11(2): 105–116.

Tindall, VR. 1987. *Jeffcoate's principles of gynaecology.* 5th ed. London: Butterworths.

Toppenberg, KS & Block, WA. 2002. 'Uterine rupture: What family physicians need to know'. *Am Fam Physician*, 66(5): 823–829. http://www.aafp.org/afp/2002/0901/p823.html (Accessed 14 October 2017).

Towler, J & Butler-Manuel, R. 1973. *Modern obstetrics for student midwives.* London: Lloyd-Luke (Medical Books).

Trounce, JR. 1983. *Clinical pharmacology for nurses.* 10th ed. Edinburgh: Churchill Livingstone.

Urden, LS, Stacy, KM & Lough, ME. 2006. *Thelan's critical care nursing: Diagnosis and management.* Philadelphia: Mosby Elsevier.

Usta, IM, Mercer, BM & Sibai, BM. 1999. 'Current obstetrical practice and umbilical cord prolapse'. *Am J Perinatol*, 16: 479–484.

UTHSCSA. nd. Labor and delivery. Maternity guide. http://familymed.uthscsa.edu/residency/maternityguide/labor%26delivery.htm (Accessed 9 October 2017).

Vago, T. 1970. 'Prolapse of the umbilical cord: A method of management'. *Am J Obstet Gynecol*, 107: 967–969.

Vance, M. 2009. 'The placenta', in *Myles textbook for midwives*, edited by D Fraser & M Cooper. 15th ed. Edinburg: Churchill Livingstone Elsevier.

Van Roosmalen, J. 1987. 'Symphysiotomy as alternative to caesarean section'. *International Journal of Gynaecology and Obstetrics*, 25: 451–458.

Velayudhareddy, S & Kirankumar, H. 2010. 'Management of foetal asphyxia by intrauterine foetal resuscitation'. *Indian J Anaesth*, 54(5): 394–399. DOI: 10.4103/0019-5049.71032. https://www.ncbi.nlm.nih.gov/pmc/articles/PMC2991648/ (Accessed 9 October 2017).

Vlok, ME & Lochner, MMM. 1983. *Manual of basic nursing.* 8th ed. Cape Town: Juta.

Waldron, BA. 1983. *Management of epidural analgesia in childbirth.* 2nd ed. Edinburgh: Churchill Livingstone.

Weber, SF. 1996. 'Cultural aspects of pain in childbirth'. *Journal of Obstetric, Gynecologic & Neonatal Nursing,* 25(1): 67–72. http://onlinelibrary.wiley.com/doi/10.1111/jogn.1996.25.issue-1/issuetoc (Accessed 9 October 2017).

WHO. 2011. *WHO Recommendations for Induction of Labour.* http://apps.who.int/iris/handle/10665/70730 (Accessed 9 October 2017).

WHO. 2015. *WHO Statement on Caesarean Section Rates.* http://apps.who.int/iris/bitstream/10665/161442/1/WHO_RHR_15.02_eng.pdf (Accessed 9 October 2017).

WHO. 2016. Stillbirths. http://www.who.int/maternal_child_adolescent/epidemiology/stillbirth/en/ (Accessed 9 October 2017).

Wikipedia. nd(a). Cardiotocography. https://en.wikipedia.org/wiki/Cardiotocography (Accessed 9 October 2017).

Wikipedia. nd(b). Labor induction. https://en.wikipedia.org/wiki/Labor_induction (Accessed 9 October 2017).

Wikipedia. 2016. Uterine inversion. https://en.wikipedia.org/wiki/Uterine_inversion (Accessed 9 October 2017).

Wikipedia. 2017a. Apgar score. https://en.wikipedia.org/wiki/Apgar_score (Accessed 9 October 2017).

Wikipedia. 2017b. Childbirth. https://en.wikipedia.org/wiki/Childbirth (Accessed 9 October 2017).

Wikipedia. 2017c. Umbilical cord prolapse. https://en.wikipedia.org/wiki/Umbilical_cord_prolapse (Accessed 9 October 2017).

Wikipedia. 2017d. Breech birth. https://en.wikipedia.org/wiki/Breech_birth (Accessed 9 October 2017).

Wikipedia. 2017e. Anaphylaxis. https://en.wikipedia.org/wiki/Anaphylaxis (Accessed 9 October 2017).

Williams, A, Adams, EJ, Tincello, DG, Alfirevic, Z, Walkinshaw, SA & Richmond, DH. 2006. 'How to repair an anal sphincter after vaginal delivery: Results of a randomised controlled trial'. *British Journal of Obstetrics and Gynaecology*, 113(8): 977–978.

Yerby, M. 2000. *Pain in childbearing. Key issues in management.* London: Bailliere Tindall.

Yue-Zhou, A. nd. CTG Interpretation. https://www.fastbleep.com/biology-notes/16/449. (Accessed 9 October 2017).

Zakaria, R, Ehringer, WD, Tsakadze, N, Li, N & Garrison, RN. 2005. 'Direct energy delivery improves tissue perfusion after resuscitated shock'. *Surgery*, 138: 195–203.

Section 6: Postnatal care

AAFP (American Academy of Family Physicians). nd. Breastfeeding (policy statement). http://www.aafp.org/about/policies/all/breastfeeding.html (Accessed 9 October 2017).

ACM (Australian College of Midwives) & NHMRC (National Health and Medical Research Council). 2012. Infant feeding guidelines for health workers. 344345. https://www.midwives.org.au/baby-friendly-health-initiative-bfhi (Accessed 20 April 2017).

Aeneil, GC. 1986. *Feeding the low-birth-weight infant.* Sydney: Experta Medica.

Angle, P & Walsh, V. 2004. 'Pain relief after ceasarian section'. *Techniques in Regional Anesthesia and Pain Management,* 5: 36–40.

Becker, GE, Cooney, F & Smith, HA. 2011. 'Methods of milk expression for lactating women'. *Cochrane Database of Systematic Reviews,* 12. http://onlinelibrary.wiley.com/doi/10.1002/14651858.CD006170.pub3/abstract (Accessed 13 October 2017).

Behr, A. 2013. Restoring breastfeeding as optimal infant feeding choice for infants through the implementation of the regulations relating to foodstuffs for infants and young children R991, 6 December 2012. What's the law got to do with it? https://www.westerncape.gov.za/assets/departments/health/regulations_991_restoring_bf_8august2013.pdf (Accessed 10 October 2017).

Belfort, MA. 2017. Overview of postpartum haemorrhage. https://www.uptodate.com/contents/overview-of-postpartum-hemorrhage (Accessed 5 September 2017).

Blair A, Cadwell, K, Turner-Maffei, C & Brimdyr, K. 2003. 'The relationship between positioning, the breastfeeding dynamic, the latching process and pain in breastfeeding mothers with sore nipples'. *Breastfeed Rev,* 11: 5–10.

Burd, I & Dozier, T. 2017. Postpartum haemorrhage. https://www.urmc.rochester.edu/encyclopedia/content.aspx?ContentTypeID=90&ContentID=P02486 (Accessed 10 October 2017).

Cadwell, K. 2007. 'Latching-on and suckling of the healthy term neonate: Breastfeeding assessment'. *J Midwifery Women's Health,* 52: 638–642.

CDC (Center for Disease Control and Prevention). 2010. WHO growth standards are recommended for use in the U.S. for infants and children 0 to 2 years of age. https://www.cdc.gov/growthcharts/who_charts.htm (Accessed 10 October 2017).

Coca, KP, Gamba, MA, Silva, RS & Abrão, AC. 2009. 'Factors associated with nipple trauma in the maternity unit'. *J Pediatr,* 85: 341–345.

Coca, KP, Gamba, MA, Silva, RS, Freitas, V & Abrão, AC. 2009. 'Does breastfeeding position influence the onset of nipple trauma?' *Rev Esc Enferm USP,* 43: 442–448.

DeLyser, F. 1983. *Jane Fonda's workout book for pregnancy, birth and recovery.* London: Penguin Books Limited.

DoH (Department of Health). nd. Road to Health. https://roadtohealth.co.za/growth-and-development/growth-calculators/ (Accessed 9 October 2017).

DoH. 2013. *Infant and Young Child Feeding Policy.* https://www.health-e.org.za/wp-content/uploads/2013/09/IYCF_Policy_2013.pdf (Accessed 2 February 2017).

DoH. 2014. *Newborn Care Charts. Routine Care at Birth and Management of the Sick and Small Newborn in Hospital.* http://www.kznhealth.gov.za/kinc/Newborn_care_charts_March_2014.pdf (Accessed 18 April 2017).

DoH. 2015. *Guidelines for Maternity Care in South Africa.* https://www.health-e.org.za/wp-content/

uploads/2015/11/Maternal-Care-Guidelines-2015_
FINAL-21.7.15.pdf (Accessed 10 October 2017).

Dongre, AR, Deshmukh, PR, Rawool, AP & Garg, BS. 2010.
'Where and how breastfeeding promotion initiatives
should focus its attention? A study from rural Wardha'.
Indian J Community Med, 35: 226–229.

Du Plessis, DW. 2008. *Juta's pocket guide to breastfeeding*.
Cape Town: Juta.

Du Plessis, DM. 2015. Guide to bottle feeding. Unpublished.
Manuscript for Baby Wise Childbirth and Parenting
Centre.

Edge, WEB. 1986. *Encyclopaedia of child care for southern
Africa*. Cape Town: David Phillips.

Giemre, P, White, V & McInnes, P. 1982. *Preparation for
parenthood, pregnancy and labour*. 2nd ed. Johannesburg:
Baby Care Co.

Henderson, P. 2009. Infant and young child feeding: Model
chapter for textbooks for medical students and allied
health professionals. Session 1: The importance of infant
and young child feeding and recommended practices.
Geneva: WHO Press.

Houston, MJ. 1984. *Maternal and infant health care*.
Edinburgh: Churchill Livingstone.

Inch, S. 2006. 'Breastfeeding problems: Prevention and
management'. *Community Pract*, 79: 165–167.

Joy, S. 2017. Postpartum depression. Medscape. http://
reference.medscape.com/article/271662-overview
(Accessed 10 October 2017).

Kalis, V, Rusavy, Z & Prka, M. 2016. 'Episiotomy', in
Childbirth trauma, edited by SK Doumouchtsis.
Springer. https://link.springer.com/
chapter/10.1007/978-1-4471-6711-2_6
(Accessed 10 October 2017).

Kent, JC, Leon, MR, Cregan, MD, Ramsay, DT, Doherty,
DA & Hartmann, PE. 2006. 'Volume and frequency of
breastfeedings and fat content of breastmilk throughout
the day'. *Pediatrics,* 117(3): e387–e395.

Kinsella, M. 2005/6. 'Pain management after ceasarian
section'. *Women's Health Medicine*, 2: 38–39.

Kuhn, L & Kroon, M. 2016. Breastfeeding and the 2015
South African guidelines for prevention of mother-to-
child transmission of HIV. http://www.scielo.org.za/pdf/
sajhivmed/v16n1/08.pdf (Accessed 10 October 2017).

Kumar, S, Kekre, NS & Gopalakrishnan, G. 2007.
'Vesicovaginal fistula: An update'. *Indian J Urol*, 23(2):
187–191. https://www.ncbi.nlm.nih.gov/pmc/articles/
PMC2721531 (Accessed 10 October 2017).

León-Cava, N et al. 2002. Quantifying the benefits of
breastfeeding: A summary of the evidence. Washington,

DC: PAHO (Pan American Health Organization). http://
www.paho.org/English/AD/FCH/BOB-Main.htm
(Accessed 10 October 2017).

Lester, B & La Gasse, L. 2004. *The Dunstan classification
of infant cries*. A Research Proposal. http://www.
dunstanbaby.com/our-research/
(Accessed 10 October 2017).

Mannan, I, Rahman, SM, Sania, A, Seraji, HR, Arifeen,
SE, Winch, PJ, Darmstadt, GL, Baqui, A & Bangladesh
Projahnmo study group. 2008. 'Can early postpartum
home visits by trained community health workers improve
breastfeeding of newborns?' *J Perinatol*, 28: 632–640.

McAdams, WD. 1990. *Nucleotides: The future beyond growth*.
Akromed. New York: Wyeth-Ayerst International.

Narramore, N. 2007. 'Supporting breastfeeding mothers on
children's wards: An overview'. *Paediatr Nurs*, 19: 18–21.

Neifert, MR. 2004. 'Breastmilk transfer: Positioning, latch-on,
and screening for problems in milk transfer'. *Clin Obstet
Gynecol*, 47: 656–675.

Nicholis, T. 2016. Puerperal infections. http://www.
healthline.com/health/puerperal-infection
(Accessed 10 October 2017).

Pettker, CM & Lockwood, CJ. 2008. Thromboembolic
disease: Diagnosis and treatment during pregnancy.
Global library of woman's medicine. http://www.glowm.
com/section_view/heading/Thromboembolic%20
Disease:%20Diagnosis%20and%20Treatment%20
During%20Pregnancy/item/165
(Accessed 10 October 2017).

Renfren, M, Fisher, C & Arms, S. 1990. *Breastfeeding: Getting
breastfeeding right for you*. Berkley, California: Celestial
Arts.

Riordan, J. 1983. *A practical guide to breastfeeding*. St. Louis:
CV Mosby.

Ryding, EL, Wiren, E, Johansson, G, Ceder, B & Dalström,
A. 2004. 'Group counselling for mothers after emergency
caesarean section. A randomised control trial of
intervention'. *Birth*, 31: 247–253.

SABR (South African Breastmilk Reserve). 2014. Bringing
milk to babies, safely. http://www.sabr.org.za/about.html
(Accessed 10 October 2017).

Sai, M, Kishore, S, Kumar, P & Aggarwal, AK. 2009.
'Breastfeeding knowledge and practices amongst mothers
in a rural population of North India: A community-based
study'. *J Trop Pediatr*, 55: 183–188.

Shering, DA & Sauls, HS. 1986. *Breastfed infant. A model for
performance*. 91st Ross Conference on Paediatric Research.
Columbus: Ross Laboratories.

Singh, R, Mailud, A & Sharma, MP. 2004. *Pattern of breast feeding and weaning at Benghazi.* 132nd meeting of the American Public Health Association. Washington DC.

Smith, JR. 2016. Postpartum hemorrhage. Medscape. http://emedicine.medscape.com/article/275038-overview (Accessed 10 October 2017).

Tait, P. 2000. 'Nipple pain in breastfeeding women: Causes, treatment, and prevention strategies'. *J Midwifery Women's Health*, 45: 212–215.

Tarwa, C & De Villiers, FPR. 2007. 'The use of the Road to Health Card in monitoring child health'. *SA Fam Pract*, 49(1): 15. http://safpj.co.za/index.php/safpj/article/viewFile/486/637 (Accessed 10 October 2017).

Ten Steps. 2017. Ten steps to successful breastfeeding. http://www.tensteps.org/ (Accessed 17 November 2017).

Thomas, V & Prangley, J. 1990. *Learn about pregnancy, labour and early baby care.* South Africa: Johnson and Johnson.

Tierz, NW & Finfley, PR. 1983. *Clinical guide to laboratory tests.* Philadelphia: WB Saunders.

Torrance, H. 2014. *A guide to finger-feeding: Information for parents and carers.* Oxford University Hospitals NHS Trust. http://www.ouh.nhs.uk/patient-guide/leaflets/files/11016Pfingerfeeding.pdf (Accessed 10 October 2017).

UNICEF (United Nations Children's Fund). nd. The baby-friendly hospital initiative. Ten steps to successful breastfeeding. https://www.unicef.org/programme/breastfeeding/baby.htm (Accessed 10 October 2017).

Whiteborn, B & Polden, M. 1984. *Postnatal exercises.* London: Century Publishing.

WHO. nd. Protecting, promoting and supporting breastfeeding: The special role of maternity services. A joint WHO/UNICEF statement. Geneva: WHO.

WHO. 1993. *Handbook of resolutions and decisions of the World Health Assembly and the Executive Board.* Volume III, 3rd ed. Geneva: WHO. http://apps.who.int/iris/bitstream/10665/79012/11/9241652098_Vol3.pdf (Accessed 30 November 2017).

WHO. 2003. *Integrated management of pregnancy and childbirth: Managing newborn problems.* Geneva: WHO.

WHO. 2007. *Evidence on the long-term effects of breastfeeding: systematic reviews and meta-analyses.* Geneva: WHO.

WHO. 2012. National infant feeding policy for maternal and neonatal services 2012. http://www.hse.ie/eng/about/Who/clinical/natclinprog/obsandgynaeprogramme/guideline19matanneoservices.pdf (Accessed 10 October 2017).

WHO. 2013. *Recommendations on postnatal care of the mother and newborn.* Geneva: WHO.

Wikipedia. nd(a). Baby friendly hospital initiative. https://en.wikipedia.org/wiki/Baby_Friendly_Hospital_Initiative (Accessed 10 October 2017).

Wikipedia. nd(b). Human milk bank. https://en.wikipedia.org/wiki/Human_milk_bank (Accessed 10 October 2017).

Wikipedia. 2016(a). Puerperal infections. https://en.wikipedia.org/wiki/Postpartum_infections (Accessed 10 October 2017).

Wikipedia. 2016(b). Postpartum haemorrhage. https://en.wikipedia.org/wiki/Postpartum_bleeding (Accessed 10 October 2017).

Wikipedia. 2017. Postpartum infections. https://en.wikipedia.org/wiki/Postpartum_infections (Accessed 10 October 2017).

Willumsum, J. 2013. *Implementation of the baby-friendly hospital initiative July 2013.* WHO. Department of Nutrition for Health and Development. http://www.who.int/elena/titles/implementation_bfhi/en/ (Accessed 10 October 2017).

Wong, AW. 2015. Postpartum infections. Medscape. http://emedicine.medscape.com/article/796892-workup (Accessed 10 October 2017).

Wood, CBS & Walker-Smith, JA. 1981. *MacKeith's infant feeding and feeding difficulties.* 6th ed. Edinburgh: Churchill Livingstone.

Section 7: Newborn care

AAP (American Academy of Pediatrics). 2017. Helping babies survive: Implementation guide. https://www.aap.org/en-us/advocacy-and-policy/aap-health-initiatives/helping-babies-survive/Pages/Implementation-Guide.aspx (Accessed 10 October 2017).

AAP & ACOG (American College of Obstetricians and Gynecologists). 2012. 'Care of the newborn', in *Guidelines for perinatal care*, edited by LE Riley & AR Stark. 7th ed. Elk Grove Village, IL: AAP.

Academy of Breastfeeding Medicine. 2010. 'Clinical Protocol Number #23: Non-pharmacologic management of procedure-related pain in the breastfeeding infant'. *Breastfeeding Medicine*, 5(6): 1–5.

Agarwal, A, Rattan, KN, Dhiman, A & Rattan, A. 2017. 'Spectrum of congenital anomalies among surgical patients at a tertiary care centre over four years'. *International Journal of Pediatrics*, Article ID 4174573. https://www.hindawi.com/journals/ijpedi/2017/4174573/ (Accessed 10 October 2017).

Allan, WC & Sobel, DB. 2004. 'Neonatal intensive care neurology'. *Semin Pediatr Neurol*, 11(2): 119–128. https://www.ncbi.nlm.nih.gov/pubmed/15259865 (Accessed 10 October 2017).

Arnold, M. 2004. 'Is the incidence of gastroschisis rising in South Africa in accordance with international trends? A retrospective analysis at Pretoria Academic and Kalafong Hospitals, 1981–2001'. *S Afr J Surg*, 42(3): 86–88. https://www.ncbi.nlm.nih.gov/pubmed/15532615 (Accessed 10 October 2017).

Aucketf, A. 1988. *Baby massage: The magic of the loving touch.* England: Thorsons.

Balaskas, J & Gordon, Y. 1990. *Waterbirth.* London: HarperCollins.

Bale, JR. 2003. *Reducing birth defects: Meeting the challenges in the developing world.* https://www.ncbi.nlm.nih.gov/books/NBK222074/?report=reader (Accessed 10 October 2017).

Blacke, J & Gregson, S. 2011. 'Kangaroo care in pre-term or low birth weight babies in a postnatal ward'. *British Journal of Midwifery*, 19(9): 568–577.

Blomqvist, YT, Frölund, L Nyqvist, KH & Rubertsson, C. 2012. 'Provision of Kangaroo Mother Care: supportive factors and barriers perceived by parents'. *Caring Sciences*, 27: 345–353.

Boston Children's Hospital. Birth defects and congenital anomalies symptoms and causes. http://www.childrenshospital.org/ (Accessed 10 October 2017).

Bruckmann, EK & Velaphi, S. 2015. 'Intrapartum asphyxia and hypoxic ischaemic encephalopathy in a public hospital: Incidence and predictors of poor outcomes'. *SAMJ*, 105(4): 298–303. http://www.samj.org.za/index.php/samj/article/view/9140 (Accessed 10 October 2017).

Caksen H, Odabaş, D, Tuncer, O, Kirimi, E, Tombul, T, Ikbal, M, Atas, B & Ari Yuca, S. 'A review of 35 cases of asymmetric crying faces'. *Genet Couns*, 2004(15): 159.

Cloherty, JP (ed). 1983. *Manual of neonatal care.* 9th ed. New York: Little Brown & Co.

Corcoran, J. 1998. 'What are the molecular mechanisms of neural tube defects?' *Bioessays*, 20: 6–8.

Culic, S. 2005. 'Cold injury syndrome and neurodevelopmental changes in survivors'. *Arch Med Res*, 36(5): 532–538.

De Onis, M & Victora, CG. 2004. 'Growth charts for breastfed babies'. *Jornal de Pediatria*, 80: 85–87. http://www.who.int/childgrowth/publications/growthcharts_br/en/ (Accessed 17 November 2017).

DoH (Department of Health). 2003. *Road to Health Chart.* https://www.westerncape.gov.za/general-publication/road-health-card (Accessed 13 October 2017).

DoH. 2013a. *Infant and Young Child Feeding Policy.* https://www.health-e.org.za/wp-content/uploads/2013/09/IYCF_Policy_2013.pdf (Accessed 10 October 2017).

DoH. 2013b. *Essential Newborn Care Quality Improvement Toolkit.* http://www.lincare.co.za/wp-content/uploads/2016/06/Essential-Newborn-Care-Quality-Improvement-Toolkit-2013-1.pdf (Accessed 10 October 2017).

DoH. 2014a. *Newborn Care Charts. Routine Care at Birth and Management of the Sick and Small Newborn in Hospital.* http://www.kznhealth.gov.za/kinc/Newborn_care_charts_March_2014.pdf (Accessed 10 October 2017).

DoH. 2014b. *Saving Mothers 2011–2013. Sixth Report on the Confidential Enquiries into Maternal Deaths in South Africa.* http://www.kznhealth.gov.za/mcwh/Maternal/Saving-Mothers-2011-2013-short-report.pdf (Accessed 10 October 2017).

DoH. 2015. *Guidelines for Maternity Care in South Africa. A Manual for Clinic, Community Health Centres and District Hospitals.* https://www.health-e.org.za/wp-content/uploads/2015/11/Maternal-Care-Guidelines-2015_FINAL-21.7.15.pdf (Accessed 10 October 2017).

Donahue, SP & Baker, CN. 2016. 'Committee on practice and ambulatory medicine. Procedures for the evaluation of the visual system by pediatricians'. *Pediatrics*, 137: 1.

Doria-Rose, VP, Kim, HS, Augustine, ETJ & Edwards, KL. 2003. 'Parity and the risk of Down's Syndrome'. *American Journal of Epidemiology*, 158(6): 503–508. https://academic.oup.com/aje/article/158/6/503/99349/Parity-and-the-Risk-of-Down-s-Syndrome (Accessed 10 October 2017).

Du Plessis, DW. 2008. *Juta's clinical guide for midwives.* Cape Town: Juta.

Ebrahim, GJ. 1979. *Care of the newborn in developing countries.* London: The Macmillan Press.

Edge, WEB. 1986. *Encyclopaedia of child care for southern Africa.* South Africa: David Phillips.

Enns, G. nd. Metabolic disease. https://www.britannica.com/science/metabolic-disease (Accessed 17 November 2017).

Feingold, M & Bossert, WH. 1974. 'Normal values for selected physical parameters: An aid to syndrome delineation'. *Birth Defects Orig Artic Ser*, 10: 1.

Fuloria, M & Kreiter, S. 2002. The newborn examination, Part I: Emergencies and common abnormalities involving the skin, head, neck, chest and respiratory and cardiovascular systems. http://www.aafp.org/afp/2002/0101/p61.html (Accessed 10 October 2017).

Gal, P. 2009. 'Patent ductus arteriosus: Indomethacin, Ibuprofen, surgery, or no treatment at all?' *J Pediatr*

Pharmacol Ther, 14(1): 4–9. https://www.ncbi.nlm.nih.gov/pmc/articles/PMC3461996/ (Accessed 10 October 2017).

Garcia, FJ & Nager, AL. 2002. 'Jaundice as an early diagnostic sign of urinary tract infection in infancy'. *Pediatrics*, 109: 5. http://pediatrics.aappublicaations.org/content/109/5/846 (Accessed 10 October 2017).

Glasser, JG. 2016. Intestinal obstruction in the newborn clinical presentation. Medscape. http://emedicine.medscape.com/article/2066380-overview (Accessed 10 October 2017).

Glick, Y & Gaillard, F. 2017. Nuchal fold thickness. Radiopedia.org. https://radiopaedia.org/articles/nuchal-fold-thickness-1 (Accessed 10 October 2017).

Goldfarb, J & Tibbetts, E. 1980. *Breastfeeding handbook.* New Jersey: Enslow.

Gupta, BK, Hamming, NA & Miller, MT. 2006. 'The eye', in *Neonatal-perinatal medicine: Diseases of the fetus and infant,* edited by AA Fanaroff, RJ Martin & MC Walsh. 8th ed. St Louis: Mosby.

Hall, DMB & Elliman, D. 2003. *Health for all children.* 4th ed. Oxford: Oxford University Press.

Hall, ES, Folger, AT, Kelly, EA & Kamath-Rayne, BD. 2014. 'Evaluation of gestational age estimate method on the calculation of preterm birth rates'. *Maternal and Child Health Journal*, 18(3): 755–762. https://link.springer.com/article/10.1007/s10995-013-1302-1 (Accessed 10 October 2017).

Hansen, TWR. 2016. Neonatal jaundice. Medscape. http://emedicine.medscape.com/article/974786-overview (Accessed 10 October 2017).

Hany, A. 2004. 'Respiratory disorders in the newborn: Identifications and diagnosis'. *Pediatrics in Review*, 26: 201–208.

Harrison, V. 2008. *The newborn baby.* 5th ed. Cape Town: Juta.

Haus, M. 1989. *Understanding allergy prevention.* 2nd ed. Sandton: Janssen Research Council.

Health, TD & Jarden, M. 2013. 'Fathers' experiences with the skin-to-skin method in the NICU: Competent parenthood and redefined gender roles'. *Journal of Neonatal Nursing*, 19: 114–121.

Henning, PA. 2002: *The newborn baby.* Pretoria: Van Schaik.

Hernandez, P & Hernandez, J. 1999. 'Physical assessment of the newborn', in *Assessment and care of the well newborn,* edited by P Thureen, J Deacon, J Hernandez & D Hall. Philadelphia: WB Saunders: 114.

Hill, MA. 2017. Gastrointestinal tract – abnormalities. https://embryology.med.unsw.edu.au/embryology/index.php/Gastrointestinal_Tract_-_Abnormalities (Accessed 10 October 2017).

Hitzeroth, HW, Niehaus, CE & Brill, DC. 1995. 'Phenylketonuria in South Africa. A report on the status quo'. *S Afr Med J*, 85(1):33–36. https://www.ncbi.nlm.nih.gov/pubmed/7784915 (Accessed 10 October 2017).

HNN (Healthy Newborns Network). 2017. Helping Babies Breathe. https://www.healthynewbornnetwork.org/partner/helping-babies-breathe/ (Accessed 10 October 2017).

Hoffman, JIE. 2013. 'The global burden of congenital heart disease'. *Cardiovasc J Afr*, 24(4): 141–145. https://www.ncbi.nlm.nih.gov/pmc/articles/PMC3721933/ (Accessed 10 October 2017).

Hudgins, L & Cassidy, SB. 2006. 'Congenital anomalies', in *Neonatal-perinatal medicine: diseases of the fetus and infant,* edited by AA Fanaroff, RJ Martin & MC Walsh. 8th ed. St Louis: Mosby: 561.

Illingworth, RS. 1987a. *The development of the infant and young child.* 9th ed. Edinburgh: Churchill Livingstone.

Illingworth, RS. 1987b. *The normal child.* 9th ed. Edinburgh: Churchill Livingstone.

Kak, LP, Johnson, J, McPherson, R, Keenan, W & Schoen, E. 2015. *Helping Babies Breathe: Lessons learned guiding the way forward.* http://cdn.laerdal.com/downloads-test/f3790/HBB_report_2010-2015_FINAL.pdf (Accessed 10 October 2017).

Kaneshiro, NK & Zieve, D. 2014. Newborn jaundice. https://medlineplus.gov/ency/article/001559.htm (Accessed 10 October 2017).

Kasap, B, Soylu, A & KavukQu, S. 2014. 'Relation between hyperbilirubinemia and urinary tract infections in the neonatal period', in *Nephrology and therapeutics. Pediatric nephrology.* https://www.omicsonline.org/open-access/relation-between-hyperbilirubinemia-and-urinary-tract-infections-in-the-neonatal-period-2161-0959.S11-009.php?aid=25010 (Accessed 7 October 2017).

Keay, AJ & Morgan, DM. 1982. *Craig's care of the newborn infant.* 7th ed. Edinburgh: Churchill Livingstone.

Kirsten, GF, Kirsten, CL, Henning, PA, Smith, J, Holgate, SL, Bekker, A, Kali, GTJ & Harvey, J. 2012. 'The outcome of ELBW infants treated with NCPAP and InSurE in a resource-limited institution'. *Pediatrics*, 129(4). http://dx.doi.org/10.1542/peds.2011-1365 (Accessed 10 October 2017).

Klett, M. 1997. 'Epidemiology of congenital hypothyroidism'. *Experimental and Clinical Endocrinology and Diabetes*, 105: 19–23. https://www.thieme-connect.com/products/ejournals/abstract/10.1055/s-0029-1211926 (Accessed 10 October 2017).

Korones, SB. 1981. *High-risk newborn infants.* 3rd ed. St Louis: CV Mosby.

Kuma, D. 2012. *Genomics and health in the developing world.* New York: Oxford University Press.

Kurinczuk, JJ, White-Koning, M & Badawi, N. 2010. 'Epidemiology of neonatal encephalopathy and hypoxic-ischaemic encephalopathy'. *Early Human Development,* 86: 329–338. https://www.researchgate.net/profile/Nadia_Badawi/publication/301092552_Epidemiology_of_neonatal_encephalopathy_and_hypoxic-ischemic_encephalopathy/links/570b41ba08ae2eb94220182d.pdf (Accessed 10 October 2017).

Lahat, E, Heyman, E, Barkay, A & Goldberg, M. 2000. 'Asymmetric crying faces and associated congenital anomalies: Prospective study and review of the literature'. *J Child Neurol,* 15: 808.

Levitt, AM & Peña, A. 2007. 'Anorectal malformations'. *Orphanet J Rare Dis,* 2: 33. https://www.ncbi.nlm.nih.gov/pmc/articles/PMC1971061/ (Accessed 10 October 2017).

Lissauer, T. 2011. 'Physical examination of the newborn', in *Neonatal-perinatal medicine: Diseases of the fetus and infant,* edited by RJ Martin, AA Fanaroff & MC Walsh. 9th ed. St Louis: Elsevier Mosby: 391–406.

Lui, SO, Hagan, D, Perin, J, Rudan, I, Lawn, JE, Cousens, S, Mathers, C & Black, RE. 2015. 'Global, regional and national causes of child mortality with projections to inform post 2015 priorities and updated systematic analysis'. *Lancet,* 385: 430–440. http://www.thelancet.com/journals/lancet/article/PIIS0140-6736(14)61698-6/abstract (Accessed 10 October 2017).

Lunze, K, Bloom, DE, Jamison, DT & Harrison, DH. 2013. 'The global burden of neonatal hypothermia: Systematic review of a major challenge for newborn survival'. *BMC Med,* 11: 24. https://www.ncbi.nlm.nih.gov/pmc/articles/PMC3606398/ (Accessed 10 October 2017).

Mahmoud, EI, Benirschke, K, Vaucher, YE & Poitras, P. 1988. 'Motilin levels in term neonates who have passed meconium prior to birth'. *Pediatric Journal, Gastro-Enterology and Nutrition,* 7: 45–90.

McKusick, VA. 1998. *Mendelian inheritance in man. A catalog of human genes and genetic disorders.* 12th ed. Baltimore, MD: Johns Hopkins University Press.

Mossey, P & Castilla, E. 2003. *Global registry and datebase of craniofacial anomalies.* Report of a WHO registry meeting on craniofacial anomalies. http://www.who.int/genomics/anomalies/en/CFA-RegistryMeeting-2001.pdf (Accessed 10 October 2017).

Moyer, A, Brown, B, Gates, E, Daniels, M, Brown, HD & Kuppermann, M. 1999. 'Decisions about prenatal testing for chromosomal disorders: Perceptions of a diverse group of pregnant women'. *Journal of Women's Health and Gender-Based Medicine,* 8: 521–531.

NaPeMMCo. 2014. *Short report 2014.* http://www.health.gov.za/index.php/shortcodes/2015-03-29-10-42-47/2015-04-30-08-18-10/2015-04-30-08-24-27?download=889:national-perinatal-morbidity-and-mortality-committee-napemmco (Accessed 17 November 2017).

Natarajan, G, Jeyachandran, D, Subramaniyan, B, Thanigachalam, D & Rajagopalan, A. 2013. 'Congenital anomalies of kidney and hand: A review'. *Clin Kidney J,* 6(2): 144–149. https://www.ncbi.nlm.nih.gov/pmc/articles/PMC4432441/ (Accessed 10 October 2017).

Neu, J. 2007. 'Gastrointestinal development and meeting the nutritional needs of premature infants'. *The American Journal of Clinical Nutrition,* 85(2): 6295–6345.

Neu, M & Robinson, J. 2010. 'Maternal holding of preterm infants during the early weeks after birth and dyad interaction at six months'. *Journal of Obstetric, Gynecologic, & Neonatal Nursing,* 39: https://www.ncbi.nlm.nih.gov/pubmed/20629927 (Accessed 10 October 2017).

Ojo, OA & Briggs, EB. 1982. *A textbook for midwives in the tropics.* 2nd ed. London: Edward Arnold.

Parsonage, S & Clark, J. 1981. *Infant feeding and family nutrition.* London: HMM.

Pattinson, RC. 2003. 'Why babies die: A perinatal survey of South Africa, 2000–2002.' *SAMJ,* 93(6): 445–450.

Pattinson, RC & Rhoda, N (for the PPIP group). 2014. *Saving Babies 2012–2013: Ninth report on perinatal care in South Africa.* Pretoria: Tshepesa Press. http://www.ppip.co.za/wp-content/uploads/Saving-Babies-2012-2013.pdf (Accessed 10 October 2017).

Permezel, M, Walker, S & Kyprianou, K. 2015. *Beischer & MacKay's obstetrics, gynaecology and the newborn.* 4th ed. Australia: Elsevier.

Powell-Hamilton, NN, Kimmel, S & DuPont, AI. 2017. Overview of birth defects. http://www.merckmanuals.com/en-pr/home/children-s-health-issues/overview-of-birth-defects/overview-of-birth-defects (Accessed 17 November 2017).

Pinheiro, PFM, Simões e Silva, AC & Pereira, RM. 2012. 'Current knowledge on esophageal atresia'. *World J Gastroenterol,* 18(28): 3662–3672. https://www.ncbi.nlm.nih.gov/pmc/articles/PMC3406418 (Accessed 10 October 2017).

Quizlet.com. 2017. Birth defects. https://quizlet.com/46325374/birth-defects-flash-cards/ (Accessed 10 October 2017).

Riddle, WR, DonLevy, SC, LaFleur, BJ, Rosenbloom, ST & Shenai, JP. 2006. 'Equations describing percentiles for birth weight, head circumference, and length of preterm infants'. *Journal of Perinatology*, 26: 556–562. http://www.nature.com/jp/journal/v26/n9/full/7211572a.html (Accessed 11 October 2017).

Rimoin, DL, Connor, JM & Pyeritz, RE. 1997. *Emery and Rimoin's principles and practice of medical genetics.* 3rd ed. New York: Churchill Livingstone.

Rioja-Mazza, D, Lieber, E, Kamath, V & Kalpatthi, R. 2005. 'Asymmetric crying faces: A possible marker for congenital malformations'. *Journal Maternal Fetal Neonatal Med*, 18: 275.

Riordan, J. 1983. *A practical guide to breastfeeding.* St Louis: CV Mosby.

Robertson-Sutton, A. 2011. *Improving newborn care in South Africa. Lessons learned from Limpopo Initiative for newborn care (LINC).* UNICEF, DoH, Save the Children. http://www.lincare.co.za/wp-content/uploads/2016/06/Improving_Newborn_Care_LINC_2011.pdf (Accessed 6 October 2017).

SAPA (South African Paediatric Association) & Johnston & Johnston Institute. 2009. *South African handbook of resuscitation of the newborn.* 3rd ed. Johannesburg.

Sears. 2013. Diarrhea. http://www.askdrsears.com/topics/health-concerns/skin-care/diarrhea (Accessed 10 October 2017).

Sengupta, S, Carrion, V, Shelton, J, Wynn, RJ, Ryan, RM, Singhal, K & Lakshminrusimha, S. 2013. 'Adverse neonatal outcomes associated with early-term birth'. *JAMA Pediatr*, 167: 1053.

Shahiana-Rashtiana, P & Kalanib, P. 2012. 'Unexplained neonatal jaundice as an early diagnostic sign of urinary tract infection'. *International Journal of Infectious Diseases*, 6(7): e487–e490. http://www.sciencedirect.com/science/article/pii/S120197121000707 (Accessed 10 October 2017).

Shore, SCL, Keet, MP & Harrison, VC. 1978. *The newborn baby.* Cape Town: Juta.

Singh, S & Madaree, A. 2016. 'Omphalocoeles: A decade in review'. *SAJCH*, 19(4). http://www.sajch.org.za/index.php/SAJCH/article/view/1149/743 (Accessed 10 October 2017).

Southgate, WM & Pittard, WB. 2001. 'Classification and physical examination of the newborn infant', in *Care of the high-risk neonate,* edited by MH Klaus & AA Fanaroff. 5th ed. Philadelphia: WB Saunders: 100.

Srivastava, V, Mandhan, P, Pringle, K, Morreau, P, Beasley, S & Samarakkody, U. 2009. 'Rising incidence of gastroschisis and exomphalos in New Zealand'. *J Pediatr Surg*, 44(3): https://www.ncbi.nlm.nih.gov/pubmed/19302857 (Accessed 10 October 2017).

Stoppard, M. 1988. *The pregnancy and birth book.* Cape Town: Timmins; Struik.

Symington, A & Pinelli, J. 2006. 'Developmental care for promoting development and preventing morbidity in preterm infants'. *Cochrane Neonatal Reviews.* https://www.nichd.nih.gov/cochrane_data/symingtona_01/symingtona_01.html (Accessed 10 October 2017).

Szpecht, D, Szymankiewicz, M, Nowak, I & Gadzinowski, J. 2016. 'Intraventricular hemorrhage in neonates born before 32 weeks of gestation: Retrospective analysis of risk factors'. *Childs Nerv Syst*, 32: 1399–1404. https://www.ncbi.nlm.nih.gov/pmc/articles/PMC4967094/ (Accessed 11 October 2017).

Tovey, DL. 1990. 'Haemolytic disease of the newborn and its prevention'. *British Medical Journal*, 300(6720): 313–316.

University of Virginia. 2017. Causes of cleft lip and palate. https://med.virginia.edu/pediatrics/about/clinical-and-patient-services/patient-tutorials/cleft-lip-palate/causes-of-cleft-lip-palate/ (Accessed 11 October 2017).

Ventura, SJ, Martin, JA, Curtin, SC, Mathews, TJ & Park, MM. 2000. 'Births: final data for 1998'. *National Vital Statistics Reports*, 48: 1–100.

Victoria State Government. Vomiting in the neonate. https://www2.health.vic.gov.au/hospitals-and-health-services/patient-care/perinatal-reproductive/neonatal-ehandbook/conditions/vomiting (Accessed 11 October 2017).

Villar, J, Cheikh Ismail, L, Victora, CG, Ohuma, EO, Bertino, E, Altman, DG, Lambert, A, Papageorghiou, AT, Carvalho, M, Jaffer, YA, Gravett, MG, Purwar, M, Frederick, IO, Noble, AJ, Pang, R, Barros, FC, Chumlea, C, Bhutta, ZA, Kennedy, SH & the International Fetal and Newborn Growth Consortium for the 21st Century (INTERGROWTH-21st). 2014. 'International standards for newborn weight, length, and head circumference by gestational age and sex: the Newborn Cross-Sectional Study of the INTERGROWTH-21st Project'. *Lancet*, 384: 857–868.

Wagle, S & Rosenkrantz, T. 2014. Hemolytic disease of newborn treatment and management. Medscape. http://emedicine.medscape.com/article/974349-treatment (Accessed 11 October 2017).

Wang, BW. 2011. Approach to vomiting. *Learn paediatrics.* http://learn.pediatrics.ubc.ca/body-systems/gastrointestinal/approach-to-vomiting/ (Accessed 11 October 2017).

WHO. 1990. *Guidelines on the Prevention and Control of Phenulketonuria.* http://apps.who.int/iris/bitstream/10665/62187/1/WHO_HDP_PKU_GL_90.4.pdf (Accessed 11 October 2017).

WHO. 2001. *Global Strategy for Infant and Young Child Feeding.* www.who.int/nutrition/publications/infantfeeding/.../index.html (Accessed 11 October 2017).

WHO. 2010. *Child Growth Standards.* http://www.who.int/childgrowth/stan dards/en/ (Accessed 11 October 2017).

WHO. 2016. Congenital anomalies. http://www.who.int/mediacentre/factsheets/fs370/en/ (Accessed 11 October 2017).

WHO. 2017. Congenital anomalies. http://www.who.int/surgery/challenges/esc_congenital_nomalies/en/ (Accessed 11 October 2017).

Wikipedia. nd. Rh disease. https://en.wikipedia.org/wiki/Rh_disease (Accessed 11 October 2017).

Wikipedia. 2017. Infant respiratory distress syndrome. https://en.wikipedia.org/wiki/Infant_respiratory_distress_syndrome (Accessed 11 October 2017).

Wood, CBS & Walker-Smith, JA. 1981. *Mackeith's infant feeding and feeding difficulties.* 6th ed. Edinburgh: Churchill Livingstone.

Woods, D, Malan, A & Van Dugteren, GR. 1988. *Notes on the newborn infant.* 2nd ed. Cape Town: University of Cape Town, Department of Paediatrics and Child Health.

Wright, NJ, Zani, A & Ade-Ajayi, N. 2015. 'Epidemiology, management and outcome of gastroschisis in Sub-Saharan Africa: Results of an international survey'. *Afr J Paediatr Surg*, 12(1): 1–6. https://www.ncbi.nlm.nih.gov/pmc/articles/PMC4955493/ (Accessed 11 October 2017).

Zaganjor, I, Sekkarie, A, Tsang, BL, Williams, J, Razzaghi, H, Mulinare, J, Sniezek, JE, Cannon, MJ & Rosenthal, J. 2016. 'Describing the prevalence of neural tube defects worldwide: A systematic literature review'. *PLoS One*, 11(4): e0151586.

Zanelli, SA. 2016. Hypoxic-ischemic encephalopathy: Differential diagnoses. Medscape. http://emedicine.staging.medscape.com/article/973501-differential (Accessed 11 October 2017).

Zhang, J, Jong, MK, Guileyardo, JM & Roberts, WC. 2015. 'A review of spontaneous closure of ventricular septal defect'. *Baylor University Medical Center Proceedings*, 28(4): 516–520. https://www.ncbi.nlm.nih.gov/pmc/articles/PMC4569244/ (Accessed 11 October 2017).

Zupan, M & Berry, GT. 2015. Galactosemia. NORD online. https://rarediseases.org/rare-diseases/galactosemia/ (Accessed 11 October 2017).

Section 8: Family planning

ARHP (Association of Reproductive Health Professionals). 2008. The single-rod contraceptive implant. http://www.arhp.org/publications-and-resources/clinical-proceedings/Single-Rod/Efficacy (Accessed 16 October 2017).

CDC (Centers for Disease Control and Prevention). 2017. Contraception. https://www.cdc.gov/reproductivehealth/contraception/index.htm (Accessed 16 October 2017).

Cook, R. 1993. 'International human rights and women's reproductive health'. *Studies in Family Planning*, Mar–Apr: 73–86. Published Population Council.

Dhont, M & Verhaeghe, V. 2013. 'Hormonal anticonception anno 2013: A clinician's view.' *Facts Views Vis Obgyn*, 5(2): 149–159. https://www.ncbi.nlm.nih.gov/pmc/articles/PMC3987360/ (Accessed 16 October 2017).

DoH (Department of Health). nd. *National Guideline for Cervical Cancer Screening Programme.* http://screening.iarc.fr/doc/SAcervical-cancer.pdf (Accessed 16 October 2017).

DoH. 2001. *National Contraceptive Policy Guidelines within a Reproductive Health Framework.* Pretoria: National DoH.

DoH. 2012. *National Contraception Clinical Guidelines. A Companion to the National Contraception and Fertility Planning Policy and Service Delivery Guidelines.* Pretoria: National DoH.

DoH. 2014. *Standard Treatment Guidelines and Essential Medicines List for South African Primary Health Care.* Chapter 7. http://www.kznhealth.gov.za/pharmacy/edlphc2014a.pdf (Accessed 16 October 2017).

Finger, WR, 1996. 'Research confirms LAM's effectiveness. Contraceptive update'. *Netw Res Triangle Park NC*, 17(1): 12–14, 24. https://www.ncbi.nlm.nih.gov/pubmed/12320442 (Accessed 16 October 2017).

Guillebaud, J. 2009. *Contraception. Your questions answered.* 5th ed. St Louis: Churchill Livingstone Elsevier.

Jonas, K, Crutzen, R, Van den Borne, B, Sewpaul, R & Reddy, P. 2016. 'Teenage pregnancy rates and associations with other health risk behaviours: A three-wave cross-sectional study among South African school-going adolescents'. *Reproductive Health*, 13: 50. https://reproductive-health-journal.biomedcentral.com/articles/10.1186/s12978-016-0170-8 (Accessed 16 October 2017).

Kaneshiro, B & Aeby, T. 2010. 'Long-term safety, efficacy, and patient acceptability of the intrauterine Copper T-380A contraceptive device'. *Int J Womens Health*, 2: 211–220. https://www.ncbi.nlm.nih.gov/pmc/articles/PMC2971735/ (Accessed 16 October 2017).

Lawrie, TA, Kulier, R & Nardin, JM. 2016. 'Techniques for the interruption of tubal patency for female sterilisation'. *Cochrane Database Syst Rev*, 5(8): CD003034. DOI: 10.1002/14651858.CD003034.pub4. https://www.ncbi.nlm.nih.gov/pubmed/27494193 (Accessed 16 October 2017).

Mandal, A. 2014. Abstinence: What is abstinence? News Medical. http://www.news-medical.net/health/What-is-Abstinence.aspx (Accessed 16 October 2017).

Massyn, H, Peer, N, Padarath, A, Barron, P & Day, C. 2015. *District Health Barometer 2014/2015*. Westville: HST. http://www.hst.org.za/publications/District%20Health%20Barometers/Complete_DHB_2014_15_linked.pdf#search=district%20health%20barometer%202014 (Accessed 16 October 2017).

Naylor, N & O'Sullivan, M. 2005. *Conscientious objection and the implementation of The Choice on Termination of Pregnancy Act 92 of 1996 in South Africa*. Cape Town: Womens Legal Centre & Ipas.

Population Reference Bureau. 2015. World Population Data Sheet. http://www.prb.org/Publications/Datasheets/2015/2015-world-population-data-sheet.aspx (Accessed 16 October 2017).

RCOG (Royal College of Obstetricians & Gynaecologists). 2015. Leading Safe Choices. Best practice in postpartum family planning. https://www.rcog.org.uk/leadingsafechoices (Accessed 16 October 2017).

SASOG (South African Society of Obstetricians and Gynaecologists). 2015. Cervical cancer screening in South Africa. http://www.sasog.co.za/images/SASOG_screening_for_cervical_cancer_November_final.pdf (Accessed 16 October 2017).

Seutalwadi, L. 2012. 'Contraceptive use and associated factors among South African youth (18–24 years): A population-based survey.' *SAJOG*, 18(2): 43–47.

Shen, J, Che, Y, Showell, E, Chen, K & Cheng, L. 2017. 'Methods of emergency contraception'. The Cochrane Collaboration. http://www.cochrane.org/CD001324/FERTILREG_methods-emergency-contraception (Accessed 16 October 2017).

Stats SA. 2015. Statistical Release. P0302. Mid-Year Population Estimates 2015. www.statssa.gov.za (Accessed 16 October 2017).

Stats SA. 2016. *South African Demographic and Health Survey (SADHS). Key Indicator Report.* http://www.mrc.ac.za/bod/SADHS2016.pdf (Accessed 16 October 2017).

Thompson, D. 2009. Good reasons for sexual abstinence. Everyday Health. http://www.everydayhealth.com/sexual-health/sexual-abstinence.aspx (Accessed 16 October 2017).

Trussell, J. 2014. 'Contraceptive efficacy'. *Glob. libr. women's med*, http://www.glowm.com/section_view/heading/Contraceptive%20Efficacy/item/374 (Accessed 16 October 2017).

Truter, A. 2011. 'n Kwantitatiewe beskrywende studie na die houding van verpleegkundiges teenoor terminasie van swangerskap binne King se sisteem teorie. Unpublished doctoral study. UNISA. http://uir.unisa.ac.za/bitstream/handle/10500/5962/thesis_truter_a.pdf?sequence=4 (Accessed 16 October 2017).

UN (Department of Economic and Social Affairs, Population Division). 2015. *Trends in contraceptive use worldwide 2015* (ST/ESA/SER.A/349). http://www.un.org/en/development/desa/population/publications/pdf/family/trendsContraceptiveUse2015Report.pdf (Accessed 16 October 2017).

WHO. 2004. Repositioning family planning in reproductive health services: Framework for accelerated action, 2005–2014. Report of the Regional Director AFR/RC54/11 Rev 1. 18 June. http://apps.who.int/iris/handle/10665/92890 (Accessed 16 October 2017).

WHO, Department of Reproductive Health and Research (WHO/RHR) and Johns Hopkins Bloomberg School of Public Health/Centre for Communication Programs (CCP), INFO Project. 2011. *Family Planning: A Global Handbook for Providers.* Baltimore and Geneva: CCP and WHO.

WHO. 2012. Safe abortion: Technical and policy guidance for health systems. 2nd edit. http://www.who.int/reproductivehealth/publications/unsafe_abortion/9789241548434/en/ (Accessed 16 October 2017).

WHO. 2013a. *Programming Strategies for Postpartum Family Planning.* http://apps.who.int/iris/bitstream/10665/93680/1/9789241506496_eng.pdf (Accessed 16 October 2017).

WHO. 2013b. *Statement for Collective Action for Postpartum Family Planning.* http://www.who.int/reproductivehealth/topics/family_planning/Statement_Collective_Action.pdf?ua=1 (Accessed 16 October 2017).

WHO. 2015. Family planning/contraception. www.who.int/entity/mediacentre/factsheets/fs351/en/ (Accessed 16 October 2017).

WHO. 2016a. Family planning. http://www.who.int/topics/family_planning/en/ (Accessed 16 October 2017).

WHO. 2016b. *Statement of Collective Action for Postpartum Family Planning.* http://www.who.int/reproductivehealth/

publications/family_planning/statmt_ppfp/en/
(Accessed 16 October 2017).

WHO. 2016c. Reproductive health. http://www.who.int/
topics/reproductive_health/en/
(Accessed 16 October 2017).

WHO. 2017. Family planning/contraception. Fact sheet.
http://www.who.int/mediacentre/factsheets/fs351/en/
(Accessed 16 October 2017).

Section 9: Perinatal and other infections in obstetrics

Alexander, J & Kowdley, KW. 2006. 'Epidemiology of
Hepatitis B – Clinical implications'. *MedGenMed*,
8(2): 13. https://www.ncbi.nlm.nih.gov/pmc/articles/
PMC1785180/ (Accessed 16 October 2017).

Ando, Y, Matsumoto, Y, Kakimoto, K, Tanigawa, T, Ekuni,
Y, Kawa, M & Toyama, T. 2003. 'Long-term follow-up
of vertical HTLV 1 infection in children breast-fed by
seropositive mothers'. *Journal of Infection*, 46: 177–179.

Berhanu, R. 2014. 'Treatment of tuberculosis during
pregnancy'. SA HIV Clinician's Society Conference.
http://www.sahivsoc.org/Files/Thurs_Rebecca_
Berhanu%20TB%20&%20pregnancy%20&%20MDR.
pdf (Accessed 16 October 2017).

Berman, SM. 2004. *Maternal Syphilis: Pathophysiology and
treatment*. Bulletin of the WHO. http://www.who.int/
bulletin/volumes/82/6/433.pdf
(Accessed 16 October 2017).

Bhowan, K, Kalk, E, Khan, S & Sherman, G. 2012.
'Identifying HIV infection in South African women: How
does a fourth generation HIV rapid test perform?' *AJLM*,
1(1). http://www.ajlmonline.org/index.php/ajlm/article/
view/4/10 (Accessed 16 October 2017).

Blumberg LH. 2015. 'Recommendations for the treatment
and prevention of malaria: Update for the 2015 season
in South Africa'. *SAMJ*, 105(3): 175–178. http://www.
kznhealth.gov.za/family/Malaria-update-SAMJ-
March2015.pdf (Accessed 16 October 2017).

Boppana, SB & Fowler, KB. 2007. 'Persistence in the
population: Epidemiology and transmission', in *Human
herpes viruses: Biology, therapy, and immunoprophylaxis*,
edited by A Arvin, G Campadelli-Fiume, E Mocarski,
PS Moore, B Roizman, R Whitley & K Yamanishi.
Cambridge: Cambridge University Press. https://www.
ncbi.nlm.nih.gov/books/NBK47423/?report=reader
(Accessed 16 October 2017).

Boshoff, L & Tooke, L. 2012. 'Congenital rubella. Is it time
to take action?' *SA Journal of Child Health*, 6(4): 106–108.

DOI: 10.7196/SAJCH.461. http://www.sajch.org.za/
index.php/SAJCH/article/view/461/345
(Accessed 16 October 2017).

Braaten, KP & Laufer, MR. 2008. 'Human papillomavirus
(HPV), HPV-related disease, and the HPV vaccine'.
Reviews in Obstet Gynecol, 1(1): 2–10. https://www.ncbi.
nlm.nih.gov/pubmed/18701931
(Accessed 16 October 2017).

Bradshaw, CS & Sobel, JD. 2016. 'Current treatment of
bacterial vaginosis. Limitations and need for innovation'.
J Infect Dis, 15(214) Supp 1: S 14–20. https://www.ncbi.
nlm.nih.gov/pmc/articles/PMC4957510/
(Accessed 16 October 2017).

Brahmbhatt, H & Gray, RH. 2003. 'Child mortality
associated with reasons for non-breastfeeding and
weaning: Is breastfeeding best for HIV-positive mothers?'
AIDS, 17: 879–885.

Brocklehurst, P & Volmink, J. 2002. 'Antiretrovirals for
reducing the risk of mother-to-child transmission of HIV
infection'. *Cochrane Database Syst Rev*, 2: CD003510.

Carlson, A, Norwitz, HER & Stiller, RJ. 2010.
'Cytomegalovirus infection in pregnancy: Should
all women be screened?' *Rev Obstet Gynecol*, 3(4):
172–179. https://www.ncbi.nlm.nih.gov/pmc/articles/
PMC3046747/ (Accessed 16 October 2017).

Caserta, MT. 2015. Congenital syphilis. http://www.
merckmanuals.com/en-pr/professional/pediatrics/
infections-in-neonates/congenital-syphilis
(Accessed 17 November 2017).

CDC (Centers for Disease Control and Prevention). 2015.
Chlamydial infections. 2015 Sexually transmitted diseases
guidelines. https://www.cdc.gov/std/tg2015/chlamydia.
htm (Accessed 16 October 2017).

CDC. 2016. Mumps vaccination. https://www.cdc.gov/
mumps/vaccination.html (Accessed 16 October 2017).

CDC. 2017a. Viral hepitatis: Perinatal transmission. https://
www.cdc.gov/hepatitis/hbv/perinatalxmtn.htm
(Accessed 16 October 2017).

CDC. 2017b. Hepatitis B. https://www.cdc.gov/vaccines/
pubs/pinkbook/hepb.html (Accessed 16 October 2017).

Chantry, CJ, Young, SL, Rennie, W, Ngonyani, M, Mashio,
C, Israel-Ballard, K, Peerson, J, Nyambo, M, Matee, M,
Ash, D, Dewey, K & Koniz-Booher, P. 2012. 'Feasibility of
using flash-heated breastmilk as an infant feeding option
for HIV-exposed, uninfected infants after 6 months of
age in urban Tanzania'. *J Acquir Immune Defic Syndr*,
60(1): 43–50. https://www.ncbi.nlm.nih.gov/pmc/articles/
PMC3380080/ (Accessed 16 October 2017).

Coovadia, HM, Rollins, NC, Bland, RM, Little, K, Coutsoudis, A, Bennish, ML & Newell, ML. 2007. 'Mother-to-child transmission of HIV-1 infection during exclusive breastfeeding in the first 6 months of life: An intervention cohort study'. *The Lancet*, 369(9567): 1107–1116. http://www.sciencedirect.com/science/article/pii/S0140673607602839 (Accessed 16 October 2017).

Creswell, J, Sahu, S, Sachdeva, KS, Ditiu, L, Barreira, D, Mariandyshev, A, Mingting C & Pillay, Y. 2014. Tuberculosis in BRICS: Challenges and opportunities for leadership within the post-2015 agenda. http://www.who.int/bulletin/volumes/92/6/13-133116/en/ (Accessed 16 October 2017).

Dabs, F, Newell, ML, Fowler, MG, Read, JS & Ghent, IAS. 2004. Working group on HIV in women and children. 'Prevention of HIV transmission through breast-feeding: Strengthening the research agenda'. *Journal of Acquired Immune Deficiency Syndrome*, 35: 67–68.

Diar, HA & Velaphi, S. 2014. 'Characteristics and mortality rate of neonates with congenital cytomegalo virus infections'. *SAJCH*, 8(4): 133–137. http://www.sajch.org.za/index.php/SAJCH/article/view/752/590 (Accessed 16 October 2017).

DoH. nd. *South Africa's National Strategic Plan for a Campaign on Accelerated Reduction of Maternal and Child Mortality in Africa (CARMMA)*. http://www.kznhealth.gov.za/family/CARMMA_South_Africa_Strategy.pdf (Accessed 16 October 2017).

DoH (Department of Health). 2010a. *The South African Antiretroviral Treatment Guidelines*. http://www.sahivsoc.org/Files/Summary_The_South_African_Antiretroviral_Treatment_2010.pdf (Accessed 16 October 2017).

DoH. 2010b. *Guidelines for Tuberculosis Prevention Therapy Among HIV-Infected Individuals in South Africa*. http://www.who.int/hiv/pub/guidelines/south_africa_hiv_tb.pdf (Accessed 16 October 2017).

DoH. 2013. *The 2013 National Antenatal Sentinel HIV Prevalence Survey South Africa*. https://www.health-e.org.za/wp-content/uploads/2016/03/Dept-Health-HIV-High-Res-7102015.pdf (Accessed 16 October 2017).

DoH. 2014. *Saving Mothers 2011–2013. Sixth Report on the Confidential Enquiries into Maternal Deaths in South Africa*. https://www.health-e.org.za/2016/05/06/report-saving-mothers-2011-2013/ (Accessed 16 October 2017).

DoH. 2015a. *Guidelines for Maternity Care in South Africa. A Manual for Clinic, Community Health Centres and District Hospitals*. https://www.health-e.org.za/wp-content/uploads/2015/11/Maternal-Care-Guidelines-2015_FINAL-21.7.15.pdf (Accessed 16 October 2017).

DoH. 2015b. *Sexually Transmitted Infections. Management Guidelines 2015. Adapted from Standard Treatment Guidelines and Essential Drugs List PHC*. Pretoria. https://www.idealclinic.org.za/docs/National-Priority-Health-Conditions/Sexually%20Transmitted%20Infections_%20Management%20Guidelines%202015.pdf (Accessed 16 October 2017).

DoH. 2015c. *National HIV Counselling and Testing Policy*. https://www.health-e.org.za/2015/07/09/guidelines-national-hiv-counselling-and-testing-hct-policy-guidelines-2015/ (Accessed 16 October 2017).

DoH. 2015d. *National Consolidated Guidelines for the Prevention of Mother-to-Child Transmission of HIV (PMTCT) and the Management of HIV in Children, Adolescents and Adults*. http://www.kznhealth.gov.za/family/HIV-Guidelines-Jan2015.pdf (Accessed 16 October 2017).

DoH. 2016. The 'last mile' plan: Elimination of MTCT in South Africa. http://www.emtct-thelastmile.co.za/ (Accessed 16 October 2017).

DoH. 2016/17. *Adult Primary Care. Symptom-Based Integrated Approach to the Adult in Primary Care*. https://www.idealclinic.org.za/docs/guidelines/Adult%20Primary%20Care%20guide%202016_2017.pdf (Accessed 16 October 2017).

Dou, H, Weiping, L, Zhoa, E, Wang, C, Zhaozhao, X & Zhou, H. 2014. 'Risk factors for candida infection of the genital tract in the tropics'. *Afr Health Science*, 14(4): 835–883. https://www.ncbi.nlm.nih.gov/pmc/articles/PMC4370062/ (Accessed 16 October 2017).

Eke, AC, Eleje, GU, Eke, UA, Xia, Y & Liu, J. 2017. 'Hepatitis B immunoglobulin during pregnancy for prevention of mother-to-child transmission of hepatitis B virus'. *Cochrane Database Syst Rev*, 11(2): CD008545. DOI: 10.1002/14651858.CD008545.pub2. https://www.ncbi.nlm.nih.gov/pubmed/28188612 (Accessed 16 October 2017).

Feucht, U, Forsyth, B & Kruger, M. 2012. 'False-positive HIV DNA PCR testing of infants: Implications in a changing epidemic'. *SAMJ*, 102(3): 149–152. http://www.samj.org.za/index.php/samj/article/view/4951/3919 (Accessed 16 October 2017).

Gardella, C. 2008. Cytomegalovirus in pregnancy. GLOWM. DOI: 10.3843/GLOWM.101. http://www.glowm.com/section_view/heading/Cytomegalovirus%20in%20Pregnancy/item/182 (Accessed 16 October 2017).

Gaydos, C & Hardick, J. 2014. 'Point of care diagnostics for sexually transmitted infections: Perspectives and advances'. *Expert Rev Anti Infect Ther*, 12(6): 657–672. https://www.

ncbi.nlm.nih.gov/pmc/articles/PMC4065592/ (Accessed 16 October 2017).

Gentile, V & Borgia, G. 2014. 'Vertical transmission of hepatitis B virus: Challenges and solutions'. *Int J Womens Health*, 6: 605–611. https://www.ncbi.nlm.nih.gov/pmc/articles/PMC4062549/ (Accessed 16 October 2017).

Gounder, CR, Wada, NI, Kensler, C, Violari, A, McIntyre, J, Chaisson, RE & Martinson, NA. 2011. 'Active tuberculosis case-finding among pregnant women presenting to antenatal clinics in Soweto, South Africa'. *Implementation and operational research: Epidemiology and prevention*. http://www.anovahealth.co.za/uploads/documents/Active_Tuberculosis_Case_Finding_Among_Pregnant17.pdf (Accessed 16 October 2017).

Helou, E, Shenoi, S, Kyriakides, T, Landry, M, Kozal, M & Barakat, LA. 2017. 'Characterizing patients with very low-level HIV viraemia: A community-based study'. *J Int Assoc Provid AIDS Care*, 16(3): 261–266. https://www.ncbi.nlm.nih.gov/pmc/articles/PMC5423832/ (Accessed 16 October 2017).

Hewitt, RG. 2002. 'Abacavir hypersensitivity reactions'. *Clinical Infectious Diseases*, 34(8): 1137–1143. https://www.ncbi.nlm.nih.gov/pubmed/11915004 (Accessed 16 October 2017).

Hilderbrand, K, Goemaere, E & Coetzee, D. 2003. 'The prevention of mother-to-child HIV transmission programme and infant feeding practices'. *South African Medical Journal*, 93(10): 779–781.

Hoosen, AA, Mphatsoe, M, Kharsany, AB, Moodley, J, Bassa, A & Bramdev, A. 1996. 'Granuloma inguinale in association with pregnancy and HIV'. *International Journal of Gynaecology and Obstetrics*, 53: 133–138.

HST. 2016. *The 90-90-90 Compendium. Volume 1: An Introduction to 90-90-90 in South Africa*. http://www.hst.org.za/publications/HST%20Publications/90-90-90%20Vol%20FINALweb31oct2016.pdf (Accessed 16 October 2017).

Jeffrey, BS & Mercer, KG. 2000. 'Pretoria pasteurization: A potential method for reduction of postnatal mother-to-child transmission of the human immunodeficiency virus'. *J Trop Pediatric*, 46(4): 219–223.

Jeffrey, B, Pullen, AE, Mokhondo, RK & Pattison, RC. 2002. *Guidelines for the implementation of Pretoria Pasteurisation in Health Care Institutions*. scholar.sun.ac.za/bitstream/10019.1/4957/3/davis_prevention_2005.pdf.tx (Accessed 17 November 2017).

Johnson, AN & Buchman, EJ. 2012. 'Puerperal infections after C section at Chris Hani Baragwanath Academic Hospital Johannesburg'. *SAJOG*, 18(3): 90–91.

http://www.sajog.org.za/index.php/SAJOG/article/view/559/312 (Accessed 16 October 2017).

Kaneel, FR (ed). 2007. *Male sexual dysfunction: Pathophysiology and treatment*. New York: CRC Press.

Kissinger, P. 2016. 'Epidemiology and treatment of Trichomoniasis'. *Curr Infect Dis Rep*, 17(6): 484. https://www.ncbi.nlm.nih.gov/pmc/articles/PMC5030197/ (Accessed 16 October 2017).

Kourtis, AP, Butera, S, Ibegbu, C, Beled, L & Duerr, A. 2003. 'Breast milk and HIV-1: Vector of transmission or vehicle of protection'. *Lancet Infect Dis*, 3(12): 786–793.

Kourtis, AP, Ibegbu, C, Nahmias, AJ, Lee, FK, Clark, WS, Sawyer, MK & Nesheim, S. 1996. 'Early progression of disease in HIV-infected infants with thymus dysfunction'. *The New England Journal of Medicine*, 335(19): 1431–1436. http://www.nejm.org/doi/pdf/10.1056/NEJM199611073351904 (Accessed 16 October 2017).

Lamont, RF, Sobel, JD, Carrington, D, Mazaki-Tovi, S, Kusanovic, JP, Vaisbuch, E & Romero, R. 2011. 'Varicella zoster virus (chickenpox) infection in pregnancy'. *BJOG*, 118(10): 1155–1162. https://www.ncbi.nlm.nih.gov/pmc/articles/PMC3155623/ (Accessed 16 October 2017).

Manicklai, S, Emery, VC, Lazarrotto, T, Boppana, SB & Gupta, RK. 2013. 'The "silent" global burden of congenital cytomegalovirus'. *Clin Microbiology Review*, 26(1): 86–102. https://www.ncbi.nlm.nih.gov/pmc/articles/PMC3553672/ (Accessed 16 October 2017).

Massyn, H, Peer, N, Padarath, A, Barron, P & Day, C. 2015. *District Health Barometer 2014/2015*. Westville: HST. http://www.hst.org.za/publications/Pages/HSTDistrictHealthBarometer.aspx (Accessed 16 October 2017).

Matuszkiewicz-Rowińska, J, Małyszko, J & Wieliczko, M. 2015. 'Urinary tract infections in pregnancy: Old and new unresolved diagnostic and therapeutic problems'. *Arch Med Sci*, 11(1): 67–77. https://www.ncbi.nlm.nih.gov/pmc/articles/PMC4379362/ (Accessed 16 October 2017).

McLean, H, Redd, S, Abernathy, E, Icenogle, J & Wallace, G. 2014. 'Manual for the surveillance of vaccine-preventable diseases'. CDC. https://www.cdc.gov/vaccines/pubs/surv-manual/chpt15-crs.html (Accessed 16 October 2017).

Meyer, AJ, Atuheire, C, Worodria, W, Kizito, S, Katamba, A, Sanyu, I, Andama, A, Ayakaka, I, Cattamanchi, A, Bwanga, F, Huang, L & Davis, JL. 2017. 'Sputum quality and diagnostic performance of GeneXpert MTB/RIF among smear-negative adults with presumed tuberculosis in Uganda'. *PLoS One* 12(7): e0180572 https://www.ncbi.nlm.nih.gov/pmc/articles/PMC5501569/ (Accessed 11 October 2017).

Mhlongo, S, Magooa, P, Müller, EE, Nel, N, Radebe, F, Wasserman, E & Lewis, DA. 2010. 'Etiology and STI/HIV coinfections among patients with urethral and vaginal discharge syndromes in South Africa'. *Sex Transm Dis*, 37(9): 566–570. DOI: 10.1097/OLQ.0b013e3181d877b7. https://www.ncbi.nlm.nih.gov/pubmed/20502394/ (Accessed 16 October 2017).

Mishra, KN, Bhardwaj, P, Mishra, A & Kaushik, A. 2011. 'Acute *Chlamydia Trachomatis* respiratory infection in infants'. *J Glob Infect Dis*, 3(3): 216–220. https://www.ncbi.nlm.nih.gov/pmc/articles/PMC3162806/ (Accessed 16 October 2017).

Moodley, D, Moodley, J, Coodavia, H, Gray, G, McIntyre, J, Hofmyer, J, Nikodem C, Hall, D, Gigliotti, M, Robinson, P, Boshoff, L, Sullivan, JL & South African Intrapartum Nevirapine Trial (SAINT) Investigators. 2003. 'A multicentered randomised controlled trial of nevirapine versus a combination of zidovudine and lamivudine to reduce intrapartum and early postpartum mother-to-child transmission of human deficiency virus type 1'. *Journal of Infectious Disease*, 187: 725–735.

Newman, L, Kamb, M, Hawkes, S, Gomez, G, Say, L, Seuc, A & Broutet, N. 2013. 'Global estimates of syphilis in pregnancy and associated adverse outcomes: Analysis of multinational antenatal surveillance data. https://doi.org/10.1371/journal.pmed.1001396 (Accessed 17 October 2017).

Ngo-Giang-Huong, N, Khamduang, W, Leurent, B,, Collins, I, Nantasen, I, Leechanachai, P, Sirirungsi, W, Limtrakul, A, Leusaree, T, Comeau, AM, Lallemant, M & Jourdain, G. 2008. 'Early HIV-1 diagnosis using in-house real time PCR amplification on dried blood spots for infants in remote and resource limited settings'. J Acquir Immune Defic Syndr, 49(5): 465–471. https://www.ncbi.nlm.nih.gov/pmc/articles/PMC3111749/ (Accessed 17 October 2017).

Nguyet-Cam, VU, Gotsch, PB & Langan, RC. 2010. 'Caring for pregnant women and newborns with Hepatitis B or C'. *Am Fam Physician*, 82(10): 1225–1229. http://www.aafp.org/afp/2010/1115/p1225.html (Accessed 17 October 2017).

PAHO (Pan American Health Organisation) & WHO. 2008. Perinatal infections transmitted by the mother to her infant. Educational material for health personnel. Latin American Center for Perinatology/Women and Reproductive Health – CLAP/SMR. http://www.paho.org/ (Accessed 17 October 2017).

Paintsil, E & Andiman, WA. 2009. 'Update on successes and challenges regarding mother-to-child transmission of HIV'. *Curr Opin Pediatr*, 21(1): 94–101. https://www.ncbi.nlm.nih.gov/pmc/articles/PMC2650837/ (Accessed 17 October 2017).

Palasanthiran, P, Starr, M, Jones, C & Giles, M. 2014. *Management of perinatal infections*. Australian Society for infectious diseases. Sydney. https://www.asid.net.au/documents/item/368 (Accessed 17 October 2017).

RCOG (Royal College of Obstetricians and Gynaecologists). 2012. *Sepsis following pregnancy. Green Top Guideline 64b*. https://www.rcog.org.uk (Accessed 17 October 2017).

Remington, JS, Klein, JP, Wilson, CB, Nizet, V & Maldonado, YA. 2011. *Infectious diseases of the fetus and newborn infant*. 7th ed. Philadelphia: Elsevier.

Salam, RA, Zuberi, NF & Bhutta, ZA. 2015. 'Pyridoxine (vit B6) supplementation during pregnancy or labour for maternal and neonatal outcomes'. *Cochrane database*, 3(6): CD000179. DOI: 10.1002/14651858. CD00179.pub3. https://www.ncbi.nlm.nih.gov (Accessed 17 October 2017).

Sherman, G. 2015. 'HIV testing during the neonatal period'. *SA Journal of HIV Medicine*, 16(1): 3. http://www.sajhivmed.org.za/index.php/hivmed/article/view/362/496 (Accessed 17 October 2017).

Shrim, A, Koren, G, Yudin, MH, Farine, D & The Maternal Fetal Medicine Committee. 2012. 'Management of varicella infection (chickenpox) in pregnancy'. *J Obstet Gynaecol Can*, 34(3): 287–292. https://www.ncbi.nlm.nih.gov/pubmed/22385673 (Accessed 17 October 2017).

Smith, M. 2009. 'The H1N1 primer for pregnant women'. *Midwifery Today*. http://www.motherbabypress.com/articles/preg_h1n1primer.asp (Accessed 17 October 2017).

Soong, D & Einarson, A. 2009. 'Vaginal yeast infection during pregnancies'. *Can Fam Physician*, 55(3): 255–256. http://www.cfp.ca/content/55/3/255/tab-article-info (Accessed 17 October 2017).

Stats SA. 2017. *Mid-year Population Estimates*. Statistical release P0302. www.statssa.gov.za/publications/P0302/P03022017.pdf (Accessed 17 October 2017).

Straface, G, Selmin, A, Zanardo, V, De Santis, M, Ercoli, A & Scambia, G. 2012. 'Herpex simplex infection in pregnancy.' *Infect Dis Obstet Gynecol*. DOI: 10.1155/2012/385697. https://www.ncbi.nlm.nih.gov/pubmed/22566740 (Accessed 17 October 2017).

Sweet, RL & Gibbs, RS. 2009. *Infectious diseases of the female genital tract*. 5th ed. Lippencot Williams and Wilkin.

TBFacts.org. 2017a. TB statistics for South Africa: National and provincial. https://www.tbfacts.org/tb-statistics-south-africa/ (Accessed 17 October 2017).

TBFacts.org. 2017b. Genexpert Test – TB diagnosis and resistance testing. https://www.tbfacts.org/xpert-tb-test/ (Accessed 17 October 2017).

TBFacts.org. 2017c. Drug resistant TB in South Africa: Hospitalization, statistics and costs. https://www.tbfacts.org/drug-resistant-tb-south-africa/ (Accessed 17 October 2017).

Tita, ATT & Andrews, WW. 2010. 'Diagnosis and management of clinical chorioamnionitis'. *Clin Perinatol*, 37(2): 339–354. https://www.ncbi.nlm.nih.gov/pmc/articles/PMC3008318/ (Accessed 17 October 2017).

University of Liverpool. 2009. HIV drug interaction checker. www.hiv-druginteractions.org (Accessed 17 November 2017).

WHO. nd. TB as global emergency. http://www.who.int/tb/publications/global-emergency/en/ (Accessed 17 October 2017).

WHO. 1999. *HIV in Pregnancy. A Review.* WHO/HS/RHR/99.15. Geneva: WHO.

WHO. 2000. *Mastitis: Causes and management.* Department of Child and Adolescent Health and Development. http://apps.who.int/iris/bitstream/10665/66230/1/WHO_FCH_CAH_00.13_eng.pdf (Accessed 17 October 2017).

WHO. 2004a. *Rapid HIV Test. Guidelines for the Use in HIV Testing and Counselling Services in Resource Constrained Settings.* http://applications.emro.who.int/aiecf/web28.pdf (Accessed 17 October 2017).

WHO. 2004b. Breastfeeding and replacement feeding practices in the context of mother-to-child transmission of HIV. An assessment tool for research. WHO/RHR/01.12 CAHL.01.21. Geneva: WHO.

WHO. 2004c. *HIV Transmission through Breastfeeding: A Review of Available Evidence.* http://www.who.int/nutrition/publications/HIV_IF_Transmission.pdf (Accessed 17 October 2017).

WHO. 2005a. Five components of DOTS. http://www.who.int/tb/dots/en/ (Accessed 17 October 2017).

WHO. 2005b. TB emergency declaration. http://www.who.int/tb/features_archive/tb_emergency_declaration/en/ (Accessed 30 November 2017).

WHO. 2006. The use of the rapid syphilis test. Special programme for research and training in tropical disease. Sponsored by UNICEF/UNDP/WORLD BANK/WHO. http://www.who.int/reproductivehealth/publications/rtis/TDR_SDI_06_1/en/ (Accessed 17 October 2017).

WHO. 2007. *HIV Transmission through Breastfeeding: A Review of Available Evidence; an Update from 2001 to 2007.*

http://who.int/nutrition/topics/Paper_5_Infant_Feeding_bangkok.pdf (Accessed 17 October 2017).

WHO. 2008. *Managing Puerperal Sepsis.* Midwifery education modules. http://www.who.int/maternal_child_adolescent/documents/4_9241546662/en/ (Accessed 17 October 2017).

WHO. 2009. Clinical management of infection with pandemic H1N1: Revised guidance. http://www.who.int/csr/resources/publications/infection_control/en/index.html (Accessed 17 October 2017).

WHO. 2010. GeneXert TB test. Diagnosis and resistant testing. https://www.tbfacts.org/xpert-tb-test/ (Accessed 17 October 2017).

WHO. 2014. *Global TB Report.* http://apps.who.int/iris/bitstream/10665/137094/1/9789241564809_eng.pdf (Accessed 17 October 2017).

WHO. 2015. *WHO Recommendations for Prevention and Treatment of Maternal Peripartum Infections.* http://apps.who.int/iris/bitstream/10665/186171/1/9789241549363_eng.pdf (Accessed 17 October 2017).

WHO. 2016a. Annex 10. WHO clinical staging of HIV disease in adults, adolescents and children. In *Consolidated guidelines on the use of antiretroviral drugs for treating and preventing HIV infection: Recommendations for a public health approach.* 2nd ed. https://www.ncbi.nlm.nih.gov/books/NBK374293/ (Accessed 17 October 2017).

WHO 2016b. *The Global Tuberculosis Report.* (WF 300). http://apps.who.int/iris/bitstream/10665/250441/1/9789241565394-eng.pdf?ua=1 (Accessed 17 October 2017).

WHO. 2016c. *The Shorter MDR-TB Regimen.* http://www.who.int/tb/Short_MDR_regimen_factsheet.pdf (Accessed 17 October 2017).

WHO. 2016d. *WHO Treatment Guidelines for Drug-Resistant Tuberculosis.* https://www.ncbi.nlm.nih.gov/books/NBK390459/ (Accessed 17 October 2017).

WHO. 2017a. The World Health Organization's infant feeding recommendation. http://www.who.int/nutrition/topics/infantfeeding_recommendation/en/ (Accessed 17 October 2017).

WHO. 2017b. Male circumcision for HIV prevention. http://www.who.int/hiv/topics/malecircumcision/en/ (Accessed 17 October 2017).

WHO & UNAIDS. 1998. *HIV in Pregnancy: A Review.* http://www.unaids.org/sites/default/files/media_asset/jc151-hiv-in-pregnancy_en_1.pdf (Accessed 18 September 2017).

Wilson, CB, Nizet, V, Maldonado, YA, Remington, JS & Klein, JO. 2016. *Remington and Klein's infectious diseases of the fetus and newborn infant.* Philadelphia: Elsevier.

Section 10: Nutrition

Burgess, A, Bijlsma, M & Ismael, C. 2009. *Community nutrition: A handbook for health and development workers.* London: Macmillan.

Caputo, C, Wood, E & Jabbour, L. 2016. 'Impact of fetal alcohol exposure on body systems: A systematic review'. *Birth Defects Research (Part C)*, 108: 174–180.

Chalmers, B. 1987. 'Dietary restriction in Pedi women during pregnancy'. *South African Medical Journal*, 70: 568.

DoH (Department of Health). 2015. *Guidelines for Maternity Care in South Africa. A Manual for Clinic, Community Health Centres and District Hospitals.* www.health-e.org.za (Accessed 17 October 2017).

Dudek, SG. 2006. *Nutrition: Essentials for nursing practice.* 5th ed. New York: Lippincott Williams.

Greenberg, JA, Bell, SJ, Guan, Y & Yu, Y. 2011. 'Folic acid supplementation and pregnancy: More than just neural tube defect prevention'. *Rev Obstet Gynecol*, 4(2): 52–59. https://www.ncbi.nlm.nih.gov/pmc/articles/PMC3218540/ (Accessed 17 October 2017).

Grodner, M, Long, S & De Young, S. 2004. *Foundations and clinical applications of nutrition: A nursing approach.* 3rd ed. New York: Mosby.

Hanretty, KP. 2010. *Obstetrics illustrated.* 7th ed. UK: Churchill Livingstone, Elsevier.

Larkby, CA, Goldschmidt, L, Hanusa, BH & Day, NL. nd. 'Prenatal alcohol exposure is associated with conduct disorder in adolescence: Findings from a birth cohort'. *J Am Acad Child Adolesc Psychiatry*, 201; 50(3): 262–271.

Lindmark, G. 2006. 'Energy/protein intake in pregnancy: RHL commentary'. *The WHO Reproductive Health Library* 9.

Montag, AC. 2016 'Fetal alcohol-spectrum disorders: Identifying at-risk mothers'. *International Journal of Women's Health*, 8: 311–323.

Moor, MC. 2009. *Nutritional assessment and care.* 6th ed. St Louis: Elsevier.

National Academy of Sciences. 2017. Dietary reference intakes: Tables and applications. http://www.nationalacademies.org/hmd/Home/Global/News%20Announcements/DRI (Accessed 17 October 2017).

NIH (National Institutes of Health). 2016. Vitamin B_6: Dietary supplement fact sheet. https://ods.od.nih.gov/factsheets/VitaminB6-HealthProfessional/ (Accessed 17 October 2017).

Papathakis, P & Rollins, N. 2005. HIV and Nutrition: Pregnant and Lactating Women. Consultation on Nutrition and HIV/Aids in Africa. Evidence, Lessons and Recommendations for Action. Durban, South Africa, 10–13 April 2005. Geneva: WHO.

Phadke, MA, Gadgil, B, Bharucha, KE, Shrotri, AN, Sastry, J, Gupte, NA, Brookmeyer, R, Paranjape, RS, Bulakh, PM, Pisal, H, Suryavanshi, N, Shankar, AV, Propper, L, Joshi, PL & Bollinger, RC. 2003. 'Replacement-fed infants born to HIV-infected mothers in India have a high early postpartum rate of hospitalization'. *Nutr*, 133(10): 3153–3157.

Rasmussen, KM & Yaktine, AL (eds). 2009. *Weight gain during pregnancy: Re-examining the guidelines.* Washington DC: The National Academies Press.

Roozen, S, Peters, G-JY & Kok, G. 2016. 'Worldwide prevalence of fetal alcohol spectrum disorders: A systematic literature review including meta-analysis'. *Alcoholism: Clinical and Experimental Research*, 40: 18–32.

Siegfried, N, Irlam, JH, Visser, ME & Rollins, NN. 2012. 'Micronutrient supplementation in pregnant women with HIV infection'. *Cochrane Database Syst Rev*, 14(3): CD009755. DOI: 10.1002/14651858.CD009755. https://www.ncbi.nlm.nih.gov/pubmed/22419344 (Accessed 17 October 2017).

Sizer, FS & Whitney, E. 2006. *Nutrition concepts and controversies.* 10th ed. Florence, KY: Thomson Wadsworth.

Viljoen, DL, Gossage, JP, Brooke, L, Adnams, CM, Jones, KL, Robinson, LK, Hoyme, E, Snell, C, Khaole, N, Kodituwakku, P, Ohene Asante, K, Findlay, R, Quinton, B, Marais, A, Kalberg, WO & May, PA. 2006. 'Fetal alcohol syndrome epidemiology in a South African community: A second study of a very high prevalence area.' *J Stud Alcohol*, 66(5): 593–604. https://www.ncbi.nlm.nih.gov/pmc/articles/PMC1414648/ (Accessed 17 October 2017).

WHO. 2013. *Guideline: Calcium Supplementation in Pregnant Women.* http://apps.who.int/iris/bitstream/10665/85120/1/9789241505376_eng.pdf (Accessed 17 October 2017).

WHO. 2016. Recommendations on antenatal care for a positive pregnancy experience. Geneva: WHO.

WHO & UNICEF (United Nations Children's Fund). 1989. *Protecting, Promoting and Supporting Breast-feeding: The Special Role of Maternity Services.* Geneva: WHO.

Zaganjor, I, Sekkarie, A, Tsang, BL, Williams, J, Razzaghi, H, Mulinare, J, Sniezek, JE, Cannon, MJ & Rosenthal, J. 2016. 'Describing the prevalence of neural tube defects worldwide: A systematic literature review'. *PloS One*, 11(4): e0151586. https://www.ncbi.nlm.nih.gov/pmc/articles/PMC4827875/ (Accessed 17 October 2017).

Section 11: Medication used in childbirth

AARC (American Association for Respiratory Care). 1994. 'Clinical Practice Guideline. Surfactant replacement therapy'. *Respiratory Care*, 39(8): 824–829.

Berkow, R, Fletcher, JA & Beers, MH (eds). 1992. *The Merck manual of diagnosis and therapy*. 16th ed. Rathway: Merck Research Laboratories.

Budd, S. nd. Briefing Paper 2. Pregnancy and labour: The evidence for the effective use of acupunture. Edited and produced by the Acupuncture Research Resource Centre. Published by the British Acupuncture Council. https://www.acupuncture.org.uk/arrc/arrc/acupuncture-in-pregnancy-and-labour-the-evidence-for-effectiveness.html (Accessed 17 October 2017).

Chisholm-Burns, MA, Wells, BG, Schwinghammer, TL, Malone, PM, Kolesar, JM, Rotschafer, JC & DiPiro, JT (eds). 2008. *Pharmacotherapy: Principles and practice*. New York: McGraw-Hill Medical.

Choonara, I & Tieder, MJ. 2002. 'Drug toxicity and adverse drug reactions in children: A brief historical review'. *Pediatic and Perinatal Drug Therapy Review*, 5(1): 12–18. https://www.researchgate.net/publication/233705675_Drug_Toxicity_and_Adverse_Drug_Reactions_in_Children_-_A_Brief_Historical_Review (Accessed 17 October 2017).

Chuntharapat, S, Petpichetchian, W & Hatthakit, U. 2008. 'Yoga during pregnancy: Effects on maternal comfort, labor pain and birth outcomes'. *Complementary Therapies in Clinical Practice*, 14: 105–115. https://www.ncbi.nlm.nih.gov/pubmed/18396254 (Accessed 17 October 2017).

Cluett, ER, Nikodem, VC, McCandlish, RE & Burns, EE. 2004. 'Immersion in water in pregnancy, labour, and birth'. Selected Cochrane Systematic Reviews. *Birth*, 31(4): 317.

DiPiro, JT, Talbert, RL, Yee, GC, Matzke, GR, Wells, BG & Posey, LM. 2002. *Pharmacotherapy: A pathophysiological approach*. 5th ed. New York: McGraw-Hill Medical.

DoH (Department of Health). 1996. *National Drug Policy for South Africa*. http://apps.who.int/medicinedocs/documents/s17744en/s17744en.pdf (Accessed 17 October 2017).

DoH. 2003. *South African Demographic and Health Survey*. Full report. https://dhsprogram.com/pubs/pdf/FR206/FR206.pdf (Accessed 17 October 2017).

DoH & MCC (Medicines Control Council). 2013. *Roadmap for Registration of Complementary Medicines*. http://www.mccza.com/documents/66d8cd937.02_Roadmap_for_CAMs_Dec13_v1.pdf (Accessed 13 October 2017).

Doyle, E & Faucher, MA. 2002. 'Pharmaceutical therapy in midwifery practice: A culturally competent approach'. *Journal of Midwifery & Women's Health,* 47(3): 122–129.

Drossou-Agakidou, V, Roilides, E, Papakyriakidou-Koliouska, P, Agakidis, C, Nikolaides, N, Sarafidis, K & Kremenopouloulos, G. 2004. 'Use of ciprofloxacin in neonatal sepsis: Lack of adverse effects up to 1 year'. *Pediatric Infectious Disease Journal*, 23(4): 346–349.

El-Chaar, G. 2003. 'Pharmaceutical care in premature infants'. *US Pharmacist*, 25: HS13–HS31.

EMC. 2017. Meronem IV 500 mg & 1 g. https://www.medicines.org.uk/emc/medicine/11215 (Accessed 17 November 2017).

Engle, WA & AAP Committee on Fetus and Newborn. 2004. 'Age terminology during the perinatal period'. *Pediatrics*, 114(5): 1362–1364. https://www.ncbi.nlm.nih.gov/pubmed/15520122 (Accessed 17 November 2017).

FDA (US Food and Drug Administration). 2009. Pregnancy and lactation labeling. http://www.fda.gov/Drugs/DevelopmentApprovalProcess/DevelopmentResources/Labeling/ucm093307.htm (Accessed 17 October 2017).

FDA. 2015a. Pregnancy and lactation labeling final rule. http://www.fda.gov./drugs/developmentapprovalprocess/developmentresources/labeling/ucm093307.htm (Accessed 17 October 2017).

FDA. 2015b. Pregnant? Breastfeeding? Better drug information is coming. http://www.fda.gov/ForConsumers/ConsumerUpdates/ucm423773.htm (Accessed 17 October 2017).

FDA. 2015c. Pregnancy, lactation, and reproductive potential: Labeling of human prescription drug and biological products—content and format: Guidance for industry. http://www.fda.gov/downloads/Drugs/GuidanceComplianceRegulatoryInformation/Guidances/UCM425398.pdf (Accessed 17 October 2017).

Feldman, DM, Carbone, J, Belden, L, Borgida, AF & Herson, V. 2007. 'Betamethasone vs. dexamethasone for the prevention of morbidity in very-low-birthweight neonates'. *American Journal of Obstetrics & Gynaecology*, 197: 284–285.

Fugh-Berman, A & Kronenberg, F. 2003. 'Complementary and alternative medicine (CAM) in reproductive-age women: A review of randomized controlled trials'. *Reproductive Toxicology*, 17: 137.

Gardner, SL, Snell, BJ & Lawrence, RA. 2002. 'Breastfeeding the neonate with special needs', in *Handbook of neonatal intensive care,* edited by GB Merenstein & SL Gardner. St. Louis: Mosby.

Gaffney, L & Smith, CA. 2004. 'Use of complementary therapies in pregnancy: The perceptions of obstetricians and midwives in South Australia'. *ANZJOG Australia and New Zealand Journal of Obstetrics and Gynecology*, 44(1): 24–29.

Gibbon, CJ (ed). 2008. *South African medicines formulary.* 8th ed. Claremont: Health and Medical Publishing Group.

Hastings-Tolsma, M & Terada, M. 2009. 'Complementary medicine use by nurse midwives in the US'. *Complementary Therapies in Clinical Practice,* 15: 212–219.

Hibbs, AM & Lorch, SA. 2006. 'Metoclopramide for the treatment of gastroesophageal reflux disease in infants: A systematic review'. *Pediatrics*, 118(2): 746–752.

Huntley, AL. 2009. 'Evidence for complementary therapies for labor pain'. *Focus on Alternative and Complementary Therapies*, 8(3): 297–301. http://onlinelibrary.wiley.com/wol1/doi/10.1211/fact.2003.00302/abstract (Accessed 17 October 2017).

Katzung, BG (ed). 2007. *Basic and clinical pharmacology.* 10th ed. New York: McGraw-Hill Medical.

Kenner, L & Lott, JW. 2007. *Comprehensive neonatal care: An interdisciplinary approach.* 4th ed. St Louis: Saunders Elsevier.

Koren, G. 2009. 'Special aspects of perinatal and pediatric pharmacology', in *Basic and clinical pharmacology*, edited by BG Katzung, SB Masters & AJ Trevor. 11th ed. New York: McGraw-Hill Medical.

McElhatton, PR. 2003. 'General principles of drug use in pregnancy'. *The Pharmaceutical Journal*, 270: 232.

Minstedt, K, Brenken, A & Kalder, M. 2009. 'Clinical indications and perceived effectiveness of complementary and alternative medicine in departments of obstetrics in Germany: A questionnaire study'. *European Journal of Obstetrics and Gynecology and Reproductive Biology*, 146: 50–54.

Mitchell, M. 2010. 'Risk, pregnancy and complementary and alternative medicine'. *Complementary Therapies in Clinical Practice*, 16(2): 109–113.

NICHD (Eunice Kennedy Shriver National Institute of Child Health and Human Development). nd. https://nichd.nih.gov/Pages/index.aspx (Accessed 17 October 2017).

Pannaraj, PS, Walsh, MD & Baker, CJ. 2005. 'Advances in antifungal therapy'. *The Pediatric Infectious Disease Journal*, 24(10): 921–922.

Paramor, L. 2005. *Sister Lilian's pregnancy & birth companion.* Cape Town: Human & Rousseau.

Pelletier, JL, Perez, C & Jacob, SE. 2016. 'Contact dermatitis in pediatrics'. *Pediatric Annals*, 45(8): e287-e292. https://

www.healio.com/pediatrics/journals/pedann/2016-8-45-8/%7Ba38755fb-2b8f-4527-bac7-fae18434c55b%7D/contact-dermatitis-in-pediatrics (Accessed 17 October 2017).

Preziosi, P. 2007. 'Age-appropriate use of drug therapy in pediatric patients'. *Journal of Chinese Clinical Medicine*, 2(9): 516–529.

Puig, M. 1996. 'Body composition and growth', in *Nutrition in pediatrics*, edited by WA Walker & HB Watkins. 2nd ed. Hamilton, Ontario: BC Decker.

Rang, HP, Dale, MM, Ritter, JM & Moore, PK. 2003. *Pharmacology.* 5th ed. Edinburgh: Churchill Livingstone.

Reiter, PD. 2002. 'Neonatal pharmacology and pharmacokinetics'. *NeoReviews*, 3(11): e229. http://neoreviews.aappublications.org/cgi/content/extract/3/11/e229 (Accessed 17 October 2017).

Sachdeva, P, Patel, BG & Patel, BK. 2009. 'Drug use in pregnancy: a point to ponder'. *Indian Journal of Pharmaceutical Sciences*, 71(1): 1–7.

Scheafer, F, Peters, P & Miller, RK. 2007. *Drugs during pregnancy and lactation. Treatment options and risk assessment.* 2nd ed. London: Elsevier.

Schellack, N. 2009. An assessment of the need for pharmaceutical care in a neonatal intensive care unit at Dr George Mukhari Hospital. Unpublished PhD dissertation. Pretoria: University of Limpopo, Medunsa Campus.

Schellack, G. 2010. *Pharmacology in clinical practice: Application made easy for nurses and allied health professionals.* 2nd ed. Cape Town: Juta.

Selli, T. 2003. Attitudes of medical practitioners regarding complementary medicine in SA. Dissertation. Johannesburg: University of the Witwatersrand. https://ujcontent.uj.ac.za/vital/access/manager/Repository/uj:8413 (Accessed 17 October 2017).

Simpson, M, Parsons, M, Greenwood, J & Wade, K. 2001. 'Raspberry leaf in pregnancy: Its safety and efficacy in labor'. *J Midwifery Womens Health*, Mar–Apr 46(2): 51–59. https://www.ncbi.nlm.nih.gov/pubmed/11370690 (Accessed 17 October 2017).

Skidmore, L. 1999. *Free desk and update. Drug guide for nurses.* 3rd ed. London: CV Mosby.

Snyman, JR (ed). 2008. *MIMS desk reference.* Volume 43. Saxonwold: MIMS.

Soliday, E & Hapke, P. 2013. 'Research on acupuncture in pregnancy and childbirth: The U.S. contribution'. *Med Acupunct*, Aug 25(4): 252–260. DOI: 10.1089/acu.2012.0950. https://www.ncbi.nlm.nih.gov/pmc/articles/PMC3746244/ (Accessed 17 October 2017).

South African medicine formulary. 7th ed. 2005. Cape Town: SAMF.

Stanway, A. 1979. *Alternative medicine. A guide to natural therapies*. London: MacDonald and Jane.

Stapleton, H. 1995. 'The use of herbal medicine in pregnancy and labour. Part II: Events after birth, including those affecting the health of babies'. *Complementary Therapy Nursing Midwifery*, 1(5): 148–153.

Taketomo, CK, Hodding, JH & Kraus, DM. 2015. *Pediatric and neonatal dosage handbook with international trade names index: A universal resource for clinicians treating pediatric and neonatal patients*. 22nd ed. Wolters Kluwer Clinical Drug Information.

Thembo, K. nd. Roadmap for registration of complementary medicines. DoH. http://www.mccza.com/documents/28190043CAMs_workshop_Feb2014_Roadmap.pdf (Accessed 17 October 2017).

Thomson, AH, Kerr, S & Wright, S. 1996. 'Population pharmacokinetics of caffeine in neonates and young infants'. *Therapeutic Drug Monitoring*, 18(3): 243–253.

Tiran, D. 2003. 'Implementing complementary therapies into midwifery practice'. *Complementary Therapies in Nursing and Midwifery*, 9: 10–13.

Tiran, D & Mack, S. 2003. 'Complementary therapies for pregnancy and childbirth – homoeopathy'. *South African Medical Journal*, 93(5): 1008–1010.

Tobin, CM, Darville, JM, Thomson, AH, Sweeney, G, Wilson, JF, MacGowan, AP & White, LO. 2002. 'Vancomycin therapeutic drug monitoring: Is there a consensus view? The results of a UK National External Quality Assessment Scheme (UK NEQAS) for Antibiotic Assays questionnaire'. *Journal of Antimicrobial Chemotherapy*, 50: 713–718.

Trounce, J. 2000. *Clinical pharmacology for nurses*. 16th ed. London: Churchill Livingstone.

Van Wyk, B & Gericke, N. 2000. *People's plants. A guide to useful plants of southern Africa*. Pretoria: Briza Publications.

Vithoulas, G. 1979. *Medicine of the new man*. New York: Arco.

Walton, AG. 2011. A healthy poke: Demystifying the science behind acupuncture. The Atlantic. https://www.theatlantic.com/health/archive/2011/09/a-healthy-poke-demystifying-the-science-behind-acupuncture/245816/ (Accessed 17 October 2017).

Wang, S, Kain, Z & White, P. 2008. 'Acupuncture analgesia: The scientific basis'. *Anesthesia & Analgesia*, February 106(2): 602–610. http://journals.lww.com/ (Accessed 17 October 2017).

Westfall, RM. 2004. 'Use of anti-emetic herbs in pregnancy: Women's choices, and the question of safety and efficacy'. *Complementary Therapies in Nursing and Midwifery*, 10: 30–36.

WHO. nd. The Anatomical Therapeutic Chemical classification system with Defined Daily Doses (ATC/DDD). http://www.who.int/classifications/atcddd/en/ (Accessed 17 October 2017).

WHO. 2003. Factsheet 134. http://www.scirp.org/(S(351jmbntvnsjt1aadkposzje))/reference/ReferencesPapers.aspx?ReferenceID=1721848 (Accessed 17 October 2017).

WHO. 2008. *Safety Issues in the Preparation of Homeopathic Medicine*. NLM classification: WB 930. http://apps.who.int/medicinedocs/documents/s16769e/s16769e.pdf (Accessed 17 October 2017).

WHO. 2012. *Use of Efavirenz during Pregnancy: A Public Health Perspective*. http://www.who.int/hiv/pub/treatment2/efavirenz/en/ (Accessed 17 October 2017).

WHO. 2013. WHO traditional medicine strategy: 2014–2023 (WHA62.13). http://www.who.int/traditional-complementary-integrative-medicine/publications/trm_strategy14_23/en/ (Accessed 17 October 2017).

Zenk, KE, Sills, JH & Koeppel, RM. 2003. *Neonatal medications and nutrition: A comprehensive guide*. 3rd ed. Santa Rosa: NICU Ink.

Index

Notes: Page numbers in *italics* refer to figures, illustrations or tables.

antenatal management 794
drugs for use in pregnancy *794*
effectiveness of 790
neonatal prophylaxis 797
side effects *789*
breastfeeding and *797*
and Caesarean section 516
CD4 cell levels 786
child mortality 43
circumcision and *784*
classifications and clinical staging of HIV
infection 786
co-infection with tuberculosis 782
counselling and testing 238, 243, 593, 793
diagnosis and tests *785*
drugs in pregnancy *842*
effects of HIV on outcomes of
pregnancy 791
effects on nutritional status 818
identification of 218
immunisation and 799
infant feeding 797
integrase inhibitors *787*
intrapartum care 795
life-threatening infections 790
maternal deaths related to 14
maternal postnatal visits at six weeks 42
neonatal care 796
Papanicolaou (Pap) smear 733
prevention of mother-to-child
transmission (PMTCT) *221*
polymerase chain reaction (PCR)
test *785, 791, 796, 796*
postpartum care 799
in pregnancy 42, 791
prevention of tuberculosis 800
support group *265*
transmission of HIV from mother to
child 15, 792, *792*
prevention best practice *793*
types of infections 783
holism 827
Homans' test 593, 607
homeopathy 826, 828
remedies in postnatal period 833
remedies in pregnancy and labour 833
hormones
female
in pregnancy 62
reproductive 57, *58*
male 62
thyroid-stimulating hormone (TSH) 300
human chorionic gonadotrophin (hCG) *see*
gonadotrophins
humane care *see* care environments
Human Genome Project *82*
human milk *see* breastfeeding; lactation
human papilloma virus (HPV) 732, 766
mucosal *766*

human placental lactogen (HPL) 63, 113
human rights, and child care 178
Human Tissue Act 65 of 1983 *442*
Human Tissue Amendment Act 51 of
1989 *452*
hyaline membrane disease (HMD) 297, 336,
359, *659*, 660 *see also* respiratory distress
syndrome (RDS)
rice grain appearance *702*
hydatidiform mole (gestational trophoblastic
disease) *96*, 114, 213, 279, 289, 319, 347
hydrocele 696
hydrocephalus 250, 687, *688*
hydrocephaly 456, *684*
hydrops fetalis 114, 345
hydrotherapy 419
hymen 48
hyperbilirubinaemia *see* jaundice
hyperemesis gravidarum
aetiology 347
cause of anaemia 301
complications of 347
definition 347
diagnosis of 347
incidence 347
pathophysiology 347
treatment and care 347
hypergalactia 148
hyperglycaemia 297
hyperplasia 208
hyperprolactinaemia 149
hyperpyrexia, cause of small-for-gestational-
age (SGA) 106
hypertension and pre-eclampsia intervention
trial at term (HYPITAT) 292
hypertension in pregnancy
assessments 243
cause of small-for-gestational-age
(SGA) 106
contributing factors 290
control of 293
management of 292
and obesity 232
placenta and *112*, 289
referral to major obstetric unit 293
signs and symptoms *295*
hypertensive disorders 289
hyperthyroidism 208, 301
hypertonic uterine contractions 409
hypertonic uterine inertia 484
hyperventilation 276, 295, 379
hypnosis 419
hypnotic drugs 420, 424
hypoglycaemia 208, 297, 300, 313, 335, 337,
659, 664, 675
hypoglycaemics, oral 299
hypoplastic left heart 692
hypotension 526
hypothalamic–pituitary–gonad axis 57
hypothalamus 57, 61, 89, 149, 214

hypothermia 300, 336, 337, 341, 637, 659, 674
cooling cap *721*
therapy *721*
hypothyroidism 208, 301
hypotonic uterine function 482, 484
hypoventilation 379
hypovolaemia 601
hypovolaemic shock 321, 332, 601
hypoxaemia 675
hypoxia
cause of perinatal death 15
definition 720
fetal 106, 114, 321, 379, 503
intrapartum 444
neonatal 118
periods of in fetus 104
of pituitary gland 58
hypoxic-ischaemic encephalopathy (HIE) 719
pathophysiology sequelae *720*
hysterectomy 604
hysterosalpingogram (HSG) 56
hysterotomy *510*

I

icterus gravis neonatorum 345
identification of newborns 448, 644
ilium 119, 121, *121*
imbelekisane 835
immaturity, cause of perinatal death 15
immune system
maternal 205
newborns
cell-mediated immunity 640
immunity through breast milk 640
passive immunity 639
immunisation
of children 29, 274, 597
HIV/AIDS and 799
of pregnant women 29, 37, 219, 238
immunoglobulins 205, 639
Rh (D) 342
immunology 756
implantation bleeding 93, 316
inborn errors 696
induction of labour (IOL)
care of obstetric woman 544
cervical ripening 541
choice of method 541
classification of 538
complications of 540
contraindications 540
differentiation from augmentation of
labour *539*
examinations *545*
incidence 538
indications for 540
intrauterine death (IUD) 362
liability of midwife 544
medical induction 542

www.ingramcontent.com/pod-product-compliance
Lightning Source LLC
Chambersburg PA
CBHW082307210326
41598CB00029B/4468